VIOLENCE

A Compendium From *JAMA*,
American Medical News,
and the Specialty Journals
of the American Medical Association

ISBN: 0-89970-493-X

Articles appearing in this compendium have appeared previously in the following issues of *The Journal of the American Medical Association:* March 4, 1992; May 6, 1992; May 20, 1992; May 27, 1992; June 3, 1992; June 10, 1992; and June 17, 1992.

The January 6, 1992, issue of *American Medical News.*

And in the June issues of the specialty journals of the American Medical Association: *American Journal of Diseases of Children, Archives of Dermatology, Archives of General Psychiatry, Archives of Internal Medicine, Archives of Neurology, Archives of Ophthalmology, Archives of Otolaryngology—Head & Neck Surgery, Archives of Pathology and Laboratory Medicine, and Archives of Surgery.*

Comments or inquiries to:

American Medical Association
Customer Service Department
515 N State St
Chicago, IL 60610

Telephone orders: 1-800-621-8335

Product No: OP350092

FOREWORD

Violence

A Compendium From *JAMA, American Medical News,* and the Specialty Journals of the American Medical Association

Murder. Arson. Drive-by-shooting. Rioting. Rape. Mugging. Stabbing. Wilding. Suicide. Assault. Incest. Spouse, Partner, Child, Elder Abuse.

A picture of American society is emerging, and it is at once both horrifying and numbing. So much so that we have been unable to stop it. We have become a society at war with itself, a nation at the mercy of a savage beast—violence.

Many of us have long recognized violence as a devastating social and public health problem. But even more of us have allowed ignorance, fear, powerlessness, and other problems that divert our attention to keep us from doing anything to resolve the problem. Certainly if violence were caused by a virus, we would have found its treatment and prevention long ago.

In an attempt to increase public and professional attention to violence, the editors of *JAMA, American Medical News,* and the American Medical Association's nine specialty journals published numerous articles on violence between January and June 1992. The best of these articles, which are collected in this Compendium, include epidemiologic studies, clinical research, government reports, case descriptions, and commentaries on a wide range of violence, from firearm homicide to abuse of children and pregnant women.

For this Compendium, we define violence as any human action resulting in injury or abuse, generally of the interpersonal variety, rather than that resulting from war or natural disasters. A pervasive, deceptive force, such violence destroys the basic, human foundation of our society and is best characterized with numbers:

- Homicide is the third leading cause of death among 15- to 24-year-olds and the leading cause of death among 15- to 24-year-old black males. The homicide rates for children and adolescents have more than doubled in the last 30 years.
- More than 1.5 million individuals in our country are victims of assault each year, and more than 650,000 women are victims of rape.
- 1.8 million women are beaten by their male partners each year, and 8% to 11% of pregnant women report being physically assaulted during pregnancy.
- Two to 4 million of our children were abused or neglected in 1991, and more than 1 million elderly were mistreated last year.

These statistics, although alarming, are probably underestimations. There is no denying that violence in America is a public health emergency—demanding immediate attention and corrective action.

These data paint a grotesque picture of a society steeped in violence, with such ubiquity and prevalence as to be seemingly accepted as inevitable. The authors and editors of this Compendium do not accept this situation as inevitable. No civilized society should be so permeated by firearm assault, homicide, rape, and child abuse. The situation is unacceptable. Prior solutions have not succeeded. New approaches are required.

We must demand unprecedented support for additional research into the causes, prevention, and treatments, for both victims and perpetrators, of all forms of violence. We need to recognize and treat violence as more than just a social aberrancy—it is a social disease. We need to educate everyone—physicians, nurses, other health professionals, students, politicians, and the public at large—about what is now known and what can now be done to address this emergency.

George D. Lundberg, MD
Roxanne K. Young
Annette Flanagin, RN, MA
C. Everett Koop, MD

Compendium Editors: George D. Lundberg, MD, Roxanne K. Young, Annette Flanagin, RN, MA, C. Everett Koop, MD
Compendium Production: M. Kathleen Berka, Thomas Handrigan, Terri Hanley, Mary C. Steermann

American Medical Association

VIOLENCE

A Compendium From *JAMA, American Medical News,* and the Specialty Journals of the American Medical Association

Articles published previously in *JAMA*

Articles published previously in *American Medical News*

Articles published previously in the Specialty Journals of the American Medical Association

VIOLENCE

Articles published previously in *The Journal of the American Medical Association*

The Cover

For the young, avant-garde painter from Christiania, it was the best of times; it was also the worst of times. It was a rise to the top of his profession; it was a fall to the depths of despair. In 1898, when he met Tulla Larsen for the first time, Edvard Munch (1863-1944) was successful and well known. Tulla was the daughter of Norway's largest wine merchant. Both were part of Christiania's bohemian intelligentsia. It would seem that Munch, deprived by tuberculosis of mother and sister in childhood and teens (*JAMA* cover December 11, 1987) would at last end his ceaseless searching and settle into some kind of stable family life of his own. But Munch's preoccupation with death, coupled with his morbid jealousy, were not easily overcome. Nor was his deep distrust of women, especially of those who might attempt to become close to him. "Should we sick people establish a new home with the poison of consumption eating into the tree of life—a new home with doomed children?" he asked. Four years later, in 1902, the whole reluctant affair with Tulla Larsen was climaxed when, in an attempt to break off with her for good, Munch shot off part of one finger of his left hand and injured another.

Munch was already drinking heavily at the time of this mysterious shooting, but his consumption of alcohol now became ever greater. He was involved in a number of public brawls. He tried several cures; none worked. His painting, obsessed from the beginning with scenes of death and dying, now began to show an alienated painter and violent death. In 1906 he painted a self-portrait with himself in a restaurant, his back turned to all except a bottle of wine (*JAMA* cover May 27, 1988). The same year he painted a woman standing beside a bed on which a man was lying. He titled it *The Murderess*. Other versions he called *The Death of Marat*. Sometimes, in this murder motif, the figures were clothed, sometimes they were naked. Sometimes the colors were as innocent as a fruit-and-flower still life. Sometimes they were as bloody as the Reign of Terror. Sometimes the scenes are barely threatening, almost intimate; at other times the scenes are overpowering. But always the relationship is that of lovers and the man is dead.

One of the many paintings based on this murder motif is *The Death of Marat I* (cover), painted in 1907, some 5 years after the final breakup with Tulla Larsen. Arne Eggum, chief curator at the National Gallery of Art/Munch Museum in Oslo, Norway, points out that, whereas the female figure was taken from a model, it clearly has Tulla Larson's features, and thus refers to that affair (Eggum A [Christophersen R, trans]. *Edvard Munch*. New York, NY: Clarkson N Potter Inc; 1985). "The male figure," he continues, "is lying on a bed which projects obliquely into the picture. The strongly perspective foreshortening of the man's figure creates an aggressive diagonal. The woman is standing rigid as a pillar of salt, strictly *en face*. The painting expresses both petrified hatred as well as a desire for contact that can never be fulfilled." Dr Eggum then calls attention to the various elements in the painting, which can be related to Munch's own notes dealing with the shooting incident: "On the table, for example, can be seen the fruit that Tulla Larsen was serving just before the shot was fired, as well as one of her magnificent hats. The impasto-painted sections, in particular the table with the still-life motif in the foreground to the right, seem to be directly inspired by the painting of Matisse, as he appeared, in the guise of an innovator, at the Fauvist exhibition in Paris in 1905. The long whiplash strokes enveloping the actual motif in a very special atmosphere may probably be regarded as expressing the artist's own reaction to the actual theme."

Also interesting is Munch's choice of title for these paintings, inasmuch as they refer to an historical event, but not as generally depicted. The incident took place in Paris on July 13, 1793, just prior to be beginning of the Reign of Terror of the French Revolution. Charlotte Corday, a royalist, sought an interview with Jean-Paul Marat, a revolutionary and influential newspaper writer, on the pretext that she would give him the names of dissidents. Finally admitted to his presence while he was in his bath, Charlotte drew a knife from beneath her dress and stabbed Marat through the heart. Charlotte was tried and guillotined 4 days later, on July 17, 1793. Marat has been immortalized in the well-known painting by the contemporary Jacques Louis David, which shows Marat slumped over in his bath. Munch has exercised his artistic license fully, keeping only the title.

Although Munch's alcoholism and violent behavior continued to worsen over the next couple of years, he finally gained permanent control over the alcohol during a stay of several months in 1909 at Dr Daniel Jacobson's clinic for nervous diseases in Copenhagen, Denmark. Upon release he immediately began work on murals for the decoration of the new University Festival Hall in Oslo. Its major work, *The Sun*, was completed in 1912, and is the backdrop for the presentation of the Nobel Peace Prize in Oslo each year on December 10 (*JAMA* cover December 8, 1989). But even though the remaining long life of Edvard Munch was outwardly calmer and much of his painting brighter, he continued to use the Marat/Corday motif almost to the end of his life. He died peacefully at his home in Ekely, outside Oslo, on the afternoon of January 23, 1944. He was 80.—M. Therese Southgate, MD

Edvard Munch (1863-1944), *Death of Marat I*, 1907, Norwegian. Oil on canvas. Courtesy of Oslo Kommunes Kunstsamlinger/Munch Museet, Oslo, Norway.

Guns, Drugs Threaten to Raise Public Health Problem of Violence to Epidemic

AS LETHAL weapons proliferate, this final decade of the 20th century is likely to be characterized by ever-increasing violence that will supplant drugs as a major public health problem and social concern.

This prediction comes from Herbert Kleber, MD, professor of psychiatry and director, Division on Substance Abuse, Columbia University College of Physicians and Surgeons, New York, NY.

In support of this position, Kleber notes that while there is little question that drug use and violence are intertwined, the use of drugs is declining. "It may not be declining as fast as we would like or in every sector, but it is declining. There is a sense that things have begun to move in the right direction."

Increased Violence Levels

"Despite this, we are seeing increased levels of violence and many of these violent episodes have nothing at all to do with drugs," says Kleber. He notes recent news reports of indiscriminate violence in schools and on the highways.

In an interview, Kleber says that "drugs are no longer as socially acceptable as they were in the 1960s. Yet, at the same time, dealers will be fighting over a shrinking drug market."

This is occurring just as much more lethal handguns are becoming readily available. As Kleber puts it, "What has changed is not just availability, although certainly weapons are more available. What has changed is the availability of better weapons."

But availability is just one factor in the violence equation, says Kleber. A second factor is the increased lethality of the weapons that are available. "Certainly the 'Saturday night specials' were cheap and available, but they were also inaccurate. These newer weapons tend to be easier to use, more accurate, and can deliver more firepower than most weapons previously in circulation. They are far more lethal and require little or no experience to use effectively," he says.

Kleber recalls that he recently fired one of these modern handguns for the first time in his life. "On a 15-yard practice range with a 9-mm repeating pistol, I was able to do a very good job at reaching the target. Not a bull's-eye every time, but very close," he says. "Considering I had never used a handgun and am not that well coordinated, I was able to do very well. One conclusion I draw from this experience is that the current technical sophistication of these weapons makes it much easier to kill somebody."

The weapons that Kleber is concerned about, such as the 9-mm repeating pistol he tested, are untouched by the present firearms legislation, he says. This deals with imported assault-type weapons such as Uzis, not with domestic handguns. In the past decade, repeating or semiautomatic pistols have largely replaced the standard six-cartridge revolver in handgun popularity, according to the Bureau of Alcohol, Tobacco, and Firearms. The modern repeating pistol can hold 10, 15, or even more cartridges. In effect, it is a handheld machine gun.

A third factor is that adolescents and young adults seem to be more ready to turn to these weapons as a way of resolving quarrels that formerly would have been dealt with by fists or, at the very worst, with knives. "There is a tendency today to solve every quarrel with guns," Kleber says.

Respect No Life

Finally, says Kleber, "Many of these individuals have no respect for their own lives, let alone the lives of others. To them, life is cheap, even their own life. They often have no vision of the future. If their life gets snuffed out, they don't feel they have lost a lot."

Kleber rejects the view that this is entirely the fault of society. After all, he says, the majority of those growing up in city slums don't use drugs or guns. "It's a slander to say young black males don't care about themselves or others, when we're really talking about a minority," he says.

Kleber, a psychiatrist with a substance abuse treatment background—he was deputy director of the Office of National Drug Policy, Washington, DC—notes the strong relationship between violence and drugs.

He cites four situations:

- The violence related to drug distribution, such as the turf battles mentioned earlier.
- The violence related to acquisition, where the addict engages in violence to get the funds to support his or her drug habit.
- The violence associated with the pharmacologic effects of a drug. Drugs such as cocaine, crack, angel dust, and the amphetamines produce irritability, paranoia, and need for action and are more likely to be associated with violence, including domestic violence, than are sedating drugs such as heroin. "This is independent of acquisition," Kleber says.
- Finally, there is indirect drug-related violence, such as auto crashes and the birth of "crack babies" to drug-addicted mothers. These elements change, depending on the level of drug use and the type of drug involved, he says.

"So," Kleber says, "if you decrease the amount of cocaine, you may not decrease the distributive violence, but you should decrease the acquisitive and pharmacologic violence because fewer people are using it." It's a complicated issue, Kleber concedes, adding: "It's a combination of gun and person, to be sure."

Kleber is reluctant to be more specific about gun control. "It's not my area of expertise," he says.

But, he adds, "I don't know if stricter gun control laws would in fact reduce gun-related violence."

As regards drugs, there are two areas of attack: Reduce the supply and increase funds for treatment. "But providing adequate funds for drug abuse treatment has been a bipartisan failure," he says. "The Republican administration has not requested adequate funds and the Democrat-controlled Congress has provided even less than the administration asked for." In the current year's budget, Congress cut by one third the funds the administration had requested for treatment.

"Sometimes it's easier to reduce access than it is to change the person," Kleber says. "Remember, we haven't changed teenagers, yet we have decreased the number of automobile deaths in this age group simply by increasing the legal drinking age."

—by Charles Marwick

Congress Acts to Resuscitate Nation's Financially Ailing Trauma Care Systems

CONGRESS may soon come to the rescue of the nation's ailing trauma care systems with a new program of federal grants to help defray uncompensated trauma care costs.

The federal assistance is aimed primarily at helping trauma centers provide medical care for undocumented aliens and for victims of drug-related violence.

The bill (HR 3698), known as the Community Mental Health and Substance Abuse Services Improvement Act of 1992, passed through the Conference Committee in May. John Liu, a legislative aide for Rep Bill Lowery (R, Calif), says quick approval by Congress and by President Bush is expected. Lowery is a major proponent of the legislation.

The dramatic increase in drug-related violence, among other factors, has strained overburdened trauma care systems in many urban areas in the United States and has forced many centers to close. Trauma care for victims of gunshot wounds is extremely expensive and many of these patients are not covered by insurance.

Uncompensated Care

"Uncompensated trauma care is the Achilles' heel of the American health care system," says Howard Champion, MD, secretary and chairman of the legislative committee for the American Trauma Society, Washington, DC. The burden of trauma care is disproportionately distributed to hospitals according to their geographic location. Unlike many other health care facilities, trauma centers cannot choose which patients they will admit, Champion says.

Like falling dominoes, each trauma care center that closes puts additional pressure on remaining trauma facilities in the area, says John T. Dailey, MPA, a researcher at the (University of) Maryland Institute for Emergency Medical Services, Baltimore.

Ideally, a person critically injured in an area of the country served by a trauma care system usually will reach a trauma center within the "golden hour"—the period of time after injury in which a patient in severe shock must be treated if he or she is likely to survive. However, Dailey says, the closure of trauma centers in the United States is creating more and more areas from which critically injured people may not be able to reach appropriate care in time.

The trauma care systems of Los Angeles, Calif, and several other cities have already collapsed, while many other systems are strained to the limit and tottering, he says.

Hanging by Fingernails

In 1986, 10 hospitals participated in Metropolitan Chicago's trauma care system. Over the next 4 years, four centers withdrew because of financial hardship.

The remaining centers are struggling with the entire patient load that keeps growing due in part to escalating drug-related violence. "The system is stretched as tight as a bow string," says John Barrett, MD, director of the Cook County Hospital Trauma Unit, Chicago, Ill. "If one more hospital is forced to close, the whole system will collapse."

According to Barrett, when Humana-Michael Reese Hospital left the system after suffering a $2 million loss in 1990, Chicago's South Side was left underserved, placing a tremendous additional burden on Christ Hospital and Medical Center, the only hospital on the South Side remaining in the trauma system. The remaining six centers, which treated approximately 10 000 trauma patients, lost a total of $12 million in 1991.

Still, the trauma system of metropolitan Chicago is working, Barrett says. Ninety-five percent of the time, the transport time from the injury scene to a level I trauma facility is within the targeted 20 minutes.

"However, we are hanging on by our fingernails," Barrett says. "It's only a matter of time before one or more of our centers will be forced to let go."

Says Barrett, the cost of caring for drug-related violence is skyrocketing. "Not only is the number of gunshot victims increasing, but their wounds are becoming more difficult and expensive to treat—thanks to the replacement of 'Saturday night specials' with higher-power, semiautomatic and automatic assault weapons," he says.

In 1982, 95% of gunshot victims treated at Cook County had been shot only once, usually with a low-velocity bullet. In 1991, 25% of gunshot victims were treated for multiple wounds, many of which were made by high-velocity bullets, Barrett reports.

Other Chicago trauma centers have equally grim statistics. According to Benn Greenspan, MPH, president and chief executive officer, Mount Sinai Hospital and Medical Center treated 502 gunshot victims in fiscal year 1991, which is 29% more than the 388 treated in 1990. The average cost of treating a trauma patient at Mount Sinai in 1990 was $12 113. Because, Medicaid only reimbursed about $4200, the hospital lost approximately $8000 per Medicaid patient, Greenspan says.

To add to the problem, most gunshot victims treated at Mount Sinai are not covered even by Medicaid, he says. While the average age of trauma patients at Mount Sinai in 1991 was 31, the average age of patients admitted for gunshot wounds was only 25, 93% of whom were male. Young males are not eligible for Medicaid, Greenspan points out.

Why So Expensive

There are additional reasons for the great cost of trauma care, says Marcia S. Mabee, PhD, senior vice president and health policy analyst for Timothy Bell and Co, Reston, Va. Trauma centers need highly specialized personnel and high-tech equipment on standby status. They also have high overtime and special training costs.

The average stay for trauma care admission in the United States is 9.9 days compared with 6.6 days for non–trauma admissions. While 19% of non–trauma patients require admission to an intensive care unit, 57% of trauma patients require a stay in an intensive care unit. Says Mabee, the average cost of a trauma admission is 2.5 to 4 times the average cost of a non–trauma admission.

Although a disproportionate percentage of patients in need of trauma care are uninsured, trauma centers must admit all patients regardless of their ability to pay. In addition, Mabee says, Medicare and Medicaid reimbursements fall far short of actual costs of trauma care.

Speaking at the recent 14th Annual R Adams Cowley National Trauma Symposium in Baltimore, Dailey reported that, in a telephone survey of state emergency medical service directors, he found 66 trauma centers had shut down between 1983 and 1989. Depending on the definition used, estimates of the number of trauma care centers in the United States range from 350 to 500, Dailey says (*J Trauma*. In press).

The American College of Surgeons and many states have their own criteria for what constitutes a trauma center.

The college recognizes three levels of trauma facilities depending on the availability of specialized equipment and medical staff for providing trauma care that is not available round the clock in most hospital emergency facilities.

According to Dailey, 15 of the closed centers were in California, most of which were clustered in the Los Angeles area; eight were in Illinois, most of which were near Chicago; and 24 were in Florida, most of which were near Miami and in central Florida.

92 Centers Closed

At the Baltimore trauma symposium, Mabee reported similarly alarming findings from a survey she conducted with the Eastern Association for the Surgery of Trauma, Washington, DC. The survey found that 92 trauma centers had closed between 1985 and 1991, leaving 457 centers in operation that were designated by the state or verified by the American College of Surgeons.

Dailey also reported the results of a mail survey he conducted of administrators and clinicians at the 66 trauma centers he found had closed. The subjects were asked to rate the impact of 26 factors on the decision to close the facility.

According to the respondents, the most significant factor was uncompensated care, followed by high operating cost and the unavailability of physicians willing to provide on-call trauma care. The mean reported financial loss incurred by the closed trauma centers during their last 12 months of operation was more than $1.2 million, Dailey reports.

It is important to note, he says, that uncompensated care was likely a significant reason for physicians' unwillingness to provide trauma care service.

That view is supported by Stephanie Kennan, Washington, DC, legislative representative for the American College of Emergency Physicians, who says that many trauma physicians either bill patients directly for services or work for groups that bill the patients. While applauding the federal initiatives to help trauma care centers, she points out that the proposed legislation does not address uncompensated physician fees, which she says significantly contributes to the shortage of physicians providing trauma care.

According to Mabee, the legislation approved by the Conference Committee authorizes funding for a new program of grants to qualified trauma centers that meet certain criteria. The centers must provide comprehensive medical care and participate in an organized system of trauma care in geographic areas heavily affected by drug-related violence.

Gunshot, Knife Wounds

They also must treat a significant number of patients for gunshot or knife wounds or other drug-related assault injuries. Priority will be given to centers that receive financial assistance from the state or other political subdivisions; that are in an area where the availability of trauma care significantly decreased due to the closure of other trauma centers; and that can show that they too are at risk of closing due to financial losses from uncompensated trauma care. Preference will also be given to centers for which a disproportionate percentage of uncompensated costs results from providing trauma care to undocumented aliens.

While Mabee says the bill is a "wonderful commitment by the federal government to save the nation's trauma care system," she is sorry the bill gives state-funded centers priority over private trauma centers. The private centers, which receive no public support despite their enormous contribution to the community, are the ones at greatest danger of closing, she says.

$225 Million Requested

The legislation calls for an appropriation of $50 million for the program in fiscal year 1992, $75 million in 1993, and $100 million in 1994. Whether Congress will appropriate these funds and where it will get them remains to be determined.

One source of funding, says Mabee, would be income derived through the Guarini-Stark amendment to the US Customs Reauthorization Bill. If adopted, the amendment would allow the first $15 million of excess unobligated funds derived from the liquidation of property seized by the US Customs Service to go into general funds, the next $30 million to fund drug treatment programs, and the remainder to support trauma care centers. Had this legislation been in effect last year, the nation's trauma center program would have received approximately $20 million, she says.

However, according to Liu, Rep Lowrey does not want the funding of trauma centers to be dependent on assets seized by the US Customs. Liu predicts that appropriation from general funds will not be a problem since the congressman is a high-ranking member of the Appropriations Committee and because the bill has many powerful cosponsors in both parties, including Rep Henry Waxman (D, Calif) and Senators Albert Gore Jr (D, Tenn), Carl Levin (D, Mich), and Lloyd Bentsen, (D, Tex), who had introduced similar legislation in the Senate.

State Initiatives

A number of states also are coming to the aid of their trauma care systems. The governor of Maryland recently signed into law an $8 surcharge on vehicle license registration to save one of the nation's best trauma systems.

According to Kimball I. Maull, MD, director of the R (the late Dr Cowley had no formal first name, only the initial) Adams Cowley Shock Trauma Center, Baltimore, the surcharge is expected to yield $26 million annually, $7 million of which will support the Maryland Institute for Emergency Medical Service Systems field operations, $11 million will support the state's Med-Evac program, $3 million will support the Shock Trauma Center, and the remainder will support training for field providers and the purchase of ambulances.

Another kind of user fee tax to help defray the costs of trauma care for gunshot victims is being proposed by Rep Barbara Flynn Currie (D, Chicago), who is chair of the Illinois House of Representatives Revenue Committee in Springfield. At a press conference held May 17 at Mount Sinai Hospital Medical Center, Chicago, Currie proposed a $20 tax on the sale of all guns in Illinois.

Firearms Industry's Share

"Although guns cost the government hundreds of millions of dollars in health care each year, the firearms industry and its consumers do not pay their fair share," Currie says. "A gun tax is the first step in reimbursing trauma centers that continue to treat gun-shot victims who are unable to cover hospital bills and carry no insurance."

News that federal and state help may be on the way appears to have boosted Barrett's spirits. "We need to hear that there's some light at the end of the tunnel to encourage hospitals to hold on and not to go out of the trauma care business," he says.

While trauma care is very expensive, it's one of the more cost-effective kinds of medicine, Barrett says. "While putting $12 million more into fighting AIDS is not likely to achieve much, it could save trauma care in Chicago and the lives of many trauma victims," he says. "Unlike the major killers that show up later in life, trauma injuries primarily affect young people, causing more years of potential life lost than heart disease and cancer combined."

—by Andrew A. Skolnick

Attacks on Homosexual Persons May Be Increasing, But Many 'Bashings' Still Aren't Reported to Police

TRAUMA SURGEON Sheldon B. Maltz, MD, says he had never even heard of antigay violence before the 12 hours it took to save Ron Cayot's life.

Three young men had jumped out of a passing car, shouting slurs at Cayot and a friend who were walking down the street in a neighborhood known for its large gay and lesbian population. There was arguing, then there were gunshots.

One bullet went into Cayot's neck, requiring reconstruction of the larynx with tissue from his clavicle. Another went into Cayot's back, through his colon, liver, and intestines, and out his abdomen, says Maltz, a critical care specialist at Illinois Masonic Medical Center, Chicago.

Two states away, Paul Carson, MD, says he "couldn't conceive of anybody doing" what his patient claims to have done. The patient, a married heterosexual truck driver, insists that his only risk for acquiring his human immunodeficiency virus (HIV) infection was cuts on his hands during the many bloody beatings he and friends systematically inflicted on randomly selected gay men over several years, "too many times to count."

"It was sort of a diversion, entertainment with friends, and they [gay men] were easy targets, was the way he talked about it," says Carson, an infectious disease fellow at the University of Minnesota, Minneapolis.

"Gay-bashing," physical assaults motivated by prejudice against homosexual persons, increased by 15% in 1991, according to reports on a total of 755 such incidents collected from community groups in five cities—Boston, Chicago, New York, Minneapolis-St Paul, and San Francisco—by the National Gay and Lesbian Task Force. Its report says that, given the geographic diversity of those cities, "it is likely that other US urban areas, and perhaps suburban and rural communities as well, are experiencing a similar upswing."

'Very Gratuitous' Violence

"In our experience, the violence is very gratuitous, and seems to be inexplicable in terms of the number of bruises on the body," says Matt Foreman, executive director of the New York City Gay and Lesbian Anti-Violence Project. Guns, even knives, are not usually the weapons of choice, but rather crowbars, clubs, and chains, he says.

"There is a lot more injury than would happen with a regular robbery" or mugging, Foreman says, adding: "With such a high level of violence, you'd almost automatically assume the guy must have asked for it, or must have been involved in some sort of real fight." But while the violence is very real, the fights tend to be anything but fair, with attackers almost always armed, outnumbering their victims, and taking them by surprise.

While some of the recently reported increase is likely due to better data collection, most such assaults still go unreported, according to groups across the country that are trying to confront the problem.

Victims are often unwilling to report the nature of the attack to police, in part because police themselves are said to sometimes verbally and physically assault gay men and lesbians. There were 146 such cases of abuse by police reported to the National Gay and Lesbian Task Force, a 29% increase, in 1991.

Physicians Not Aware

Foreman says physicians sometimes may not believe patients who say they have been "gay-bashed," not necessarily because of prejudice against homosexuals, but because "we're always looking for rational reasons."

Physicians who treat these victims are often not told how the injuries occured because the patient fears "secondary victimization," says Gregory M. Herek, PhD, a psychology professor at the University of California, Davis.

"Physicians frequently assume that their patients are heterosexual" unless specifically told otherwise, says Herek. Physicians may also convey an insensitivity that will make victims of antigay violence less likely to reveal their sexual orientation, he says.

Gay and lesbian patients may worry that physicians will "treat them badly" because they are homosexual "or that this might get on their medical chart, which could have a lot of negative implications for them in the future," as employment and other forms of discrimination against gay men and lesbians are legal in more than 40 states. "If something shows up in the newspaper identifying them as the target of a gay attack, that can set them up for a lot of other harassment and discrimination from other people that has nothing at all to do with the original assault," says Herek.

For these reasons, some physicians advise against automatically encouraging victims to go to the police. In Michigan, Terry S. Stein, MD, says some of his own patients have been abused by police, and feels that filing a police report may be "unwise unless there is some assurance that the police are not going to victimize them again."

Physicians "need to be sensitive to the potential trauma and fear that a gay or lesbian person is experiencing, and not simply encourage them to report this without some thoughtful working through of what the outcome would be," says Stein, a professor of psychiatry at the Michigan State University College of Human Medicine, East Lansing.

However, not reporting these crimes "perpetuates the silence that has so long supported violence against lesbians and gay men," says Bill Dineen, a vice president of the Pink Angels Antiviolence Project, a volunteer group that patrols the neighborhood where Cayot was shot. "As far as the police department is concerned, if a crime doesn't get reported it didn't happen, and nothing gets done about it."

Dineen adds that police in the district patrolled by the Pink Angels are now very "committed to following up on the information we give them." The same is beginning to be true in many areas where community groups have worked with police.

Pierre Ludington, MD, president of the gay-oriented American Association of Physicians for Human Rights in San Francisco, says that, "in this city, the police are very sensitive to it, and will chase perpetrators down as quickly as they chase perpetrators of anything down."

Sexual Assaults Not Believed

Herek says physicians tend to be especially insensitive to gay men and lesbians in cases of sexual assault.

"There's an unwillingness to believe that a man, especially a gay man, can be sexually assaulted," Herek says. Physicians often "act as though this is something the victim brought on himself."

Herek says that, "in reality, in a great many cases of male/male sexual assault, it is heterosexual males who use sexual assault as just another way of degrading their victim. It really drives home the idea that rape is a crime of violence instead of passion when you see it being perpetrated by heterosexual men against gay men."

Lesbian victims of sexual assault often are asked questions in the emergency department "that tend to assume that they are heterosexual," with disapproval and disbelief when the woman says she is not on any form of birth control, says Herek. When a rape is a lesbian's first sexual contact of any kind with a man, it "can create a lot of psychological problems beyond what other women who have been raped would face," he adds.

Causes Deep-seated, Understudied

The questions of who perpetrates these violent acts and why, and why they seem to be increasing, have not been studied in a rigorous way. Rochelle Klinger, MD, professor of psychiatry at the Medical College of Virginia, Richmond, and member of the American Psychiatric Association Committee on Gay, Lesbian and Bisexual Issues, says she had trouble finding anything directly on antigay violence in the psychiatric literature during a recent search. Most information is in anecdotal accounts in the lay press, with some in academic articles on the more general issue of homophobia, she says.

"There is a lot of research about the stigmatization process in which society condones homophobia. That is the first step," says Klinger. "Then certain individuals take that to the furthest step, which is to actually be violent against gay men and lesbians."

Michigan State's Stein says causes are "rooted in both individual and societal prejudice. Many people perceive that aspects of antigay and antilesbian violence are "legitimized" by failure to prohibit discrimination against homosexuals and by failure of the courts to respond to the violence "in a way that gives a clear message that it is wrong."

"There isn't the same kind of moral outrage that is attached to racial and anti-Semitic violence," says Foreman. "As society increasingly condemns other forms of hate-motivated violence, it usually doesn't condemn antigay violence" to the same degree.

In 1991, for example, of nearly 600 cases followed through the courts by the New York antiviolence group, only two resulted in convictions. The lack of or weak official condemnation by the courts, schools, churches, and news media "keeps this going," says Foreman.

'Window of Acceptability'

"That's part of the explanation for the rise in antigay violence. There is still this window of acceptability," says Foreman.

There are attempts to close that window. Several state and local jurisdictions have included sexual orientation in laws mandating stiffer penalties for hate crimes (although some have explicitly excluded it).

A similar bill has been introduced in Congress. The 1990 federal Hate Crimes Statistics Act directs the Federal Bureau of Investigation (FBI) to collect data on sexual orientation and other bias-related crimes.

Only 26 states are submitting data so far. But the FBI hopes to publish its first report this fall, says Uniform Crime Reports instructor Bernie Dryden.

Perpetrator motives "are something we'd have a hard time understanding," says Carson, who found it "very hard to talk about" the violence his HIV-positive patient said he had committed. "A couple times in my office afterwards, he was crying about this stuff. I don't know if it was because of remorse or the realization of how he looked to other people."

One theory is that perpetrators may perceive themselves as enforcing society's gender rules or as defending their own masculine identity, says Foreman, noting that attacks often occur in the presence of such persons' female friends.

(Carson says his patient was "very upset" at the implication in some press accounts that latent homosexuality might have been behind his behavior.)

Perpetrators 'Different'

Those who carry out antigay violence are "different from normal perpetrators of violent crime," says Foreman, more often being middle class, able to afford their own attorneys, and looked at leniently by judges because they seldom have prior records.

Herek says some attackers are motivated by "deep-seated hostility or hatred," but many seem to participate because of more situational influences, like peer pressure.

A "classic pattern for violence against lesbians and gay men on the street is a group of late adolescent or young adult males, one of whom perhaps has strong feelings of wanting to go out and beat up some 'fags' or 'queers,' and that person cajoles the other members of the group. There is a feeling of a need to prove themselves to their friends, and so they go along with it," says Herek. "Perhaps they would not have initiated it themselves, but obviously they don't have strong feelings against it or they wouldn't have gone along with it."

Herek says that, unlike racially motivated attacks, which are more likely when the victim inadvertently wanders into the wrong neighborhood, perpetrators of antigay attacks go to gay areas seeking out victims. "That implies some sort of predisposition or premeditation, but it seems frequently that that may be the motive of just one or a couple members of the group, and the others are along for the ride."

The widespread belief that gay men especially are "not formidable foes" may also be a factor, he says, although "it's interesting that the perpetrators usually don't take any chances. They usually outnumber the victim and often carry weapons. There's no chance of a fair fight occurring."

That might also partly explain the increase of physical assaults, as gay men and lesbians are increasingly visible and may be increasingly likely to confront harassment. Dineen says that Ron Cayot's verbal response to a verbal assault "is indicative of where our community is. No, we are not acceptable targets and, no, we are not going to sit idly by and allow you to demean us or try to limit our expression or our sense of dignity and confidence just because you're uncomfortable with it."

Whether expressing that sentiment in verbal confrontation with someone hurling insults on the street is a good idea "depends on whether or not they have a gun," says Dineen, suggesting that a safer alternative is to step back, take a full description of the perpetrators and report it to police and antiviolence community groups.

Prevention in Physician's Office

Foreman says physicians may be able to play an important role in preventing antigay violence.

Adolescents account for 80% of all attacks, according to the New York Police Department's data. "Many are coming to grips with their own sexuality—not to say that gay-bashers are in fact gay, but that there are sexual identity issues that they act out" to prove that they are not gay or that they are a "real man."

"If physicians working with adolescents when sexuality issues come up would say that being gay is nothing bad or abnormal to be condemned or cured, that would be a big help," says Foreman.

Carson acknowledges that he can never prove that his patient acquired his HIV infection via gay-bashing. While there "clearly are some documented cases where trauma from infected blood seemed to transmit the virus," Carson says he doubts that it is "a real significant risk."

Yet he reported the case in a letter to the *Lancet* (1991;337:731) because "if anything will give pause to people maybe doing that sort of violence, it was worth it."—by Paul Cotton

CDC Investigators Explore New Territory in Aftermath of Unrest in Los Angeles

GOING WHERE apparently no epidemiologists have ever gone before, a team from the Centers for Disease Control (CDC) in Atlanta, Ga, has taken the public health approach to the most extreme outbreak in the ongoing epidemic of urban violence.

Seven investigators descended on Los Angeles, Calif, as the riots there ebbed. "Our mission," says Mark Rosenberg, MD, "was first to assess the injuries that occurred as a result of the disturbance and second to work with the community to help them develop ways of starting and supporting long-term approaches to youth violence prevention."

Violence, says Rosenberg, who is director of the Injury Control Division at the CDC, should be susceptible to the same public health approach used to eradicate smallpox and reduce the incidence of heart disease—epidemiologic research to better define risk factors, followed by the development, implementation, and evaluation of interventions.

Need to Act Quickly

As with acquired immunodeficiency syndrome (AIDS), there is no magic bullet vaccine, and "it is clear we need to change behaviors to make an impact on preventing its spread," says Rosenberg. And, as with AIDS, the situation is so urgent that "we need to get out and try a variety of programs and approaches, and try them quickly," he says, even before it is known which if any will actually work.

Two approaches in particular are being studied in pilot programs. One tries to teach young people not to be violent. The second involves intervening with victims of violence while they still are in the emergency department.

"We've identified some programs we think will work, and want to share these with affected communities throughout the country," says Rosenberg. "It's very important to tell people that there are things they can do."

That very notion, he says, "in and of itself is important in giving people a sense that they're not powerless, that they do not have to be passive victims, and that they can make a difference in their communities, their families, and their own lives."

The theory behind emergency department intervention, says Rosenberg, is that people who come in with injuries from violence are frequently perpetrators of violence. They may go back out on the street to "get even," or else get involved in the same types of activities that resulted in their initial injury.

Prevention in the Hospital

"If you can get to these people in the hospital when they have an injury, you may be able to teach them about the risks certain activities entail, about ways to resolve disputes without violence, or even the wisdom of walking away from fights," says Rosenberg. "The theory is compelling, and we'd like to try it."

Some emergency medicine physicians are rather skeptical, though.

"I've gotten to the point that I don't even bother asking what happened because I never get straight answers anyway," says neurosurgeon Leslie Geiger, MD. Geiger practices at Daniel Freeman Hospital in Inglewood, Calif, and helped patch up Reginal Denny, the truck driver whose near-fatal beating during the first hours of rioting in Los Angeles was televised worldwide.

Bruce Bulias, MD, who works in the emergency department at Daniel Freeman, says such a program "on the surface sounds nice," and might work "in a select group, maybe." But he says that "we have enough work down here just dealing with violence after it occurs, without worrying about what's going on out there and trying to prevent it."

Rosenberg says he believes that intervention in the emergency department may work. But he acknowledges that evaluation of such programs' effectiveness can be even harder than getting them up and running.

"You have to get it in place and done well so it has a chance of succeeding. You have to reach enough people so it might have a measurable impact. And you have to stick with the program and its evaluation long enough to detect the impact, if it has one," he says.

Unfortunately, Rosenberg concedes, such evaluation "may take many years. And we don't think we have time to wait."

Few Programs, Fewer Resources

Yet, while Rosenberg stresses the need for quick action, in Los Angeles right now there do not seem to be the resources "to get anything implemented quickly," says Maricella Hammett, MPH, a CDC health scientist. And for now, there does not seem to be all that much to implement.

After meeting with health leaders, public health researchers, state and local health officials, criminal justice representatives, community-based organizations, and even gang leaders and members, Hammett says, "we didn't really come up with a whole lot as far as what could be done right now."

What they did come up with, she says, "is a better understanding of the problems in Los Angeles and what we need to be thinking about if we're interested in reducing violence."

That might entail providing services to children at risk, and not just the recreational activities traditionally offered to occupy otherwise idle young hands. Instead, "more broad-based programs," including tutoring after school, mentoring by successful adults in the community, and self-esteem–building support systems for both children and parents are needed, Hammett says.

Mentoring programs seem particularly, though for reasons unknown, to decrease violent behavior, says Alex E. Crosby, MD, a CDC epidemiologist who also went to Los Angeles. "That's not necessarily medical care, but it is care for the community.

How to Handle Hopelessness

Other aspects are much harder to get a handle on. "Unemployment, racism, hopelessness, exposure to violence—all those things are directly associated with violent behavior," says Hammett.

She notes that unemployment, for example, is not in the purview of public health. Yet, she adds, "it's really hard to implement anything without dealing with problems such as these. All we can do at this point is to continue to gain a better understanding of the community, their perception of what they feel their problems are, and come together to talk about how to deal with those things."

Reed Tuckson, MD, president of the Charles R. Drew University of Medicine and Science in the Watts area of Los Angeles, says: "You must look at what occurred here from every element of life."

Tuckson says this extends "from the way people make a living to their education to how our institutions work and don't work—the level of respect and dignity as human beings. The causes relate very fundamentally to a community of people who absolutely feel hopeless and totally frustrated because of a history of insult, racism, disenfranchisement, and unfair financial practices of banks and other entrepreneurial institutions. They're frustrated simply trying to get through each day."

Inadequate health care contributes to the frustration, he adds. Both Drew and the Martin Luther King Medical Center were created in response to Los Angeles' 1965 Watts riots. They are "on the front lines in the health care fight, taking care of a population that is overwhelmingly uninsured in a hospital that receives grossly inadequate support," Tuckson says. "The hospital asked to take care of the people with the highest burdens of disease is given fewer resources than probably any other in the country. There is a fundamental incompatability there."

He adds that "it kills me when officials talk about how we have the finest health care system in the world, and that we don't want a Canadian system where people have to wait for certain procedures, as if people are not waiting in lines now for everything."

Tuckson says many of the urban poor "lack a concept of the possibility of a meaningful future, any sense that things will be better, that there's any chance for you to make it, and any chance that anybody's going to give a damn whether you make it or not."

Tuckson also cites the cumulative "psychic consequences" of violence among people in the community, and against them by police: "Each of those episodes has a consequence, and adds to the frustration."

"Put all that stuff together and let it simmer over time, and it doesn't matter much what the incident is that triggers unrest," he says. "Tensions are so high that the trigger is pulled by itself."

True Community Leaders Are Key

Key to addressing such problems, says Hammett, is finding true community leaders, not so much representatives of community organizations but "people who live directly in the communities affected by violence who are respected by that community. We have to figure out who they are, and how we can involve them."

One such leader, she suggests, is Paul Guidry, MD, who was born, raised, and is practicing in South Central Los Angeles—the epicenter of the recent unrest.

With a tenuous truce among gangs in the aftermath of the unrest, Guidry sees "an opportunity here with this window in history to markedly improve our whole country, a chance for the ones left out of our country's expansion to come back on board." He estimates that there are 1 million gang members throughout California, all disenfranchised members of society who are "right now at this point in time all reaching out, wanting to just be able to live the American dream."

However, this opportunity will be wasted, Guidry predicts, if the approach to solutions is decided by outsiders and implemented from the top down.

So far, says Guidry, "the same people who got us into this mess in the first place are the ones being allowed to make the decisions on how we keep it from happening again. Those people have not sat down with the people on the street to reach common ground. They just assume they know the problem. If they had known the problem in the beginning we wouldn't be where we are now."

If "we don't get any grassroots, from-the-bottom-up type structuring, the anger is going to boil up again, but it's going to lash out well outside the affected communities," Guidry cautions.

"This [riot] was a very small tremor" compared to what could occur next time, he says. "You've got people who have no fear. They've been shot multiple times, lived under poverty, had no hope. They're not afraid of the National Guard or the military or the police, and they're very well armed."

Riots, or revolt, as he terms the recent unrest, "are very negative and very destructive. It is a lot easier, just like with preventive medicine, to prevent things than to come in and try to get them cured."

Military Attack?

Richard Wigod, MD, president of the Los Angeles County Medical Association, says he advocates "a military attack" on areas with high degrees of crime and gang violence. "I don't see how society can tolerate much more of this kind of thing. We need to somehow make a sweep through those neighborhoods, take all the weapons we can find, and take some of these people off the streets somehow."

While uncomfortable with the possible trampling of constitutional rights, "what's happening is chaos," says Wigod.

Such an approach, says Guidry, would be like "pouring gasoline on a fire. Even if you cleaned everything up and took every gun away, you still haven't improved the root cause problems.

"That seige mentality, treating us in these communities not as citizens but as an enemy such as Iraq, that will never cure anything. It wouldn't take long to buy more guns, and we would be in the same mess again, only with the animosity even more bitter.

"The solution is not quasi-military. The solution is equal opportunity."

Tuckson also says that the "good guys/bad guys" discussion "drives me nuts. It is horrible to riot and loot, but you'll have a hard time trying to understand it if you write them off as bad people and take them to jail.

"To deny that there are legitimate reasons for the unrest does not help in terms of treatment and intervention."

Guidry outlines six principles for addressing the situation:

1. Confronting what he sees as "blatant racism" of the law enforcement and judicial systems.
2. Putting the needs of US citizens before those of other countries.
3. Rebuilding the infrastructure of American cities.
4. Investing in education, jobs, and industry so those in lower socioeconomic classes are "not forced into the drug and crime trades as their only option."
5. Establishing health care "for the masses, so one's medical prognosis does not have to be worse for poor blacks."
6. Getting the news media to stop negative stereotypical portrayals of minorities.

Guidry says that the resources to be allocated for rebuilding Los Angeles might even be adequate "so long as they go from the bottom up, and not from the top down. With the trickle-down theory we've been dealing with since the early 1980s, nothing has trickled down, it's a drought at the bottom."

'Opportunity for Medicine'

Tuckson says that all of medicine "now has the opportunity, the responsibility, and the obligation to make use of our networks and collaborations as health professionals facing these crises. Those trying to fight on the front lines need the help of those who have access to resources."

At some point, he says, "we have to say to each other that, while we're training plastic surgeons to go work on Rodeo Drive, maybe we can find a way to be of some assistance to those trying to work on the front lines in places where the rest of us really don't want to go."

That, says Tuckson, "is a moral commitment that we have as part of the profession."

Some such help is already provided through collaborations with the University of California at Los Angeles. Talks are under way with several federal agencies, and Tuckson says he has received an "astounding" array of calls from people throughout American medicine, yet he warns against any "Pollyana sense that it's going to happen magically. It's going to be very hard."

—by Paul Cotton

Hospital Staff, Victims, Families Cope With Life-Altering Effects of Violence

THE WRONG PLACE at the wrong time. That's where victims of urban violence say they were when tragedy struck.

If their luck changes, they may find themselves afterward in the right place to reclaim a life that has been altered forever by traumatic injury, often from a gun or a knife. This is a story about some of the staff at one of these places and a few of the victims of this country's war against itself.

The Rehabilitation Institute of Chicago (RIC) is not only highly esteemed in Illinois, but the *U.S. News & World Report* "America's Best Hospitals" survey rated it first in the nation (August 5, 1991). It is one of 135 rehabilitation hospitals and 672 rehabilitation units in general hospitals in the United States.

Such facilities used to exist primarily to help patients of all ages who were injured in motor vehicle, diving, and other accidents. Now, the ones located in cities are hard pressed to take care of all the younger members of the community who have been disabled deliberately—often permanently—by the violent acts of their peers.

Untold Stories

"Every time I turn on the news or go to a movie, the emphasis is on the perpetrators of violence," says physiatrist Vinod Sahgal, MD, director of the Brain Trauma Program at RIC. "None of those who dramatize this whole issue take the time to depict what happened to the victim—and to the victim's family."

He says he deplores the fact that presentations involving violence tend to leave viewers "fixated" on its exciting aspects, while ignoring the inevitable results. "It's very easy to write about the crime," says Sahgal. "The hard thing is to make the victim's side of the story as dramatic."

Sahgal's own workdays are full of this quieter drama. The brief newspaper story recounting yet another not-quite-deadly assault is quickly forgotten.

The victim, the physician recounts, may be one of his patients, "an upper-middle-class black social worker who labored for years to make life better for residents of a public housing development until one day a couple of them, under the influence of cocaine, battered her to a pulp."

Brought to RIC, the woman lingers comatose for months. After her condition is stabilized under a care regimen for persons in a persistent vegetative state created by the Brain Trauma Program staff, her husband takes her home, where he will devote his life to her care.

But Sahgal's responsibility hasn't ended. Eventually the patient's insurance entitlements run out, the family can no longer manage, and the physician must write detailed letters to the third-party payer. Not entertaining, he says, never seen on prime-time TV, but this is the real drama spawned by the decline of civility in American society.

Eighty percent of patients in a persistent vegetative state go home from RIC after technology has saved their lives. "Does anybody know," Sahgal asks rhetorically, "what happens to the relatives of these people?"

Patients like the social worker, with no remaining cognitive function, are at one end of the spectrum seen in the program. Then there are victims of violence who are in a locked-in state. Unable to move or speak, they are nevertheless aware of everything. Still others are severely injured but have some residual function.

Emergency departments save lives, Sahgal says, "and I provide a backup so that this life is maximized to its potential. My responsibility is to provide a structure for the survivors of accident or assault."

Sahgal has been associated with RIC for 27 years, ever since his student days at Northwestern University Medical School, with which it is affiliated. "When I went into this work," he says, "I thought we were going to be dealing with purely automobile accidents; maybe one or two bad societal issues. But now it's a very ugly scene. It's very hard for me to be making a living by taking care of these situations."

It's not that Sahgal feels sorry for himself. A man of deep compassion, he is trying to convey the sense of frustration aroused by cases that continually increase in number and savagery.

In addition to street crime, often fueled by drugs, including alcohol, he says, "there is violence which is brought from the community into the house. Right now, I have here two mothers who were beaten by their sons because they refused to give their children money to go and buy crack cocaine. And I have one son who became so belligerent and threatening to his family that the family ganged up and beat him on the head."

Battered wives and children, adolescents, and husbands, too, however tragic, are nothing new, and this is one form of violence that cuts across social and economic lines. But regarding his patients in general, says Sahgal, "the higher the socioeconomic group, the lower the incidence of perpetrated violence. And vice versa."

Because RIC is a private, not-for-profit institution, it accepts patients from all financial levels "with physical disabilities that affect their ability to perform activities of daily living." This makes for a mix of adults and children of varied background with differing diagnoses. Still, one has only to enter the lobby where patients in wheelchairs sit chatting or awaiting visitors, or look in on the common areas of head injury or spinal cord injury floors, to note the preponderance of young black males.

Sitting Ducks in the City

"If somebody wants to shoot you, they'll likely come in a van, especially with a side door they can slide open real quick," says Deshawn Brown, a 17-year-old who seems to know what he's talking about. As he got off a bus last November, Brown was shot through the spine by a 28-year-old man he had told not to bother Brown's young cousin.

A junior in high school whose favorite subject is history, Brown says he later read the newspapers for the day he was shot. "Three other guys in Chicago got shot that day too," he says. "Killed."

After 2 weeks in Chicago's Cook County Hospital, Brown was moved to RIC, where he says he "worked real

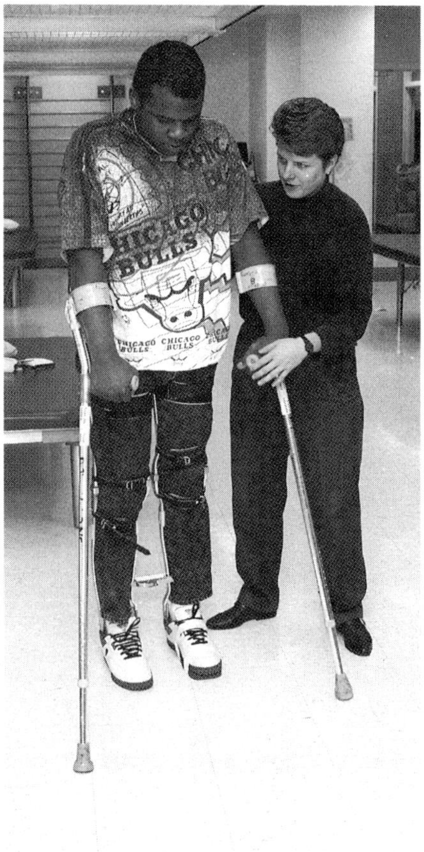

Rehabilitation Institute of Chicago

Deshawn Brown tries walking with his new braces, assisted by physical therapist Julie DeWerd.

hard and got an early discharge." A tall, strong young man with an engaging smile and his hair styled in the latest finger wave, Brown lives with his mother, stepfather, and younger brother in a suburb south of the city.

He visits RIC as an outpatient three times a week to work out and strengthen his arm muscles. His goal is to "first get my braces, then get a job."

Pondering the circumstances that put him in the hospital, Brown says, "I remember they used to have fistfights. Now it's drive-bys or shootouts. People just don't care anymore."

Another patient interviewed in the Robert R. McCormick Physical Therapy Treatment Area is a 16-year-old Chicago South Sider. The victim of a drive-by shooting near his home last September, during the first week of his junior year in high school, this young man now attends a wheelchair-accessible school and visits RIC three times a week.

"Around my house," says the all-too-typical teenager, "there's no fighting, just shooting." As in Brown's case, he says, the two men who shot him were soon caught. One was 25 years old, the other 23. The alleged perpetrators haven't been tried yet.

Accident Creates Activists

As accustomed as Chicagoans, like other urban residents, have become to these stories, sometimes the age of perpetrators of violence—as well as the victims—can still astonish. On March 10, the city reeled from the news that an 8-year-old boy had shot a 3rd-grade classmate in a West Side elementary school.

The boy carried two guns to school in a bookbag, allegedly sold one to the school-bus driver, then later is said to have pulled the other out in the classroom and shot Michelle Rodriguez in the back.

According to Bonnie and William Sanchez, the little girl's mother and stepfather, and police who took the boy into custody, they had "never seen anybody so cool." The boy is scheduled to undergo psychiatric evaluation to determine whether he can stand trial, which would be as a juvenile offender.

The bullet injured Michelle's third vertebra. After surgeons at Chicago's Children's Memorial Hospital operated and her condition was stabilized, the child found herself, like older gunshot victims, in the Spinal Cord Injury Program at RIC. The winsome little girl made excellent progress and recently walked out and home, wearing a brace and continuing to go to a local hospital for physical therapy.

The incident has made ardent gun control advocates out of her parents. Bonnie Sanchez says they knew the neighborhood was dangerous—street gangs have taken over one nearby playground for shooting sprees and no one walks around heedlessly after dark—but "even with all this going on, it never entered my mind that one of my kids could get shot in school. That would be the last place I would think of."

Now, William Sanchez takes time off from his construction job and Bonnie finds babysitters for Michelle and her two sisters and brother at home so the parents can travel to Springfield, the state capital, and testify for gun control legislation introduced by Sen William Marovitz (D, Chicago).

"Before the accident happened to Michelle," Sanchez says, "we were against guns, but we didn't know what we could do about it. Now people are helping us make a difference. I think if everybody who feels the same way would work for this, we could all make a difference."

He and Bonnie speak as one on the main point: "This incident isn't over for us until something is done about gangbangers getting hold of guns and using them without getting severely punished. The little kids see the big kids doing it. That little boy who shot Michelle brought those guns from home, from his older brother. A lot of young punks have semiautomatic weapons that even the police aren't allowed to have. We need to put an end to all these kids having guns."

Gunshot Injuries Going Up

Gary Yarkony, MD, director of the Spinal Cord Injury Program at RIC, would like to see a decrease in the number of injuries resulting from gunshot wounds, as well as the ones from accidents and "another weapon of violence, only bigger—the automobile." From June 1990 to December 1991, firearms accounted for 27% of the admissions to his program (after 34% from motor vehicle accidents and 30% from falls).

"The injuries are difficult enough for the patient to adapt to," Yarkony says, "but they also disrupt the lives of the relatives. The patients have suddenly become dependent upon their parents or children, husbands or wives. Then they have to deal with, 'Why am I the victim of random, senseless violence?' "

In Detroit, Mich, gunshot wounds have become the leading cause of spinal cord injury, Yarkony says. In Chicago, they aren't the leading cause overall, but they are probably the leading cause of paraplegia. The inner-city population in which spinal cord injury from firearms is most common also has problems that make rehabilitation generally more difficult—although some members bring unusual strengths to bear.

As an example of the difficulties, says Yarkony, although RIC does not require private insurance, the fact that most of the young, inner-city victims of guns are dependent on public aid creates problems with such things as billing for attendant care and replacing wheelchairs as they deteriorate. "There's no chance at all for any home renovations or modifications to make their daily life easier," he says.

Then, there are problems with leaving the rehabilitation setting and returning to an environment where nutrition, care, and comfort are minimal. "You can't heal a pressure sore if you don't have adequate nutrition, or there's no one to help turn you when you're in bed, or you've got a high injury above C-6 and are poikilothermic and you can't adjust the temperature in your apartment."

Poor people also find accessible housing hard to come by. They may have to wait until the public housing authority has an apartment available.

"Many victims of inner-city violence have no insurance," Yarkony points out. "Public aid is willing to keep people in

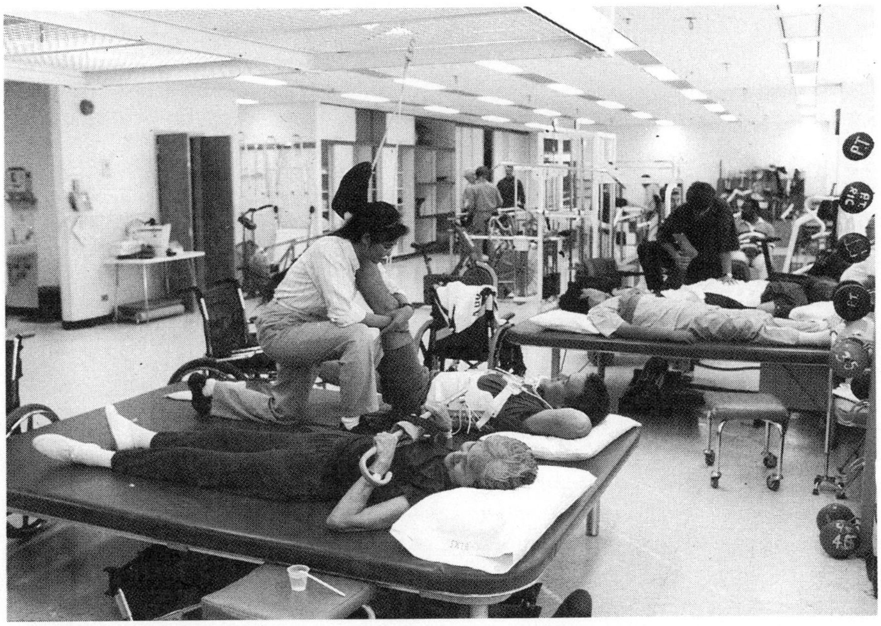

Rehabilitation Institute of Chicago

The physical therapy treatment area is a bustling part of the rehabilitation program for patients with spinal cord injury. Many of the participants are outpatients who visit several times each week.

the hospital as long as they go to therapy and are progressing, but if you run into a situation where they're not progressing in therapy but you don't have everything in line to get them home, that's where you run into trouble. All the problems anyone has with spinal cord injury are exacerbated for the inner-city population," he concludes.

While they are at RIC, everyone with a spinal cord injury (similar to people with brain trauma) is treated by a team consisting of nurses, a nurse-therapist who serves as a resource person, social worker, psychologist, physiatrist, and occupational, physical, vocational, and recreational therapists. The team meets in conference once every 2 weeks, so everyone is aware of the patient's problems—and progress—in other areas.

"I think you'll notice that the atmosphere here is a lot brighter than you would expect," says Frank Mordini, PhD, a psychologist in the Spinal Cord Injury program, and he's right. The decor is colorful and paintings hang on many walls.

Everything is geared to answer the questions Mordini states as, "How can you, as a disabled person, fit back into your world? How can you reintegrate your self-concept and feel good about yourself?"

"You're not going to do your traditional psychotherapy here," Mordini says. "These individuals [inner-city youths] would not have sought out psychological help at any time in their life. Now they're in rehabilitation and part of their rehab is everyone sees the psychologist. Their feeling is, 'I've lost everything and now I don't want anybody messing with my mind, the only thing I have left. Nobody's going to start playing games with my mind, so I don't want to see a psychologist.'

"Also, they're not used to talking about their feelings. They're used to action. They've dealt with their emotions through action. So they have a hard time with the psychologist, but you understand that and work with it. After what's happened to them, these people are very angry. The most important thing is to depersonalize the anger and build trust of the staff, on whom the patients are totally dependent."

Differing Reactions

Mordini says the reaction to their disability of the young inner-city men (and while there are some women, there are many more men) is a little different from some other groups. Many gang members see the injury as a badge of courage, he says: "They've kind of done their thing and the wheelchair represents that." Others feel even more vulnerable to the violence in the community that put them into the hospital.

Life in the inner city equips some patients with a kind of resiliency, Mordini says. "Dealing with hardships is just part of their lives. They know they're going to go on, and it's just going to be another part of life, another shot at them. There's no discrepancy between their world view and what happened to them, so in some ways it's easier for them to adjust to their new life."

Robert Heilbronner, PhD, a specialist in neuropsychology, works with patients who have suffered head injury. His patients have, in many ways, a rougher road to travel than do Mordini's, maneuvering in their wheelchairs or struggling to walk with their braces. He tends to view them differently, too.

Heilbronner says, "A brain injury often occurs in people who are basically masochistic—but I don't mean in the sexual sense. I mean they haven't learned how to look out for their best interests. They engage in a lot of risk-taking, unhealthy activities that will likely lead to a brain injury or something else that is going to cause pain for them."

Rehabilitation for such people is difficult. Mentioning the usually cited contributory factors—impoverished home environments, lack of adult male supervision—that lead to gang membership and its frequently damaging results, Heilbronner says, "We have many people who are not introspective or adept at talking about their emotions. Many times we just have to let them go. Many of these people were drinkers and drug users before their injury, and they become worse after it. Many who were not substance abusers become abusers."

He says the traditional treatment approaches won't work for these people because of their impaired cognitive function. However, some recovery programs are trying to develop dual diagnoses of "traumatic brain injury plus substance abuse," and to direct their programs specifically to these people.

Little known to the public at large but sobering to therapists, says Heilbronner, is the finding that a person who has had one head injury is four times as likely as the general population to have a second one. "If they have had two severe head injuries," he says, "and believe me, we see them, they are eight times as likely to have others."

Heilbronner and other members of an interdisciplinary team try to help survivors of brain injury adjust to their lives after they may have lost most of what makes life worth living: "thinking ability, psychosocial skills, physical functions, income, family members, self-esteem."

He emphasizes that the obvious impairments—slow thinking, difficulty in walking and talking, problems with memory—are not as great impediments to patients' readjustment to society as are their psychological and emotional reactions and changes in behavior.

Less than 10% of people with brain injury return to work without formal rehabilitation, Heilbronner says. Family and marital problems are common.

The psychologist says he thinks the most effective therapy is done on an outpatient basis, in groups of half a dozen or so similarly afflicted people meeting daily, for about 6 months. "They're confronted with their deficits but they're also being supported," he says.

Some people make remarkable comebacks. Heilbronner talks about a young woman accountant, badly injured in a fall, who not only recovered but decided to switch her career to occupational therapy and work to help others. And Sahgal's office is crowded with paintings, sculpture, and other objects made by his patients.

Yet, "there aren't a lot of success stories," says Heilbronner. "People do the best they can at any moment, given their developmental history, current environmental constraints, and current brain function. You can't expect more of them than they're capable of."

What Do Paraplegics Sound Like?

"You learn to do the best you can with what you have," says 25-year-old Patricia Filardi, who didn't know what she would become capable of after hoodlums stabbed her in the back of the neck, nearly severing her spinal cord, almost 2 years ago. It was early in the evening on Halloween.

After attacking Patti Filardi as she parked her car on a quiet residential street on Chicago's West Side—on her way to visit her grandfather—the two men tried but failed to drag her into the car, then threw her into the street and ran over her hand as they drove away in her car. They have not been caught.

Today, Patti doesn't shrink from her memory of the dreadful incident, but blessed with a remarkably positive nature (as well as abundant good looks and supportive family and friends), she looks confidently toward the future.

She speaks particularly of the support of her cousin, Shari Schabowski, MD, who was a medical student at the time Patti entered the hospital and is now a first-year resident in emergency medicine at Henry Ford Hospital in Detroit. From the first night, when Shari insisted on staying in the intensive care unit and spent 3 hours washing the blood out of her cousin's luxuriant blonde hair, the two young women have never given up on Patti's future.

Reflecting on her life since she was forced to stop teaching aerobics and start learning to experience the world from a seated position, Patti says a major adjustment is having to rely on others. "Society stresses independence. When you're a child you want to reach independence. Then something like this happens to you and you're totally dependent again. It's a big change."

Also, one has to plan the simplest things carefully. "It could take you any-

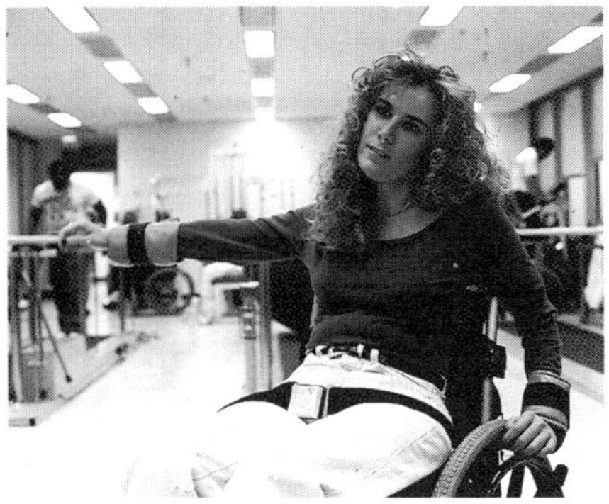

Rehabilitation Institute of Chicago

Patricia Filardi practices "ranging" in an attempt to maximize her physical ability.

where from 20 minutes to an hour to get dressed," she says, "and you have to say to yourself, 'Will I have enough endurance after I get myself dressed and up and out the door to go to school, to go to work, to get on with everything else?'

"Sometimes you have to weigh your priorities and decide, 'Would I rather have someone help me get dressed and have it take 5 minutes, and have endurance for the rest of the day, or would I rather do it myself?' "

Patti's endurance has improved as time goes on, she says. She does go to school and plans to become an architect. She goes to work at the same job she had before: as a receptionist (using typing sticks to augment the limited motion of her fingers) in the Orthopedics Department at Northwestern Medical Faculty Foundation.

And as for everything else, she says, "I still go out. I love to meet people. I love to eat." However, says this model-slim woman, "You have to watch your weight. You always want to look your best. And you have to stay healthy, too. The heavier you get the harder it is to push your wheelchair."

Watching Patti Filardi chat with the others working out in the physical therapy center, one is impressed with how far she's come from the person who "had a very big problem with most of the patients who were here when I came in, because they were young black men. I was totally terrified of them because of the ones who hurt me. There were a lot of patients on the floor who were in gangs or had been in gangs and would talk about violence. That was how they had become injured."

Now, she says, "I have friends here who are young and are black. But it's taken a lot of time to cope with it."

Some things Patti is still working on are overcoming fear of being alone and vulnerable and fear of physical contact. She's doing pretty well at learning to be more patient with herself, she says, adding quietly, "You have to be more patient with others now all the time."

Most important, she says, "You don't want people to feel sorry for you. I think if you're friendly and you talk to people and you educate them, they'll learn about people with disabilities."

Her faith in humanity was put to the test recently when Patti tried to place a telephone order for tickets to a Chicago Bulls game and requested wheelchair seating. After a lengthy process of being shunted from one ticket seller to another, she finally got one who said, "No problem."

But then the ticket seller asked, "By the way, what do you need wheelchair seating for?" When Patti replied, "I'm in a wheelchair," he said, "Well, you don't sound like that."

"And then I wondered," reflects Patti wryly, "what does someone in a wheelchair sound like?"

'Think First'

High school students throughout the United States are beginning to hear some thought-provoking stories from people in wheelchairs. The speakers are paralyzed young men and women who take part in a national program, developed by neurosurgeons, known as "Think First." The program aims to alert students to risky behavior and motivate them to change it through encounters with their disabled peers.

"In order to get people to change their behavior—to avoid hanging with gangs or riding with drunk drivers, for example—they must realize that the consequences of that behavior are severe," says Julie Sells, OT, coordinator of RIC's Injury Prevention Program as well as its "Think First" program. "These kids have got to realize that they're not just going to die if they get shot or get in a car accident, for example, and then it's all going to be over. They've got to see that brain injuries and spinal cord injuries can lead to disabilities that you may live with for a lifetime."

One of her most effective speakers, says Sells, is Andrell Dorsey, a young man who was caught in gang crossfire as he was shooting hoops in a park about 4 years ago. Living today with a bullet in his neck (because removing it is considered too dangerous), Dorsey sits in his wheelchair at Chicago area junior high and high school assemblies and tells students about his experiences at RIC. He also says, "I stayed out, I didn't listen to my mama, and I was at the wrong place at the wrong time." He tries to impress on his listeners that they can, at least in some measure, control their own luck. Dorsey tells teenagers, "I want you all to start thinking while you still have a choice."—by Marsha F. Goldsmith

Adolescents May Experience Home, School Abuse; Their Future Draws Researchers' Concern

OF ALL THE TYPES of family violence, abuse of adolescents is perhaps one of the most overlooked. Many people, including professionals, assume that the majority of victims of child abuse are small children. Identification and treatment programs tend to focus on the very young.

But research in recent years is beginning to paint a picture of adolescence that is more abuse-ridden than early childhood. According to statistics compiled by the National Center on Child Abuse and Neglect, Washington, DC, adolescents experience a disproportionately high level of child abuse, including the most severe abuse that results in serious injuries and death.

Youths aged 12 to 17 years constitute 38% of the child population, yet 47% of the victims of all forms of child maltreatment fall into this age group. Teenagers aged 15 to 17 years represent 19% of the child population, yet they experience 27% of the serious injuries and 23% of the fatalities due to child abuse (National Center on Child Abuse and Neglect. *Executive Summary: National Study of the Incidence and Severity of Child Abuse and Neglect.* Washington, DC: US Dept of Health and Human Services; 1982).

A large-scale study conducted within recent years has further defined the extent and types of abuse that adolescents experience within the family. Mildred Daley Pagelow, PhD, adjunct research professor of sociology at California State University, Fullerton, surveyed 1025 college students at three state university campuses in Southern California about their experience of family violence during adolescence. Pagelow first presented her findings at the 1988 annual meeting of the Pacific Sociological Association.

And recently, in a separate but complementary study, 3357 middle and senior high school students in an Indiana school district were surveyed about their approval of hitting family members, fellow students, and girlfriends and boyfriends under various scenarios. The students were predominantly white (African-Americans were the largest minority, at 12%), and from working- and middle-class families in Anderson, Ind (population, 65 000).

Sociologist Barbara Carson, PhD, and Diane Daane, JD, both assistant professors of criminal justice and criminology at Ball State University, Muncie, Ind, presented their findings at the 1992 annual meeting of the American Sociological Association.

The studies reveal a high level of interfamily abuse and approval of abuse during adolescence within these groups. The data also raise serious questions about the effects of abuse in the home, the role of physical punishment, and the possibility that family violence might be perpetuated by this generation of future parents.

Violence Against Children

Of the college students Pagelow surveyed, 42% said their fathers physically assaulted them as adolescents, and 49% said their mothers assaulted them. Mothers tended to use the milder forms of violence, such as slapping. Fathers kicked, punched, choked, and beat up their children more often than did the mothers.

An open-ended item produced numerous comments about parental abuse. About half of the students referred to emotional abuse and neglect. Many adolescents were shaken or whipped with objects commonly used to "punish" children, such as belts, straps, sticks, boards, and wooden spoons, Pagelow reports.

One mother "pulled [her daughter's] hair out." One father twisted his son's ear, and another father hit his daughter's head on her sister's head. "To some," Pagelow says, "these may seen to be mild forms of punishment for children aged 12 or over, yet the fact that the victims vividly remembered them years later shows that they were abusive events in their younger lives."

Violence Between Siblings

Both studies examined violence between siblings—perhaps the most common form of violence within families. Of the students Pagelow surveyed who had siblings living at home at age 12 years, almost half were victims or aggressors of "violent acts of kicking and punching." Ten percent said their siblings beat them up, and 4% said their siblings threatened them with a knife or gun, or used a knife or gun against them.

In Carson and Daane's survey of middle and senior high school student attitudes, 74% of the students approved of hitting one's sibling if one is reacting to being hit first. Forty-three percent approved of hitting if the sibling breaks one's stereo, 38.5% approved if the sibling makes fun of the student in front of friends, and 24.8% approved if there is an argument and the other sibling "does not listen to reason."

"Violence between children is so commonplace," Pagelow says, "that it is looked at as 'normal' childhood behavior. Parents take it for granted that 'kids will be kids,' and tend to ignore sibling violence. Yet it can have long-lasting effects."

In individual interviews with students, Pagelow found that parents often "hotly defended" the aggressive child and were either unaware or refused to believe that their children behaved violently toward one another, especially when weapons were involved.

Pagelow found in her study that more violence occurs between siblings than any other type of interfamily violence. Straus, Gelles, and Steinmetz, in their 1980 book, *Behind Closed Doors: Violence in the American Family,* also reported this finding in a survey of parents. The authors also found that families with sons-only consistently have more sibling violence than families with daughters-only. This difference increases as the children mature, until it is twofold by ages 15 through 17 years.

Violence Between Spouses

It is not difficult to imagine where these children may have learned to use violence. Thirty-one percent of the students surveyed by Pagelow said their fathers had been abusive to their mothers, and 24% said their mothers had been abusive to their fathers. Regarding the most severe forms of abuse, 7% of the fathers of these students beat up their mothers, 3% threatened them with weapons, and 1.2% used a knife or gun.

In her survey, Pagelow used a modified conflict tactic scale that listed eight categories of behavior termed "psychological violence" and nine categories termed "physical violence." Except in one of the psychological abuse items, "cried," the students said their fathers were more violent than their mothers in all types of behavior.

Ten percent of the fathers and 7% of the mothers kicked or punched the other; 5% of the fathers and 1% of the mothers choked the other.

In Carson and Daane's survey, a small but significant percentage of adolescents approved of hitting one's spouse under certain circumstances. For example, 9.6% of the students approved of a husband hitting his wife if she "would not listen to reason," 7.2% approved if she embarrassed him in front of his friends, 6.5% approved if she wrecked the car, and 22.6% approved if she hit him first.

Although the percentages in most of these scenarios are small, Carson says they should not be quickly dismissed. Because of the large sample size, a rate as low as 6.5% represents 215 students within the Anderson school district who feel it is appropriate for a husband to hit his wife if she wrecks the car.

Approval of a wife hitting her husband was even greater. More than 12% said a wife could hit her husband if he would not listen to reason, 11.8% if he embarrassed her in front of her friends, 8.4% if he wrecked the car, and 59.4% if he hit her first.

Carson and Daane were surprised at the high percentage of students who approved of a wife hitting her husband within the context of "self-defense." They have concluded that this represents an "implicit tolerance of violence against women." That is, giving a woman approval to hit back in self-defense in no way provides for her defense, they explain. If both men and women are free to exchange blows with one another, it is invariably the woman who will sustain the most serious injuries. In many situations, hitting back could increase the woman's risk for violence.

Hitting back does not resolve the conflict, they add, and besides, no person deserves to be hit, be they male or female.

Violence Against Peers

Carson and Daane also questioned the students about their approval of hitting one's girlfriend or boyfriend. With the exception of the scenario where one does not listen to reason, the adolescents gave more approval to violence in dating relationships than between married couples.

The finding reflects an overall observation by these researchers that there is more widespread approval of the use of force in situations that are especially relevant to the lives of these students, compared with situations that involve older adults.

The approval rating was even higher when the students were asked about hitting another student. Almost one third said they approved of hitting another student if the student embarrassed them, 29.3% said they approved if another student wrecked their car, 33.6% approved of hitting a student to defend one's "group" or clique, and 58.5% approved of hitting if a slur had been made against their parents.

The high approval of violence between students was particularly alarming given that 34% of the students approved of students carrying knives in school, and 14.1% (450 students) said they felt it was appropriate, at least sometimes, to carry guns in school.

Interventions For Those At Risk

Overall, Carson says her survey revealed about 400 to 500 students out of approximately 3300 in the Anderson middle and senior high school system who approve of violence in a wide range of contexts. "These kids are being taught this somewhere," she says. "Odds are they are witnessing or being a victim of violence at home. There is strong research that shows that exposure to violence affects attitudes about violence."

Also worrisome is the possible relationship between approval of violence and engaging in violence. Research in this area does not support a completely causal relationship, Carson says, but people who approve of violence are more likely to engage in violence.

Carson and Daane's study was commissioned by the Anderson Mayor's Commission on Domestic Violence. In their report to the commission, the researchers endorsed educational programs in conflict mediation, which are now under way.

They also advocated group counseling sessions for "victims," the term they used to describe the several hundred students who they suspect are experiencing or witnessing violence at home based on the students' high approval of violence.

The researchers also suggest that students be exposed to adults who tell them that no form of hitting is appropriate and that there are better ways to resolve problems and express anger.

Counteracting Violence

"As a society, we rank very high in our approval of violence," Carson says, "and a lot of forces out there teach kids that it's okay to use violence. We must make a strong commitment to prohibit violence in the home, or else the [anti-violence] message is just not going to get through."

Carson and Daane advocate establishing the home as a "no hitting zone." This prohibits hitting between all family members, including corporal punishment.

In *Behind Closed Doors*, Straus demonstrates a relationship between the age of last spanking and the probability of engaging in child abuse as an adult. The later into adolescence a person was spanked, Straus says, the more likely that person will abuse his or her children.

In one study, Carson says, 40% of the parents who used corporal punishment said they used it when they had had a bad day, and that "it had nothing to do with the child's behavior."

Five countries now prohibit all forms of corporal punishment in schools and homes. They are Sweden, Norway, Finland, Switzerland, and Austria. Sweden was the first, in 1979. "They did it because they wanted to lower their rates of child abuse," Carson says, "and it worked."

Most industrialized nations have banned corporal punishment in schools, according to the National Coalition to Abolish Corporal Punishment in Schools. Exceptions include the United States, South Africa, and parts of Canada and Australia.

As of May 1992, 29 US states allow corporal punishment, although many cities within these states ban the practice. (See also pp 3205-3208.)

Indiana still allows corporal punishment in schools, Carson says. "Counselors tell me they find it difficult to persuade abusive parents to stop hitting their children when the parents point out that teachers are hitting them as well."

Power and Powerlessness

Pagelow notes that her sample of college students may not be representative of adolescents nationwide. If anything, it may underrepresent the typical adolescent's experience of abuse. Researchers have noted that the 40% of the population who attend college are more bright, motivated, upwardly mobile, mentally healthy, and affluent than those who don't attend college.

If this assumption is correct, Pagelow says, it is difficult to imagine that the other 60% would have grown up in less violent homes.

Pagelow says that many theories have emerged regarding adolescent maltreatment. Of these, she writes, "power–powerlessness and scapegoating seem to have great explanatory power for all types of abuses in the family. In this model, abusers perceive themselves as lacking power in their general environment but powerful in relationship to others in their family units."

When abusers exert their power over family members to compensate for powerlessness elsewhere, they are scapegoating, Pagelow says. "They find weaker targets who cannot retaliate to use as scapegoats against which to displace their hostilities."

"Parents who psychologically and physically abuse their adolescents may be fearful of losing their own youth at the same time that their youngsters are demanding more independence," Pagelow says. Some parents, feeling powerless against the situation, "lash out against

(Continued on p 3131.)

(Continued from p 3128.)
their relatively powerless children."

Likewise, "siblings may attack each other because their targets are weaker and less able to retaliate than parents or teachers who deny them privileges and other adults who make them feel powerless," Pagelow says.

In the 1983 book *The Dark Side of Families*, Finkelhor comments further: "the most common patterns of family abuse are not merely for the more powerful to abuse the less powerful, but for the *most* powerful to abuse the *least*.

"This is an interesting commonality: Abuse tends to gravitate toward the relationships of greatest power differential."—by Teri Randall

ACOG Renews Domestic Violence Campaign, Calls for Changes in Medical School Curricula

REFERRING TO domestic violence as a "sickness to which no civilized country should be subjected," the president of the American College of Obstetricians and Gynecologists (ACOG) has announced his college's renewed commitment to address the needs of battered women.

Speaking at the college's annual meeting, ACOG president Richard F. Jones III, MD, described a four-part program that emphasizes both physician and patient education.

Several other medical organizations, representing more than 150 000 physicians and 30 000 nurses, also have agreed to become involved. They are the American College of Emergency Physicians, the American Academy of Family Physicians, the American Academy of Pediatrics, and the Organization for Obstetricians, Gynecologists, and Neonatal Nurses.

A Commitment for Education

As part of this program, both graduate and undergraduate medical training programs have agreed to include the issue of domestic violence in their curricula.

The committee within ACOG that publishes the recommended instructional objectives for medical students—the Association of Professors of Gynecology and Obstetrics—plans to place in its next edition "special emphasis" on the identification of battered women, appropriate interventions, and legal issues, says George Wilbanks, MD, immediate past president of the committee.

The next edition is about 1 year from publication, says Wilbanks, who is also professor and chair of obstetrics and gynecology at Rush Medical College of Rush University, Chicago, Ill.

In addition, members of the Council on Resident Education in Obstetrics and Gynecology, ACOG's organization of residency program directors, will discuss at their annual retreat next month how to increase faculty and resident surveillance of domestic violence. Council member Robert Resnik, MD, says the meeting is the "first step" in increasing the awareness of program directors and people involved in the training of those who will be providing health care for women. Resnik is also professor and chair of the Department of Reproductive Medicine, University of California, San Diego.

Revised Board Examinations

The American Board of Obstetrics and Gynecology has also agreed to look for meaningful ways to examine physicians on this topic during their written and oral board examinations, Jones says.

The campaign will encourage physicians to become advocates for resources needed by battered women. There are only 1300 shelters in the 3200 counties of the United States, Jones says, and—because of this deficiency—only one out of four battered women gets the assistance needed.

"More money is spent on animal shelters than on women's shelters," Jones adds. "It is simply appalling."

Physicians also will be encouraged to lobby for laws to protect battered women—on the federal, state, and local level.

ACOG will also produce an array of written materials for health professionals with the "most up-to-date information" about resources for battered women. And it will strive to increase public awareness and make the 800 toll-free hot line number for battered women (1-800-333-SAFE) "as familiar as 911."

Shock of Recognition

Jones says he had no idea how often his patients experienced violence at home until, about 2 years ago, he changed the questions he asked them. "When I saw a woman with black and blue marks in my office, I used to ask her how she got them. This gave her the obvious opportunity to say 'I'm clumsy,' or 'I live with a big dog who jumps on me,' or 'I take aspirin so I bleed easily.'"

About 2 years ago, Jones began to ask directly, "Have you been hit or harmed any time in the past year?" "Are you in any danger?" or "Is someone doing this to you?".

One of the first times he used these questions, a patient he had seen for years started crying and told him that her husband beat her every Monday, Wednesday, and Friday with a plastic baseball bat.

Jones was "stunned" by the responses he received. "Whereas, in the past, I would confront a case of battering a few times a year, now I was confronting these cases two or three times a week.

"I had viewed myself as a reasonably perceptive, reasonably kind and caring physician—and I had missed all this. And, if I had missed all this, surely others have as well."

Ask Every Patient

Jones says he now asks every patient about risk for abuse, usually during the review of systems.

This campaign is a continuation of work started in 1985 by Luella Klein, MD, past president of ACOG, and chair of the panel on spouse abuse at the Surgeon General's Workshop on Violence and Public Health.

Out of that workshop, ACOG developed guidelines for the identification of domestic violence and for appropriate interventions. These guidelines were incorporated into a Technical Bulletin entitled *The Battered Woman* that was widely distributed in 1989.

Jones says obstetricians and gynecologists have "a double reason for addressing the problem. The first is to protect our patients themselves. The second is to protect their unborn children during pregnancy, because, as brutal as it seems, recent studies show that pregnancy itself may incite violence by the husband or partner.

"Clearly, we have the opportunity and, I believe, the moral and professional obligation to face this problem head on. It's time to renew our commitment to this issue."—by Teri Randall

From the Centers for Disease Control

Leads From the Morbidity and Mortality Weekly Report
Atlanta, Ga

Firearm-Related Deaths— Louisiana and Texas, 1970-1990

MMWR. 1992;41:213-215, 221

IN 1990, firearm-related injuries surpassed motor-vehicle crashes as the leading cause of death from injuries in both Louisiana and Texas, and from 1979 through 1987, these states ranked third and fifth, respectively, for age-adjusted firearm-related death rates.[1] (In both state analyses, a firearm-related death was defined as any death with the underlying cause listed as codes E922.0-E922.9, E955.0-E955.4, E965.0-E965.4, E970, or E985.0-E985.4 in the International Classification of Diseases [ICD], 8th and 9th revisions; a motor-vehicle-related death was defined as any death with the underlying cause listed as codes E810.0-E825.0 in the ICD, 8th and 9th revisions.)

Because firearm-related injuries are a major cause of death in Louisiana and Texas, the Louisiana Disability Prevention Program, Louisiana Office of Public Health, and the Injury Control Program, Epidemiology Division, Texas Department of Health, used death certificates to examine patterns in firearm-related mortality. This report summarizes the analysis of death certificate data for firearm-related mortality in these two states.

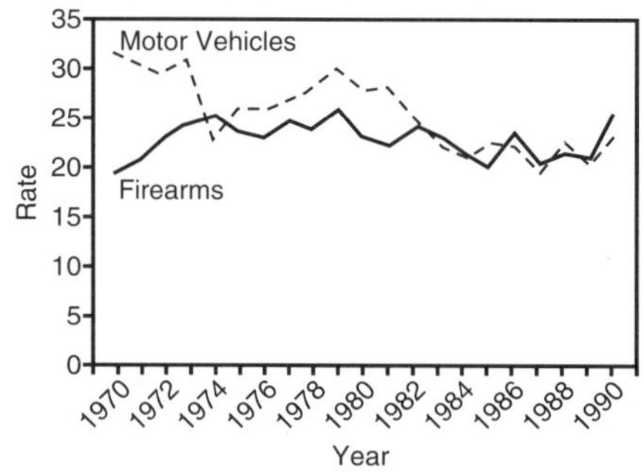

Fig 1.—Rates of firearm- and motor-vehicle-related deaths*—Louisiana, 1970-1990.

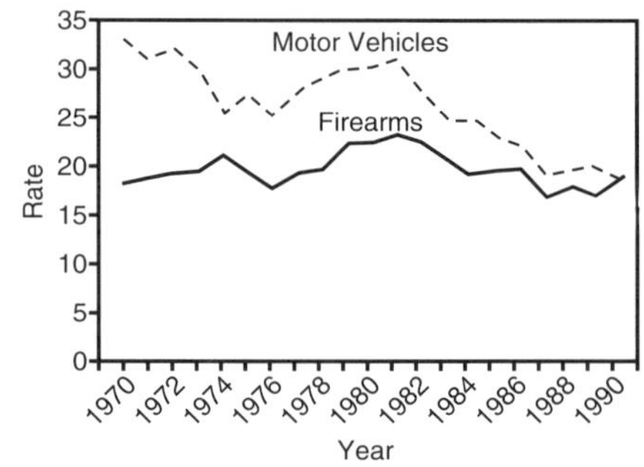

Fig 2.—Rates of firearm- and motor-vehicle-related deaths*—Texas, 1970-1990.

Louisiana

In Louisiana, firearm-related deaths have been the leading cause of injury-related mortality for 4 of the 5 years from 1986 through 1990. From 1970 through 1990, motor-vehicle-related death rates declined by 30% (from 32.4 per 100 000 population to 22.6 per 100 000) while the rate for firearm-related deaths fluctuated. Firearm-related death rates—including homicide and suicide—increased most for black males (42%) from 1970 through 1990 (from 54.1 per 100 000 to 76.7 per 100 000). Although the overall firearm-related death rate did not increase as dramatically among white males (16% during 1970-1990), the firearm-related suicide rate for white males increased 47%.

From 1985 through 1990, 5647 persons died as a result of firearm-related injuries; of these deaths, 2677 (47%) were suicides, 2591 (46%) were homicides, 321 (6%) were classified as unintentional, 19 (0.3%) resulted from legal intervention, and 39 (0.7%) were of unknown intent. In 1990, males were 5.5 times more likely to die from firearm-related injuries than were females (43.7 per 100 000 and 7.9 per 100 000, respectively); blacks were 2.2 times more likely to die from firearm-related injuries than were whites.

Texas

During 1990, firearm-related injuries surpassed motor-vehicle crashes as the leading cause of injury-related mortality in Texas,[2] the first state to report this pattern to CDC. From 1964 through 1989, deaths resulting from motor-vehicle crashes had been the leading cause of injury mortality in Texas. Although death rates for motor-vehicle crashes decreased by 42% from 1970 through 1990 (from 32.5 per 100 000 population to 18.8 per 100 000), the firearm-related death rate remained relatively constant.

From 1985 through 1990, 19 184 persons died from firearm-related injuries; of these deaths, 9286 (48%) were suicides, 8581 (45%) were homicides, 1028 (5%) were classified as unintentional, 114 (1%) resulted from legal intervention, and 175 (1%) were of unknown intent.[2] Males were five times more likely to die from firearm-related injuries than were females (31.3 per 100 000 versus 6.2 per 100 000). Age-specific rates were highest for persons aged 25-34 years (28.9 per 100 000). Blacks were 1.9 times more likely to die from firearm-related injuries than were Hispanics or whites (32.3 per 100 000 versus 17.4 per 100 000 and 16.8 per 100 000, respectively). The firearm-related death rate was highest for black males (57.1 per 100 000).

Reported by: DW Lawrence, MPH, EAG Hooten, MSPH, JB Mathison, MD, Disability Prevention Program; LJ Hebert, MD, Office of Public Health, Louisiana Dept of Health and Hospitals. D Zane, MS, MJ Preece, Injury Control Program; P Patterson, MD, Family Health Svcs; E Svenkerud, MD, Epidemiology Div, D Perrotta, PhD, Environmental Epidemiologist, Texas Dept of Health. Div of Injury Control, National Center for Environmental Health and Injury Control, CDC.

CDC Editorial Note: The trends that led to the emergence of firearm-related deaths as the leading cause of injury-related mortality in Louisiana and Texas are similar to those for the United States. Since 1966, the death rate for motor-vehicle crashes (measured as deaths per 100 million vehicle miles of travel) in the United States has declined substantially[3] and has been associated with a combination of interventions, including the construction of safer highways and vehicles, reductions in the levels of alcohol-impaired driving, lower speed limits, and increased use of safety belts, motorcycle helmets, and child passenger restraint devices.[4] In comparison, during 1970-1990, the firearm-related death rate has fluctuated; however, these rates have been higher than at any time since the 1920s.[5]

States, local communities, and school systems have employed a variety of strategies to prevent firearm-related injuries and deaths. An important element of many of these strategies is to inhibit, restrict, or reduce immediate access to firearms in the general population or in specific locations. For example, in 1976, the District of Columbia banned the purchase, sale, transfer, or possession of handguns by civilians. An evaluation of this regulation found that it was associated with a 25% reduction in firearm-related homicides, a 23% reduction in firearm-related suicides, and an estimated 47 lives saved per year.[6] In some states and localities, firearms are prohibited from being carried in public; in Detroit and in Massachusetts, legislation that increased the penalty for violating such laws reduced the occurrence of firearm-related homicides.[7,8] In some school systems, methods used to deter students from bringing firearms on school grounds include random locker searches, walk-throughs with metal detectors, and policies requiring that students use only clear plastic or mesh bookbags so that weapons cannot be readily hidden.[9]

Community efforts to prevent firearm-related deaths should use other measures in addition to reducing access to firearms. Suicide may be prevented by improved identification and referral of persons at increased risk (e.g., those suffering from clinical depression or who exhibit suicidal behavior). Efforts to prevent homicide may include reduction of the incidence of interpersonal violence through behavioral and other interventions (e.g., conflict resolution training and mentoring programs).[10] The reduction of mortality from motor-vehicle crashes in Louisiana and Texas illustrates how public health approaches can be used to control and prevent injury. The application of such approaches to firearm-related injury holds the potential for decreasing the morbidity and mortality associated with this problem.

References

1. CDC. Injury mortality atlas of the United States, 1979-1987. Atlanta: US Department of Health and Human Services, Public Health Service, CDC, 1991.
2. Zane DF, Preece MJ, Patterson PJ, Svenkerud EK. Commentary: firearm-related mortality in Texas (1985-1990). Tex Med 1991;87:63-5.
3. National Highway Traffic Safety Administration. Fatal Accident Reporting System-1990: a review of information on fatal traffic crashes in the United States. Washington, DC: US Department of Transportation, National Highway Traffic Safety Administration, 1991; publication no. DOT-HS-807-794.
4. Transportation Research Board. Safety research for a changing highway environment. Washington, DC: National Research Council, 1990:13-35. (Special Report no. 229).
5. Wintemute GJ. Firearms as a cause of death in the United States, 1920-1982. J Trauma 1987;27:532-6.
6. Loftin C, McDowall D, Wiersema B, Cottey TJ. Effects of restrictive licensing of handguns on homicide and suicide in the District of Columbia. N Engl J Med 1991;325:1615-20.
7. Deutsch SJ, Alt FB. The effect of the Massachusetts' gun control law on gun-related crimes in the city of Boston. Evaluation Quarterly 1977;1:543-68.
8. O'Carroll PW, Loftin C, Waller JB, et al. Preventing homicide: an evaluation of the efficacy of a Detroit gun ordinance. Am J Public Health 1991;81:576-81.
9. National School Safety Center. Weapons in schools—NSSC resource paper. Malibu, California; National School Safety Center, 1990.
10. National Committee for Injury Prevention and Control. Injury prevention: meeting the challenge. New York: Oxford University Press, 1989.

Physical Fighting Among High School Students—United States, 1990

MMWR. 1992;41:91-94

DURING 1986, interpersonal violence caused an estimated 2.2 million injuries and more than 20 000 deaths in the United States.[1,2] Physical fighting, a common form of interpersonal violence among adolescents, is a prominent cause of injuries and homicides in this age group.[3] This article presents self-reported data about the prevalence and incidence of physical fighting among high school students in the United States during 1990.

The national school-based Youth Risk Behavior Survey (YRBS) is a component of the Youth Risk Behavior Surveillance System, which periodically measures the prevalence of priority health-risk behaviors among youth through representative national, state, and local surveys.[4] The 1990 YRBS used a three-stage sample design to obtain a representative sample of 11 631 students in grades 9-12 in the 50 states, the District of Columbia, Puerto Rico, and the Virgin Islands. Students were asked: "During the past 30 days, how many times have you been in a physical fight in which you or the person you were fighting were injured and had to be treated by a doctor or a nurse?" and "Who did you fight with the last time you were in a physical fight?" In this report, incidence rates describe the number of times per 100 students that physical fights occurred during the 30-day period. (The incidence rate was calculated by adding the number of times each student reported being involved in a physical fight during the 30 days preceding the survey and dividing this sum by the total number of students. The number of physical-fighting episodes per student was then multiplied by 100 to determine the incidence rate per 100 students. Students who replied that they had fought two or three times were assigned a physical fighting frequency of 2.5; four or five times, 4.5; and six or more times, 6.)

Because students were not asked the location of these fights, the extent to which physical fights occurred on school premises was not determined.

Nearly 8% of all students in grades 9-12 reported that, during the 30 days preceding the survey, they had been in at least one physical fight that resulted in an injury requiring treatment by a doctor or nurse. Of these students, 53.3% said they had fought one time; 27.8%, two or three times; 10.1%, four or five times; and 10.1%, six or more times. Male students (12.2%) were significantly more likely than female students (3.6%) to report having been in a fight.

An estimated 18 physical-fighting incidents occurred per 100 students per month. However, the incidence of physical fighting was four times higher for male students (28 incidents per 100 students) than for female students (7 incidents per 100). The incidence was highest for black male students (47 incidents per 100), followed by Hispanic male students (35 incidents per 100) and white male students (22 incidents per 100).

TABLE 1. Percentage of high school students who reported being in a physical fight,* by race/ethnicity† and sex—United States, Youth Risk Behavior Survey, 1990§

Race/Ethnicity	Male		Female		Total	
	%	(95% CI¶)	%	(95% CI)	%	(95% CI)
White	10.1	(8.3-12.0)	2.4	(1.9-2.9)	6.2	(5.3-7.2)
Black	17.6	(13.6-21.6)	7.7	(4.9-10.4)	12.5	(9.5-15.5)
Hispanic	16.2	(12.4-20.0)	4.4	(2.1-6.7)	10.0	(7.7-12.2)
Total	**12.2**	**(10.6-13.8)**	**3.6**	**(3.0-4.3)**	**7.9**	**(7.0-8.9)**

*During the 30 days preceding the survey, in which at least one person required treatment by a doctor or nurse.
†Numbers from racial/ethnic groups other than white and black were too small to provide separate estimates; however, the totals include all races.
§Unweighted sample size=11,631 students.
¶Confidence interval.

Students who reported four or more physical fights during the 30 days preceding the survey (1.6% of all students) accounted for nearly half (46.4%) of all physical fights.

Among students who were involved in a physical fight, the most recent physical fight was more likely to have been with an acquaintance (family member, friend, or date) (57.3%; 95% confidence interval [CI]=54.8%-59.8%) than with a stranger (32.1%; 95% CI=29.7%-34.5%). Male students (40.2%; 95% CI=37.6%-43.0%) reported physical fights with strangers significantly more often than female students (18.6%; 95% CI=14.6%-22.4%).

TABLE 2. Thirty-day incidence* of physical fighting, by race/ethnicity† and sex—United States, Youth Risk Behavior Survey, 1990§

Race/Ethnicity	Male		Female		Total	
	Incidence	(95% CI¶)	Incidence	(95% CI)	Incidence	(95% CI)
White	22	(15-29)	4	(3-6)	13	(10-17)
Black	47	(29-66)	16	(6-26)	31	(19-44)
Hispanic	35	(24-46)	11	(0-22)	22	(14-30)
Total	**28**	**(23-33)**	**7**	**(5-9)**	**18**	**(15-21)**

*Per 100 students. Students who reported fighting (i.e., having been in a physical fight in which at least one person required treatment by a doctor or nurse) two or three times were assigned a fighting frequency of 2.5; four or five times, 4.5; and six or more times, 6.

†Numbers from racial/ethnic groups other than white and black were too small to provide separate estimates; however, the totals include all races.

§Unweighted sample size=11,631 students.

¶Confidence interval.

Reported by: Div of Injury Control, National Center for Environmental Health and Injury Control; Div of Adolescent and School Health, National Center for Chronic Disease Prevention and Health Promotion, CDC.

CDC Editorial Note: Preventing physical fighting among young persons should be an important public health strategy to prevent injuries and deaths from violence. Homicide is the second leading cause of death for persons aged 15-24 years,[5] and nonfatal violence often precedes fatal violence among young persons.[6] The demographic patterns of physical fighting in this report are consistent with those characterizing homicide: the prevalence of both is greater among males and minorities than females and nonminorities, and both physical fighting and homicide occur most frequently among persons who know each other.[7] These similarities suggest that physical fighting is part of a spectrum of violent behavior that may result in homicide.

One of the national health objectives for the year 2000 (objective 7.9) is to reduce by 20% the incidence of physical fighting among adolescents aged 14-17 years.[5] To achieve this objective, the incidence rate determined by the 1990 YRBS must be reduced from 18 episodes per 100 students per month to 14 or fewer episodes. Strategies that may reduce interpersonal violence include decreasing the cultural acceptance of violence[8]; decreasing aggressive behavior among parents and their children[9]; reducing the exposure of children and adolescents to violence in the media[10]; and improving the recognition, management, and treatment of adolescent victims and those at high risk for assaults.[8]

Many experts in the prevention of violence recommend that emphasis also should be placed on helping schools and other agencies that serve youth to teach nonviolent conflict resolution skills as a means of preventing violence (objective 7.16).[5] Educational interventions for adolescents who have not yet established patterns of physical-fighting behavior may reduce the need for more extensive rehabilitative efforts later (i.e., through juvenile detention centers, correctional facilities, or in-school disciplinary programs). Most of the recommended strategies to reduce physical fighting among adolescents require greater cooperation among educational programs and other services in public health, criminal justice, education, and social service agencies.

References

1. Bureau of Justice Statistics. Injuries from crime: special report. Washington, DC: US Department of Justice, Bureau of Justice Statistics, 1989; publication no. NCJ-116811.
2. CDC. Homicide surveillance: high-risk racial and ethnic groups—blacks and Hispanics, 1970-1983. Atlanta: US Department of Health and Human Services, Public Health Service, 1986.
3. University of California at Los Angeles, CDC. The epidemiology of homicide in the city of Los Angeles, 1970-79. Atlanta: US Department of Health and Human Services, Public Health Service, CDC, 1985.
4. Kolbe LJ. An epidemiologic surveillance system to monitor the prevalence of youth behaviors that most affect health. Health Education 1990;21:44-8.
5. Public Health Service. Healthy people 2000: national health promotion and disease prevention objectives—full report, with commentary. Washington, DC: US Department of Health and Human Services, Public Health Service, 1991:235-9; DHHS publication no. (PHS)91-50212.
6. Luckenbill DF. Criminal homicide as a situated transaction. Social Problems 1977;25:176-86.
7. Federal Bureau of Investigation. Uniform crime reports for the United States, 1990. Washington, DC: US Department of Justice, 1991.
8. National Committee for Injury Prevention and Control. Injury prevention: meeting the challenge. Am J Prev Med 1989;5(suppl):192-203.
9. Widom CS. The cycle of violence. Science 1989;244:160-6.
10. National Institute of Mental Health. Television and behavior: ten years of scientific progress and implication for the eighties; summary report. Vol 1. Rockville, Maryland: National Institute of Mental Health, 1982.

From the Surgeon General, US Public Health Service

A Medical Response to Violence: Violence in the United States is a public health emergency. I commend the American Medical Association for sponsoring this ongoing series of articles on violence. The papers contained in this issue of *JAMA* cover many aspects of violence in our nation and offer recommendations for action. The medical community must take a strong, visible leadership role in the effort to end the epidemic of violence. Such leadership may help us to significantly reduce the rates of violence and create a safer, healthier society.

It is truly remarkable to see the phenomenal improvement in health status that has occurred in this country during the last 100 years. Our nation has made incredible strides in combating diseases that once took an enormous toll; polio, smallpox, diphtheria, and dysentery are only a few of the dread diseases now considered controllable. Even the fight against heart disease, the leading killer of Americans, has seen a sustained and dramatic drop in mortality rates since 1950. Heart disease mortality figures have declined 15%; the age-adjusted mortality rate has declined by 40%. What remarkable progress!

Despite these significant gains, however, we still face deadly assaults on the health of Americans. This issue of THE JOURNAL addresses one of these current health threats—violence. Although violence is not a disease in the "classic" sense, its impact on personal and public health is as profound as that of many physiologic ills—perhaps more so. Whatever definition we use, violence has become a problem of epidemic proportion in our society.

Homicide has become the 10th leading cause of death in the United States; suicide is the eighth leading cause of death. In 1989 alone, the last year for which complete statistics are available, 22 909 people died from homicide; 30 232 people died at their own hands. It is indeed a sad commentary that the United States has the highest homicide rate of any Western industrialized country.

Violence is found at alarming rates in many aspects of our daily lives. Each year, it is estimated that more than 1.5 million individuals are victims of assault; more than 650 000 women are victims of rape; 1.5 to 2.5 million children are abused or neglected; and 700 000 to 1.1 million elderly Americans are abused or neglected.

The impact of such violence on the health of our nation's youth and minorities is particularly worrisome. Homicide is now the second leading cause of death among 15- to 24-year-olds and the leading cause of death among 15- to 34-year-old black males. It is a tragic reality that the populations of young black American males face a homicide rate that is at least 8 times greater than that of their white counterparts of comparable age.

Suicide has become the third leading cause of death for 15- to 34-year-old Americans and the second-leading cause of death for 15- to 24-year-old Native Americans. These rates are growing. Homicide rates among the young are at their highest level of this century. The homicide rates for children and adolescents have more than doubled in the past 30 years. Since 1950, the suicide rate among children and adolescents has nearly tripled; in fact, in 1989, the suicide rate among our country's young was the highest it has ever been.

Physicians and other health professionals are firsthand witnesses to the consequences of violence. From the victim of a gunshot wound in the operating room to the abused child or adult seen in a physician's office or emergency department, across the country we see, diagnose, treat, mend, patch, console, and care for the victims of violence and their families thousands of times each day.

What must we do to curtail this epidemic? Clearly, given the complexity of the problem, there is no single solution. But that cannot and must not deter our search for creative solutions from within the public health community. Violence is a multifaceted problem that results from many social and economic factors; poverty, racism, disregard for human life, family and community disintegration, denial of educational opportunity, peer pressure, and absence of positive values all contribute to the epidemic's spread.

Violence cannot be curbed by talking alone. If we are to succeed in stemming the epidemic of violence, we must first address the social, economic, and behavioral causes of violence. We must try to improve living conditions for millions of Americans. We must try to provide the economic and educational opportunities for our youth that racism and poverty destroy. Health care must become affordable and accessible for all Americans. We must help the educational system to instill the values that hold our society together. We must maintain and strengthen our families.

Just as we health professionals have done for other health problems, we have a clear duty to take a leadership role in the antiviolence movement. We must press for changes in economic conditions and insist on expanded access to health care. When required to do so, we must report the acts of violence that we are called upon to treat. We must work to make our society more compassionate, fair, and just. As physicians, we have the duty to inform and educate our patients and the public about the causes and effects of violence. Such a duty requires that we advocate the establishment of violence prevention programs in schools, clinics, churches, and other community centers. We must open and maintain channels with other disciplines and professions involved in efforts to end violence. We must establish coalitions with parents, educators, law enforcement personnel, social service workers, clergy, community leaders, government officials, and other health care professionals, and we must continue to fight this plague as a nation.

In short, we need to change the way we view each other and treat each other. We must offer a strong sense of community, not a feeling of alienation. We must encourage recognition of the importance of each individual and teach the politics of inclusion, not exclusion. We must offer hope and take the necessary steps to make that hope a reality. As health professionals, the prevention of violence by using public health methods in our communities is as much our responsibility as is the treatment of its victims.

—by Antonia C. Novello, MD, MPH
Surgeon General
Public Health Service,
John Shosky, PhD
Consultant to the Surgeon General,
and Robert Froehlke, MD
Division of Epidemiology
Michigan State Department of
Public Health, Lansing

Editor's Note: Inquiries may be directed to John Shosky, Office of the Surgeon General, Department of Health and Human Services, Room 718-E, 200 Independence Ave SW, Washington, DC 20201; telephone (202) 245-7163.

A Medical Response to Domestic Violence: Domestic violence is an extensive, pervading, and entrenched problem in the United States. It is an outrage to women and the entire American family.

Health care providers must take an active, vigorous role in identifying this serious recurrent public health problem. This is not just a "minor dispute" between spouses or loved ones. It is a violation of our criminal laws and a callous disregard for human life. If we do not help to break the cycle of abuse, it will reflect itself in the next generation.

Estimates suggest that at least 2 to 4 million women each year are physically abused. Six out of every 10 married couples have experienced violence at some time during their marriage, according to one survey. Domestic violence may touch as many as one fourth of all American families.

One study found violence to be the second leading cause of injuries to women, and the leading cause of injuries to women ages 15 through 44 years (*Am J Epidemiol.* 1991;134:59-68). That study, conducted for a 1-year period by the Philadelphia Injury Prevention Program, examined injuries to women resulting in emergency department visits or death.

The authors found that falls were reported to be the leading cause of death overall, and that rates of falls were highest among young women 25 through 34 years of age. Such high rates of falls among young women should make health care providers suspicious that some of these so-called "fall injuries" are actually sustained in beatings—after all, other studies have determined that fall injuries are highest in the elderly, not in able-bodied women.

Violence often occurs at the hands of people the victim knows well. According to the Uniform Crime Report of the Federal Bureau of Investigation (FBI), 30% of women killed in the United States die at the hands of a husband or boyfriend. In 1990, more than 800 women were killed by their husbands; 400 more were killed by their boyfriends.

In 1990, the National Crime Survey estimated that, for the years 1979 through 1987, at least 626 000 violent victimizations of women were committed by husbands or boyfriends each year.

Prevention of the abuse of women must not focus solely on legal marriages; to do so will miss abuse that occurs during dating, abuse that happens in nontraditional relationships, and abuse that happens in relationships that have been terminated through separation and divorce. For example, one study conducted in Atlanta found that more than one fifth of intimate violence incidents involved prior or estranged partners, and more than one fifth involved nonspousal partners.

What is the profile of the abuser? Unfortunately, the causes of abuse are complex and sometimes defy prediction. Yet, in many cases the perpetrator is a male intimate, often one who feels threatened or alienated in some way. Alcohol and/or illegal drug use are often involved, and guns and other weapons are frequently present.

Pregnancy does not exempt women from being abused. From 4% to 8% of women going to prenatal clinics were abused during pregnancy. Patterns of abuse seem to vary. For some women, battering begins or is exacerbated during pregnancy, whereas, for others, it stops altogether.

Sadly, domestic violence may be underreported. Many women fail to report acts of violence. Often there are strong social or familial pressures to abstain from reporting, not to mention fear of reprisal, or denial.

One essential solution is for physicians to increase their awareness. More than half of the victims of assaults by intimates are seriously injured. At least 25% report receiving medical care. One in 10 is treated in a hospital or emergency department. It is estimated that 35% of women who visit hospital emergency departments are there for symptoms of ongoing abuse. Unfortunately, as few as 5% of the victims of domestic violence are so identified.

We must recognize not only that abuse is common, but that it escalates in severity within relationships. This means that there are chances for physicians to intervene before domestic violence reaches life-threatening levels. As a profession, we have not produced a sterling record of success in this area. We must overcome our own denial and apathy.

It is known that if women are asked about violence directly and routinely, in a way that isn't threatening, they will discuss their abuse, particularly if they feel safe and if they feel the health care provider really wants to know. Therefore, we should ask about psychological or physical abuse in the home in order to make referrals to appropriate agencies or to professional counselors.

We must also work with other health care professionals, community leaders, and government officials to standardize protocols to screen trauma patients in the hospital emergency department. This technique has been found to substantially increase the ability of health care personnel to correctly identify battered women. I commend the Joint Commission on the Accreditation of Health Care Organizations for recently passing accreditation standards for the care of abuse victims.

In addition, the Public Health Service (PHS) has developed a framework for actions to deal with domestic violence, one that involves developing guidelines to assist communities in implementing programs aimed at preventing violence, and aiding communities to design and implement multifaceted community violence prevention programs. The PHS is also conducting scientific research to evaluate specific preventive interventions. The PHS is also training staff, community leaders, and health professionals in violence prevention.

Finally, physicians must step forward and help establish broad-based community coalitions to enhance awareness of domestic violence. We must assume the leadership role that is incumbent on us as professionals and compassionate citizens of this country.

As health professionals, we must make every effort to end domestic violence. Women must be able to live their lives free from violence, both inside and outside the home. Our awareness, our intolerance of violence, and our active intervention can greatly diminish the license for domestic abuse. As professionals, we can make a remarkable difference.

—by Antonia C. Novello, MD, MPH
Surgeon General,
US Public Health Service;
Mark Rosenberg, MD, PhD
and Linda Saltzman, PhD
National Center for Environmental
Health and Injury Control,
Centers for Disease Control,
Atlanta, Ga;
and John Shosky, PhD
Consultant to the Surgeon General

Editor's Note: Inquiries may be directed to John Shosky, Office of the Surgeon General, Department of Health and Human Services, Room 718-E, 200 Independence Ave SW, Washington, DC 20201; telephone (202) 245-7163.

From the Assistant Secretary for Health, US Public Health Service

Reducing Youth Violence—The Physician's Role: The United States set a new murder record in 1991, for the second year in a row. The estimated 24 020 slayings recorded last year topped by about 2.5% the 23 440 murders in 1990. In the absence of effective intervention, law enforcement experts expect this tragic trend to continue, as a recent Senate Judiciary Committee report put it, "for many years to come."

While not the whole story, easy access to firearms figures prominently in the growing violence, and our children and young people are being hit particularly hard. Homicide is the second leading cause of juvenile injury deaths—second only to motor vehicle crashes. And gunshot wound is the cause of death about 75% of the time.

Suicide is the third-ranked cause of injury death in children and a serious public health concern, with rates for persons aged 15 to 19 years nearly doubling over the past two decades, from 5.9 suicides per 100 000 youngsters in 1970 to 11.3 per 100 000 in 1988. Guns were used in 61.2% of the suicides in 1988.

A recent Justice Department report, "Teenage Victims," noted that teenagers are more likely than adults to be victims of violent crime. Over the period of 1985 through 1988, a national crime survey reported an average of 67 of 1000 teens, compared with 26 of 1000 adults, were victims of rape, robbery, or assault each year. Teenaged victims described their attacker as an acquaintance almost twice as often as adults did.

For many children today, violence is not a drama that unfolds on television or film. It's a reality that they have known since birth and witness routinely on the streets of their neighborhoods and even in their own homes. Often, they are the victims. In 1986, nearly 4000 children younger than 19 years died of gunshot wounds, accounting for 12% of all deaths in that age group. If the cause was polio or untreated appendicitis, physicians would be taking action. Is there not a role for physicians in this epidemic?

As a native of a western state and, now, a resident of the Washington, DC, area, I can appreciate how different backgrounds and conditions foster different views of the violence problem and the part that guns play in it. As a physician, I have yet another view: I see, in youth violence, an epidemic as frustrating as the acquired immunodeficiency syndrome and as debilitating as such past scourges as polio. I see a domestic destruction of more young people than died in many of our military actions. And I see a great need for physicians and other citizens to find areas of agreement on how to fight this enemy.

Those areas of accord do exist. Few would claim, for example, that minors should have access to loaded weapons at home or that they should be permitted to carry them on the streets or to take them to school. We should all be able to agree that children and firearms are a dangerous and impermissible combination. That is why our health objectives for the year 2000 call for reducing the inappropriate storage of firearms, weapon-carrying by adolescents, and weapon-related injury deaths in this country.

Can we find other niches of agreement? As individual physicians, we certainly can emphasize to parents and to our young patients the risks of firearms. Perhaps questions about home access to a handgun can have as much predictive value as questions about alcohol and tobacco use.

Louis W. Sullivan, MD, secretary of the US Department of Health and Human Services, has urged physicians to foster a culture of character that emphasizes the nonviolent resolution of conflict, personal responsibility, and community service.

Fighting is a prominent cause of injuries among high school students and often precedes homicides.

Recognizing that adolescents, particularly boys, are prone to this kind of violent behavior, we can offer counsel on the difference between standing up for oneself and being foolhardy. We can speak up for the old virtues of counting to 10, of staying sober and under control, and of walking away from dangerous situations.

We can push to raise the penalties for carrying weapons on school grounds, and we can speak out to make sure that liquor stores and bars are not selling alcoholic beverages to underage juveniles.

We can try to bridge opposing points of view and seek areas of agreement. For example, some who reject the National Rifle Association's opposition to all gun control can support its emphasis on gun safety.

More than 1 million children are abused and neglected in the United States each year. Abuse in the home, a serious problem in and of itself, quite often propels children into the streets, where violence is both a danger and a temptation.

Physicians and other health professionals—who see the addicted mother-to-be, the battered child, and the teenaged victim—sometimes are uniquely situated to intervene. The American Medical Association's new Physicians' Campaign Against Family Violence will help them do so and may reduce by-product youth violence, as well.

We also must do our best to expand horizons. In Annapolis, Md, last summer, the city's housing authority teamed up with students from St Mary's College and the Marine Trades Association of Maryland in a program called "Sail Into Life" that brought together the sailing crowd and youngsters from the public housing projects.

Every Wednesday, the kids were taken out on the 50-foot *Gem*. Under the watchful eye of the boat's skipper and the volunteer students from St Mary's, these children learned about sailing, teamwork, the Chesapeake Bay, and much more—including themselves. The young sailors also took swimming and drown-proofing lessons, completed a boating safety course, and visited boat yards.

This program—and others that inspire and fire up children—can help them realize that there are other things out there to reach for besides a gun.

—by James Mason, MD, DrPH
Assistant Secretary for Health
Head of the Public Health Service
and Robert Proctor
Writer, Office of Communications

Editor's Note: Inquiries may be directed to Bill Grigg, Office of Communications, US Public Health Service, Room 719-H, 200 Independence Ave SW, Washington, DC 20201; telephone (202) 245-6867.

Abstracts

CHILD ABUSE NEGL — Oxford, England

Intra- and Extrafamilial Child Homicide in Sweden 1971–1980

Over the 10-year period studied, a total of 96 children under 15 years of age were killed in Sweden. This number constituted an average annual rate of 0.6 per 100,000 children. The violence, most frequently involving strangulation, shooting, and stabbing, was largely directed at young children. The pattern of child homicide was mainly characterized by intrafamilial violence, especially in connection with the suicide of a parent-perpetrator. Extrafamilial homicides were rare and only committed by male perpetrators. Cases of child abuse by a parent and cases of sexual abuse were infrequent. By psychiatric examination after the crime, only 10 perpetrators out of 47 examined were found not mentally ill.

(1991;15:45-55) Lis K. H. Somander and Lennart M. Rammer. Reprint requests to Lis K. H. Somander, Department of Forensic Medicine, Faculty of Health Sciences, University of Linköping, S-581 85 Linköping, Sweden.

N ENGL J MED — Boston, Mass

Effects of Restrictive Licensing of Handguns on Homicide and Suicide in the District of Columbia

Background. Whether restricting access to handguns will reduce firearm-related homicides and suicides is currently a matter of intense debate. In 1976 the District of Columbia adopted a law that banned the purchase, sale, transfer, or possession of handguns by civilians. We evaluated the effect of implementing this law on the frequency of homicides and suicides.

Methods. Homicides and suicides committed from 1968 through 1987 were classified according to place of occurrence (within the District of Columbia or in adjacent metropolitan areas where the law did not apply), cause (homicide or suicide), mechanism of death (firearms or other means), and time of occurrence (before or after the implementation of the law). The number of suicides and homicides was calculated for each month during the study period, and differences between the mean monthly totals before and after the law went into effect were estimated.

Results. In Washington, D.C., the adoption of the gun-licensing law coincided with an abrupt decline in homicides by firearms (a reduction of 3.3 per month, or 25 percent) and suicides by firearms (reduction, 0.6 per month, or 23 percent). No similar reductions were observed in the number of homicides or suicides committed by other means, nor were there similar reductions in the adjacent metropolitan areas in Maryland and Virginia. There were also no increases in homicides or suicides by other methods, as would be expected if equally lethal means were substituted for handguns.

Conclusions. Restrictive licensing of handguns was associated with a prompt decline in homicides and suicides by firearms in the District of Columbia. No such decline was observed for homicides or suicides in which guns were not used, and no decline was seen in adjacent metropolitan areas where restrictive licensing did not apply. Our data suggest that restrictions on access to guns in the District of Columbia prevented an average of 47 deaths each year after the law was implemented.

(1991;325:1615-1620) Colin Loftin et al, Violence Research Group, Institute of Criminal Justice and Criminology, University of Maryland at College Park, 2220 Lefrak Hall, College Park, MD 20742-8235.

Edited by Jeanette M. Smith, MD, Contributing Editor.

J TRAUMA — Baltimore, Md

The Role of Early Surgical Intervention in Civilian Gunshot Wounds to the Head

Surgical management of gunshot wounds of the head has remained a controversial issue in the care of civilian patients. In an attempt to determine who might benefit from aggressive surgical intervention, we examined 89 patients over a 3-year period who had suffered cranial gunshot wounds and had at least one computed tomographic scan of the head after admission. Patients were divided into those receiving early (<24 hours) surgical intervention (ES, n=27), late (>24 hours) surgical intervention (LS, n=6) or no surgical intervention (NS, n=56). Overall mortality was 63%. Ten of 27 patients (37%) in the ES group died compared with 46 of 56 patients (82%) in the NS group ($p<0.0001$). Glasgow Coma Scale (GCS) scores in the ES group averaged 7.86±4.72 and in the NS group 5.59±4.42 ($p<0.05$). The GCS scores in the LS group (all of whom survived) were significantly higher than those of the other two groups, 12.17±4.10. The number of patients with GCS scores of 3 or 4 on admission was significantly less in the ES (41%) than in the NS group (66%, p=0.035) and survival was better with surgery (36%) than without (3%, p= 0.007). Patients with mass lesions (clot, ventricular blood) were more often found in the ES group (17/27) than in the NS group (18/56) (p =0.008). Patients with bihemispheric injuries fared better with surgery (7 of 14 survivors) than without (2 of 33 survivors, p=0.0003). Only one infectious complication (brain abscess) was encountered in the LS group. No delayed intracranial complications in survivors in the NS group were seen. From this review early surgical intervention seemed to result in better survival but was frequently undertaken in those patients who were less neurologically impaired and who manifested evidence of mass lesions on scanning. There was evidence to suggest that even pessimistic situations (severe neurologic deficit, bihemispheric injuries) might benefit from aggressive management.

(1992;32:398-400) Thomas S. Helling et al, 4320 Wornall Rd, Kansas City, MO 64111.

J THORAC CARDIOVASC SURG — St Louis, Mo

Penetrating Thoracic Wounds Caused by Plastic Bullets

Thoracic penetrating injuries caused by a new plastic bullet were studied to determine the nature of the wounds and the appropriate management. Twenty-six casualties from the Israeli-Palestinian conflict (Intifada) were included. The organs most commonly involved were lung (n=21), bony chest wall (n=9), heart (n=3), and diaphragm. Bleeding was at least moderate in 20 patients, amounting in all patients to an average of 975 ml. Thoracotomy was required in 11 patients (42%) mainly because of cardiac injury (n=3) and aortic or other arterial bleeding (n=3). Simple oversewing of severed organs (n=8) or ligation of bleeding vessels (n=3) was satisfactory. Two patients died (7.7% mortality); one after major liver resection; the other was dead on arrival. We conclude that plastic bullets have a linear course unless displaced by the bony chest wall, when they tend to fragment and cause simple fractures. Fired from a presumed range of at least 70 m, plastic bullets behave like low-velocity missiles, and tissue destruction is minimal. Management should be similar to that of civilian thoracic penetrating trauma.

(1992;103:381-385) Alon Yellin et al, Department of Thoracic Surgery, The Sheba Medical Center, Tel Hashomer 52621, Israel.

J FAM VIOL — New York, NY

Hostility and Stress as Mediators of Aggression in Violent Men

This research investigated hypothesized differences on the Buss-Durkee Hostility Inventory between five groups of men who varied in terms of being violent toward female cohabitants, nonfamily members, or no one, and in terms of marital satisfaction. Other measures, such as stress and childhood abuse data, were employed to interpret the findings. A two-way MANCOVA (group by race) with six sociodemographic covariates revealed significant differences on three Hostility Inventory subscales. The maritally violent men had significantly higher total Hostility than any of the other groups and were significantly discriminable from the other groups. Nonetheless, the beliefs and behaviors of violence-prone individuals overlap to some degree. A cognitive-behavioral model with stimulus variables of life stressors, intervening variables of hostility and negative stress reactions, and response variables of different forms of aggression served as a framework for interpreting the results.

(1991;6:217-241) Ola W. Barnett et al, Social Science Division, Seaver College/Pepperdine University, Malibu, CA 90263.

AM J EPIDEMIOL — Baltimore, Md

Incidence Rates of Firearm Injuries in Galveston, Texas, 1979–1981

Firearm injury mortality rates have been characterized in various settings, but little is known of the total magnitude of firearm injury, including morbidity. The authors determined population-based incidence rates of firearm injury among residents of Galveston, Texas, from 1979–1981 by using police, emergency department, hospital, emergency medical services, medical examiner, and vital records to identify 239 firearm injury cases. Vital records, medical examiner, and police records each identified more than 95% of the fatalities, but police records (sensitivity=98%) were better than emergency department or hospital records (sensitivity=82% and 28%, respectively) for identifying all nonfatal cases. The annual age-adjusted incidence rate of firearm injury was 128 per 100,000 persons. Black males, with the highest firearm injury rate (459 per 100,000 persons), were injured at 46 times the rate of white females (10 per 100,000 persons). The overall case fatality rate was 30%, including 25% of the assaults/homicides, 81% of the parasuicides/suicides, and 0% of the unintentional injuries. On the basis of the case fatality rates, an estimated 140,000 firearm injuries occur in the United States annually. The case fatality rate for penetrating head injuries was 80% versus 48% for chest injuries and 6% for all other parts of the body. The results are discussed with respect to policy recommendations for reducing firearm injuries.

(1991;134:511-521) Roberta K. Lee et al, University of Texas School of Nursing, University of Texas Medical Branch J-29, Galveston, TX 77550.

OPHTHALMOLOGY — Philadelphia, Pa

Vitreoretinal Traction and Perimacular Retinal Folds in the Eyes of Deliberately Traumatized Children

The pathophysiology of perimacular folds in eyes of deliberately traumatized children is disputed. The authors reviewed the clinical and forensic records and systemic and ocular findings at autopsy of three children with perimacular retinal folds who died after being violently shaken. Two of the children suffered direct head trauma in addition to being shaken; one patient was violently shaken without any physical or forensic evidence of direct head trauma. No direct ocular trauma was detected. In each case, the vitreous had partially separated from the retina but remained attached to the internal limiting membrane at the apices of the folds and the vitreous base, implicating traction in the pathogenesis of these folds. Although some intraocular findings in deliberately traumatized children may be explained by direct head injury, the possibility of both direct head trauma and shaking must be considered. Perimacular folds may develop without direct ocular or head trauma and may constitute evidence supporting violent shaking.

(1991;98:1124-1127) Stephen J. Massicotte et al. Reprint requests to Robert Folberg, Room 233 MRC, University of Iowa, Iowa City, IA 52242.

ARCH SURG — Chicago, Ill

Anatomic Considerations in Penetrating Gluteal Wounds

A retrospective study of 81 patients with penetrating gluteal wounds was performed to determine if the site of penetration was useful in predicting the likelihood of associated vascular or visceral injury. There were 53 gunshot wounds and 28 stab wounds, including one impalement. The gluteal region was divided into upper and lower zones by determining whether entry occurred above or below the greater trochanters. Sixty-six percent of all penetrating gluteal wounds entered the upper zone. Thirty-two percent of patients with upper zone penetration had associated vascular or visceral injury. Only one of 27 patients with lower zone penetration sustained major injury. The site of entry plays a critical role in determining the likelihood of serious injury associated with penetrating gluteal wounds. Wounds penetrating above the greater trochanters demand thorough evaluation, especially gunshot wounds.

(1992;127:407-410) David W. Mercer et al, Department of Surgery, Temple University School of Medicine, Philadelphia, Pa.

MIL MED — Washington, DC

Etiological Characteristics of Abusive Husbands

This study compared abusive husbands with nonabusive, marital discordant husbands using six measures to ascertain certain etiological characteristics of abusers. Both groups completed the Jenkins Activity Survey for measuring type A behavior, the Short Michigan Alcoholism Screening Test, the Index of Self-Esteem, the Spence-Helmrich Attitudes Toward Women Scale, the Index of Marital Satisfaction, and a simple rating scale to access their perceptions of their wives' physical attractiveness. As predicted, abusers evidenced significantly higher type A behaviors, higher problem drinking behaviors, more rigid attitudes toward women, lower marital satisfaction, and rated their wives as less attractive than did nonabusers. Inconsistent with the literature, however, no significant differences were discovered between the self-esteem of abusers and nonabusers.

(1991;156:670-675) David Farley Hurlbert et al, Darnall Army Community Hospital, Fort Hood, Tex.

Prediction of Suicide in Military Medical Facilities

The scope of the suicide problem is briefly reviewed and the distinction between actuarial and clinical prediction is discussed. Three approaches to the process of clinical prediction are (1) use of multiple predictors; (2) use of objective rating scales, and (3) psychodynamic formulation of risk. These are discussed and specific suggestions are offered for incremental implementation in military medical facilities depending on availability of psychiatric resources. The major warning signs of suicidal behavior are outlined and recommendations offered for training of ward personnel.

(1992;157:139-141) Capt Richard N. Carrera, Department of Psychology, University of Miami, PO Box 248185, Coral Gables, FL 33124.

S AFR MED J Cape Town, South Africa

Sexually Transmitted Disease Surveillance in a Child Abuse Clinic

The sexually transmitted disease surveillance system instituted at the Child Abuse and Neglect (CAN) clinic of the Transvaal Memorial Institute for Child Health and Development was evaluated after 1 year. The presenting complaint of the vast majority of the 227 patients was sexual abuse. In more than half (52%), child abuse was medically proven, and it was highly suspected in another 18%. In only 6% did no abuse take place. About half the patients suffered non-penetrative sexual abuse, 40% penetrative abuse and 10% suffered non-sexual abuse.

Smears for gonorrhoea were positive in 2 out of 152 patients; for *Chlamydia* in 1 out of 140; for *Gardnerella and Trichomonas* in 2 and 1 case, respectively. Syphilis serology yielded 3 positive results out of 162, and hepatitis B, 6 out of 143. No positive results were found in tests for HIV and herpes.

With the exception of hepatitis B tests, all positive results occurred in children considered on clinical grounds to have medically proven or highly suspected sexual abuse.

These results will allow modification of the surveillance system and testing of those children more likely to test positive, while doing fewer tests overall.

(1992;81:84-86) F. P. R. De Villiers et al, Child Abuse Clinic, Transvaal Memorial Institute for Child Health and Development, and University of the Witwatersrand, Johannesburg, South Africa.

AM J PSYCHIATRY Washington, DC

The Role of Violence in Decisions About Hospitalization From the Psychiatric Emergency Room

Objective: The authors evaluated the relationship between violent behavior and decision making about hospitalization from the psychiatric emergency room.

Method: The medical charts of 321 patients evaluated in an urban psychiatric emergency room during a 4-week period were reviewed retrospectively. Violent behavior was defined as physical attacks on persons or fear-inducing behavior before or during the evaluation in the emergency room; and its value in predicting hospitalization decisions was assessed with logistic regression analyses that also included 12 demographic, clinical, and contextual variables.

Results: A model predicting hospitalization decisions was developed and cross-validated. Although violent patients were more likely to be hospitalized than nonviolent patients, clinical variables such as diagnosis and overall severity of psychiatric impairment were more important than violent behavior in predicting hospitalization decisions.

Conclusions: Despite legal pressures to focus on overt behaviors such as violence as a basis for liability prevention and civil commitment, clinicians in this study did not allocate inpatient resources to preventively detain persons unlikely to benefit from treatment. Rather, they hospitalized the most severely disturbed patients, with diagnoses such as schizophrenic and manic disorders for which a widely accepted therapeutic armamentarium exists. The results are consistent with clinical recommendations that in the evaluation of the violent patient, attention needs to be given to the underlying disorder, since violent behavior itself can result from diverse causes only some of which require inpatient psychiatric treatment.

(1992;149:207-212) Dale E. McNiel et al, 401 Parnassus Ave, San Francisco, CA 94143-0984.

Edited by Jeanette M. Smith, MD, Contributing Editor.

OPHTHALMOLOGY Philadelphia, Pa

Ocular Findings at Autopsy of Child Abuse Victims

The incidence of retinal hemorrhage in child abuse victims was studied in cadavers of children that underwent autopsy in the Los Angeles County Coroner's office. One hundred ninety consecutive cases of childrens' eyes received at Doheny Eye Institute from 1985 to 1989 were included in the study. Retinal hemorrhage is the most common form of eye damage due to child abuse and is more likely to occur in infants who have been shaken than after blunt trauma to the head. Accordingly, retinal involvement is seen more frequently in younger children. The mechanism of retinal hemorrhage is unknown, but the authors' evidence suggests that it is not a direct result of submeningeal hemorrhage. The retinal hemorrhages are found most frequently in the bipolar and nerve fiber layers. They may be severe and widespread or small, scattered foci; both forms are indicative of abuse type injury. Any child who is comatose or who has other unexplained neurologic symptoms should have a thorough eye examination with the pupils dilated with emphasis on studies of the retina.

(1991;98:1519-1524) Ralph S. Riffenburgh and Lakshmanan Sathyavagiswaran. Reprint requests to Dr Riffenburgh, Doheny Eye Institute, 1355 San Pablo St, Los Angeles, CA 90033.

ANN PEDIATR Paris, France

Sexual Abuse in Children in Cameroon

Reports of sexual abuse in children are infrequent in the French-speaking nations of black Africa. This study was undertaken to determine the incidence of sexual abuse in children in Yaounde, describe the profile of victims, and identify factors associated with sexual abuse. Seventeen female rape or attempted rape victims were enrolled over an 8-month period. Most (57.05%) were 7 to 15 years of age and lived in underprivileged neighborhoods. Genital bleeding (12 cases), hymenal tears (14 cases) and/or perineal tears were the main lesions found. Most of the rapists were young adults (19-45 years old in 70.5% of cases) who were neighbors, relatives or friends of the family, and single (58.82%). The motivations of the rapists were unclear. This medicosocial reality which is new in Cameroon needs attention.

(1992;39:111-114) P. O. Koki Ndombo et al, Section Pédiatrie, CUSS, Yaounde, Cameroon.

SOUTH MED J Birmingham, Ala

Stress and Suicide in Police Officers: Paradigm of Occupational Stress

All occupations are associated with stress, but certain occupations are significantly more stressful than others. Stress is not always harmful. It is the individual's reaction to stress that determines the outcome, ie, whether the individual will adapt or become maladaptive. Individuals who feel they can control events or are in control of their lives are better able to handle stress than individuals who believe they are the victims of fate or chance and who feel powerless and helpless. For those individuals who feel powerless or helpless, suicide may be a means of taking control over their helplessness. Police officers, who are subject to extraordinary stress, present a paradigm for the study and treatment of stress in other occupations.

(1992;85:233-243) Francis L. McCafferty et al, 31314 Center Ridge Rd, Westlake, OH 44145.

AM J OBSTET GYNECOL — St Louis, Mo

Colposcopy to Establish Physical Findings in Rape Victims

Objective: Conventional rape examination protocols have been poor in yielding positive genital findings (10% to 30% typically). We report our experience with a revised protocol employing colposcopy to perform genital examinations of victims and to document findings.

Study Design: Physical examinations were performed on rape victims seen by San Luis Obispo County's Suspected Abuse Response Team between 1985 and 1990, and the results were reviewed for this study.

Results: Of 131 patients seen within 48 hours and who experienced penile penetration, 114 (87%) had positive findings. Colposcopic magnification allowed examiners to characterize these findings as acute mounting injuries, typically seen at 3, 6, and 9 o'clock on the posterior fourchette and consisting chiefly of lacerations, ecchymosis, and swelling.

Conclusions: An examination protocol that includes colposcopy may be the most reliable means to document and characterize genital findings in rape victims and to evaluate whether findings may be linked to a reported sexual assault.

(1992;166:83-86) Laura Slaughter and Carl R. V. Brown. Reprint requests to Dr Slaughter, SART, 1551 Bishop, Bldg A, Suite 110, San Luis Obispo, CA 93401.

J ADOLESC HEALTH — New York, NY

Child Abuse and Mental Health Among Adolescents in Dependent Care

Do adolescents in dependent care who have been abused or neglected demonstrate more mental health problems than their nonabused peers? This study examined relationships of child abuse, depression, and self-esteem among 82 adolescents (mean age 14.5 years, 52% male, 82.9% white) living in a dependent care facility. Of these, 32 adolescents were victims of child abuse or neglect. Upon admission, 54 adolescents were identified as depressed on the Beck Depression Inventory. Initial scores on the depression and self-esteem instruments did not differ by age, race, or history of maltreatment, though trends among subtypes of abuse were identified. Females had significantly lower self-esteem and tended toward more depression. Repeat evaluation 6 months after admission revealed significant improvement in both depression and self-esteem scores for the entire sample. As a group, however, the maltreated adolescents did not demonstrate significant improvement in depression, and a history of neglect was associated with less improvement. Depression in this dependent care sample was common, however, we did not identify the maltreated adolescents as having significantly more problems with self-esteem or depression. For some adolescents, dependent care may be an appropriate and helpful alternative.

(1992;13:121-127) Roberta A. Hibbard et al, Department of Pediatrics, Indiana University Medical Center, 702 Barnhill Dr, Indianapolis, IN 46202.

Physical and Sexual Abuse as Predictors of Substance Use and Suicide Among Pregnant Teenagers

In order to better define risk factors for perinatal substance abuse, data from 352 pregnant teenagers enrolled in a comprehensive prenatal clinic were analyzed. Fifteen years was the average age, 82% were of minority descent, and all were receiving public assistance. At their first visit, a social worker obtained information on their home environment, family history, education, peer relationships, physical and mental health, and history of substance use. Following the interview, all teens were given a complete prenatal examination, including drug toxicology screening. The results indicate relatively low rates of substance use based on toxicology at the time of enrollment (3.6%). Self-reported rates of substance use prior to awareness of conception varied from 23% for tobacco to 17% for alcohol and marijuana; 7% of the subjects reported use of illicit substances after conception was confirmed. In addition, 80 of the 352 subjects acknowledged having been physically or sexually abused and 40 admitted to having suicidal ideation or actions. A comparison of those teenagers who had been physically or sexually abused with the remaining cohort revealed significant differences on marijuana ($p < 0.01$) and cocaine ($p < 0.05$) use prior to awareness of conception and on prior suicidality ($p < 0.0001$). A positive history of physical or sexual abuse delineated a subset of pregnant teenagers who were at high risk for self-destructive behaviors. Teenagers in prenatal clinics should be screened, not only for current and past substance use, but also for sexual and physical abuse, domestic violence, and suicidal thoughts and actions.

(1992;13:128-132) Mahin Bayatpour et al, Department of Pediatarics, Valley Medical Center, 445 S Cedar Ave, Fresno, CA 93702.

J FAM VIOLENCE — New York, NY

Knowledge of Spouse Abuse in the Community: A Comparison Across Locations

Of concern to many who study criminality of all kinds is the high level of known abuse in a climate of noninvolvement by others. The research reported in this paper clearly indicates that noninvolvement in spousal assault cases is not dependent on low levels of knowledge of the problem, as many people admit to being aware of its occurrence among relatives, friends, and neighbors. This knowledge does vary, however, by location of the respondents with strong effects of nonmetropolitan residents expressing greater knowledge of the occurrence of this violence than people living in urban areas. We find this in the context of lower levels of self-reported victimization. It could be that these lower levels reflect a reluctance on the part of nonmetropolitan women to admit to researchers that they are victims of this problem. Or it could suggest that these women have access to a more intricate network of support from friends and family who become involved in discussing this problem with the victims and helping them to reduce its incidence.

(1991;6:303-317) Leslie W. Kennedy et al, Department of Sociology, University of Alberta, Edmonton, Alberta, Canada T6G 2H4.

Low and High Deviance Analogue Assessment of Parent-Training With Physically Abusive Parents

This study examined the utility of a parent-training program which included training to facilitate generalization to high-demand child-management situations, and employed structured analogue assessments of parent discipline performance in high-demand situations. A single-subject design was used to evaluate the effects of intervention with three physically abusive parents. The use of parenting skills was observed during free-play assessments (in clinic and home) with their child and two home-simulation assessments (low- and high-deviance) with clinical assistants enacting scripted child behaviors. Results support the effectiveness of the parent-training package and the use of low- and high-demand home-simulation assessments. Attempts to assess the impact of treatment on child management related to high-demand situations is particularly important given that these situations may function as antecedents to abuse behavior. The findings contribute to the literature on parent-training with physically abusive parents and suggest directions for future research and practice.

(1991;6:279-301) Virginia M. MacMillan et al, Department of Psychology, West Virginia University, Morgantown, WV 26506-6040.

Parricide

Following a review of the literature on parricide, family violence theory is briefly explored regarding its applicability to understanding the parricidal family. Characteristics of the adult perpetrator, including the role of the victim, is discussed and two cases illustrating successful prevention are presented. Finally, two case illustrations are presented and the issue of preventive intervention based on the psychoeducation model is discussed.

(1991;6:375-394) Christina E. Newhill, School of Social Work, University of Pittsburgh, Pittsburgh, PA 15260.

J FAM VIOLENCE — New York, NY

The Relationship of Abuse and Witnessing Violence on the Child Abuse Potential Inventory With Black Adolescents

A number of social and psychological factors present in most adolescent parents place them at high risk for abusive behavior toward their children. However, current child abuse potential measures do not include adolescent samples as part of the psychometric data base. Consequently, the purpose of this study was twofold: (1) to investigate whether a Black adolescent sample would perform differently than an adult nonabusing sample on the Child Abuse Potential Inventory (CAP), and (2) to examine the relationship between history of abuse or witnessing violence to scores on the CAP. Results revealed that Black adolescents scored significantly higher than the adult normative sample on the CAP; consequently, cutoff scores need to be empirically established for adolescents. Additional analyses indicated that a history of abuse, as well as a history of witnessing violence, are associated with a high potential for abuse.

(1991;6:351-363) Trisha R. Miller et al, Department of Psychology, St Louis University, 221 N Grand Blvd, St Louis, MO 63103.

CHILD ABUSE NEGL — Oxford, England

Child Sexual Abuse Prevention: Evaluation and One-Year Follow-up

Because of the high incidence and negative psychological consequences of child sexual abuse, prevention programs have been developed and implemented nationwide. Few programs, however, have been comprehensively evaluated. In this multimodal study, a 3-session adaptation of the *Feeling Yes, Feeling No* curriculum was provided to 286 third and fourth graders from four schools whose responses were compared to 113 delayed-treatment control children from two schools. Program impact was assessed using a knowledge scale, the State-Trait Anxiety Inventory for Children, a videotape vignettes measure, a parent questionnaire, and disclosure data. Treatment children exhibited significantly greater knowledge and better ability to discriminate safe from unsafe situations on the video measure than control children at posttesting. These gains were maintained at 6-week follow-up testing. There were no differences in treatment and control children's self-reported anxiety or parents' reports of negative emotional/behavioral consequences, which were minimal. Over 5% of participating children reported ongoing or past sexual abuse. In the One-Year Follow-Up Study, children's knowledge gains and prevention skills scores on the video measure were maintained at one-year follow-up. A 1-session "booster shot" program further enhanced children's safety discrimination skills on the video measure.

(1991;15:123-138) Ann Hazzard et al, Box 26065, Grady Memorial Hospital, 80 Butler St, SE, Atlanta, GA 30335.

'Don't Shake the Baby': The Effectiveness of a Prevention Program

The suggestion has been made that a systematic approach to informing all parents of newborns about the danger of shaking a baby is needed. The purpose of this study was to determine whether an educational campaign about the dangers of shaking a baby could influence parental knowledge, and would be perceived as helpful by new parents. A total of 15,708 parents of newborns in one urban county received a "Don't Shake the Baby" packet over a one year period. Moms ranged in age from 14 to 44 years, and 90% were white. A response postcard in the educational packet was returned to 3,293 parents (21%). More than three-fourths of respondents said the information was helpful to them, and 49% indicated that subsequent to reading the materials, they were less likely to shake their babies. Ninety-one percent said they thought other parents of newborns should read the material.

(1992;16:11-18) Jacy Showers, Research Institute, 615 Copeland Mill Rd, Suite 2E, Westerville, OH 43081.

Teachers' Knowledge, Attitudes, and Beliefs About Child Abuse and Its Prevention

In considering the great responsibility placed upon teachers to involve themselves in child abuse prevention, education, and detection, the National Committee for Prevention of Child Abuse (NCPCA) conducted a nationwide survey of teachers from 40 school districts in 29 randomly selected counties. The survey explores teachers' knowledge, attitudes, and beliefs about child abuse and its prevention. Five hundred and sixty-eight teachers responded, revealing that while the majority of teachers confront child abuse among their students, they are provided insufficient education on how to address it. Other findings are reported with respect to teachers' reporting behavior, potential barriers to reporting, child assault prevention programs, and corporal punishment in schools.

(1992;16:229-238) Nadine Abrahams et al. Reprint requests to Deborah Daro, 332 S Michigan Ave, Suite 1600, Chicago, IL 60604.

PEDIATRICS — Evanston, Ill

Genital Injuries Resulting From Sexual Abuse: A Longitudinal Study

Three children who incurred genital injuries as a result of sexual assaults were followed up on a longitudinal basis to document the anatomical changes which ensued. The subjects, who were 4 months, 4 years 5 months, and 9 years of age, were followed up for periods ranging from 14 months to 3 years. A multimethod examination approach and a 35-mm camera mounted on a colposcope were used to examine and record their injuries. Signs of the acute damage disappeared rapidly, and the wounds healed without complications. Following the resolution of the acute injuries, the changes created by the trauma remained relatively stable throughout the prepubertal years. The most persistent findings were irregular hymenal edges and narrow rims at the point of the injury. Over time the jagged, angular margins smoothed off. Disruption of the hymen exposed underlying longitudinal intravaginal ridges whose hymenal attachments created mounds or projections. There was little apparent scar formation. Even the injuries to the posterior fourchettes healed with minimal scar tissue and left only the slightest evidence of the trauma. With the onset of puberty, the hymenal changes in the oldest subject were obscured by the hypertrophy of this membrane. An examination technique which used a Q-tip to separate the redundant tissues demonstrated that the signs of trauma had survived.

(1992;89:307-317) John McCann et al, University of California, Davis Medical Center, Department of Pediatrics, 2516 Stockton Blvd, Sacramento, CA 95817.

Legal Proof of Child Sexual Abuse in the Absence of Physical Evidence

Child sexual abuse criminal court cases from a 12-month period were reviewed to determine the frequency and significance of physical evidence in legally "proven" felony cases with penetration. One hundred fifteen consecutive cases were reviewed, and 87 (76%) had resulted in conviction of the perpetrator on felony charges. Charges of vaginal rape were made in 88 cases, and oral and/or anal sodomy in 67 cases. Physical evidence was present in only 23% of all cases that resulted in felony convictions. Felony convictions were obtained in 67 (79%) of 85 cases without physical evidence and in only 20 (67%) of 30 cases with physical evidence. Eight of the 10 cases without physical evidence that did not result in conviction involved victims younger than 7 years of age. Cases involving the youngest victims had a significantly lower conviction rate (12 of 23), despite a very high frequency (13 of 23) of physical evidence ($P<.0005$). Physical evidence was neither predictive nor essential for conviction. Successful prosecution, particularly in cases involving the youngest victims, depended on the quality of the verbal evidence and the effectiveness of the child victim's testimony.

(1991;88:506-511) Allan R. De Jong and Mimi Rose. Reprint requests to Dr De Jong, Thomas Jefferson University Hospital, Suite 270, 909 Walnut St, Philadelphia, PA 19107.

Letters

Firearm Access and Suicide

To the Editor.—I would like to make some comments regarding the small-scale study of adolescent suicide in western Pennsylvania, even though the basic recommendation—that access to firearms by suicidal teenagers should be restricted by parents—is not controversial.

First, projecting from the authors' data, overall gun ownership levels in the households of suicidal (including attempts and completions) and nonsuicidal teenagers in a psychiatric hospital were at most 45%, but hunting license information and other data suggest that household gun ownership levels are significantly higher in the nontroubled teenaged population of western Pennsylvania. Although the study is too small-scale to be conclusive, the suggestion that household gun ownership is positively associated with mentally healthy teenagers is certainly worthy of more study.

Second, while the small-scale study—a sampling of 67 suicides over a 2-year period in the western section of a large and populous state—attempted to find all teen suicides, suicides may be undercounted by 25% to 50%, in the guise of automobile accidents, for example, but not firearms, since fortunately, there are too few gun-related accidents for misdiagnoses to alter suicide data significantly. As a result, both gun use and household gun ownership may be significantly exaggerated.

Third, with such a tiny sample, there is no basis for the study's conclusion that storing guns "locked" is an inadequate means of reducing teenage access. There were three suicides in households where guns were stored locked, and there was no detail on what that meant. Locking guns can range from a penny's worth of plastic through the operating mechanism to enclosure in a $10,000 safe.

Fourth, the study went well beyond its statistical data in endorsing an incompetently conducted study of suicide in Vancouver, British Columbia, and Seattle, Wash, which pretended the Canadian gun law somehow reduced suicide *only* among teenagers and young adults, with no impact on the overall rate. Furthermore, it ignored the rather telling fact that the suicide rate was higher overall and among almost all age and ethnic groups in the gun-restrictive Canadian city, and did not compare the suicide rates from the periods before and after the passage of the restrictive law.

The only scientific effort to measure the impact of the Canadian law on suicide found a substitution of other means but no improvement in the suicide rate.

Paul H. Blackman, PhD
National Rifle Association
Washington, DC

1. Brent DA, Perper JA, Allman CJ, Moritz GM, Wartella ME, Zelenak JP. The presence and accessibility of firearms in the homes of adolescent suicides: a case-controlled study. *JAMA.* 1991; 266:2989-2995.
2. Rosenberg ML, Davidson LE, Smith JC, et al. Operational criteria for the determination of suicide. *J Forensic Sci.* 1988;33:1445-1456.
3. Sloan JH, Rivara FP, Reay DT, Ferris JAJ, Kellerman AL. Firearm regulations and rates of suicide: a comparison of two metropolitan areas. *N Engl J Med.* 1990; 322:369-373.
4. Rich CL, Young JG, Fowler RC, Wagner J, Black NA. Guns and suicide: possible effects of some specific legislation. *Am J Psychiatry.* 1990; 147:342-346.

In Reply.—Dr Blackman raises concerns about the size of the study as limiting the ability to draw firm conclusions. However, this study is a replication of a previously published comparison of 27 suicides and 56 suicidal adolescents. The fact that *both* studies yielded the same results strengthens the ability to draw the conclusion that the availability of firearms is a risk factor for adolescent suicide.

Blackman raises an interesting hypothesis, "that household gun ownership is positively associated with mental health in teenagers." I am not sure if Blackman is suggesting that there are salutary properties associated with firearm ownership, or whether those families with psychiatrically ill adolescents are less likely to have a gun available in the home. Both the suicide victims and suicide attempters were psychiatrically ill, but the rate of firearm ownership was higher in families of suicide victims, suggesting that there is no relationship between psychiatric illness in an adolescent and gun availability.

The questions about the underascertainment of suicide and its possible effects on our results is a good one. In a previous study, we described a rate of underascertainment of adolescent suicide of 25% from 1960 through 1983 in Allegheny County, Pennsylvania, but from 1978 through 1983, the rate of underascertainment was only 11%. While it is theoretically possible that certain automobile accidents are disguised suicides, previous psychological autopsy studies among adults indicate that only 1% to 2% of single-passenger vehicular accidents are in fact suicides.

Blackman raises two questions about our conclusions about the method of storage. First, the definition of *locked*, and second, the statistical power to draw the conclusion that we did. We defined *locked* as any barrier to access that required substantial force in the absence of a key. As we state in the "Comment" section, when the samples in the present and previous studies are combined, more restrictive storage *did* seem to convey some protective effect. However, the size of the effect attributable to the method of storage was small compared with the effect of the availability. Therefore, the risk of having the gun available appeared to be greater than the benefit of "safe" storage.

Blackman is correct that the study by Rich et al showed that a Canadian firearm law had no impact on the suicide rate, and we cited this study in our original article. Recently, Loftin et al found a 23% reduction in the suicide rate in Washington, DC, subsequent to the enactment of a more restrictive firearm-ownership law. As for the 1990 study by Sloan et al, space does not permit a rebuttal of Blackman's criticism except to say that we viewed it as an elegant, rather than an "incompetently performed," study.

In summary, Blackman is apparently in agreement with the basic conclusion of our article, that access to firearms should be restricted for suicidal teens. The most efficient means for attaining this end still remains a matter for scientific debate.

David A. Brent, MD
University of Pittsburgh School of Medicine
Western Psychiatric Institute and Clinic
Pittsburgh, Pa

Joshua A. Perper, MD, LLB, MSc
Chief Coroner, Allegheny County
Pittsburgh, Pa

1. Brent DA, Perper JA, Goldstein CE, et al. Risk factors for adolescent suicide: a comparison of adolescent suicide victims with suicidal inpatients. *Arch Gen Psychiatry.* 1988;45;581-588.
2. Brent DA, Perper JA, Allman CJ, Moritz GM, Wartella M, Zelenak JP. Alcohol, firearms, and suicide among youth: temporal trends in Allegheny County, Pennsylvania, 1960-1983. *JAMA.* 1987;257:3369-3372.
3. Schmidt CW, Shaffer JW, Zlotowitz HI, Fisher RS. Suicide by vehicular crash. *Am J Psychiatry.* 1977;134:175-178.
4. Rich CL, Young JG, Fowler RC, Wagner J, Black NA. Guns and suicide: possible effects of some specific legislation. *Am J Psychiatry.* 1990; 147:342-346.
5. Loftin C, McDowall D, Wiersema B, Cottey TJ. Effects of restrictive licensing of handguns on homicide and suicide in the District of Columbia. *N Engl J Med.* 1991; 325:1615-1620.
6. Sloan JH, Rivara FP, Reay DT, Ferris JAJ, Kellerman AL. Firearm regulations and rates of suicide: a comparison of two metropolitan areas. *N Engl J Med.* 1990; 322:369-373.

Final Exit and the Risk of Suicide

To the Editor.—Critics of the controversial book *Final Exit* have cautioned that it may encourage and facilitate suicide among individuals with treatable psychiatric disorders. Even among the infirm elderly and those with serious medical disorders, suicide is often secondary to potentially remediable psychological factors rather than intractable pain or inexorable death. With its lurid examples, explicit instructions, and vigorous advocacy for suicide, *Final Exit* may have an especially pernicious effect on adolescents, who, with their high rates of attempted and completed suicide, appear susceptible to imitative influences and cultural factors that glorify or destigmatize suicide. The following case report illustrates the potential dangers of facilitating adolescent suicidality.

Two 14-year-old girls, A and B, were referred by their school principal for emergency psychiatric assessment after each accused the other of being suicidal. Girl A had recently purchased *Final Exit*, brought it to school, and gave it to B, who in turn circulated it to several other students. Both girls had significant prior risk factors for suicidality.

Girl A was a bright, melodramatic girl, who liked poetry and worried about existential matters. She reported often feeling depressed, experiencing insomnia, trouble concentrating, and anhedonia. She reported trouble getting along with her family, who in turn described her as oppositional and manipulative, with escalating behavioral problems. A family history of substance abuse was highlighted by a close relative's death from a drug overdose 3 years earlier. Girl A denied overt suicidal ideas, but often imagined her own funeral in great detail, including all the people who would be present.

Girl B, a talkative, emotionally intense girl, had a more extensive history of suicidal thoughts and manipulative gestures. She often felt aggrieved toward her family. Three weeks prior to evaluation, following a fight with her family, she called up all her friends to tell them good-bye, implying she was going to kill herself. Two years earlier she had taken 4 to 5 acetaminophen tablets without telling anyone. At evaluation, however, she denied currently feeling suicidal and claimed that it was A, rather than herself, who had voiced suicidal thoughts.

Girl A initially denied knowing *Final Exit* was a "suicide book," but later stated that she bought it for B, who had talked with her about suicide. During the evaluation, A spontaneously remarked that she felt the book "shouldn't be available to society." She expressed relief at being able to leave her copy of the book in the emergency department.

Following emergency evaluation and crisis intervention, both girls were referred for extended individual and family outpatient treatment.

Although both girls denied having a suicide pact, they appeared caught up in a shared adolescent "culture of suicide" in which the exchange of confidences concerning suicidal fantasies and plans came to be an increasingly important part of their friendship and peer group. The recent notoriety and easy accessibility of the book *Final Exit* appears to have become an element in the evolution of these teenagers' mutually reinforcing self-destructive fantasies.

Excessive interest by an adolescent in such suicide manuals warrants careful evaluation. Further data on the impact of such works on vulnerable adolescents are needed.

Phillip B. Chappell, MD
Robert A. King, MD
Yale Child Study Center
New Haven, Conn
Michael Enson, CISW
Clifford W. Beers Guidance Clinic
New Haven, Conn

1. Humphry D. *Final Exit.* Eugene, Ore: The Hemlock Society; 1991.
2. Miles SH, reviewer. *JAMA.* 1991;266:2150. Review of: *Final Exit: The Practicalities of Self-Deliverance and Assisted Suicide for the Dying.*
3. Conwell Y, Caine ED. Rational suicide and the right to die: reality and myth. *N Engl J Med.* 1991;325:1100-1102.
4. American Association of Suicidology. Press release, August 16, 1991, Denver, Colo.
5. Shaffer D, Garland A, Gould M, Fisher P, Trautman P. Preventing teenage suicide: a critical review. *J Am Acad Child Adolesc Psychiatry.* 1988; 27:675-687.

The Violence Our Violent Country Does to Others

To the Editor.—In this year of the 500th anniversary of the Columbus' landing in America, I'd like to offer some ideas on violence in the Americas, rather than just violence in the United States.

I am a public health physician who was born and raised in Latin America, but I have had all of my medical training in the United States.

It seems to me that with an ethnocentric view of sociological problems in this country, it is easy to forget the violent effects of our own society on neighboring countries. Thus, it is common to read nowadays about the epidemiology of homicide, rape, suicide, and abuse of elders, spouses, and children.

While all of these are problems that affect all societies, is it not true that maybe there is another type of violence, which we could describe as the violence of one culture against another? What I propose we should think about is how our super-advanced culture may be provoking violence in other parts of this hemisphere.

Some of the ways may be rather subtle.

For example, American pharmaceutical companies test their products not yet approved by the US Food and Drug Administration in Puerto Rico and other Latin American countries. Is this not prejudice or a form of violence against other lives? Or are those lives south of the border less valuable than those directly regulated by the Food and Drug Administration? We export agricultural chemicals (such as pesticides) that are no longer approved by the Environmental Protection Agency for use in these countries, and many crops are treated with such chemicals. We export cigarettes to other countries and promote a habit there that has been condemned by many surgeons general of the United States. Is this not also violence inflicted by one culture on another?

Finally, the greed for drugs that are illegal in this country can be seen as stimulating some of the native economies of Latin America, but more consistently and importantly as promoting a reign of turbulence, of narcoguerrillas, and of urban violence in countries such as Peru and Colombia.

Every year, *JAMA* dedicates an issue to the remembrance of the Hiroshima/Nagasaki holocaust. Yet there is a more subtle and ongoing morbidity and mortality that we ourselves provoke.

Should we not remember the first principle of Hippocratic medicine—at least, do no harm?

Henry T. Wasserman, MD, MPH
Coral Gables, Fla

1. Last J. *Maxcy-Rosenau-Last Public Health and Preventive Medicine.* 13th ed. New York, NY: Appleton-Lange;1991:1035-1064.

Books

Violence

Deadly Consequences, by Deborah Prothrow-Stith, 269 pp, $22.50, ISBN 0-06-016344-5, New York, NY, HarperCollins, 1991.

> Maybe we should erect a black marble slab and start compiling the names of all those like Arnulfo Williams whose lives are wasted by violence. Covering the slab with names will not take long. Every day more than 60 Americans die in homicides. About 450 a week. About 1900 a month. 23,000 a year. 46,000 in two years.
>
> In two years we would have a solemn memorial covered with names, just like the Vietnam Memorial in Washington, DC. Mourners could come and weep. Mothers and fathers could express their anguish. Children could find a legacy, small but powerful, as they trace their fingers over the names of the fathers taken from them. Only this memorial would be different. Very soon the names would spill over, and you would need another memorial, and another and another to report the names of the endless stream of fatalities.

So says Deborah Prothrow-Stith, an internist subspecializing in adolescent medicine, who served for a time as Commissioner of Health for the Commonwealth of Massachusetts and now is an assistant dean at the Harvard School of Public Health. Her book *Deadly Consequences,* written with professional writer Michaele Weissman, is subtitled "How Violence is Destroying Our Teenage Population and a Plan to Begin Solving the Problem."

Sensitized to the issue of inner-city violence during a surgical clerkship in medical school, the author "wanted to understand the forces that sent so many teenagers to the emergency room cut up, shot up, bleeding and dead." She views violence as a public health problem. "Over time, employing an array of interventions, the public health approach can change people's attitudes, and in the long run, their destructive behavior. We have done this with cigarettes . . . we have done this with drunk driving . . . we have done this with exercise and diet . . . I believe we can do the same thing for violence," she says.

Unfortunately, *Deadly Consequences* provides more exhortation than enlightenment. Consciousness-raising, particularly directed toward members of the medical profession, is a major theme. We physicians are castigated for our lack of will to reduce homicide and other forms of violence. Speaking of her emergency room experience, Prothrow-Stith says, "I believed that the lack of outrage doctors expressed in the face of so much mayhem represented, in a sense, society's acquiescence. So long as 'they' were killing each other, nobody seemed to mind."

Is our society and our profession so blind to the violence issue? I think not. No one watching the nightly television news needs convincing that kids in urban ghettos are killing each other. No one reading Claude Brown's *Manchild in the Promised Land* or viewing the remarkable film *Boyz N the Hood* need wonder about the origins of ghetto violence. Would that the remedy be as simple as expressing more outrage. Banging the drum more loudly does not necessarily bring about the desired results.

The book's greatest strength is its focus on violence with the greatest potential for prevention, that which occurs between individuals who know each other. Special emphasis is appropriately placed on attempts to deter violent behavior in children. Prothrow-Stith contends that aggression is a learned behavior that can be unlearned. She calls on schools to teach children how to manage conflict and anger in a nonviolent manner. Some interesting examples of "violence prevention curricula" are described. It would be nice to see some evaluation of their effectiveness. "Would that the remedy be as simple as expressing more outrage."

The weakest point is the book's failure to describe the political terrain, however rocky, that must be traversed to bring about significant improvements. A scant two pages, for example, are devoted to efforts to curtail the widespread availability of handguns. Defining violence as a public health problem akin to cigarette smoking, drunk driving, and overeating will appeal to the same folks who feel that physicians hold some special expertise in efforts to prevent nuclear war. I feel we do not possess such expertise. I do feel, however, that physicians should speak up along with other concerned citizens to advocate for adequate employment opportunities, housing, and education for ghetto children. The killings will stop only when their deadly consequences are perceived to have an impact, not only on "them," but on all the rest of us in the United States.

Abraham B. Bergman
Harborview Medical Center
Seattle, Wash

Family Violence

When a Child Kills: Abused Children Who Kill Their Parents, by Paul A. Mones, 331 pp, $21, ISBN 0-671-67420- X, New York, NY, Pocket Books, 1991.

The author, Paul Mones, is an attorney who specializes in defending children who kill their parents. This book, which is based on his work as a consultant to other lawyers on about 100 cases in 30 states, describes the lives of eight teenagers who committed parricide. His straightforward and graphic style provides the reader with a poignant understanding of these teenage victims of child abuse and family violence.

The teenagers described in this book suffered from an extreme form of child abuse, which typically included physical, mental, and, frequently, sexual abuse from a very young age, by the parent who was eventually killed. Mones accurately emphasizes that the word *abuse* minimizes what these children were forced to endure. Terms such as *torture, soul murder, deprivation,* and *survival* are key concepts in understanding the consequences of this abuse. The fundamental contradiction in these cases (ie, the child still loves the abusing parent), which is reflective of the psychodynamics of child abuse, is made more understandable by the unfolding of the teenagers' painful stories in each section of this book.

Two introductory chapters present a very readable historical account concerning the recognition of child abuse as a medically diagnosable syndrome, as first discussed in the landmark 1962 *JAMA* article by Kempe et al, "The Battered-Child Syndrome." Relevant studies about family violence are reviewed, and the reasons for underreporting the incidence of family violence are described. The evolution of legal protection for children in the United States is chronicled, beginning with the intervention by the Society for the Prevention of Cruelty to Animals in New York City in 1874 when a young girl was found starving and chained to her bed.

The book has six sections based on the nature of the parricide (boys who kill their fathers, patricide committed by daughters, girls who kill their mothers, matricide committed by sons, children who kill both parents, and children who hire others to kill their parents). Each section is preceded by several introductory pages that summarize statistical and cultural information relevant to the specific type of parricide being reviewed. For example, the reader learns that there have been more than 300 parricides per year since 1976, with sons generally committing over 90% of the offenses. The majority of the parricides are patricides, and the rarest form of parricide is matricide committed by daughters. A weakness in these introductory pages is the superficial descriptions of various theoretical models, which attempt to explain the reasons underlying the specific type of parricide (eg, why do sons kill their fathers?).

Mones provides the reader with insight into the legal strategies needed in preparing and trying parricide cases. Defense attorneys need to assume the role of a prosecutor attempting to try the dead for their abusive crimes against their children in life. The attorney must then resume the role of defense attorney and prove that, but for the abuse, the parricide would not have occurred. These strategies require the defense attorney to educate judges and juries about relevant cultural, psychological, and systems issues in child abuse cases. For example, Mones points out that society may have some tolerance for understanding events leading to a son killing his father but often finds a similar action leading to the death of a son's mother to be totally unacceptable and not understandable. Inadequacies in social services, child protection teams, and the criminal justice system are exposed.

A final chapter and appendix effectively describe the plight of children who have killed their parents. The limitations of the legal system in dealing with such children are highlighted. An appendix provides useful information for the lay public concerning how individuals can make a difference in preventing or stopping child abuse.

The target audience for this book appears to be the educated lay public, although attorneys and physicians will likely find it helpful in becoming more sensitized to child abuse issues. The physician who wants a more scientific presentation of similar issues will find *Juvenile Homicide*, edited by Benedek and Cornell (Washington, DC, American Psychiatric Press, 1989), more useful, although less specific concerning the issue of parricide.

Jeffrey L. Metzner, MD
Kempe National Center
Denver, Colo

Loaded Guns in the Home

Analysis of a National Random Survey of Gun Owners

Douglas S. Weil, ScM, David Hemenway, PhD

Objective.—To identify factors associated with keeping guns loaded. Four hypotheses were tested: that people are more likely to keep their firearms loaded if (1) the primary reason for owning a gun is protection, (2) the gun is a handgun, (3) there are no children in the household, or (4) the gun owner has not received training in the proper use of firearms.

Design and Setting.—A random national telephone survey of gun owners conducted in December 1989. A screening question was used to identify individuals as gun owners. Participants were called at home.

Participants.—605 individuals (approximately two thirds of the population contacted) participated in the survey. All were 18 years and older, most were men (64%), and a few were nonwhite (12%). The majority owned more than one gun (77%).

Results.—Three of the four hypotheses were substantiated by the data. Handgun owners (odds ratio [OR], 2.17; 95% confidence interval [CI], 1.67 to 2.82), individuals who owned a firearm principally for protection (OR, 1.65; 95% CI, 1.30 to 2.11), and people who lived in households without children (OR, 1.42; 95% CI, 1.13 to 1.82) were all more likely to keep a gun loaded than other individuals. Instruction in the proper use of firearms did not seem to affect the probability of keeping guns loaded (OR, 0.86; 95% CI, 0.69 to 1.07).

Conclusions.—The spontaneous nature of many firearm deaths has led to speculation that a substantial proportion of firearm-related morbidity and mortality could be prevented if easy access to loaded weapons were reduced through appropriate storage practices. Our findings show that a significant proportion of gun owners disregard basic safety procedures. However, without information on the specific content of safety instruction, we cannot say that education about safe storage practices is ineffective.

(*JAMA*. 1992;267:3033-3037)

RESEARCH that links the availability of loaded firearms to gun violence tends to be more descriptive than analytic. However, the spontaneity with which deadly violence occurs has lent support to the contention that easy access to a loaded gun may be an important risk factor for both homicide and suicide as well as unintentional shootings.

Many homicides and suicides appear to be the result of impulsive behavior. Homicides frequently occur during arguments, often domestic, when emotions run high and when one or both parties have been drinking.[1,2] Individuals who take their own lives often do so when confronting a severe but temporary crisis.[3] For example, young male suicide victims (for whom the suicide rate tripled between 1950 and 1980) were not generally depressed but acted on impulse in response to "trouble at home, in school, and with the police."[4]

The US General Accounting Office (GAO) reported that 1501 unintentional firearm deaths occurred in 1988. Over 70% involved a handgun, and most occurred in or near the home.[5] Several studies estimate that there are four to six nonfatal injuries for every fatal accidental shooting.[6-9] Among those killed unintentionally in 1988 were 277 children 15 years and younger.[5] Pediatric morbidity and mortality due to accidental gunshot wounds are often the result of spontaneous happenings that occur when children find and play with a loaded gun. This fact has led researchers to suggest that failure to prevent access to these weapons may be an important risk factor for injury.[6,10-14]

As a result of the spontaneous or impulsive nature of many firearm fatalities, it is logical to expect that "a substantial portion of these events might be prevented if immediate access to lethal weapons was reduced, in particular through appropriate storage of guns and ammunition."[15] Thus, one goal of Healthy People 2000 is a 20% reduction in the "proportion of people who possess weapons that are inappropriately stored and therefore dangerously available."[15]

A recent national survey found that firearms were present in 46% of households and that one in four households had a handgun.[16] Over half of the handgun owners surveyed said that their guns were currently loaded. These findings are consistent with those of a smaller study in which 55% of gun owners questioned claimed they always kept their weapons loaded; 10% said that their guns were "loaded, unlocked and within reach of children."[10]

According to virtually all experts, including the National Rifle Association and the Sporting Arms and Ammunition Manufacturer's Institute, the safe handling of a firearm requires that guns be stored unloaded in a locked area separate from the ammunition.[17,18] Many gun owners apparently do not follow this advice.

Society's ability to address the problem of firearm-related fatalities could

From the Department of Health Policy and Management, Harvard School of Public Health, Boston, Mass.

Reprint requests to Department of Health Policy and Management, Harvard School of Public Health, Fourth Floor, Kresge, 677 Huntington Ave, Boston, MA 02115 (Mr Weil).

be improved by research into the storage of guns.[8]

We lack routinely collected information on behavioral risk factors (e.g. gun storage and accessibility to loaded weapons) that contribute to firearm associated morbidity and mortality. Information on these factors would help to establish the characteristics of persons with easy access to guns so that high-risk groups could be targeted for intervention. In addition, such information would help evaluate efforts aimed at preventing firearm injury, reducing access, and altering unsafe storage practices.[4]

This study analyzes a national random sample of gun owners to identify factors associated with keeping guns loaded. Four principal hypotheses are tested: that, all else equal, people are more likely to keep their firearms loaded if (1) the primary purpose for owning a gun is protection from crime, (2) the gun is a handgun, (3) there are no children in the household, and (4) the owner has not received instruction in the proper use of firearms.

METHODS

Data Origin and Potential Sources of Bias:

The data used were obtained from a random national telephone survey of gun owners 18 years and older. The survey, sponsored by *Time* magazine and Cable News Network, was conducted December 15 through 22, 1989, by Yankelovich Clancy & Shulman Inc. Telephone numbers were randomly generated to ensure that households with both listed unlisted numbers were included. Respondents were not identifiable to the researchers by name or address. Participants were asked a screening question; approximately one in three individuals declined to answer this screening question, with no significant drop in participation for the remaining questions.

Surveys that sample the population are subject to sampling error. Results may differ from what would be obtained if the whole population were interviewed. For a survey of 600 respondents, the results are subject to an error margin of ±4 percentage points for each question because of chance variation in the sample.

Telephone surveys are subject to systematic error. Individuals without telephones or those who work unusual hours may not be represented. In 1986, 7% of all people in the United States (including more than 15% of all blacks and 27% of people living below the poverty line) lived in households that did not have a telephone.[19]

Registered gun owners have been shown to provide generally valid responses to questions about gun ownership.[20] However, the same may not be true for owners of unregistered weapons. Individuals who own guns illegally or for illegal purposes may be reluctant to admit ownership. Gun owners under the age of 18 years were not surveyed.

The imprecise wording of some questions might cause measurement error or incorrect interpretation of the results. For example, respondents were asked, "Do you sometimes keep your gun loaded, always keep it loaded, or never keep it loaded?" It is not immediately clear how someone with more than one weapon would answer this question, particularly if one gun were always loaded and another never loaded.

Finally, while respondents were asked why they purchased their gun, they were not asked why they kept it loaded. A primary goal of this study is to help determine who keeps loaded weapons.

Outcome Variable

A dichotomous dependent variable was created by separating individuals who never kept their gun(s) loaded from those who did keep a gun loaded some of the time or always. A second model, which excludes individuals who sometimes kept their guns loaded, was analyzed to determine whether the predicted odds ratios were sensitive to the treatment of this intermediate response group.

Individuals who kept their gun(s) both unlocked and loaded create the greatest potential for injury. Therefore, we created an alternate dependent variable that compares people whose firearms are loaded and unlocked with all other gun owners. Our principal results were unchanged when using this variable. We report the findings of the model that uses keeping a firearm loaded as the outcome of interest so that we can show the relationship between keeping a gun locked and keeping it loaded.

Predictors

The four key indicator variables examined were (1) type of gun, (2) reason for owning a gun, (3) presence of children in the home, and (4) training in the proper use of guns. To capture the effect of gun type, respondents who owned a handgun were placed into one category, and everyone else was put into the reference group. Individuals who owned both a handgun and a long gun were placed in the handgun category.

Individuals who owned their gun(s) primarily "for protection from crime," were distinguished from the subjects in the reference group that contains all other responses (hunting, target shooting, gun collection, work, other, and not sure).

Respondents were also categorized by whether or not they lived with children. Ninety-five people could not directly be assigned to either category. However, using responses from other questions, it was possible to determine that 73 of these individuals lived alone and that nine were married and living only with their spouses. These 82 people (86%) were put in the "no children" category, and the rest were put in the reference group. The results of the analysis do not appreciably differ by the assignment of the remaining 13 people.

Two questions in the survey concerned respondents' training in the use of firearms. The first asked whether the individual had been given instruction. Those who had received training were asked, "Where did you get this training—from someone you knew, from a class, from military training, or in some other way?" People who said that they received training from the military or a class were put into one category. All other individuals, including those who said that they had not received any training, were put into the reference category. Informal instruction may be more similar to military or classroom training than to a lack of training. Hence, an analysis was also conducted comparing individuals with any form of instruction in the proper use of guns with those with no training.

Background Variables

Various factors that might confound the relationship between the possession of a loaded firearm and any of the four predictors were incorporated into the model. Included among these variables were demographic characteristics such as the gun owner's age, race, sex, level of education achieved, and the region of the country where the respondent lives.

Other factors that might be associated with both the outcome and one or more predictors are the number of guns owned, whether or not they were kept locked up when not in use, and the location where they were stored (eg, in the bedroom). Respondent's income is another potential confounder. However, 20% of the participants (n=119) declined to provide information about their income, so the variable is not included in the final model. A sensitivity analysis was conducted to determine whether the presence of income in the model affects the results.

There is no established theory that suggests the functional form for many of the potential confounding variables. Alternative forms were tested to determine whether the principal results were sensitive to the way these background variables were specified. For example, the number of guns owned could be treated as a continuous or dichotomous variable. It could also be treated as several dichotomous variables. We tried various forms and none altered our results.

Multivariate logistic regression is used to estimate the odds ratio (OR) of keeping a gun loaded for individuals with a given characteristic (eg, they were handgun owners) relative to individuals without that characteristic while simultaneously controlling for the other variables in the model.

RESULTS

The sample consisted of 605 individuals; most were men (75%), few were nonwhite (12%). Each respondent owned at least one gun, with the majority owning more than one (77%). The most commonly owned type of firearm was a rifle (72%), while 61% of the respondents owned a handgun. The weapons were typically kept unloaded at all times. However, more than one third of the gun owners kept their gun(s) loaded either all of the time (25%) or some of the time (12%). Furthermore, 53% of the people surveyed did not keep their firearms locked up.

Simple crosstabulations indicate that owning a handgun, purchasing the weapon for protection, and having no children in the household are all positively correlated with keeping a gun loaded; training in the proper use of firearms is not significantly correlated with the dependent variable (Table 1). Similar results are found in multiple logistic analysis (Table 2). Only 583 observations are included in this analysis, since information concerning one or more of the variables of interest is missing for 22 individuals.

Table 1.—Crosstabulations of Possible Predictors of Private Ownership of a Loaded Gun and Associated χ^2 Statistics

Factor	No.*	Sometimes or Always Keep Gun Loaded, %	χ^2
Handgun†			
Owns a handgun	364	51	81.18‡
Does not own a handgun	227	15	
Purpose§			
Protection from crime	162	63	64.20‡
Other	432	27	
Children in house§			
No	358	42	8.11‖
Yes	236	30	
Training§			
Military or class	311	36	0.59
None or other	283	38	
Region§			
Southern¶	260	50	31.37‡
Other	334	27	
Race§			
White	523	35	6.46‖
Nonwhite	71	50	
Locked up#			
Yes	267	33	2.62**
No	319	40	
Age, y††			
≤34	228	34	1.25
≥35	361	39	
No. of guns owned§			
≤2	257	33	3.05**
≥3	337	40	
Where stored§			
Bedroom	255	39	0.61
Other	339	36	
Education††			
≤High school	320	36	0.35
>High school	296	35	

*N=605 in the sample population.
†Fourteen observations were missing.
‡$P<.001$.
§Eleven observations were missing.
‖$P<.01$.
¶The southern region included Alabama, Arkansas, Delaware, Florida, Georgia, Kentucky, Louisiana, Maryland, Mississippi, North Carolina, Oklahoma, South Carolina, Tennessee, Texas, Virginia, and West Virginia. The other region included all remaining states. Alaska, Hawaii, and Washington, DC, are not represented in the sample.
#Nineteen observations were missing.
**$P<.1$.
††Sixteen observations were missing.

The strongest predictor of respondents who possess a loaded firearm was the type of gun owned. Handgun owners were more than twice as likely as other individuals to keep their guns loaded at least some of the time (OR, 2.17; 95% confidence interval [CI], 1.67 to 2.82).

Among the people surveyed, individuals who owned their weapons primarily for protection from crime were 65% more likely to keep their firearms loaded than individuals who owned their guns for other purposes (OR, 1.65; 95% CI, 1.30 to 2.11). People who did not live with children were over 40% more likely to report that they kept their weapons loaded than gun owners living in households with children (OR, 1.42; 95% CI, 1.13 to 1.82).

Other factors associated with the maintenance of a loaded firearm are geographic location, race, and whether or not the gun was locked up when not in use. Individuals who lived in the South and those who were not white were more likely to keep their guns loaded. People who did not lock up their guns were also more likely to keep them loaded.

Of the four main hypotheses, the only one that cannot be substantiated is the proposed association between training in the proper use of guns and the likelihood that a gun will be kept loaded. In the study population, instruction did not seem to affect the probability of keeping guns loaded (OR, 0.86; 95% CI, 0.69 to 1.07). The result holds whether the variable is any training or only military or classroom instruction.

If the income variable is included in the model, the principal findings are unaffected. Furthermore, the results do not appreciably differ when subjects who kept their guns loaded only some of the time are excluded from the analysis.

COMMENT

Handguns are the most common type of firearm involved in gunshot deaths in the home, whether accidental or intentional.[12,21] The most common reason given for owning a handgun is protection from crime,[10,22] yet only a small percentage of firearm deaths in the home are the result of a incident requiring self-protection.[21,23] Unfortunately, no study seems to link specific shooting incidents with the reason for owning a gun.

This study does not include data on shootings. However, it does link gun type and purpose of gun ownership to the likelihood of keeping a gun loaded. Handgun owners and individuals who own firearms for protection are more likely than other gun owners to keep their weapons loaded. The tendency to keep ammunition in the gun may help explain the large number of injuries associated

Table 2.—Factors Associated With Keeping a Gun Loaded*: Interpreting the Fitted Logistic

Factor	Logistic Regression Results, Odds Ratio (95% Confidence Interval)†
Handgun	
1=owns a handgun	2.17 (1.67-2.82)
0=other	
Purpose	
1=protection from crime	1.65 (1.30-2.11)
0=other	
Children living in home	
1=no	1.43 (1.13-1.82)
0=yes	
Training	
1=formal (military or other)	0.86 (0.69-1.07)
0=none or informal	
Region‡	
1=southern states	1.61 (1.31-1.98)
0=other	
Race	
1=nonwhite	1.37 (1.01-1.86)
0=white	
Locked up when stored	
1=no	1.23 (1.01-1.54)
0=yes	
Age, y§	
30s	
1=30-39	1.24 (0.92-1.66)
0=other	
40s	
1=40-49	1.10 (0.80-1.52)
0=other	
50s	
1=≥50	1.11 (0.83-1.48)
0=other	
Sex	
1=male	1.06 (0.82-1.36)
0=female	
No. of guns owned∥	
2 or 3	
1=own 2 or 3 guns	0.83 (0.62-1.11)
0=other	
4 or more	
1=own 4 or more guns	1.19 (0.88-1.62)
0=other	
Where stored	
1=bedroom	0.92 (0.75-1.14)
0=other	
Education¶	
College	
1=attended college	1.20 (0.97-1.49)
0=other	
Postgraduate	
1=have postgraduate degree	0.90 (0.54-1.48)
0=other	

*1=store gun loaded some or all of the time, 0=never store gun loaded.
†N=583 for the logistic regression result; 22 observations were missing.
‡The southern region included Alabama, Arkansas, Delaware, Florida, Georgia, Kentucky, Louisiana, Maryland, Mississippi, North Carolina, Oklahoma, South Carolina, Tennessee, Texas, Virginia, and West Virginia. The other region included all remaining states. Alaska, Hawaii, and Washington, DC, are not represented in the sample.
§The reference group consisted of all individuals between the ages of 18 and 29 years.
∥The reference group consisted of all individuals who owned only one gun.
¶The reference group consisted of all individuals who had not been to college.

with accidental discharges and intentional shootings not justified by self-defense needs.

Research suggests that easy access to a loaded gun may be a risk factor for accidental firearm injuries among children[11,12,14] and may be a contributing factor for adolescent suicide.[24] Among the gun owners surveyed, those with children in the home were less likely to keep their guns loaded. Nonetheless, it appears that many families with children do keep loaded guns in the home (30%), even though experts, such as the American Academy of Pediatrics,[13] warn of the danger.

Increased attention has been given to the potential of design modification as a way of reducing the morbidity and mortality associated with firearms discharges.[5,12,25,26] According to the GAO, two devices, a childproof safety mechanism and a mechanism that indicates whether a gun is loaded, could reduce accidental firearm fatalities by approximately 31%. However, noting that "a majority of the accidents . . . examined involved some violation of safe gun-handling standards," and noting the large number of weapons already privately owned, the GAO suggests the need for "proper education in the use and handling of firearms."[5]

We did not discover any study that linked instruction in the use of guns to the safe handling of these weapons by their owners. One study that looked at unintentional firearm fatalities among children did note that the victim and the gun owner (most often the victim's parent) were unlikely to have received any training in gun safety procedures.[11] Furthermore, the authors note that, even after an accident, guns often remained accessible and safety rules were not observed.

Safety instruction does not necessarily lead to the observation of safety rules. The results of this analysis indicate that training, even if provided by the military or in a formal class, is not associated with safe gun-handling procedures as they relate to keeping guns loaded. One possible explanation is that important safety information is omitted from the training. Another possible explanation is that this information is insufficiently emphasized, particularly for individuals who have purchased a firearm for protection. Unfortunately, the survey did not collect information on the specific content of the safety instruction received, so we cannot determine whether education about safe storage practices is ineffective based on this analysis.

In the study population, nonwhite individuals were more likely than whites to keep their guns loaded (OR, 1.37; 95% CI, 1.01 to 1.86). One possible explanation is that blacks and other racial minorities feel less secure in their homes than whites. Violent crime, such as robbery, rape, and aggravated assault, is committed against members of black households at a rate 1½ times higher than the rate among white households,[27] and nonwhites are several times more likely than whites to be homicide victims.[28]

Among the individuals surveyed, those who did not keep their weapons locked up were more likely than other individuals to keep their weapons loaded (OR, 1.23; 95% CI, 1.01 to 1.54). This pairing of hazardous behaviors creates the greatest risk of injury. While such behavior runs counter to the theory of risk compensation,[29] it is probably to be expected. Many people who own firearms for protection may believe they need ready access to a weapon that is both loaded and unlocked.

The South has high rates of homicide, gun homicide, and gun ownership compared with other regions of the country.[30,31] This study indicates that southerners are also more likely to keep their firearms loaded.

The are several limitations to this analysis. The information in the data set is derived from self-reports rather than observational data. This could be a problem if, for instance, respondents were unable to recall whether their guns were loaded. Indeed, the GAO report suggests that a contributing factor in many accidental firearm fatalities is the victim's belief that the gun was not loaded when it was.[5] Self-report data are also subject to inaccuracies if respondents are embarrassed to tell the truth. For example, some individuals living with small children may not want to admit to keeping a loaded gun in the house.

The generalizability of the survey may also be limited by two factors. First, racial minorities account for a small percentage of respondents. Telephone surveys tend to underrepresent low-income and minority groups, and this appears to be the case in the present study. Second, the survey excluded gun owners under 18 years old, yet many young people own guns.

CONCLUSION

J. Warren Cassidy, formerly executive vice-president of the National Rifle Association, wrote that gun owners in America are "safe, sane and courteous in their use of guns."[32] The large number of gun-related assaults, homicides, suicides, and accidental shootings raises questions about this assertion. Our findings show that a significant proportion of gun owners disregard basic safety procedures. Over one third of the gun owners surveyed kept their weapons loaded, and more than half kept them unlocked. People who owned handguns or owned their guns for protection from crime were the most likely to keep their guns loaded. The presence of children in the home was a modifying factor. However, a significant number of gun owners with children reported that their guns(s) were neither unloaded nor locked up. One of the most interesting finding of this analysis is that instruction in the proper handling of firearms was not associated with whether a gun was kept loaded when not in use.

This work was partially supported by the Harvard Injury Control Center, Boston, Mass, funded by the Centers for Disease Control, Atlanta, Ga.

We thank Eric Rimm, ScD, and Sara Solnick, ScM, for their assistance in the development of this report.

References

1. Zimring FE. Is gun control likely to reduce violent killings? *Chicago Law Rev.* 1968;35:721-737.
2. Federal Bureau of Investigation. *Uniform Crime Reports for the United States, 1985.* Washington, DC: US Dept of Justice; 1986.
3. Seiden RH. Suicide prevention: a public health/public policy approach. *Omega.* 1977;8:267-275.
4. Rosenberg ML, Mercy JA. Introduction. In: Rosenberg ML, Feneley MA, eds. *Violence in America: A Public Health Approach.* New York, NY: Oxford University Press; 1991:3-13.
5. *Many Deaths and Injuries Caused by Firearms Could Be Prevented.* Washington, DC: US General Accounting Office; 1991. Publication GAO/PEMD-91-9.
6. Rivara FP, Stapleton FB. Handguns and children: a dangerous mix. *J Dev Behav Pediatr.* 1982; 3:35-38.
7. Jagger J, Dietz PE. Death and injury by firearms: who cares? *JAMA.* 1986;255:3143-3144.
8. Cook PJ. *The Technology of Personal Violence: A Review of the Evidence Concerning the Importance of Gun Availability and Use in Violent Crime, Self Defense, and Suicide.* Washington, DC: National Academy Press. In press.
9. Wright JD, Rossi PH, Daly K. *Under the Gun: Weapons, Crime, and Violence in America.* Hawthorne, NY: Aldine Publishing Co; 1983.
10. Patterson PJ, Smith LR. Firearms in the home and child safety. *AJDC.* 1987;141:221-223.
11. Heins M, Kahn R, Bjordnal J. Gunshot wounds in children. *Am J Public Health.* 1974;64:326-330.
12. Wintemute GJ, Teret SP, Kraus JF, Wright MA, Gretchen B. When children shoot children: 88 unintentional deaths in California. *JAMA.* 1987; 257:3107-3109.
13. Keck NJ, Istre GR, Coury DL, Jordan F, Eaton AP. Characteristics of fatal gunshot wounds in the home in Oklahoma: 1982-1983. *AJDC.* 1988;142:623-626.
14. Ordog GJ, Wasserberger J, Schatz I, et al. Gunshot wounds in children under 10 years of age: a new epidemic. *AJDC.* 1988;142:618-622.
15. *Healthy People 2000: National Health Promotion and Disease Objectives.* Washington, DC: US Dept of Health and Human Services; 1990:236. Publication PHS 91-50212.
16. *Handgun Ownership in America.* Princeton, NJ: The Gallup Organization; 1991. Distributed by the *Los Angeles Times* Syndicate, May 29, 1991.
17. Zimring FE, Hawkins. *The Citizen's Guide to Gun Control.* New York, NY: MacMillan Publishers Ltd; 1983.
18. *Firearms Safety Depends on You.* Riverside, Conn: Sporting Arms & Ammunition Manufacturer's Association Inc; 1987.
19. Thornberry OT, Massey JT. Trends in United States telephone coverage across time and subgroups. In: Groves RM, Biemer PP, Lyberg LE, Massey JT, Nichols WL II, Waksberg J, eds. *Telephone Survey Methodology.* New York, NY: John Wiley & Sons Inc; 1988:25-49.
20. Kellermann AL, Rivara FP, Banton J, Reay D, Flinger CL. Validating survey responses to questions about gun ownership among owners of registered handguns. *Am J Epidemiol.* 1991;131:1080-1084.
21. Kellermann AL, Reay DT. Protection or peril? an analysis of firearm-related deaths in the home. *N Engl J Med.* 1986;314:1557-1560.
22. Barlow B, Niemirska M, Gandhi RP. Ten years' experience with pediatric gunshot wounds. *J Pediatr Surg.* 1982;17:927-932.
23. Rushforth NB, Hirsch CS, Ford FB, Adelson L. Accidental firearm fatalities in a metropolitan county (1958-1973). *JAMA.* 1975;100:499-505.
24. Brent DA, Perper JA, Goldstein CE, et al. Risk factors for adolescent suicide: a comparison of adolescent suicide victims with suicidal inpatients. *Arch Gen Psychiatry.* 1988;45:581-588.
25. Hemenway D, Weil DS. Phasers on stun: the case for less lethal weapons. *J Policy Analysis Manage.* 1990;9:94-98.
26. Wintemute GJ, Teret SP, Kraus JF. The epidemiology of firearm deaths among residents of California. *West J Med.* 1987;46:374-377.
27. Moore M, Trojanowicz RC, Kelling GC. *Crime and Policing: Perspectives on Policy.* Washington, DC: National Institute of Justice, US Dept of Justice; 1988. Publication GPO 1988-202-045:80044.
28. *Centers for Disease Control Home Surveillance Report 1970-1978.* Atlanta, Ga: Centers for Disease Control; 1983.
29. Hemenway D. Risk compensation. In: *Prices and Choices.* Cambridge, Mass: Ballinger Publishing Co; 1988:249-258.
30. Gastil R. Violence, crime and punishment. In: Wilson CR, Ferris W, eds. *Encyclopedia of Southern Culture.* Chapel Hill, NC: University of North Carolina Press; 1989:1469-1513.
31. *National Data Program for the Social Sciences: The NORG General Social Survey: Questions and Answers.* Chicago, Ill: University of Chicago; 1986.
32. *Time.* January 29, 1990:16.

Urban High School Youth and Handguns

A School-Based Survey

Charles M. Callahan, MD, MPH, Frederick P. Rivara, MD, MPH

Objective.—To determine the prevalence of handgun ownership among urban high school youth and investigate associations with socioeconomic status, ethnicity, and deviant behaviors.

Design.—Survey of half of the Seattle, Wash, public high schools, which enroll 50% of the school district's 11th-grade students (N=970).

Main Outcome Measures.—Self-reports of handgun ownership, perceived access to handguns, racial/ethnic identity, social status (Hollingshead's Two Factor Index of Social Position), and social deviance (Seattle Self-Report Instrument) were determined.

Results.—Thirty-four percent of the students reported easy access to handguns (47% of males, 22% of females) and 6.4% reported owning a handgun (11.4% of males, 1.5% of females). Reported firearm experiences indicated a high rate of handgun utilization: 33% of handgun owners had fired at someone, 9.7% of female students reported a firearm homicide or suicide in family members or close friends, and 6% of male students reported carrying a handgun to school sometime in the past. Handgun ownership was more common among students who reported deviant behaviors. Adjusting for age, gender, and racial/ethnic group and controlling for covariation among the problem behaviors, gang membership (odds ratio [OR], 8.8; 95% confidence interval [CI], 3.7 to 20.8), sentencing by a judge (OR, 4.6; 95% CI, 1.3 to 15.5), selling drugs (OR, 3.7; 95% CI, 1.8 to 7.8), suspension or expulsion from school (OR, 3.5; 95% CI, 1.7 to 7.0), and assault and battery (OR, 2.5; 95% CI, 1.1 to 5.9) were associated with handgun ownership. However, 22% of male handgun owners did not report any of the above behaviors.

Conclusion.—The availability of handguns to the urban high school students surveyed is pervasive, and it is not limited to high-risk groups.

(*JAMA*. 1992;267:3038-3042)

FIREARM injuries among American youth are a nationwide tragedy and an international embarrassment.[1] The frequency and lethality of firearm injuries have resulted in this method of dying now being among the leading causes of death for various groups of young people. In 1988, firearms accounted for 20% of all deaths among 15- to 24-year-olds. Over three fourths of adolescent homicides and slightly more than half of adolescent suicides are firearm related, with the majority the result of handguns.[2] It is estimated that for every firearm fatality, there are 2.4-fold more nonfatal firearm injuries,[3] often with serious morbidity.[4]

From the Department of Pediatrics, University of Washington, Seattle. Dr Callahan is now with Children's Hospital and Medical Center, Seattle.

Reprint requests to Harborview Injury Prevention and Research Center, 325 Ninth Ave, ZX-10, Seattle, WA 98104 (Dr Callahan).

Despite the frequent association of firearms, especially handguns, with serious adolescent injuries, little is known about which adolescents have access to handguns and who decides to acquire one. The purposes of the present article are to determine the self-reported extent of handgun access and ownership among a population of urban high school students; to discover the self-reported reasons for ownership; and to relate access and ownership to socioeconomic status, ethnicity, and deviant behavior.

METHODS

Sample Population

During a 6-week period in the winter of 1990-1991, we conducted a cross-sectional survey of 11th-grade students in the Seattle (Wash) Public School District. In the city of Seattle, 73% (2244/3088) of all 11th-grade students attend public schools and the remainder attend private schools.[5] The dropout rate for 11th graders attending public schools during the 1988-1989 school year was 15.3%.[6]

All 10 high schools were approached, and the decision for school participation was made by individual principals. Five of the 10 principals agreed to participate in the study.

This study was approved by the Human Subjects Review Committee of the University of Washington and the Research Office of the Seattle Public School District.

Survey

Data were collected by means of an anonymous questionnaire administered by one person (C.M.C.) during a required history course in each school. Following written notification, passive consent by the parents was presumed unless telephone contact was made with the research team or school.

The 76-item questionnaire measured self-reported deviant behavior, socioeconomic status (SES), drug/alcohol use, educational aspirations, driving behavior, group memberships, social activities, the availability and use of firearms, and injuries to self and family members.

Deviant behaviors were ascertained using 34 of the original 69 questions from the Seattle Self-Report Instrument. This instrument, developed in 1975 and validated in 14 000 youth, related self-reported socially deviant behaviors with police contacts.[7] In our study, students were asked to check any of the deviant acts they had done in the past 3 years.

Social status was measured with Hollingshead's Two Factor Index of Social Position[8] based on student report of the occupation and highest grade of education of household wage earners. The wage earner in the home with the highest occupational and educational scores was coded. Weighted partial scores of the occupational and educational levels of the wage earner were combined to generate a social class from I (highest) to V (lowest).

The principal outcome variable was handgun ownership, which included personal ownership and shared ownership with friends. Perceived access to hand-

Table 1.—Demographic Characteristics of the Study Population

	Respondents*	
	No.	%
Gender	938	
M		49
F		51
Racial/ethnic group	967	
White		47
Asian/Pacific Islander		21
Chinese		(5)
Southeast Asian		(8)
Filipino		(5)
Japanese		(1)
Pacific Islander		(3)
African American		17
Others		15
Hispanic		(2)
Native American/Alaskan Native		(1)
Multiracial/ethnic		(4)
Other		(8)
Social class†	702	
I		29
II		30
III		24
IV		14
V		3

*Number with missing data=970−No.
†Social class by Hollingshead's score.[8]

Table 2.—Demographic Characteristics of the Schools

	Surveyed	Not Surveyed
No. of schools	5	5
Enrollment	1119	1125
Racial/ethnic group, %		
African American	20	18
Asian/Pacific Islander	24	38
White	49	37
Other	7	7
Grade point average	2.6	2.7
Graduation rate, %	89	88
Suspension/expulsion rate, %	13	16
Weapon confiscations*		
Guns	0.1	0.5
Knives	1.7	3.6
All†	4.3	7.7

*Weapons confiscated per 100 students, school year 1990/1991.
†Guns, knives, stars, ammunition, etc.

guns was also examined. Handgun access was coded as easy if the student selected "I already have one" or "I could get one in a few days"; other responses were coded as difficult. Internal consistency of responses to handgun questions with similar content was assessed.

Data Analysis

Bivariate analyses were conducted using the Yates corrected χ^2 statistic or two-tailed Fisher's Exact Test. The prevalence ratio (PR) (eg, prevalence of easy access in students reporting a behavior divided by the prevalence of easy access in students denying that behavior) was one effect measure. Epi-Info software[9] generated PRs with Taylor series 95% confidence intervals (CIs).[10] The relative rarity of handgun ownership permitted the use of the odds ratio to estimate the relative risk of handgun ownership among different groups of students.[11] The odds ratio with Cornfield's 95% CIs represents the ratio of the odds of handgun ownership in those with a selected behavior to the odds of ownership in those without the behavior. Logistic regression analysis (SPSS-PC 4.01, SPSS Inc, Chicago, Ill) generated adjusted odds ratios, controlling for age, gender, racial/ethnic group, and other problem behaviors.

RESULTS

Demographic Characteristics

Students.—Of the 1119 students enrolled in the five participating schools, 970 (87%) were surveyed. During the survey, 132 students (12%) were absent, one parent actively withheld permission, and 16 students refused to participate.

Almost half of the sample was male (Table 1). The mean age of the students was 16.3 (±0.7) years. Forty-seven percent of the participants described themselves as white and 17% as African American. For purposes of analysis, Asians and Pacific Islanders were combined (21%) and Hispanics, Native Americans/Alaskan Natives, multiracial/ethnic students, and others were combined. Because 17% of the students were unwilling or unable to report the occupation and 15% the education level of the primary wage earner in their home, data on SES were missing for 27%. Data on SES were more likely to be missing for minority racial/ethnic groups (SES missing values were as follows: whites, 14%; African Americans, 33%; Asians/Pacific Islanders, 48.5%; and others, 30%) and in students receiving subsidized school lunches (missing data for 60% [72/119] of students with subsidized lunch vs 23% [190/821] of students with self-pay lunch).

Internal consistency of responses to questions relating to firearm use was high. All 28 students who reported shooting at someone also reported having easy access to handguns, and the eight students who reported firing at someone in their home also reported elsewhere in the questionnaire as having shot at someone.

Study Schools.—In comparing the five schools surveyed with the schools that did not participate (Table 2), more whites and fewer Asians/Pacific Islanders were enrolled in the surveyed schools. The mean grade point averages and the graduation rates for the two groups of schools were similar. The suspension and expulsion rate was 3% lower in the surveyed schools. The number of weapons (guns, knives, and/or any type) confiscated during the preceding school year was higher in the nonparticipating schools.

Access to Handguns

Overall, 34% of the students perceived handguns to be easily accessible (Table 3). Male students were twice as likely as female students to report easy access to handguns. Easy access to handguns was almost twice as common for African Americans as for Asians/Pacific Islanders, with whites falling between these two groups. The highest prevalence of easy access was reported by African-American male students (59%). Easy access to handguns was most common in the lowest social class (class V) and least common in the highest social class (class I). Handguns were perceived to be easily accessible by more than 50% of male youths in all social classes except the highest class, in which 36% reported easy access.

When students who perceived handguns to be easily accessible (n=321) were asked where they would acquire a handgun, 31% said they would obtain it from a friend, 18% would buy one on the street, 13% already owned one, 8% specified a gun shop, and 7% would obtain it from home. Overall, only 22% doubted they would ever need one.

Handgun Ownership

Handgun ownership was reported by 6.4% of students (Table 3). Of the 60 handgun owners, 51 (85%) reported personal ownership and nine (15%) had shared ownership with friends. Male students were eight times as likely to report ownership as female students. Statistically similar rates of handgun ownership were reported by African Americans and Asians/Pacific Islanders when compared with whites.

The relationship between social class and handgun ownership was similar to that for access. Handgun ownership was more common in the lowest social class (20%) and least common in the highest social class (3.1%). However, social class could not be determined for 28% (17/60) of the handgun owners, thus limiting further comparisons. Students who reported hearing gunfire in their neighborhoods

Table 3.—Factors Associated With Handgun Access and Ownership

	Easy Access		Ownership	
	No. of Respondents	%	No. of Respondents	%
No.	954	34	937	6.4
Gender				
M	457	47*	446	11.4*
F†	467	22	462	1.5
Racial/ethnic group				
African American	159	49*	154	11.0
Asian/Pacific Islander	194	25‡	196	4.1
White†	454	34	444	6.3
Other	144	30	140	5.0
Social class				
I† (highest)	201	24	195	3.1
II	209	40§	208	8.2‡
III	165	43*	163	6.7
IV	99	41§	97	5.2
V (lowest)	21	57§	20	20.0§
Neighborhood gunfire				
Never†	837	32	824	5.2
Sometimes	80	44‡	78	11.5‡
Often	37	65*	34	23.5*
Expect to attend college				
No	83	43	83	15.6§
Yes†	867	33	850	5.5

*$P<.001$.
†Reference group for pair-wise comparisons.
‡$P<.05$.
§$P<.01$.

often (at least one or two times per week) reported a fourfold higher rate of handgun ownership compared with students from neighborhoods where gunfire was never heard.

The prevalence of handgun ownership did not vary significantly by participation in school sports, church membership, or employment. Students who did not expect to attend college reported a threefold greater prevalence of handgun ownership than students expecting to attend college.

For the 31 students who *owned* a handgun only (29 either shared the handgun or owned long guns in addition to handguns), the median age of acquiring a handgun was 15.0 years (range, 11 to 16 years). The handgun was received as a gift for 29%, all but one of which were from parents. Twenty-two percent acquired their handgun from a friend; 19% bought it from someone on the street and 6% from a gun store. Seven (22%) of the 31 students chose "other" as a source category.

Among the handgun owners, only 27% (16/60) selected hunting or target shooting as the primary reason for owning *any firearm*.

Firearm Experiences

Almost half (46%) of handgun owners, 4% of all 11th-grade students, and 6.6% of male students had carried a handgun to school at some time. Three percent of students, 5% of male students, 9% of students with easy access to handguns, and 33% of handgun owners indicated they had shot at another person.

Serious firearm injuries (including homicide or suicide and excluding war-related injuries) to family members or close friends were reported by 9.7% (46/475) of all female students and 5.0% (23/463) of all male students (PR, 1.9%; 95% CI, 1.2% to 3.2%). More than one quarter (20/74) of African-American female students reported serious firearm injuries to family members or close friends.

Problem Behaviors and Handgun Availability

The availability of handguns, in terms of either perceived easy access or actual ownership, was more common in students who reported problem behaviors (Table 4).

The strongest associations with handgun access were gang membership (PR, 2.8; 95% CI, 2.4 to 3.2), selling drugs (PR, 2.7; 95% CI, 2.3 to 3.2), interpersonal violence (ie, robbery [PR, 2.6; 95% CI, 2.2 to 3.2], assault and battery [PR, 2.7; 95% CI, 2.3 to 3.1], striking a teacher [PR, 2.4; 95% CI, 1.8 to 3.1]), conviction for crimes (PR, 2.5; 95% CI, 2.0 to 3.1), and either suspension or expulsion from school (PR, 2.1; 95% CI, 1.8 to 2.5).

The association between handgun ownership and problem behaviors is presented in Table 5. The crude odds ratios for owning a handgun are significant for all behaviors listed. The strongest associations are seen with students reporting the more deviant behaviors (ie, gang membership, sentencing by a judge, selling drugs, assault and battery) and being suspended or expelled from school. Controlling for age, gender, and racial/ethnic group with logistic regression and a forward stepwise method for entering the problem behaviors, the adjusted odds ratios reflect the independent effect contributed by the individual behavior, simultaneously adjusting for the other four behaviors. Problem driving behaviors, chemical abuse, and other school-related behaviors did not increase the odds of gun ownership once gang membership, court sentencing, selling drugs, assault, and school suspensions or expulsions were entered into the equation. Although gang members of the same age, gender, and race were 8.8-fold more likely to own a handgun than non–gang members, it is important to realize that only 37% of handgun owners were gang members. Further, 22% (13/60) of the handgun owners did not report any of the five problem behaviors that were independently associated with handgun ownership.

For nearly all problem behaviors, the crude odds ratios were considerably higher for female compared with male students, indicating that few female students without deviant behaviors owned handguns. For example, the crude odds ratios for female handgun owners who reported selling drugs, gang membership, assault and battery, or being sentenced by a judge were 61, 36, 22, and 13, respectively (vs crude odds ratios for males of 7.3, 17.7, 9.1, and 11.9, respectively). Although the rarity of female handgun ownership prevents more precise estimation of the association in this sample, all seven female handgun owners reported at least two of the deviant behaviors, in contrast to 22% of male handgun owners who reported no deviant behaviors.

COMMENT

Data from this report indicated that many urban high school students have easy access to handguns and that handgun ownership is not uncommon. The firearm experiences of these students were not limited to mere perceptions of ready access. The reported frequency of carrying weapons, discharging firearms, and firearm injuries among family members or close friends suggests that handguns are not only accessible but frequently used.

Ecological studies by Wintemute and others[12-15] have suggested an association of the high rates of homicide, suicide, and unintentional deaths from firearms with high local and regional rates of gun ownership. The availability of handguns has been shown to increase the risk of urban

Table 4.—Problem Behaviors Associated With Handgun Access and Ownership

Problem Behavior	Easy Access		Ownership	
	No. of Respondents	%	No. of Respondents	%
Deviant behavior				
Gang member				
Yes	47	87	44	52
No	907	31	893	4
Sentenced by judge				
Yes	23	83	22	50
No	931	33	915	5
Assault and battery				
Yes	60	83	58	38
No	894	31	879	4
Robbery				
Yes	29	86	29	41
No	925	32	908	5
Sold drugs				
Yes	84	81	83	32
No	870	30	854	4
School				
Striking teacher				
Yes	19	79	19	37
No	935	33	918	6
Suspensions				
Yes	137	62	133	23
No	817	29	804	4
"High" in school				
Yes	189	61	184	12
No	765	27	753	5
Driving				
Motor vehicle violations				
>2	42	64	42	17
1	81	48	80	12
None	819	31	801	5
Driving "high"				
Yes	134	55	130	12
No	820	31	807	5
Chemical abuse				
Beer				
≥Monthly	263	53	256	10
≤Few times	691	27	681	5
Cocaine				
Ever	21	71	20	20
Never	933	33	917	6
Marijuana				
≥Monthly	97	62	96	17
<Few times	857	31	841	5

homicide in all age groups[16] and to be a significant risk factor for urban suicide in the 15- to 24-year-old age group.[17]

Previous publications about adolescent problem behaviors have either ignored or minimally considered handgun availability.[18-21] A recent study of adolescents and firearms by Sadowski et al[22] focused on nonurban youth, a population that differs in the types of firearms acquired and in which recreational use of long guns predominates. Sadowski et al reported that 4.9% of rural youth owned a handgun. Male students had a rate of handgun ownership ninefold greater than female students, and school dropouts were three times more likely to own a handgun. Neither race nor SES was associated with handgun ownership. Sadowski et al reported associations of handgun ownership with hunting and the possession of long guns. In our study, this association was less apparent.

We explored the association of handgun ownership with many problem behaviors. Chance associations are possible with the number of comparisons made, but the magnitude of the odds ratios and the consistency of the associations of handgun ownership with the correlated problem behaviors make chance an unlikely explanation for the associations found.

Although direct validation and reliability of responses about behaviors or attitudes were not possible due to the anonymous nature of the survey, the findings in our study are comparable with other reports. The higher rate of African-American firearm injuries among close friends or family members found in our survey is congruent with national race-specific mortality data. A recent report from the Centers for Disease Control and its 1990 nationwide school-based Youth Risk Behavior Survey noted that 20% of all students in grades 9 through 12 reported carrying a weapon to school at least once in the month preceding the survey.[23] Of those carrying weapons, 20.8% reported carrying a firearm. They concluded that approximately one student in 20 had carried a firearm, usually a handgun, to school in the month prior to the survey.

The 1987 National Adolescent Student Health Survey,[24] a school-based survey that included 5560 10th graders, reported that 41% of male and 24% of female 10th graders could obtain a handgun. In the National Adolescent Student Health Survey, 2.9% of 10th-grade male students had carried a handgun to school during the past year compared with our finding that 6.6% of 11th-grade male students had carried a handgun to high school at least once.

Although death during adolescence is uncommon, violent causes (homicide and suicide) are among the most common reasons for death. By studying an urban population and focusing on handguns, our intention was to further the understanding of this more common mechanism of injury among the youth most at risk.[25-27]

While handgun ownership was strongly associated with problem behaviors in the Seattle public schools surveyed, handguns were not restricted to any one social class or racial/ethnic group or restricted to students who reported deviant behaviors. Students have handguns for various reasons and obtain them from numerous sources.

Both access to handguns and handgun ownership are related to problem behaviors, and the strongest associations are seen with the more deviant behaviors. Despite these associations, our data and the scope of adolescent firearm injuries in the United States suggest that the availability of handguns to urban youth is not restricted to the more deviant individuals but extends into the mainstream.

The major limitation of this study is the lack of a random sample that would permit us to generalize our findings to the total population of Seattle public school 11th-grade students. However, it seems reasonable to conclude that the effect measures from this study are likely to be underestimates for the Seattle School District, the city of Seattle, and urban centers in general. In light of the higher disciplinary rates and rate of weapons confiscation in the nonparticipating schools, exclusion of those five schools may have lowered the true prevalence of handgun ownership and the associations with deviant behaviors. Students who

Table 5.—Handgun Ownership and Problem Behaviors: Crude and Adjusted Odds Ratios (ORs)*

Problem Behavior	Crude OR (95% CI)	Adjusted OR (95% CI)†
Deviant behavior		
Gang member	25.3 (12.2-52.7)	8.8 (3.7-20.8)
Sentenced by judge	17.7 (6.7-46.5)	4.6 (1.3-15.5)
Assault and battery	13.5 (6.9-26.3)	2.5 (1.1-5.9)
Robbery	12.6 (5.3-29.9)	NS
Sold drugs	12.0 (6.5-22.2)	3.7 (1.8-7.8)
School		
Striking teacher	9.5 (3.2-27.4)	NS
Suspensions	7.5 (4.2-13.4)	3.5 (1.7-7.0)
"High" in school	2.8 (1.5-4.9)	NS
Driving		
Motor vehicle violations		
>2	3.5 (1.2-8.7)	NS
1	2.5 (1.1-5.5)	NS
Driving "high"	2.4 (1.3-4.6)	NS
Chemical abuse		
Cocaine	3.8 (0.9-12.4)	NS
Marijuana	3.6 (1.9-7.0)	NS
Beer	2.3 (1.3-4.1)	NS

*CI indicates confidence interval; and NS, not significant after adjustment.
†Adjusted for age, racial/ethnic group, gender, and other deviant behaviors.

are found carrying a firearm in Seattle schools are uniformly expelled; other high-risk individuals (ie, frequently absent students, school dropouts, and incarcerated youth) were not surveyed. Moreover, victims of firearm injuries, the seriously disabled or fatally injured, are excluded from such a school-based survey. Data about handguns in private schools are not available.

The prevalence of handguns among high school students in Seattle is likely to be lower than in other urban centers. During 1986 through 1988, Seattle had lower rates of adolescent male firearm homicide for both whites (3.8/100 000) and African Americans (48.5/100 000) when compared with the national average for urban areas (9.0 and 82.3/100 000, respectively) (Lois Fingerhut, MA, National Center for Health Statistics, oral communication, May 15, 1991). Firearm suicide rates specific to urban centers are not available, but the firearm suicide rate among 15- to 24-year-olds in King County (which includes Seattle) (7.38/100 000) is slightly lower than the national average (8.0/100 000).[2]

Previous work that compared adolescents' self-report of deviant behaviors with actual police and court records indicated high correlations, except among the more deviant minority male youth, who underreported their criminal behavior.[7] Kellerman et al[28] demonstrated the validity of self-reported handgun ownership among recent adult purchasers of handguns in Seattle and Memphis (Tenn). The validity of self-reported handgun ownership in adolescents is unknown.

CONCLUSION

Despite federal regulations restricting the sale of handguns to adolescents, the high school students surveyed reported that handguns are accessible and acquisition is neither difficult nor uncommon. In view of the high rate of firearm homicide and suicide among adolescents, this access to handguns must be addressed.[29,30] Similar to the adult segment of society, certain adolescents will feel a need or desire to own a handgun and there appear to be few barriers to ownership. Parents, school administrators, teachers, and health care providers should view handgun availability as a major threat to the health of high school age youth.

This study was funded by a National Institutes of Health National Research Service Award (5T32 PE1002) and by a grant from the Centers for Disease Control (R49/CCR 002570).

We are indebted to the students, history teachers, and principals of the Seattle School District. We are grateful to Thomas Koepsell, MD, MPH, and David Klein for helpful editorial review and frequent discussions. We wish to recognize the patience and secretarial expertise of Marie Spaugy, and we wish to thank Arthur Kellermann, MD, MPH, Katherine Christoffel, MD, MPH, and Garen Wintemute, MD, MPH, for review and critique of earlier versions of the manuscript.

References

1. Fingerhut LA, Kleinman JC. International and interstate comparisons of homicide among young males. *JAMA.* 1990;263:3290-3295.

2. Fingerhut LA, Kleinman JC, Godfrey MS, Rosenberg H. Firearm mortality among children, youth and young adults 1-34 years of age, trends and current status: United States, 1979-88. *Monthly Vital Stat Rep.* 1991;39(11):1-15.

3. Lee RK, Waxweiler RJ, Dobbins JG, Paschetag T. Incidence rates of firearm injuries in Galveston, Texas, 1979-1981. *Am J Epidemiol.* 1991;134:511-521.

4. Graham PM, Weingarden SI. Victims of gun shootings: a retrospective study of 36 spinal cord injured adolescents. *J Adolesc Health Care.* 1989;10:534-536.

5. Krohn B. *Washington Education Directory 1990-1991.* Seattle, Wash: Barbara Krohn & Associates; 1990.

6. Anderson C, Vaughan R, Haynes D. *Data Profile District Summary 1989-1990.* Seattle, Wash: Seattle Public Schools; 1989.

7. Hindelang MJ, Hirshehi T, Weis JG. *Measuring Delinquency.* Beverly Hills, Calif: Sage Publications; 1981:123.

8. Hollingshead AB, Redlich F. *Social Class and Mental Illness.* New York, NY: John Wiley & Sons Inc; 1958:387-397.

9. Dean AD, Dean JA, Burton AH, Dicker RC. *Epi-Info Version 5.* Stone Mountain, Ga: USD Inc; 1990.

10. Kleinbaum DG, Kupper LL, Morgenstern H. *Epidemiologic Research: Principles and Quantitative Methods.* Belmont, Calif: Wadsworth Publishing Co; 1982:296-300.

11. Hulley SB, Cummings SR. *Designing Clinical Research.* Baltimore, Md: Williams & Wilkins; 1988: 206.

12. Wintemute GJ. Firearms as a cause of death in the United States, 1920-1982. *J Trauma.* 1987;27: 532-536.

13. Markush RE, Bartolucci AA. Firearms and suicide in the United States. *Am J Public Health.* 1984; 74:123-127.

14. Boyd JH, Moscicki EK. Firearms and youth suicide. *Am J Public Health.* 1986;76:1240-1242.

15. Ford AB, Rushforth NB, Rushforth N, Hirsch CS, Adelson L. Violent death in a metropolitan county, II: changing patterns in suicides (1959-1974). *Am J Public Health.* 1979;69:459-464.

16. Sloan JH, Kellerman AL, Reay AT, et al. Handgun regulations, crime, assaults and homicide: a tale of two cities. *N Engl J Med.* 1988;319:1256-1262.

17. Sloan JH, Rivara FP, Reay AT, Ferris JA, Kellerman AL. Firearm regulations and rates of suicide: a comparison of two metropolitan areas. *N Engl J Med.* 1990;322:369-373.

18. Dryfoos JG. *Adolescents at Risk: Prevalence and Prevention.* New York, NY: Oxford University Press Inc; 1990.

19. Jessor R, Chase JA, Donovan JE. Psychosocial correlates of marijuana use and problem drinking in a national sample of adolescents. *Am J Public Health.* 1980;70:604-613.

20. Irwin CE, Millstein SG. Biopsychosocial correlates of risk-taking behaviors during adolescence. *J Adolesc Health Care.* 1986;7:825-965.

21. Tonking R. Adolescent risk-taking behavior. *J Adolesc Health Care.* 1987;8:213-220.

22. Sadowski LS, Cairns RB, Earp JA. Firearm ownership among non-urban adolescents. *AJDC.* 1989;143:1410-1413.

23. Centers for Disease Control. Weapon-carrying among high-school students—United States, 1990. *MMWR.* 1991;40:681-684.

24. American School Health Association, et al. *The National Adolescent Student Health Survey.* Oakland, Calif: Third Party Publishing Co; 1989.

25. Gausche M, Seidel J, Henderson DP, et al. Violent death in the pediatric age group: rural and urban differences. *Pediatr Emerg Care.* 1989;5:64-67.

26. Wintemute GJ, Teret SP, Kraus JF, Wright MW. The choice of weapons in firearm suicides. *Am J Public Health.* 1988;78:824-826.

27. Christoffel KK, Christoffel T. Handguns as a pediatric problem. *Pediatr Emerg Care.* 1986;2:75-81.

28. Kellerman AL, Rivara FP, Banton J, Reay D, Fligner CL. Validating survey responses to questions about gun ownership among owners of registered handguns. *Am J Epidemiol.* 1990;131:1080-1084.

29. Christoffel KK. Toward reducing pediatric injuries from firearms: charting a legislative and regulatory course. *Pediatrics.* 1991;88:294-305.

30. Council on Scientific Affairs, American Medical Association. Firearm injuries and deaths: a critical public health issue. *Public Health Rep.* 1989;104: 111-119.

Weapon Involvement and Injury Outcomes in Family and Intimate Assaults

Linda E. Saltzman, PhD; James A. Mercy, PhD; Patrick W. O'Carroll, MD, MPH; Mark L. Rosenberg, MD, MPP; Philip H. Rhodes, MS

Objective.—To compare the risk of death and the risk of nonfatal injury during firearm-associated family and intimate assaults (FIAs) with the risks during non–firearm-associated FIAs.

Design.—Records review of police incident reports of FIAs that occurred in 1984. Victim outcomes (death, nonfatal injury, no injury) and weapon involvement were examined for incidents involving only one perpetrator.

Setting.—City of Atlanta, Ga, within Fulton County.

Participants.—Stratified sample (n=142) of victims of nonfatal FIAs, drawn from seven nonfatal crime categories, plus all fatal victims (n=23) of FIAs.

Main Outcome Measures.—Risk of death (vs nonfatal injury or no injury) during FIAs involving firearms, relative to other types of weapons; risk of nonfatal injury (vs all other outcomes, including death) during FIAs involving firearms, relative to other types of weapons.

Results.—Firearm-associated FIAs were 3.0 times (95% confidence interval, 0.9 to 10.0) more likely to result in death than FIAs involving knives or other cutting instruments and 23.4 times (95% confidence interval, 7.0 to 78.6) more likely to result in death than FIAs involving other weapons or bodily force. Overall, firearm-associated FIAs were 12.0 times (95% confidence interval, 4.6 to 31.5) more likely to result in death than non–firearm-associated FIAs.

Conclusions.—Strategies for limiting the number of deaths and injuries resulting from FIAs include reducing the access of potential FIA assailants to firearms, modifying firearm lethality through redesign, and establishing programs for primary prevention of violence among intimates.

(*JAMA*. 1992;267:3043-3047)

THE PUBLIC health approach to violence prevention incorporates strategies not only for reducing the occurrence of violent events, but also for reducing the likelihood of death or nonfatal injury when such events do occur.[1] A critical issue in the public debate over appropriate policies for preventing injuries in violent situations is the extent to which the involvement of particular weapon types alters the likelihood of injurious outcomes. Research on assault[2] has found that the involvement of firearms increases the likelihood that assault incidents will result in homicide. Research on robbery suggests, however, that although a gun's involvement in a robbery may increase the risk of homicide,[3] victims of robberies committed with guns are *less* likely to sustain nonfatal injuries than are victims of robberies in which guns are not involved.[4,5] No study to date has examined how the involvement of firearms or other weapons affects the risk of death or nonfatal injury during violence among intimates. Many investigators believe that family and intimate assaults (FIAs) are often the impulsive results of violent arguments rather than being premeditated acts. For such FIAs, access to lethal weapons may be an important determinant of the incident's outcome. We analyzed data from a study of FIAs in a large, urban community[6] to estimate (1) the probability of death resulting from FIAs, given differences in the types of weapons involved in the incidents, and (2) the probability of nonfatal injury resulting from FIAs, given differences in weapon involvement.

METHODS

Incident reports from the Bureau of Police Services for the city of Atlanta, Ga, for 1984 were reviewed to identify fatal and nonfatal FIAs, as has been described in greater detail elsewhere.[6,7] Cases had to meet all of the following criteria: (1) the incident was classified as a homicide or as a nonfatal incident involving one or more of the following: physical contact between parties, use of a weapon, threat with a weapon, or explicit verbal threat of bodily harm; (2) the victim's residence and the site of the incident were within the city of Atlanta and within Fulton County; (3) the incident involved only one perpetrator; or (4) the victim and perpetrator were emotionally intimate when the incident

From the Division of Injury Control, National Center for Environmental Health and Injury Control, Centers for Disease Control, Atlanta, Ga.

Presented at the American Public Health Association meeting, Atlanta, Ga, on November 12, 1991.

Reprint requests to Centers for Disease Control, 1600 Clifton Rd, Mailstop F-36, Atlanta, GA 30333 (Dr Saltzman).

occurred or had been at some earlier time. Emotionally intimate relationships included, for example, marriage, boyfriend-girlfriend relationships, terminated nonspousal and spousal partnerships, and other relationships among family members and relatives.

All homicides that occurred during the study period and that met the above criteria (n=23) were included. These homicides represented nearly one fifth of all homicides that occurred in Atlanta during the study period. Nonfatal FIAs (n=142) were drawn from a stratified sample of incidents from seven nonfatal crime categories (rape, robbery, assault, disorderly conduct, family and children offenses, sex offenses, and other).

Outcomes for victims were coded as death, nonfatal injury, or no injury. Weapons were considered "involved" whether the perpetrator actually used them or only brandished them. Weapon involvement was coded "firearm," "knife or other cutting instrument," or "bodily force or noncutting/nonfirearm weapon." "Bodily force or noncutting/nonfirearm weapon" included involvement of objects other than firearms or knives (eg, a blunt object or rock) or use of bodily force in the absence of other weapons. (Bodily force alone was involved in 4% [n=1] of fatal incidents and 50% [n=71] of nonfatal incidents.) Three nonfatal incidents (2%) in which perpetrators made verbal threats of bodily harm but used no weapons are also included in this category.

When incidents involved weapons in combination with bodily force (17% [n=4] of fatal incidents and 13% [n=19] of nonfatal incidents), we coded for whichever weapons were involved, since bodily force was potentially present during all incidents. For three nonfatal incidents that involved more than one weapon plus bodily force, we coded only for the most lethal weapon involved (two firearms, one knife or other cutting instrument).

We used the weapon and injury outcome data to examine two specific questions: (1) What is the risk of death (vs nonfatal injury or no injury) during FIAs involving firearms relative to other types of weapons? (2) What is the risk of nonfatal injury (vs all other outcomes, including death) during FIAs involving firearms relative to other types of weapons?

To determine the risk of nonfatal injury or of death, all nonfatal incidents in a given crime category were weighted to reflect the estimated incidence for that crime category. The weights for nonfatal victims varied from about 20 to 40; all homicides were weighted 1. Estimated variances for the probability of death also took the weights into account.

Table 1.—Number of Deaths and Estimated Number of Nonfatal Outcomes,* by Weapon Type, Family and Intimate Assault, Atlanta, Ga, 1984

Weapon Type	Outcome, % (No.)			
	Death	Nonfatal Injury	No Injury	Total
Firearm	3.9 (14)	45.2 (163)	50.9 (183)	**100 (360)**
Knife or other cutting instrument	1.3 (5)	62.7 (244)	36.0 (140)	**100 (389)**
Bodily force or noncutting/nonfirearm weapon	0.2 (4)	69.3 (1667)	30.5 (735)	**100 (2406)**

*The numbers of deaths for each weapon type are actual counts. The numbers of incidents with nonfatal injuries and the numbers of incidents with no injuries are estimates.

We then estimated the probabilities of death or of nonfatal injury given the involvement of different weapon types.[8] For example, for incidents involving firearms:

$$p\,(\text{nonfatal injury, firearm incidents}) = \frac{\sum_{i=1}^{n} w_i d_i}{\sum_{i=1}^{n} w_i}$$

where d_i=1 if person i suffered a nonfatal injury, d_i=0 if person i did not suffer a nonfatal injury (ie, death or no injury), and w_i = weight for person i.

Confidence intervals for the probabilities were computed first on a transformed scale, in this case the logit scale [$\log(p/1-p)$], then transformed back to the original scale. This method provides more accurate confidence intervals than intervals computed on the original scale, especially when the estimated probability is small as was the case here for the probability of death.

When comparing two weapon categories, we estimated the relative risks by taking the ratio of the two estimated probabilities. We computed the confidence intervals for the relative risks on the log scale, that is, log [p(firearm)/p (knife or other cutting instrument)] and then transformed the result back to the ratio scale.

The estimated variance of the log relative risk for the two estimated probabilities p_1 and p_2 was obtained using the delta method or Taylor series[9] with the following formula:

$$\text{Var}\left(\log\frac{\hat{p}_1}{\hat{p}_2}\right) = \frac{1}{\hat{p}_1}^2\text{Var}(\hat{p}_1) + \frac{1}{\hat{p}_2}^2\text{Var}(\hat{p}_2)$$

RESULTS

Weapon-specific victim outcomes are presented in Table 1. Less than 1% of all FIAs resulted in death. The percentage with fatal outcomes was greatest when firearms were involved. Death was least likely when neither firearms nor knives were involved. By contrast, nearly half the incidents involving firearms resulted in nonfatal injury, whereas nearly two thirds of the FIAs involving knives or other cutting instruments and more than two thirds of those involving other weapons or bodily force resulted in nonfatal injuries. National Crime Survey data analysis[10,11] indicates that armed offenders do not always use their weapons to injure their victims. For example, an offender with a firearm may push, hit, or kick the victim. However, in all but two incidents in this study, the injuries sustained were those expected from the types of weapons involved (eg, a gunshot wound when a firearm was involved). The two exceptions were a nonfatal incident involving a knife in which the victim was injured but suffered no cuts and another nonfatal incident in which the victim suffered cuts although a firearm was involved.

Table 2 shows risk of death (vs nonfatal injury or no injury) and risk of nonfatal injury (vs all other outcomes including death) expressed per 1000 weapon-specific incidents, with associated 95% confidence intervals. The FIAs that involve firearms have the highest risk of death (39.0 per 1000 incidents), whereas FIAs involving bodily force or noncutting/nonfirearm weapons have the lowest risk (1.7 per 1000 incidents). However, firearm-associated FIAs have the lowest risk of nonfatal injury (452.3 per 1000 incidents), whereas FIAs involving bodily force or noncutting/nonfirearm weapons have the highest risk (692.9 per 1000 incidents).

Table 3 shows the risk of death for FIAs involving firearms, relative to FIAs involving other types of weapons. The FIAs that involve firearms are three times more likely to result in death than FIAs involving knives or other cutting instruments, and they are 23 times more likely to result in death than FIAs involving bodily force or noncutting/nonfirearm weapons. Overall, FIAs involving firearms are 12 times more likely to result in death than all nonfirearm FIAs. The confidence interval for the estimated relative risk comparing firearm-associated FIAs with FIAs that involve knives

Table 2.—Risk of Death or Nonfatal Injury by Weapon Type, Family and Intimate Assault, Atlanta, Ga, 1984

Weapon Type	Risk per 1000 Weapon-Specific Incidents (95% Confidence Interval)	
	Death	Nonfatal Injury
Firearm	39.0 (19.0-76.0)	452.3 (247.3-675.1)
Knife or other cutting instrument	12.8 (5.0-34.0)	626.9 (402.4-807.8)
Bodily force or noncutting/nonfirearm weapon	1.7 (0.6-4.5)	692.9 (596.2-776.4)
Total nonfirearm weapons	3.2 (1.6-6.4)	683.8 (594.8-761.4)

Table 3.—Risk of Death or Nonfatal Injury During Firearm-Associated FIAs, Relative to Non–Firearm-Associated FIAs, Atlanta, Ga, 1984*

Weapon Types Compared	Relative Risk (95% Confidence Interval)	
	Death	Nonfatal Injury
Firearms vs knives or other cutting instruments	3.0 (0.9-10.0)	0.7 (0.4-1.3)
Firearms vs bodily force or noncutting/nonfirearm weapons	23.4 (7.0-78.6)	0.7 (0.4-1.1)
Firearms vs all nonfirearms	12.0 (4.6-31.5)	0.7 (0.4-1.1)

*FIA indicates family and intimate assault.

or other cutting instruments includes 1; the confidence intervals for the other relative risks do not.

The relative risk of nonfatal injury for firearm-associated FIAs relative to non–firearm-associated FIAs are also shown in Table 3. Regardless of the weapon category with which they are compared, firearm-associated FIAs have a lower risk of nonfatal injury (relative risk = 0.7). For each relative risk the confidence interval includes 1.

COMMENT

Weapon-Specific Differences in the Risk of Fatal FIAs

We found clear evidence that firearm-associated FIAs are much more likely to result in death than non–firearm-associated FIAs. This finding is consistent with results from studies of other types of violence: case fatality rates for assaults, robberies, and other violent altercations are much higher when the assailants use firearms than when such incidents involve cutting instruments, blunt objects, or body parts.[2,12] Our analysis of National Crime Survey data[13] and vital statistics mortality data[14] also confirms that case fatality rates are higher when firearms are involved.

Two interpretations have been advanced to explain this weapon-specific difference in the risk of death during other types of violent altercations, and these interpretations may be applied to our consideration of FIAs. First, it has been suggested that violent altercations involving firearms will result in death more frequently than altercations without firearms simply because, all other things being equal, firearms are more deadly than other weapons.[2,12] Inherent in this interpretation is the assumption that most people who kill their family members or intimates with a firearm would be unable or unwilling to exert the greater physical or psychological effort required to kill with another, typically available weapon. The implication of this first interpretation is that limiting immediate access to firearms or redesigning firearms so that they are less lethal or less easily loaded and fired might have a substantial impact on reducing mortality from such incidents.

The second interpretation is that the higher case fatality rates for violent altercations involving firearms reflect the relatively higher prevalence of assailants with a clear and sustained intent to kill among those who use firearms.[15] That is to say, people who intend to kill another person choose firearms because of their relatively greater deadliness compared with other weapons. Under this interpretation, it is conceivable that a determined assailant without a firearm but with a clear and sustained homicidal intent would exert whatever other greater efforts would be required to kill the intended victim. In contrast to the first interpretation, the implication of this interpretation is that reduced access to firearms during FIAs would not substantially reduce the number of homicides because assailants with clear and sustained intent to kill would substitute other weapons to achieve the same destructive goal.

Both interpretations grant that killing with a firearm is easier than killing with most other, typically available weapons. Therefore, the magnitude of the preventive effect of limiting ready access to firearms will depend largely on the proportion of assailants who are involved in fatal firearm-associated FIAs and who (if no firearm were available) would have such a clear and sustained homicidal intent that they would use some other weapon and still succeed in killing their victim. Unfortunately, there are no data available with which to determine that proportion.

There is no reason to believe, however, that even among people with determined homicidal intent, homicidal efforts will always be successful when other weapons must be substituted for firearms. Granting that some persons, in the absence of firearms, would commit homicide using alternate weapons, we find no evidence to suggest that a substantial proportion of fatal FIAs involve persons with such sustained, cold-blooded homicidal intent. Indeed, studies of male batterers and anecdotal reports suggest that many FIAs (fatal and nonfatal) are a spontaneous response to conflict or anger and frequently occur without premeditation or planning.[16-18]

In addition, some indirect evidence shows that assailants who use firearms are not more likely to have a clear intent to kill than those who use knives. Zimring[2] investigated a series of attacks involving guns or knives, using the location and number of wounds inflicted as a basis for judging the assailant's intent. In these attacks, which typically involved relatives and acquaintances, a greater percentage of attackers with knives than with guns appeared to be intent on killing.[2] Finally, to date, researchers have found no evidence of compensatory increases in homicides involving other weapons when firearm access is restricted.[19-22]

Regardless of which of the two interpretations dominates in explaining weapon-related patterns in the risk of death, reduced access to firearms is likely to result in fewer homicides because killing is easier with firearms. However, the magnitude of the preventive effect of reduced access would be greater for homicides committed impulsively than for those marked by sustained homicidal intent. Given the available evidence, we interpret weapon-specific differences in the risk of death from FIAs as due primarily to the first interpretation—the greater lethality of firearms. This interpretation suggests two preventive approaches.

First, if access to loaded firearms were reduced, fatal FIAs might be prevented because assailants would be forced to substitute weapons less certain to kill. Many different strategies could be used to reduce firearm access. Innovative strategies should be explored, such as police confiscation of firearms used during FIA incidents, restriction of firearm purchase or acquisition by persons subject to domestic violence restraining orders or protective orders (as is the case in California[23]), or restriction of firearm acquisition or purchase by convicted spouse abusers—both misdemeanants and felons. Strict enforcement of existing laws prohibiting threats to kill or threats with weapons and of laws prohibiting firearm ownership by convicted felons should decrease firearm access for FIA perpetrators. In addition, educational interventions might be designed to disseminate information about concrete steps to reduce immediate access, such as separate locked storage for firearms and ammunition. Public information campaigns could be designed to communicate important research findings about the danger of keeping loaded firearms in the home,[24] so that the public can make more informed decisions about owning or purchasing firearms for protection.

Second, the design of firearms could be modified to decrease their lethality.[25] For example, handguns could be designed to be less easily loaded and fired. They could also be designed to shoot something other than bullets (eg, electricity, tranquilizers, or anesthetics). In 1986, the Attorney General of the United States held the Conference on Less Than Lethal Weapons[26] to lay the groundwork for developing useful, safe technology for less than lethal weapons; efforts are still under way in this regard.

Weapon-Specific Differences in the Risk of Nonfatal FIAs

In this study we found that the presence of a firearm lowered the risk of nonfatal injury relative to other weapons, although this effect was not statistically significant. Research on violent encounters indicates that the risk of nonfatal injury is significantly lower when firearms are involved, relative to other weapons.[4,5,10] This finding has been interpreted to suggest that when firearms are involved in a violent incident, intimidated victims may minimize their risk of injury by avoiding physical altercations with their assailants. This finding also suggests that a strategy of reducing the access of potential FIA assailants to firearms may come at the cost of increased nonfatal injuries.

The Predominance of Nonfatal FIAs

Although intervening to reduce fatal injuries is highly desirable, expanded emphasis should also be placed on preventing FIAs from occurring in the first place. More than 99% of FIAs do not result in death, and in addition to injuries, nonfatal FIAs have other serious consequences. Battered women are at increased risk for psychosocial and other health problems, including depression, alcohol and other drug problems, suicide attempts, and child abuse.[27-32] In addition, FIAs may contribute to the intergenerational transmission of violence.[33,34] Effective primary prevention strategies will reduce not only nonfatal injuries but also fatal injuries. Such strategies may need to emphasize attitude and behavior change by potential assailants, rather than relying on environmental modifications, since FIAs frequently involve the use of readily available household objects and bodily force.

Many different preventive strategies have been proposed for reducing the incidence of FIAs.[35] These include comprehensive community-based programs; teaching children and adolescents nonviolent alternatives for dealing with stress and anger[36,37]; devising ways to prevent dating violence, which is a possible precursor to adult violence among intimates[38,39]; targeting the news and entertainment media's role in legitimizing violence[40]; and increasing training for health care providers in identifying and referring women at risk of being abused (including the use of standardized protocols),[35,41-43] because some researchers believe that a series of family violence incidents may eventually escalate to violence resulting in serious injury or death.[44] Early identification and referral of persons at risk may allow for an intervention before situations escalate.

The Impact of Biases in Risk Estimates

Risk estimates presented in this study could be biased by our reliance on data that relate only to incidents that come to police attention. It is well known that nonfatal FIAs are underreported to police.[45,46] We have therefore overestimated, to some extent, the risk of death in both firearm and nonfirearm FIAs. Data from the National Crime Survey for the years 1979 to 1986 indicate, however, that FIA events that involve firearms are much more likely to be reported to police than those that involve other weapons, and that FIA events that involve nonfatal injuries are much more likely to be reported to police than those involving no injury.[47] These data suggest that we overestimated the risk of death to a greater extent for non–firearm-associated FIAs than for firearm-associated FIAs. Therefore, in Table 3, we have underestimated the relative risk of death comparing firearm-associated with non–firearm-associated FIAs. In addition, these underreporting patterns do not appear to have introduced any substantial bias into our estimates of the risk of nonfatal injury in firearm-associated FIAs relative to non–firearm-associated FIAs.

CONCLUSION

We estimate that FIAs involving firearms are at least 12 times more likely to result in death than FIAs involving all other types of weapons. Reducing the access of potential FIA assailants to firearms and reducing firearm lethality through redesign represent potentially effective prevention strategies. Simultaneously, efforts to reduce the overall incidence of FIAs through primary prevention must be expanded. All three of these prevention strategies must be evaluated for efficacy.

For this report we used data from the study of Family and Intimate Assaults in Atlanta, Ga, supported under a collaborative agreement between the Centers for Disease Control and the Georgia Department of Human Resources (U50/CCU400931-01-1), with the additional collaboration of the Fulton County (Georgia) Health Department and the Atlanta Department of Public Safety. Additional support was provided through an interagency agreement (86-IJ-R-200) with the National Institute of Justice.

The following were members of the Collaborative Working Group for the Study of Family and Intimate Assaults in Atlanta: (1) Atlanta Department of Public Safety: George Napper, PhD, Ardith Peters, PhD, Guy O. Seymour, PhD, and Jack Mallory, MSW; (2) Fulton County Health Department: William R. Elsea, MD, MPH, Robert J. Finton, MSPH, and Richard F. Lyles, PhD; (3) Georgia Department of Human Resources: R. Keith Sikes, DVM, MPH, Project Director; Jane C. Carr, RN, Assistant Project Director; Sandra S. Huguley, MA, Senior Research Associate; and Anne Becker, Lois Ellison, Steve Erickson, Theresa Irby, Debbie Lester, Kathy Marth, William D. Patterson, MA, Terrie Sterling, MA, MS, and Angela Wine, Research Associates; and (4) Centers for Disease Control: Linda E. Saltzman, PhD, Project Officer; James A. Mercy, PhD; Mark L. Rosenberg, MD, MPP; Richard J. Waxweiler, PhD; and Harvey F. Davis, Jr, MPH.

We thank Garen J. Wintemute, MD, MPH, Colin Loftin, PhD, and Kenneth E. Powell, MD, MPH, for their helpful comments on a draft of this article.

References

1. Mercy JA, O'Carroll PW. New directions in violence prediction: the public health arena. *Violence Victims*. 1988;3:285-301.
2. Zimring F. Is gun control likely to reduce violent killings? *Univ Chicago Law Rev*. 1968;35:721-737.
3. Cook PJ. Robbery violence. *Criminal Law Criminol*. 1987;78:357-376.
4. Cook PJ. The effect of gun availability on violent crime patterns. *Ann Am Acad Political Soc Sci*. 1981;455:63-79.
5. Conklin J. *Robbery and the Criminal Justice System*. Philadelphia, Pa: JB Lippincott; 1972.
6. Saltzman LE, Mercy JA, Rosenberg ML, et al. Magnitude and patterns of family and intimate assault in Atlanta, Georgia, 1984. *Violence Victims*. 1990;5:3-17.
7. Saltzman L, Mercy JA, Rhodes, PH. Identification of nonfatal family and intimate assault incidents in police data. *Am J Public Health*. In press.
8. Cochran WG. *Sampling Techniques*. 3rd ed. New York, NY: John Wiley & Sons Inc; 1977.

9. Cox DR, Hinkley DV. *Theoretical Statistics*. London, England: Chapman & Hall Ltd; 1974.
10. Rand M, DeBerry M, Klaus P, Taylor B. *The Use of Weapons in Committing Crimes*. Washington, DC: US Dept of Justice; 1986. Bureau of Justice Statistics Special Report.
11. Rand MR. *Handgun Crime Victims*. Washington, DC: US Dept of Justice; 1990. Bureau of Justice Statistics Special Report.
12. Cook PJ. The technology of personal violence. In: Tonry M, ed. *Crime and Justice: A Review of Research*. 14th ed. Chicago, Ill: University of Chicago Press; 1991:1-71.
13. *Criminal Victimization in the United States, 1988*. Washington, DC: US Dept of Justice; 1990.
14. National Center for Health Statistics. *Vital Statistics Mortality Data, Compressed Mortality Files*. Hyattsville, Md: Centers for Disease Control; 1988.
15. Wolfgang ME. *Patterns in Criminal Homicide*. Philadelphia: University of Pennsylvania Press; 1958.
16. Adams DC, McCormick AJ. Men unlearning violence: a group approach based on the collective model. In: Roy M, ed. *The Abusive Partner: An Analysis of Domestic Battering*. New York, NY: Van Nostrand Reinhold Co; 1982:170-197.
17. Campbell J. Misogyny and homicide of women. *Adv Nurs Sci*. 1981;3:67-85.
18. Goetting A. Men who kill their mates: a profile. *J Fam Violence*. 1989;4:285-296.
19. Sloan JH, Kellerman AL, Reay DT, et al. Handgun regulations, crimes, assaults, and homicide: a tale of two cities. *N Engl J Med*. 1988;319:1256-1262.
20. Hedeboe J, Charles AV, Nielsen J, et al. Interpersonal violence: patterns in a Danish community. *Am J Public Health*. 1985;75:651-653.
21. Baker SP. Without guns, do people kill people? *Am J Public Health*. 1985;75:587-588.
22. Sproule CF, Kennett DJ. Killing with guns in the U.S.A. and Canada 1977-1983: further evidence for the effectiveness of gun control. *Can J Criminol*. 1989;31:245-251.
23. Assembly Bill No. 108, 1991, Cal Stat ch 953.
24. Kellermann AL, Reay DT. Protection or peril? an analysis of firearm-related deaths in the home. *N Engl J Med*. 1986;314:1557-1560.
25. Webster DW, Chaulk CP, Teret SP, Wintemute GJ. Reducing firearm injuries. *Issues Sci Technol*. Spring 1991:73-79.
26. Sweetman S. *Report on the Attorney General's Conference on Less Than Lethal Weapons*. Washington, DC: National Institute of Justice, US Dept of Justice; 1987.
27. Stark E, Flitcraft A, Zuckerman D, Grey A, Robison J, Frazier W. *Wife Abuse in the Medical Setting: An Introduction for Health Personnel*. Washington, DC: Office of Domestic Violence; 1981. Monograph No. 7.
28. Koss MP, Koss PG, Woodruff WJ. Deleterious effects of criminal victimization on women's health and medical utilization. *Arch Intern Med*. 1991;151: 342-347.
29. Stets JE, Straus MA. Gender differences in reporting marital violence and its medical and psychological consequences. In: Straus MA, Gelles RJ, eds. *Physical Violence in American Families: Risk Factors and Adaptations to Violence in 8,145 Families*. New Brunswick, NJ: Transaction Publishers; 1989:151-165.
30. Saunders DG. Family violence. *Emerg Care Q*. 1991;7:51-61.
31. Follingstad DR, Neckerman AP, Vormbrock J. Reactions to victimization and coping strategies of battered women: the ties that bind. *Clin Psychol Rev*. 1988;8:373-390.
32. Haber JD, Rogers A. Abused women and chronic pain. *Am J Nurs*. 1985;85:1010-1012.
33. Hotaling GT, Sugarman DB. An analysis of risk markers in husband to wife violence. *Violence Victims*. 1986;1:101-124.
34. Widom CS. The cycle of violence. *Science*. 1989; 244:160-166.
35. National Committee for Injury Prevention and Control. *Injury Prevention: Meeting the Challenge*. New York, NY: Oxford University Press Inc; 1989.
36. Levy B. *Skills for Violence-Free Relationships: Curriculum for Young People Ages 13-18*. Santa Monica: Southern California Coalition on Battered Women; 1984.
37. Family Violence Curriculum Project. *Preventing Family Violence: A Curriculum for Adolescents*. Boston: Massachusetts Dept of Public Health; 1984.
38. Billingham RE. Courtship violence: the patterns of conflict resolution strategies across seven levels of emotional commitment. *Fam Relations*. 1987;36:283-289.
39. Parrot A. *Acquaintance Rape and Sexual Assault Prevention Training Manual*. 2nd ed. Ithaca, NY: Dept of Human Service Studies, College of Human Ecology, Cornell University; 1986.
40. Gelles RJ, Cornell CP. *Intimate Violence in Families*. 2nd ed. Newbury Park, Calif: Sage Publications; 1990.
41. McLeer SV, Anwar RAH. The role of the emergency physician in the prevention of domestic violence. *Ann Emerg Med*. 1987;16:1155-1161.
42. *Healthy People 2000: National Health Promotion and Disease Prevention Objectives: Full Report, With Commentary*. Washington, DC: Public Health Service; 1991.
43. Centers for Disease Control. Education about adult domestic violence in U.S. and Canadian medical schools, 1987-88. *MMWR*. 1989;38:17-19.
44. Straus MA. Domestic violence and homicide antecedents. *Bull N Y Acad Med*. 1986;62:446-465.
45. Teske RHC Jr, Parker ML. *Spouse Abuse in Texas: A Study of Women's Attitudes and Experiences*. Huntsville, Tex: Survey Research Program, Criminal Justice Center, Sam Houston State University; 1983.
46. Schulman MA. *A Survey of Spousal Violence Against Women in Kentucky*. Washington, DC: US Dept of Justice; 1979.
47. US Dept of Justice, Bureau of Justice Statistics. *National Crime Surveys: National Sample, 1979-1987, Revised Questionnaire* [computer file]. 5th ICPSR ed. Ann Arbor, Mich: Inter-university Consortium for Political and Social Research [producer and distributor]; 1991. Conducted by the US Dept of Commerce, Bureau of the Census.

Firearm and Nonfirearm Homicide Among Persons 15 Through 19 Years of Age

Differences by Level of Urbanization, United States, 1979 Through 1989

Lois A. Fingerhut, MA; Deborah D. Ingram, PhD; Jacob J. Feldman, PhD

Objective.—To examine trends (1979 through 1989) and current status in firearm and nonfirearm homicide rates by level of urbanization among persons 15 through 19 years of age.

Design.—The Compressed Mortality File, a county-level mortality and population database maintained by the National Center for Health Statistics, Centers for Disease Control, Hyattsville, Md, and the 1980 Human Resource Profile County Codes are used to analyze age-, sex-, and race-specific firearm and nonfirearm homicide rates by urbanization level.

Setting.—United States, 1979 through 1989.

Subjects.—Black and white males and females 15 through 19 years of age whose underlying cause of death was either firearm homicide (E965.0 through E965.4 or E970) or nonfirearm homicide (E960 through E964, E965.5 through E969, or E971 through E978) in the *ICD-9* (*International Statistical Classification of Diseases, Injuries, and Causes of Death, Ninth Revision*).

Main Outcome Measures.—Urbanization level–specific firearm and nonfirearm homicide rates.

Results.—The 1989 firearm homicide rate in metropolitan counties was nearly five times the rate in nonmetropolitan counties (13.7 vs 2.9 deaths per 100 000 population). Firearm homicide rates were highest in core metropolitan counties, 27.7 per 100 000 population; rates were higher for black males than for any other race-sex group in each of five county urbanization strata for 1979 through 1989. Nonfirearm homicide rates are considerably lower, with smaller urban differentials; the rate in metropolitan counties was 1.4 times the rate in nonmetropolitan counties (2.6 vs 1.8 per 100 000 population). From 1979 through 1984, firearm homicide rates declined in each of the county strata. From 1984 through 1987, firearm homicide rates increased, and from 1987 through 1989 they increased rapidly, from 23% to 35% per year in the four metropolitan strata. From 1979 through 1989, nonfirearm homicide rates declined or remained stable.

Conclusions.—Large urbanization differentials in firearm homicide and smaller differentials in nonfirearm homicide are identified. Firearm homicide rates are highest and increasing the fastest among black teenage males in the core, fringe, and medium metropolitan strata.

(*JAMA*. 1992;267:3048-3053)

FROM 1979 through 1989, the firearm homicide rate for persons 15 through 19 years of age in the United States increased 61%, from 6.9 to 11.1 deaths per 100 000 population, a larger increase than for any other 5-year age group (unpublished data from the Compressed Mortality File [CMF], National Center for Health Statistics, Centers for Disease Control, Hyattsville, Md). During this same period, the nonfirearm homicide rate decreased 29%, from 3.4 to 2.4 deaths per 100 000 population. Thus, the increase observed in the total homicide rate among 15- through 19-year-olds during the period 1979 through 1989 resulted solely from increases in firearm homicides. Furthermore, firearm homicide, the second-leading cause of death for all 15- through 19-year-olds, has been increasing more rapidly than any other cause of death (Fig 1).

While other studies have presented firearm and nonfirearm homicide rates by age, race, and sex at the national and state levels,[1-3] the present study extends this work by focusing on differences in firearm and nonfirearm homicide among black and white 15- through 19-year-olds by level of urbanization. Urbanization levels are used to stratify counties by size and relationship to a primary central city. Stratifying by level of urbanization can identify important differentials in mortality that can foster the formulation of intervention strategies. This analysis is a step forward in identifying those areas in greatest need of violence prevention programs.

DATA AND METHODS

This analysis is restricted to white and black persons 15 through 19 years of age. This analysis does not include Asian or Native American persons, since the age-specific county population estimates needed to calculate death rates for these persons are only available for census years. While both white and black persons can be of Hispanic origin, Hispanic persons were not analyzed separately because of the lack of age-specific county population estimates. Throughout this article, the word "teenagers" is used interchangeably with persons 15 through 19 years of age.

The data are from the Compressed Mortality File (CMF), a county-level national mortality and population database maintained by the Office of Analysis and Epidemiology, National Center for Health Statistics (NCHS), Centers for Disease Control. The CMF uses death records from the NCHS National Vital Statistics System (NVSS). Death records in the NVSS are collected by the states and tabulated by the NCHS,

From the Office of Analysis and Epidemiology, National Center for Health Statistics, Centers for Disease Control, Hyattsville, Md.

Reprint requests to Office of Analysis and Epidemiology, National Center for Health Statistics, Room 1080, 6525 Belcrest Rd, Hyattsville, MD 20782 (Ms Fingerhut).

with cause of death information coded in accordance with the International Classification of Diseases (ICD). The population estimates are from the Bureau of the Census. For the period 1981 through 1989, the Bureau of the Census intercensal population estimates are used rather than postcensal estimates.

Firearm homicides are defined in the *International Statistical Classification of Diseases, Injuries, and Causes of Death, Ninth Revision (ICD-9)*,[4] as codes E965.0 through E965.4 or E970. Nonfirearm homicide includes *ICD-9* codes E960 through E964, E965.5 through E969, or E971 through E978.

The 1980 Human Resource Profile county codes (HRPC) were used to categorize counties by level of urbanization.[5] These codes group all US counties by the official 1973 metropolitan-nonmetropolitan designation. The codes have been updated through 1980 and are available for public use on the Area Resource File, maintained by the Bureau of Health Professions. The following definitions of county urbanization strata are used in this analysis.

Metropolitan counties are composed of *core* counties that contain the primary central city of a Metropolitan Statistical Area (MSA) with a 1980 population of 1 million or more. *Fringe* counties are the counties of MSAs with 1980 populations of 1 million or more. *Medium* counties are counties of MSAs with 1980 populations of 250 000 to 999 999. *Small* counties are counties of MSAs with 1980 populations under 250 000. *Nonmetropolitan* counties are those that are not part of an MSA.

In this analysis, total and race- and sex-specific annual firearm and nonfirearm homicide rates are calculated for the five urbanization strata for 1979 through 1989. Differences between death rates are considered significant at $P \leq .05$ using a two-tailed *t* test of the difference between rates. Unless otherwise stated, all comparisons made in the text are statistically significant at $P = .05$.

Plots of the firearm homicide rates in each of the urbanization strata showed a decline from 1979 through 1984, an increase from 1984 through 1987, and a faster increase from 1987 through 1989. Nonfirearm homicide rates generally declined for the entire 1979 through 1989 period. Therefore, three trend lines were fit to the firearm homicide rates (1979 through 1984, 1984 through 1987, and 1987 through 1989) and one trend line was fit to the nonfirearm homicide rates. Weighted least-squares regression was used to fit a line to the logarithm of the death rates for each period. The weight used was the number of deaths. A χ^2 test was used to assess goodness of fit.

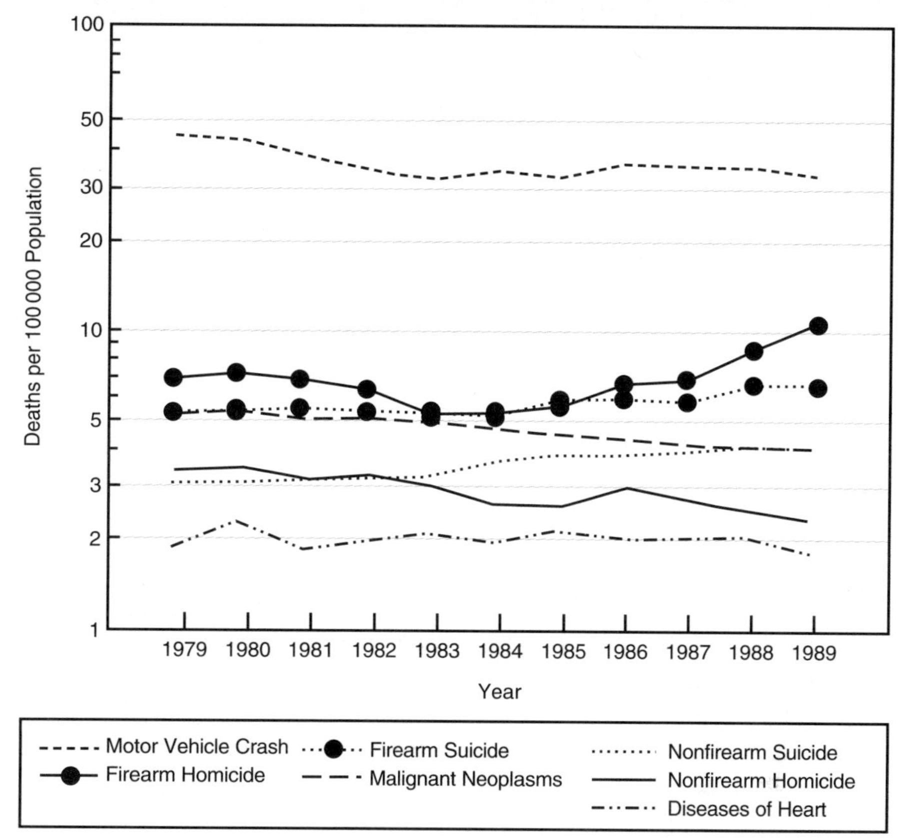

Fig 1.—Leading causes of death among persons 15 through 19 years of age, 1979 through 1989 (from the Compressed Mortality File of the National Center for Health Statistics, Centers for Disease Control).

Table 1.—Firearm and Nonfirearm Homicide Rates by Urbanization Strata Among Persons 15 Through 19 Years of Age, 1989*

Urbanization Strata	Homicide Rates per 100 000 Population (SE)				
	All†	Black Males	White Males	Black Females	White Females
			Firearm Homicide		
Total	11.1 (0.2)	85.3 (2.5)	7.5 (0.3)	8.6 (0.8)	1.7 (0.2)
Metropolitan	13.7 (0.3)	100.9 (3.0)	9.0 (0.4)	10.0 (0.9)	2.0 (0.2)
Core	27.7 (0.8)	143.9 (5.0)	21.5 (1.1)	13.4 (1.5)	3.0 (0.4)
Fringe	4.9 (0.4)	54.0 (5.9)	3.0 (0.5)	5.4 (1.9)	1.0 (0.3)
Medium	7.5 (0.4)	63.1 (4.6)	3.5 (0.5)	7.5 (1.6)	2.0 (0.3)
Small	5.7 (0.6)	48.2 (6.7)	4.3 (0.7)	5.8 (2.4)	1.3 (0.4)
Nonmetropolitan	2.9 (0.3)	15.5 (2.5)	3.0 (0.4)	2.1 (0.9)	1.0 (0.2)
			Nonfirearm Homicide		
Total	2.4 (0.1)	8.4 (0.8)	1.9 (0.2)	3.1 (0.5)	1.5 (0.1)
Metropolitan	2.6 (0.1)	8.7 (0.9)	2.2 (0.2)	3.4 (0.6)	1.6 (0.2)
Core	4.0 (0.3)	10.4 (1.4)	3.8 (0.5)	4.4 (0.9)	1.9 (0.3)
Fringe	1.9 (0.2)	6.4 (2.0)	1.3 (0.3)	2.7 (1.4)	2.0 (0.4)
Medium	1.9 (0.2)	7.4 (1.6)	1.6 (0.3)	2.4 (0.9)	1.1 (0.3)
Small	1.5 (0.3)	6.5 (2.5)	1.6 (0.7)	1.9 (1.3)	1.5 (0.5)
Nonmetropolitan	1.8 (0.2)	7.1 (1.7)	0.9 (0.2)	1.7 (0.9)	1.3 (0.3)

*From the Compressed Mortality File of the National Center for Health Statistics, Centers for Disease Control.
†Includes races not shown separately.

For some of the race-sex-urbanization strata, trend lines could not be fit because the rates are based on small numbers of deaths and are too unstable. A χ^2 test was used to determine whether the slopes were significantly different from zero. The average annual percentage change in the death rates for a given time period is $100(e^b - 1)$, where "b" is the slope estimate of the regression line for the particular time period. In the figures that accompany the trend section of this analysis, the death rates are plotted on a logarithmic rather than a linear scale. For a given rate change, eg, from 2 to 3 per 100 000 population or from 20 to 30 per 100 000 population, the logarithmic scale emphasizes that the relative change is the same—50%. Not all percentage increases are of practical importance even though they may be statistically significant. For example, a large percentage change in a low rate may not be highlighted in the text.

RESULTS

Current Status by County Strata, 1989

The 1989 firearm homicide rate among all 15- through 19-year-olds in metropolitan counties was nearly five times the rate in nonmetropolitan counties, 13.7 vs 2.9 deaths per 100 000 population (Table 1). Within metropolitan counties, the rate was four to six times higher in the core counties, 27.7 per 100 000 population, than in the fringe, medium, or small county strata. The metropolitan-nonmetropolitan differential in the 1989 nonfirearm homicide rate was much smaller, 2.6 vs 1.8 deaths per 100 000 population. Within metropolitan counties, the nonfirearm homicide rate in the core county stratum (4.0 per 100 000 population) was two to three times the rates in the other metropolitan strata.

While the primary focus of this analysis is on urbanization strata variation in firearm and nonfirearm homicide, the race-sex differentials within each stratum are large, necessitating separate analyses of the strata by race and sex. At each urbanization level, firearm homicide rates are highest for black males and lowest for white females (Table 1). While the total firearm homicide rate for white males is similar to the rate for black females, within the urbanization strata this relationship is not consistent. The total nonfirearm homicide rate is also highest for black males and lowest for white females. Within the urbanization strata, rates for black males are also highest. For the other race-sex groups, however, significant differences in nonfirearm homicide rates could generally not be detected because the rates are based on relatively small numbers of deaths and, hence, have relatively large standard errors.

Urbanization Differences by Race and Sex, 1989

The black teenage male firearm homicide rate in 1989 in metropolitan counties was 6.5 times the rate in nonmetropolitan counties (100.9 vs 15.5 per 100 000 population) (Table 1). Within metropolitan counties, the firearm homicide rate for these teenagers in the core county stratum (143.9 per 100 000 population) was two to three times the rates in the fringe, medium, or small metropolitan strata (48 to 63 per 100 000 population).

The firearm homicide patterns observed for white males were similar to

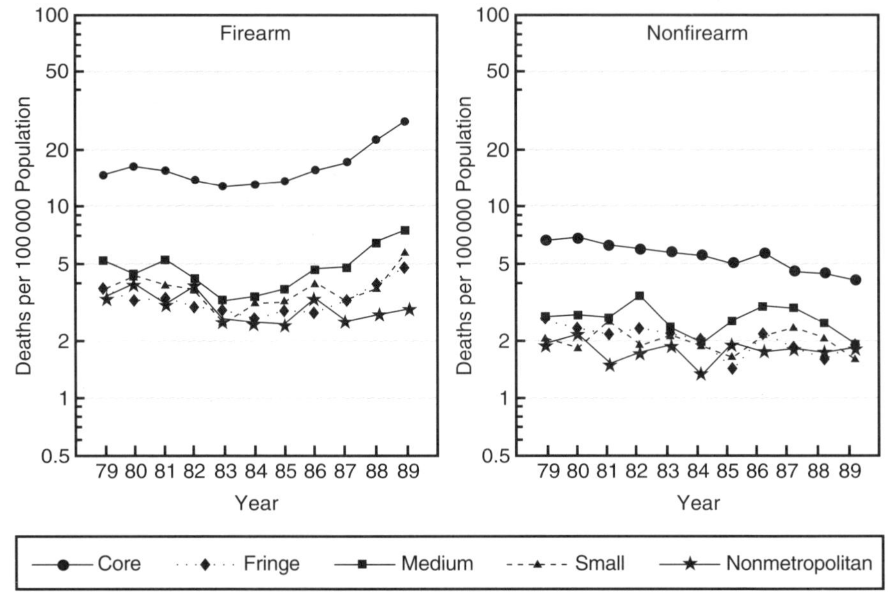

Fig 2.—Homicide rates by urbanization strata among persons 15 through 19 years of age, 1979 through 1989 (from the Compressed Mortality File of the National Center for Health Statistics, Centers for Disease Control).

Table 2.—Average Annual Percentage Change in Firearm and Nonfirearm Homicide Rates by Urbanization Strata, by Race and Sex, 1979 Through 1989*

Urbanization Strata/ Race and Sex	Average Annual Change in Rate, %			
	Firearm Homicide			Nonfirearm Homicide, 1979-1989
	1979-1984	1984-1987	1987-1989	
Core metropolitan	−4.1†	9.5†	27.8†	−4.6†
Black male	−7.5†‡	15.8†	27.8†	−3.2†
Black female	−7.7†	14.0†	13.9	−3.5†
White male	−10.9†‡	2.3	30.0†	−7.0†
White female	2.8	−15.3†	32.6†	−3.4†
Fringe metropolitan	−6.3†	7.2	23.2†	−3.4†
Black male	−3.3	16.4†	41.5†	−0.2
Black female	−5.1	−13.4	28.9	−3.0
White male	−8.2†	3.6	2.1	−5.5†
White female	−9.9†	−2.0	10.9	−2.7
Medium metropolitan	§	13.5†	23.9†	§
Black male	−9.0†	25.5†	33.5†	1.0
Black female	−1.7	10.2	5.8	−1.9
White male	−7.8†	§	§	−4.9†
White female	−11.5†	16.0	38.3†	−0.7
Small metropolitan	−6.6†	2.2	34.5†	−1.0
Black male	−4.5	7.9	72.0†	0.4
Black female	−27.0†	31.7	−6.7	2.9
White male	−3.7	−9.1	27.0	§
White female	−17.7†	15.3	−3.0	−2.9
Nonmetropolitan	§	3.8	7.7	−1.0
Black male	−12.3†	23.9†	7.8	2.5
Black female	1.7	19.5	−16.6	4.6
White male	§	§	8.6	−5.7†
White female	0.6	§	5.3	−1.4

*From the Compressed Mortality File of the National Center for Health Statistics, Centers for Disease Control.
†Significantly different from zero.
‡1980-1984.
§Data were too unstable to fit a trend line.

those for black males, although the rates were considerably lower. The 1989 firearm homicide rate for white males in metropolitan counties was three times the rate in nonmetropolitan counties (9.0 vs 3.0 per 100 000 population) and was also higher in the core metropolitan counties (21.5 per 100 000 population) than in the other metropolitan strata (3 to 4 per 100 000 population).

The patterns observed for black teenage females were similar to those for the males; the firearm homicide rate in metropolitan counties was five times the rate in nonmetropolitan counties (10.0 vs 2.1 per 100 000 population). The core county stratum rate was about twice the rates in other metropolitan strata (13.4 vs 5 to 7 per 100 000 population).

Among white teenage females, the 1989 firearm homicide rates were lower than for any of the other race-sex groups. However, there remains the similar pattern of higher rates in metropolitan than nonmetropolitan counties (2.0 vs 1.0 per 100 000 population), with the rate in core counties higher than those in the other metropolitan strata.

Nonfirearm homicide rates were lower than firearm homicide rates in every urbanization stratum for black and white teenage males. For black females, the nonfirearm homicide rates were lower than the firearm homicide rates in the core and medium strata and were similar in the fringe, small, and nonmetropolitan strata. The pattern observed for white females was similar (with one exception) to that for black females; the nonfirearm homicide rate was higher than the firearm homicide rate in the fringe stratum.

Among black males and among black and white females, there were no within–urbanization strata differences in nonfirearm homicide. Among white males, the nonfirearm homicide rate in the core stratum was higher than in the other strata.

Trends by County Strata, 1979 Through 1989

Firearm homicide rates in 1989 were higher than in 1979 in the core, fringe, medium, and small metropolitan strata. In the nonmetropolitan stratum, the rate in 1989 was not significantly different from the rate in 1979. In contrast, nonfirearm homicide rates in 1989 were lower than in 1979 in the core and medium strata and similar to the 1979 rates in the fringe, small, and nonmetropolitan strata.

From 1979 through 1984, firearm homicide rates generally declined, on average, 4% to 7% per year in the core, fringe, and small metropolitan strata (Fig 2 and Table 2). In the medium and nonmetropolitan strata, the rates were too unstable to fit a trend line. In contrast, from 1984 through 1987, firearm homicide rates increased, on average, 10% per year in the core stratum and 14% per year in the medium metropolitan stratum and remained stable in the other strata (Fig 2 and Table 2). From 1987 through 1989, annual increases in the four metropolitan strata were considerably steeper than from 1984 through 1987, ranging from 23% to 35%. In the nonmetropolitan stratum, the annual increase was not significantly different from zero.

The trend in nonfirearm homicide rates was one of decline throughout most of 1979 through 1989. The nonfirearm homicide rate declined an average of 5% per year in the core stratum and 3% per year in the fringe stratum, and remained stable in the small and nonmetropolitan strata. The rates in the medium stratum were too unstable to fit a trend line.

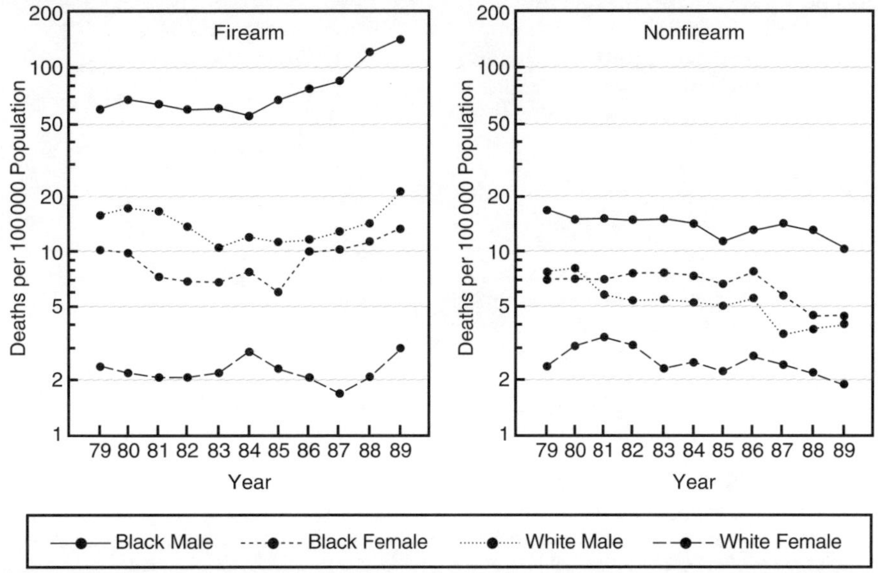

Fig 3.—Homicide rates in core metropolitan counties among persons 15 through 19 years of age, 1979 through 1989 (from the Compressed Mortality File of the National Center for Health Statistics, Centers for Disease Control).

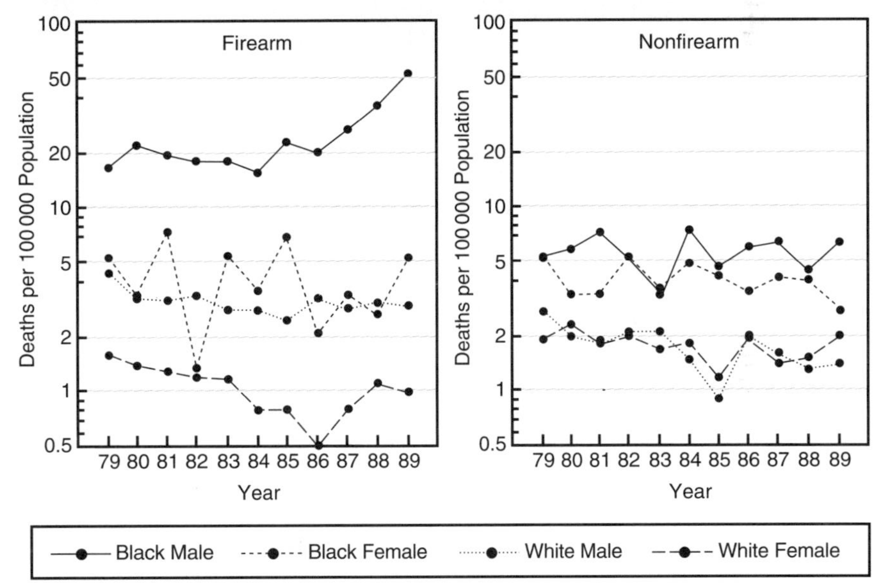

Fig 4.—Homicide rates in fringe metropolitan counties among persons 15 through 19 years of age, 1979 through 1989 (from the Compressed Mortality File of the National Center for Health Statistics, Centers for Disease Control).

Race- and Sex-Specific Trends by County Strata, 1979 Through 1989

From 1979 through 1984, firearm homicide rates in the *core* stratum declined 8% per year among black females (Fig 3 and Table 2). For black and white males, trend lines were fit for the period 1980 through 1984; firearm homicide rates declined 8% and 11% per year, respectively. In contrast, from 1984 through 1987, large annual increases were observed for black teenagers (14% to 16% per year), and a large decrease (15% per year) was observed for white females. In the most recent period, 1987 through 1989, annual increases in firearm homicide rates, averaging about 30% per year, occurred among black males, white males, and white females. (Since the firearm homicide rates in the core stratum are so much higher than in any of the other strata, the vertical scale in Fig 3 is different from the scales in Figs 4 through 7).

Average annual declines in firearm homicide rates from 1979 to 1984 in the *fringe* stratum were observed for white teenagers (8% to 10%) (Fig 4 and Table 2). From 1984 through 1987 and from 1987 through 1989, firearm homicide rates for black males increased 16% and 42% per year, respectively.

In the *medium* stratum, average annual declines of 8% to 12% from 1979 through 1984 were observed for black and white males and for white females (Fig 5 and Table 2). The rate for black males increased 26% per year from 1984 through 1987 and 34% per year from 1987 through 1989. An equally large increase (38% per year) was observed for white females from 1987 through 1989.

In the *small* metropolitan stratum, firearm homicide declined precipitously from 1979 through 1984 among black and white females, 27% and 18% per year, respectively (Fig 6 and Table 2). From 1987 through 1989, the rate for black males increased at a rate of 72% per year.

Annual declines from 1979 through 1984 in firearm homicide in *nonmetropolitan* counties were observed for black and white males (Fig 7 and Table 2). Among black males, the rate increased 24% per year from 1984 through 1987.

Nonfirearm homicide rates declined faster for white males (5% to 7% per year) than for the other race-sex groups in the core, fringe, medium, and nonmetropolitan strata. In the core stratum, nonfirearm homicide rates declined about 3% per year for black teenagers and for white females. In the other strata, the annual percentage changes were not significantly different from zero.

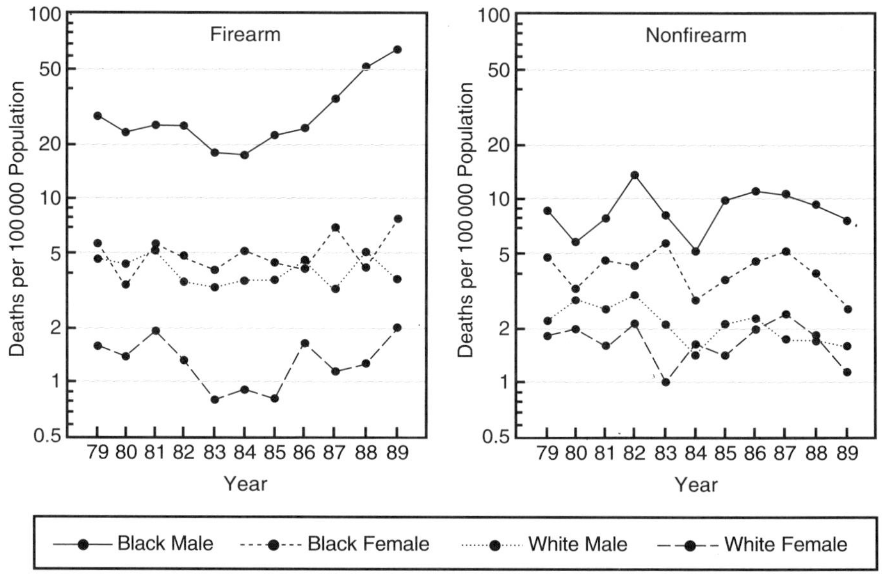

Fig 5.—Homicide rates in medium metropolitan counties among persons 15 through 19 years of age, 1979 through 1989 (from the Compressed Mortality File of the National Center for Health Statistics, Centers for Disease Control).

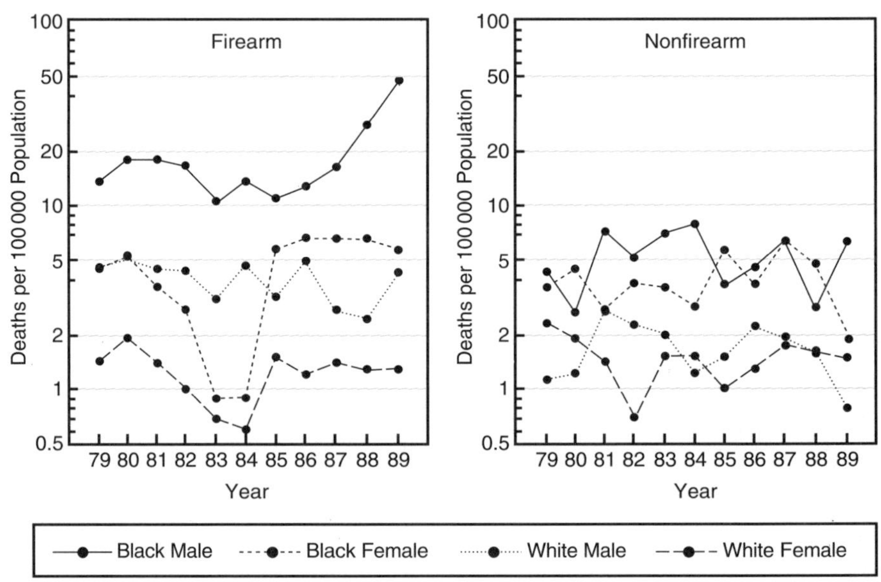

Fig 6.—Homicide rates in small metropolitan counties among persons 15 through 19 years of age, 1979 through 1989 (from the Compressed Mortality File of the National Center for Health Statistics, Centers for Disease Control).

COMMENT

In 1986, firearm homicide became the second-leading cause of death for all 15- through 19-year-olds, and the death rate for this cause is increasing (Fig 1). This analysis has shown that teenage firearm homicide rates are highest in the core stratum, much lower in the fringe, medium, and small metropolitan strata, and lowest in the nonmetropolitan stratum. The firearm homicide rate for all teenagers in the core county stratum in 1989 was 10 times the rate in the nonmetropolitan strata, 27.7 vs 2.9 deaths per 100 000 population. For the leading cause of teenage death, motor vehicle crashes, the core-nonmetropolitan relative difference was considerably smaller (and in the opposite direction) (Fig 8).

In summary, this study has identified, among teenagers, large urbanization differentials in firearm homicide and smaller differentials in nonfirearm ho-

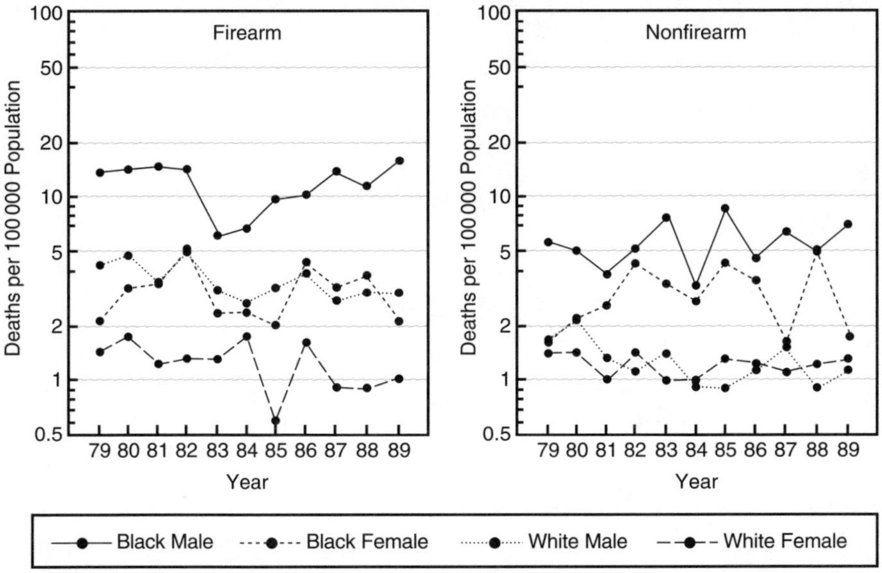

Fig 7.—Homicide rates in nonmetropolitan counties among persons 15 through 19 years of age, 1979 through 1989 (from the Compressed Mortality File of the National Center for Health Statistics, Centers for Disease Control).

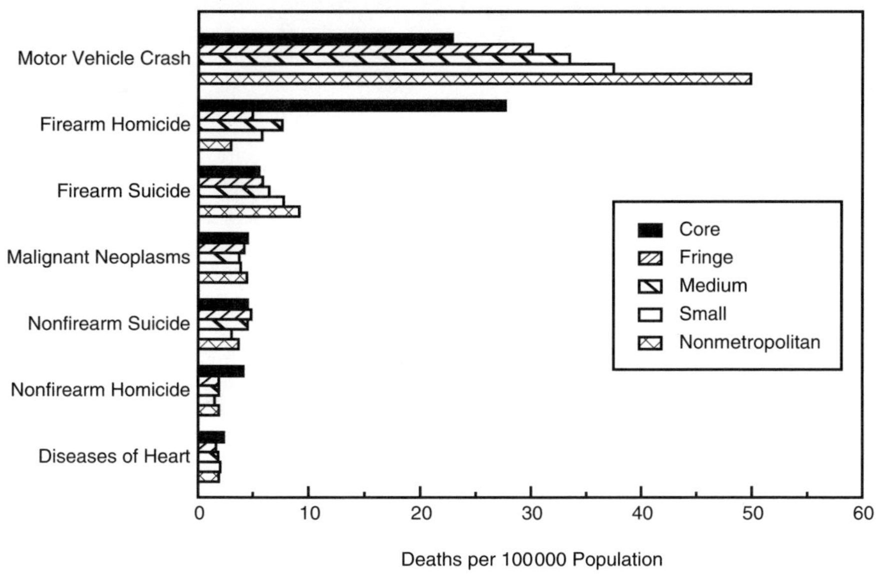

Fig 8.—Leading causes of death by urbanization level among persons 15 through 19 years of age in 1989 (from the Compressed Mortality File of the National Center for Health Statistics, Centers for Disease Control).

micide. Following a general decline in firearm homicide from 1979 through 1984, the rates increased, with larger increases since 1987. As a result of the increases, the 1989 firearm homicide rates in the metropolitan strata were about twice as high as the 1984 rates. In the nonmetropolitan stratum, the 1989 rate was similar to the rate in 1984. Firearm homicide rates for black males have been the highest across each of the strata, with the rates in core counties strikingly higher than for any other race-sex-urbanization group. While the urbanization differentials are generally the same for nonfirearm homicide, the rates continue to be much lower and have been declining.

It is important to remember that, even though the firearm homicide rates in the fringe, medium, small, and nonmetropolitan strata are so much lower than in the core stratum, they are still very high compared with firearm homicide rates in other countries. Even the firearm homicide rates in the nonmetropolitan stratum (where the rates are the lowest) are substantially higher than in many other industrialized nations.[3] For example, the firearm homicide rate for white teenage males in nonmetropolitan counties, 3 per 100 000 population, was 10 times the average firearm homicide rate for young adult males in 12 industrialized countries.[3,6] The current levels and the recent rates of increase in firearm homicide in each of the strata are unacceptably high and need to be reduced.

It is relatively easy to speculate about the reasons for the recent and rapid increases in firearm homicide among teenagers. Factors are likely to include increased use of crack cocaine, changes in the types and lethality of firearms, urban poverty, and myriad sociologic factors. Because it is also likely that risk factors will vary by locale, strategies for reducing firearm homicide must be established at subnational levels.

We have shown that firearm homicide rates are highest and increasing the fastest among black teenage males in the core, fringe, and medium metropolitan strata. A more focused analysis is needed to identify counties within these strata where the rates are highest and increasing the fastest. This is necessary in the effort to develop appropriate intervention strategies. If individual counties with particularly high rates and large increases in firearm homicide are identified, programs can be implemented where they are needed the most. In an era of budget constraints, knowing where to spend intervention dollars is crucial. Given the increasing trends, surveillance of firearm homicide at the county level is necessary, since counties that have low rates may become counties with high rates. Keeping track of such changes is a key step in the process of slowing and eventually reversing the increasing trend of teenage firearm homicide.

References

1. Fingerhut LA, Kleinman JC, Godfrey E, Rosenberg H. Firearm mortality among children, youth, and young adults 1-34 years of age, trends and current status: United States, 1979-88. *Monthly Vital Stat Rep.* 1991;39:1-16. No. 11.
2. Fingerhut LA, Kleinman JC. Firearm mortality among children and youth. In: *Advance Data From Vital and Health Statistics.* Hyattsville, Md: National Center for Health Statistics; 1989:1-8. No. 178.
3. Fingerhut LA, Kleinman JC. International and interstate comparisons of homicide among young males. *JAMA.* 1990;263:3292-3295.
4. World Health Organization. *Manual of the International Statistical Classification of Diseases, Injuries, and Causes of Death, Based on the Recommendations of the Ninth Revision Conference, 1975.* Geneva, Switzerland: World Health Organization; 1977.
5. *User Documentation for the ODAM Area Resource File as of March 1990.* Rockville, Md: Bureau of Health Professions; 1990.
6. *World Health Statistics Annual 1989 and 1990.* Geneva, Switzerland: World Health Organization; 1989-1990.

Firearm Homicide Among Black Teenage Males in Metropolitan Counties

Comparison of Death Rates in Two Periods, 1983 Through 1985 and 1987 Through 1989

Lois A. Fingerhut, MA; Deborah D. Ingram, PhD; Jacob J. Feldman, PhD

Objective.—To identify US counties (1) that had either significantly high or significantly low firearm homicide rates among black males 15 through 19 years of age in 1983 through 1985 and in 1987 through 1989, and/or (2) that experienced a significant increase in the firearm homicide rate between 1983 through 1985 and 1987 through 1989.

Design.—Using the Compressed Mortality File, a county-level mortality and population database maintained by the National Center for Health Statistics, Centers for Disease Control, Hyattsville, Md, county-level firearm homicide rates are analyzed.

Setting.—Eighty counties with a population of at least 10 000 black males 15 through 19 years of age in 1987 through 1989.

Subjects.—Black males 15 through 19 years of age whose underlying cause of death was classified as firearm homicide (E965.0 through E965.4, or E970) in the *ICD-9 (International Statistical Classification of Diseases, Injuries, and Causes of Death, Ninth Revision)*.

Main Outcome Measure.—County-specific firearm homicide rate.

Results.—In 1983 through 1985 and in 1987 through 1989, seven and 13 counties, respectively, were identified that had significantly high firearm homicide rates. Firearm homicide rates were significantly high in both time periods in the following counties: Los Angeles, California; Wayne, Michigan; Kings, New York; St Louis City, Missouri; and Baltimore City, Maryland. Firearm homicide rates increased significantly between 1983 through 1985 and 1987 through 1989 in 34 of the 80 counties. Twenty counties had significantly low rates in both time periods. Several counties with low rates in 1983 through 1985 experienced significant increases and by 1987 through 1989 were among those with high rates.

Conclusions.—Surveillance of firearm homicide rates at the county level in counties with high and with low rates is a necessary first step in the development of successful violence prevention programs. Those counties where rates are high and increasing are the counties that are in greatest need for intervention strategies. Knowledge of the incidence of nonfatal firearm injuries is also needed.

(*JAMA*. 1992;267:3054-3058)

From the Office of Analysis and Epidemiology, National Center for Health Statistics, Centers for Disease Control, Hyattsville, Md.

Reprint requests to the Office of Analysis and Epidemiology, National Center for Health Statistics, Room 1080, 6525 Belcrest Rd, Hyattsville, MD 20782 (Ms Fingerhut).

FIREARM homicide is the leading cause of death among black males 15 through 19 years of age in the United States, and has been since 1969 (Compressed Mortality File, National Center for Health Statistics, Centers for Disease Control, Hyattsville, Md, 1989 update). From 1987 through 1989, the firearm homicide rate among black males 15 through 19 years of age increased 71% to 85.3 deaths per 100 000 population, while the death rate from motor vehicle crashes (the second leading cause of death among black teenage males) fell 3% to 26.5 per 100 000 population (Fig 1).

In 1989, the firearm homicide rate among black males 15 through 19 years of age in metropolitan counties was 6.5 times the rate in nonmetropolitan counties (100.9 deaths compared with 15.5 deaths per 100 000 population). The rate in core counties (the largest metropolitan counties in which the primary central city is located) was two to three times the rates in the other metropolitan strata[1]. From 1987 through 1989, firearm homicide rates among 15- through 19-year-old black males increased considerably in metropolitan counties.[1]

While firearm homicide is a public health problem of national dimensions, intervention programs are more likely to be successfully implemented at the local level. This analysis identifies counties in the United States that had either significantly high or significantly low firearm homicide rates among black males 15 through 19 years of age in the period 1983 through 1985 and in the period 1987 through 1989, and/or experienced a significant increase in the fire arm homicide rate between 1983 through 1985 and 1987 through 1989. Knowing which specific counties have high rates and/or fast increases in their rates should assist injury prevention specialists de-

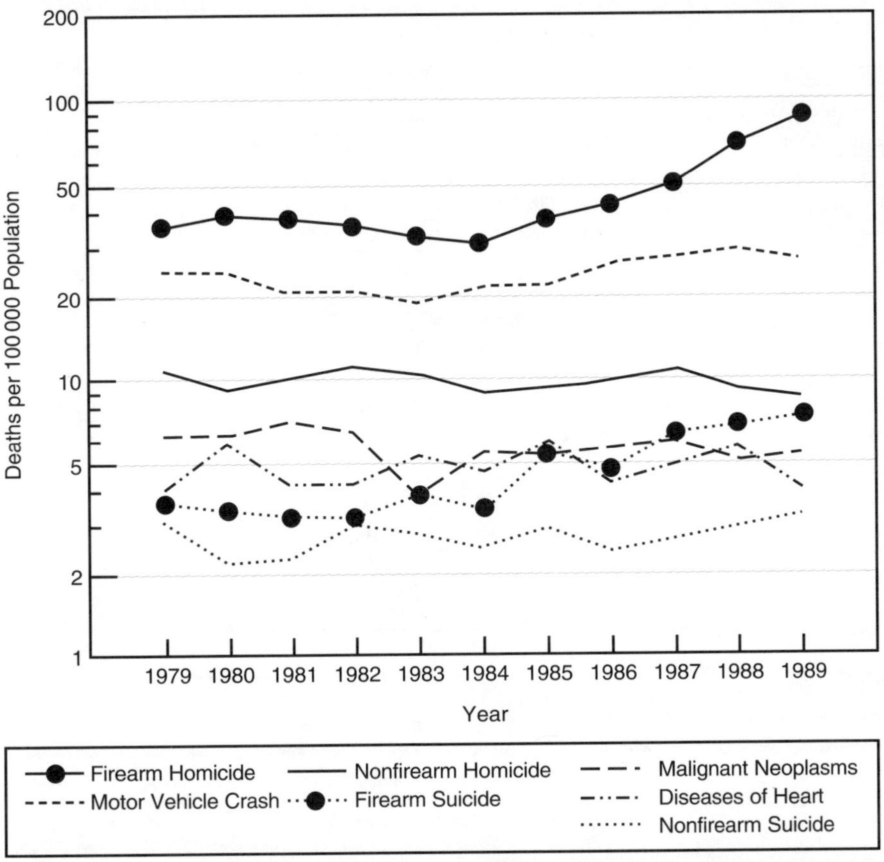

Fig 1.—Leading causes of death for black males 15 through 19 years of age, 1979 through 1989. (from the Compressed Mortality File of the National Center for Health Statistics, Centers for Disease Control).

velop more effective prevention programs and stimulate interaction among communities.

DATA AND METHODS

This analysis is restricted to black males 15 through 19 years of age. Throughout this article, the word "teenager" is used interchangeably with persons 15 through 19 years of age. The data are from the Compressed Mortality File, a county-level national mortality and population database maintained by the Office of Analysis and Epidemiology, National Center for Health Statistics, Centers for Disease Control, Hyattsville, Md. The Compressed Mortality File uses death records from the National Center for Health Statistics, National Vital Statistics System. Intercensal population estimates are from the Bureau of the Census. Firearm homicides are defined in the *International Statistical Classification of Diseases, Injuries, and Causes of Death, Ninth Revision*,[2] as codes E965.0 through E965.4 or E970.

Eighty of the 3075 counties in the United States with a population of at least 10 000 black males 15 through 19 years of age for the 3-year period 1987 through 1989 were selected for analysis. All 80 counties were metropolitan counties. Metropolitan counties as defined by the Office of Management and Budget are counties within a metropolitan statistical area.

Three years of population and mortality data were combined to provide relatively stable estimates. Two time periods were chosen for this analysis, 1983 through 1985 and 1987 through 1989. Based on a previous analysis, firearm homicide rates among teenagers declined from 1979 through 1984; thus, the period 1983 through 1985 is considered the end of this decline.[1] The period 1987 through 1989 is the most recent 3 years of national data available.

To determine whether an individual county's firearm homicide rate was significantly high for the period 1987 through 1989 compared with the rate for all 80 counties combined, we estimated the probability that the observed number of firearm homicides would occur in that county. To do this, a simulation was carried out with 1000 iterations. For each iteration, the observed number of firearm homicides in the 80 counties was distributed randomly among the counties in proportion to their black male 15- through 19-year-old populations. For each county, this procedure generated a distribution of firearm homicides with a mean approximately equal to the expected number of firearm homicides for the county. A county's observed number of firearm homicides was compared with the simulated distribution. If the county's observed number of firearm homicides or a larger number occurred in fewer than 5% of the iterations, the county's firearm homicide rate was significantly higher than the combined counties' rate. Conversely, the county's rate was significantly lower if the observed number or a smaller number of firearm homicides occurred in less than 5% of the iterations. The same procedure was carried out for the 1983 through 1985 period as well.

To determine whether there was a significant increase in firearm homicide between 1983 through 1985 and 1987 through 1989, a two-tailed t test of the difference between individual county rates for each period was calculated. Differences between death rates are considered significant if $P \leq .05$.

RESULTS

The black teenage male population in the 80 counties included 67% of all black teenage males residing in metropolitan counties in 1987 through 1989. In addition, these 80 counties accounted for 87% of the 2733 firearm homicide victims who had been residents of metropolitan counties during 1987 through 1989. The firearm homicide rate for black males 15 through 19 years of age in 1987 through 1989 in the 80 counties was 104.0 deaths per 100 000 population, about 30% higher than the rate in all metropolitan counties (80.4 per 100 000 population).

For the period 1987 through 1989, firearm homicide rates in the 80 counties were rank ordered and firearm homicide rates for black males 15 through 19 years of age in the top 25% (20 counties) of all 80 counties were considered high (Fig 2). Firearm homicide rates in 13 of the 20 counties were significantly higher than the rate for all 80 counties (Fig 2, asterisked counties). The firearm homicide rates in these 13 counties ranged from 129 deaths per 100 000 population to 227 deaths per 100 000 population. Note that only one county (Suffolk, Massachusetts) had a firearm homicide rate that was as high as the 13 counties, but not significantly different from the total.

In 1983 through 1985, the black teenage male firearm homicide rate for the

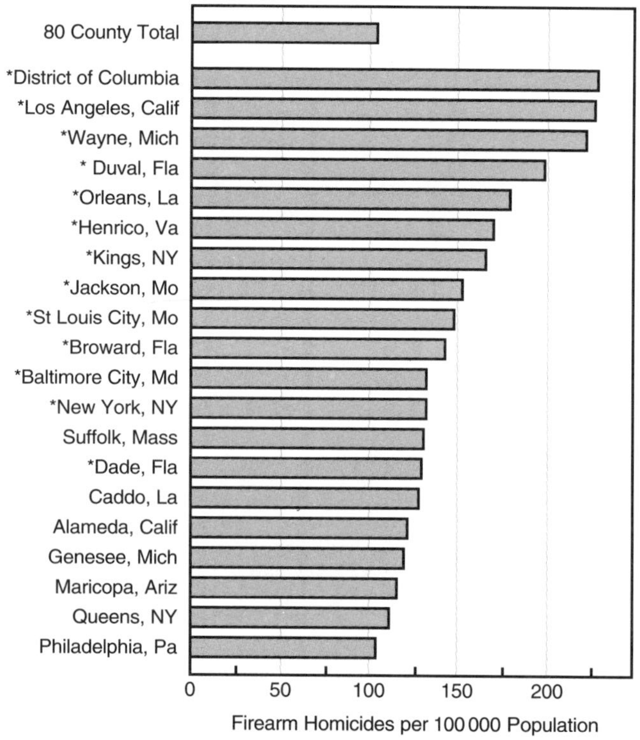

Fig 2.—Firearm homicide in counties ranked in top 25% among the 80 selected counties for black males 15 through 19 years of age, 1987 through 1989. An asterisk indicates that the firearm homicide rate was significantly high (from the Compressed Mortality File of the National Center for Health Statistics, Centers for Disease Control).

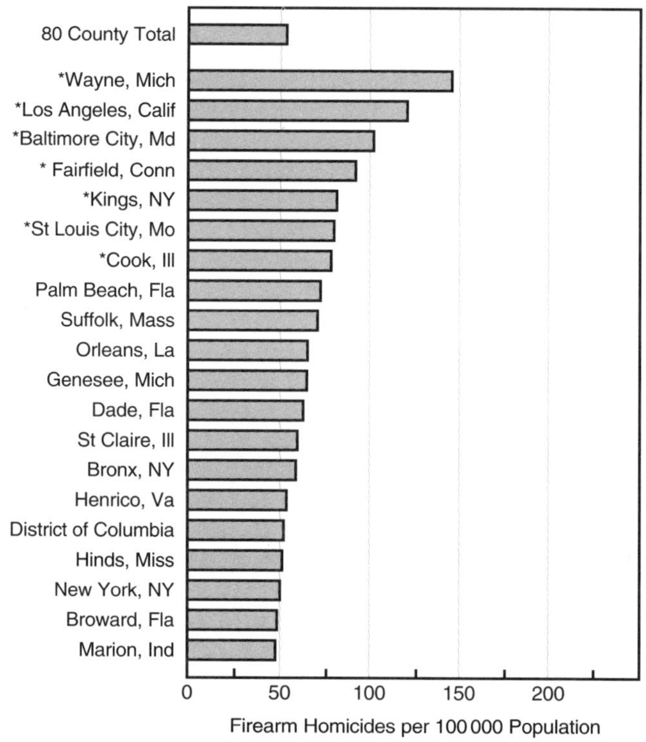

Fig 3.—Firearm homicide in counties ranked in top 25% among the 80 selected counties for black males 15 through 19 years of age, 1983 through 1985. An asterisk indicates that the firearm homicide rate was significantly high (from the Compressed Mortality File of the National Center for Health Statistics, Centers for Disease Control).

80 counties was 52.6 per 100 000 population, about 30% higher than for all metropolitan counties during that period. The firearm homicide rates in the 20 counties with rates in the highest quartile are shown in Fig 3. In 1983 through 1985, seven of these counties had significantly high firearm homicide rates compared with the rate for all 80 counties in 1983 through 1985 (Fig 3, asterisked counties). Firearm homicide rates in the seven counties ranged from 78 deaths to 145 deaths per 100 000 population. The rates in these seven counties ranked highest regardless of statistical significance.

Firearm homicide rates in the following five counties were significantly high in both 1983 through 1985 as well as in 1987 through 1989: Los Angeles, California; Wayne, Michigan; Kings, New York; St Louis City, Missouri; and Baltimore City, Maryland. The number of firearm homicides in these five counties accounted for 41% of all black teenage male firearm homicides in metropolitan counties in 1983 through 1985 and for 30% in 1987 through 1989.

Counties with significantly low firearm homicide rates were also identified. In 1987 through 1989, 36 of the 80 counties had firearm homicide rates among black teenage males that were lower than expected (Fig 4). Firearm homicide rates in these counties ranged from less than 10 deaths per 100 000 population to 89 deaths per 100 000 population. In 1983 through 1985, 28 of the 80 counties had firearm homicide rates that were significantly low, with rates ranging from less than 10 deaths to 39 deaths per 100 000 population (Fig 5). Twenty of the counties had significantly low rates in both time periods.

TRENDS

From 1983 through 1985 to 1987 through 1989, the firearm homicide rate increased significantly in 34 of the 80 counties (Table). (In four of these 34 counties there were no firearm homicides in 1983 through 1985 and there were seven to 12 firearm homicides in 1987 through 1989. In order to calculate a percentage change in the rates for these four counties, we assumed that each county had one firearm homicide in the earlier period.) Within this relatively short time frame, firearm homicide rates in 18 of the 34 counties more than tripled and in 10 of these 18 counties the rates jumped by factors of more than six.

Of the 20 counties with firearm homicide rates in the top quartile in 1987 through 1989, the rates increased significantly in all but three counties (Baltimore City, Maryland; Suffolk, Massachusetts; and Genesee, Michigan). Of those in the top quartile in 1983 through 1985, firearm homicide rates in 11 counties increased significantly. Of the seven counties with significantly high rates, increases were not significant in three counties (Fairfield, Connecticut; Baltimore City, Maryland; and Cook, Illinois). Three counties (Wayne, Michigan; Los Angeles, California; and St Louis City, Missouri) had significantly high firearm homicide rates in both time periods and significant increases in their firearm homicide rates. In four counties with significantly low rates in both time periods (Shelby, Tennessee; Richmond, Georgia; Jefferson, Kentucky; and Franklin, Ohio) significant increases were observed in their rates; three of these had no firearm homicides in 1983 through 1985.

COMMENT

This analysis has identified metropolitan counties with high firearm homicide rates, with low firearm homicide

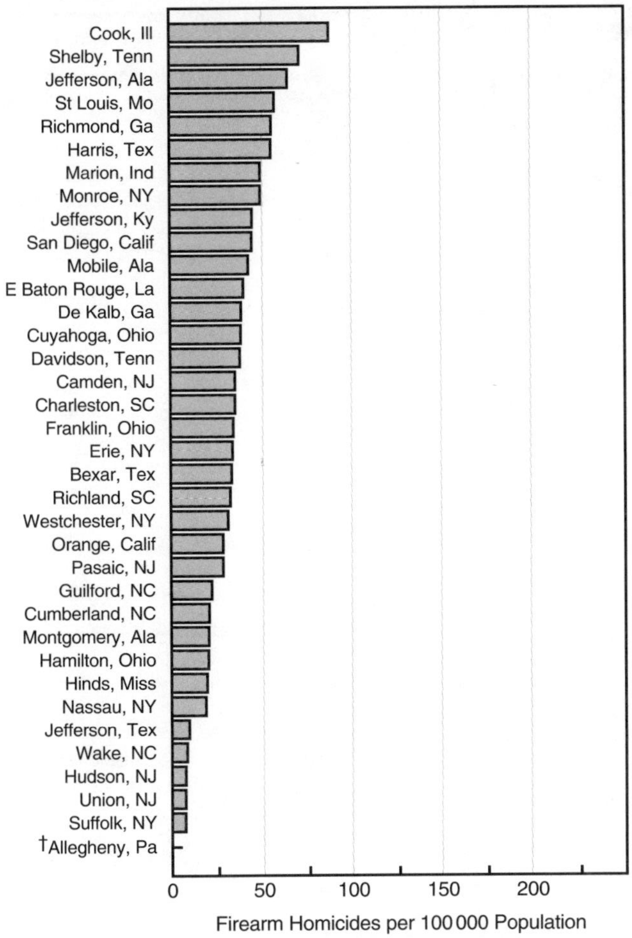

Fig 4.—Firearm homicide rates in counties with significantly low rates among the 80 selected counties for black males 15 through 19 years of age, 1987 through 1989. A dagger indicates that the homicide rate was zero (from the Compressed Mortality File of the National Center for Health Statistics, Centers for Disease Control).

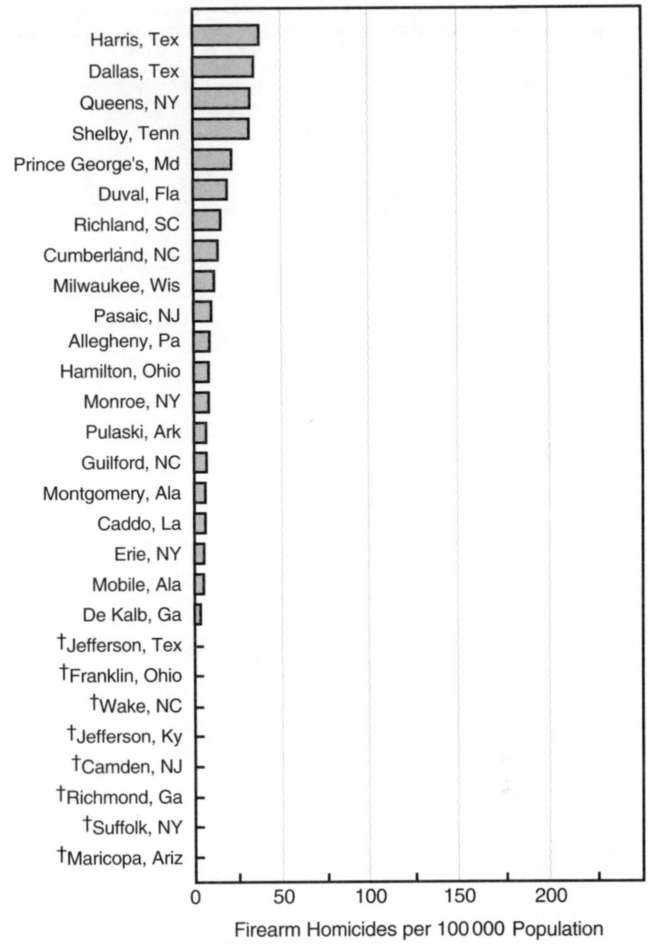

Fig 5.—Firearm homicide rates in counties with significantly low rates among the 80 selected counties for black males 15 through 19 years of age, 1983 through 1985. A dagger indicates that the homicide rate was zero (from the Compressed Mortality File of the National Center for Health Statistics, Centers for Disease Control).

rates, and those where rates have recently been increasing among black males 15 through 19 years of age. Those where the rates are high and increasing are the counties that are in greatest need for violence intervention strategies. Thirteen counties were identified as having significantly high firearm homicide rates in 1987 through 1989; five of the counties also had high rates in 1983 through 1985: Los Angeles, California; Wayne, Michigan; Kings, New York; St Louis City, Missouri; and Baltimore City, Maryland. In 34 of the 80 counties, firearm homicide rates increased significantly from 1983 through 1985 to 1987 through 1989. In 18 of those, the rate more than tripled. From a programmatic perspective, it is not important to compare the individual firearm homicide rates in those counties with significantly high rates. The critical point is that firearm homicide rates in these counties are in excess of the expected rate.

Counties with low rates of firearm homicide in 1987 through 1989 also warrant the attention of violence prevention teams. In Cook County, Illinois, with the largest population of black teenage males of all counties, the firearm homicide rate in 1987 through 1989 was significantly low. In 1983 through 1985, the rate in Cook County was significantly high compared with the rate for the 80 counties for that period. Between the two time periods, the rate did not increase significantly. In five counties (Cuyahoga, Ohio; San Diego, California; Jefferson, Alabama; Marion, Indiana; and St Louis, Missouri) the firearm rates in 1987 through 1989 were significantly low, were not significantly different in 1983 through 1985, and did not increase between the two periods.

Counties with currently low rates of firearm homicide or nonsignificant increases should not be complacent in their approach to prevention. Counties must be on the alert not only for increases in firearm homicides, but for events that may lead to a series of homicides. In the public health approach, we can think of "crime waves" just as we think of outbreaks of illness. Firearm homicide rates in 1983 through 1985 were significantly lower than expected in four counties: Duval, Florida; Caddo, Louisiana; Maricopa, Arizona; and Queens, New York. By 1987 through 1989, firearm homicide rates in those counties had increased significantly and were ranked in the upper quartile, with the rate in Duval County being significantly high. In addition, in 1983 through 1985, firearm homicide rates were similar to the total 80-county rate in seven counties: Orleans, Louisiana; Henrico, Virginia; Jackson, Missouri; Broward, Florida; Dade, Florida; New York, New York; and in the District of Columbia; by 1987 through 1989, firearm homicide rates in those

Firearm Homicide Rates and Ratio of Rates in Counties With Significant Increases in Rates for Black Males 15 Through 19 Years of Age, 1983 Through 1985 and 1987 Through 1989*

	Rate per 100 000 Population		
County, State	1983-1985	1987-1989	Ratio
Caddo, La	6.7	126.6	18.9
Pulaski, Ark	8.0	90.3	11.3
Duval, Fla	18.9	197.8	10.5
DeKalb, Ga	4.3	39.0	9.1
Mobile, Ala	5.8	42.4	7.3
Milwaukee, Wis	11.9	73.3	6.2
Jackson, Mo	32.1	152.0	4.7
District of Columbia	51.9	227.2	4.4
Prince George's, Md	20.5	85.9	4.2
Alameda, Calif	33.0	121.0	3.7
Queens, NY	32.6	110.4	3.4
Hillsborough, Fla	28.9	92.2	3.2
Henrico, Va	53.6	169.4	3.2
Tarrant, Tex	23.8	74.1	3.1
Broward, Fla	48.8	143.1	2.9
Fulton, Ga	35.7	101.4	2.8
San Bernardino, Calif	33.6	92.4	2.8
Orleans, La	65.0	178.3	2.7
New York, NY	49.7	132.2	2.7
Dallas, Tex	34.6	90.2	2.6
Essex, NJ	37.6	95.2	2.5
Philadelphia, Pa	41.5	103.4	2.5
Mecklenburg, NC	41.5	102.4	2.5
Shelby, Tenn	31.3	72.5	2.3
Dade, Fla	62.7	129.3	2.1
Kings, NY	80.7	164.9	2.0
Los Angeles, Calif	119.3	226.0	1.9
St Louis City, Mo	79.2	148.2	1.9
Bronx, NY	59.1	92.7	1.6
Wayne, Mich	145.1	220.8	1.5
Maricopa, Ariz	10.8†	114.9	10.6
Richmond, Ga	7.5†	55.6	7.4
Jefferson, Ky	6.3†	45.1	7.2
Franklin, Ohio	5.0†	34.6	6.9

*From the Compressed Mortality File of the National Center for Health Statistics, Centers for Disease Control.
†Rate calculated assuming there was one firearm homicide rather than the observed zero deaths.

counties were significantly high.

Surveillance of homicide at the county level is necessary in the development of successful violence prevention programs. However, it is only a first step. Knowledge of the incidence of nonfatal injuries is also needed. Having the additional information on firearm morbidity at the county level would allow us to know, for example, if the high number of firearm homicides in a particular county resulted from poor emergency medical care or, conversely, if the number would have been even higher if quality emergency medical care didn't exist. For example, emergency medical care in Wayne County, Michigan, and Los Angeles County, California, is likely to be high quality; thus, it is reasonable to assume that the number of firearm homicides in those counties underestimates the incidence of firearm violence. A locality's level of violence, after all, should be measured by nonfatal as well as fatal assaultive injuries; patterns of firearm assaultive injury may not be the same as patterns of firearm homicide. There are currently no reliable cause-specific injury morbidity estimates at the national level and relatively few localities across the country have begun to address this issue. Criminal justice data can be used to approximate the risk of injury. Among black teenagers in 1988, there were an estimated 3900 aggravated assault victims per 100 000 population,[3] close to 100 times the rate for black teenage firearm homicide.

In conclusion, firearm homicide is the leading cause of death for black males 15 through 19 years of age. It claims close to 1000 of their lives annually. These children live in a relatively small number of counties in the United States; it behooves us to protect their lives.

References

1. Fingerhut LA, Ingram DD, Feldman JJ. Firearm and nonfirearm homicide among persons 15 through 19 years of age: differences by level of urbanization, United States, 1979 through 1989. *JAMA.* 1992;267:3048-3053.
2. World Health Organization. *Manual of the International Statistical Classification of Diseases, Injuries, and Causes of Death, Based on the Recommendations of the Ninth Revision Conference, 1975.* Geneva, Switzerland: World Health Organization; 1977.
3. US Bureau of Justice Statistics. *Criminal Victimization in the United States 1988: A National Crime Survey Report.* Washington, DC: US Bureau of Justice; 1990. Publication NCJ-122024.

Death in the City

An American Childhood Tragedy

Leland Ropp, MD; Paul Visintainer, PhD; Jane Uman, MPH; David Treloar, MD

Objective.—To look at trends in mortality and homicide rates in a specific metropolitan area, comparing the urban and suburban mortality trends.

Design.—Descriptive study of mortality rates. Linear regression determined whether changes in mortality rates over time represented significant trends.

Setting.—Industrial metropolitan area in the United States, population, 2 337 891.

Participants.—Pediatric deaths (1 to 18 years of age) in a 9-year period. Population characteristics: 36% black, 64% white, 50% each urban and suburban.

Main Outcome Measures.—Pediatric mortality rates for 1980 through 1988, grouped by urban vs suburban, age, gender, and race. Rates calculated using national census figures and plotted over time.

Results.—There was a 50% increase in all-cause mortality in the urban pediatric population as compared with no change or a slight decline in the suburban and national populations. The increase was found in the black urban population. Homicide showed the largest increase (252%). Firearm-related homicides accounted for the majority of homicide deaths.

Conclusions.—(1) There were significant differences in mortality between the urban and suburban pediatric populations. (2) The increase in homicides, specifically firearm homicides, in the urban population accounted for the increase in overall mortality rates. (3) The increase in homicide rates was significant only for the 10- to 14-year-old males and the 15- to 18-year-old male and female portions of the black urban population. (4) Firearm homicides have become epidemic in the black urban population we studied.

(*JAMA*. 1992;267:2905-2910)

ACCURATE figures on mortality rates among children and adolescents are essential in planning appropriate public health and emergency health care policies. The National Center for Health Statistics (NCHS) tracks mortality rates. Individual authors, using their data, report trends or changes in rates on a regular basis.[1]

Since 1900 there has been a marked decrease in childhood mortality across all age groups. This is primarily due to the decrease in deaths caused by infectious diseases. There still remain substantial differences in the rate of decline with respect to age, gender, and race.[2]

Data from the NCHS on pediatric mortality rates show that homicide remains a major cause of death for blacks, regardless of gender. Nationally, homicide is the leading cause of death for black males and females 15 to 19 years of age.[2] For black males, aged 10 to 14 years, homicide has ranked either third or fourth as a cause of death for several years. Large disparities in homicide rates exist by gender and race. Males generally have higher rates than females, and blacks usually have higher rates than whites for all pediatric age groups. Changes in rates of homicide and the association with prevalence of guns are widely discussed topics in public health literature.[1-7]

The experience of health professionals working in inner-city emergency departments would suggest that the trends in pediatric mortality may be quite different locally from those projected at the national level. Homicide is widely perceived as a problem in American cities. However, NCHS data in the *Vital and Health Statistics Reports* have shown homicide rates in children only by geographic location at the county and state level. Information is regularly published on mortality rates at the city or county level, only for children less than 1 year of age. Furthermore, while the homicide problem in adolescent black males has received considerable attention,[1-3] younger children are perceived to be relatively immune from homicide and thus have received little attention, in comparison.

The purpose of this article is to examine the trends in pediatric homicide rates within a defined metropolitan region. Since national data may not reflect regional trends due to the aggregation of data, this study will present data on age-, race-, and gender-specific patterns of pediatric mortality, as well as trends related to firearm-related homicides. National data should be used to determine national policy, but local or regional data

This article is one of a number of articles on violence that will appear in upcoming issues of THE JOURNAL. The reader is referred to the June 10, 1992, issue, which will be dedicated to studies of violence.

From the Division of Pediatric Emergency Medicine (Drs Ropp and Treloar) and the Division of Biostatistics and Research Epidemiology (Dr Visintainer and Ms Uman), Henry Ford Hospital, Detroit, Mich.

Reprint requests to Emergency Department, Henry Ford Hospital, 2799 W Grand Blvd, Detroit, MI 48202 (Dr Ropp).

is necessary to determine local or regional policy. This additional data on all causes of mortality and specifically homicides will allow more effective planning of public health interventions, targeting specific age groups within specific demographic groups and areas.

METHODS

Wayne County, Michigan, was used as the metropolitan population base to examine trends in childhood mortality. The population was evenly divided in 1980 between the city of Detroit (urban population, 1 203 339) and suburban Wayne County (population, 1 134 552). Although both areas experienced declines in their populations during the 1980s, the distribution of the pediatric populations between the areas remained virtually unchanged in 1990. The pediatric population of the city of Detroit declined by 17.7% between 1980 (353 714) and 1990 (291 293). The suburban population showed a similar decline of 18.3% (319 104 to 260 653). The proportion of black children in Detroit increased from 76.3% in 1980 to 84.7% in 1990. The suburban pediatric population remained overwhelmingly white during the decade (92.3% in 1980 and 91.6% in 1990). Crime rates, average income, and other measures of the social environment indicate that social and economic stress are higher in Detroit than the remainder of Wayne County.[8]

The mortality data for all children in Wayne County, aged 1 to 18 years, were obtained from the Michigan Department of Health Center for Health Statistics death certificate records for the years 1980 through 1988. The causes of death for all external causes (motor vehicle accidents, suicide, homicides, fire), *International Classification of Diseases, Ninth Revision* (*ICD-9*)[9] E codes 800 through 999.9, are filled in by the Wayne County medical examiner, a forensic pathologist. The death certificates are coded by the Department of Health for cause of death using the *ICD-9* codes. The E codes 960 through 969 are specific types of homicide. Firearm homicides are E codes 965 through 965.4. Legal interventions, E codes 970 through 978, are not included in our homicides. The death certificates are classified by location of death rather than city of residence.

Pediatric deaths were classified by age group (1 to 4 years, 5 to 9 years, 10 to 14 years, and 15 to 18 years), sex, race (white, black), and location (city of Detroit vs suburban Wayne County). Population denominators for the same categories were obtained from the US Department of Commerce, Census Bureau, National Census, for 1980 and 1990.[8] Population bases for interim years were estimated by averaging the change in the age-, sex-, race-, and location-specific numbers from 1980 to 1990 over the 10-year period.

All mortality rates are reported as cases per 100 000 population. Crude rates and rates that are collapsed over time are age-adjusted to the 1980 Detroit pediatric population (age groups: 1 to 4 years, 5 to 9 years, 10 to 14 years, and 15 to 18 years). The regression equation with mortality rate as the dependent variable and year as the independent variable tested whether the slope of the fitted line deviates either positively or negatively from zero (no trend over time). Variables for age group, sex, race, and location, as well as interactions between these variables and year, were included in regression models to identify differences in average mortality rates and determine significant differences in trends among subgroups of the population. We note that mortality rates presented in this article represent "true" population rates and are not subject to sampling error.[10]

RESULTS

During the 9-year period covering 1980 through 1988, the all-cause mortality rate for children (1 to 18 years of age) increased almost 50% for the urban population. In 1980 the mortality rate was 49.48 per 100 000 population, while in 1988, the mortality rate had risen to 73.20 per 100 000 population. Conversely, the all-cause mortality rate for children in the suburban areas remained stable. The suburban mortality rate was 32.9 per 100 000 population in 1980 and 27.9 per 100 000 population in 1988.

Gender- and race-specific all-cause mortality rates for urban and suburban pediatric populations are shown in Fig 1, top and bottom, respectively. Black urban males showed a consistent and highly significant increase in all-cause mortality over the interval ($P<.0001$). The rate increased 74% from a low of 68.5 per 100 000 population in 1980 to 119.2 per 100 000 population in 1988. Although not nearly as striking, black urban females showed a significant 50% increase in the all-cause mortality rate over the interval. The rate increased from 29.9 per 100 000 population in 1980 to 44.7 per 100 000 population in 1988 ($P=.016$) for black females residing in the urban population (city of Detroit). Neither white males or white females in the urban population nor any gender- or race-specific suburban group showed any significant change in all-cause mortality during the 9-year interval.

Figure 2 presents the pediatric deaths due to homicides compared with all other causes of deaths for the urban population collapsing across gender, age, and race categories. The nonhomicide death rate showed a nominal 11% increase from 40.71 per 100 000 population in 1980 to 45.28 per 100 000 population in 1988 ($P=.083$). In contrast, the homicide rate showed a highly significant 252% increase over the period increasing from 8.76 per 100 000 population in 1980 to 30.84 per 100 000 population in 1988 ($P<.0001$). Consequently, the proportion of the total pediatric death rate explained by the homicide rate increased substantially. In 1980, the homicide rate accounted for about 18% of the total urban all-cause mortality rate. In 1988, this proportion increased to approximately 41%.

Focusing on homicide rates among pediatric subgroups in Detroit, black males had significantly higher homicide rates than females ($P=.001$), and homicide rates increased significantly with increasing age group ($P<.001$). Adjusting for rate differences by gender and age group, there was a significant increase in homicide rates from 1980 through 1988 ($P=.03$). The age- and gender-specific homicide rates for black urban youths from 1980 through 1988 are shown in the Table. The increase for males in the 10- to 14-year-old age group was about two deaths per 100 000 population per year ($P=.01$), whereas the increase for males in the 15- to 18-year-old age group was about 25 deaths per 100 000 population per year ($P=.001$). For females, a significant increasing trend in homicides occurred only for the 15- to 18-year-old age group ($P=.03$). The rate of increase during the interval was about 2.5 deaths per 100 000 population.

Figure 3 examines the homicide rates by comparing the 15- to 18-year-old black urban males with the black suburban males and the white urban and suburban males. There is a significant rise in homicides, 54.4 per 100 000 population to 185.85 per 100 000 population ($P=.0008$), from 1980 through 1988 in only the black urban subgroup. The fluctuations in the homicide rate over time in the suburban black population, $P=.99$, reflects the relatively small population base, approximately 2500 individuals, from which these rates were derived.

The relationship between firearm and other types of homicide is shown in Fig 4 for the 15- to 18-year-old black urban male population. The graph clearly demonstrates an overwhelming preponderance of gun involvement. The rate of firearm-related homicides increased from 54.4 per 100 000 population in 1980 to 168.3 per 100 000 population in 1988 ($P=.001$), increasing about 22 deaths per year. In contrast, homicides not involv-

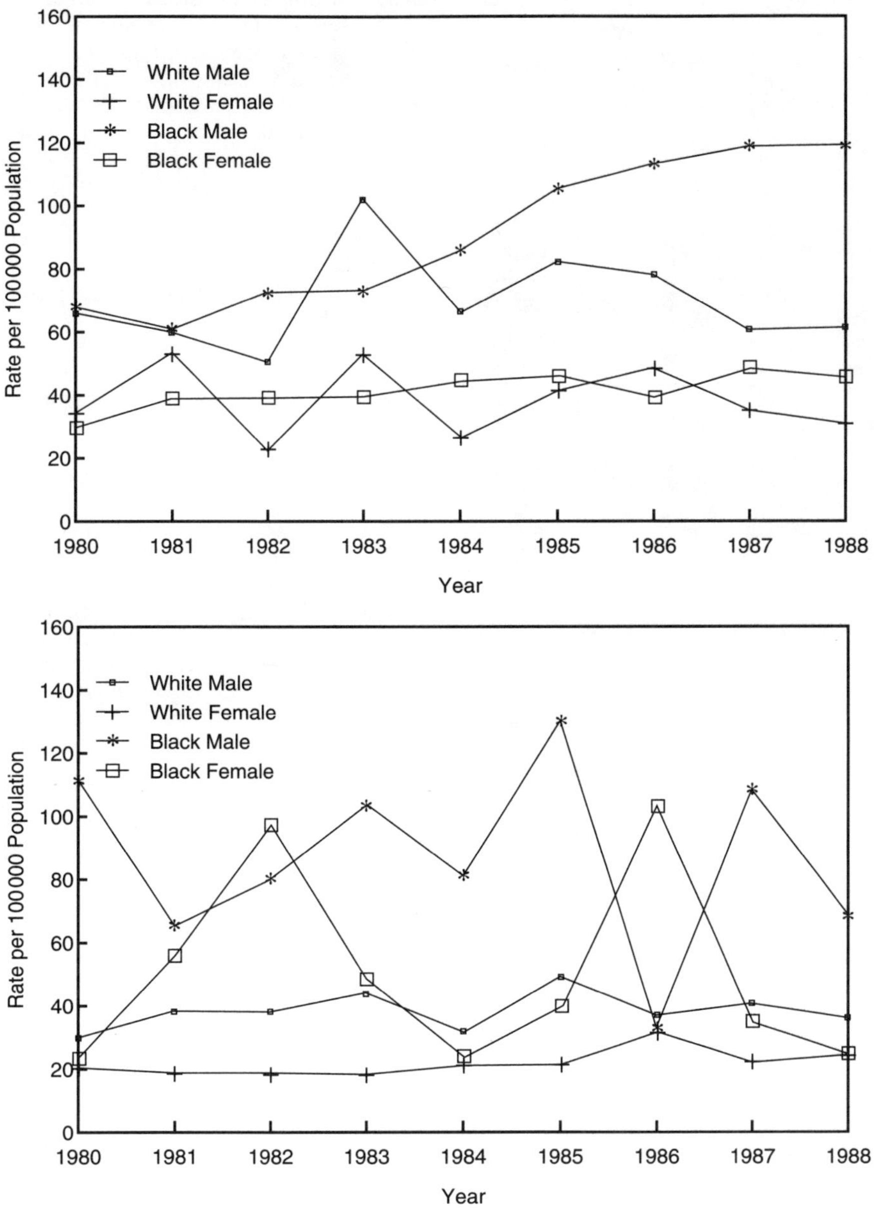

Fig 1.—Top, Urban pediatric all-cause mortality rate by gender and race, 1980 through 1988, age-adjusted to 1980 urban total pediatric population. Bottom, Suburban pediatric all-cause mortality rate by gender and race, 1980 through 1988, age-adjusted to 1980 urban total pediatric population.

ing firearms showed a marginal increase of two per 100 000 population each year and only a slightly positive trend (*P*=.11). Thus, the increasing trend in the homicide rate among 15- to 18-year-old black urban males could be attributed almost entirely to firearm homicides.

In 1988, homicides were the leading cause of death for black males aged 5 years and older. In each of the three age groups (5 to 9 years, 10 to 14 years, and 15 to 18 years), homicides accounted for 30%, 41%, and 62% of the total deaths, respectively. For females, homicides ranked as the leading cause of death in the 10- to 14- and 15- to 18-year-old age groups, accounting for 36% and 32% of all deaths, respectively, in 1988. In all other age groups, homicide was one of the top two causes of death in 1988.

COMMENT

Death rates have shown a steady downward trend for all age groups of children (1 to 19 years of age) in the United States since 1900. The decrease in mortality in the early part of the century was due to decreases in death due to natural causes. National Center for Health Statistics figures showed a 37% decrease from 1970 through 1985 in the death rate for children aged 1 to 4 years, 50% for children aged 5 to 9 years, 25% for children aged 10 to 14 years, and 27% for children aged 15 to 19 years.[2]

However, national trends in mortality rates can obscure trends in rates occurring in smaller restricted geographic areas. For this reason, we examined the pediatric mortality rates and trends (1 through 18 years of age) within Wayne County, Michigan, ie, Detroit municipality vs the remainder of Wayne County. The urban population showed an increase in mortality rates of 50% over the 9-year period, 1980 through 1988. This is in contrast to the suburban Wayne County population, which showed a nonsignificant decrease of 15% in childhood mortality rates over the identical 9-year period, with a resulting 160% difference in childhood mortality rates in our urban and suburban populations in 1988.

Natural causes of death accounted for 90% of childhood (1 to 19 years of age) deaths in 1900, 80% in 1934, but by 1985 accounted for only 36% of childhood deaths.[2] In Wayne County, Michigan, deaths due to natural causes accounted for a slightly higher percentage (45%) of all deaths in 1985 for both the urban and suburban populations. However, due to the rise in deaths from external causes, by 1988, natural causes of death comprised only 25% of all deaths in the urban population, while remaining 46% in the suburban population.

Deaths due to all external causes combined decreased nationally for all age groups (1 to 19 years of age) in the period from 1968 through 1985.[2] The only specific external causes of death to show slight increases nationally have been homicide and suicides.[2] Nationally, homicides showed a slight increase for children under 15 years of age through 1985, but has never ranked higher than third or fourth for any specific age, gender, or race age group under 15 years of age.[1] The homicide rate in the black 15- to 19-year-old males showed a decrease from 1970 through 1978 (65 per 100 000 population to 39 per 100 000 population).[2] Since then, homicides have risen nationally to 79.5 per 100 000 population in 15- to 19-year-old black males by 1988.[10] Homicide became the leading cause of death for black females 15 to 19 years of age in 1971 and has remained three to five times higher than for white females.[2]

In this study, the increase in the urban all-cause mortality rate over the 9-year interval appears to be due largely to an increase in homicide rates. Homicide rates increased 252%, whereas death rates for all other causes combined increased 11% during the interval. There was a substantial rise in ho-

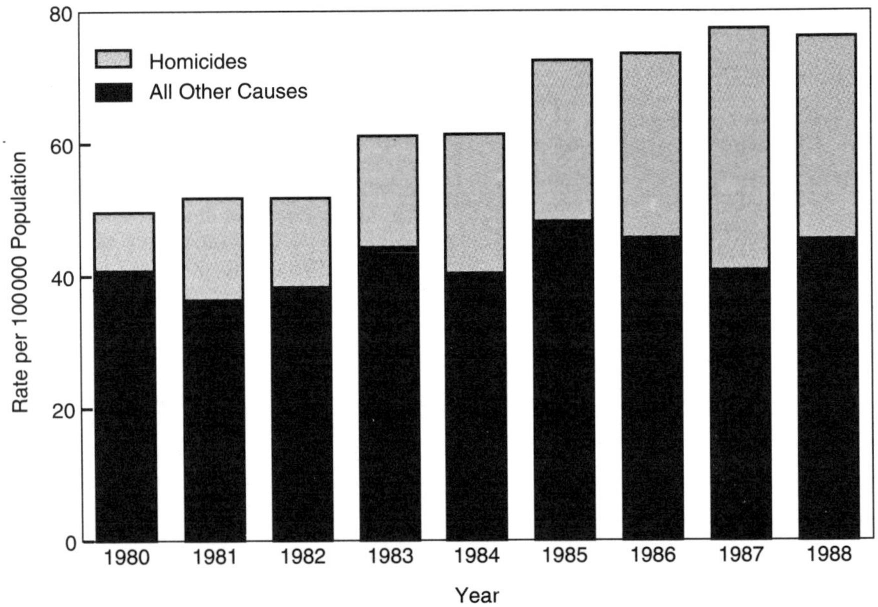

Fig 2.—Urban pediatric mortality rate, homicide vs all other causes of death rates, 1980 through 1988, age-adjusted to 1980 urban total pediatric population.

Urban Homicide Rates per 100 000 Population Among Blacks, by Age Group and Gender, 1980 Through 1989

Age Group, y/Gender	Year 1980	1981	1982	1983	1984	1985	1986	1987	1988	P*
1-4										
M	3.70	3.66	7.24	3.58	17.71	3.50	3.47	10.29	10.18	.35
F	3.78	14.96	11.10	10.99	10.87	3.59	14.20	10.54	10.43	.72
5-9										
M	0.0	0.0	5.22	10.65	2.72	0.0	0.0	8.69	17.77	.12
F	5.09	5.18	2.64	0.0	5.50	2.81	2.87	0.0	2.99	.21
10-14										
M	10.22	12.98	15.82	8.04	16.35	16.62	22.55	17.21	32.11	.01
F	2.59	7.89	5.34	2.72	13.79	5.61	2.86	8.72	14.79	.18
15-18										
M	54.43	71.71	68.55	96.33	117.42	180.26	201.83	272.46	185.85	<.001
F	6.65	23.32	6.68	20.09	30.21	16.82	30.36	30.44	27.13	.03

*Test of trend.

micide rates in the urban population, with increases in the black 15- to 18-year-old males (240%), 15- to 18-year-old black females (300%), and 10- to 14-year-old males (200%). Homicide was the leading or second ranked cause of death in all pediatric age groups in our urban black population by 1988.

In 15- to 18-year-old males, firearm-related homicides increased at a rate of about 22 deaths per 100 000 population per year. Other types of homicide increased, on average, two deaths per 100 000 population per year.

The rise in childhood mortality rate in our urban population could be attributed almost entirely to increasing homicide rates and primarily homicide by gun. Unlike the national figures, there was no decrease in deaths due to homicide in the early 1980s and since 1984 there has been an explosive rise in the rate of homicides.

There are several limitations to the interpretations of these data that should be noted. First, age, gender- and race-specific estimates of the Wayne County pediatric population were based on data from the 1980 and 1990 census estimates. Changes from 1980 to 1990 were interpolated over the intervals. It is likely that our mortality rates will differ slightly from those derived from sample estimates. However, these differences are likely to be small and have a negligible effect on the trends presented here.

A second limitation concerns the variability in rates arising from small numbers of deaths or small population denominators. For instance, we assume there is no sampling variability in these rates (ie, the entire population of deaths and persons at risk have been enumerated). However, a change from one year to the next of one or two deaths may represent a large change in the death rate for specific subgroups of the pediatric population (ie, 15- to 18-year-old black suburban males). We note that large variability in mortality rates over time would make detection of significant trends more difficult.

Although previous studies have shown substantial misclassification of cause of death for some diseases,[11] classification of homicides appears to be extremely accurate. Moyer et al [12] found the sensitivity and specificity of coding for homicides to be greater than 95% for a sample of adults. We expect the coding accuracy would be similarly high in this population because of the high visibility afforded pediatric homicides and because all external causes of death are reviewed and coded by medical examiners who are forensic pathologists.

The classification of death certificates by location would potentially allow some deaths in the urban numbers to be suburban children who died in the city or vice versa. Children with injuries or deaths that occurred in the suburbs would generally be taken to suburban hospitals, but the possibility exists that they would be stabilized and then transferred to urban hospitals where the death occurred.

With respect to these limitations, we believe that the trends in pediatric homicides in the Detroit area focus on a serious problem that will continue to grow. The influence of firearms on pediatric homicide rates is clear. These data are consistent with previous reports suggesting an association between firearms and pediatric fatalities. For instance, homicide violence has been noted to be the second leading cause of death due to injury after motor vehicle accidents in children.[13] In 1990, Beaver et al[14] looked at pediatric firearm fatalities in Maryland and found 48% to be due to handguns. Copeland[15] found an increased incidence of firearm fatalities among children 14 years of age and younger in Dade County, Florida, with 70% of the firearms owned by a family member and handguns accounting for 70% of the injuries. Wood and Mercy[16] found unintentional firearm-related fatalities were highest in low-income areas. A study of firearm injuries in Galveston, Tex, showed a fatality rate of 30% and an increased incidence in black males.[17]

Several studies have looked at the prevalence of firearms in the population and its relationship to homicide and other violent crime. In a study comparing homicide rates in Seattle, Wash, and Vancouver, British Columbia, Sloan et al[6]

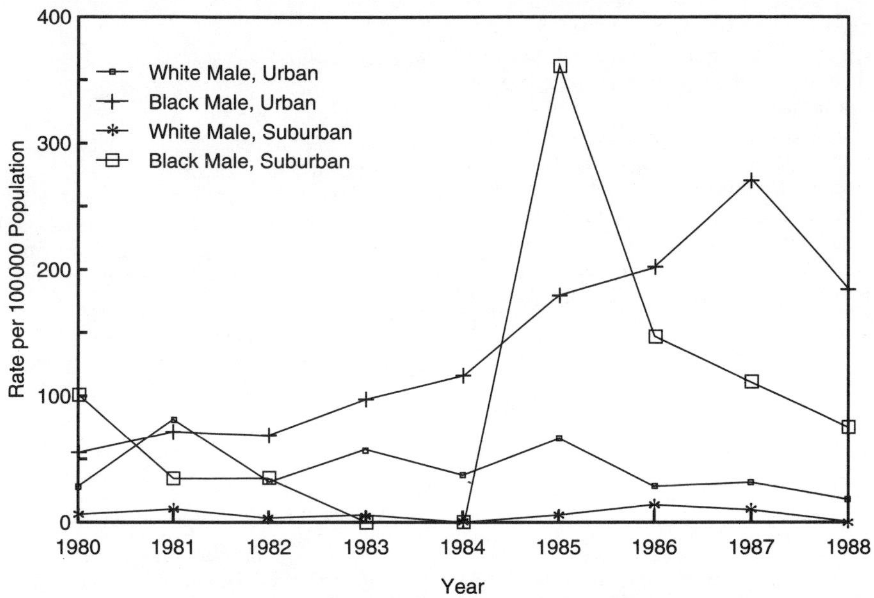

Fig 3.—Homicide rate in urban vs suburban 15- to 18-year-old males by race, 1980 through 1988.

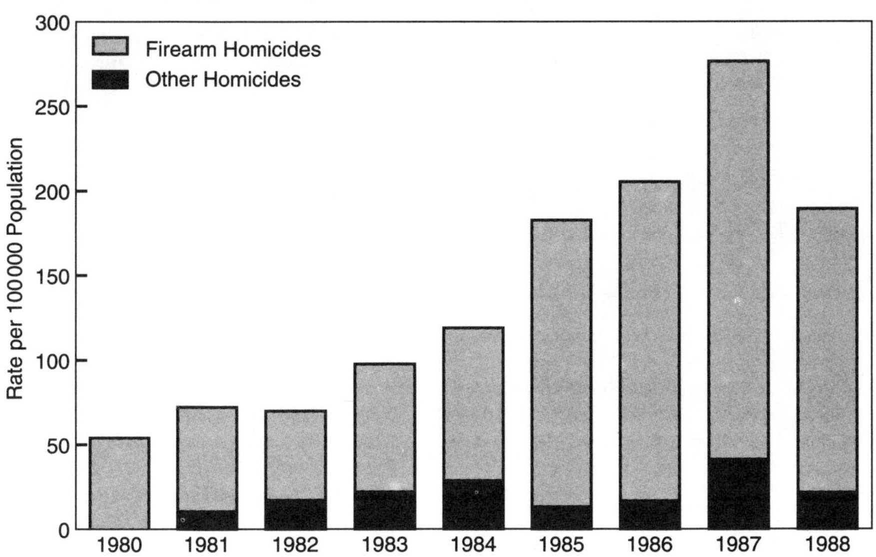

Fig 4.—Urban black males, 15 to 18 years of age, firearm homicide vs other types of homicide rates, 1980 through 1988.

reported that while all other violent crimes were similar in incidence, the relative risk for death by homicide was 1.63 for Seattle compared with Vancouver, with the excess risk due to the 4.8-fold difference in murder using a handgun. A similar study compared northeastern Ohio with a similar region in Denmark. The rate of homicide in Denmark was one-fifth the rate in Ohio.[18] In both studies, the difference was a restrictive gun control law and limited availability of handguns in the general population. In another study, the introduction of a restrictive law on handguns was associated with a significant reduction in both the homicide and suicide rates in the District of Columbia, despite the ready availability of firearms in neighboring states.[19] However, the effectiveness of firearm restriction on homicide rate reduction has been questioned by a recent study that looked at homicide rates in Canada and neighboring states after excluding large cities from the analysis.[20]

The significant increase in homicides in older childhood groups compared with younger children reflects different homicide patterns. Older children's mortalities are more often due to firearms and occur during arguments, participation in criminal activity, and poor supervision in adult environments. Homicides in younger children are more often due to abuse by parents and caretakers and less likely due to firearms.[21-23] Firearm availability is therefore less likely to affect homicides rates in this age group. Firearm homicide in young children is more likely a random occurrence, possibly leading to the high degree of variability in rates when compared with the systematic increase that occurred in the older children over the same time period in our study.

The fact that there were large variations in homicide rates in the suburban 15- to 18-year-old black male population, but no overall trend, does not support those individuals who have postulated a subculture of violence in the black population. Our study, however, does support those individuals who have postulated a relationship between poverty, family breakdown, and other problems in the urban environments.

Our study does not answer the question of whether effective gun control legislation would reduce pediatric homicides. However, these data clearly emphasize two points: (1) that homicides explain a rapidly growing proportion of the total pediatric mortality rate and (2) that guns, in particular, are involved in a disproportional large number of homicide deaths. Baker[4] elegantly summed up the argument by noting that "people without guns injure people: guns kill them." In Detroit, this could be paraphrased as "people with guns kill black children."

The American Academy of Pediatrics, in a recent policy statement on firearms, recommends several steps including removing handguns from children's environments by steps, including restrictions on the purchase and possession of firearms up to and including a ban, gun education courses, preventive safety counseling for parents, and reducing the romanticization of guns.[24] The American College of Emergency Physicians recommends several steps relating to handguns, including mandatory waiting periods, screening, and education prior to the purchase of a handgun, as well as increased penalties for the commission of crimes using a handgun.[25] Christoffel[26] has outlined steps toward reducing pediatric injuries from firearms through a legislative and regulatory course.

Clearly, in our urban population, with homicide as the leading or second leading cause of death in all age groups of black children, we have an epidemic that requires a concerted public health approach. The study by Fingerhut and Kleinman[3] in 1990 confirms that this is a national problem in the 15- to 24-year-old black male age group. The fact that these trends may be specific to the Detroit area and potentially other large urban areas and differ from national data highlights the importance of examining regional trends.

Such data are necessary to tailor interventions and meet public health goals. Secretary of Health and Human Services Sullivan[27] notes that it will require a broad-based approach addressing issues including poverty, drug and alcohol abuse, and working to keep our families together. He states that we need to develop "a culture of character" and teach respect and concern for others and skills such as conflict resolution. With a broad-based approach, we may be able to reduce violence among children and adolescents and meet specific goals for reducing homicides that are outlined in Healthy People 2000.[28]

CONCLUSIONS

1. There were significant differences in mortality between the urban and suburban pediatric populations.

2. The increase in homicides, specifically homicide by gun in the urban population, accounted for the increase in overall mortality rates.

3. The increase in homicides was significant for only the 10- to 14-year-old male and 15- to 18-year-old male and female subgroups of the black urban population.

4. Homicide by gun is an epidemic in the black urban population we studied.

References

1. Fingerhut L, Kleinman J. Mortality among children and youth. *Am J Public Health.* 1989;79:899-901.
2. Fingerhut L, Kleinman J. Trends and current status in childhood mortality. *Vital Health Stat 3.* Washington, DC: US Dept of Health and Human Services; January 1989:1-44.
3. Fingerhut L, Kleinman J. International and interstate comparisons of homicide among young males. *JAMA.* 1990;263:3292-3295.
4. Baker S. Without guns, do people kill people? *Am J Public Health.* 1985;75:587-588.
5. Rockett I, Smith G. Homicide, suicide, motor vehicle crash, and fall mortality: United States' experience in comparative perspective. *Am J Public Health.* 1989;79:1396-1400.
6. Sloan JH, Kellerman A, Reay D, et al. Handgun regulations, crime, assaults, and homicide: a tale of two cities. *N Engl J Med.* 1988;319:1256-1262.
7. Christoffel K. Release of the forum on firearms and children report. In: *Proceedings of the Medical/Science Writers Conference, July 18, 1990, New York.* Elk Grove Village, Ill: American Academy of Pediatrics; 1990.
8. *State and Metropolitan Area Data Book, 1986.* Washington, DC: US Bureau of the Census; 1986.
9. *International Classification of Diseases; Ninth Revision.* Washington, DC: US Dept of Health and Human Services; 1980. US Public Health Service publication PHS 80-1260.
10. Fingerhut L, Kleinman J, Godfrey E, Rosenberg H. Firearm mortality among children, youth, and young adults 1-34 years of age, trends and current status: United States, 1979-1988. *Monthly Vital Stat Rep.* 1991;39:1-15.
11. Gittelsohn A, Royston P. Annotated bibliography of cause-of-death validation studies: 1958-1980. *Vital Health Stat 2.* Hyattsville, Md: National Center for Health Statistics; 1982:1-42. Publication PHS 82-1363.
12. Moyer LA, Boyle CA, Polluck DA. Validity of death certificates for injury-related causes of death. *Am J Epidemiol.* 1989;130:1024-1032.
13. Guyer B, Ellers B. Childhood injuries in the United States. *AJDC.* 1990;144:649-652.
14. Beaver B, Moore V, Peclet M, Haller A, Smialek J, Hill JL. Characteristics of pediatric firearm fatalities. *J Pediatr Surg.* 1990;25:97-100.
15. Copeland A. Childhood firearms fatalities: the metropolitan Dade County experience. *South Med J.* 1991;84:175-178.
16. Wood N, Mercy J. Unintentional firearm-related fatalities, 1970-1984. *MMWR CDC Surveill Summ.* 1988:37:1:47-52.
17. Lee R, Waxweiler R, Dobbins J, Paschetag T. Incidence rates of firearm injuries in Galveston, Texas, 1979-1981. *Am J Epidemiol.* 1971;134:511-521.
18. Hedeboe J, Charles AV, Nielson J, et al. Interpersonal violence: patterns in a Danish community. *Am J Public Health.* 1985;75:651-653.
19. Loftin C, McDowall D, Wiersema B, Cottey T. Effects of restrictive licensing of handguns on homicide and suicide in the District of Columbia. *N Engl J Med.* 1991;325:1615-1620.
20. Centerwall BS. Homicide and the prevalence of handguns: Canada and the United States, 1976 to 1980. *Am J Epidemiol.* 1991;134:1245-1260.
21. Jason J. Childhood homicide spectrum. *AJDC.* 1983;137:578-581.
22. Christoffel KK, Anzinger NK, Amari M. Homicide in childhood: distinguishable patterns of risk related to developmental levels of victims. *Am J Forensic Med Pathol.* 1983;4:129-137.
23. Paulson JA, Rushforth NB. Violent death in children in a metropolitan county: changing patterns of homicide, 1958-1982. *Pediatrics.* 1986;78:1013-1020.
24. Policy statement: firearm injuries affecting the pediatric population. *AAP News.* 1992;8:22-23.
25. ACEP's position on weapons. *ACEP News.* 1990;9:4.
26. Christoffel K. Toward reducing pediatric injuries from firearms: charting a legislative and regulatory course. *Pediatrics.* 1991;88:294-305.
27. Sullivan L. Violence as a public health issue. *JAMA.* 1991;265:2778.
28. *Healthy People 2000: National Health Promotion and Disease Prevention Objectives.* Washington, DC: US Dept of Health and Human Services, Public Health Service; 1990.

Primary Care Physicians' Response to Domestic Violence

Opening Pandora's Box

Nancy Kathleen Sugg, MD, MPH, Thomas Inui, MD, ScM

Objective.—To explore primary care physicians' experiences with domestic violence victims to determine the barriers to problem recognition and intervention in the primary care setting.

Design.—Ethnography, a qualitative research method involving the use of open-ended, semistructured interviews.

Setting.—An urban health maintenance organization serving a predominantly white, middle-income population.

Participants.—Thirty-eight physicians, predominantly family practitioners (89%), were interviewed.

Results.—Analysis of the interviews revealed that physicians found exploring domestic violence in the clinical setting analogous to "opening Pandora's box." Their issues include lack of comfort, fear of offending, powerlessness, loss of control, and time constraints.

Conclusion.—This study revealed several barriers that physicians perceived as preventing them from comfortably intervening with domestic violence victims. These issues need to be addressed in training programs. Further studies should be done to assess generalizability of these findings to other groups of physicians.

(*JAMA*. 1992;267:3157-3160)

THE IMPACT of repetitive violence on an individual's health often brings domestic violence into the medical setting. Since it is believed that the majority of medical visits related to domestic violence are not in the form of overt trauma, but present as multiple somatic complaints or stress-related illnesses, primary care physicians are in a key position to offer referral for intervention.[1] Although the term *domestic violence* is used to describe the use of violence against a variety of household members, this study focuses on primary care physicians' response to violence between intimate partners or spouses.

The landmark prevalence study for the general population was conducted in 1975.[2] In a nationwide random sample of couples, 28% were found to have experienced violence at some point in their history. Furthermore, 3.8% of women living in couples had experienced severe violence in the year of the study. When extrapolated to the general population, this represents 1.8 million women per year being battered; if divorced or separated women are included, this estimate is 3 to 4 million women per year.[3]

In the medical literature, most of the prevalence data are from emergency department studies. One survey[4] of emergency department patients found that 22% of both men and women had experienced at least one episode of domestic violence. McLeer and Anwar[5] found that when an appropriate trauma history was obtained, 30% of female trauma cases were a result of domestic violence.

Recently, concern about physician responsiveness to domestic violence has been expressed.[6] Several studies have shown that even with knowledge of the underlying cause of the trauma, many physicians fail to respond to the battering. One study[7] found that in 40% of the cases where physicians interacted with battered women in an emergency department setting, physicians made no response to the abuse. In another emergency department that had a protocol for domestic violence, in 92% of the domestic violence cases, physicians failed to give any referral or follow-up for abuse.[8]

Little information is available on the prevalence of domestic violence in the primary care setting or on the primary care physicians' response to domestic violence. This study explores primary care physicians' experiences with and attitudes about domestic violence to determine the barriers to effective intervention in a primary care setting.

METHODS

The goal of this study was to uncover the barriers to domestic violence intervention from within the physician's frame of reference, as opposed to verifying the investigators' a priori hypotheses about the barriers. For this reason, ethnography was the chosen research method. Ethnography is a qualitative research method that seeks to generate hypotheses through analysis of narrative data obtained by in-depth interviews. One of us (N.K.S.) conducted all the interviews after studying ethnographic techniques and training with a medical anthropologist.

The study consisted of semistructured, open-ended interviews with 38 primary care physicians between August 1990 and February 1991. The study was approved by the Human Subjects Review Committee at the University of Washington, Seattle, and informed consent was obtained from all participants. Physicians were asked to describe domestic violence cases they had managed. Probe questions were asked concerning the physicians' role in identifying and intervening in domestic violence cases and also the physicians' own personal experiences of violence or abuse. The interviews lasted approximately 1 hour and were audiotaped. Demographic information was obtained at the end of the interviews. Brief field notes were made after the interviews, and the tapes transcribed.

From the Division of General Internal Medicine, University of Washington, Seattle. Dr Sugg was a fellow in the Robert Wood Johnson Clinical Scholars Program, Seattle, when this work was completed.

The views expressed in this article do not necessarily reflect the views of the Robert Wood Johnson Foundation.

Reprint requests to Harborview Medical Center, 325 Ninth Ave, Seattle, WA 98104 (Dr Sugg).

The Study Site

A large, urban health maintenance organization (HMO) was chosen as the site of the study. The HMO had several attributes that made it an optimal study site, including a large primary care physician staff, an orientation toward disease and injury prevention, and a research group interested in the prevalence of domestic violence. There was no protocol in place for dealing with intimate-partner violence at the time of this study. The HMO served an enrollee population that was predominantly white and middle-income, with the majority of enrollees having received some education beyond high school.

The Participants

Primary care physicians serving in six of seven satellite clinics associated with the urban hospital were selected for the study. One clinic was excluded from the study because of the familiarity of the clinic staff with the investigator. At the onset of the study, the intent was to interview 35 to 40 subjects. The physicians were sent letters describing the study and requesting participation. Of the 58 physicians who received the letter, 41 (71%) agreed to participant, eight (14%) refused to participate, and nine (14%) could not be reached after multiple telephone attempts. Three physicians who agreed to participate were not interviewed because of schedule conflicts. Of the 38 physicians who were interviewed, 63% were men and 37% were women, which was representative of the male-to-female primary care provider ratio at the institution. The age range was from 33 to 58 years old, with a mean of 41 years. The study group was 89% white, 8% Asian, and 3% black. Eighty-two percent of the physicians were married, and 87% had children. The group consisted of 34 family practitioners and four internists. Time since graduation from medical school ranged from 4 to 29 years, with a mean and median of 15 years.

Analysis

Multiple readings of the transcripts were performed to identify major ideas or themes revealed in the physicians' words, phrases, metaphors, and examples. Important and frequently expressed ideas or themes were then studied for patterns of connection and grouped into broader categories, for example, issues of power, issues of privacy, and issues of time constraints. The dominant ideas and patterns of connection were compared between various subgroups of physicians, such as men and women, abused and nonabused.

Validity

Method of analysis and review of results were critiqued by two independent medical anthropologists. Peer review of hypothesis formation and data analysis was formally accomplished in work-in-progress sessions with nine physicians who were not study participants and not staff members of the HMO study site. Member group review was accomplished by distributing the final results to all physicians who participated in the study and asking for their critiques. Of the five participants who responded with critiques, none expressed concern regarding the accuracy of the findings.

RESULTS

Repeatedly, the image of opening Pandora's box[1] was used by physicians to describe their reaction to exploring domestic violence with patients. Eighteen percent of physicians used the phrase, "Pandora's box." (According to Greek mythology, Pandora was the first woman. Her creation was part of Zeus' revenge against Prometheus for providing mankind with fire. She single-handedly opened a box and unleashed the spites of aging, labor, sickness, insanity, passion, and vice into the world.[9]) Eight percent used analogous phrases such as "opening a can of worms."

> I think that some physicians, and I do the same thing, if you are very busy and have lots of patients waiting, you just don't ask a question that you know is going to open a Pandora's box. Even if it crosses your mind, you don't ask.

This metaphor suggests the fear of unleashing a myriad of evils. By examining the comments of the respondents, these "evils" begin to take the shape of "too close for comfort," "fear of offending," "powerlessness," "loss of control," and "tyranny of the time."

Too Close for Comfort

The close identification that physicians have with their patients may preclude them from considering the possibility of domestic violence in their differential diagnosis. Close identification was a major theme for 39% of physicians in this study. Physicians who came from white, middle-class backgrounds, with no experience of domestic violence, often assumed that their patients with similar characteristics would likewise not be at risk for violence.

> Maybe you're dealing with, presuming you're a woman with a husband and two kids, a professional, you're so similar to me, we probably both drive Suburbans, both go skiing, we all don't abuse the children. . . . And then maybe you get a young black woman in with two little kids, unemployed, having a headache or God knows what, you might bring it up because it is chaos, social chaos. Although, I guess both women could be abused.

Although most physicians intellectually acknowledged that domestic violence cuts across all races, classes, and ethnic groups, the socioeconomic status of the patient was clearly used as a marker for determining whether abuse was likely.

> Now the kind of patients that I take care of are probably somewhat less at risk for that . . . while, primarily these are, at least in this clinic, white, middle-class folks. And obviously there is domestic violence in white middle-class folks, but it's not rampant. And I see it very seldom.

Many physicians also admitted that they were more likely to ask patients of lower socioeconomic status about abuse.

> We have a unique population here in that it's poorer, inner-city population, fairly substantial Afro-American population. So I think we see the majority of domestic violence in that group. I think we are looking for it more there too. We're more tuned in to it.

Among women physicians, the close identification with patients created another problem. Uncovering domestic violence among patients similar to them would expose some of these physicians to their own fear of vulnerability and lack of control.

> I think it's that I tend to identify with these people too much. If they are getting beaten up and don't have control over the situation, maybe that could happen to me. . . . And if it is some lady who doesn't speak much English because she came from Ethiopia, well, that's one of those people. But if it's a PhD who teaches . . . which is what I used to do before I went to medical school, that gets pretty close.

The diagnosis of abuse may also be hindered when physicians too closely identify with abused patients due to their own past experience of abuse or violence. When asked about a previous history of child abuse or physical violence with an intimate partner, 14% of male physicians and 31% of female physicians acknowledged their own experience. As a group, abused physicians could not be distinguished from nonabused physicians in their major themes or patterns of responses.

Fear of Offending

Fear of offending the patients was one of the strongest fears expressed by physicians. Over half (55%) revealed concern regarding offending the patient. This fear often originated in the physician's discomfort with areas that are culturally defined as private.

> The second factor is the fear of offending the patient. I don't ask a married woman if she has

lesbian thoughts. It just doesn't occur to me even though I might ask sexual preference of other patients. Again, out of context, where I'm not really thinking of domestic violence, it's sort of a sensitive private area that I might not explore unless I really need to.

The uncertainty of whether patients would consider domestic violence a legitimate area to probe was distressing to physicians.

It's the same kind of hesitance that I have or feeling of comfort I have in dealing with people's sexual preference. I'm not wanting to touch on something that they are uncomfortable dealing with too. It has to do with both of us, our levels of comfort. And also I don't want to be nosing into somebody's business if they don't want me nearby.

Physicians felt that by even broaching the subject of violence, the patient would take offense at the implications of the question. However, many male physicians voiced an even stronger fear that if they were to inquire about violence, it would be viewed as a betrayal of trust by the patient and endanger the physician-patient relationship.

I guess it is because you are asking about behavior that the great majority of people would find abhorrent. Tough questions about sexual preference or anything else, some people get the worrisome thought that by asking the question, the patient is going to think that you think that he does that. He is going to think, "I'm not like that, Doc. What must you think of me?" That, you worry, does violence to your relationship.

It is of interest that even though female physicians expressed concern about offending the patient, none suggested that inquiring would jeopardize the physician-patient relationship.

The fear of offending the alleged batterer may underlie some physicians expressing the need to judge the truth of the situation and the discomfort they felt if the truth was not clear.

With children I have an automatic sense of vulnerability. With domestic violence I have enough of a sense of uncertainty about the vulnerability and the dynamics between the two.... Whenever I thought it was clear-cut and began to explore it with the partner, it quickly became more complex and not as clear-cut, and so I would, I guess, with even the little experience I have had with it, have been left in doubt about the clarity of who is vulnerable and who isn't.

A patient responding positively to a physician's question concerning whether abuse had occurred did not establish the diagnosis of abuse for some physicians. These physicians felt they needed to get unbiased information and go to persons other than the patient to get the truth. The language used to express the concern of truth took on a legal tone for some physicians.

Well, one thing is the credibility of the witness. Some people will say things that I may not tend to believe, I may not have reason to believe them. And in that setting I may well contact some other family member or something to see if I have some confirmation of the problem, with the permission of the patient if I can get it.... Because for some people there may be secondary gain in trying to say something.

It appears that to suggest the diagnosis of domestic violence is to "accuse" the partner of being a batterer. When this weight of judgment is placed on the diagnosis, full "truth" is required by some physicians. For some physicians, blame needed to be assigned, and a "true victim" and "true perpetrator" needed to be identified. Anything less clear-cut was unsettling.

Powerlessness

Many of the physicians (50%) voiced frustration and feelings of inadequacy when discussing what would constitute appropriate interventions.

Well, it doesn't seem to make any difference to me if you have a skull fracture because a tree fell on you or a baseball bat fell on you. It is still a skull fracture. It needs to be dealt with. And you try to prevent another occurrence. If it is a baseball bat that a spouse used, then that seems to be a legitimate cause for concern. But the problem is, what the hell do you do about it?

Many pointed to the complexity of the problem and the fact that they had no "tools" to help.

I think we tend to look more on the technical side of medicine, things we can help, like appendicitis. Domestic violence is a big morass which we will never escape. I get a headache thinking about it. And that attitude translates into the type of care we give those patients.

There was a strong sense of powerlessness when physicians described their inability to "fix it." Many pointed to their lack of training on this issue, with 61% revealing that they had no training on intimate-partner violence in medical school, residency, or continuing medical education courses, as opposed to 8% who expressed that they had received good training in this area.

Loss of Control

Forty-two percent of physicians expressed the frustration that although they would intervene with advice or referral to resources, ultimately the control of the outcome was in the hands of the patient. Until the patient was motivated to change, these physicians felt their attempts at intervention were useless.

I try to refer to resources. But that is part of my sense of impotence. I can't give this woman a job. I can't hold her hand. I can't do it for her.

Many physicians were frustrated by their inability to control the patient's behavior, and the patients' inability to control the circumstances of their lives. This need to gain control and expediently solve the problem was one of the major obstacles to physicians' willingness to address domestic violence.

And the fact is I am not sure I'd have any effect anyway. I certainly find that most of my advice on smoking and alcohol and other self-destructive behaviors has no effect on people and it gets very frustrating. And to see this as rarely as I do, I get the feeling that it would be another one of those frustrating situations where I get involved and invest myself and yet have nothing come of it.

This issue of control was most prominent when physicians described their frustration with the repetitive nature of domestic violence. This reaction was most marked among female physicians.

I get to the point where I feel discouraged because I feel like, with someone that's in ... an abusive situation, until that person's ready to take care of it, I'm banging my head against the wall. I'm doing it over and over and over again, and it's like my own abuse in a sense.... At what point do I just say "We'll take up your hypertension today, and I'm sorry your family life isn't going so well"?

The Tyranny of the Time Schedule

The majority of physicians (71%) identified the time constraints of a busy primary care practice as the major deterrent for asking about violence in the home. Their greatest fear was that this is one more issue that will consume more of their scarce time.

You don't open a Pandora's box for the same reason you don't generally ask people, "Do you have sexual problems?" Not because it is not important, but because you don't have time to do that. You literally don't have time to deal with all this.

The majority of the physicians interviewed felt that domestic violence was of such low prevalence in their patient population that pursuing it was not a good investment of time.

Well, I think in part because you still see it rarely. You know, it's not the major medical issue that you see in your practice. It might be there much more than you realize, but it is not a confrontation in your practice. There are so many topics that this one is low on my list of how yielding, I mean, how much yield do you get to spend 5 minutes, 3 minutes on this.

Several physicians voiced frustration with the overwhelming role physicians were being asked to play.

In the case of being a primary care provider and being expected to deal with the total person and the total body and you have 30 minutes, you can't ask all the questions.

Outliers

There were two physicians who stood out from the rest because of their level of comfort in dealing with domestic violence. They differed from their colleagues in several ways. They identified domestic violence cases often in their practice. They had a comfortable, neutral, business-as-usual approach to asking questions about violence. They perceived their role as validating a patient's feelings, discussing safety issues, and referring patients to appropriate resources. They also saw the time frame for change as a prolonged course and were not concerned with the idea of a quick fix. One physician had encountered several abused patients early in his clinical career and had experienced positive outcomes when the issue was addressed in the medical setting. A sense of personal competence developed through subsequent reading on abuse and experience with abused patients. The other physician had a previous history of abuse for which he had received counseling. His own recovery was his evidence that intervention had a significant effect.

COMMENT

The issues raised by the physicians in this study have broad implications. The close identification of physicians with patients of their own socioeconomic background can generate a denial that leads to two dangerous consequences. First, abused patients from higher socioeconomic groups will not be identified because they will not be asked. Second, the misconception that domestic violence is predominantly a product of poverty will be perpetuated through selective questioning of lower socio-economic groups.

If physicians have a personal experience of violence, the impact of that experience is likely to influence their ability to broach the issue with patients. As was revealed in this small group, violence with intimate partners and child abuse are experiences that are not unknown to physicians. It is interesting to note that no clear difference in the pattern of response was found between abused and nonabused physicians. Further research is necessary to understand how a previous history of abuse influences a physician's ability to diagnose and intervene with domestic violence.

The fear of offending the patient is embedded in the cultural construct of what is private. Not wanting to overstep the bounds of what is private, yet acknowledging that domestic violence has medical consequences, leaves the physician wary of how to approach the issue. It is the same tension that had to be overcome in addressing such issues as cigarette smoking, alcohol and drug use, and sexual preference.

When physicians encounter instances of domestic violence, they may feel ineffective in their ability to intervene. Some physicians felt they had no power because their tools were limited to medications or surgeries, and these were clearly inappropriate approaches to "fixing" of domestic violence. Other physicians felt they did have tools in the form of emotional support and/or appropriate referrals, but were frustrated by their inability to control whether a patient accepted what they offered. This is an area where the deficit in training is most evident. Physicians need to be educated in appropriate intervention strategies and need to become knowledgeable about the expected time course of change so that issues of power and control become less problematic.

The time element was the most pervasive and driving fear. It magnified the other fears mentioned by the physicians. Problems that could be offensive or have no easy answers may not be delved into because of time pressure. Higher priority will likely be given to the organic causes of disease that can be expediently dealt with in the time frame that has emerged for medical practice. Given the number of illnesses that do not fall neatly into 20 minutes, it may be necessary to re-examine the clinical time schedule that has evolved.

The data generated by ethnography provide information on the dilemmas confronting physicians, from within the physicians' frame of reference and in the physicians' language. This type of information is crucial in designing educational programs. It is clear from this study that educating physicians to intervene more effectively in domestic violence is not simply a matter of providing facts. As with all health issues that encompass elements of both medicine and social work, education on domestic violence must include examining and reshaping the internal barriers that may hinder physicians' clinical skills. Describing the actual educational approach to these issues is beyond the scope of this paper but is an area in great need of further research and development.

Several limitations to this study should be cited, since most medical researchers will not be familiar with ethnographic research. First, the nature of qualitative research is to explore what is present, as opposed to counting how often something is present. The percentages given in this study cannot be used to determine the prevalence of a belief, but only to give the frequency of expression of the dominate themes. The statement that 71% of physicians identified time as an issue does not mean that 39% did not think time is an issue but that the comments of 39% did not reveal time to be a dominant theme.

Next, "reliability" and "validity" are not concepts that can be directly taken from quantitative research and applied to qualitative research. These concepts, it has been suggested, are represented in the qualitative research domain by concerns about "trustworthiness."[10] Would another investigator examine our data and discover the same themes? Probably, but not certainly. This issue was dealt with explicitly by peer review, the process by which dominant themes were reviewed and confirmed by physicians not involved in this study. Do the results accurately reflect the beliefs of the physicians studied? We believe they do. The group member review, where the results were reviewed by all the study participants, supports this belief.

Finally, would all physicians produce the same themes if given the opportunity? We do not know. Qualitative research results are not assuredly generalizable. The in-depth nature of the study method does not lend itself to large sample sizes, nor are the participants chosen randomly. The information obtained is true to the locale studied. Further study by survey or widely dispersed focus groups would be needed to produce generalizable information. The subject matter is serious enough to merit such an effort since the course of domestic violence tends to be repetitive and to escalate in severity, making early diagnosis and intervention necessary to prevent severe injury or death. The issues raised in this study need to be addressed for physicians to develop a nonthreatening approach to domestic violence that will no longer raise the specter of Pandora's box.

References

1. Stark E, Flitcraft A, Zuckerman D, Gray A, Robison J, Frazier W. *Wife Abuse in the Medical Setting: An Introduction for Health Care Personnel.* Washington, DC: Office of Domestic Violence; 1981. Monograph 7.
2. Straus M, Gelles R, Steinmetz SK. *Behind Closed Doors: A Survey of Family Violence in America.* New York, NY: Doubleday; 1980.
3. Stark E, Flitcraft A, Frazier W. Medicine and patriarchal violence: the social construct of a 'private' event. *Int J Health Serv.* 1979;9:461-493.
4. Goldberg CA, Tomlanovich MC. Domestic violence victims in the emergency department. *JAMA.* 1984;251:3259-3264.
5. McLeer SV, Anwar R. A study of battered women presenting in an emergency department. *Am J Public Health.* 1989;79:65-66.
6. Randall T. Domestic violence intervention calls for more than treating injuries. *JAMA.* 1990;264:939-944.
7. Kurz D. Emergency department responses to battered women: resistance to medicalization. *Soc Probl.* 1987;34:69-81.
8. Warshaw C. Limitations of the medical model in the care of battered women. *Gender Soc.* 1989;3:506-517.
9. Graves R. *The Greek Myths.* Mt Kisco, NY: Moyer Bell Limited; 1986.
10. Lincoln Y, Guba E. *Naturalistic Inquiry.* Beverly Hills, Calif: Sage Publications; 1985.

Attitudes of Primary Care Physicians Toward Corporal Punishment

Kenelm F. McCormick, MD

Objective.—The purpose of this study was to determine whether or not family physicians and pediatricians support the use of corporal punishment. The frequency with which these physicians offer anticipatory guidance on discipline was also studied.

Design.—Self-report survey, mailed to study participants.

Participants.—The sample for this study was 800 family physicians and 400 pediatricians, randomly selected from the Ohio State Medical Board's roster of family physicians and pediatricians. Physicians with a subspecialty were excluded. Participants who did not return their surveys received a second, and if necessary, a third mailing of the survey. After three mailings, a total of 619 physicians (61%) completed a survey.

Main Outcome Measure.—Participants were considered to support corporal punishment if they would tell a parent in their medical practice that spanking would be an appropriate response to any one of a series of childhood misbehaviors presented in the survey.

Results.—Of family physicians, 70% (95% confidence interval [CI], 66% to 75%) support use of corporal punishment. Of pediatricians, 59% (95% CI, 52% to 66%) support corporal punishment. Of pediatricians, 90% (95% CI, 86% to 94%) indicated that they include discipline issues either always or most of the time when providing anticipatory guidance to parents. Significantly fewer family physicians (52%; 95% CI, 47% to 57%) indicated that they discuss discipline either always or most of the time when providing anticipatory guidance ($P<.01$).

Conclusions.—Most family physicians and pediatricians support the use of corporal punishment in spite of evidence that it is neither effective nor necessary, and can be harmful. Pediatricians offer anticipatory guidance on discipline more often than family physicians.

(*JAMA*. 1992;267:3161-3165)

INTERPERSONAL violence is a major health problem that needs to be addressed by physicians.[1-4] The genesis of violent behavior involves many factors. Many social and behavioral scientists assert that childhood experiences with violence are part of the underpinnings of violence and tolerance of violence in adults.[5,6] Corporal punishment is a common experience that children have with interpersonal violence.[6,7] Corporal punishment contributes to the problem by serving as a model of problem solving using interpersonal violence.[8-10] For the child, parental use of corporal punishment validates the use of violence in resolving disputes.[5,9-14] Corporal punishment can be a harmful practice that frequently escalates to abuse.[11,15] Not only a problem in promoting violence, there is evidence that corporal punishment is ineffective and even counterproductive as a child-raising strategy.[8-10,16-20] The use of corporal punishment decreases the likelihood that more effective parent-child interaction will take place. Corporal punishment and other power-assertive discipline practices result in inferior development of moral reasoning.[13]

From the Barberton (Ohio) Citizen's Hospital, Family Practice Residency, and the Society of Teachers of Family Medicine, Violence Education Task Force, Kansas City, Mo.

Reprint requests to Barberton Citizen's Hospital, Family Practice Residency, 155 Fifth St NE, Barberton, OH 44203 (Dr McCormick).

THE CASE AGAINST CORPORAL PUNISHMENT AND FOR ITS ALTERNATIVES

In reviewing the literature on punishment in humans, Johnston[21] sets out some requirements for its effective use. A few of them are (1) the intensity of the punishment should be as great as possible each time it is delivered; (2) the punishment should be delivered after each occurrence of the undesired behavior; (3) alternative, rewarded, unpunished behaviors must be available; and (4) there should be no avenue for unauthorized escape from punishment. In reviewing the literature on punishment as applied to corporal punishment in schools, Bongiovanni[22] found that these requirements and others would be impractical within the school setting. In particular, Bongiovanni notes that the requirement for intense punishment puts the punished child at considerable risk for physical injury. Few school districts would be willing to take such a risk. While Bongiovanni addressed the use of corporal punishment in schools, there is no reason to suppose that parents, who rarely receive formal training in parenting, should be able to apply corporal punishment more effectively or less dangerously than school officials. It is ironic that the risks of corporal punishment are such that no investigator is likely to find support for an experimental protocol in which some children receive effective levels of physical punishment and some do not.

A mechanism by which intergenerational transmission of violence may take place is observational, incidental learning. In one study, preschool children engaged in another task were allowed to observe adult models performing an arbitrary behavior.[23] Control subjects did not observe the behavior. Later, the children who had observed the behavior reproduced it, while control subjects did not. In a similar study, preschool children observed adults modeling unusual, aggressive behavior while control subjects did not.[24] Children in the experimental group spontaneously reproduced the novel, aggressive behavior while controls did not. Flanders[25] reviewed literature on imitative learning and found that such learning could generalize across different models, different physiological drives, and different stimulus situations. Carlson[26] presented school-age children with vignettes of peer misdeeds and asked the children what the best response of the wrongdoer's parents should be. Children were most likely to recommend physical discipline when the misdeed was aggressive, and much more likely to do so when the misdeed involved aggression against a family member. According to Carlson, these results suggest that the family is a training ground for violence, especially for violence against other family members. Owens and Straus[27] analyzed the data from a national survey on violence done in 1968. They found a moderate correlation between childhood experience of interpersonal violence and adult approval of interpersonal violence. Unfortunately, this analysis did not control for the severity of the violence experienced as a child, lumping all experience of any corporal punishment with abuse. Lefkowitz et al[28] investigated the effects of parental punishment practice on the behavior and attitudes of adults in a longitudinal design. The punishment practices of parents of a group of 8-year-old children were determined, and the children were interviewed 10 years later, as young adults. The analysis showed that parental punishment practice influenced the attitudes of the young adults toward punishing children, and in some subgroups, aggressive behavior in the adults. However, the authors note that several other sociocultural and individual variables accounted for most of aggressive behavior.

It is important to dig deeper than statistics on documented physical abuse to identify the danger in corporal punishment. Berger et al[15] interviewed college students about their childhood experience with physical punishment. Using what they believed to be a very stringent definition of abuse, the authors found that 9% of the subjects had been physically abused in the name of punishment. A surprising number of the abused subjects did not identify themselves as abused. Using physical marks such as welts and bruises to define abuse, Graziano and Namaste[11] found a similar (10.6%) prevalence of abuse in the name of punishment in interviewed college students. Berkowitz et al[29] have shown in an experimental design that aversive conditions may stimulate the production of aggressive behavior, even when the target of the aggression is not the cause of the aversive conditions. In fact, much of what passes for ordinary corporal punishment is not punishment at all, but aversively stimulated aggression against the child.[30] The goal of aversively stimulated aggression is to inflict pain.[31] Given that the real goal of much corporal punishment is to inflict pain, not to punish, it is not surprising that much corporal punishment is abusive. Societal permission to use corporal punishment is the child's ticket to victimization.

The purpose of discipline is to teach children how to behave; the purpose of punishment is to reduce children's misbehavior. When corporal punishment is used, the motivation for behaving well is avoidance of pain rather than good behavior for its own sake. Hoffman and Saltzstein[32] used indexes of guilt, internalized moral judgment, acceptance of responsibility for actions, and consideration for others to measure the moral development of seventh-graders as affected by parental disciplinary practice. The authors compared power assertion parenting techniques (including corporal punishment) with love withdrawal and induction (focusing children's attention on the harmfulness of their behavior). They found that frequent use of power assertion techniques resulted "considerably consistently" in less advanced moral development compared with induction. In this study, mild corporal punishment was not considered separately from other power assertions, but was clearly the main thrust in classifying parental practices. It must be noted that the association of parental practices with moral development was strong in middle-class children, but not clear in the lower class. The authors suggest that more socializing influences come from outside the home in the lower class. In a longitudinal, prospective study spanning 19 years, McCord[33] found that aggressive parents raised more expressive and antisocial children. Punitive parents raised more egocentric and antisocial children. McCord postulated that expressive action, including doing physical violence, was normalized for the children of aggressive parents.

Many proponents of corporal punishment argue that it is necessary and that its abandonment will result in less disciplined children. Some cite their experience with children who are not physically punished and are not well-behaved. Farley et al[34] interviewed officials of 36 school districts in which corporal punishment had been eliminated. Only one school district reported increased problems because corporal punishment was eliminated. Although a large majority of American youngsters are subjected to corporal punishment, a considerable number are not.[11,15] Studies of the consequences of corporal punishment such as those cited above[27,28,32-34] provide no support for the notion that children who are not physically punished behave inferiorly to those who are physically punished.

In spite of evidence that corporal punishment is not a useful discipline technique, parents and physicians will be unwilling to give it up if there are no alternatives. Many studies have shown that effective alternatives to corporal punishment exist and can be learned by parents.[35-39] Published studies vary from case reports of one subject using extinction[40] to a controlled experimental design with 32 subjects using time-out to modify behavior.[41]

In summary, evidence for the futility and harm of corporal punishment spans the research of a variety of disciplines from laboratory psychology to education to medicine. Also, the literature of these disciplines is poor in work that supports the use of corporal punishment. Although the use of mild corporal punishment (such as spanking) by parents has not been studied often, application of principles derived from the work of investigators in a variety of fields shows that the practice can be damaging and unnecessary.

Since corporal punishment can be harmful, and effective alternatives exist, its use should be discouraged by physicians. Several national organizations, including the American Academy of Pediatrics, have taken at least limited stands against the use of corporal punishment.[8,16,42-45] These organizations are not always supported in their objections to corporal punishment by the people they represent. In a study of pediatricians' attitudes toward use of corporal punishment in schools, only 13% indicated strong disagreement with the use of corporal punishment.[46] In another study, only 10% of pediatricians and family physicians agreed that light spanking was inappropriate as a disciplinary measure.[47] A survey of psychologists found that the majority used corporal punishment in their own homes.[48]

Small, mobile contemporary families allow little opportunity for young people to learn parenting skills by observation and practice with younger siblings. Thus, young parents often turn to the family physician or pediatrician for advice on child-raising issues. Common behavioral concerns and questions, including discipline questions and problems, were the most frequent behavioral issues encountered in a study of pediatrics in family practice.[49] Many behavioral problems may be avoided or more effectively managed if parents have skills to deal with the problems before they occur.[17,50,51] Thus, anticipatory guidance on discipline should be considered an essential part of the family physician's or pediatrician's preventive medicine program for young families.

The purpose of this study was to determine what family physicians' and pediatricians' attitudes are toward corporal punishment. The frequency with which these physicians offer anticipatory guidance on discipline was also studied.

METHODS

Subjects

The sample for this study was 800 family physicians and 400 primary care pediatricians randomly selected from the Ohio State Medical Board's roster of licensed physicians.[52] The study population (948 pediatricians and 1902 family physicians) was meant to include physicians who spend a significant amount of time taking care of children, and who may frequently receive questions from parents about discipline problems. Physicians identified as pediatricians or family physicians with a subspecialty (eg, pediatric gastroenterologist) were excluded.

Study Design

A self-report survey was used for the study. Subjects were asked to complete the survey and return it in a preaddressed, stamped envelope. A cover letter accompanied the survey and assured respondents of response confidentiality. To maximize the response rate, the survey was remailed to nonresponders about 4 weeks after the first mailing. A third mailing was done 4 weeks after the second. The first round of surveys was mailed in February 1991; data collection was completed in the first week of June 1991.

The date of return of each survey was noted to identify any differences between early and late responders. To identify potential bias due to nonresponders, the sex, age, and practice location of the respondent family physicians was compared with data on all Ohio family physicians provided by the American Academy of Family Physicians.[53,54] Similar data were not available for pediatricians.

Study Instrument

In the survey, the term *spanking* was used. Spanking was explicitly defined as only "mild spanking" (striking of the child's buttocks or hand with an open hand, lightly, leaving no mark except transient redness). The term was specifically meant to exclude practices that might be considered abusive. The survey included questions about the physicians' demographic characteristics and practice location and questions about the physicians' approach to the practice of corporal punishment.

The survey presented respondents with nine scenarios of childhood misbehavior, three different behaviors for three ages. The scenarios were meant to sample respondents' opinion about corporal punishment in various age groups as well as in response to dangerous, trivial, and aggressive misbehaviors. Subjects were asked to state whether they would advise a parent in their practice that spanking is an appropriate response for each combination of misbehavior and age. The survey also asked respondents to indicate how often they include discipline-related issues when providing anticipatory guidance.

The survey instrument was the product of multiple revisions tested on small groups of family practice residents and faculty and pediatric residents. The original survey attempted to identify attitudes toward corporal punishment more directly. Subjects were asked to state whether they felt spanking was "definitely," "probably," "probably not," or "definitely not" a useful strategy in child-raising. The results of this survey were difficult to interpret because many subjects stated that they objected to spanking, but noted certain circumstances in which they would approve of it. The circumstances cited most often were "difficult-to-control" children and grave misbehavior. Also, the age of the child was a factor.

Since the stated question in this investigation was to find out whether the study group supports the use of corporal punishment, the survey was constructed to account for individuals who find any reason to use corporal punishment. To tap attitudes, the survey asked respondents to state what they would advise parents under a variety of circumstances.

Analysis

Respondents who indicated that they would advise parents that spanking was appropriate in any one or more of the survey scenarios were classified as supporting corporal punishment. Several physicians indicated in written comments that they were not opposed to corporal punishment, although they would not advise it in any of the scenarios presented. These individuals were classified as not opposed to corporal punishment. Practice location was considered urban if the practice was located in an Ohio county that is part of a metropolitan statistical area.[55]

To detect any effect related to physicians' age, respondents were assigned to two age groups, less than 40 years and 40 years or older. Logistic regression analysis was used to detect age-related differences that might be confounded by parenthood status. Survey data were tabulated and statistics calculated using standard statistical software packages.[56,57]

RESULTS

A total of 183 surveys were undeliverable or excluded from analysis because the respondent was not a family physician or primary care pediatrician. Six hundred nineteen surveys were returned for a response rate of 61%. One hundred ninety-seven (59%) pediatricians and 422 (61%) family physicians returned surveys. Surveys returned from the first mailing numbered 431; 128 surveys were returned in the second mailing and 60 surveys were returned in the third mailing. No differences were detected in attitudes and characteristics of physicians who responded in the second and third mailing.

The number of physicians who support the use of corporal punishment was 413 (67%; 95% confidence interval [CI], 63% to 70%). Of pediatricians, 116 (59%; 95% CI, 52% to 66%) support the use of corporal punishment. Of family physicians, 297 (70%; 95% CI, 66% to 75%) indicated that they support the use of corporal punishment. The difference in attitude between pediatricians and family physicians was significant ($P<.01$).

The Table shows the percentage of family physicians and pediatricians who would support the use of corporal punishment in each situation presented in the survey. Although a minority of respondents supported corporal punishment in any single situation, a majority indicated support for corporal punishment in at least one scenario. Only 128 (21%) respondents indicated support for corporal punishment in more than three of the situations presented in the survey.

Percent of Physicians Who Would Support Spanking in a Given Situation

	Age, y					
	2		5		8	
Situation	Pediatricians	Family Physicians	Pediatricians	Family Physicians	Pediatricians	Family Physicians
Child refuses to go to bed at the usual, established time	4	9	6	20	5	16
Child runs into the street without looking	46	44	33	46	16	29
Child hits one of his or her playmates	9	18	10	31	8	25

Inspection of the Table shows that, for all children's ages, support for corporal punishment is greatest when the misbehavior is one that is dangerous to the child (running into the street). Of physicians who would support corporal punishment, 172 (42%) would support it for the dangerous misbehavior only. Pediatricians and female physicians are more likely than family physicians and male physicians to support corporal punishment only for dangerous misbehavior ($P<.01$).

Support for corporal punishment was least when the misbehavior is relatively minor (not going to bed on time). There was considerable support for use of corporal punishment in response to an aggressive misbehavior in all children's age groups. For instance, 31% of family physicians would support corporal punishment for a 5-year-old child who hits one of his or her playmates. Pediatricians were significantly less likely than family physicians to support corporal punishment for aggressive misbehavior ($P<.01$).

Of physicians supporting corporal punishment, 90% have one or more children of their own, 23% are female, and 25% practice in a rural setting. Of physicians who do not support corporal punishment, 93% have children, 25% are female, and 22% practice in a rural setting. There was no significant difference between physicians supporting or not supporting corporal punishment for these characteristics. Physicians less than 40 years of age are less likely to have children of their own (85%) than older physicians (96%). For family physicians, there was no difference between the average age, sex, and practice location of the Ohio family physician population compared with respondents.

Significantly more support for corporal punishment was found among physicians younger than 40 years (72%) compared with physicians 40 years or older (63%, $P<.05$). Subsequently, respondents were assigned to age groups in decades: less than 40 years, 40 to 49 years, 50 to 59 years, 60 to 69 years, and more than 69 years old. A χ^2 analysis for trend with advancing age was calculated for these age groups. This analysis did not show a linear age effect. Logistic regression analysis did not find parenthood status to be a confounding variable in analyzing the effect of physician age on attitude toward corporal punishment.

Of pediatricians, 90% (95% CI, 86% to 94%) indicated that they discuss discipline-related issues either always or most of the time when providing anticipatory guidance to parents. Only 52% (95% CI, 47% to 57%) of family physicians offer such guidance always or most of the time. This difference between pediatricians and family physicians was statistically significant ($P<.01$). Female physicians offer anticipatory guidance always or most of the time (81%) more often than male physicians (59%, $P<.01$).

There was a significant difference in anticipatory guidance practice between physicians who would support the use of corporal punishment and those who would not. Physicians opposed to corporal punishment stated that they offer anticipatory guidance more frequently than those who support corporal punishment ($P<.01$).

COMMENT

An important recommendation of the Surgeon General's Workshop on Violence and Public Health[14] was: "... the cultural acceptance of violence be decreased by discouraging corporal punishment at home, forbidding corporal punishment at school... (because these) are models and sanctions of violence." The purpose of this study was to find out whether physicians who are responsible for the primary health care of children support the use of corporal punishment by parents. The study suggests that the majority of these physicians support the use of corporal punishment in the home.

Pediatricians are less likely to support the use of corporal punishment than family physicians. Pediatricians are also less likely to support corporal punishment for misbehavior that is not dangerous to the child or for aggressive misbehavior. This may reflect the amount of training these physicians receive in residency regarding childhood development and child-raising issues. It also may reflect the amount of involvement of the groups' professional academies in promoting the abandonment of the practice of corporal punishment.

An age-related difference in attitude toward corporal punishment was noted. Physicians in the youngest age group are more likely than older physicians to support the use of corporal punishment. They are also less likely than older physicians to have children; but parenthood status, itself, is not related to attitude toward corporal punishment. The increased support for corporal punishment in the younger age group is not easily accounted for. Perhaps this finding really does, indirectly, reflect parenthood status. Physicians in the younger age group who have children are more likely to have young children. Because misbehavior in young children is not as readily dealt with by cognitive methods, these physicians may be more supportive of the use of corporal punishment.

Also, younger physicians who do not have children may have spent less time thinking critically about discipline methods than older physicians who have had to confront childhood misbehavior in their own children. In this survey, several physicians commented that they had used corporal punishment on their own children, had found the method lacking, and did not recommend it to parents in their medical practice.

A large block of physicians would only support the use of corporal punishment in response to a misbehavior that is dangerous to the child. Although it may seem encouraging that many physicians are uncomfortable enough with corporal punishment to limit its use to extreme circumstances, this finding reflects a stubborn persistence of the myth that corporal punishment is appropriate, effective, and the best alternative for dealing with childhood misbehavior. Female physicians are more likely to limit support for corporal punishment to dangerous situations. This finding may reflect society as a whole in demonstrating a greater readiness in men to solve problems with violence.[58,59]

Pediatricians are more likely to provide anticipatory guidance on discipline to parents in their practices. A difference was also noted in anticipatory guidance between male and female physicians. That pediatricians offer anticipatory guidance more often than family physicians may reflect the greater amount of training they receive on developmental and child-raising issues. With less training, many family physicians may be reluctant to offer advice on behavioral issues spontaneously. Behavioral science training in family practice residencies has been found lacking by at least one study.[49] However, this lack has also been noted in pediatric training programs.[50] It is unclear why female physicians offer anticipatory guidance more often than male physicians.

Certain cautions are warranted in interpreting the results of this study. Nonresponders (39%) represent a significant proportion of this study's sample. No attempt was made to survey nonresponders to see if their attitudes toward corporal punishment differ systematically from responders. Comparing the first with later waves of responders may be a way of estimating bias due to nonresponse.[60] In this study, no significant difference in attitude toward corporal punishment or anticipatory guidance practice was found in comparing the responses of subjects in the first, second, and third mailings. Also, for family physicians, certain demographic characteristics of the population were available. No difference in these characteristics was found when comparing the family physician respondents with the Ohio family physician population. Thus, at least with regard to these characteristics, the respondents are representative of the population.

The definition of corporal punishment used in this survey was meant to exclude any practice that most people would consider abusive. In addition, the definition was limited to the common practice of spanking. It is possible that some physicians would consider even this mild practice too severe. Some physicians may not have indicated their support for corporal punishment, even though they would support a milder or different form of the practice.

The survey was constructed to present a representative sample of childhood misbehaviors, but the situations presented do not exhaust the possible misbehaviors for which corporal punishment may be administered. Indeed, a few physicians included written comments indicating that they could support corporal punishment for some behaviors, but not for the ones described in the survey. As a result, it is possible that the number of physicians who support corporal punishment is underestimated by this survey.

The subjects in this study are Ohio family physicians and pediatricians. Attitudes toward corporal punishment and anticipatory guidance practices of these physicians may differ from those of physicians in other regions of the United States.

CONCLUSIONS

According to Wessel,[10] "A physician, educator, or other professional child care worker who inflicts or sanctions corporal punishment, even with parental permission, misjudges his or her professional role and responsibility." In this study, most primary care pediatricians and family physicians were found to support the use of corporal punishment in childhood discipline. This opinion is held in spite of considerable evidence that corporal punishment is neither necessary nor beneficial in child-raising. The opinion is also held contrary to the official position of scientific and professional groups. Also, only about half of family physicians include discussion of discipline issues when providing anticipatory guidance to parents.

Interpersonal violence is a source of great suffering in terms of emotional and physical health in this country. The cycle of violence begins in early childhood with the use of corporal punishment. Corporal punishment teaches the use of violence as a problem-solving method. A contribution to ending the cycle of violence would be made if parents abandoned corporal punishment in favor of effective, nonviolent disciplinary techniques. Family physicians and pediatricians can contribute by teaching and encouraging parents to use such techniques. Unfortunately, most physicians still believe that corporal punishment is appropriate. Family medicine and pediatrics educators can help end the cycle of violence by teaching residents about appropriate discipline techniques and by encouraging the inclusion of such issues when providing anticipatory guidance to parents.

This study was supported by a grant from the Ohio Academy of Family Physicians Foundation, Columbus.

References

1. Merz B. Family violence and the physician. *Am Med News.* January 6, 1992:3.
2. Hendricks-Matthews M. The role of family physicians in violence reduction. *Ohio Fam Physician News.* 1989;41:22.
3. Hulley SB. Control of unintended injuries and those due to violence. In: Wyngaarden JB, Smith LH Jr, eds. *Cecil Textbook of Medicine, I.* 18th ed. Philadelphia, Pa: WB Saunders Co; 1988:40-42.
4. Sullivan L. Violence as a public health issue. *JAMA.* 1991;265:2778.
5. Gelles RJ. An exchange/social control theory. In: Finkelhor D, Gelles RJ, Hotaling GT, Straus MA, eds. *The Dark Side of Families: Current Family Violence Research.* Beverly Hills, Calif: Sage Publications; 1983:151-165.
6. Straus MA. Ordinary violence, child abuse, and wife-beating: what do they have in common? In: Finkelhor D, Gelles RJ, Hotaling GT, Straus MA, eds. *The Dark Side of Families: Current Family Violence Research.* Beverly Hills, Calif: Sage Publications; 1983:213-234.
7. Korsch BM, Christian JB, Gozzi EK, Carlson PV. Infant care and punishment: a pilot study. *Am J Public Health.* 1965;55:1880-1888.
8. American Psychological Association. Policy statement of the American Psychological Association. *Am Psychol.* 1975;30:632.
9. Hyman IA, Bongiovanni A, Friedman RH, McDowell E. Paddling, punishment, and force: where do we go from here? *Child Today.* September-October 1977;6:17-23.
10. Wessel MA. The pediatrician and corporal punishment. *Pediatrics.* 1980;66:639-641.
11. Graziano AM, Namaste KA. Parental use of physical force in childhood discipline: a survey of 679 college students. *J Interpers Violence.* 1990;5:449-463.
12. Green JL. Parenting skills and discipline. In: Hoekelman RA, ed. *Primary Pediatric Care.* St Louis, Mo: CV Mosby Co; 1987:606-609.
13. Herzberger SD. Social cognition and the transmission of abuse. In: Finkelhor D, Gelles RJ, Hotaling GT, Straus MA, eds. *The Dark Side of Families: Current Family Violence Research.* Beverly Hills, Calif: Sage Publications; 1983:317-329.
14. *Surgeon General's Workshop on Violence and Public Health: Report.* Rockville, Md: US Dept of Health and Human Services, Public Health Service; 1985. US Dept of Health and Human Services publication HRS-D-MC 86-1.
15. Berger AM, Knutson JF, Mehm JG, Perkins KA. The self-report of punitive childhood experiences of young adults and adolescents. *Child Abuse Negl.* 1988;12:251-262.
16. American Public Health Association, Governing Council. Policy statements. *Am J Public Health.* 1980; 70:308-309.
17. Christophersen ER. The pediatrician and parental discipline. *Pediatrics.* 1980;66:641-642.
18. National Education Association. *Report of the Task Force on Corporal Punishment.* Washington, DC: National Education Association; 1972.
19. Poole SR, Ushkow MC, Nader PR, et al. The role of the pediatrician in abolishing corporal punishment in schools. *Pediatrics.* 1991;88:162-167.
20. Straus MA. Some social antecedents of physical punishment: a linkage theory interpretation. *J Marriage Fam.* 1971;33:658-663.
21. Johnston JM. Punishment of human behavior. *Am Psychol.* 1972;27:1033-1054.
22. Bongiovanni AF. An analysis of research on punishment and its relation to the use of corporal punishment in the schools. In: Hyman IA, Wise JH, eds. *Corporal Punishment in American Education: Readings in History, Practice, and Alternatives.* Philadelphia, Pa: Temple University Press; 1979:351-372.
23. Bandura A, Huston AC. Identification as a process of incidental learning. *J Abnorm Soc Psychol.* 1961;1:311-318.
24. Bandura A, Ross D, Ross SA. Transmission of aggression through imitation of aggressive models. *J Abnorm Soc Psychol.* 1961;63:575-582.
25. Flanders J. A review of research on imitative behavior. *Psychol Bull.* 1968;69:316-337.
26. Carlson, BE. Children's beliefs about punishment. *Am J Orthopsychiatry.* 1986;56:308-312.
27. Owens DJ, Straus MA. The social structure of violence in childhood and approval of violence as an adult. In: Hyman IA, Wise JH, eds. *Corporal Punishment in American Education: Readings in History, Practice, and Alternatives.* Philadelphia, Pa: Temple University Press; 1979:107-125.
28. Lefkowitz MM, Huesmann R, Eron LD. Parental punishment: a longitudinal analysis of effects. *Arch Gen Psychiatry.* 1978;35:186-191.
29. Berkowitz L, Cochran S, Embree M. Physical pain and the goal of aversively stimulated aggression. *J Pers Soc Psychol.* 1981;40:687-700.
30. Thyer B. Punishment-induced aggression: a possible mechanism of child abuse? *Psychol Rep.* 1987; 60:129-130.
31. Emery RE. Family violence. *Am Psychol.* 1989; 44:321-328.
32. Hoffman M, Saltzstein H. Parent discipline and child's moral development. *J Pers Soc Psychol.* 1967; 5:45-57.
33. McCord J. Parental behavior in the cycle of aggression. *Psychiatry.* 1988;51:14-23.
34. Farley AC, Kreutter KJ, Russel RR, Blackwell S, Finklestein H, Hyman IA. The effects of eliminating corporal punishment in the schools: a preliminary study. *Inequality Educ.* 1978;23:57-60.
35. Alevisos KJ. The effects of verbalizing contingency in time-out procedures. *J Behav Ther Exp Psychiatry.* 1975;6:253-255.
36. Bernal ME. Behavioral feedback in the modification of brat behaviors. *J Nerv Ment Dis.* 1969;148: 375-385.
37. Drabman RS, Jarvie G. Counseling parents of children with behavior problems: the use of extinction and time-out techniques. *Pediatrics.* 1987;59:78-85.
38. Drabman R, Spitalnik R. Social isolation as a punishment procedure: a controlled study. *J Exp Child Psychol.* 1973;16:236-249.
39. Forehand R, Roberts MW, Doleys DM, Hobbs SA, Resick PA. An examination of disciplinary procedures with children. *J Exp Child Psychol.* 1976; 21:109-120.
40. Williams CD. The elimination of tantrum behavior by extinction procedures. *J Abnorm Soc Psychol.* 1959;59:269.
41. Gardner HL, Forehand R, Roberts M. Time-out with children: effects of an explanation and brief parent training on child and parent behaviors. *J Abnorm Child Psychol.* 1976;4:277-288.
42. American Academy of Pediatrics, Committee on Psychological Aspects of Child and Family. The pediatrician's role in discipline. *Pediatrics.* 1983;72:373-374.
43. American Academy of Pediatrics, Committee on School Health. Corporal punishment in schools. *Pediatrics.* 1984;73:258.
44. American Academy of Pediatrics, Committee on School Health. Corporal punishment in schools. *Pediatrics.* 1991;88:173.
45. Corporal punishment in schools. *Am J Psychiatry.* 1989;146:1524.
46. Kelly PC, Weir MR, Fearnow RG. Pediatrician's views: latchkey children, corporal punishment. *Tex Med.* 1987;83:40-42.
47. Morris JL, Johnson CF, Clasen M. To report or not to report: physicians' attitudes toward discipline and child abuse. *AJDC.* 1985;139:194-197.
48. Anderson KA, Anderson DE. Psychologists and spanking. *J Clin Child Psychol.* Fall 1976:46-49.
49. Poole SR. Pediatric behavioral science in family practice. *J Fam Pract.* 1983;16:365-374.
50. Christophersen ER. Anticipatory guidance on discipline. *Pediatr Clin North Am.* 1986;33:789-798.
51. Erickson MT. Common behavior problems of childhood. In: Gabel S, Erickson MT. *Child Development and Developmental Disabilities.* Boston, Mass: Little Brown & Co Inc; 1980:411-432.
52. *Roster of Registered Physicians, Osteopathic Physicians, and Podiatrists in the State of Ohio.* 10th ed. Columbus, Ohio: State Medical Board of Ohio; 1990.
53. *Active Member Practice Profile for Chapter Ohio.* Kansas City, Mo; American Academy of Family Physicians: July 2, 1991.
54. *Demographic Characteristics by Membership Type for Chapter Ohio.* Kansas City, Mo; American Academy of Family Physicians: July 2, 1991.
55. US Bureau of the Census. *Statistical Abstract of the United States: 1989.* 109th ed. Washington, DC: US Dept of Commerce; 1989.
56. Dean AD, Dean JA, Burton AH, Dicker RC. *Epi Info, Version 5: A Word Processing, Database, and Statistics Program for Epidemiology on Micro-computers.* Stone Mountain, Ga: USD Inc; 1990.
57. *BMDP Statistical Software.* Los Angeles, Calif: BMDP Statistical Software Inc; 1988.
58. Goodwin J. Family violence: principles of intervention and prevention. *Hosp Community Psychiatry.* 1985;36:1074-1079.
59. Greenblat CS. A hit is a hit is a hit . . . or is it? approval and tolerance of the use of physical force by spouses. In: Finkelhor D, Gelles RJ, Hotaling GT, Straus MA, eds. *The Dark Side of Families: Current Family Violence Research.* Beverly Hills, Calif: Sage Publications; 1983:235-260.
60. Keller K, Podell RN. The survey in family practice research. *J Fam Pract.* 1975;2:449-453.

Parental Alcohol Use, Problem Drinking, and Children's Injuries

Polly E. Bijur, PhD, MPH; Matthew Kurzon, MS; Mary D. Overpeck, MPH; Peter C. Scheidt, MD, MPH

Objective.—Millions of US children are exposed to parents who are problem drinkers, yet there is little evidence about the effect of parental alcohol consumption on children's health. The aim of this study was to assess the association between children's injuries and parental drinking.

Design.—Survey of a nationally representative sample of the US population by household interview.

Participants.—12 360 children and parents from single-family households, with data from the Alcohol and Child Health supplements to the 1988 National Health Interview Survey.

Main Outcome Measure.—Serious injuries—injuries resulting in hospitalization, surgical treatment, missed school, one half day or more in bed.

Results.—Children of mothers categorized as problem drinkers had 2.1 times the risk of serious injury as children of mothers who were nondrinkers (95% CI, 1.3 to 3.5). Other measures of mothers' alcohol consumption (ie, average, maximum, and self-rated consumption) were unrelated to child injuries, as were all measures of fathers' drinking. Children of women who were problem drinkers married to men rated as moderate or heavy drinkers had a relative risk of serious injury of 2.7 (95% CI, 0.8 to 8.6) compared with children of nondrinkers.

Conclusion.—Children of women who are problem drinkers have an elevated injury risk; children with two parents who are problem drinkers are at higher risk. Further research is needed on potential mechanisms and interventions. Primary prevention might be enhanced if physicians elicited information about parental drinking, helped secure appropriate treatment, and participated in public health efforts to reduce the deleterious effects of alcohol.

(*JAMA*. 1992;267:3166-3171)

THE EMERGENCE of injuries as the premier threat to child health and the pervasive use of alcohol by many elements of American society invite examination of a relationship between these two factors, particularly in light of the deadly role alcohol is known to play in adult injuries.[1-3] It has been estimated that 7 million US children live with an alcoholic parent,[4] and 18.1% of US adults report having lived with an alcoholic or problem drinker when they were children.[5] The psychological and social consequences to children of exposure to alcoholic parents have been well documented, and a number of studies have linked child abuse and neglect to parental alcoholism.[6-10] Identifying and clarifying an association between parental alcohol abuse and child injuries could provide a valuable focus for further research on potential mechanisms and interventions, promote policy that would affect prevention and treatment of adult alcohol-related problems, and help modify public attitudes toward alcohol consumption.

Few studies have focused on the association between parental alcohol use/abuse and child injuries. One study of alcohol-related motor vehicle deaths in North Carolina[11] found that 70% of children in these crashes were passengers in cars in which drivers had been drinking, many of whom were presumed to be the victims' parents. Two studies have examined rates of nonfatal injuries to children of alcoholic parents, and both found 1½ to three times the rate of injuries to the children of alcoholics compared with similar children.[12,13]

The 1988 National Health Interview Survey (NHIS) afforded a unique opportunity to examine the association between parental alcohol use and child injuries on a national scale by the inclusion of a supplement on adult alcohol practices (NHIS-Alcohol) and one on child health (CHS).

It was hypothesized (1) that the relationship would be stronger between mother's alcohol consumption/problems and child injuries than between father's alcohol consumption/problems and child injuries because children spend more time with mothers than with fathers; (2) that young children would be at the highest risk, as younger children are assumed to be most vulnerable to lapses in supervision; and (3) that the association would be strongest in socially disadvantaged family settings, due to an accumulation of stressors and a lack of resources to adequately cope with multiple sources of stress.

SUBJECTS AND METHODS

The data for this study were collected through household interviews by the US Bureau of the Census for the National Center for Health Statistics (NCHS).[14] The NHIS-Alcohol was administered to

From the Department of Pediatrics, Albert Einstein College of Medicine, Bronx, NY (Dr Bijur and Mr Kurzon); and the National Institute of Child Health and Human Development, Rockville, Md (Ms Overpeck and Dr Scheidt).

Presented in part at the 60th Annual Meeting of the Society for Pediatric Research, New Orleans, La, April 30, 1991.

Reprint requests to Department of Pediatrics, Albert Einstein College of Medicine, Room 920, Rose F. Kennedy Center, Bronx, NY 10461 (Dr Bijur).

one randomly selected adult aged 18 years or more in each of 43 809 families sampled by the NHIS, a response rate of 90%. The CHS data were obtained on 17 110 children under 18 years. Data about the selected child's injuries were elicited from an adult in each family.

Children were included in these analyses (1) if they lived in a one-family household, (2) if the adult who completed the NHIS-Alcohol could be identified as the child's mother or father figure, and (3) if there were CHS data on injuries. The CHS data were provided by the mother or mother figure for 91% of the children included in these analyses. Both supplements were completed in 15 700 households. Seventy-nine percent of the households (N=12 360) had children who met all the criteria; 7782 of the children had mothers who were the NHIS-Alcohol respondents and 4578 had fathers who were the respondents. The larger number of mothers who were NHIS-Alcohol respondents is due to the higher proportion of single-parent families headed by women.

Alcohol Measures

Four measures of the NHIS-Alcohol respondents' alcohol use were derived from the NHIS-Alcohol data. Only current drinkers (12 drinks or more in the year before the interview) were asked the questions used for these measures. Current nondrinkers were divided into two categories: (1) nondrinkers (abstainers and infrequent lifetime drinkers) and (2) former drinkers (<12 drinks in the year before the interview but ≥12 drinks in any previous year).

Problem Drinking.—Current drinkers answered 41 self-administered questions about the number of times they had alcohol-related problems in the past year (0, 1, 2 or 3, or ≥4 times) (eg, tried to cut down or stop drinking and found you couldn't do it? driven a car after having too much to drink? unable to remember some of the things you did while drinking?). While the NHIS-Alcohol questions were designed to operationalize the criteria for alcohol use disorders in the *Diagnostic and Statistical Manual of Mental Disorders, Revised Third Edition* (*DSM-III-R*),[15] there was no simple way to derive the diagnoses because the frequency of problems did not directly relate to the qualitative terms used in the *DSM-III-R* manual, and the items could not be clearly assigned to the individual criteria by either factor analysis or expert judgment. Two scales were derived by summing items that measured two broad areas of alcohol problems: (1) alcohol control and addiction and (2) interference with functioning. Respondents who scored at or above the 90th percentile on one or both scales were categorized as having no problems; the remainder were categorized as having some problems. Male and female respondents were separately categorized. A statistically derived cutpoint of the 90th percentile was adopted as straightforward and easily replicated.

Quantity of Ethanol.—Data on the frequency and amount of alcohol consumed in the most recent 2-week period in which the respondents drank were combined into a measure of the average amount of ethanol consumed, modeled on an approach used by Williams et al.[16] The amounts were categorized as follows: (1) light drinker—estimated daily consumption, 0.3 to 6.4 mL; (2) moderate drinker—estimated daily consumption, 6.5 to 29 mL; and (3) heavy drinker—estimated daily consumption, 30 mL or more.

Maximum Number of Drinks.—Respondents were classified as those reporting one or more occasions of drinking one to four drinks, five to eight drinks, and nine or more drinks in the year before the interview.

Self-perceived Rating.—The NHIS-Alcohol respondents who were current drinkers were asked, "Do you now consider yourself to be a heavy, moderate, light, very light, or occasional drinker?" As fewer than 2% of the respondents considered themselves to be heavy drinkers, the heavy and moderate categories were combined. All the NHIS-Alcohol respondents were asked to rate the drinking of other adults in the household as heavy, moderate, light, very light, or occasional; quit drinking; or never drank.

Injuries

The CHS respondents were asked if the index child had experienced an accident, injury, or poisoning that required medical attention in the year before the interview. Injuries were excluded if they (1) occurred more than 12 months before the interview or (2) resulted from misadventures or complications of medical care or adverse effects of drugs in therapeutic use or were the late effects of injuries (*ICD-9* [*International Statistical Classification of Diseases, Injuries, and Causes of Death, Ninth Revision*] E codes 870 through 879, 929, and 930 through 949).[17] Serious injury episodes were defined as injuries resulting in one half day or more in bed, any time missed from school, one or more nights in the hospital, or surgical treatment. In addition, injuries were classified by place of occurrence, circumstance (eg, motor vehicle crash), and type of injury, regardless of severity. There were 2063 injury episodes in the year prior to the interview; 720 of them were categorized as serious. Serious injuries were used as the major outcome because preliminary analyses showed them to be less subject to biased recall and likely to have more impact on children, families, and society than all injuries. The most common serious injury was laceration requiring sutures (38.6%), followed by fractures (18.1%). Head injuries accounted for 6.8% of the serious injuries.

Covariates

Two demographic variables, age and race of the parent, were strongly associated both with problem drinking and children's injuries. Family composition (two- or one-parent household) was associated with problem drinking and has been shown to be associated with total injuries[18] and was also used as a covariate.

Statistical Analysis

Annual rates of injuries per 100 children were calculated by dividing the number of injuries by the number of children and multiplying by 100. As the outcome of interest was a measure of child health, child weights provided by the NCHS were used to adjust the rates for the nonequal probability of sample selection and to allow calculation of national estimates. The adult person weights were used to describe the distribution of the adult alcohol respondent characteristics. The sample sizes reported in the tables reflect the actual number of subjects in each of the groups. Adjusted rates and SEs of the rates were calculated using Proc Regress within SUDAAN, which takes the complex sample of the NHIS and CHS into account.[19] Relative risks (RRs) were calculated by dividing rates in each group by the rate of injuries in the comparison group, most often the nondrinkers. The 95% confidence intervals (CIs) around the RRs were calculated using a formula based on the method of Katz et al.[20,21]

RESULTS

Description of Sample

The women who were problem drinkers were less likely to be black and to live in two-parent families than the nondrinkers (Table 1). They were also younger and had fewer children than the nondrinkers. Current drinkers who were not problem drinkers had more education and higher incomes than the other respondents. Similarly, men who were problem drinkers were younger and had fewer children than nondrinkers, and a smaller proportion of problem drinkers was black compared with non-

Table 1.—Selected Social and Demographic Characteristics of Female NHIS Alcohol Supplement Respondents by Problem Drinking*

	Problem Drinking Scale					
	Nondrinker	Former Drinker	No Problems	Some Problems	Problem Drinker	Total
Race, %						
B	17.1	10.7	10.6	10.5	11.1	13.1
W	72.9	84.4	84.9	85.3	85.1	85.1
Other	10.0	4.9	4.5	4.2	3.9	3.9
Family structure, %						
Two-parent family	78.8	81.7	80.4	78.2	68.5	78.5
Single-parent family	19.7	17.1	18.2	20.2	29.6	20.0
Other	1.4	1.3	1.4	1.5	1.9	1.5
Education, %						
≤12 y	68.9	59.5	52.3	51.5	65.0	61.4
>12 y	31.1	40.5	47.7	48.5	35.0	38.6
Income, %						
<$20 000/y	38.3	30.1	22.3	24.4	34.2	31.4
$20 000/y to $34 999/y	31.0	33.9	26.7	27.1	30.0	30.2
≥$35 000/y	30.8	36.0	51.0	48.5	35.8	34.2
Mean age, y	36.5	34.8	36.1	34.0	32.6	35.4
Mean No. of children	1.99	1.86	1.82	1.89	1.81	1.90
No. of respondents†	2875	1562	1586	811	948	7782

*Proportions and means reflect adult person weights. NHIS indicates National Health Interview Survey.
†The number of respondents varies because of missing data.

Table 2.—Serious Injuries to Children by Measures of Parental Alcohol Consumption and Problem Drinking

	Mothers			Fathers		
	N	Annual Serious Injury Rate to Children, per 100*	Relative Risk† (95% Confidence Interval)	N	Annual Serious Injury Rate to Children, per 100*	Relative Risk† (95% Confidence Interval)
Nondrinkers	2875	4.5	1.0	640	6.0	1.0
Former drinkers	1562	7.4	1.5 (1.1 to 2.1)	880	5.5	0.8 (0.5 to 1.4)
Current drinkers						
Problem drinking						
No problems	1586	6.0	1.2 (0.9 to 1.7)	1394	5.0	0.8 (0.5 to 1.2)
Some problems	811	6.7	1.4 (1.0 to 2.1)	1080	6.2	1.0 (0.6 to 1.6)
Problem drinkers	948	10.0	2.1 (1.3 to 3.5)	584	6.0	1.0 (0.5 to 1.6)
Quantity of ethanol per day, mL						
0.3 to 6.4	2228	7.4	1.5 (1.1 to 2.2)	1431	4.9	0.8 (0.5 to 1.3)
6.5 to 29	920	7.3	1.5 (1.0 to 2.3)	1140	5.8	1.0 (0.5 to 1.5)
≥30	197	5.9	1.2 (0.6 to 2.3)	487	7.5	1.2 (0.6 to 2.0)
Maximum No. of drinks per day						
1 to 4	2303	7.4	1.5 (1.1 to 2.2)	1292	4.9	0.8 (0.4 to 1.3)
5 to 8	733	6.8	1.4 (0.9 to 2.2)	935	4.8	0.7 (0.4 to 1.2)
≥9	309	7.7	1.6 (0.9 to 2.9)	831	7.6	1.2 (0.7 to 2.0)
Self-rating						
Very light	2142	7.7	1.6 (1.1 to 2.3)	1448	5.5	0.9 (0.5 to 1.4)
Light	757	6.0	1.3 (0.9 to 1.9)	792	5.1	0.9 (0.4 to 1.5)
Moderate/heavy	432	7.8	1.6 (1.0 to 2.8)	796	6.4	1.1 (0.6 to 1.7)

*Serious injuries are those that resulted in one-half day or more in bed, missed school, hospitalization, or surgery. These are crude rates.
†Relative risks are adjusted for race, family composition, and age of mother.

drinkers (data not shown). However, due to the way the sample was selected, 97% of the male respondents lived in two-parent households while only 79% of the female respondents lived in two-parent households.

Parental Alcohol Consumption, Problems, and Child Injuries

Children of women classified as problem drinkers had 2.1 times the risk of serious injury of children of women who did not drink alcohol after adjustment for race, family composition, and mother's age (Table 2). These RRs were statistically distinguishable from an RR of 1.0 ($P<.05$). Children of women who formerly drank alcohol but did not drink in the year before the interview were also at excess risk of serious injuries. There was a statistically significant dose-response relationship ($P<.001$) between the number of alcohol-related problems women have and the risk of child injury. The children of mothers who were problem drinkers had a number of serious injuries two thirds greater than that of children of mothers who were current drinkers but who reported having no problems on the problem drinking scale (10 vs six injuries per 100 children; 95% CI, 1.0 to 2.7).

None of the other measures of maternal alcohol consumption had a clear-cut dose-response relationship with child injuries or a relationship indicating a threshold level of consumption beyond which children were at increased risk.

None of the measures of father's drinking or alcohol-related problems was associated with increased risk of child injuries when the comparison was with nondrinkers. Compared with the rates of serious child injury in the lowest category of the current drinkers (ie, no problems on the problem drinking scale, 0.3 to 6.4 mL of ethanol consumed per day, maximum number of drinks per day of 1 to 4, self-perceived rating of very light drinking), the children of the drinkers in the highest categories of these measures had 20% to 60% more injuries (quantity of ethanol consumed: RR, 1.5, 95% CI, 0.9 to 2.5; maximum number of drinks: RR, 1.6, 95% CI, 1.0 to 2.5; self-rating of drinking: RR, 1.2, 95% CI, 0.7 to 1.8).

A series of analyses was performed to elucidate the differential relationship between maternal and paternal drinking and child injuries. To assess whether the differential association was due to more time spent with the mother, the relationship was examined separately for women who were employed vs those not employed outside the home. It was hypothesized that, if exposure were a salient factor, children of women who were problem drinkers not employed outside the home would be at higher risk of injuries than children of employed mothers. Contrary to this hypothesis, the RRs were similar in both groups (employed outside the home: RR, 2.2, 95% CI, 1.1 to 4.5; not employed outside the home: RR, 2.1, 95% CI, 1.2 to 3.6).

In this data set, 48.9% of married women categorized as problem drinkers were married to men rated as moderate or heavy drinkers, while only 13.0% of the men who were problem drinkers rated their wives as moderate or heavy drinkers. Therefore, it is possible that the stronger relationship between the mother's alcohol-related problems and child injuries was due to exposure to problem drinking in both parents, whereas the impact of the father's drinking may be modified by mothers who drink less than their spouses. This was investigated by analyzing the injuries of children of respondents married to

Table 3.—Serious Injuries to Children by Parental Problem Drinking and by Rating of Spouse's Drinking

	Nondrinker/Quit/ Very Light or Light Drinker			Moderate/Heavy Drinkers		
Parental Problem Drinking	N	Annual Serious Injury Rate to Children, per 100*	Relative Risk† (95% Confidence Interval)	N	Annual Serious Injury Rate to Children, per 100*	Relative Risk† (95% Confidence Interval)
Mother						
Nondrinkers	1581	4.5	1.0	191	5.1	1.0
Problem drinkers	243	6.9	1.5 (0.7 to 3.7)	233	13.7	2.7 (0.8 to 8.6)
Father						
Nondrinkers	550	5.1	1.0	8	31.1	1.0
Problem drinkers	400	4.6	0.9 (0.5 to 1.7)	60	11.1	‡

*Serious injuries are those that resulted in one-half day or more in bed, missed school, hospitalization, or surgery. These are crude rates.
†Relative risks are adjusted for race, family composition, and age of mother.
‡The relative risk was not calculated because of the small number in the contrast category.

Table 4.—Serious Injuries to Children by Mothers' Problem Drinking and by Mothers' Education and Children's Age and Sex

	N	Annual Serious Injury Rate to Children, per 100*	Relative Risk† (95% Confidence Interval)
Mother's education			
≤12 y			
Nondrinkers	1999	4.7	1.0
Problem drinkers	630	7.5	1.6 (1.0 to 2.5)
>12 y			
Nondrinkers	876	4.2	1.0
Problem drinkers	318	15.0	3.4 (1.4 to 7.8)
Child's age			
0 to 4 y			
Nondrinkers	847	3.5	1.0
Problem drinkers	324	7.8	2.1 (1.0 to 4.5)
5 to 12 y			
Nondrinkers	1216	3.0	1.0
Problem drinkers	404	9.0	2.7 (1.0 to 4.9)
13 to 17 y			
Nondrinkers	812	8.3	1.0
Problem drinkers	220	15.1	1.8 (0.6 to 5.1)
Sex			
Boys			
Nondrinkers	1504	5.8	1.0
Problem drinkers	484	10.1	1.7 (1.0 to 2.9)
Girls			
Nondrinkers	1371	3.2	1.0
Problem drinkers	464	9.9	2.9 (1.3 to 6.5)

*Serious injuries are those that resulted in one-half day or more in bed, missed school, hospitalization, or surgery. These are crude rates.
†Relative risks are adjusted for race, family composition, and age of mother.

spouses rated as moderate or heavy drinkers separately from those of children of respondents married to spouses not rated as moderate or heavy drinkers (Table 3). The RR of serious child injuries in the children of 233 women who were problem drinkers married to men who were rated as moderate or heavy drinkers (RR, 2.7) was substantially higher than the analogous RR for women married to men who were not moderate or heavy drinkers (RR, 1.5). The rate of serious injuries in the children of 60 men categorized as problem drinkers married to moderate- or heavy-drinking mothers was 11.1 per 100, higher than the rate of serious child injuries in children of all mothers who were categorized as problem drinkers (10.0 per 100).

Children of single mothers who were problem drinkers had an RR of serious injuries of 2.3 (95% CI, 1.2 to 4.3), higher than the risk for children of women married to nondrinkers or light drinkers but lower than the RR for children of two parents who both may be problem drinkers.

Socioeconomic Status (SES), Child's Age, and Sex as Modifiers of the Alcohol-Injury Relationship

To assess whether children with parents who are problem drinkers and who have lower SES are at increased risk of injuries, the analyses were stratified by education of the alcohol respondent, highest occupation in household, and income. Children of mothers with 12 years or less of education had a lower risk of injury associated with their mother's alcohol problems than children of mothers with more than 12 years of education (Table 4). Similarly, children of mothers in the lowest categories of occupation and income had a lower risk of injury associated with alcohol than those in the higher categories (data not shown). Compared with low-SES mothers who did not drink, the low-SES mothers who were problem drinkers were significantly more likely to be single (χ^2=27.8, P<.001) and to have moved more often (χ^2=25.7, P=.01). Both these factors may be barriers to seeking medical care that could result in lower rates of reported injuries. The association between father's problem drinking and child injuries was unaffected by these stratifications. No group was at higher or lower risk than any other group (data not shown).

The relationship between mother's problem drinking and child injuries was not strongest in the preschool children, as originally hypothesized (Table 4), nor was it stronger in preschool children who were cared for by their mothers and thus had more exposure to their mother's problem drinking than children cared for by other people or who were in preschool (data not shown).

Mother's problem drinking appears to be associated with an increase in the injury rate for girls, making it comparable to that of sons of problem drinkers. Because the girls with nondrinking mothers had a significantly lower rate of injuries than boys with nondrinking mothers (t=2.4, P=.02), the point estimate of the RR of injuries to girls associated with mother's problem drinking was substantially higher than the risk to boys, although the CIs have some overlap.

Nature, Circumstance, and Place of Injury by Maternal Alcohol Problems

Compared with children of mothers classified as nondrinkers, the children of problem drinkers had a higher risk of all types of injuries except burns (data not shown). They were at particularly high risk of sustaining head injuries (RR, 5.1, 95% CI, 1.4 to 17.8) and fractures (RR, 2.8, 95% CI, 1.4 to 5.8).

Children of mothers who were problem drinkers had a lower rate of motor vehicle–related injuries than children of nondrinkers (RR, 0.55, 95% CI, 0.3 to 1.2). In contrast, the children of problem drinkers had substantially more injuries involving bicycles, skateboards, and roller skates (RR, 2.2, 95% CI, 1.1 to 4.1) and dog and insect bites (RR, 5.7, 95% CI, 1.3 to 24.4) than children of nondrinkers.

While children of problem drinkers had more injuries at home than children of nondrinkers (RR, 1.6, 95% CI, 1.2 to 2.1), their risk of injuries occurring in recreational areas (RR, 3.4, 95% CI, 1.7 to 6.7) and in the street (RR, 2.2, 95% CI, 0.8 to 6.0) was even greater.

COMMENT

These data suggest that maternal alcohol-related problems have a strong association with serious child injuries. The father's alcohol consumption and problem drinking appear to be unrelated to risk of child injuries compared with nondrinkers and weakly associated compared with light current drinkers.

While it was hypothesized that the mother's drinking would be more strongly associated with child injuries than the father's drinking because children spend more time with their mothers, two analyses did not support this view. First, the children of women who were unemployed and who were problem drinkers were not at higher risk than similar children whose mothers were employed. Second, preschool-aged children who were cared for by their mothers did not have a higher risk of injuries associated with maternal alcohol problems than preschool-aged children who were in day care or nursery school or being cared for by someone else.

A more likely explanation of the different association in men and women is that the effect of the mother's problem drinking is due in large part to the presence of two parents in the household who may both be problem drinkers. Ample evidence exists that there is significant family dysfunction in families of alcoholics[6] that may lead to increased injury risk for children exposed to two parents with problem drinking through the inability of the family to provide both a safe physical environment and a nurturing emotional environment. The lower risk of injuries for children of parents who are problem drinkers but who are married to spouses who are not problem drinkers suggests that a parent without alcohol-related problems can offset the risk of injuries associated with his or her spouse's drinking. The spouse without problem drinking can do this by providing emotional support,[22,23] by positive role modeling, and/or by assuming responsibilities for supervision and parenting. Children of single mothers with problem drinking also have higher risks of injuries than children of both men and women with problem drinking who are married to spouses without problem drinking, which may reflect the lack of a spouse who could offset the risk associated with maternal alcohol problems.

The implication that the mother's drinking is more strongly related to child injuries than the father's drinking must be viewed cautiously for several reasons. First, the differential association could be an artifact of the self-reports of alcohol consumption and alcohol-related problems. Male respondents tend to report fewer physical and psychological symptoms than women, regardless of alcohol consumption.[24,25] Thus, the similar rates of injuries to children of men classified as heavy or problem drinkers and to children of men in other categories of the alcohol variables may reflect male respondents' unwillingness to report alcohol-related problems, resulting in misclassification of problem drinkers. Second, use of nondrinkers as the comparison group could bias the findings, as abstention and infrequent lifetime drinking are less normative behavior in men than women. In this sample, only 14% of the men were classified as nondrinkers vs 38% of the women (using adult weights). The comparison of the highest alcohol consumption and problem drinking categories with the categories reflecting light drinking avoids some of the inferential problems associated with comparisons with nondrinkers. These analyses revealed excess injury risk of 25% to 60% associated with the father's alcohol consumption, suggesting a moderate effect of father's drinking, and a continued excess risk of 67% associated with the mother's problem drinking.

The use of survey data to assess the relationship between alcohol use/abuse and injuries may introduce some sources of bias not found in data from medical providers while avoiding other biases from medical record data. Survey methodology has the advantage of providing data from a variety of sources (eg, emergency departments, clinics, private physicians, inpatient hospital services) without being subject to the vagaries of data-collection methods in multiple sites of care. It has the disadvantage of being subject to different reporting styles, underreporting of intentional injuries, and imperfect recall. It is known that longer recall periods lead to a predictable decrease in the number of injuries reported and that less severe injuries are more subject to memory decay than more serious ones.[26] While there are no methodological studies of reporting children's injuries by degree of alcohol use or abuse, it is possible that respondents who are problem drinkers are less able and/or less willing than other respondents to recall children's injuries. This systematic difference would lead to an observed rate of injuries in children of problem drinkers that underestimates the magnitude of the relationship. Therefore, the true risk to children of problem drinkers may be larger than indicated by this report.

The lack of a relationship between mother's drinking and child injuries in families of lower SES was an unexpected finding. The higher frequency of moves and single-parent family status in low-SES problem drinkers plus other, unmeasured factors, such as proximity of health services, all may serve as barriers to seeking medical care for child injuries by women with multiple social problems.

If a primary mechanism linking mother's use of alcohol to child injury is through direct supervision, one would expect preschool-aged children to be at highest risk, as found by Chafetz et al[12] and Putnam.[13] Contrary to these findings, in the present study, the youngest children did not have the highest risk of serious injury associated with maternal problem drinking. This result suggests that the effect of maternal problem drinking on the quality of the mother-child relationship or on child behavior may be more important than interference with direct supervision. The higher risk of bicycle, skateboard, and other recreational injuries and of animal and insect bites may reflect a wider exposure to high-risk activities and environments without proper safety considerations.

While the point estimates of relative risk in this study indicate that mothers' problem drinking may affect their daughters' injury risk more than that of their sons, the overlapping CIs suggest that this conclusion should be viewed cautiously. The finding that girls' risk of injury may be more strongly affected by mothers' drinking is, however, consistent with the health maintenance organization (HMO)–based study of Putnam.[13] Girls have fewer injuries than boys, which may be due to less exposure to hazards or a lower frequency of high-risk behaviors.[27,28] The effect of maternal alcohol problems may be a more salient contributor to the injuries of girls than boys because of the absence of other, competing risk factors and exposures for the girls' injuries.

These nationally representative data strongly suggest that children of women who are problem drinkers have an elevated risk of experiencing serious injuries and that children exposed to two parents with alcohol problems are at even higher risk. These data have several implications. Physicians who treat both parents and children need to be cognizant of the potential role played by parental problem drinking. The data suggest that the primary prevention of injuries might be enhanced if physicians included questions about parental alcohol use in the social history and encouraged adults with alcohol-related problems to seek treatment. The association between parental drinking and child injuries might be used as a motivation for behavioral change, as parents may respond more readily to messages concerning the effect of their behavior on their children's health than to messages about the impact on their own health. Further research that would elucidate the potentially causal links between parental alcohol use and children's injuries could be used to design intervention strategies. Finally, physician support is also needed for measures designed to reduce consumption and abuse on the societal level, such as extension of liability for injuries to advertisers and manufacturers and limiting the times and days of sales. Efforts on both the individual and societal levels are necessary components of a comprehensive and effective injury-control program.

This work was supported in part by grant R01-HD25416-02 from the National Institute of Child Health and Human Development. We thank Yossi Harel, PhD, and Deborah Hasin, PhD, for their comments on the research and Van Parsons, PhD, for assistance with the statistical analysis and programming.

References

1. Lowensfels AB, Miller TT. Alcohol and trauma. *Ann Emerg Med.* 1984;13:1056-1060.
2. Waller JA. 'Accident' proneness: fact or fiction. In: *Injury Control: A Guide to the Causes and Prevention of Trauma.* Lexington, Mass: Lexington Books; 1985:467-472.
3. Reilly EL. Role of alcohol use and abuse in trauma. *Adv Psychosom Med.* 1986;16:17-30.
4. National Institute on Alcohol Abuse and Alcoholism. Children of alcoholics: an interview with the NIAAA director. *Alcohol Health Res World.* 1984; 8:1-3.
5. Schoenborn CA. *Exposure to Alcoholism in the Family: United States, 1988.* Hyattsville, Md: National Center for Health Statistics; 1991. Advance Data No. 205.
6. Kammeier ML. Adolescents from families with and without alcohol problems. *Q J Stud Alcohol.* 1971;32:364-372.
7. El-Guebaly N, Oxford D. The offspring of alcoholics. *Am J Psychiatry.* 1977;134:357-365.
8. Orford J. Alcohol and the family: an international review of the literature with implications for research and practice. *Res Adv Alcohol.* 1990;10: 81-153.
9. Kaplan SJ, Pelcovitz D, Salzinger S, Ganeles D. Psychopathology of parents of abused and neglected children and adolescents. *J Am Acad Child Psychiatry.* 1983;22:238-244.
10. Famularo R, Stone K, Barnum R, Wharton R. Alcoholism and severe child maltreatment. *Am J Orthopsychiatry.* 1986;56:481-495.
11. Margolis LH, Kotch J, Lacey JH. Children in alcohol related motor vehicle crashes. *Pediatrics.* 1986;77:870-872.
12. Chafetz ME, Blane HT, Hill MJ. Children of alcoholics: observations in a guidance clinic. *Q J Stud Alcohol.* 1971;32:687-698.
13. Putnam S. Parental alcoholism as a risk factor in adolescents' injury rates: an HMO study. Presented at the American Medical Conference on Unintentional Injuries in Adolescents; November 6, 1987; Chicago, Ill.
14. Adams PF, Hardy AM. Current estimates from the National Health Interview survey: United States 1988. *Vital Health Stat.* 1989;10:173.
15. American Psychiatric Association, Committee on Nomenclature and Statistics. *Diagnostic and Statistical Manual of Mental Disorders, Revised Third Edition.* Washington, DC: American Psychiatric Association; 1987.
16. Williams GD, Dufour M, Bertolucci D. Drinking levels, knowledge, and associated characteristics: 1985 NHIS findings. *Public Health Rep.* 1986;101: 593-598.
17. World Health Organization. *Manual of the International Statistical Classification of Diseases, Injuries, and Causes of Death, Based on the Recommendations of the Ninth Revision Conference, 1975.* Geneva, Switzerland: World Health Organization; 1977.
18. Dawson, DA. Family structure and children's health and well being. *J Marriage.* 1991;53:573-584.
19. Shah BV, LaVange LM, Barnwell BG, Killinger JE, Wheeless SC. *SUDAAN: Procedures for Descriptive Statistics User's Guide.* Research Triangle Park, NC: Research Triangle Institute; 1989.
20. Kleinbaum DG, Kupper LL, Morgenstern H. *Epidemiologic Research.* Belmont, Calif: Lifetime Learning Publications; 1982:298.
21. Katz D, Baptista J, Azen SP, Pike MC. Obtaining confidence intervals for the risk ratio in cohort studies. *Biometrics.* 1978;34:469-474.
22. Obuchowska I. Emotional contact with the mother as a social compensatory factor in children of alcoholics. *Int Ment Health Res Newslett.* Winter 1974;16:2-4.
23. Clair D, Genest M. Variables associated with the adjustment of offspring of alcoholic fathers. *J Stud Alcohol.* 1987;48:345-355.
24. Linden W, Paulhus D, Dobson K. Effects of response styles on the report of psychological and somatic distress. *J Consult Clin Psychol.* 1986;54: 309-313.
25. Beyer JM, Trice HM. A retrospective study of similarities and differences between men and women employees in a job-based alcoholism program from 1965-1977. *J Drug Issues.* 1981;11:233-266.
26. *Optimum Recall Period for Reporting Persons Injured in Motor Vehicle Accidents.* Rockville, Md: National Center for Health Statistics; 1972. US Dept of Health, Education, and Welfare publication HSM 72-1050. Vital and Health Statistics, ser 2, No. 50.
27. Rivara FP, Bergman AB, LoGerfo JP, Weiss NS. Epidemiology of childhood injuries, II: sex differences in injury rates. *AJDC.* 1982;136:502-506.
28. Bijur P, Golding J, Haslum M, Kurzon M. Behavioral predictors of injury in school-age children. *AJDC.* 1988;142:1307-1312.

Television and Violence

The Scale of the Problem and Where to Go From Here

Brandon S. Centerwall, MD, MPH

IN 1975, Rothenberg's Special Communication in *JAMA*, "Effect of Television Violence on Children and Youth," first alerted the medical community to the deforming effects the viewing of television violence has on normal child development, increasing levels of physical aggressiveness and violence.[1] In response to physicians' concerns sparked by Rothenberg's communication, the 1976 American Medical Association (AMA) House of Delegates passed Resolution 38: "The House declares TV violence threatens the health and welfare of young Americans, commits itself to remedial actions with interested parties, and encourages opposition to TV programs containing violence and to their sponsors."[2]

Other professional organizations have since come to a similar conclusion, including the American Academy of Pediatrics and the American Psychological Association.[3] In light of recent research findings, in 1990 the American Academy of Pediatrics issued a policy statement: "Pediatricians should advise parents to limit their children's television viewing to 1 to 2 hours per day."[4]

Rothenberg's communication was largely based on the findings of the 1968 National Commission on the Causes and Prevention of Violence[5] and the 1972 Surgeon General's report, *Television and Growing Up: The Impact of Televised Violence*.[6] Those findings were updated and reinforced by the 1982 report of the National Institute of Mental Health, *Television and Behavior: Ten Years of Scientific Progress and Implications for the Eighties*, again documenting a broad consensus in the scientific literature that exposure to television violence increases children's physical aggressiveness.[7] Each of these governmental inquiries necessarily left open the question of whether this increase in children's physical aggressiveness would later lead to increased rates of violence. Although there had been dozens of laboratory investigations and short-term field studies (3 months or less), few long-term field studies (2 years or more) had been completed and reported. Since the 1982 National Institute of Mental Health report, long-term field studies have come into their own, some 20 having now been published.[8]

In my commentary, I discuss television's effects within the context of normal child development; give an overview of natural exposure to television as a cause of aggression and violence; summarize my own research findings on television as a cause of violence; and suggest a course of action.

TELEVISION IN THE CONTEXT OF NORMAL CHILD DEVELOPMENT

The impact of television on children is best understood within the context of normal child development. Neonates are born with an instinctive capacity and desire to imitate adult human behavior. That infants can, and do, imitate an array of adult facial expressions has been demonstrated in neonates as young as a few hours old, ie, before they are even old enough to know cognitively that they themselves have facial features that correspond with those they are observing.[9,10] It is a most useful instinct, for the developing child must learn and master a vast repertoire of behavior in short order.

Whereas infants have an instinctive desire to imitate observed human behavior, they do not possess an instinct for gauging a priori whether a behavior ought to be imitated. They will imitate anything,[11] including behaviors that most adults would regard as destructive and antisocial. It may give pause for thought, then, to learn that infants as young as 14 months of age demonstrably observe and incorporate behaviors seen on television (Fig 1).[12,13] (Looking ahead, in two surveys of young male felons imprisoned for committing violent crimes, eg, homicide, rape, and assault, 22% to 34% reported having consciously imitated crime techniques learned from television programs, usually successfully.[14])

As of 1990, the average American child aged 2 to 5 years was watching over 27 hours of television per week.[15] This might not be bad, if young children understood what they are watching. However, up through ages 3 and 4 years, many children are unable to distinguish fact from fantasy in television programs and remain unable to do so despite adult coaching.[16] In the minds of such young children, television is a source of entirely factual information regarding how the world works. Naturally, as they get older, they come to know better, but the earliest and deepest impressions were laid down when the child saw television as a factual source of information about a world outside their homes where violence is a daily commonplace and the commission of violence is generally powerful, exciting, charismatic, and efficacious. Serious violence is most likely to erupt at moments of severe stress—and it is precisely at such moments that adolescents and adults are most likely to revert to their earliest, most visceral

From the Department of Psychiatry and Behavioral Sciences, University of Washington, Seattle. Dr Centerwall is currently in private practice.
Reprint requests to 611 33rd Ave E, Seattle, WA 98112 (Dr Centerwall).

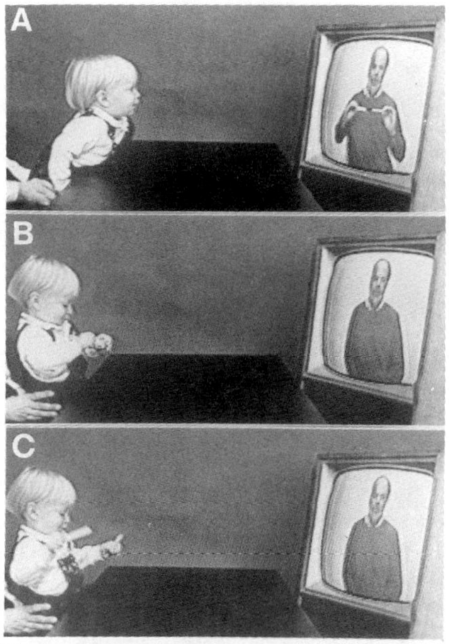

Fig 1.—This series of photographs shows a 14-month-old boy learning behavior from a television set. In photograph A the adult pulls apart a novel toy. The infant leans forward and carefully studies the adult's actions. In photograph B the infant is given the toy. In photograph C the infant pulls the toy apart, imitating what he had seen the adult do. Of infants exposed to the instructional video, 65% could later work the toy, as compared with 20% of unexposed infants ($P<.001$) (reprinted with permission from Meltzoff[12]).

sense of what violence is and what its role is in society. Much of this sense will have come from television.

Not all laboratory experiments and short-term field studies demonstrate an effect of media violence on children's behavior, but most do.[17,18] In a recent meta-analysis of randomized, case-control, short-term studies, exposure to media violence caused, on the average, a significant increase in children's aggressiveness as measured by observation of their spontaneous, natural behavior following exposure ($P<.05$).[19]

NATURAL EXPOSURE TO TELEVISION AS A CAUSE OF AGGRESSION AND VIOLENCE

In 1973, a small Canadian town (called "Notel" by the investigators) acquired television for the first time. The acquisition of television at such a late date was due to problems with signal reception rather than any hostility toward television. Joy et al[20] investigated the impact of television on this virgin community, using as control groups two similar communities that already had television. In a double-blind research design, a cohort of 45 first- and second-grade students were observed prospectively over a period of 2 years for rates of objectively measured noxious physical aggression (eg, hitting, shoving, and biting). Rates of physical aggression did not change significantly among children in the two control communities. Two years after the introduction of television, rates of physical aggression among children in Notel had increased by 160% ($P<.001$).

In a 22-year prospective study of an age cohort in a semirural US county (N=875), Huesmann[21] observed whether boys' television viewing at age 8 years predicted the seriousness of criminal acts committed by age 30. After controlling for the boys' baseline aggressiveness, intelligence, and socioeconomic status at age 8, it was found that the boys' television violence viewing at age 8 significantly predicted the seriousness of the crimes for which they were convicted by age 30 ($P<.05$).

In a retrospective case-control study, Kruttschnitt et al[22] compared 100 male felons imprisoned for violent crimes (eg, homicide, rape, and assault) with 65 men without a history of violent offenses, matching for age, race, and census tract of residence at age 10 to 14 years. After controlling for school performance, exposure to parental violence, and baseline level of criminality, it was found that the association between adult criminal violence and childhood exposure to television violence approached statistical significance ($P<.10$).

All Canadian and US studies of the effect of prolonged childhood exposure to television (2 years or more) demonstrate a positive relationship between earlier exposure to television and later physical aggressiveness, although not all studies reach statistical significance.[8] The critical period of exposure to television is preadolescent childhood. Later variations in exposure, in adolescence and adulthood, do not exert any additional effect.[23,24] However, the aggression-enhancing effect of exposure to television is chronic, extending into later adolescence and adulthood.[8,25] This implies that any interventions should be designed for children and their caregivers rather than for the general adult population.

These studies confirm what many Americans already believe on the basis of intuition. In a national opinion poll, 43% of adult Americans affirm that television violence "plays a part in making America a violent society," and an additional 37% find the thesis at least plausible (only 16% frankly disbelieve the proposition).[26] But how big a role does it play? What is the effect of natural exposure to television on entire populations? To address this issue, I took advantage of an historical experiment—the absence of television in South Africa prior to 1975.[8,25]

TELEVISION AND HOMICIDE IN SOUTH AFRICA, CANADA, AND THE UNITED STATES

The South African government did not permit television broadcasting prior to 1975, even though South African whites were a prosperous, industrialized Western society.[8] Amidst the hostile tensions between the Afrikaner and English white communities, it was generally conceded that any South African television broadcasting industry would have to rely on British and American imports to fill out its programming schedule. Afrikaner leaders felt that that would provide an unacceptable cultural advantage to the English-speaking white South Africans. Rather than negotiate a complicated compromise, the Afrikaner-controlled government chose to finesse the issue by forbidding television broadcasting entirely. Thus, an entire population of 2 million whites—rich and poor, urban and rural, educated and uneducated—was nonselectively and absolutely excluded from exposure to television for a quarter century after the medium was introduced into the United States. Since the ban on television was not based on any concerns regarding television and violence, there was no self-selection bias with respect to the hypothesis being tested.

To evaluate whether exposure to television is a cause of violence, I examined homicide rates in South Africa, Canada, and the United States. Given that blacks in South Africa live under quite different conditions than blacks in the United States, I limited the comparison to white homicide rates in South Africa and the United States and the total homicide rate in Canada (which was 97% white in 1951). Data analyzed were from the respective government vital statistics registries. The reliability of the homicide data is discussed elsewhere.[8]

Following the introduction of television into the United States, the annual white homicide rate increased by 93%, from 3.0 homicides per 100 000 white population in 1945 to 5.8 per 100 000 in 1974; in South Africa, where television was banned, the white homicide rate decreased by 7%, from 2.7 homicides per 100 000 white population in 1943 through 1948 to 2.5 per 100 000 in 1974 (Fig 2). As with US whites, following the introduction of television into Canada the Canadian homicide rate increased by 92%, from 1.3 homicides per 100 000 population in 1945 to 2.5 per 100 000 in 1974 (Fig 3).

For both Canada and the United States, there was a lag of 10 to 15 years between the introduction of television and the subsequent doubling of the ho-

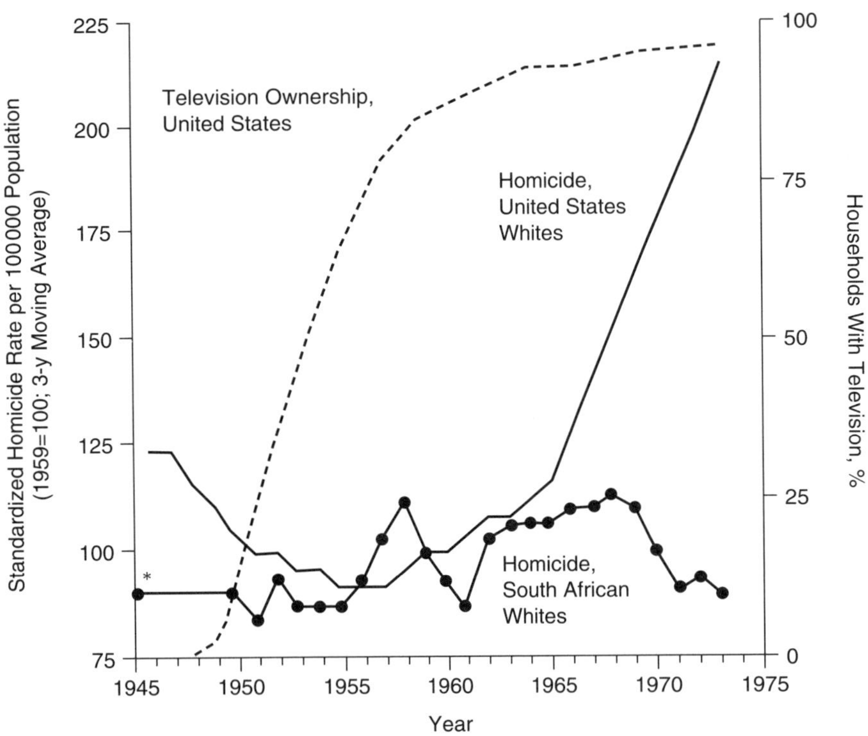

Fig 2.—Television ownership and white homicide rates, United States and South Africa, 1945 through 1973. Asterisk denotes 6-year average. Note that television broadcasting was not permitted in South Africa prior to 1975 (from Centerwall[8] and reprinted by permission of Academic Press).

micide rate (Figs 2 and 3). Given that homicide is primarily an adult activity, if television exerts its behavior-modifying effects primarily on children, the initial "television generation" would have had to age 10 to 15 years before they would have been old enough to affect the homicide rate. If this were so, it would be expected that, as the initial television generation grew up, rates of serious violence would first begin to rise among children, then several years later it would begin to rise among adolescents, then still later among young adults, and so on. And that is what is observed.[8]

In the period immediately preceding the introduction of television into Canada and the United States, all three countries were multiparty, representative, federal democracies with strong Christian religious influences, where people of nonwhite races were generally excluded from political power. Although television broadcasting was prohibited prior to 1975, white South Africa had well-developed book, newspaper, radio, and cinema industries. Therefore, the effect of television could be isolated from that of other media influences. In addition, I examined an array of possible confounding variables—changes in age distribution, urbanization, economic conditions, alcohol consumption, capital punishment, civil unrest, and the availability of firearms.[8] None provided a viable alternative explanation for the observed homicide trends. For further details regarding the testing of the hypothesis, I refer the reader to the published monograph[8] and commentary.[25]

A comparison of South Africa with only the United States (Fig 2) could easily lead to the hypothesis that US involvement in the Vietnam War or the turbulence of the civil rights movement was responsible for the doubling of homicide rates in the United States. The inclusion of Canada as a control group precludes these hypotheses, since Canadians likewise experienced a doubling of homicide rates (Fig 3) without involvement in the Vietnam War and without the turbulence of the US civil rights movement.

When I published my original paper in 1989, I predicted that white South African homicide rates would double within 10 to 15 years after the introduction of television in 1975, the rate having already increased 56% by 1983 (the most recent year then available).[8] As of 1987, the white South African homicide rate had reached 5.8 homicides per 100 000 white population, a 130% increase in the homicide rate from the rate of 2.5 per 100 000 in 1974, the last year before television was introduced.[27] In contrast, Canadian and white US homicide rates have not increased since 1974. As of 1987, the Canadian homicide rate was 2.2 per 100 000, as compared with 2.5 per 100 000 in 1974.[28] In 1987, the US white homicide rate was 5.4 per 100 000, as compared with 5.8 per 100 000 in 1974.[29] (Since Canada and the United States became saturated with television by the early 1960s [Figs 2 and 3], it was expected that the effect of television on rates of violence would likewise reach a saturation point 10 to 15 years later.)

It is concluded that the introduction of television in the 1950s caused a subsequent doubling of the homicide rate, ie, long-term childhood exposure to television is a causal factor behind approximately one half of the homicides committed in the United States, or approximately 10 000 homicides annually. Although the data are not as well developed for other forms of violence, they indicate that exposure to television is also a causal factor behind a major proportion—perhaps one half—of rapes, assaults, and other forms of interpersonal violence in the United States.[8] When the same analytic approach was taken to investigate the relationship between television and suicide, it was determined that the introduction of television in the 1950s exerted no significant effect on subsequent suicide rates.[30]

To say that childhood exposure to television and television violence is a predisposing factor behind half of violent acts is not to discount the importance of other factors. Manifestly, every violent act is the result of an array of forces coming together—poverty, crime, alcohol and drug abuse, stress—of which childhood exposure to television is just one. Nevertheless, the epidemiologic evidence indicates that if, hypothetically, television technology had never been developed, there would today be 10 000 fewer homicides each year in the United States, 70 000 fewer rapes, and 700 000 fewer injurious assaults.[25,31]

WHERE TO GO FROM HERE

In the war against tobacco, the tobacco industry is the last group from whom we expect any meaningful action. If someone were to call on the tobacco industry to cut back tobacco production as a matter of social conscience and out of concern for the public health, we would regard that person as being at least simple-minded, if not frankly deranged. Oddly enough, however, people have persistently assumed that the television industry operates by a higher standard of morality than the tobacco industry—that it is useful to appeal to its social

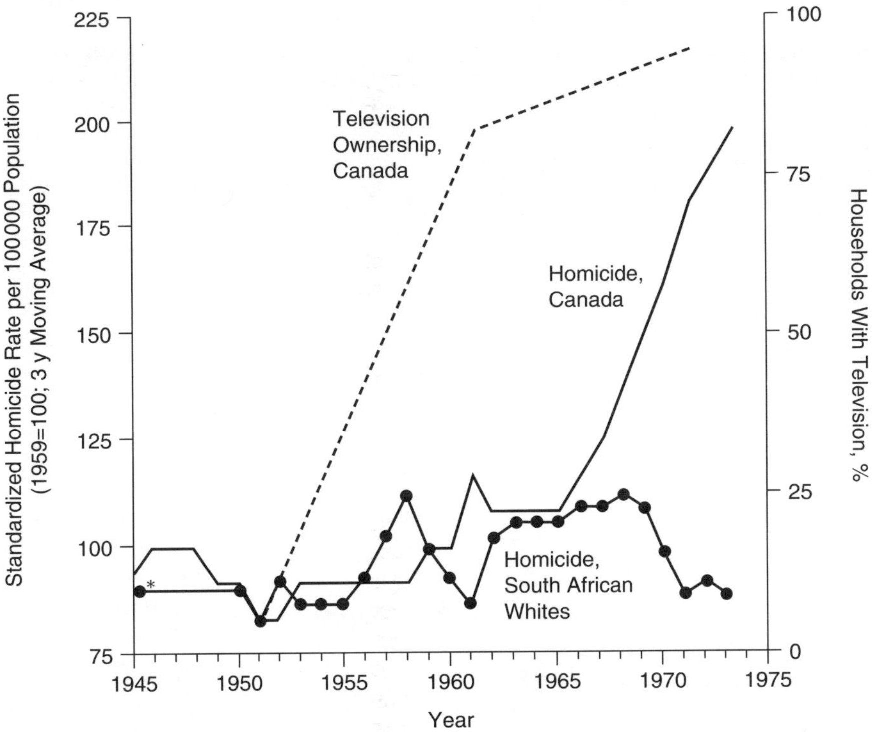

Fig 3.—Television ownership and homicide rates, Canadians and white South Africans, 1945 through 1973. Asterisk denotes 6-year average. Note that television broadcasting was not permitted in South Africa prior to 1975 (from Centerwall[8] and reprinted by permission of Academic Press).

conscience. This was true in 1969 when the National Commission on the Causes and Prevention of Violence published its recommendations for the television industry.[32] It was equally true in 1989 when the US Congress passed a television antiviolence bill that granted television industry executives the authority to confer on the issue of television violence without being in violation of antitrust laws.[33] Even before the law was fully passed, the four networks stated that they had no intention of using this antitrust exemption to any useful end and that there would be no substantive changes in programming content.[34] They have been as good as their word.

Cable aside, the television industry is not in the business of selling programs to audiences. It is in the business of selling audiences to advertisers. Issues of "quality" and "social responsibility" are entirely peripheral to the issue of maximizing audience size within a competitive market—and there is no formula more tried and true than violence for reliably generating large audiences that can be sold to advertisers. If public demand for tobacco decreases by 1%, the tobacco industry will lose $250 million annually in revenue.[35] Similarly, if the television audience size were to decrease by 1%, the television industry would stand to lose $250 million annually in advertising revenue.[35] Thus, changes in audience size that appear trivial to you and me are regarded as catastrophic by the industry. For this reason, industry spokespersons have made innumerable protestations of good intent, but nothing has happened. In over 20 years of monitoring levels of television violence, there has been no downward movement.[36,37] There are no recommendations to make to the television industry. To make any would not only be futile but create the false impression that the industry might actually do something constructive.

The American Academy of Pediatrics recommends that pediatricians advise parents to limit their children's television viewing to 1 to 2 hours per day.[4] This is an excellent point of departure and need not be limited to pediatricians. It may seem remote that a child watching television today can be involved years later in violence. A juvenile taking up cigarettes is also remote from the dangers of chronic smoking, yet those dangers are real, and it is best to intervene early. The same holds true regarding television-viewing behavior. The instruction is simple: For children, less TV is better, especially violent TV.

Symbolic gestures are important, too. The many thousands of physicians who gave up smoking were important role models for the general public. Just as many waiting rooms now have a sign saying, "This Is a Smoke-Free Area" (or words to that effect), so likewise a sign can be posted saying, "This Is a Television-Free Area." (This is not meant to exclude the use of instructional videotapes.) By sparking inquiries from parents and children, such a simple device provides a low-key way to bring up the subject in a clinical setting.

Children's exposure to television and television violence should become part of the public health agenda, along with safety seats, bicycle helmets, immunizations, and good nutrition. One-time campaigns are of little value. It needs to become part of the standard package: Less TV is better, especially violent TV. Part of the public health approach should be to promote child-care alternatives to the electronic baby-sitter, especially among the poor who cannot afford real baby-sitters.

Parents should guide what their children watch on television and how much. This is an old recommendation[32] that can be given new teeth with the help of modern technology. It is now feasible to fit a television set with an electronic lock that permits parents to preset which programs, channels, and times they wish the set to be available for; if a particular program or time of day is locked, the set won't turn on for that time or channel.[38] The presence of a time-channel lock restores and reinforces parental authority, since it operates even when the parents are not at home, thus permitting parents to use television to their family's best advantage. Time-channel locks are not merely feasible, but have already been designed and are coming off the assembly line (eg, the Sony XBR).

Closed captioning permits deaf and hard-of-hearing persons access to television. Recognizing that market forces alone would not make closed-captioning technology available to more than a fraction of the deaf and hard-of-hearing, the Television Decoder Circuitry Act was signed into law in 1990, requiring that, as of 1993, all new television sets (with screens 33 cm or larger, ie, 96% of new television sets) be manufactured with built-in closed-captioning circuitry.[39] A similar law should require that eventually all new television sets be manufactured with built-in time-channel lock circuitry—and for a similar reason. Market forces alone will not make this technology available to more than a fraction of households with children and will exclude poor families, the ones who suffer the most from violence. If we can make television technology available that will benefit 24 million deaf and hard-of-hearing Americans,[39] surely we can do no less for the benefit of 50 million American children.[35]

Unless they are provided with information, parents are ill-equipped to judge which programs to place off-limits. As a final recommendation, television programs should be accompanied by a violence rating so parents can gauge how violent a program is without having to watch it. Such a rating system should be quantitative and preferably numerical, leaving aesthetic and social judgments to the viewers. Exactly how the scale ought to be quantified is less important than that it be applied consistently. Such a rating system would enjoy broad popular support: In a national poll, 71% of adult Americans favor the establishment of a violence rating system for television programs.[40]

It should be noted that none of these recommendations impinges on issues of freedom of speech. That is as it should be. It is not reasonable to address the problem of motor vehicle fatalities by calling for a ban on cars. Instead, we emphasize safety seats, good traffic signs, and driver education. Similarly, to address the problem of violence caused by exposure to television, we need to emphasize time-channel locks, program rating systems, and education of the public regarding good viewing habits.

Figure 1 was provided by A. N. Meltzoff, University of Washington, Seattle.

References

1. Rothenberg MB. Effect of television on children and youth. *JAMA.* 1975;234:1043-1046.
2. American Medical Association. *Proceedings of the House of Delegates, June-July, 1976.* Chicago, Ill: American Medical Association; 1976:280.
3. Zylke JW. More voices join medicine in expressing concern over amount, content of what children see on TV. *JAMA.* 1988;260:1831-1832.
4. American Academy of Pediatrics, Committee on Communications. Children, adolescents, and television. *Pediatrics.* 1990;85:1119-1120.
5. Baker RK, Ball SJ, eds. *Violence and the Media: A Staff Report to the National Commission on the Causes and Prevention of Violence.* Washington, DC: US Government Printing Office; 1969.
6. Surgeon General's Scientific Advisory Committee on Television and Social Behavior. *Television and Growing Up: The Impact of Televised Violence.* Washington, DC: US Government Printing Office; 1972.
7. Pearl D, Bouthilet L, Lazar J, eds. *Television and Behavior: Ten Years of Scientific Progress and Implications for the Eighties.* Rockville, Md: National Institute of Mental Health; 1982.
8. Centerwall BS. Exposure to television as a cause of violence. In: Comstock G, ed. *Public Communication and Behavior.* Orlando, Fla: Academic Press Inc; 1989;2:1-58.
9. Meltzoff AN, Moore MK. Newborn infants imitate adult facial gestures. *Child Dev.* 1983;54:702-709.
10. Meltzoff AN, Moore MK. Imitation in newborn infants: exploring the range of gestures imitated and the underlying mechanism. *Dev Psychol.* 1989;25:954-962.
11. Meltzoff AN. Infant imitation after a 1-week delay: long-term memory for novel acts and multiple stimuli. *Dev Psychol.* 1988;24:470-476.
12. Meltzoff AN. Imitation of televised models by infants. *Child Dev.* 1988;59:1221-1229.
13. Meltzoff AN. Memory in infancy. In: Squire LR, Byrne J, Nadel L, Roediger H, Schacter D, Thompson R, eds. *Encyclopedia of Learning and Memory.* New York, NY: Macmillan Publishing Co Inc; 1992.
14. Heller MS, Polsky S. *Studies in Violence and Television.* New York, NY: American Broadcasting Company; 1976.
15. AC Nielsen Company. *Nielsen Report on Television 1990.* Northbrook, Ill: Nielsen Media Research; 1990.
16. Flavell JH. The development of children's knowledge about the appearance-reality distinction. *Am Psychol.* 1986;41:418-425.
17. Andison FS. TV violence and viewer aggression: a cumulation of study results, 1954-1976. *Public Opinion Q.* 1977;41:314-331.
18. Hearold S. A synthesis of 1043 effects of television on social behavior. In: Comstock G, ed. *Public Communication and Behavior.* Orlando, Fla: Academic Press Inc; 1986;1:65-133.
19. Wood W, Wong FY, Chachere JG. Effects of media violence on viewers' aggression in unconstrained social interaction. *Psychol Bull.* 1991;109:371-383.
20. Joy LA, Kimball MM, Zabrack ML. Television and children's aggressive behavior. In: Williams TM, ed. *The Impact of Television: A Natural Experiment in Three Communities.* Orlando, Fla: Academic Press Inc; 1986:303-360.
21. Huesmann LR. Psychological processes promoting the relation between exposure to media violence and aggressive behavior by the viewer. *J Soc Issues.* 1986;42(3):125-139.
22. Kruttschnitt C, Heath L, Ward DA. Family violence, television viewing habits, and other adolescent experiences related to violent criminal behavior. *Criminology.* 1986;24:235-267.
23. Milavsky JR, Kessler RC, Stipp HH, Rubens WS. *Television and Aggression: A Panel Study.* Orlando, Fla: Academic Press Inc; 1982.
24. Hennigan KM, Del Rosario ML, Heath L, Cook TD, Wharton JD, Calder BJ. Impact of the introduction of television on crime in the United States: empirical findings and theoretical implications. *J Pers Soc Psychol.* 1982;42:461-477.
25. Centerwall BS. Exposure to television as a risk factor for violence. *Am J Epidemiol.* 1989;129:643-652.
26. Harris L. Too much TV violence. *Harris Survey.* August 4, 1977.
27. Central Statistical Service. *Deaths: Whites, Coloureds and Asians, 1987.* Pretoria, South Africa: Government Printer; 1989.
28. World Health Organization. *World Health Statistics Annual, 1989.* Geneva, Switzerland: World Health Organization; 1989.
29. National Center for Health Statistics. *Vital Statistics of the United States, 1987.* Hyattsville, Md: US Department of Health and Human Services; 1990.
30. Centerwall BS. Young adult suicide and exposure to television. *Soc Psychiatry Psychiatr Epidemiol.* 1990;25:149-153.
31. Johnson JM, DeBerry MM Jr. *Criminal Victimization 1989: A National Crime Survey Report.* Washington, DC: US Department of Justice; 1990.
32. National Commission on the Causes and Prevention of Violence. *To Establish Justice, To Insure Domestic Tranquility: Final Report of the National Commission on the Causes and Prevention of Violence.* Washington, DC: US Government Printing Office; 1969:187-207.
33. Dietz WH, Strasburger VC. Children, adolescents, and television. *Curr Probl Pediatr.* 1991;21:8-31.
34. Clark KR. Antiviolence law won't bring much change, networks say. *Seattle Times.* August 10, 1989:F12.
35. US Bureau of the Census. *Statistical Abstract of the United States: 1991.* Washington, DC: US Government Printing Office; 1991.
36. Signorielli N, Gross L, Morgan M. Violence in television programs: ten years later. In: Pearl D, Bouthilet L, Lazar J, eds. *Television and Behavior: Ten Years of Scientific Progress and Implications for the Eighties.* Rockville, Md: National Institute of Mental Health; 1982:158-173.
37. Gerbner G, Gross L, Morgan M, Signorielli N. *The Violence Profile: Enduring Patterns.* Philadelphia, Pa: Annenberg School of Communication; 1989.
38. Surgeon General's Northwest Conference on Interpersonal Violence. *Report.* Seattle, Wash: US Public Health Service; 1987:93-94.
39. DuBow S. The Television Decoder Circuitry Act—TV for all. *Temple Law Rev.* 1991;64:609-618.
40. Los Angeles Times Poll. Television sex and violence. Poll 196, September 19, 1989. In: Opinion Research Service. *American Public Opinion Data.* Louisville, Ky: Opinion Research Service; 1989.

Origins and Clinical Relevance of Child Death Review Teams

Michael J. Durfee, MD; George A. Gellert, MD, MPH, MPA; Deanne Tilton-Durfee

Interagency child death review teams have emerged in response to the increasing awareness of severe violence against children in the United States. Since 1978, when the first team originated in Los Angeles, Calif, child death review teams have been established across the nation. Approximately 100 million Americans or 40% of the nation's population now live in counties or states served by such teams; most have been formed since 1988. Multiagency child death review involves a systematic, multidisciplinary, and multiagency process to coordinate and integrate data and resources from coroners, law enforcement, courts, child protective services, and health care providers. This article provides an introduction to the unique factors and magnitude of suspicious child deaths, and to the concept and process of interagency child death review. Future expansion of this process should lead to more effective multiagency case management and prevention of future deaths and serious injuries to children from child abuse and neglect.

(*JAMA*. 1992;267:3172-3175)

OVER 1000 American children die each year of intentional injuries at the hands of a caretaker (P. W. McClain, MS, J. J. Sacks, MD, MPH, R. D. Froehlke, MD, A. D. Ewigman, MD, oral communication, April 1992).[1] Most are infants or young toddlers.[2-4] No single health, social service, law enforcement, or judicial system exists to track and comprehensively assess the circumstances of child deaths.[5] This article describes the expanding national implementation of interagency multidisciplinary child death review teams in response to the critical need for systematic evaluation and case management of suspicious child deaths.

From the Los Angeles (Calif) County Department of Health Services (Dr Durfee), Orange County Health Care Agency, Santa Ana, Calif (Dr Gellert), and Los Angeles County (Calif) Interagency Council on Child Abuse and Neglect (Ms Tilton-Durfee).

Reprint requests to Department of Health Services, County of Los Angeles, 313 N Figueroa St, Los Angeles, CA 90012 (Dr Durfee).

MAGNITUDE OF THE PROBLEM

It is difficult to estimate the incidence of fatal child abuse using traditional data systems.[6] Available statistics reflect varied levels of competence in detection, evaluation, and recording of child deaths and variation in definitions used by different agencies. The National Committee for Prevention of Child Abuse, which annually surveys all states, reported a national incidence of 1383 child abuse fatalities for 1991.[1] The National Committee for Prevention of Child Abuse survey does not utilize a rigorous case definition and excludes cases not known to social service departments or other child abuse agencies. The Centers for Disease Control uses vital statistics and Federal Bureau of Investigation *Uniform Crime Reports* to arrive at an annual national figure of about 2000 child fatalities from abuse or neglect (P. W. McClain, MS, J. J. Sacks, MD, MPH, R. D. Froehlke, MD, A. D. Ewigman, MD, oral communication, April 1992). In Los Angeles County, California, 14 years of multiagency child death review suggests that the numbers will increase as abuse-related fatalities are more accurately identified and reported.

UNIQUE FACTORS IN CHILD DEATH

Death scene investigators evaluating adult victims may follow protocols fairly objectively. First responders to an imminent or actual child death scene, however, may be swept up in an intense focus on providing life support for the victim and emotional support for the victim's family. Even when it becomes apparent at the hospital that the circumstances of death are suspicious, delays may occur before an investigator returns to the scene of the event, or investigators may visit only the hospital and request that the medical staff interpret the death.

Criminal investigation of a child death caused by a caretaker is unique for investigators, since the perpetrator is legally responsible for the child and has continuous access to the victim. This contrasts with the majority of adult homicides where the victim and perpetrator are not cohabiting at the time the injury causing death is perpetrated. Child deaths may also result from the neglect of children by caretakers who are expected to provide for the child victim's biological needs. The concept of not feeding, protecting, or otherwise providing for the unique needs of a young child may be difficult to comprehend for a homicide detective with no child abuse training.

Most suspicious child deaths occur among very young children. Studies of "fatal child abuse" or of "homicide by

Table 1.—Evolution of Child Death Review Teams in the United States*

State	Status of First Team: Year	Location	Present Status†: State	Local	Population Covered by Teams, in Millions
California	1978	Los Angeles County	x	x	29.8
South Carolina	1985	State	x		3.5
Missouri	1986	Boone County	x	x	5.1
Oregon	1986	State	x	x	2.8
Minnesota	1987	State	x	x	4.4
Ohio	1988	Franklin County		x	1.0
Colorado	1988	State	x	x	3.3
Florida	1989	Local/state	x	x	12.9
Illinois	1989	Cook County		x	5.6
Vermont	1989	State	x		0.6
Georgia	1990	State/local	x	x	6.5
Iowa	1990	State	x		2.8
Indiana	1991	Marion County		x	1.0
Maryland	1991	State	x		4.8
New Hampshire	1991	State	x		1.1
New Mexico	1991	State	x		1.5
North Carolina	1991	State/local	x	x	6.6
Washington	1991	Spokane County	x	x	4.9
Hawaii	1992	Honolulu County		x	0.8
Maine	1992	State	x		1.2
Oklahoma	1992	State	x		3.1
Total					**103**

*States having state and/or local teams including (1) interagency teams including health, human and social services, and criminal justice representatives; (2) inclusive intake of potentially suspicious child deaths from coroners' or health databases, or from local referral; and (3) team review of cases.
†Status as of April 1992.

caretaker" indicate that 50% of the victims are under 1 year of age.[2-4] These young victims may have no previous records or only medical records that are not frequently accessed as part of the death investigation. Autopsies of young children require a specialized understanding of pediatrics, pathology, child abuse, and forensic investigation. Few jurisdictions have such experts. Autopsies may be conducted by physicians with no formal pathology training, much less specialization in forensic pathology.[7] Radiological and laboratory equipment for clinical or forensic tests may make a diagnosis possible,[8,9] but these tests may be unavailable locally or may not be ordered to reduce costs.

The above factors contribute to inappropriate surveillance, potential underreporting, misclassification, and mismanagement of child deaths. Case management is further confounded by problems in interagency communications. An extreme example of a case lost in multiple systems involved a 10-month-old infant whose family had 52 agency contacts before the child was eventually beaten to death. Contacts included law enforcement, child protective services, hospital emergency departments, public health nurses, and a psychiatric emergency team. Most individual agency actions appeared reasonable, but no single agency had a comprehensive and collective record of contacts with the family.

HISTORY OF CHILD DEATH REVIEW TEAMS

Child abuse prevention and intervention are relatively new phenomena. "Child abuse" was not indexed in *Index Medicus* until 1965 and "infanticide" was not indexed until 1970. Much of the limited medical literature on fatal child abuse has been published within the last 3 years. The preponderance of medical and other data are available only from uncirculated sources.[10-12]

Los Angeles County began the nation's first interagency child death review team involving criminal justice and health and human service professionals in 1978. This team evolved from the experience of clinical teams conducting "death review" rounds on internal medicine wards. Weekly review of all adult deaths on a busy hospital service demonstrated the educational benefits of a systematic review of death as a way to improve services to the living. Child death review adapted the process of review to the premature deaths of children in the community. By April 1992, interagency, multidisciplinary child death review teams drawing cases systematically from agency referrals, coroner–medical examiner records, or vital statistics had been established at the state and/or local level in 21 states (Table 1), covering 100 million Americans or 40% of the nation's population.

CHILD DEATH REVIEW TEAMS

Multiagency child death review teams lend greater clarity and coherence to case management and help define intraagency and interagency problems. The core team includes at least five members with representatives from the coroner–medical examiner's office, law enforcement agencies, prosecuting attorneys (municipal, district, or state), child protective services, pediatricians with child abuse expertise, and health professionals, including public health nurses.[13-15]

In most states, the coroner–medical examiner or health department supplies a list of child death cases selected through an established protocol designed to include all deaths with suspicious causation. Colorado and Missouri state teams and some local teams review all child deaths from any cause.[12,16] Confidentiality of medical records is maintained within the team process. The medical examiner or other medical professionals interpret autopsy findings and medical history for nonmedical team members. Law enforcement assumes the role of case manager if criminal investigation is warranted. Prosecutors educate the team on criminal law pertaining to individual cases and pursue litigation as appropriate. Child protective services provides records from previous contacts with the victim's family and coordinates efforts to protect surviving siblings. Medical professionals access and interpret clinical records of trauma or physical neglect, educate the team on pertinent medical issues, and may assist in referrals for direct health care evaluation and services for surviving family members. Public health specialists may provide vital records and can develop epidemiological risk profiles of families for early detection and prevention of child death and serious injury.

Other team members can include representatives from mental health agencies, fire department emergency medical personnel, probation and parole departments,[14] substance abuse treatment providers, local school and preschool educators, sudden infant death syndrome experts, and state or local child advocates. Private hospitals may participate if they are actively involved with child abuse prevention or have involvement in a case under review.[13,14]

Most team members are employed at the direct service level, although senior managers and political appointees may be a part of some mandated state teams. Most teams have grown in the number and diversity of members during the first year of reviewing cases.

Teams may function at the state and/or local jurisdictional level. Some large

Table 2.—Potential Outcomes/Impact of Interagency Child Death Review

Improvement of the following:

(1) Interagency communication for management of death cases and for management of future nonfatal cases.
(2) Accuracy of and capability for criminal, civil, and social intervention for families with fatalities.
(3) Intervention with surviving and at-risk siblings, including counseling and follow-up.
(4) Profile of families at risk for fatal or severe abuse and neglect.
(5) Intraagency and interagency systems using cases to audit the total health and social service systems and to minimize misclassification of cause of child death.
(6) Evaluation of the impact of specific risk factors, including substance abuse, domestic violence, and previous child abuse.
(7) Interagency services to high-risk families.
(8) Data collection for surveillance of deaths and for study of categories of death such as bathtub drownings or burns.
(9) Relationship with mass media and use of media to educate the public about child abuse prevention.
(10) Intercounty and interstate communications regarding child death.

states have local teams but no state teams. The trend is toward establishing both local and state teams (Table 1). Missouri became the first state to establish a complete functioning network of state and local teams in all jurisdictions (March 1992). The various teams began through individual initiative, state-initiated legislation, or administrative mandate. Some county teams gather in regional clusters and the southern states scheduled the first regional multistate meeting in South Carolina in April 1992. Most teams function with little or no specific funding; resources for team management come from the member agencies. A few teams receive additional funding for staff support. All teams save costs through increased effectiveness of interventions and reduced duplication of efforts.

Table 2 summarizes several of the potential outcomes of multiagency child death review. Few data are currently available but should become more so in the next few years. One of the first tangible changes in case outcome in Los Angeles County occurred in 1983. Seven child death cases chosen from a systematic team review from 1981 through 1983 that were designated as natural or accidental in causation were modified at a coroner's inquest to "death at the hands of another." Several of these cases resulted in criminal actions and referrals of surviving siblings for protective services. Another case reviewed by the team was reclassified from homicide to natural death.

The multiagency team process is more vigorous than the single agency process, more capable of clearly identifying a case that is suspicious, and more able to deal with special challenges, such as the difficulty of identifying the perpetrator out of multiple caretakers, separating out physical findings that confuse the determination of cause of death,[17] or distinguishing sudden infant death syndrome from suffocation.[18] The results are more focused, more complete, and the process is more accountable. Outcome reports from the team add to that accountability.

Child death review also creates an opportunity for a systematic review of agency actions (and inactions). This has been particularly important with respect to improving and integrating interagency communications, and allowing agencies the opportunity to address deficits in their own systems. Surviving siblings can be identified and referred for protection, evaluation, and service. Health professionals with previous contacts with the child or family can improve their clinical judgment and case management skills by learning retrospectively from the follow-up information obtained through child death review.

Small case numbers in rural counties and the ability of the involved agencies to focus extensively on each case offers an opportunity for some teams to develop specifically targeted local preventive actions for childhood injury. Such action may involve various multiagency prevention programs, including child safety seats for automobiles, drowning prevention, and suicide prevention.

Law enforcement, child protective services, coroner's investigators, and public health nursing team members all conduct home visits and investigations. These professionals thereby possess outreach capability for families that are beyond the coverage of mainstream community medical systems. Team education allows such professionals to become a resource for detecting and referring medical and social problems that predispose a family to violence. High-risk problems that may be detected include pregnancies involving maternal substance abuse, pregnant women exposed to domestic violence, failure-to-thrive infants, and homes lacking basic child safety measures.

SPECIAL POPULATIONS

Other special populations could benefit from review, including spousal homicides with surviving children, child siblings as perpetrators, children killing parents, and homicides of disabled adults and the dependent elderly by family members. The team process may be extended to live children with the addition of children with severe nonfatal injuries.

Child and adolescent suicides with a history of prior child abuse represents another potential population for multiagency review and management. In Los Angeles County, 28% of all suicides under the age of 18 years in 1989 (n=43) were found to have a history of previous child protective services. The incidence of previous child abuse was inversely related to age (85% of 14-year-olds).[4] This has resulted in the formation of a multiagency task force to address child and adolescent suicide.

The Los Angeles County coroner investigates approximately 40 fetal deaths annually from a countywide total of over 1000 fetal deaths per year. Most of the coroner's cases appear to result from maternal substance abuse, usually cocaine. Several fetal deaths each year result from homicide or assault of a pregnant woman.[4] Fetal deaths traditionally receive intervention only at the hospital. Team intervention with fetal deaths from maternal substance abuse may include a public health nurse referral to help the mother and other family members prevent such behavior in the future. Fetal deaths from assaults on the mother may be followed by criminal justice investigation and prosecution.

SIGNIFICANCE FOR MEDICAL PROFESSIONALS

The child death review team is an activity with significant impact on basic health care. Physicians and other health professionals contribute to and benefit from the child death review team process. Physicians assure that medical records are made available to review teams, explain and interpret medical findings for nonmedical team members, and assist with case referral and management. Participating clinicians may improve their access to other agencies and thereby achieve a broader base for health care service provision to children, and increase their sensitivity for management of high-risk families.

Medical team members are exposed to extensive clinical material, including Munchausen syndrome by proxy,[19,20] sudden infant death syndrome, apnea and suffocation,[18] drowning,[21] burns,[22] neglect,[23] abdominal trauma,[24] neonaticide,[25] shaken baby syndrome,[26,27] and head trauma.[28] Clinical pathological conferences, even for unusual presentations, may include child abuse in the differential diagnosis.[29]

Medical team members have special value as liaisons with other health care providers who cared for the child before the incident that caused death. Occasionally, previous caretakers will have noted injuries or family problems that may assist in defining a pattern of abusive behavior. Previous caretakers may also have failed to report suspected child abuse or neglect and may benefit from peer support and consultation.

FUTURE ISSUES AND CONCLUSIONS

The US Advisory Board on Child Abuse and Neglect has made specific recommendations to the Secretary of Health and Human Services about the development of child death review teams[30] and held a national hearing on fatal child abuse in Los Angeles in April of 1992. The US Department of Health and Human Services is heading an interagency task force to address implementation of this process nationally. The US Public Health Service objectives for the year 2000 include recommendations for state-level child death review teams in 45 states.[31] The task for the 1990s will be to build a national network of teams and to integrate that network with health care providers to establish a prevention system for families and children before they are injured or killed.

Child death review began initially as a method to address suspected child abuse or neglect fatalities. Many teams have expanded this focus to address all coroners' cases including suicide, accidental deaths, and natural deaths. Prevention of child abuse fatalities involves early detection of families at risk and coordinated multiagency intervention directed at those risk factors. Factors that elevate risk in a particular locality can be identified through the study of past child deaths. The team process facilitates more competent and predictable intervention through agencies that have learned to work together more effectively.

The interagency child death review team is clearly an idea whose time has come. Child death review teams have grown rapidly in the last 3 years with little or no external funding and limited national leadership. Federal and state funding and support of child death review teams would greatly facilitate the expansion of review across the nation. A national data registry could quantify and demonstrate the impact on detection, management, and prevention of fatal child abuse on an ongoing basis.

References

1. Daro D, McCurdy K. *Current Trends in Child Abuse Reporting and Fatalities: The Results of the 1991 Annual Fifty State Survey.* Chicago, Ill: National Committee for the Prevention of Child Abuse; 1992.
2. Christoffel K. Violent death and injury in US children and adolescents. *AJDC.* 1990;144:697-706.
3. Division of Injury Control, Center for Environmental Health and Injury Control, Centers for Disease Control. Childhood injuries in the United States. *AJDC.* 1990;144:627-646.
4. Los Angeles County Interagency Council on Child Abuse and Neglect. *Child Death Review Team Report.* Los Angeles, Calif: Los Angeles County Interagency Council on Child Abuse and Neglect; 1990, 1991.
5. Durfee M. Fatal child abuse: intervention and prevention. *Protecting Child.* Spring 1989:9-12.
6. Anderson TL, Wells SJ. *Data Collection for Child Fatalities: Existing Efforts and Proposed Guidelines.* Washington, DC: American Bar Association Center on Children and the Law and the American Academy of Pediatrics; 1992.
7. Lundstrom M, Sharpe R. Getting away with murder. *Public Welfare.* Summer 1991:18-29.
8. Kleinman PK, Blackbourne SD, Marks SC, Karellas A, Belanger PL. Radiological contributions to the investigation and prosecution of cases of fatal infant abuse. *N Engl J Med.* 1989;320:507-511.
9. Riffenburgh RS, Lakshmanan S. The eyes of child abuse victims: autopsy findings. *J Forensic Sci.* 1991;36:741-747.
10. Smith P, Durfee M. *Child Death Review: A Review of Unpublished Reports by States.* Los Angeles, Calif: Los Angeles County Dept of Health Services; 1991.
11. *A Report of Oregon Fatalities due to Abuse and Neglect, 1985-89.* Salem, Ore: State of Oregon, Dept of Human Resources, Child Protective Services Program; 1990.
12. *Colorado Child Fatality Review Committee Annual Report and Conference Proceedings.* Denver, Colo: Colorado Child Fatality Review Committee; 1991.
13. *California Protocol for Child Death Review Teams.* Sacramento, Calif: California Dept of Justice; 1988.
14. Granik LA, Durfee M, Wells SJ. *Child Death Review Teams: A Manual for Design and Implementation.* Washington, DC: American Bar Association and the American Academy of Pediatrics; 1992.
15. Kaplan SR, Granik LA. *Child Fatalities Investigative Procedures Manual.* Washington, DC: American Bar Association and the American Academy of Pediatrics; 1992.
16. Strangler GJ, Kivlahan C, Knipp M. How can we tell when a child dies from abuse? Missouri's new law will help answer that question. *Public Welfare.* Fall 1991;5-11.
17. Levin AW. Ocular manifestations of child abuse. *Ophthalmol Clin North Am.* 1990;3:249-262.
18. Meadows R. Suffocation, recurrent apnea, and sudden infant death. *J Pediatr.* 1990;117:351-357.
19. Sullivan CA, Francis GL, Bain MW, Hartz J. Munchausen syndrome by proxy: 1990 a portent for problems? *Clin Pediatr.* 1990;29:587-590.
20. Kravitz RM, Wilnott RW. Munchausen syndrome by proxy presenting as factitious apnea. *Clin Pediatr.* 1990;29:587-590.
21. Griest KJ, Zumwalt RE. Child abuse by drowning. *Pediatrics.* 1989;83:41-46.
22. McLoughlin E, McGuire A. The causes, cost, and prevention of childhood burn injuries. *AJDC.* 1990;144:677-683.
23. Margolin L. Fatal child neglect. *Child Welfare.* 1990;4:309-319.
24. Fossum RM, Descheneaux KA. Blunt trauma of the abdomen in children. *J Forensic Sci.* 1991; 36:47-50.
25. Saunders E. Neonaticides following 'secret' pregnancies: seven case reports. *Public Health Rep.* 1989;104:368-372.
26. Alexander R, Sato Y, Smith W, Bennet T. Incidence of impact trauma with cranial injuries ascribed to shaking. *AJDC.* 1990;144:724-726.
27. Spaide RF, Swengel RM, Scharre DW, Mein C. Shaken baby syndrome. *Am Fam Physician.* 1990; 41:1145-1152.
28. Apolo JU. Bloody cerebrospinal fluid: traumatic tap or child abuse? *Pediatr Emerg Care.* 1987;2: 93-95.
29. Reece RM. Unusual manifestations of child abuse. *Pediatr Clin North Am.* 1990;37:905-921.
30. US Advisory Board on Child Abuse and Neglect. *Creating Caring Communities: Blueprint for an Effective Federal Policy on Child Abuse and Neglect.* Washington, DC: US Advisory Board on Child Abuse and Neglect; 1991.
31. *Healthy People 2000: National Health Promotion and Disease Prevention Objectives.* Washington, DC: US Dept of Health and Human Services, Public Health Service; 1990.

Male Victims of Sexual Assault

Gary H. Lipscomb, MD; David Muram, MD; Pat M. Speck, RN; Brian M. Mercer, MD

Objective.—To compare the demographics, physical findings, and assault characteristics of incarcerated, sexually assaulted men with those of nonincarcerated, sexually assaulted men.

Design.—Case series of 99 adult male victims of sexual assault evaluated over a 3-year period.

Setting.—Memphis Sexual Assault Resource Center, a nonhospital-based clinic that serves as the primary resource for sexually assaulted victims in the Memphis and Shelby County, Tennessee, area.

Participants.—All adult male victims of sexual assault evaluated at the Memphis Sexual Assault Resource Center during the study period were included in the study. Ninety-nine victims were studied, including 80 incarcerated men and 19 men from the community.

Results.—The victims of sexual assault in the community group were older than the victims in the incarcerated group. Apart from the age difference and weapon use, there were no statistically significant differences between the incarcerated and nonincarcerated victims.

Conclusions.—The similarities between the two groups suggest that sexual assault of men may not be unique to prisons, and all men are potential victims. Further studies are required to better understand these crimes and to develop education and prevention programs.

(*JAMA*. 1992;267:3064-3066)

CRIMES of sexual assault are prevalent in today's society and affect both men and women, regardless of their age or socioeconomic class.[1] While the actual number of victims remains unknown, there is an overwhelming consensus that many assaults remain unreported by victims.[2] While many organizations have been advocating on behalf of female victims of rape, society has chosen to largely ignore male victims of sexual assault, preferring to presume that such assaults occur only as isolated events affecting primarily prison inmates.[2-4] The few published reports describing sexual assaults on male victims estimate that 0.5% to 3% of inmates are sexually assaulted.[5] Data on nonincarcerated men are lacking. What data have been reported deal primarily with child victims of sexual abuse.[6] In this study, we compare the demographics, physical findings, and assault characteristics of adult male, sexually assaulted victims who were incarcerated and nonincarcerated adult male victims.

Materials and Methods

The study was conducted at the Memphis Sexual Assault Resource Center (MSARC). The MSARC is a nonhospital-based clinic that serves as the primary resource for sexually assaulted victims in the Memphis and Shelby County, Tennessee, area. Personnel are available 24 hours a day to provide medical services and to collect specimens for forensic evaluation. Victims enter the system through self-referral or referral from the police or local hospitals. A nurse from the MSARC performs a sexual assault examination in the receiving hospital's emergency department if the patient's medical condition precludes travel to the MSARC. All services are free of charge to the patient. Victims are encouraged but not required to notify authorities of the assault. The center routinely examines male victims assaulted in the community as well as the victims from the city or county penal system.

Records were reviewed for all male victims of sexual assault who were 15 years of age or older and seen at the MSARC between January 1, 1988, through December 12, 1990. The state of Tennessee considers victims of sexual assault who are 15 years of age and older as adults and does not refer these individuals to the Department of Human Services for further follow-up. Therefore, for the purpose of this report, we chose to include all victims 15 years of age or older as adults. Data collected via standardized protocol included the physical findings, demographics of the victims and assailants (if known), type of assault, history of previous assault, assailant's relationship to the victim, use of weapon, self-reported mental illness, location of assault, and number of assailants. Victims were not questioned about sexual orientation or, in the case of inmates, the reason for incarceration. Statistical analysis was performed for the entire study group and separately for inmates and noninmates using the two-tailed Pearson χ^2 test and the Student's t test where appropriate. A P value of $<.05$ was considered significant.

Results

During the study period, 1752 adults were evaluated at the MSARC. From these adults there were 99 (5.7%) male victims who made up the study group. Eighty victims were inmates from the Shelby County penal system, and the

From the Department of Obstetrics and Gynecology, University of Tennessee, Memphis (Drs Lipscomb, Muram, and Mercer), and the Memphis (Tenn) Sexual Assault Resource Center (Ms Speck).

Reprint requests to Department of Obstetrics and Gynecology, University of Tennessee, 853 Jefferson Ave, Room E102, Memphis, TN 38103 (Dr Lipscomb).

Demographics of the Victims and Characteristics of the Assaults

	Inmates, No. (%) (n=80)	Community, No. (%) (n=19)
Age, y		
<18	1 (1.2)	3 (15.8)
18-20	31 (38.8)	5 (26.3)
21-30	43 (54.0)	6 (31.6)
31-40	5 (6.2)	3 (15.8)
>40	0 (0.0)	4 (21.1)
Trauma scale*		
0	60 (75.0)	11 (58)
1	18 (22.5)	8 (42.1)
2	2 (2.5)	0 (0.0)
3	0 (0.0)	0 (0.0)
4	0 (0.0)	0 (0.0)
Assailants, No.		
1	25 (31.2)	9 (47.4)
2	23 (28.8)	5 (26.3)
3	16 (20.0)	3 (15.8)
4	8 (10.0)	1 (5.3)
>4	7 (8.8)	1 (5.3)
Weapon use		
None	54 (67.5)	6 (31.6)
Guns	0 (0.0)	5 (26.3)
Knives	18 (22.5)	5 (26.3)
Blunt objects	7 (8.8)	1 (5.3)
Assault type		
Anal only	30 (37.5)	9 (47.4)
Oral only	10 (12.5)	5 (26.3)
Anal/oral	30 (37.5)	4 (21.0)
Assailant/victim, race		
White/white	0 (0.0)	0 (0.0)
White/black	1 (1.2)	1 (5.3)
Black/white	23 (28.8)	5 (26.3)
Black/black	45 (56.2)	10 (52.6)
Multiple/white†	0 (0.0)	1 (5.3)
Multiple/black†	0 (0.0)	1 (5.3)
Unknown	10 (12.5)	1 (5.3)

*0 indicates none; 1, mild (bruises, abrasions); 2, moderate (cuts, bites); 3, extreme (medical treatment required); and 4, life-threatening.

†Multiple indicates black and white assailants (no other races present).

remaining 19 assaults occurred within the community. All of the assaults involved male assailants except one rape of a man in the community by two women during a robbery and extortion attempt.

Assaults on nonincarcerated men occurred in a wide variety of sites and locations within the community with no one area predominating. Only two nonincarcerated victims knew their assailants, and in both instances the assault occurred following recreational drug use by both the victim and assailant. Ten (53%) of 19 victims were abducted and taken to other sites where the assault actually occurred.

The demographics of the victims and the characteristics of the assaults are shown in the Table. As this table demonstrates, inmates were younger overall (mean age, 23.3 years; range, 17 to 39 years) than victims assaulted in the community (mean age, 30.5 years; range, 15 to 62 years). Only three victims were younger than 18 years—two aged 17 years and one aged 15 years. One of theses three (a 17-year-old victim) was an inmate. This difference in age was statistically significant at a value of $P<.04$.

There was no statistical difference between the two groups with regard to the presence or absence of trauma incurred during the assault. Victims were often assaulted by more than one assailant, but contrary to common belief, prisoners were no more likely to be assaulted by multiple assailants than were nonincarcerated victims. Weapons of some type were commonly employed in the attacks. As one might suspect, weapons were less common in prison ($P<.01$). However, this difference was solely attributable to the lack of firearms in prison. There was no difference in the use of knives (or other sharp objects) or clubs by the two groups. Blacks accounted for the majority of victims and the majority of assailants in both groups. There were no differences noted between inmates and noninmates in the racial composition of assailants and victims.

Of the 99 victims, 16 reported a history of mental or psychiatric illness. Seventeen patients also reported previous sexual victimization. Seven patients reported both a history of mental illness and previous sexual victimization. Although there were no differences between inmates and noninmates in self-reported mental illness or prior victimization, there was a significant association of mental illness with prior sexual assault in general ($P<.01$). In those patients revealing the dates of previous victimization, nine of 10 were victimized during adulthood.

Comparison between the incarcerated and nonincarcerated victims showed no significant difference in any variable studied, except for the use of weapons and the age of the victims.

Comment

The current study describes a relatively large series of adult male victims of sexual assault. Even though the majority of patients in the current series were inmates in a correctional facility, the number of patients assaulted within the community is comparable with other reports of noninstitutionalized male victims.[7-13] None of the victims in this series sustained injuries serious enough to require medical attention. Injuries were not limited to the perineal area but were the result of beatings the victims sustained during the assault. These findings correspond to our experience with female victims of sexual assault and suggest that in most instances the threat of physical force or injury is enough to subdue the victim. Only two patients, both inmates, sustained more than minor bruises and abrasions during the assault, and these two victims did not require medical attention. While these injuries may have occurred when the victims were subdued, it is also possible that the beatings represent the settling of other disputes in the prison.

All of the assaults except one were committed by other men. Sexual assault of men by women is extremely rare, but has been previously reported.[14] In this particular instance, the assault was documented by photographs taken by an armed female accomplice during a robbery. The assailants threatened to deliver the photographs to the victim's wife if the robbery was reported.

Weapons were used in most of the assaults occurring in the community compared with only one third of assaults occurring in jail. Interestingly, if firearms were excluded, there was no difference in the use or type of weapon used by the two groups. In the less confined community situations, a potential victim may be able to flee an unarmed assailant. The presence of a weapon, particularly firearms, would discourage such attempts. Within the confines of a prison, physical threat alone may be enough to intimidate that potential victim into submission.

As a group, the victims of sexual assault that occurred in the community were older than the victims in the incarcerated group. Although this age difference was statistically significant ($P<.04$), it probably reflects the relatively young age of prisoners in general. There was no specific age that put either incarcerated or nonincarcerated victims at an increased risk of assault.

The Shelby County area has a large black population and the penal population is primarily black. Since violent crimes are most often committed by and against poor members of ethnic minorities, it is not surprising that blacks accounted for the majority of victims and the majority of assailants. Moss et al[5] have suggested that the sexual assault of men, at least in prison, may be part of a racial power struggle. These conclusions were primarily based on unpublished data from the 1970s indicating that minority groups were almost exclusively the aggressor against white victims. Our data suggest that rather than being racially motivated, the demographics of both the perpetrators and male victims of sexual assault may be more similar to that of other violent crimes.

In the present series, the correlation of mental illness with repeat sexual assault raises the possibility that such mental illness places an individual at an increased risk for repeated assault. This increased risk may be the result of the victims' risk-taking behaviors, or because these individuals are perceived as being easy targets. However, since the definition of mental illness was left to each victim, the exact nature of this "illness" is unknown. It is uncertain what percentage of the general population would respond affirmatively to this question. Without further definition of the term *mental illness*, a meaningful comparison of the incidence of mental illness in our group as compared with the overall population in prison or the community cannot be made. More detailed studies would be needed to establish the actual relationship, if any, between mental illness and risk for sexual assault.

Victims from the community were not only sexually assaulted but also voluntarily chose to seek medical and/or therapeutic help. Only a small percentage of women actually report sexual assault.[2] Similarly, most assaults on men in the community are probably not reported to the authorities and are therefore not investigated. This may reflect the victim's fear of being labeled a homosexual or intense embarrassment about being a victim of sexual assault. However, the incarcerated patient may have been brought into a hospital for a medical evaluation not by his own choosing, thus disproportionately increasing the number of inmates in any series. In a prison setting where an assailant and his victim continue to live in close proximity, the victim may report an assault to receive protection from further assaults. Therefore, this sample of victims may not be representative of all sexually assaulted men and may, in fact, represent a very skewed subset of sexually assaulted men.

Apart from the age differences and weapons used, which reflect differences distinctive to the prison environment, there were no significant differences between the incarcerated and nonincarcerated victims in our group of patients. The similarities between these two groups would suggest that the sexual assault of men may not be due to conditions unique to a prison, and all men are potential victims. Goth and Burgess[9] have suggested that the sexual assault of men, like sexual assault of women, is not a sexually motivated crime, but rather a crime of aggression. In their series, many offenders who assaulted men were relatively indiscriminate regarding the sex of their victim. They chose their victim based on presumed vulnerability and availability rather than sex. In a community environment, women are likely to be perceived as more vulnerable than men and, thus, more likely to become victims. Despite the similarities, the current series includes only a few victims who were assaulted in the community and appears to justify previously accepted impressions that most male victims of sexual assault are inmates.

Very little is known about the long-term sequelae in men following sexual assault. Further studies are required to better understand these crimes and to develop education and prevention programs. In the meantime, we must develop a support system to provide counseling for victims who demonstrate emotional distress.

References

1. Kemp C. Sexual abuse, another hidden pediatric problem. *Pediatrics.* 1978;62:382-386.
2. Goth A, Birnbaum H. *Men Who Rape.* New York, NY: Plenum Press; 1979.
3. Brownmiller S. *Against Our Will.* New York, NY: Simon & Schuster Inc Publishers; 1975.
4. Burgess A, Holmstrom L. Rape trauma syndrome. *Am J Psychiatry.* 1974;131:981-986.
5. Moss C, Hosford R, Anderson W. Sexual assault in prison. *Psychol Rep.* 1979;44:823-828.
6. Geist RF. Sexually related trauma. *Emerg Med Clin North Am.* 1988;6:439-466.
7. Anderson C. Males as sexual assault victims: multiple levels of trauma. *J Homosex.* 1981-1982; 7:145-162.
8. Davis A. Sexual assaults in the Philadelphia prison system and sheriff's vans. *Transaction.* 1968; 6:8-16.
9. Goth N, Burgess W. Male rape: offenders and victims. *Am J Psychiatry.* 1980;137:806-810.
10. Goyer PF, Eddleman HC. Same-sex rape of nonincarcerated men. *Am J Psychiatry.* 1984;141: 576-579.
11. Kaufman A, Divasto P, Jackson R, Vorhees D, Christy J. Male rape victims: noninstitutionalized assault. *Am J Psychiatry.* 1980;137:221-223.
12. Mezey G, King M. The effects of sexual assault on men: a survey of 22 victims. *Psychol Med.* 1989; 19:205-209.
13. Sagrin E. Prison homosexuality and its effect on post-prison sexual behavior. *Psychiatry.* 1976; 39:245-257.
14. Masters WH. Sexual dysfunction as an aftermath of sexual assault of men by women. *J Sex Marital Ther.* 1986;12:35-45.

Assessing for Abuse During Pregnancy

Severity and Frequency of Injuries and Associated Entry Into Prenatal Care

Judith McFarlane, DrPH; Barbara Parker, PhD; Karen Soeken, PhD; Linda Bullock, MS

Objective.—To assess the occurrence, frequency, and severity of physical abuse during pregnancy and associated initiation of prenatal care.

Design.—Stratified, prospective cohort analysis.

Setting.—Public prenatal clinics in Houston, Tex, and Baltimore, Md.

Participants.—Total population-based sample of 691 black, Hispanic, and white pregnant women. All of the women were urban residents and most of the Hispanic women were Mexican American. All participants were invited into the study at the first prenatal visit and were followed up until delivery.

Main Outcome Measure.—Identification of abuse status.

Results.—A three-question Abuse Assessment Screen detected a 17% (1/6) prevalence of physical or sexual abuse during pregnancy, which is more than double all previous published reports. When evaluated against nationally tested research instruments, the three-question screen that was asked at the first prenatal visit was sensitive and specific to abuse status. Abuse was recurrent, with 60% of abused women reporting two or more episodes of assault. Location of abuse focused on the head. Frequency and severity of abuse and potential danger of homicide was appreciably worse for white women. Abused women were twice as likely as nonabused women to begin prenatal care during the third trimester.

Conclusions.—A simple clinical assessment screen completed by the health care provider in a private setting and with the male partner absent is as effective as research instruments in identifying abused women. Straightforward, routine clinical assessment is recommended as essential in preventing potential trauma, interrupting existing abuse, and protecting health.

(*JAMA*. 1992;267:3176-3178)

PHYSICAL abuse during pregnancy has recently been recognized as a significant risk to the health of both mother and infant.[1-3] Depending on the population surveyed and the number of questions asked, reports of abuse during pregnancy vary from 3% to 8%.[4-9] Limitations of reported studies include lack of data on the severity or frequency of the injury and association of abuse with entry into prenatal care. Many previously sampled populations were predominantly of one ethnic or racial group. To our knowledge, the effectiveness of direct clinical assessment for abuse compared with research interview questionnaires has not been evaluated.

From the Texas Woman's University, Houston (Dr McFarlane and Ms Bullock); the University of Maryland, Baltimore (Drs Parker and Soeken). Ms Bullock is a student at the University of Otago (New Zealand).

Reprint requests to Texas Woman's University, 1130 M. D. Anderson Blvd, Houston, TX 77030 (Dr McFarlane).

Methods

To determine the frequency and severity of physical abuse during pregnancy and associated entry into prenatal care, 691 black, Hispanic, and white pregnant women in public prenatal clinics in Houston, Tex, and Baltimore, Md, were assessed for abuse using the Abuse Assessment Screen (AAS) (Table 1). Following appropriate approval by institutional review boards at both sites and completion of informed consent procedures, screening questions were asked in a private setting by the woman's primary care provider. Women who answered yes to questions 2, 3, or 4 were considered abused. Following assessment, all women (both abused and nonabused) completed the Conflict Tactics Scale (CTS)[10] and the Index of Spouse Abuse (ISA).[11] Abused women were administered a Danger Assessment Screen (DAS) to determine their potential danger of homicide.[12] All instruments were offered in English and Spanish and were readministered during the second and third trimesters. All women were offered written information on the cycle of violence and community resources for law enforcement, safe shelter, and legal aid.

The CTS measures self-reported frequency of violent tactics within a relationship during the past year. Four subscales are measured, including verbal reasoning (eg, discussion and arbitration); verbal aggression (eg, swearing and threatening to hit); minor violence (eg, pushing, shoving, and slapping); and severe violence (eg, kicking, hitting, and using a knife or gun). In the current study, internal consistency reliability (coefficient α) was .80. Construct validity has been supported by significant and substantial correlation between CTS scores and variables in other independent studies.[13,14] Percentile norm data exist for the CTS based on data obtained from national probability sampling in 1979 and 1985.[15,16]

The ISA is a 30-item, self-report scale designed to measure the severity or magnitude of physical (ISA-P) and nonphysical (ISA-NP) abuse inflicted on a woman by her male partner. In the current study, the internal consistency reliability (coefficient α) was .95 for the instrument as a whole, was .87 for the ISA-P subscale, and was .93 for the ISA-NP subscale.

Finally, the DAS was administered to assist the abused women to determine their potential danger of homicide. The DAS has assessed reliability of .71 and a correlation of .75 with the ISA-P subscale and .49 with the severe-abuse subscale of the CTS.

All data were obtained by self-report. Reports of abuse were not validated with emergency department or police reports. The results described herein may not be generalizable to populations other than those surveyed.

Results

The demographic characteristics, abuse status, and entry into prenatal care of the 691 pregnant women are presented in Table 2. Most women were between the ages of 20 and 29 years, with 31%

Table 1.—Determination of Frequency and Severity of Physical Abuse During Pregnancy

Abuse Assessment Screen (Circle YES or NO for each question)

1. Have you ever been emotionally or physically abused by your partner or someone important to you? .... YES NO

2. Within the last year, have you been hit, slapped, kicked, or otherwise physically hurt by someone? .... YES NO

   If YES, by whom (circle all that apply)

   Husband Ex-husband Boyfriend Stranger Other Multiple

   Total No. of times ________

3. Since you've been pregnant, have you been hit, slapped, kicked, or otherwise physically hurt by someone? .... YES NO

   If YES, by whom (circle all that apply)

   Husband Ex-husband Boyfriend Stranger Other Multiple

   Total No. of times ________

   Mark the area of injury on a body map

   Score each incident according to the following scale:

   1=Threats of abuse, including use of a weapon
   2=Slapping, pushing; no injuries and/or lasting pain
   3=Punching, kicking, bruises, cuts, and/or continuing pain
   4=Beaten up, severe contusions, burns, broken bones
   5=Head, internal, and/or permanent injury
   6=Use of weapon, wound from weapon

   (If any of the descriptions for the higher number apply, use the higher number)

4. Within the last year, has anyone forced you to have sexual activities? .... YES NO

   If YES, by whom (circle all that apply)

   Husband Ex-husband Boyfriend Stranger Other Multiple

   Total No. of times ________

5. Are you afraid of your partner or anyone you listed above? .... YES NO

Table 2.—Characteristics of 691 Pregnant Women

Characteristics	Black, % (n=267)	Hispanic, % (n=236)	White, % (n=188)	Total, % (n=691)
Age, y				
13-19	31	30	31	31
20-29	55	57	59	57
≥30	14	13	10	12
Married	7	62	40	35
Below poverty level	94	96	97	95
Parity, primigravida	24	36	39	32
Physical–sexual abuse				
Within last year	29	20	29	26
During pregnancy	19	14	19	17
Within last year and during pregnancy	58	50	58	55
Entered prenatal care at third trimester				
Abused	26	19	15	21
Nonabused	14	7	12	11

being teenagers. Using the three-question AAS, 17% of women (1/6) reported abuse during pregnancy. Abused women were twice as likely to begin prenatal care during the third trimester. Frequency, severity, and perpetrator of abuse is presented in Table 3. Abuse was recurrent, with 60% of abused women reporting two or more episodes of violence. White women experienced the most episodes of abuse.

Severity was scored for each episode of abuse using the scale on the AAS. Although each episode may have involved a variety of assaults (eg, slapping, punching, cuts, and burns), only the most severe abuse reported was assigned to the episode. Each woman was counted only once. When compared with black and Hispanic women, white women experienced more severe episodes of abuse. Some severity data are missing because the information was initially collected on a separate form and, consequently, was missed. The index was moved to the AAS, which yielded more complete data.

Consistent with reported marital status, the perpetrator of abuse was almost always someone the woman knew intimately. Multiple perpetrators tended to be reported by teenagers, who cited both a boyfriend and parent as abusive. Location of the abuse during pregnancy focused on the head, regardless of ethnicity. Entire body abuse was more likely to be experienced by Hispanics and whites, with a combination of assaults (eg, head and torso or head and extremities) reported more frequently by blacks.

To evaluate the three-item AAS as compared with the 30-item ISA, subscale scores on ISA-P and ISA-NP were plotted for women classified as abused or nonabused using the three-item AAS. Women who were identified as abused on the three-question AAS also scored significantly higher on the ISA. This analysis confirmed that when compared with research instruments, three straightforward screening questions yielded valid and specific identification of abuse.

Finally, there was a similar pattern of abuse by ethnic groups on the ISA, CTS, and DAS (Table 4). White women scored higher than black or Hispanic women on all subscales, except the minor violence subscale of the CTS.

Comment

When a cohort of 691 black, Hispanic, and white pregnant women were assessed for abuse with three clinical questions, one in six women reported physical or sexual abuse. The three clinical questions gave results similar to those obtained with carefully validated research instruments.

Abuse was recurrent, with 60% of abused women reporting two or more episodes of violence. Frequency and severity of abuse during pregnancy, as well as potential danger for homicide, were appreciably worse for white women. Scores on the CTS, ISA, and DAS were consistent by ethnicity. White women scored the highest on each instrument (ie, they repeatedly experienced the most abuse) and black women scored the lowest (ie, they repeatedly experienced the least abuse); Hispanics consistently scored higher than blacks and lower than whites. These findings are similar to those of Berenson et al,[6] who found that prevalence of reported physical abuse was 3.5 times higher among white than Hispanic or black women.

Although physical abuse has never been directly implicated or measured as a barrier to prenatal care, in this study abused women were twice as likely to begin prenatal care during the third trimester. Physical abuse, with the associated perpetrator behaviors of power and control endemic to the cycle of violence, may function during pregnancy as a barrier to accessing prenatal care through forced avoidance.

This study documents a level of physical abuse during pregnancy that was

Table 3.—Frequency, Severity, and Perpetrator of Abuse During Pregnancy

	Black, % (n=52)	Hispanic, % (n=32)	White, % (n=36)	Total, % (n=120)
Frequency of abuse				
Once	50	28	28	37
2-3	23	35	28	28
4-14	15	28	33	24
≥15	6	6	8	7
Missing data	6	3	3	4
Severity of abuse, score				
1=Threats, including use of weapon	10	0	0	3
2=Slapping, pushing (no lasting pain)	36	50	27	38
3=Punching, kicking, bruises, cuts	17	25	36	20
4=Beaten up, contusions, burns	10	3	3	5
5=Head injury, internal injury	0	3	6	3
6=Use of weapon, wound from weapon	2	0	3	2
Missing data	25	19	25	23
Perpetrator of abuse				
Husband, ex-husband	6	50	33	30
Boyfriend	58	41	44	48
Stranger	4	0	2	2
Other (family member, neighbor)	23	3	17	14
Multiple	6	3	3	4
Missing data	4	3	0	2

Table 4.—Mean Subscale Scores on the Index of Spouse Abuse (ISA), Conflict Tactics Scale (CTS), and Danger Assessment (DA) by Abuse and Ethnicity*

	Abused			Nonabused		
	Black	Hispanic	White	Black	Hispanic	White
No. of women	78	48	56	188	188	132
Scale						
ISA-P	12.20	18.86	22.72	1.97	1.91	3.0
ISA-NP	20.48	27.69	32.16	5.78	5.77	7.6
No. of women	73	41	52	180	171	121
Scale						
CTS reason	6.67	5.85	11.15	12.13	10.06	13.83
CTS verbal	33.04	41.46	46.69	11.56	7.64	16.02
CTS minor	9.29	15.83	15.10	1.53	0.34	0.92
CTS severe	6.74	9.80	12.06	0.73	0.05	0.38
No. of women	71	39	46	...	...	...
Scale						
DA	2.72	4.06	4.40	...	...	...

*ISA-P indicates physical abuse; and ISA-NP, nonphysical abuse. In CTS subscale, reason=reasoning; verbal=verbal aggression; minor=minor violence; and severe=severe violence.

more than twice as high as previous reports in the literature. A possible reason for the higher reported rate is that the women were interviewed by their primary care provider with whom they would have return visits, and the women may have felt safe revealing their abuse history to a clinician they would see again. Additionally, the women in the present study were interviewed during each trimester, and some women who were not abused on the first visit reported abuse later in the pregnancy.

The implications of our study are simple and straightforward. Three assessment questions asked in a private setting identified that one in six pregnant women in this population had been abused. When compared with nationally tested research interview questionnaires, the AAS, when administered by the primary provider, is valid and reliable. In a related study, self-report for abuse was measured against primary provider assessment. Approximately 8% of women self-reported abuse on a standard medical history intake form, but when asked the same abuse assessment questions by a health care provider, 29% of the women reported abuse.[17] Once identified, the abused woman warrants education, advocacy, and referral. Recommended strategies for intervening for abuse during pregnancy have been put forward.[18-22]

Typically, pregnancy is the only time that healthy women come into frequent contact with health care providers. This study documents that three simple clinical screening questions can reliably identify abused women. Assessment for abuse during pregnancy must be standard care for all pregnant women.

This study was supported by grant R49/CCR603514-01 from the Division of Injury Epidemiology and Injury Control, Centers for Disease Control, Atlanta, Ga.

We wish to acknowledge Josephine Ryan, DNSc, and Laura Smith McKenna, DNSc, for editorial assistance on earlier drafts of the manuscript.

References

1. American College of Obstetricians and Gynecologists. *The Abused Woman.* Washington, DC: American College of Obstetricians and Gynecologists; 1988.
2. American College of Obstetricians and Gynecologists. *The Battered Woman.* Washington, DC: American College of Obstetricians and Gynecologists; 1989.
3. US Dept of Health and Human Services. *Surgeon General's Workshop on Violence and Public Health.* Washington, DC: Public Health Service; 1986.
4. Hillard PJ. Physical abuse in pregnancy. *Obstet Gynecol.* 1985;66:185-190.
5. Helton A, McFarlane J, Anderson E. Battered and pregnant: a prevalence study. *Am J Public Health.* 1987;77:1337-1339.
6. Berenson A, Stiglich N, Wilkinson G, Anderson G. Drug abuse and other risk factors for physical abuse in pregnancy among white non-Hispanic, black, and Hispanic women. *Am J Obstet Gynecol.* 1991; 164:491-499.
7. Schei B, Bakketeig LS. Gynaecological impact of sexual and physical abuse by spouse: a study of a random sample of Norwegian women. *Br J Obstet Gynaecol.* 1989;96:1379-1383.
8. Campbell J, Poland M, Waller J, Ager J. Correlates of battering during pregnancy. *Res Nurs Health.* In press.
9. Amaro H, Fried L, Cabral H, Zuckerman B. Violence during pregnancy and substance use. *Am J Public Health.* 1990;80:575-589.
10. Straus M. Measuring intrafamily conflict and violence: the Conflict Tactics (CT) Scales. *J Marriage Fam.* 1979;41:75-88.
11. Hudson W, McIntosh S. The index of spouse abuse: two quantifiable dimensions. *J Marriage Fam.* 1981;43:873-888.
12. Campbell J. Nursing assessment for risk of homicide with battered women. *Adv Nurs Sci.* 1986; 8:36-51.
13. Steinmetz SK. *The Cycle of Violence: Assertive, Aggressive, and Abusive Family Interactions.* New York, NY: Praeger Publishers; 1977.
14. Jorgensen SK. Societal class heterogamy, status striving, and perception of marital conflict: a partial replication and revision of Pearlin's contingency hypothesis. *J Marriage Fam.* 1977;39:653-689.
15. Straus M, Gelles R, Steinmetz S. *Behind Closed Doors: Violence in the American Family.* New York, NY: Anchor Books; 1981.
16. Straus M, Gelles R. Societal change and change in family violence from 1975 to 1985 as revealed by two national surveys. *J Marriage Fam.* 1986;48:465-479.
17. McFarlane J, Christoffel K, Bateman L, Miller V, Bullock L. Assessing for abuse: self-report versus nurse interview. *Public Health Nurs.* 1991;8:245-250.
18. McFarlane J. Battering during pregnancy: tip of an iceberg revealed. *Women Health.* 1989;15:69-83.
19. McFarlane J. Violence during teen pregnancy: health consequences for mother and child. In: Levy B, ed. *Dating Violence: Young Women in Danger.* Seattle, Wash: Seal Press; 1991.
20. McFarlane J. Battering in pregnancy. In: Sampselle CM, ed. *Violence Against Women: Nursing Research, Education, and Practice Issues.* New York, NY: Hemisphere; 1991.
21. Parker B, McFarlane J. Nursing assessment of the battered pregnant woman. *Matern Child Nurs J.* 1991;16:161-164.
22. Lazarro M, McFarlane J. Establishing a screening protocol for abused women. *J Nurs Adm.* 1991; 21:24-28.

Cocaine Use, Risk Taking, and Fatal Russian Roulette

Peter M. Marzuk, MD; Kenneth Tardiff, MD, MPH; Dennis Smyth, MD; Marina Stajic, PhD; Andrew C. Leon, PhD

Objective.—To examine the association between recent cocaine use and risk taking, particularly in the form of playing Russian roulette, a paradigm for extreme risk-taking behavior.

Design.—A case-control study.

Cases and Controls.—The prevalence of cocaine use among all Russian roulette fatalities (N=14) was compared with a demographically similar, randomly selected sample (N=54) of all suicides by handgun during a contemporaneous 4-year period in New York City, NY.

Results.—Recent use of cocaine, the most common drug found at autopsy, was detected in 64% of Russian roulette fatalities and in 35% of the control group ($P<.05$). All Russian roulette fatalities were male and usually young and unemployed. Blacks and Hispanics accounted for 80% of all cases and were overrepresented compared with their numbers in the general population.

Conclusion.—In some populations cocaine may be associated with life-threatening risk-taking behaviors.

(*JAMA*. 1992;267:2635-2637)

COCAINE use has been associated with fatal accidents, suicides, and homicides.[1,2] With the exception of alcohol, no other drug of abuse is so closely linked to violent premature death. The way in which cocaine mediates an increased risk of both intentional and unintentional injuries and death is uncertain. However, one possibility is that use of this drug increases the propensity for engaging in risk-taking activities. A quintessential example of extreme risk-taking behavior is Russian roulette. This is a deadly game of chance in which an individual spins the cylinder of a revolver containing one or more bullets, places the gun to his head, and pulls the trigger. A previous article reported that 58% of Russian roulette victims had alcohol or other drugs present at the time of autopsy, but the authors did not identify which drugs were involved.[3]

In contrast, individuals with intent to die who shoot themselves in a suicide attempt are usually not engaging in risk taking since the probability of death is near certain. To investigate the role of cocaine in life-threatening risk-taking behavior, we compared the prevalence of recent use of this drug among all Russian roulette fatalities with that of a demographically similar, randomly selected sample of handgun suicide controls.

Methods

The study used a case-control design. All deaths caused by firearms occurring in New York City from 1984 through 1987 that were not certified as homicides by the New York City Medical Examiner were reviewed. The review included police, medical examiner, and on-scene investigations, previous hospital records, if available, and autopsy and toxicology reports.

Cases were considered those individuals who had died of a self-inflicted firearm injury incurred while playing Russian roulette, as previously described. A total of 15 cases, all males ranging in age from 15 to 51 years, were identified over the 4-year period. The manner of death was usually certified as "circumstances undetermined, Russian roulette" and not classified as suicide.

Toxicological analyses were performed in 14 cases (93%). In one case, the subject died several weeks after the fatal injury following a prolonged hospital stay, thereby prohibiting determination of drug use at the time of injury. In all other cases death was instantaneous. Thus, the study sample consisted of 14 Russian roulette cases.

The prevalence of cocaine use among cases was compared with the prevalence of cocaine use in a suicide control group that consisted of individuals who were certified as having died instantaneously by gunshot wounds to the head with handguns during the same 4-year period. The control group was chosen from a larger sample of all such individuals to reflect the age and gender characteristics of the case group. The size of the control group (N=56) was designed to be four times the number of cases, as a selection ratio of four to one (controls to cases) nearly optimizes the statistical power in a case-control study.[4] Thus, from a total sample of 304 males between the ages of 15 and 55 years who committed suicide with handguns, a control group of 56 individuals was selected using a computerized random number generator. Toxicological analysis was unavailable in two of these subjects; thus, the total control group comprised 54 individuals.

Toxicological analyses included assay for benzoylecgonine, the principal metabolite of cocaine, and ethanol, as well as screening for a number of other drugs.

This article is one of a number of articles on violence that will appear in upcoming issues of THE JOURNAL. The reader is referred to the June 10, 1992, issue, which will be dedicated to studies of violence.

From the Departments of Psychiatry (Drs Marzuk, Tardiff, and Leon) and Public Health (Dr Tardiff), Cornell University Medical College, New York, NY; and the Office of Chief Medical Examiner, City of New York, and Department of Forensic Medicine, New York (NY) University School of Medicine (Drs Smyth and Stajic).

Reprint requests to Department of Psychiatry, Cornell University Medical College, 1300 York Ave, New York, NY 10021 (Dr Marzuk).

Blood and urine samples were obtained at autopsy and stored at 4°C until assay. Benzoylecgonine was screened in urine samples using a homogeneous enzyme immunoassay.

Results were considered positive if benzoylecgonine was detected at concentrations of 0.3 mg/L or greater. Analysis was repeated on positive samples. In addition, positive urine samples underwent substantiation of results in blood for cocaine and/or metabolites by radioimmunoassay. Ethanol analysis was performed by head space gas chromatography. Results were considered positive if blood ethanol concentration was 2 mmol/L or higher. Cases in which blood ethanol concentrations were 7 mmol/L or greater underwent gas chromatography to assess concentrations. Acidic and basic drugs were analyzed using either thin-layer chromatography or gas liquid chromatography.

Chi-square tests were used to determine significant differences in prevalence rates across groups. When at least one expected frequency was less than 5, a Fisher's Exact Test was used instead. Mean ages of cases and controls were compared using Student's *t* test. All tests were two-tailed with an α level of .05.

Results

During the 4-year period spanning 1984 through 1987, 15 cases of fatal Russian roulette occurred in New York City. All such deaths were among males ranging in age from 15 to 51 years (mean age, 31.3 years). Black and Hispanic males accounted for 80% of these deaths and were markedly overrepresented in the series compared with their numbers in the general population. Most players were unmarried (66%) and unemployed (53%). In only one case was there a known history of previous suicidal ideation or attempts. None of the individuals left suicide notes.

More than three quarters of all Russian roulette deaths were witnessed by at least two or more persons. Of note, the witness group usually comprised males of similar age who outnumbered female witnesses by ratios ranging from 2:1 to 6:1.

There were no statistically significant differences between the Russian roulette group and the control group in mean age, sex, or race-ethnicity. Overall, drugs or alcohol were detected in 78.6% of cases and 61.1% of controls (P=.35). However, the prevalence of recent cocaine use among Russian roulette fatalities (64.3%) was almost twice that of the control sample (35.2%) (P<.05). Both the prevalence of alcohol use and the conjoint prevalence of these drugs did not differ between groups. Cocaine was the only drug detected in 29% of cases. Other drugs were detected in only three cases and included phencyclidine, meperidine, propoxyphene, and phenytoin.

Russian roulette was played under at least two circumstances. In one scenario, an individual engages in risk taking as part of a fatalistic gamble. This pattern is illustrated by one middle-aged man in the series, who had a negative toxicological analysis for cocaine and who played the game at home, alone, whenever he was confronted with a serious problem. Witnesses reported that he frequently remarked that if he survived, it would be a "divine sign" he was meant to live and would be able to overcome his problems, and if he died, he "would not have to worry about his problems anymore." Viewed this way, Russian roulette is analogous to the concept of suicide attempts as fatalistic gambles of various probabilities of lethal outcome.[5]

Many players in this series, particularly cocaine users, were neither fatalistic nor suicidal. According to witnesses and family members interviewed in medical examiner and police investigations, none of the cocaine-using players reported recent suicidal intent, left suicide notes, or had a history of frank suicidal behavior. Rather, cocaine users appeared to engage in an extreme risk-taking "ordeal" to enhance their self-esteem in the presence of other males. For example, several players in the cocaine-using group repeatedly challenged other men to play the game. One man tossed live bullets at other men urging them to join. Another claimed this was the way for an individual to "prove he is a man." In several cases, the game was played during ongoing gambling with cards.

Comment

This study demonstrates a strong association between recent cocaine use and one form of extreme risk-taking behavior, Russian roulette. Cocaine and/or metabolites were detected in nearly two thirds of all victims of this deadly game and were nearly twice as likely to be found at autopsy compared with suicide controls. If suicidal individuals with self-inflicted firearm injuries to the head can be presumed not to be taking risks, as death is a virtual certainty, this study suggests that cocaine use may alter risk-taking propensity in some individuals.

All cocaine users have some degree of risk-taking propensity as they subject themselves to a variety of dangers including negotiating a "deal" for the drug, unpredictable or untoward pharmacologic side effects, and social or legal consequences that may include marital disruption, job dismissal, arrest or conviction. However, the way in which cocaine may induce some users to engage in life-threatening higher-stakes risks is unknown.

At the outset, it should be pointed out that the presence of cocaine metabolites in urine establishes use of the drug only in the previous 48 to 72 hours.[6] Eyewitness accounts suggest that some of these individuals were using cocaine immediately prior to death. Others may have used the drug several hours or even days before death, which occurred long after acute effects had subsided. One possibility, then, is that cocaine produces in some users an immediate grandiose euphoria and sense of invincibility that seriously distorts the perception of risk. In several cases, for example, witnesses reported that victims remarked that they were impervious to bullets and would not be harmed.

Cocaine acting alone or in concert with alcohol may distort the level of acceptable risk. Chronic cocaine use results in marked depletion of several neurotransmitters including serotonin, a deficiency state linked to violent impulsive behaviors.[7,8] Most cocaine users are also heavy alcohol consumers. In this series alone, 21% of victims had both drugs detected at autopsy. Alcohol intoxication has been associated with acceptance of greater subjective risk.[9] Polysubstance abuse has also been associated with increased risk taking.[10]

The demographic findings of this study are similar to those of a large study of Russian roulette victims in the Miami, Fla, area.[3] In both studies, victims were likely to be young, male, and black or Hispanic, and to have died in the presence of similarly aged peers. The cocaine-using players in the present study were particularly likely to die amidst a peer group with a male-to-female ratio of 2:1 or greater. This finding underscores the point made by Fishbain et al[3] that the presence of others may not have deterred, but rather enhanced risk-taking behaviors.

A number of studies have postulated a "risk-shift" phenomenon, operant in groups, in which group decisions about risk-taking behavior are more dangerous than decisions reached by individuals alone.[11] Individuals with low self-esteem may also take larger risks than persons with higher self-esteem in the presence of others.[12] Thus, some cocaine users who suffer from chronic lowered esteem might be particularly vulnerable to assuming larger risks in group settings. This pattern may explain, in part, the association of violence and gang warfare among adolescent street gangs who use cocaine, since subordinate gang members may rise in the gang hierarchy by assuming life-threatening risks.

Conclusions

What, then, are the clinical implications of this study? First, a history of cocaine use should prompt the clinician to inquire about a person's access to and use of firearms. Second, while this study establishes a link between cocaine use and only one type of extreme risk-taking activity, we believe it may be useful for clinicians to inquire specifically about other dangerous behaviors in cocaine users who present for treatment. However, only additional studies will conclusively establish whether cocaine-induced alterations in risk-taking propensity may explain some of the morbidity associated with such risky endeavors as reckless fast driving, promiscuous sex, gambling, fighting, and dangerous sports and hobbies. It is also uncertain whether this same mechanism explains, in part, the association of cocaine use with fatal accidents and homicides. If other similar behaviors appear to be linked to drug use, the development of risk-taking profiles may ultimately serve as a useful clinical marker to identify individuals most likely to die violent premature deaths.

This study was supported in part by a Readers Digest Research Fellowship (Dr Marzuk). We thank Charles Hirsch, MD, Chief Medical Examiner of the City of New York, and his staff for their assistance as well as Isadora Johnson for manuscript preparation.

References

1. Tardiff K, Gross EM, Wu J, Stajic M, Millman R. Analysis of cocaine positive fatalities. *J Forensic Sci.* 1989;34:53-63.
2. Marzuk PM, Tardiff K, Leon AC, Stajic M, Morgan EB, Mann JJ. Prevalence of recent cocaine use among motor vehicle fatalities in New York City. *JAMA.* 1990;263:250-256.
3. Fishbain DA, Fletcher JR, Aldrich TE, Davis JM. Relationship between Russian roulette deaths and risk-taking behavior: a controlled study. *Am J Psychiatry.* 1987;144:563-567.
4. Cole P. Introduction. In: Davis W, ed. *Statistical Methods in Cancer Research: The Analysis of Case Control Studies.* Lyon, France: International Agency for Research on Cancer, World Health Organization; 1980.
5. Weiss JM. The gamble with death in attempted suicide. *Psychiatry.* 1957;20:17-25.
6. Ambre J, Fischman M, Ruo T. Urinary excretion of cocaine, benzoylecgonine, ecgonine methyl ester in humans. *J Anal Toxicol.* 1988;34:53-63.
7. Brown GL, Goodwin FK. Cerebrospinal fluid correlates of suicide attempts and aggression. *Ann N Y Acad Sci.* 1986;487:175-188.
8. Dackis CA, Gold MS. New concepts in cocaine addiction: the dopamine depletion hypothesis. *Neurosci Biobehav Rev.* 1985;9:447-469.
9. Teger AI, Katkin ES, Pruitt DG. Effects of alcoholic beverages and their congener content on level and style of risk-taking. *J Pers Soc Psychol.* 1969;11:170-176.
10. Adlaf EM, Smart RG. Risk-taking and drug use behavior: an examination. *Drug Alcohol Depend.* 1983;11:287-296.
11. Kogan N, Wallach MA. Risk-taking as a function of the situation, the person, and the group. In: Mandler G, Mussen P, Kogan N, Wallach M, eds. *New Directions in Psychology, III.* New York, NY: Holt Rinehart & Winston; 1967:111-278.
12. Cohen PA, Sheposh VP. Audience and level of esteem as determinants of risk-taking. *Pers Soc Psychol Bull.* 1977;11:119-122.

The Epidemiology of Murder-Suicide

Peter M. Marzuk, MD; Kenneth Tardiff, MD, MPH; Charles S. Hirsch, MD

Objective.—To review the epidemiology, patterns, and major determinants of murder-suicide and to discuss the clinical and research strategies for identifying the individuals at greatest risk for this type of violence.

Data Sources.—Data were obtained from English-language articles based on searches using MEDLINE (from 1966), PsychINFO (from 1967), and EMBASE (from 1974) programs. In addition, relevant articles, books, and monographs identified from the reference list of retrieved articles were reviewed.

Study Selection.—Case-control studies, descriptive epidemiologic surveys, and case series were chosen for review.

Data Extraction.—Because of the limited scope of the pertinent research literature, all data relevant to the incidence, demographics, circumstances, and precipitants of murder-suicide were summarized by the authors.

Data Synthesis.—Murder-suicide occurs with an annual incidence of 0.2 to 0.3 per 100 000 person-years and accounts for approximately 1000 to 1500 deaths yearly in the United States. The annual incidence of these events is relatively constant across industrialized nations and has not significantly changed over several decades. The principal perpetrators are young males with intense sexual jealousy, depressed mothers, or despairing elderly men with ailing spouses. The principal victims are female sexual partners or consanguineous relatives, usually young children. Clinical depression, specific motivations such as male sexual proprietariness or maternal salvation fantasies, and a history of previous suicide attempts are important in explaining underlying psychopathological mechanisms.

Conclusions.—Murder-suicide occupies a distinct epidemiological domain that overlaps with suicide, domestic homicide, and mass murder. These events may be categorized into one of only several phenomenologic typologies that share similar demographics, motivations, and circumstances. Despite the disruption of families and communities caused by murder-suicide, there are no standardized operational definitions, validated taxonomic systems, or national surveillance networks for these events, all of which are needed to develop prevention strategies.

(*JAMA*. 1992;267:3179-3183)

MURDER-SUICIDE is a dramatic, violent event in which an individual commits homicide and shortly thereafter commits suicide. Although these incidents are infrequent, they probably account for 1000 to 1500 combined suicide and homicide deaths annually in the United States alone, placing their mortality on par with other diseases such as pulmonary tuberculosis (1467 deaths), viral hepatitis (1290 deaths), influenza (1943 deaths), and meningitis (1156 deaths).[1] Because many murder-suicides result in the death or injury of family members and sometimes mass murder, they cause countless additional morbidity, family trauma, and disruption of communities. On the basis of our review of the limited literature, we believe these events occupy a distinct epidemiologic domain that overlaps with simple suicide, domestic homicide, and mass murder. We review the incidence of these events, propose a clinical typology, examine underlying psychopathologic mechanisms, discuss clinical implications, and suggest research strategies for the future.

From the Section of Public Health Research in Psychiatry, Department of Psychiatry (Drs Marzuk and Tardiff) and the Department of Public Health (Dr Tardiff), Cornell University Medical College, New York, NY; and the Office of Chief Medical Examiner, New York, and the Department of Forensic Medicine, New York University School of Medicine, NY (Dr Hirsch).

Reprint requests to Department of Psychiatry, Cornell University Medical College, 1300 York Ave, New York, NY 10021 (Dr Marzuk).

DEFINITION

Review of many studies of murder-suicide suggests that there is, as of yet, no standardized operational definition for this phenomenon. The principal variability in defining a case lies in the specification of both the level of evidence needed to ascertain that a homicide has been committed by the subject, and the interval between the homicide and the suicide. In our view, a murder-suicide has occurred when, on the basis of medical examiner review, a person has committed a homicide (codes E960 through E969 of the *International Statistical Classification of Diseases, Ninth Revision* [*ICD-9*][2]) and subsequently commits suicide (*ICD-9* codes E950 through E959) within 1 week of the homicide. The interval between events is important to specify in any operational definition to distinguish the group in which suicide appears to be phenomenologically and motivationally linked with a prior homicide from a group of violent individuals with a history of recklessness, assaults, or murder who ultimately die by suicide. The few studies that have specified intervals reported a range from 1 day to 3 months.[3-5]

We continue to use the term *murder-suicide* in accordance with the predominant nomenclature in the literature, although we recognize that generically *homicide-suicide* is more applicable. Murder is a degree of homicide defined by statute in each of the United States, whereas suicide is not a legal term. However, the requirement that an individual be convicted of murder prior to suicide is far too restrictive, as the time interval between homicide and suicide in most of these events is less than 24 hours, and no trial is ever held. Thus, we have excluded individuals who only assault others prior to suicide and conversely, those who commit homicide but fail to complete a suicide attempt, even though such groups may show etiologic overlap with true murder-suicides. Unusual cultural variants of multiple murder that frequently precede suicide were not considered.[6] Individuals who accidentally kill others and then commit suicide were also excluded.

Murder-suicide perpetrators also need to be distinguished phenomenologically from two much less commonly encountered offenders: mass murderers (an offender who willfully injures five or more persons, of whom three or more are killed) and serial murderers (an offender who kills others in three or more separate incidents).[7]

INCIDENCE

Because of the lack of a national surveillance system and variations in operational criteria used to define an "event," the annual incidence of murder-suicide in the United States is difficult to determine. However, the few American studies conducted over the past three decades suggest an annual incidence of 0.20 to 0.30 per 100 000 persons in certain localities.[3-5,8,9] A *Time* magazine survey of all deaths by firearms in 1 week in the United States uncovered 11 incidents of firearm-related murder-suicides, accounting for a total of 22 deaths.[10] If this 7-day period is at all representative of an average week, one would predict at least 572 suicides of this type and more than an equal number of homicides annually. Thus, a conservative estimate places the mortality of these events at 1000 to 1500 deaths per year nationally.

In a review of 17 studies spanning different periods from 1900 through 1979 and involving 10 nations, Coid[11] found that the incidence of murder-suicide was remarkably constant, averaging 0.20 to 0.30 per 100 000 (range, 0.04 in Scotland to 0.40 among Israeli Western Jews) although the countries studied showed marked variation in overall suicide and homicide rates. However, he found that murder-suicides as a percentage of all homicides differed dramatically across nations. In nations with high homicide rates, murder-suicides accounted for a relatively small proportion of total homicides. For instance, Philadelphia, Pa, with a high homicide rate in 1948 through 1952, and Denmark, with a low rate in 1960, had virtually identical murder-suicide rates (0.21 to 0.22 per 100 000). Yet, murder-suicide accounted for 3.6% of all homicides in Philadelphia and 42% of homicides in Denmark.[12,13] In the United States in the 1980s, it is likely that murder-suicides represented 1.5% of all suicides and 5% of all homicides annually.

CLINICAL TYPOLOGIES

Any taxonomic system used to classify murder-suicides must span a range of motives, circumstances, and demographics. Thus, it is difficult in most typologies to separate presumed motives from other characteristics such as victim-offender relationships. However, the motivations and demographics seem so linked that they allow construction of an exclusive categorical typology that accounts for the vast majority of documented murder-suicides. Nevertheless, it would be naive to assume that murder-suicide is unique and shares no characteristics with other forms of fatal violence or that this typology is exhaustive.

A proposed classification system that categorizes murder-suicides by type of victim-offender relationships and by class of common precipitants or motives is shown in the Table. This typology, which requires empiric validation, is descriptive and, admittedly, does not address the complex etiology of these events. Nevertheless, these categories may be useful in providing the clinician with a relatively simple mental construct for assessing the risk of this type of violence.

As the Table indicates, murder-suicides span a range of victim-offender relationships and motives. However, we will focus on the four most common profiles that are potentially preventable and are likely to be encountered by a wide range of clinicians including emergency physicians, psychiatrists, marital counselors, family practitioners, and internists. These include spousal murder-suicides either due to jealousy or declining health; filicides; and familicides. In addition, the widely publicized but uncommon extrafamilial retaliators, who account for some of the worst mass murders in the United States, are discussed.

Proposed Clinical Classification of Murder-Suicide Based on Victim-Offender Relationship (Type) and Principal Motive or Precipitant (Class)*

Type of Relationship
I. Spousal or Consortial†
Perpetrator
1. Spouse
2. Consort
Type of Homicide
i. Uxoricidal (spouse-killing)
ii. Consortial (murder of lover)
II. Familial‡
Perpetrator
1. Mother
2. Father
3. Child (under 16 y)
4. Other adult family member (over 16 y)
Type of Homicide
i. Neonaticide (child <24 h)
ii. Infanticide (child >1 d, <1 y)
iii. Pedicide (child 1 through 16 y)
iv. Adult family member (>16 y)
III. Extrafamilial§
Class
A. Amorous jealousy
B. "Mercy killing" (because of declining health of victim or offender)
C. "Altruistic or extended suicides" (includes salvation fantasies of rescue and escape from problems)‖
D. Family financial or social stressors
E. Retaliation
F. Other
G. Unspecified

*Classification of murder-suicides is specified by type (Roman numeral) with subtype of perpetrator (number) and subtype of homicide (lower case Roman numeral) as well as by letters to denote principal motives or precipitants. The classification can include mixed types of victims and multiple motives of offenders. Examples using the typology, including a "mixed type," include the following: (1) A husband who killed his wife out of suspicions of infidelity would be coded type I(1)i-A; (2) a mother who killed her 2-year-old son (maternal filicide) to "rescue" him from a perceived ruinous world would be coded type II(1)iii-C; (3) an adult who kills his adult brother for unknown motives would be coded type II(4) iv-G; and (4) a man who kills his wife and his 6-month-old son and 2-year-old daughter because he suspects his wife of infidelity and is under severe financial pressures represents a mixed category and would be coded type I(1)i/II(2)ii,iii/A,D.

†Principal victim-offender relationship is spouse or lover.

‡Principal victim-offender relationship is consanguineal (blood relative) or other familial, nonmarital relationship.

§Principal victim-offender relationship not marital, consortial, or familial, and includes friends, acquaintances, and strangers.

‖See discussion of filicide-suicide in "Clinical Typologies" for a full explanation.

Spousal Murder-Suicide (Amorous Jealousy)

The most common type (IA) (Table), which represents one half to three fourths of all murder-suicides in the United States, usually involves amorous jealousy that is also known as "psychotic," and "morbid jealousy."[3-5,14-16] Typically, a male between the age of 18 and 60 years develops suspicions or knowledge of his girlfriend's or wife's infidelity, becomes enraged, and both murders her and commits suicide, usually using firearms. This pattern forms the central plot of many literary classics and operas including *Othello*, *Wozzeck*, and *Luisa Miller*.[17] In one variant, the murder-suicide offender may kill the rival lover as well, thus completely destroying a lover's triad (triadic death).[15]

The "infidelity" may be real or perceived and delusional, and thus ranges from ruminative or obsessional to psychotic. The latter case constitutes the "Othello syndrome," in which delusions of infidelity are accompanied by irritability, despondency, and aggression.[18] While some murder-suicides occur shortly after the onset of "malignant jealousy," more often there has been a chronically chaotic relationship fraught with jealous suspicions, verbal abuse, and sublethal physical violence.[5,14,19] The triggering event is often the female's rejection of her lover and her immediate threat of withdrawal or estrangement.

In the United States, slightly less than half of spousal homicides are perpetrated by wives, usually in self-defense following chronic abuse by husbands.[20] In contrast, over 90% of murder-suicides involving couples are perpetrated by men.[9] Thus, women who kill their husbands are much less likely than their male counterpart perpetrators to commit suicide. From 19% to 26% of male spouse murderers committed suicide compared with 0% to 3% of their female counterparts.[12,21,22]

Sexual jealousy arising from male sexual proprietariness, which fuels many simple male-perpetrated spousal homicides is even more prominent in analogous murder-suicides.[23] For example, recent estrangement of partners increases both the risk of male-perpetrated spousal homicide and murder-suicide.[3,19] In Canada, 35.3% of men who killed estranged wives committed suicide compared with only 21.6% of nonestranged spousal murderers.[21]

Spousal Murder-Suicide (Declining Health)

This group (type I[1]i-B) usually comprises elderly men who have either poor health, ailing spouses, or both, who shoot their wives and then commit suicide.[3,13,24] Often, suicide notes describe the inability of one or both partners to cope with declining health or loneliness, or inform the family of wills, burial plots, and insurance. These cases resemble "mercy killings" or simple suicide pacts among the elderly in which both individuals, usually by poisoning themselves, are certified as suicides.[25,26] These offenders also resemble the profile of the "elderly white male suicide," who is usually widowed or separated, depressed, and in poor health and despair. A newer variant includes persons with AIDS who are murdered by their lover or spouse, who then commits suicide.

Filicide-Suicide

In the United States, at least half of all pedicides (children aged 1 through 16) and infanticides (children under the age of 1 year) are perpetrated by parents.[27,28] Whereas the percentage of strangers who murder children and then commit suicide is small, 16% to 29% of mothers and 40% to 60% of fathers commit suicide immediately after murdering their children (filicide).[27-30]

The age- and sex-related risk of filicide-parental suicides is unknown. Boys and girls appear to be at nearly equivalent risk.[31] In simple child killing, mothers are more likely to kill infants than are fathers,[29,32,33] but as children age, the child's risk of dying at the hands of his or her mother or father (while lower than in infancy) appears to equalize or even reverse.[21,32] Among filicide-suicides, few mothers who commit neonaticide (murder of an infant less than 1 day old) ever commit suicide,[33] and only 2.3% of mothers and 10.5% of fathers who committed infanticide committed suicide.[21] Thus, among type II familial murder-suicides, the most commonly encountered subtypes are the maternal (type II[1]iii) and paternal (type II[2]iii) murderers of children over the age of 1 year and less than 16 years (pedicides).

Typically, the murderous mother beats, suffocates, stabs, strangles, drowns, gases, or throws the child from the window and uses a similar method for suicide.[27,28] Firearms, rarely used by mothers, are more commonly used by murderous fathers.[27]

The most important diagnosis in maternal filicide-suicides is depression, often with psychotic features.[28,34-36] The depressed suicidal mother may psychotically perceive her infant as an "extension" of herself, and both deaths, in effect, represent an "extended" suicide.[32,35,37,38] In maternally perpetrated murders of children who are older than 1 year but usually under age 5, the primary motive appears to be a "deluded altruism."[13,28,29,32,39] In effect, the mother perceives the child as solely dependent on her for care and sees a need to escape and "save" herself and her children from a painful, ruinous world.

Familicide-Suicide

Clinicians encountering the depressed senior male of a household should consider the risk of familicide-suicide. This prototype, best conceptualized in the Table as a mixed type I(1)i/type II(2)i-iv with mixed motives, resembles Dietz's "family annihilator."[40] Typically, the senior male who is depressed, paranoid, or intoxicated kills every member of his family including his spouse (type Ii), children (type IIi-iii), other relatives (type IIiv), and sometimes pets. The victims are usually shot, stabbed, or strangled. Occasionally, the house is set on fire. In another variant, adult-dependent children who are physically or mentally disabled are killed[41] along with the spouse.

In the United States, the perpetrators of familicide are almost exclusively male.[21] Often the precipitants include cumulative financial, marital, or other social stresses on the family. Suicide notes suggest the murderers often see themselves as "altruistically" delivering the family from continued hardships.[15] In other cases, the perpetrator suspects marital infidelity.[34,42] Some investigators have stressed "dependent-protective" motives.[14] That is, the senior male commands a relationship in which he perceives that only he can satisfy the needs of the victims. When this relationship is threatened, he erupts in a frustrated homicidal-suicidal rage.

Extrafamilial Murder-Suicide

These persons comprising type III E (Table) include disgruntled individuals who probably have paranoid and narcissistic traits who believe they have been slighted in some way.[43] They may have been dismissed from employment or passed over for a job promotion, denied monetary compensation such as insurance or disability or a bank loan, or perceive themselves as humiliated by others or deprived of appropriate recognition.[43] Seeking vengeful vindication, they usually kill employers, teachers, physicians, or bankers with a firearm prior to turning the gun on themselves. In this type of murder-suicide, while there are specific targets, many bystanders including police may be killed when the perpetrator either is thwarted from reaching the target or sprays the target's area with bullets.[44]

DEMOGRAPHICS

Demographic characteristics of victims and offenders largely reflect the predominant typological category of murder-suicide within nations. It is uncertain why nations display a comparable annual incidence of overall murder-suicides, yet vary in the distribution of these events across typological categories. In the United States where amorous jealousy probably accounts for the majority of all murder-suicides, the typical offender is married, involved in a love relationship, or recently estranged. The mean age of offenders in three US studies was 39.6 years, and an average of 93% to 97% of offenders were male and 50% to 86% were white.[3,5,8,14,15,43] The principal method of both homicide and suicide was firearms, which were used in 80% to 94% of cases,[3,5,14,15,43] but all means, including aircraft, have been described.[45-47] From 84% to 90% of cases involved only one victim.[3,5,14,15] Compared with offenders, over 85% of all victims are female. Offenders and victims are usually of the same race.[12] Most victims (>65%) were spouses or lovers of male offenders, who spanned all ages, but on average were several years younger than the offender.[43]

Murder-suicides in England show different demographic patterns.[13] While spousal killings (type I) are important, maternal filicide-suicides (type II[2]iii) represent a significant percentage of all cases.[13] Thus, females accounted for 40% of offenders and males accounted for 30% of victims. Almost half of all victims were under age 16, a quarter were under age 5. Sixty-nine percent of male offenders killed a spouse or girlfriend alone, and 17.2% killed children alone or children with spouses. Ninety-two percent of female offenders killed their own children or the spouse and the children. Only 5.0% of females killed a spouse or lover alone.

A DISTINCT DOMAIN

To elucidate etiology, one may ask whether murder-suicide more closely resembles a suicide with a homicidal component or a homicide with a suicidal component. Several lines of evidence suggest that these events occupy a distinct epidemiological domain that displays similarities to and differences from both types of violence.

First, the short time span, often minutes, between the murder and suicide suggests that neither act is "incidental" to the other.[48,49] That is, it is unlikely that murder-suicide is primarily a homicide, in which the murderer commits suicide after several hours of remorseful brooding. Many of these events were carefully planned as a unified two-stage sequential act. In several studies, 15% to 30% of offenders left notes, often detailing the motives behind both the suicide and the homicide,[5,14] and in other studies, victims were stalked by the murderer.[15,49]

Second, whereas suicide is distributed across all ages from adolescence to old age for both men and women, murder-suicide is confined principally to young and middle-aged men with marital, common-law, or live-in relationships with women, with smaller concentrations among premenopausal mothers and elderly men. Two factors believed to protect against suicide, marriage and parenting, are apparently crucial to the dynamics of murder-suicide.[50-52]

Third, compared with all homicide offenders in the United States, the murder-suicide offender is more likely to be white, male, older, married, to have murdered females, and unlikely to have a prior arrest record.[4,12,14,53] Because most homicides in the United States involve same-sex disputes or robbery or drug dealing,[54,55] these differences largely disappear when one compares male offenders with male spouse killers or female offenders with maternal child killers.

Whereas homicide victims span all ages of men and women and are related to the killer in a range of ways, including family members, acquaintances, employers, police, or strangers, with few exceptions, virtually all victims of murder-suicide are either female sexual partners or blood relatives, usually children. Men almost never commit suicide immediately after killing unrelated men. Compared with men, women are very unlikely to commit suicide after murdering anyone other than children. Thus, murder-suicide differs from both homicide and suicide in that it is committed against specific family targets by members of a very distinct group with demographics that differ from the typical suicide or homicide offender.

BIOPSYCHOSOCIAL DETERMINANTS

The biological, psychological, and social determinants of murder-suicide remain to be elucidated. However, any psycho-pathological mechanism postulated to explain murder-suicide must include diagnoses, motives, and a preexisting suicide propensity.

Almost all individuals who commit suicide are found to have a mental illness.[56] There are, unfortunately, few studies of murder-suicide with designs that allow the reliable assessment of the psychiatric diagnosis of offenders immediately prior to the event. Nevertheless, we believe the most convincing unifying diagnosis common to all subtypes of murder-suicide is depression. In one study that used the psychological autopsy method comparing 12 cases of spousal (couples) murder-suicide with 24 cases of spousal (couples) murder alone, 75% of the murder-suicide offenders met criteria established by the *Diagnostic and Statistical Manual of Mental Disorders, Revised Third Edition*[57] for a depressive disorder, compared with none of the simple spousal murderers.[9] In West's[13] study, which involved review of police and coroner's records as well as reports from family doctors and social workers, depressive disorders represented, by far, the largest category of mental illness, accounting for over 36% of all cases. Other studies consistently emphasize the role of depression in spousal murder-suicide.[16,42,58-62] Depression was also considered to be a critical ingredient in filicide-suicides.[21,28,29,32,34]

Some studies have stressed the importance of psychosis.[19,45,63,64] Many suicidal murderers have well-circumscribed delusions of jealousy,[13,16] paranoia,[65] or rescue,[15,28,37] but few studies have systematically situated the delusions within the larger diagnostic context of depression, schizophrenia, or paranoid disorders.

Few studies have examined the role of drugs or alcohol in these events. In several, 12% to 50% of offenders[3,5,8,14,15,39,66] and 14% to 29% of victims[5,43] had alcohol detectable in their blood at autopsy. In another study, the prevalence of detectable blood alcohol levels at autopsy was significantly greater in homicide (50%) than murder-suicide offenders (33%) and in simple homicide victims (37%) than in murder-suicide homicide victims (0%).[9] Thus, it is unlikely that alcohol or drug abuse differentiates these events from other homicides or suicides.

The intent of offenders spans a spectrum from predominantly homicidal to suicidal. In some spousal and extrafamilial retaliatory types, there are homicidal motives arising from male sexual proprietariness and revenge, respectively. In both, there are strong elements of possessiveness and control.[66,67] The killing of ailing spouses resembles mercy killing. The murders of blood relatives either in child killing or familicide appear to represent "extended" suicides.[13]

Because most individuals with either depression or these specific motives do not commit suicide, diagnosis and motives alone are insufficient to explain murder-suicides. In recent years, many investigators have argued the presence of a suicidal and violent propensity, an amalgam of maladaptive psychological traits best conceived of as "impulsivity," perhaps with an underlying deficit in serotonergic functioning.[68-71] Thus, only individuals with a suicidal trait who are concurrently in a state of depression may be at high risk of suicide. There are, to date, no biological studies that have specifically examined murder-suicides, in which one would predict low serotonergic activity in offenders. Other lines of evidence, however, do suggest that many offenders had made previous suicide attempts.[13]

Whether murder-suicide offenders also have a preexisting "violent tendency" is uncertain. Most case histories from several studies suggest that male offenders, while less likely than murderers to have an arrest record, do have a history of domestically perpetrated violence and chronic spouse abuse.[3-5,9,19] It has not been established whether mothers who commit suicide after killing their children had a history of violence or child abuse.

CLINICAL MANAGEMENT

As with the prediction of simple suicide, any evaluation of murder-suicide risk is likely to overpredict mortality. That is, there will be a large number of individuals who conform to a "deadly epidemiologic profile" who will never die in a murder-suicide. However, these types discussed should underscore the importance of evaluating homicide potential in depressed individuals with the same conscientious detail as suicide risk.[9,60,72] Intervention strategies might include immediate removal of firearms from the home, marital or crisis counseling, procurement of additional help for parental caretaking responsibilities, mobilization of other family members to observe the patient, and intensive treatment of mental illness, including hospitalization.

RESEARCH STRATEGIES

Research on murder-suicide is severely limited. Because these events have an extremely low base rate, studies must be largely retrospective in design and conducted either over large geographic areas or long time spans. Thus, most investigations to date have been case series that have relied on limited medical examiner or police reports. Only a few have used a more extensive database including interviews with treating physicians, social workers, family members, or review of hospital records. Even this "psychological autopsy" method, which is successfully used to investigate homicides and suicides, is limited because both the offender and the person most likely to be aware of the immediate precipitants are dead.

We believe that there should be a four-phase research strategy. First, public health officials, forensic psychiatrists, epidemiologists, medical examiners, and other experts should formulate a standardized operational definition of murder-suicide.

Second, a national surveillance network should be established to count murder-suicides and other "linked violent events" such as mass murders and suicide pacts. This would provide more definitive incidence figures, reveal temporal and geographic trends, and allow assessment of the role of the news media in triggering these events.

Third, data accrued from a national population base would facilitate the conceptualization and validation of a taxonomic system, which is critical to the conducting of further studies.

Fourth, psychological autopsy studies involving interviews of families, physicians, and others and that use suicides, accidents, or homicides as controls are needed to assess the role of antemortem diagnosis, psychosocial precipitants, medical illnesses, and a history of suicidality or violence. Postmortem brain studies, particularly of the serotonergic system, might identify underlying neurotransmitter imbalances. Treatment trials of "survivors," particularly young children who lose both parents to murder-suicide, are also needed.[73] Such studies are essential to refine the profile of the individuals at greatest risk, to identify causative psychopathologic mechanisms, and to devise prevention strategies.

This work was supported in part by an Aaron Diamond Foundation (New York, NY) award and National Institute on Drug Abuse (Rockville, Md) grant 1 RO1 DA06534-01 to Drs Tardiff and Marzuk.

The authors thank Patricia Tomasulo, MLS, and the staff of the Payne Whitney Library, New York, NY, and Malvin Vitriol, MLS, of the Milton Helpern Library of Legal Medicine of the Institute of Forensic Medicine, New York, NY, for their assistance. We also thank Isadora Johnson for manuscript preparation.

References

1. US Dept of Health and Human Services. *Vital Statistics of the United States, 1988.* Hyattsville, Md: US Dept of Health and Human Services; 1991:2.
2. World Health Organization. *Manual of the International Statistical Classification of Diseases, Injuries, and Causes of Death, Based on the Recommendations of the Ninth Revision Conference, 1975.* Geneva, Switzerland: World Health Organization; 1977.
3. Currens S, Fritsch T, Jones D, et al. Homicide followed by suicide—Kentucky, 1985-1990. *MMWR.* 1991;40:652-653, 659.
4. Palmer S, Humphrey JA. Offender-victim relationships in criminal homicide followed by offender's suicide, North Carolina, 1972-1977. *Suicide Life Threat Behav.* 1980;10:106-118.
5. Allen NH. Homicide followed by suicide: Los Angeles, 1970-1979. *Suicide Life Threat Behav.* 1983; 13:155-165.
6. Teoh JI. The changing psychopathology of amok. *Psychiatry.* 1972;35:345-351.
7. Dietz PE. Patterns in human violence. In: Hale RE, Frances AJ, eds. *American Psychiatric Association Annual Review.* Washington, DC: American Psychiatric Press Inc; 1987;6:465-490.
8. Wolfgang ME. An analysis of homicide-suicide. *J Clin Exp Psychopathol.* 1958;19:208-218.
9. Rosenbaum M. The role of depression in couples involved in murder-suicide and homicide. *Am J Psychiatry.* 1990;147:1036-1039.
10. Leviton J, Riley M. 7 deadly days. *Time.* July 17, 1989:31-52, 57-61.
11. Coid J. The epidemiology of abnormal homicide and murder followed by suicide. *Psychol Med.* 1983; 13:855-860.
12. Wolfgang ME. *Patterns in Criminal Homicide.* Oxford, England: Oxford University Press; 1958.
13. West DJ. *Murder Followed by Suicide.* Cambridge, Mass: Harvard University Press; 1967.
14. Berman AL. Dyadic death: murder-suicide. *Suicide Life Threat Behav.* 1979;9:15-23.
15. Selkin J. Rescue fantasies in homicide-suicide. *Suicide Life Threat Behav.* 1976;6:79-85.
16. Shepherd M. Morbid jealousy: some clinical and social aspects of a psychiatric symptom. *J Ment Sci.* 1961;107:687-753.
17. Fegetter G. Suicide in opera. *Br J Psychiatry.* 1980;136:552-557.
18. Enoch MD, Trethowan WH. The Othello syndrome. In: Enoch MD, Trethowan WH, eds. *Uncommon Psychiatric Syndromes.* Chicago, Ill: Year Book Medical Publishers Inc; 1979.
19. Dorpat TL. Suicide in murderers. *Psychiatry Digest.* 1966:51-55.
20. Mercy JA, Saltzman LE. Fatal violence among spouses in the United States, 1976-85. *Am J Public Health.* 1989;79:595-599.
21. Daly M, Wilson M. *Homicide.* New York, NY: Aldine DeGruyter; 1988.
22. Wilbanks W. *Murder in Miami.* Lanham, Md: University Press of America; 1984.
23. Daly M, Wilson M. Evolutionary social psychology and homicide. *Science.* 1988;242:519-524.
24. Fishbain DA, Goldberg M, Rosomoff RS, Rosomoff HL. Homicide-suicide and chronic pain. *Clin J Pain.* 1989;5:275-277.
25. Fishbain DA. Suicide pacts and homicide. *Am J Psychiatry.* 1986;143:1319-1320.
26. Rosenbaum M. Crime and punishment—the suicide pact. *Arch Gen Psychiatry.* 1983;40:979-982.
27. Adelson L. Pedicide revisited: the slaughter continues. *Am J Forensic Med Pathol.* 1991;12:16-26.
28. Myers SA. Maternal filicide. *AJDC.* 1970;120: 534-536.
29. Rodenburg M. Child murder by depressed parents. *Can Psychiatr Assoc J.* 1971;16:41-48.
30. Wilkey I, Pearn J, Petric G, Nixon J. Neonaticide, infanticide and child homicide. *Med Sci Law.* 1982;22:31-34.
31. Lester D. Murdering babies: a cross-national study. *Soc Psychiatry Psychiatr Epidemiol.* 1991;26:83-85.
32. Resnick PJ. Child murder by parents: a psychiatric review of filicide. *Am J Psychiatry.* 1969;126: 73-82.
33. Resnick PJ. Murder of the newborn: a psychiatric review of neonaticide. *Am J Psychiatry.* 1970; 126:58-64.
34. Harder T. The psychopathology of infanticide. *Acta Psychiatr Scand.* 1967;43:196-245.
35. Bourget D, Bradford JM. Homicidal parents. *Can J Psychiatry.* 1990;35:233-237.
36. Bourget D, Bradford JM. Affective disorder and homicide: a case of familial filicide: theoretical and clinical considerations. *Can J Psychiatry.* 1987;32: 222-225.
37. Browne WJ, Palmer AJ. A preliminary study of schizophrenic women who murdered their children. *Hosp Community Psychiatry.* 1975;26:71-75.
38. D'Orban PT. Women who kill their children. *Br J Psychiatry.* 1979;134:560-571.
39. Somander LK, Rammer LM. Intra- and extrafamilial child homicide in Sweden 1971-1980. *Child Abuse Negl.* 1991;15:45-55.
40. Dietz PE. Mass, serial and sensational homicide. *Bull N Y Acad Med.* 1986;62:477-491.
41. Fink WL, Roth LH. Altruistic murder-suicide: a case report and clinical indications. *Hosp Community Psychiatry.* 1979;30:558-559.
42. Goldney RD. Family murder followed by suicide. *Forensic Sci.* 1977;9:219-228.
43. Copeland AR. Dyadic death—revisited. *J Forensic Sci Soc.* 1985;25:181-188.
44. Lester D. Murder followed by suicide in those who murder police officers. *Psychol Rep.* 1987;60: 1130.
45. Lew EO. Homicidal hanging in a dyadic death. *Am J Forensic Med Pathol.* 1988;9:283-286.
46. Marcikic M, Mandic N. Homicide-suicide by stabbing. *Am J Forensic Med Pathol.* 1990;11:312-315.
47. Goldney RD. Homicide and suicide by aircraft. *Forensic Sci Int.* 1983;21:161-163.
48. Cavan R. *Suicide.* Chicago, Ill: University of Chicago Press; 1928:254-262.
49. Santoro JP, Dawood AW, Ayral G. The murder-suicide: a study of postaggressional suicide. *Am J Forensic Med Pathol.* 1985;6:222-225.
50. Gottlieb P, Kramp P, Gabrielsen G. The practice of forensic psychiatry in cases of homicide in Copenhagen, 1959 to 1983. *Acta Psychiatr Scand.* 1987;76: 514-522.
51. Gove W. Sex, marital status and mortality. *Am J Sociol.* 1973;79:45-67.
52. Lester D. Benefits of marriage for reducing risk of violent death from suicide and homicide for white and non white persons: generalizing Gove's findings. *Psychol Rep.* 1987;61:198.
53. Gudjonsson GM, Petursson M. Homicide in Nordic countries. *Acta Psychiatr Scand.* 1990;82:49-54.
54. Tardiff K. Patterns and major determinants of homicide in the United States. *Hosp Community Psychiatry.* 1985;36:632-639.
55. Jason J, Strauss LT, Tyler CW. A comparison of primary and secondary homicides in the United States. *Am J Epidemiol.* 1983;117:309-319.
56. Buda M, Tsuang MT. The epidemiology of suicide: implications for clinical practice. In: Blumenthal SJ, Kupfer DJ, eds. *Suicide Over the Life Cycle.* Washington, DC: American Psychiatric Press Inc; 1990:17-37.
57. Committee on Nomenclature and Statistics, American Psychiatric Association. *Diagnostic and Statistical Manual of Mental Disorders, Revised Third Edition.* Washington, DC: American Psychiatric Association; 1987.
58. Hansen JP, Bjarnason O. Homicide in Iceland 1946-1970. *Forensic Sci.* 1974;4:107-117.
59. Hirose S. Depression and homicide. *Acta Psychiatr Scand.* 1979;59:211-217.
60. Rosenbaum M, Bennett B. Homicide and depression. *Am J Psychiatry.* 1986;143:367-370.
61. Lester D, Perdue W, Brookhart D. Murderers who have attempted suicide. *Psychol Rep.* 1974;35: 238.
62. Fishbain DA, Rao VJ, Aldrich TE. Female homicide-suicide perpetrators: a controlled study. *J Forensic Sci.* 1985;30:1148-1156.
63. Virkkunen M. Suicide linked to homicide. *Psychiatr Q.* 1974;48:276-282.
64. Wong M, Singer K. Abnormal homicide in Hong Kong. *Br J Psychiatry.* 1973;123:295-298.
65. Lesco PA. Murder-suicide in Alzheimer's disease. *J Am Geriatr Soc.* 1989;37:167-168.
66. Lindqvist P. Criminal homicide in Northern Sweden 1970-1981: alcohol intoxication, alcohol abuse, and mental disease. *Int J Law Psychiatry.* 1986;8:19-37.
67. Danto BL. Suicide among murders. *Int J Offender Ther Comp Criminol.* 1978;22:140-148.
68. Mann JJ, Stanley M, eds. *Psychobiology of Suicidal Behavior.* New York, NY: New York Academy of Science; 1986.
69. Brown GL, Ebert MH, Goyer PF, et al. Aggression, suicide, and serotonin: relationships of CSF amine metabolites. *Am J Psychiatry.* 1982;139:741-746.
70. Linnoila M, Virkkunen M, Scheinin M, Nuutila A, Rimon R, Goodwin FK. Low cerebrospinal fluid 5-hydroxyindoleacetic acid concentration differentiates impulsive from non-impulsive violent behavior. *Life Sci.* 1983;33:2609-2614.
71. Van Praag H, Plutchik R, Apter A, eds. *Violence and Suicidality: Perspectives in Clinical and Psychological Research.* New York, NY: Brunner/Mazel Inc; 1990.
72. Batt JC. Homicidal incidence in the depressive psychoses. *J Ment Sci.* 1948;94:782-792.
73. Blom GE, Etkind SL, Carr WJ. Psychological interventions after child and adolescent disasters in the community. *Child Psychiatry Hum Devel.* 1991; 21:257-267.

Assault Weapons as a Public Health Hazard in the United States

Council on Scientific Affairs, American Medical Association

MOST of the scientific research relating to firearms and their effects on public health has concentrated on handguns. Despite the severity of the firearm problem in this country, and the wealth of publicity associated with it, more scientific investigation is needed on all firearm injuries[1] and those due to special classes of guns like assault weapons. The purpose of this report is to review what is known about assault weapons and their impact on public health and to discuss legislation to restrict the sale and private ownership of assault weapons. This report adds to the information provided by Substitute Resolution 264 (A-89), Restriction of Assault Weapons, which states that "the AMA [American Medical Association] supports appropriate legislation that would restrict the sale and private ownership of large-clip, high-rate-of-fire automatic and semiautomatic firearms, or any weapon that is modified or redesigned to operate as a large-clip, high-rate-of-fire automatic or semiautomatic weapon."

DEFINING ASSAULT WEAPONS

Traditionally, firearms have been split into two broad categories: long guns, which are fired from the shoulder (rifles and shotguns); and handguns, which are designed to be fired with one hand (revolvers and pistols).[2] The term *assault rifle* originated during World War II and refers to military weapons capable of automatic fire and having detachable magazines that hold 20 or more cartridges.[3] Assault weapons were developed to utilize firepower, in order to reduce the reliance on marksmanship in military settings. Currently, the term includes both automatic and semiautomatic firearms designed for killing people and generally considered to be of little use for hunting or trap and skeet shooting. *Automatic* and *semiautomatic* refer to the operating mechanism of a firearm and can apply to either long guns or handguns; there are semiautomatic rifles and semiautomatic pistols.[2] Semiautomatic hunting rifles are precisely aimed and fired from the shoulder, while assault weapons are meant to be spray-fired from the hip.[4] Both automatic and semiautomatic firearms can be spray-fired. Holding down the trigger of an automatic firearm results in a continuous stream of bullets until the ammunition magazine is emptied. In the case of a semiautomatic firearm, each trigger pull releases a single bullet, loads the next bullet, and permits rapid, sustained firing until the magazine is emptied.[4]

Not all semiautomatic firearms are assault weapons.[2] According to Sugarmann and Rand, "assault weapons are merely one type of semiautomatic firearm that can be distinguished by specific design characteristics."[5] Proponents who seek to regulate or ban assault weapons contend that assault weapons can be distinguished from other semiautomatic weapons by attached "combat hardware," such as silencers, folding stocks, bayonets, large-capacity magazines, short barrels, pistol grips on rifles or shotguns, or threaded barrels for accommodating flash suppressors.[4] They may also be differentiated by the ease with which they convert to fully automatic weapons and by their use in organized crime and narcotics cases. Opponents of a ban argue that some of these features may also apply to semiautomatic firearms used for hunting and sport,[6] and they feel that banning semiautomatic assault weapons is the first step toward banning all semiautomatic firearms.[2]

Assault weapons are difficult to define in legal terms,[2] and the lack of a precise definition may be the greatest obstacle to successful legislation against assault weapons. Confusion exists about weapons terminology: terms like *assault*, *paramilitary*, and *semiautomatic* are considered to be synonyms, when they are not.[2] Current legislative efforts to control the ownership and use of assault weapons have focused on semiautomatic weapons; therefore, the remainder of this report will concentrate on semiautomatic firearms used as assault weapons. For the purposes of this report the term *semiautomatic assault weapons* refers to the semiautomatic firearms that were permanently banned from importation into the United States in July 1989 and those domestically manufactured firearms identified in legislation such as that proposed by Sen Dennis DeConcini (D, Ariz) (S 747, Antidrug, Assault Weapons Limitation Act of 1989)[7] and Rep Fortney (Pete) Stark (D, Calif) (HR 1190, Semiautomatic Assault Weapons Act of 1989).[8]

PREVALENCE OF POSSESSION AND USE IN CRIME

Approximately 200 million firearms are owned by private citizens in the United States.[9] Since gun manufacturers are not required to give out their sales figures, and reports do not usually differentiate between standard long guns and assault weapons, a reliable estimate of how many of these guns are assault weapons is not available.[2] The best estimate may be the sum of the number of assault weapons legally imported into the United States and

Members of the Council on Scientific Affairs at the time of the report included the following: Yank D. Coble, Jr, MD, Jacksonville, Fla; A. Bradley Eisenbrey, MD, PhD, Royal Oak, Mich, Resident Representative; E. Harvey Estes, Jr, MD, Durham, NC, Vice Chairman; Mitchell S. Karlan, MD, Beverly Hills, Calif; William R. Kennedy, MD, Minneapolis, Minn; Michael P. Moulton, San Antonio, Tex, Medical Student Representative; Patricia Joy Numann, MD, Syracuse, NY; William C. Scott, MD, Tucson, Ariz, Chairman; W. Douglas Skelton, MD, Macon, Ga; Richard M. Steinhilber, MD, Cleveland, Ohio; Jack P. Strong, MD, New Orleans, La; Henry N. Wagner, Jr, MD, Baltimore, Md; William R. Hendee, PhD, Secretary; William T. McGivney, PhD, Assistant Secretary; Sharon B. Buchbinder, RN, MA, and Sona Kalousdian, MD, MPH, staff authors.

From the Council on Scientific Affairs, American Medical Association, Chicago, Ill.

This report was submitted to the House of Delegates of the American Medical Association at the June 1990 annual meeting as an informational report of the Council on Scientific Affairs.

This report is not intended to be construed or to serve as a standard of medical care. Standards of medical care are determined on the basis of all the facts and circumstances involved in an individual case and are subject to change as scientific knowledge and technology advance and patterns of practice evolve. These reports reflect the views of scientific literature as of June 1990.

Reprint requests to the Council on Scientific Affairs, American Medical Association, 515 N State St, Chicago, IL 60610 (Jerod M. Loeb, PhD).

the number of assault weapons that are domestically produced. This estimate depends on which models of semiautomatic weapons are considered to be assault weapons. If assault weapons are defined as the 49 models that were temporarily banned from importation by the Bush administration in March 1989, plus those made domestically, then the US Treasury Department's Bureau of Alcohol, Tobacco, and Firearms (BATF) estimates that there are 1 million assault weapons in private hands in the United States.[10] Another BATF estimate is much higher—2 to 3 million—when 1.5 million M-1 semiautomatic Garands are included.[11] These weapons were used by the US military, and surplus Garands have been sold at a special price by the US Army to National Rifle Association members.[12] They are not included among the weapons banned by President Bush and are now widely used in high-power–rifle competition.

In 1987, according to the Federal Bureau of Investigation's (FBI's) Uniform Crime Reports, 1.3 million crimes against individuals were reported, and 361 000 involved a firearm. A total of 35 100 trace requests were filed during that same year.[13] Requests to trace the ownership of a gun are submitted by police departments to the BATF. These requests may be filed to trace firearms known to have been used in crimes or found at crime scenes or to identify stolen weapons. Police departments around the country differ in the frequency with which they request traces and the crime characteristics and gun attributes that may prompt a request.[13] The sample of firearms for which traces are requested is not likely to be representative of all firearms used in crimes. Despite these limitations, trace requests submitted to the BATF form the only national database of its kind.

In 1989, Stewart and Alexander of the Cox Newspaper Bureau analyzed gun trace requests to estimate the approximate prevalence of assault weapon use by criminals. They examined 42 758 requests submitted to the BATF during the period January 1, 1988, through March 27, 1989.[13] Among all firearms traced, pistols (29% of all traces) and revolvers (33%) were traced most frequently by law enforcement agencies.[13] Using a list of 64 models, which included the 49 banned weapons and the US-made weapons listed in S 386 (introduced by Sen Howard Metzenbaum [D, Ohio]), Stewart and Alexander concluded that one of every 10 firearm traces involves an assault weapon.[13]

An analysis of the major types of crimes for which gun traces were submitted revealed that assault weapons were involved in 12.4% of gun traces related to narcotics crimes and 30% of traces related to organized crime.[13] Ninety percent of the assault weapons traces involved only 10 models: six rifles, three pistols, and one shotgun. In a comparison of nine major US cities, Los Angeles, and Miami, had the highest percentages of assault weapons traces (19% and 18%, respectively); Washington, DC, had 13%, and Detroit, and New York City both had 11%. Two thirds of traced assault weapons were domestically manufactured.[13]

Two pieces of evidence suggest that the number of assault weapons in the United States increased between 1986 and 1988. First, the percentage of firearm trace requests for assault weapons grew from 6% in 1986 and 1987 to 10% in 1988 and the first 3 months of 1989.[13] Second, the number of importation requests for semiautomatic weapons has also grown: 40 000 in 1987, 44 000 in 1988, and 114 000 in the first 3 months of 1989,[14] which was immediately before the Bush administration's temporary importation ban.

Although the proliferation of semiautomatic weapons has been documented, the reasons for the increase have not. In 1984, President Reagan removed importation restrictions on Chinese military surplus weapons, which made the relatively inexpensive AK-47 ($300) readily available.[15] In addition, a renewed interest in the Vietnam War, along with the availability of cheap ammunition, and the frequent appearance of assault weapons on television ("The A-Team" and "Miami Vice"), in movies (*Rambo* and films with Chuck Norris and Arnold Schwarzenegger), and in weapons magazines, have probably all had a role in increasing their popularity.[15] In 1987, the US toy industry spent more than $40 million on advertising new war toys that included water and dye-pellet versions of the Uzi and AK-47.[15]

INCIDENCE OF DEATH AND INJURY

The actual numbers of deaths and injuries caused by assault weapons are not known. While the FBI's Uniform Crime Reports tabulate the number of reported homicides by types of firearms used, there is not a separate category for assault weapons.[16] The reported number of firearm homicides was 11 084 in 1988,[16] and 8.1% of the gun traces for homicides during the same period were assault weapons.[13] Even given the limitations of these data, these figures may still be used to give a crude approximation of the number of reported homicides due to assault weapons: 898. This figure is similar to the number of homicides in which rifles (764) or shotguns (1117) were used and is considerably lower than the number of homicides due to handguns (8278) in the same year.[16] Statistics on firearm suicides and unintentional firearm deaths, as compiled by the National Center for Health Statistics, are not subdivided according to type of firearm. It is unlikely that assault weapons are responsible for many of these deaths, as Wintemute et al[17] have shown that revolvers and pistols are the weapons of choice in firearm suicides.

Perhaps the most succinct depiction of the assault weapon problem was made by the California Attorney General's Office: "The danger of the semiautomatic assault weapon is not yet the frequency with which it is used in crime or the volume which exist compared to other types of guns. Rather the danger is the potential each semiautomatic assault weapon confers upon an individual to kill and wound a large number of people."[18]

During the past year, the medical and lay press have reported on an epidemic of drug-related violence.[19] Semiautomatic weapons have been described as the weapon of choice for drug gangs,[18,20] and officials have noticed their use has increased in areas where crack cocaine is endemic.[18] In Los Angeles, at least 20% of those seen in emergency departments for injuries from assault weapons were innocent bystanders who became victims of drive-by shootings.[21] One South Bronx, NY, hospital has determined that 75% of all the trauma cases it treats are drug-related.[22] Clearly, the injuries from assault weapons are taxing hospital emergency departments in large urban areas.[19,21-25] For this reason, military trauma physicians are being recruited to relieve the work load at the Washington (DC) Hospital Center[26] and at Martin Luther King Hospital in Los Angeles.[25] In return, these surgeons receive practical experience in treating combat wounds.[26]

Wounds from high-velocity assault weapons resemble the wounds inflicted in the Vietnam War: they are often multiple and massive,[21] and immediate treatment is critical to survival. High-velocity bullets may set up shock waves and cause cavitation effects, resulting in unpredictable damage at sites far from the wound tract.[27] With low-velocity assault weapons, multiple wounds still occur, but the damage is localized to the tissues adjacent to the wound tract, and the full extent of the injury can usually be determined at the time of surgery.[27] A spokesman for the Hospital Council of Southern California has stated that mortality rates from high-velocity bullet wounds are four to five times higher than those from low-velocity bullet wounds and stab wounds.[21]

The estimated cost of treating a case of penetrating trauma (like that from an assault weapon) varies from $15 000 to $20 000.[19,23,25] A stay in intensive care is not unusual[19,25] and may cost as much as $150 000,[25] and patients may require a long rehabilitation.[25] These patients need a tremendous amount of care and can be a burden on hospitals.[21] Most gunshot wound patients are not covered by private insurance, and their costs are reimbursed by government insurance programs or are uncompensated. Thus, the public bears a major share of the cost.[19,23] The hospitals that belong to the trauma system in Chicago lost an average of $6000 per trauma patient in 1987 and 1988. According to the Chicago Department of Health, this corresponds to $10 million of uncompensated care charges for each of these years.[24] It is easy to see how this can affect the fiscal viability of hospitals and trauma systems[19,21] and force hospitals to drop out of trauma networks.

The number of deaths from assault weapons can be estimated, but again, no reliable data are available on how many of the victims were treated before dying, or how many were injured and survived. Estimated costs for treating firearm injuries in general are available, however; Martin et al[28] conducted a population-based study of all patients hospitalized for firearm injuries during 1984 at San Francisco (Calif) General Hospital, the region's only trauma center. The cost (total hospital costs, not including professional fees) for the initial hospitalizations for the 131 patients in the study was $905 809, for a mean cost of $6915 per patient.[28] Eighty-six percent of these costs were paid from public sources, which is a much larger percentage than the costs paid from public sources for all hospitalizations combined.[28]

The total number of firearm injuries have been estimated by applying the ratio of firearm deaths in San Francisco to the total number of firearm deaths in the United States for 1984.[28] This analysis assumes that the San Francisco ratio is similar to the ratio of injuries to deaths in the rest of the country and that the severity of injuries is also similar. When their mean cost is multiplied by the injury estimate, then the national cost for first hospitalizations due to firearm injuries was $429 million in 1984.[28] Total direct costs (hospitalizations, professional fees, rehabilitation, physical therapy, and long-term-care costs) are probably greater than $1 billion per year, and the associated indirect costs would be twice this figure.[28]

Data sources for firearm injuries in general are fragmented and incompatible with each other,[29] so it is not surprising that reliable data are not available for the number of assault weapons, the numbers of deaths and injuries resulting from the use of assault weapons, and the costs associated with them. Health care provision systems, especially emergency departments and trauma centers, need to collect epidemiological data on the incidence of assault weapons injuries and the costs associated with victims' health care, in order to enable informed decisions about assault weapons and the public's health.

PUBLIC OPINION

In January 1989, Patrick Purdy opened fire with an AK-47 assault rifle on a Stockton, Calif, school yard, firing approximately 120 rounds in about 2 minutes. Five children were killed, and 28 children and one teacher were wounded.[20] Public outrage focused attention on assault weapons, which were available under the same restrictions as ordinary rifles.[20]

In February 1989, *Time* magazine reported the results of a *Time*/Cable News Network poll in which 86% of respondents felt that crime is getting worse, and 84% felt that firearm violence is becoming a bigger problem in the United States.[30] In the same survey, while 84% of those polled said that people have a right to own guns, two of three people felt that existing laws make it too easy to buy guns, and 89% favored a 2-week waiting period in order to conduct a background check. Fifty-one percent of those polled would make civilian ownership of semiautomatic weapons illegal,[30] and 77% favored the mandatory registration of semiautomatic weapons.[31] Opinion was evenly divided as to whether stricter gun control laws would reduce the amount of violence in the country.[30] Two weeks later in another poll, a higher percentage (72%) of all respondents favored a federal ban on the manufacture, sale, and possession when the phrase "semiautomatic assault guns such as the AK-47" was included. Even two thirds of gun owners favored a ban on these weapons.[32]

Several law enforcement organizations have endorsed banning the manufacture and sale of assault weapons. These include the International Association of Chiefs of Police, the National Sheriffs' Association, the National Association of Black Law Enforcement Executives, the Police Executive Research Forum, the National Association of Police Organizations, and the Fraternal Order of Police.[4] The Board of Governors of the American Bar Association has called for laws to restrict private ownership of assault weapons.[33] Former Sen Barry Goldwater, a life member of the National Rifle Association, has said that there is no reason to use automatic or semiautomatic weapons for hunting and that "they have no place in anybody's arsenal. If any SOB can't hit a deer with one shot, then he ought to quit shooting."[34]

REGULATION OF ASSAULT WEAPONS

Baker et al[35] have identified four times in a "gun's life span" when legal regulation can occur: (1) the time of manufacture or importation, (2) the time of sale or transfer, (3) the period of possession, and (4) the period of use. The most stringent regulation occurs during the time a gun is used. Possession is also regulated, in an attempt to keep guns out of the hands of criminals. They note that laws against possession are hard to enforce and are of little value once the gun is in an individual's hands. States have laws, which vary greatly from state to state, dealing with the sale of guns, and there are federal requirements for gun manufacturers and importers.[35]

Automatic weapons have been regulated since 1934, largely in response to the use of submachine guns in violent crime during the prohibition era.[3] These weapons must be registered, and an FBI criminal record check and a $200 transfer tax are required to transfer ownership.[2,4] In 1986, federal legislation outlawed the future production and importation of automatic weapons.[2,4] In 1989, President Bush banned the importation of certain semiautomatic weapons. Federal law does not specifically regulate semiautomatic weapons, but treats them like other handguns, shotguns, and rifles,[2] and it does not prohibit the domestic manufacture of semiautomatic assault weapons.[4] According to the BATF, the majority of semiautomatic assault weapons that are used in crimes were originally purchased legally.[4]

The 1968 Gun Control Act gave the BATF the authority to ban the importation of any weapon that is not "generally recognized as particularly suitable or readily adaptable to sporting purposes."[36] In March 1989, prompted by the Stockton killings and publicity on the use of "sporting" semiautomatic weapons for violent crime, the Bush administration temporarily banned the importation of 49 foreign-made rifles that had been considered sporting weapons.[37] No pistols were banned, so some manufacturers have redesigned banned rifles as pistols.[38,39] The US manufacturers increased production of domestic counterparts to the banned weapons and reportedly made up for the lost imports.[40] In any event, the BATF has reported that 75% of the assault weapons in this country are made domestically,[37,40] so a ban on imports should not have a marked effect on the overall supply.

In an effort to determine what types of firearms are currently used for sporting purposes, the BATF sent out 3000 questionnaires to competitive shooting clubs, licensed hunting guides, state fish and game commissioners, editors of hunting and gun publications, and hunting association executives.[37] Based on these results and the BATF's analysis of weapon characteristics (eg, barrel length, caliber, and safety devices)[5] that are common to assault weapons, 43 assault weapons were permanently banned from importation into the United States in July 1989.[37]

Several AMA-supported bills that dealt with assault weapons were introduced in the 101st Congress in 1989 and

1990. The legislation that came closest to enactment was S 747, introduced by Senator DeConcini.[7] This bill sought to prohibit importation, domestic manufacture, and sale of a specific set of *new* weapons, but would not have affected weapons that were lawfully owned before its enactment or purchases by government entities. The Secretary of the Treasury would have been able to recommend other weapons for ban, but such additions required congressional approval. An additional 5-year prison sentence would have been given to those convicted of using or carrying assault weapons in violent crimes or drug trafficking.[7] The bill also called for a study of the legislation's effectiveness. If enacted, the law would have been automatically repealed after 3 years. The US Senate Committee on the Judiciary initially reported the bill in July 1989, by a vote of seven to six with one abstention.[41]

While no action was taken on S 747, similar provisions were incorporated in the Senate's comprehensive, or omnibus, crime bill, S 1970, introduced by Sen Joseph R. Biden, Jr (D, Del).[41] In the spring of 1990, gun control advocates turned back attempts by gun control opponents to delete the assault weapons ban from the crime package; first by a vote of 48 to 52 on the Senate floor, and then, on a vote to reconsider, by one vote (49 to 50). Later in the year, in order to pass a comprehensive anticrime bill, Senate conferees agreed to delete these provisions in exchange for the House's agreement to delete racial protections for death penalty defendants.[41] The AMA supported HR 4225, the Restricted Weapons Act of 1990, which was introduced by Rep William J. Hughes (D, NJ).[42] HR 4225 would have expanded the Secretary of the Treasury's existing authority to include domestically made semiautomatic rifles that did not meet the "sporting purposes" test. Within 60 days of enactment, the Secretary of the Treasury would have been required to publish a list of banned weapons. Weapons that were legally owned by individuals at the time of the list's publication would not have been affected. Although scheduled for consideration, the House of Representatives did not consider this bill before the close of the 101st Congress.

Some state and local governments have already proposed or enacted their own legislation to regulate assault weapons.[43] California prohibits the sale of specific assault weapons throughout that state. Maryland and Virginia have restricted possession,[43,44] and some cities, like Stockton[44] and Denver,[45] have either banned the guns or required registration. Other states and cities have bills pending,[5,43] but there is not a consensus on exactly which weapons should be included.

BARRIERS TO LEGISLATION

The single greatest barrier to the enactment of federal legislation restricting or banning access to semiautomatic assault weapons is a precise definition of the weapons. Establishing objective criteria is proving difficult for legislators, as expressed by the differences in specific weapons listed in the various federal, state, and local bills that have been passed or are pending.

In his testimony to the Senate Judiciary Committee in May 1989, Edward Ezell, PhD, curator of the National Firearms Collection at the Smithsonian Institution's National Museum of American History, emphasized that the central issue in any gun control argument is the balance between the private ownership of firearms (an individual right) and the question of public safety (the common good),[46] or in this instance, individual rights vs public health. Cost must also be a primary consideration, since taxpayers bear most of the costs associated with firearms injuries.[28] The AMA will continue to monitor the impact of assault weapons on public health and to support appropriate legislation to reduce this impact and save lives and scarce health care dollars.

References

1. Mercy JA, Houk VN. Firearm injuries: a call for science. *JAMA.* 1986;255:3143-3144.
2. *Assault Weapons and Accessories in America.* Washington, DC: Educational Fund to End Handgun Violence and New Right Watch; September 1988.
3. *Assault Rifle Fact Sheet 1: Definitions and Background.* Washington, DC: Institute for Research on Small Arms in International Security; March 24, 1989.
4. *Assault Weapon Questions & Answers.* Washington, DC: Handgun Control Inc; 1990.
5. Sugarmann J, Rand K. *Assault Weapons: Analysis, New Research, and Legislation.* Washington, DC: Violence Policy Center; March 1989.
6. *The Truth About Semi-Autos.* Washington, DC: National Rifle Association–Institute for Legislative Action; December 1989.
7. S 747, Antidrug, Assault Weapons Limitation Act of 1989. Introduced by Sen Dennis DeConcini (D, Ariz), April 11, 1989, referred to Committee on the Judiciary.
8. HR 1190, Semiautomatic Assault Weapons Act of 1989. Introduced by Rep Fortney (Pete) Stark (D, Calif), March 1, 1989, referred to the Committees on the Judiciary and Ways and Means.
9. *NRA Firearms Fact Card-1990.* Washington, DC: National Rifle Association–Institute for Legislative Action; 1990.
10. Bureau of Alcohol, Tobacco, and Firearms, US Treasury Department. Cited by: Stewart J, Alexander A. Assault weapons muscling in on the front lines of crime. *Atlanta Journal Constitution.* May 21, 1989:A1.
11. Bureau of Alcohol, Tobacco, and Firearms, US Treasury Department. Cited by: Stewart J, Alexander A. Judge to rule anew on army sales of assault weapons to NRA members. *Atlanta Journal Constitution.* October 14, 1989:A19.
12. Stewart J, Alexander A. Judge to rule anew on army sales of assault weapons to NRA members. *Atlanta Journal Constitution.* October 14, 1989:A19.
13. Stewart J, Alexander A. Assault weapons muscling in on the front lines of crime. *Atlanta Journal Constitution.* May 21, 1989:A1.
14. Lamar JV. Gunning for assault rifles. *Time.* March 27, 1989:39.
15. Stewart J, Alexander A. 'Miami Vice' the trendsetter in assault weapons. *Atlanta Journal Constitution.* September 17, 1989:A13.
16. *Crime in the United States, 1988.* Washington, DC: Federal Bureau of Investigation, US Dept of Justice; 1989.
17. Wintemute GJ, Teret SP, Kraus JF, Wright MW. The choice of weapons in firearm suicides. *Am J Public Health.* 1988;78:824-826.
18. *Assault Weapons: Background Paper.* Sacramento: California Attorney General's Office; February 1989.
19. Wagner L. Hospitals feeling trauma of violence. *Mod Healthcare.* February 5, 1990:23-32.
20. Church GJ. The other arms race. *Time.* February 6, 1989:20-26.
21. Pinkney DS. ERs seeing more 'war wounds' caused by assault weapons. *Am Med News.* April 14, 1989:3,42-45.
22. Goldfarb B. Hospitals endure a drug war assault. *USA Today.* March 19, 1990:D1.
23. McCarthy C. Guns and drugs are stretching emergency rooms to the limit. *Washington Post.* February 21, 1989:14, health section.
24. Kim H. Trauma networks look for rescue. *Mod Healthcare.* February 5, 1990:33-36.
25. Gross J. Epidemic in urban hospitals: wounds from assault rifles. *New York Times.* February 21, 1989:A1.
26. Ver Berkmoes R. Medical outpost in an urban war zone. *Am Med News.* April 28, 1989:37,40-42.
27. Feuchtwanger MM. High velocity missile injuries: a review. *J R Soc Med.* 1982;75:966-969.
28. Martin MJ, Hunt TK, Hulley SB. The cost of hospitalization for firearm injuries. *JAMA.* 1988;260:3048-3050.
29. Jagger J, Dietz PE. Death and injury by firearms: who cares? *JAMA.* 1986;255:3143-3144.
30. Barrett LI. Have weapons, will shoot. *Time.* February 17, 1989:22.
31. *Assault Weapons: Polling Data.* Washington, DC: Handgun Control Inc; September 1990.
32. Gallup G. *Federal Ban on Assault Guns Backed by Large Majority.* Princeton, NJ: Gallup Poll; March 19, 1989.
33. Stewart J, Alexander A. ABA leadership endorses limits on civilian access to military assault weapons. *Atlanta Journal Constitution.* June 22, 1989:A6.
34. Conconi C. Personalities. *Washington Post.* April 4, 1989:E3.
35. Baker SP, Teret SP, Dietz PE. Firearms and the public health. *J Public Health Policy.* 1980;1:224-229.
36. Gun control controversy. *Congressional Digest.* May 1986:134.
37. Stewart J, Alexander A. US slams the door on 43 models of foreign guns. *Atlanta Journal Constitution.* July 8, 1989:A1.
38. Stewart J, Alexander A. Foreign, US gun makers try end run on Bush ban. *Atlanta Journal Constitution.* October 2, 1989:A3.
39. LA Times/Washington Post Service. New gun menace hits US. *News-Sun.* January 17, 1990:B2.
40. Johnson K. Assault rifles: despite curb, no shortage. *New York Times.* September 16, 1989:8,10.
41. Inside Congress, 5: assault weapons. *Congressional Q.* November 24, 1990:3914-3915.
42. HR 4225, Restricted Weapons Act of 1990. Introduced by Rep William J. Hughes (D, NJ), March 8, 1990, referred to the Committee on the Judiciary.
43. Calhoun D. From controversy to prevention: building effective firearm policies. *Injury Prevention Network Newslett.* Winter 1989-90;7:12-19.
44. Stewart J, Alexander A. Threats target assault guns foes. *Atlanta Journal Constitution.* June 18, 1989:A1.
45. Gun registration begins in Denver. *New York Times.* November 16, 1989:B14.
46. *Hearings Before the Constitution Subcommittee of the Senate Committee on the Judiciary,* 101st Cong, 1st Sess (1989) (testimony of Edward C. Ezell, PhD, curator of the National Firearms Collection at the Smithsonian Institution's National Museum of American History).

Violence Against Women

Relevance for Medical Practitioners

Council on Scientific Affairs, American Medical Association

Evidence collected over the last 20 years indicates that physical and sexual violence against women is an enormous problem. Much of this violence is perpetrated by women's intimate partners or in relationships that would presumably carry some protective aura (eg, father-daughter, boyfriend-girlfriend). This violence carries with it both short- and long-term sequelae for women and affects both their physical and psychological well-being. The high prevalence of violence against women brings them into regular contact with physicians; at least one in five women seen in emergency departments has symptoms relating to abuse. However, physicians frequently treat the injuries only symptomatically or fail to recognize the injuries as abuse. Even when recognized, physicians are often without resources to address the needs of abused women. This report documents the extent of violence against women and suggests paths that the physician community might take to address the needs of victims.

(*JAMA*. 1992;267:3184-3189)

THE TWO decades since the 1960s witnessed a new national awareness of violence faced by women. Prior to the 1970s, the focus was on the danger of assault or rape by strangers or acquaintances. Violence in the family was thought to be infrequent and to result from psychopathology in the individuals involved rather than being viewed as a society-wide problem. Only in the past 15 years have systematic data on the prevalence and outcomes of intimate violence been gathered and responses been so wide-ranging, involving advocacy, medical care, mental health, criminal justice, and academic communities.[1,2] Major research and policy initiatives now address aggression occurring within families. Rape laws have been amended to protect victims of assault by marital partners. Nearly every state has established new legislation addressing violence between adult partners, and federal legislation on violence against women is pending.

The medical community—along with the criminal justice system—is the most likely to see women victims and as such constitutes a frontline of identification and intervention. However, physicians and other medical staff are rarely provided with training or specific protocols to aid in dealing with these cases. The cost of the failure to identify and intervene in violence is incalculable, particularly in violence by intimates, since assaults tend to be repeated over time, produce more injuries than assaults by strangers, and have complicated sequelae with implications for further morbidity.

This report reviews the following (overlapping) forms of violence against women: rape, physical and sexual assaults by marital or dating partners, and the long-term effects of child sexual molestation.

RAPE

In traditional definitions, rape was defined as the forcible carnal knowledge of a female against her will and was generally restricted to vaginal-penile penetration. In the last two decades, legal definitions of rape have undergone extensive revisions: many statutes now define rape as the "nonconsensual sexual penetration of an adolescent or adult obtained by physical force, by threat of bodily harm, or when the victim is incapable of giving consent by virtue of mental illness, mental retardation, or intoxication."[3] These definitions typically include other types of sexual penetration as well as attempts to commit rape.

Incidence and Prevalence of Rape

According to Federal Bureau of Investigation crime reports, 92 486 rapes of women were reported to police in 1988. However, officials consider rape to be vastly underreported. Estimates based on the National Crime Survey, which includes incidents not necessarily reported to the police, are nearly twice as high, even though the National Crime Survey contains no specific questions on sexual assault and therefore likely misses many cases.[4]

Prevalence studies using epidemiologic methods yield more reliable estimates. Such studies now indicate that at least 20% of adult women, 15% of college women, and 12% of adolescent girls have experienced sexual abuse and assault during their lifetimes.[5] Estimates for African American women are even higher.[6] Children are most at risk from assaults by family members and other caretakers, while adolescents and young adult women are most at risk for acquaintance and date rape and least at risk from someone unknown to them.

From the Council on Scientific Affairs, American Medical Association, Chicago, Ill.

This report was prepared for the Council on Scientific Affairs by Angela Browne, PhD, from the Department of Psychiatry at the University of Massachusetts, Worcester.

This is a substantially shortened version of a report prepared for the American Medical Association Council on Scientific Affairs. The recommendations in the report were adopted as policy by the House of Delegates at its December 1991, meeting. The text of the full report is available by writing to the Department of Mental Health, American Medical Association, 515 N State St, Chicago, IL 60610.

This report is not intended to be construed or to serve as a standard of medical care. Standards of medical care are determined on the basis of all the facts and circumstances involved in an individual case and are subject to changes as scientific knowledge and technology advance and patterns of practice evolve. This report reflects the views of scientific literature as of August 1991.

Reprint requests to Group on Science and Technology, American Medical Association, 515 N State St, Chicago, IL 60610 (Roger Brown, PhD).

Both young adult and older women are more vulnerable to sexual assaults by marital or ex-marital partners than to rape by acquaintances, other family members, or strangers combined.

Impacts on Psychological and Social Well-being

Initial Effects.—Initial reactions to sexual assault include shock, numbness, withdrawal, and denial. Victims of stranger attacks typically fear their assailant will return and further harm them. Victims of attacks by acquaintances or intimates are often stunned that someone known to them or someone they trusted could attack them in this manner. In initial presentations to police or medical staff, victims may appear unnaturally calm and detached (although some physical signs such as shaking or lowered skin temperature are usually present); or they may be crying or angry.

Typically, there is a lessening of initial symptoms after the first 2 weeks, and the victim may enter a denial phase in which there is an outward appearance of adjustment. However, studies suggest a period, occurring from 2 weeks to several months postassault, in which symptomatology returns and may intensify.[7] It is at this time that the victim may begin a pattern of help-seeking for these symptoms, without informing those she contacts of the rape experience that underlies them.

Long-term Effects.— Research documents that aftereffects of rape are persistent and long lasting. Victims often react with chronic anxiety and feelings of vulnerability, loss of control, and self-blame long after the assault.[8,9] Long-term reactions include anxiety, nightmares, catastrophic fantasies, feelings of alienation and isolation, sexual dysfunctions, and physical distress.[10] Moreover, women who have been raped tend to score high on almost every kind of measure of psychological distress.[11] Rape victims who were as much as 16 years postassault were found to have consistently higher levels of fear and anxiety than women without rape experiences. Other long-term effects include mistrust of others, phobias, depression, hostility, and somatic symptoms.[9] Suicidal thoughts are reported in between 33% and 50% of victims; in a community sample of women not seeking treatment, between 17% and 19% of rape victims made suicide attempts.[8,12]

The complex of effects in the aftermath of rape often meets the criteria for the diagnosis of posttraumatic stress disorder (PTSD). Hallmarks of PTSD include psychic numbing, intrusive reexperiencing of the trauma, avoidance of stimuli associated with the trauma, and intense psychological distress. Women with prior victimization histories evidence especially severe aftereffects.[13] Although it is often assumed that women who are the victims of stranger rapes are more severely traumatized than those victimized by persons they know, in comparing victims on measures of depression and anxiety, women assaulted by family members or dates experience as severe levels of distress as women assaulted by acquaintances or strangers.[14]

Impacts on Physical Health and Well-being

Immediate medical concerns after rape include injury, infection, and documentation. Physical effects of trauma may include soreness, bruising, and rectal bleeding. Gastrointestinal irritability, fatigue, tension headaches, intense startle reactions, and disturbed sleeping and eating patterns also often are noted.[10]

Ongoing health concerns include gynecological trauma, risk of pregnancy, and the potential for contracting infections or sexually transmitted diseases. The risk of human immunodeficiency virus infection is of increasing concern to rape victims and those who treat them and contributes to the sense of fear and irreparable damage. Victims may also seek to escape the pain of rape's aftereffects through alcohol and drugs, further disrupting physical and psychological well-being.

Special Considerations for Health Care Providers

Rape victims appear to be frequent users of medical services in the months and years postassault. In one study, visits to physicians increased 18% in the year of the assault, 56% in the following year, and 31% the year after, compared with previctimization levels.[15] Nearly all victims made visits to primary-care physicians in each of the 2 years after the assault.[16]

Although most emergency departments have established protocols for rape victims who are seen soon after the incident and who acknowledge that they have been raped, only a small minority of victims seek this type of assistance. Other victims present to private physicians or emergency departments with complaints based on the symptoms, but do not disclose that an assault has occurred. Still others do not present until months after the incident, but then contact the medical community repeatedly over time. Early identification of rape trauma by medical staff can help demystify nonspecific medical complaints and enable the physician to make appropriate referrals to help sources to assist with rape recovery.

Specific protocols that take into account the victim's relationship to the assailant will also contribute to the effectiveness of treatment. Women are more likely to be sexually assaulted by their intimates than by strangers. These victims are less likely to formally report the assault and thus are unlikely to be assisted under established protocols. Even given rape disclosure, established procedures may not provide medical staff with guidance on what to do if the assailant is present in the emergency department or physician's office. Medical protocols should take this into account and develop procedures for cases of intimate violence.

PARTNER VIOLENCE

Studies now document that women in the United States are more likely to be assaulted and injured, raped, or killed by a current or ex-male partner than by all other types of assailants combined.[17-20] In a 1985 survey of intact couples, nearly one out of every eight husbands had carried out one or more acts of physical aggression against their female partner during the survey year.[21] Over one third of these assaults involved severe aggression such as punching, kicking, choking, beating up, or using a knife or a gun. In an average 12-month period in the United States, approximately 2 million women are severely assaulted by male partners.[18,21,22]

As with other types of intimate violence, figures based on national surveys are marked underestimates. Such surveys typically do not include the very poor, those who do not speak English fluently, or individuals who are institutionalized, hospitalized, homeless, or incarcerated at the time the survey is conducted. National researchers agree that the true incidence of partner violence is probably double the above estimates: 4 million severely assaulted women per year. Studies on prevalence suggest that from one fifth to one third of all women will be physically assaulted by a partner or ex-partner during their lifetime.[23] Further, victims of violence by intimates are much more likely to be reassaulted within 6 months than are those attacked by nonintimates.[18]

Risks of Partner Violence for Women and Men

Although some surveys suggest nearly equal participation rates (ie, that about as many women as men have perpetrated at least one act of aggression), there is no measure of acts that are undertaken in self-defense. In general, men perpetrate more aggressive actions against their female partners than women do against their male partners, and men perpetrate more severe actions and are more likely to perpetrate multiple aggressive actions against their partner during a single incident than are women against male partners.[21,22]

In combination with men's greater average physical strength, these factors lead to quite different outcomes for women and men. Women are much more likely to be injured by their male partners than men are by their female partners.[24] Over 80% of all assaults against spouses and ex-spouses result in injuries, compared with 54% of the victims of stranger violence; victims of marital violence also have the highest rates of internal injuries and unconsciousness.[25]

Homicide figures for the United States also demonstrate the differential risk for women and the severity of physical outcomes of partner assault. From 1976 through 1987, the deaths of approximately 38 648 people over the age of 15 years resulted from one partner killing another (including married, common-law, divorced, or dating partners). Of these deaths, 61% of the victims were women and 39% were men.[26] Over one half of women murdered in the United States are killed by a current or former male partner. From 1976 through 1984, there was a decrease of more than 25% in the overall numbers of women killing male partners.[20] This drop was linked with the presence of domestic violence legislation and other services for abused women. This decrease has not been matched by a similar decline in men killing female partners, however.

Dynamics of Violence Against Wives

Types of partner abuse against women reported in epidemiologic surveys range from being slapped, punched, kicked, or thrown bodily to being scalded, choked, smothered, or bitten. Typical assaultive episodes often involve a combination of assaultive acts, verbal abuse, and threats.[27] The repetition of aggression in families is facilitated by the fact that victims are readily available, the amount of time at risk is high, assaults can be carried out in private, and wife assault is a relatively low-risk behavior for the aggressor.

Characteristics of Persons Involved in Marital Violence

National random samples document the diverse socioeconomic backgrounds of victims. However, empirical studies have not found characteristics that differentiate women who are victimized from women who are not. In a review of 52 studies with comparison groups, only one of 42 potential risk markers for women—witnessing parental violence as a child or adolescent—was consistently associated with becoming a victim of marital violence.[28] Studies also suggest that being sexually abused as a child leaves a woman more at risk for revictimization in later life.[29] Although studies from special populations stress symptomology, the symptoms that most battered women exhibit appear most likely to be sequelae of the violence rather than its antecedents.[1,28] Some commonalities have been found among male abusers, however. Men who assault female partners are more likely to have witnessed or experienced violence in childhood, to abuse alcohol, to be sexually assaultive to their wives, and to be at risk for violence against children than are men in comparison groups of nonabusive males.[28]

Impacts on Psychological and Social Well-being

As would be expected, women victims of a partner's violence have many of the same reactions as victims of other types of trauma. During assaults, the primary focus is on self-protection and survival. Reactions of shock, denial, withdrawal, confusion, psychological numbing, and fear are common. During and after an assault, a victim may offer little or no resistance, in an attempt to minimize the threat of injury or renewed aggression.

Like rape victims, long-term reactions in women abused by male partners include fear, anxiety, fatigue, sleeping and eating disturbances, intense startle reactions, and physical complaints. Abused women may become dependent and suggestible and find it difficult to make decisions alone. Effects of trauma are exacerbated by the fact that the aggressor is someone they may love, trust, and depend on. Unlike the victims of strangers, victims of marital violence have legal, financial, and role relationships with their assailants, confounding their decisions on what to do about the violence as well as the psychological sequelae. Perceptions of vulnerability, loss, and betrayal or hopelessness may be especially severe. There is also a high prevalence of depression, and suicide attempts are common.[30] Violence at home typically leaves no place in which defenses can be let down.

Impacts on Physical Health and Well-being

Injuries range from bruises, cuts, black eyes, concussions, broken bones, and miscarriages to permanent injuries such as damage to joints, partial loss of hearing or vision, and scars from burns, bites, or knife wounds. Typical injury patterns include contusions or minor lacerations to the head, face, neck, breast, or abdomen. These are often distinguishable from accidental injuries, which are more likely to involve the periphery of the body. In a hospital-based study, victims of domestic violence were 13 times more likely to sustain injury to breast, chest, or abdomen than accident victims.[31] Abused women are also more likely to have multiple injuries than accident victims.[32] When this pattern of injuries is seen in a woman, particularly in combination with evidence of old injury, physical abuse should be suspected.

Primary care complaints include chronic headaches, abdominal pains, muscle aches, recurrent vaginal infections, sleep and eating disorders, and depression. Victims may also begin to abuse alcohol or prescription drugs, although, in studies of general populations, alcohol abuse does not distinguish battered women from nonvictimized women. Recent research also suggests an association with delayed physical effects, particularly arthritis, hypertension, and heart disease (C. Corrao, unpublished data, 1985).

Special Considerations for Health Care Providers

Victims' Use of Health Care Services.—In studies of emergency department visits, 22% to 35% of women presenting with any complaint were there because of symptoms relating to partner abuse.[33] One project estimated that 21% of all women using emergency surgical services were there for sequelae of domestic violence, one half of all injuries presented by women occurred in the context of partner abuse, and over one half of all rapes of women over the age of 30 had been perpetrated by an intimate partner.[34] Rates are even higher in special-care populations. Abused women are likely to present with depression, anxiety, family/marital/sexual problems, and vague medical complaints. Due to the ongoing and injurious nature of domestic violence against women, abused women may visit physicians repeatedly, with increasingly severe physical trauma. Stark and Flitcraft[31(p302)] found that nearly one battered woman in five had presented at least 11 times with trauma; another 23% had brought six to 10 abuse-related injuries to the attention of clinicians. However, in most cases, the victimization history underlying these injuries was never identified.

Battering During Pregnancy.—Victims of a partner's violence during pregnancy face the risk of especially severe outcomes.[35] The 1985 National Family Violence Survey found that 154 out of every 1000 pregnant women were assaulted by their mates during the first 4 months of pregnancy, and 170 per 1000 women were assaulted during the fifth through the ninth months.[36] Approximately 37% of obstetric patients, across class, race, and educational lines, are physically abused while pregnant.[37] Such assaults can result in placental separation, antepartum hemorrhage, fetal fractures, rupture of the uterus, liver, or spleen, and preterm labor.[35] Because of the high incidence of assault against pregnant women, those providing pre- and postnatal care have an excellent opportunity to identify this abuse and reduce the potential negative outcomes.[38(p6)]

MARITAL RAPE

Although a neglected topic in the areas of both family violence and medicine, empirical research has shown that marital rape is an integral part of marital violence.[19,39,40] Marital rape has been reported in relationships in which no other forms of physical abuse occur. However, it seems to be most frequent as a form of aggression in relationships in which other violent behaviors are ongoing.[19] Sexual assault is reported by 33% to 46% of women victims who are being physically assaulted by their partners.[23] In severely abusive relationships, violent, forcible sexual assault may occur as often as several times a month.

Sexual abuse is an extremely serious form of marital violence. It is possible to inflict an intense level of physical pain over a long period and to cause a wide range of injuries, from superficial bruises and tearing to internal injuries and scarring. The psychological impact of assault by an intimate can also be extreme. Victims of marital rape suffer many of the same reactions as other rape victims and are likely to exhibit particularly severe sequelae, both emotionally and physically (including very severe depression and suicidality). Yet, except for child sexual molestation, this type of violence is least likely to be reported by victims. An awareness of the potential for forcible sexual assault in marriage, particularly in cases in which other types of physical abuse have been identified, will enable the clinician to sensitively assess the cause of observed symptoms.

COHABITING AND DATING VIOLENCE

Recent investigations have found a high prevalence of physical assault among dating and cohabiting couples as well. As with other types of intimate violence, the risk of injury is quite different for women and men. In one study of college students, women were four times as likely to sustain moderate to severe injuries as a result of dating violence as were males.[41] Self-reported motivations for perpetrating dating violence also differ. Whereas most women give self-defense or retaliation as their motivation, male respondents were most likely to report that the purpose of their violence was to "intimidate," "frighten," or "force the other person to do something." Violence as a response to sexual denial was also frequently reported by males.

Sexual Assault in Dating Relationships

Rape victimization for females is highest in the 16- through 19-year age group and next highest in the 20- through 24-year age group, with overall rates about four times as high as the mean for all women.[42] A survey of over 6000 college students found that 42% of women students reported some type of sexual assault, including forcible sexual contact, attempted rape, and completed rape.[10] Rapes and attempted rapes involved greater levels of violence than did nonsexual assaults in dating relationships. Surprisingly, rates of rape victimization did not vary significantly based on whether the school was large or small, or located in an urban, metropolitan, or rural area.

Reported levels of both nonsexual and sexual physical assaults against girls or women by nonmarital intimate partners have increased during the past 15 years. Although some of this may be due to greater sensitivity to the topic, severe types of violence against women do appear to be increasing. For example, although the rate of homicide victimization for male partners in dating or living-together relationships has varied unsystematically, the rate of females killed by dating or cohabiting partners increased sharply from 1976 through 1987.[26]

Considerations for Health Care Providers

Violence in dating relationships traditionally has been considered relatively unserious, with few services or protocols designed to address it. However, recent evidence on the prevalence, morbidity, and increasing number of male-perpetrated homicides in these relationships requires serious attempts to identify violence between nonmarried intimates and to effectively intervene. Screening techniques to assess for current or past victimization should be used for all categories of female patients, regardless of demographic or relational circumstances.

SEXUAL MOLESTATION IN CHILDHOOD

A history of childhood sexual molestation is highly associated with enduring physical and psychological sequelae, so that a lack of knowledge regarding this history may confuse the medical and psychological picture. Long-term effects in victims can be pronounced.

Long-term Effects

Impacts on Psychological and Social Well-being.—Effects of child sexual molestation include impacts on emotions, self-perception, and social functioning.[43] Adult survivors are more likely to report depression and to have been hospitalized for depression than are other types of victims or nonvictims. A high incidence of self-destructive behavior, both suicidal ideation and deliberate self-harm (eg, cutting, burning, or otherwise inflicting self-injury) has also been found in adult survivors of child sexual assault, distinguishing them even within clinical populations. This includes an exceptionally high prevalence of suicide attempts. Symptoms of anxiety, including chronic and severe sleep disorders, anxiety attacks, chronic fearfulness, and hypervigilance, also frequently are noted, along with disturbances in adult sexual pleasure and comfort.[29] Some survivors of child sexual molestation also report a general sense of alienation persisting into adulthood, as well as difficulty trusting others, relating to women and men, and parenting.[29]

Approximately one fifth of child sexual abuse victims evidence serious long-term psychological effects.[29] These may include disassociative responses as well as other PTSD indicators such as numbing of affect, chronic states of arousal, nightmares, and flashbacks. Victims who have experienced abuse by fathers or stepfathers, whose assaults involved genital contact, and whose molestation involved force, appear to be at especially high risk for severe long-term sequelae.[29] Perhaps most troubling is the increased risk of women who have been sexually abused as children to be revictimized later in life by both strangers and intimates. In one random-sample study, 33% to 68% of the victims later experienced a rape (depending on the seriousness of the childhood abuse they suffered), compared with 17% of women who were not child victims.[44] Victims of child sexual abuse also are more likely later to be physically abused by husbands or other adult partners.[44]

Impacts on Physical Health and Well-being.—Somatic disorders include abdominal pain, headaches, and eating disorders (eg, anorexia or bulimia). Adult victims may also evidence the effects of venereal disease. In a study of children, sexual victimization resulted in the transmission of venereal disease in 13% of 409 victims.[45] Female victims of child sexual assault also are at higher risk for substance abuse and the development of alcoholism than women without this childhood history.[46]

Special Considerations for Health Care Providers

A history of child sexual molestation in patients is almost always masked by other presenting problems. Further, medical and psychological symptomatology may be compounded by revictimization experiences. Indications that a history of child sexual abuse should be explored include (1) symptoms of PTSD without an apparent history of current or past rape, dating violence, partner abuse, or other trauma; (2) evidence of ongoing severe depression—especially if accompanied by self-harm and suicide attempts; (3) evidence of sexual dysfunction or unusual anxiety involving sexual activities or exposure of the body (possibly including medical, and especially gynecological, examinations); (4) early onset of alcohol or drug abuse; (5) a childhood history of running away; and (6) a history of repeated physical or sexual victimization.

PSYCHOPATHOLOGY VS THE EFFECTS OF TRAUMA

Clinicians in medical settings suggest that, in many cases, a diagnosis of PTSD is often the most accurate for victims of intimate violence.[10,32] The "most common traumata" suggested in the *Diagnostic and Statistical Manual of Mental Disorders, Revised Third Edition*[47] for PTSD is "a serious threat to one's life or physical integrity, or a serious threat or harm to one's children." Further, the presence of ongoing physical or sexual abuse is listed under the "extreme stressor" category. The only category more severe is reserved for "catastrophic" events and includes captivity as a hostage and concentration-camp experiences. Regardless, for behaviors to be seen as posttraumatic stress reactions, the trauma must be known—something that is not possible if a detailed victimization history is not obtained and effects are interpreted in isolation. In one study of adult women with sexual molestation histories, two thirds met the diagnostic criteria for PTSD. However, none had received that diagnosis and, in most cases, dealing with the impact of the childhood trauma was not even considered in their treatment.[48]

IMPLICATIONS FOR POLICY AND PRACTICE

Physicians and other health care providers rarely probe for the underlying causes of the injuries they treat,[31] but a treatment plan based primarily on the treatment of symptoms is ineffective for a victim of violence, particularly if assaults are ongoing and thus sequelae continually recur. Treating only the symptoms initiates a cycle of patient contacts with medical and mental health service providers, with the attendant risks of increasingly severe and debilitating sequelae for the patient, as well as exhaustion of resources within the system providing care. A more effective response over time is for medical professionals to routinely screen for victimization—including intimate physical and sexual assault—in their initial and ongoing assessments and to develop treatment plans that address the cause of the trauma as well as its manifestations.[33,49] Often, knowledge of a history of victimization provides a starting point from which to disentangle a confusion of presenting complaints and symptoms.

Guidelines for Medical Settings

Structured resources within a medical setting will greatly facilitate effective interventions. Basic components for targeted responses to violence against women include the following.

1. Training to develop an awareness of risk factors, indicators, estimated prevalence, sequelae, and considerations for the medical context. Training should include becoming familiar with assessment procedures risk assessment, safety planning, and procedures for linking victims to resources. Training on interpersonal violence should be incorporated into core curricula for undergraduate, graduate, and continuing education for those in the health professions.

2. Protocols to assess for current or past victimization as a routine part of obtaining a medical/psychiatric history. Procedures should give specific guidance, based on the type of abuse and the individuals at risk (eg, for a victim of a stranger vs marital or date rape; or for a woman victim with a child who is also at risk).

3. Response staff within the medical setting if possible. Staff would follow up with patients and act as a link with both in-house and community resources. Other tasks would include the identification of high-risk and repeat cases and coordination of triage efforts for intensive intervention with special-risk cases.

4. Referral sources within the community or area for women victims of violence. Medical settings should develop linkages with a variety of area resources including battered women's shelters and crisis services, rape crisis centers and services, services for adult survivors of child sexual abuse, legal services for women victims, treatment programs for men who abuse female partners, and services for abusive parents. The maintenance of reciprocal relations with this network will benefit patients, and medical personnel will no longer be required to carry the full burden of intervention.

Health Care Goals for Women Victims of Violence

Treatment goals for women victims of violence include the attainment of physical health, mental health, and safety from further harm. By incorporating routine questions for assessment, sensitive responses to disclosure, and effective referrals to resources into standard procedures, physicians will take an active role in finding solutions to the effects of violence on their patients.

Routine Screening. — Screening should be carried out at the entry points of contact between women and medical care (eg, primary care, emergency services, obstetric and gynecologic services, psychiatric services, and pediatric care). Guidelines for obtaining information on a trauma history, identifying coping mechanisms, and assessing the potential for further danger are provided by McLeer and Anwar,[49] Patten and colleagues,[50] and the American College of Obstetricians and Gynecologists.[38]

Validation of the Experience.—An explanation that many people experience physically aggressive actions from their intimates, that often they are afraid to tell anyone about it, and that such experiences can have painful and even dangerous sequelae should accompany assessments for victimization and characterize professional responses to disclosure. In discussing physicians' responses to abused women, Anne Flitcraft, MD, notes that "the very acknowledgment that domestic violence is going on, and that you and she agree it is a serious problem, is a very powerful and therapeutic first step."[33]

Record Keeping.—Archival studies of medical records note that victimization histories, if noted at all, are typically included with a list of symptoms or behavioral problems. More specific documentation—including indications of a trauma history from the initial screening, a description of symptomatology potentially linked to the victimization, and referrals made—provides a basis for later review of treatment plans. Such records are also useful to assess progress or to indicate the need for more intensive interventions at a later contact with the patient.

Referral.—After disclosure of victimization, referral should be made as quickly as possible to specially trained staff within the setting or to outside resources. Whenever possible, these resources should be "trauma-specific" (eg, rape victims would be referred to those with expertise in rape crisis and/or marital or date rape and abused women would be referred to those with expertise in domestic violence). Particularly in cases of domestic violence in which victims are still with their abusers, protocols need to address the following: (1) the handling of referrals when the assailant is on the premises; (2) procedures for response if the immediate need of the patient is for protection; and (3) the context in which ongoing abuse and threat is to be addressed. Referring a victim to counseling with her assailant is potentially dangerous. The victim may resist discussing the issues or completely deny that a problem exists in an attempt not to anger her partner or further endanger herself.

RECOMMENDATIONS FOR POLICY

The Council on Scientific Affairs recommends the following:

1. That the American Medical Association, working with members of the Federation and other relevant organizations, undertake a campaign to alert the health care community to the widespread prevalence of violence against women—that the effects of such violence are likely seen on a regular basis—and to sensitize them to the needs of victims of violence.
2. That physicians routinely incorporate screening leading to identification of female patients who are or have been victims of violence.
3. That physicians give due validation to the experience of victimization and of observed symptomatology as possible sequelae.
4. That physicians record a patient's victimization history, observed trauma potentially linked to the victimization, and make appropriate referrals.
5. That physicians, after diagnosing a violence-related problem, refer patients to appropriate medical or health care professionals and/or community-based trauma-specific resources as soon as possible.
6. That training on interviewing techniques, risk assessment, safety planning, and procedures for linking to resources be incorporated into undergraduate, graduate, and continuing medical education programs.
7. That the American Medical Association collect and disseminate protocols on identifying and treating victims of violence and develop, in conjunction with other relevant organizations, guidelines for treatment in which protocols are absent.

References

1. Fagan J, Browne A. Violence between spouses and intimates. In: Reiss AJ, Roth JA, eds. *Understanding and Controlling Violence.* Washington, DC: National Academy Press. In press.
2. Schechter S. *Women and Male Violence.* Boston, Mass: South End Press; 1982.
3. Searles P, Berger RJ. The current status of rape reform legislation: an examination of state statutes. *Wom Rights Law Reporter.* 1987;9:25-43.
4. Koss MP. The women's mental health research agenda: violence against women. *Am Psychol.* 1990; 45:374-380.
5. Koss MP. Hidden rape: sexual aggression and victimization in a national sample of students in higher education. In: Burgess AW, ed. *Rape and Sexual Assault.* New York, NY: Garland Publishing; 1988;2:3-25.
6. *Hearings Before the Select Committee on Children, Youth, and Families of the House of Representatives*, 101st Cong, 2nd Sess (1990) (testimony of Gail E. Wyatt, PhD).
7. Forman B. Psychotherapy with rape victims. *Psychotherapy: Theory, Research, and Practice.* 1980;17:304-311.
8. Kilpatrick DG, Veronen LJ, Best VL. Factors predicting psychological distress among rape victims. In: Figley CR, ed. *Trauma and Its Wake.* New York, NY: Brunner/Mazel; 1985.
9. Resick P, Calhoun K, Atkeson B, Ellis E. Adjustment in victims of sexual assault. *J Consult Clin Psychol.* 1981;49:705-712.
10. Koss MP, Harvey M. *The Rape Victim: Clinical and Community Approaches to Treatment.* Beverly Hills, Calif: Sage Publications; 1991.
11. Resick P. Sex-role stereotypes and violence against women. In: Franks V, Rothblum ED, eds. *The Stereotyping of Women: Its Effects on Mental Health.* New York, NY: Springer Publishing Co Inc; 1983.
12. Resick PA, Jordan CG, Girelli SA, Hutter CK, Marhoefer-Dvorak S. A comparative outcome study of behavioral group therapy for sexual assault victims. *Behav Ther.* 1989;19:385-401.
13. Sorenson SB, Golding JM. Depressive sequelae of recent criminal victimization. *J Trauma Stress.* 1990;3:1154-64.
14. Koss MP, Dinero TE, Seibel C, Cox S. Stranger, acquaintance, and date rape: is there a difference in the victim's experience? *Psychol Women Q.* 1988; 12:1-24.
15. Koss MP, Koss P, Woodruff WJ. Relation of criminal victimization to health perceptions among women medical patients. *J Consult Clin Psychol.* 1990;58:147-152.
16. Koss MP, Woodruff WJ, Koss PG. Deleterious effects of criminal victimization on women's health and medical utilization. *Arch Intern Med.* 1991;151: 342-347.
17. Finkelhor D, Yllo K. *License to Rape: Sexual Abuse of Wives.* New York, NY: Holt Rinehart & Winston; 1985.
18. Langan PA, Innes CA. *Preventing Domestic Violence Against Women.* Washington, DC: US Dept of Justice, Bureau of Justice Statistics; 1986.
19. Russell DEH. *Rape in Marriage.* New York, NY: Macmillan Publishing Co Inc; 1982.
20. Browne A, Williams KR. Exploring the effect of resource availability and the likelihood of female-perpetrated homicides. *Law Soc Rev.* 1989;23:75-94.
21. Straus MA, Gelles RJ, eds. *Physical Violence in American Families: Risk Factors and Adaptions to Violence in 8,145 Families.* New Brunswick, NJ: Transaction Publishers; 1990.
22. Straus MA, Gelles RJ, Steinmetz S. *Behind Closed Doors: Violence in the American Family.* Garden City, NY: Anchor Press; 1980.
23. Frieze IH, Browne A. Violence in marriage. In: Ohlin L, Tonry M, eds. *Family Violence: Crime and Justice, A Review of Research.* Chicago, Ill: University of Chicago Press; 1989:163-218.
24. Stets JE, Straus MA. Gender differences in reporting of marital violence and its medical and psychological consequences. In: Straus MA, Gelles RJ, eds. *Physical Violence in American Families: Risk Factors and Adaption to Violence in 8,145 Families.* New Brunswick, NJ: Transaction Publishers; 1990:151-165.
25. Lentzner HR, DeBerry MM. *Intimate Victims: A Study of Violence Among Friends and Relatives.* Washington, DC: US Dept of Justice, Bureau of Justice Statistics; 1980.
26. Browne A, Williams KR. Gender, intimacy, and lethal violence: trends from 1976-1987. *Gender and Society.* In press.
27. Browne, A. *When Battered Women Kill.* New York, NY: Macmillan/Free Press; 1987.
28. Hotaling GT, Sugarman DB. An analysis of risk markers in husband to wife violence: the current state of knowledge. *Violence Victims.* 1986;1:101-124.
29. Browne A, Finkelhor D. The impact of child sexual abuse: a review of the research. *Psychol Bull.* 1986;99:66-77.
30. Stark E, Flitcraft A. Violence among intimates: an epidemiological review. In: Van Hasselt VB, Morrison RL, Bellack AS, Hersen M, eds. *Handbook of Family Violence.* New York, NY: Plenum Press; 1988:293-318.
31. Stark E, Flitcraft A, Frazier W. Medicine and patriarchal violence: the social construction of a 'private' event. *Int J Health Serv.* 1979;9:461-493.
32. Burge SK. Violence against women as a health care issue. *Fam Med.* 1989;21:368-373.
33. Randall T. Domestic violence intervention calls for more than treating injuries. *JAMA.* 1990;264: 939-940.
34. Stark E, Flitcraft A, Zuckerman D, Grey A, Robison J, Frazier W. *Wife Abuse in the Medical Setting: An Introduction for Health Personnel.* Washington, DC: Office of Domestic Violence; 1981. Monograph 7.
35. Saltzman LE. Battering during pregnancy: a role for physicians. *Atlanta Med.* 1990;64:45-48.
36. Gelles RJ. Violence and pregnancy: are pregnant women at greater risk of abuse? *J Marriage Fam.* 1988;50:841-847.
37. Helton A, McFarlane J, Anderson E. Battered and pregnant: a prevalence study. *Am J Public Health.* 1987;77:1337-1339.
38. American College of Obstetricians and Gynecologists. *The Battered Woman.* Washington, DC: American College of Obstetricians and Gynecologists; 1989. Technical bulletin 124.
39. Walker LE. *The Battered Woman Syndrome.* New York, NY: Springer Publishing Co Inc; 1984.
40. Fagan J, Friedman E, Wexler S, Lewis V. *The National Family Violence Evaluation: Final Report, Volume I: Analytical Findings.* San Francisco, Calif: URSA Institute; 1984.
41. Makepeace JM. Gender differences in courtship violence. *Fam Relations.* 1986;36:383-388.
42. Bureau of Justice Statistics. *Criminal Victimization in the United States, 1982.* Washington, DC: US Dept of Justice; 1984.
43. Gold E. Long-term effects of sexual victimization in childhood: an attributional approach. *J Consult Clin Psychol.* 1986;54:471-475.
44. Russell DEH. *The Secret Trauma: Incest in the Lives of Girls and Women.* New York, NY: Basic Books Inc Publishers; 1986.
45. White KN, Snyder J, Bourne R, Newberger EH. *Treating Child Abuse and Family Violence in Hospitals.* Lexington, Mass: Lexington Books; 1989.
46. Miller BA, Downs WR, Gondoli DM, Keil A. The role of childhood sexual assault in the development of alcoholism in women. *Violence Victims.* 1987;2:57-172.
47. American Psychiatric Association, Committee on Nomenclature and Statistics. *Diagnostic and Statistical Manual of Mental Disorders, Revised Third Edition.* Washington, DC: American Psychiatric Association; 1987.
48. Craine P. Cited by: Gondolf EW. *Psychiatric Responses to Family Violence: Identifying and Confronting Neglected Danger.* Lexington, Mass: Lexington Books; 1990.
49. McLeer SV, Anwar RA. The role of the emergency physician in the prevention of domestic violence. *Ann Emerg Med.* 1987;16:1155-1161.
50. Patten SB, Gatz YK, Jones B, Thomas DL. Post-traumatic stress disorder and the treatment of sexual abuse. *J Nat Assoc Soc Workers.* 1989; 34:197-203.

Physicians and Domestic Violence

Ethical Considerations

Council on Ethical and Judicial Affairs, American Medical Association

DOMESTIC violence, spouse abuse, and battering all refer to the victimization of a person with whom the abuser has or has had an intimate/romantic relationship.[1,2] These three terms are used interchangeably throughout this article. Domestic violence may take the form of physical, sexual, and psychological abuse, is generally repeated, and often escalates within relationships.[3-7]

Most evidence indicates that domestic violence is predominantly perpetrated by men against women.[8-11] Some evidence suggests that women are as likely to use violence against male partners as men are against female partners.[12] However, these research findings have been criticized on various counts as misleading.[13(p312),14(pp181-183),15] In particular, it is clear that the impact on the health of female victims of domestic violence is generally much more severe than the impact on the health of male victims.[3,14,16] Battering is also known to occur in gay and lesbian relationships, but there has been little research in this area.

Women in the United States are more likely to be victimized, through assault, battery, rape, or homicide, by a current or former male partner than by all other assailants combined.[3] The rate of injury to women from battering surpasses that of car accidents and muggings combined.[1,2,17,18] Just over one half of all women murdered in the United States are killed by male partners, and 12% of murdered men are killed by female partners.[14(p204)] Other documented sequelae include various medical complaints, miscarriages, abortion, drug and alcohol abuse, attempted suicide, and mental illness.[2(p1413),13,19]

PHYSICIANS' ETHICAL DUTY TO DIAGNOSE AND TREAT FAMILY VIOLENCE

Beneficence and Nonmaleficence

The medical ethical principle of beneficence requires physicians to intervene in cases of domestic violence. Some may argue that physicians' ethical obligations to patients who are battered are limited to treating the bodily manifestations—injuries and other symptoms. In doing more, physicians will step out of their medical role. However, in their book on beneficence, noted bioethicists Edmund Pellegrino and David Thomasma[20(p10)] describe physicians' duties as going beyond simply addressing the physical injury or disease of their patients:

> The aim of medicine is to address not only the bodily assault that disease or an injury inflicts but also the psychological, social, even spiritual dimensions of this assault. To heal is to make whole or sound, to help a person reconvene the powers of the self and return, as far as possible, to his [or her] conception of a normal life.

Treating only the injuries and symptoms of abuse will not address the ongoing family violence that is at the root of its victims' health problems. When physicians do not diagnose abuse, it is most likely to continue and will often escalate. One study found that approximately one in five battered women presenting to physicians had sought medical attention for injuries from abuse 11 times previously.[1]

The ethical principle of nonmaleficence—do no harm—also directs physicians to diagnose domestic violence. When a diagnosis of abuse is missed, treatment is likely to be inappropriate and potentially harmful. For example, it has been documented that physicians often prescribe medications for battered women, usually pain medications or mild tranquilizers, which are contraindicated for abuse victims because they are at an increased risk for suicide and drug or alcohol abuse.[21(pp252-253)] Further, such drugs may hamper the victim's alertness, making her more vulnerable to assault.[22(p100)]

Failing to diagnose abuse may also further the victim's sense of entrapment and thereby contribute to victimization.[13] Often when battered women seek help from others including the police, health care providers, friends, and family, they are met with denials of the seriousness of the abuse.[2,21,23(p119)] Victims also often encounter blame, misinformed advice, and punitive responses when they seek help.[23(p119)] Inability to find help often causes victims to feel that there is no escape from the violence. These feelings of helplessness and entrapment are associated with the psychosocial problems caused by abuse.[2,13,23] When physicians

From the Council on Ethical and Judicial Affairs, American Medical Association, Chicago, Ill.

This report is an abridged version of Report B, "Physicians and Family Violence: Ethical Considerations," adopted by the House of Delegates of the American Medical Association at the 1991 Interim Meeting.

Reprint requests to Health Law Division, American Medical Association, 515 N State St, Chicago, IL 60610 (David Orentlicher, MD, JD).

Members of the Council on Ethical and Judicial Affairs include the following: Oscar W. Clark, MD, Gallipolis, Ohio, Chair; John Glasson, MD, Durham, NC, Vice Chair; Allison M. August, Chicago, Ill; John A. Barrasso, MD, Casper Wyo; Charles H. Epps, MD, Washington, DC; Robert McQuillan, MD, Kansas City, Mo; Charles W. Plows, MD, Anaheim, Calif; George T. Wilkins, Jr, MD, Edwardsville, Ill; David Orentlicher, MD, JD, Chicago, Ill, Secretary and staff author; Kristen A. Halkola, Chicago, Ill, Associate Secretary and Staff author; Anita K. Schweickart, Chicago, Ill, Staff Associate and principal staff author.

disregard signs of abuse, they contribute to victims' sense of entrapment and further their patients' health risks.[2,13,23]

Physicians are particularly well situated to intervene in cases of domestic violence because persons who are in violent relationships often visit physicians for injuries and other symptoms related to their abuse.[2,24] Between 22% to 35% of women presenting with complaints in emergency departments are suffering from injuries or symptoms caused by ongoing abuse.[1,25] Battered women also often visit primary care physicians for a variety of medical complaints, such as abdominal pains, headaches, and sleep disorders.[21] Twenty-five percent of female emergency psychiatric patients are battered by a male partner,[17] and up to 64% of female psychiatric inpatients are abused as adults.[26] Physicians who specialize in gynecology and obstetrics are also likely to come into contact with battered women. Pregnancy in particular appears to be a high risk factor for abuse.[2,27]

Although the solutions to domestic violence extend into social, legal, and political realms, in which physicians may have limited influence, physicians can provide a number of important interventions. Currently, the American Medical Association is developing protocols for the detection and management of domestic violence. Probably the most important contribution physicians can make to ending abuse and protecting the health of its victims is to identify and acknowledge the abuse.[21] Identifying domestic violence can initiate the process by which people may get the necessary assistance to find safety. Other primary responsibilities include providing sensitive support, clearly documenting the abuse, providing information about options and resources, and, with the patient's consent, making necessary referrals. Physicians must also facilitate an assessment of the level of danger faced at home. When danger is present, physicians must participate in efforts to secure a safe place, including offering hospitalization, if necessary, for patients when there are no available shelters.

Physicians' Failure to Diagnose and Treat Family Violence

A number of studies have shown that physicians often fail to diagnose abuse when signs and symptoms are present. In one study, emergency department physicians identified one in 35 of their female patients as battered, while a review of the medical charts indicated that in fact, one in four were likely to have been battered.[21] Another study found that physicians' discharge diagnoses correctly indicated spouse abuse in only 8% of the cases in which explicit information about abuse (eg, patient statements about abuse) or very strong indications of abuse were recorded in the medical chart.[28] As the author of the study noted, "physicians in other clinical situations would not discharge a patient from the emergency room with a potentially life-threatening condition."[28(p510)] Not surprisingly, in a survey that asked 1000 abused women to rate the effectiveness of various professionals in addressing their abuse, health care professionals had the lowest rating, ranking behind battered women's shelters, lawyers, social service workers, police, and clergy.[29]

Barriers to Diagnosing and Treating Family Violence

Lack of Knowledge and Training.—One barrier to detecting and treating family violence is a lack of knowledge and training. For example, physicians are usually not trained to recognize and correctly interpret behaviors associated with spouse abuse. As a result of their abuse, battered women often make frequent visits to their doctor or an emergency department for complaints or symptoms that do not appear to have an organic basis. Physicians often respond by judging the patient to be neurotic. In a review of physicians' records, researchers found statements labeling women as "neurotic," "hysterical," "a crock," and "a hypochondriac" significantly more frequently when the patient was at risk for abuse than not.[21]

Societal Misconceptions.—Physicians share a number of pervasive societal misconceptions about domestic violence that undermine the medical response to battering.[30] The most harmful of these misconceptions include the following: (1) domestic violence is rare; (2) violence does not occur in relationships that appear "normal"; (3) domestic violence is a private matter that should be resolved without outside intervention; and (4) battered women are responsible for their abuse.

The belief that domestic violence is rare stems from the traditional view of the family as a safe haven from the troubles of the outside world. There is now extensive evidence that families and other intimate relationships are often anything but safe. Physicians' lack of awareness of the prevalence of domestic violence contributes to their reluctance to consider abuse in the differential diagnosis and to disbelieve that abuse has occurred even when the signs are evident.

The attitude that domestic violence does not occur in seemingly "normal" or "healthy" relationships causes physicians to miss diagnoses of abuse. In particular, it is often assumed that abusers can be easily identified as pathological and excessively violent. Physicians may be especially likely to disbelieve that abuse has occurred when they know and like the suspected abuser. However, abuse occurs in seemingly normal families and abusers often appear indistinguishable from other people and often do not behave violently in other circumstances.[2(p1417),31] In fact, abusive partners may appear especially concerned or attentive when they accompany victims to receive medical care (because they feel remorseful, do not want to be suspected of abuse, or do not want the patient to be seen alone).

Similarly, many believe battering only occurs in certain racial and socioeconomic groups. Abuse appears to be more frequent among blacks than whites. However, evidence also suggests that this difference may reflect a greater likelihood of black women to report their abuse than white women.[13] Socioeconomic differences in prevalence figures for domestic violence may also contribute to perceived racial differences. One study found that within similar income levels, blacks were less likely than whites to experience domestic abuse.[32] Domestic violence appears to be more prevalent among people with lower income levels.[13] However, the most rigorous study found only a 3% difference between the incidence of abuse of lower-income women and middle-income women.[33] At any rate, it is clear that domestic violence cuts across racial and class categories.

Another common misconception is that domestic violence is a private matter and should be resolved within the relationship.[24] Battered women are often advised to try to work out their difficulties themselves.[23(p119)] Unfortunately, without assistance, continuing to live in an abusive relationship can be the most dangerous course for victims, since abuse is usually repeated and often escalates in severity. Similarly, battered women may be advised to seek marriage counseling. However, marriage counseling is contraindicated because the safety of the victim is not prioritized and she remains vulnerable to continued abuse.[34]

Physicians may believe that victims themselves would prefer to be left alone. Physicians are often reluctant to broach the subject with patients who show signs of potential abuse. Studies on spouse abuse have documented that physicians generally do not ask in-depth questions about how victims were injured, or who caused the injuries.[28] However, evidence suggests that battered women expect their physicians to initiate discussions about abuse, and that they will respond to their physician's inquiries, if asked directly in an empathetic and nonjudgmental way.[35]

Another societal misconception about domestic violence is that women are responsible for their victimization.[24] They may be blamed for provoking the abuse, enjoying the abuse, not leaving the relationship, not pressing criminal charges, and/or being resistant to interventions. These beliefs are based on misconceptions about the dynamics of domestic violence. Many barriers prevent victims from leaving abusive relationships or pressing criminal charges. These barriers include the presence of children in the home, fear of retaliation, not having a safe place to go, financial dependency and/or a lack of job skills, emotional ties, denial, self-blame, hope that the situation will improve, and feelings of helplessness caused by abuse.

The blaming of victims may enter into the medical response to domestic violence subtly. Physicians may perceive that the woman is the source of the problem if she does not act on their advice to end the relationship, go to a shelter, or file for a protection order. Ending victimization can be a lengthy process, particularly when there are few options.[24] Perceiving battered women as noncompliant or problematic may cause physicians to discontinue their care or to fail to intervene in future cases of abuse. Therefore, patience and support from physicians can be important to individuals in abusive relationships.

Lack of Resources for Victims of Abuse.—One of the primary aims when treating victims of family violence is to help bring victims into contact with resources such as shelters, social services, legal assistance, and support groups. However, often such resources are limited or are not available.

As part of a grass-roots movement, battered women's shelters have greatly expanded in number over the last two decades.[36] Shelters often provide and coordinate numerous services for battered women and their children, including child care, legal advocacy, job training, welfare services, support groups, and counseling. However, battered women's programs do not exist in many areas.[37] The services that do exist are generally poorly funded.[36] Battered women's shelters are almost always filled to capacity and, as a result, must turn many women away.[36,38]

SPECIAL ETHICAL CONSIDERATIONS

Confidentiality

In opinion 5.05,[39] the Council on Ethical and Judicial Affairs states that physicians have an ethical obligation to maintain patient confidentiality. Confidentiality is necessary so that patients feel free to make full disclosure of relevant information about their health.

When a patient is subject to domestic violence, the need for patient trust in the physician is especially important since patients may feel embarrassed, ashamed, or afraid to reveal that they have been battered. Furthermore, the safety of the patient may be jeopardized if the physician discloses a diagnosis of abuse to the patient's spouse or partner. Therefore, abuse must be discussed with the patient in privacy and safety. Spouses, partners, or other third parties, including the police, should not be notified of an abuse diagnosis without the expressed consent of the patient. When physicians are required to report serious assaults or injuries inflicted by weapons, they should discuss their legal obligations with the patient, explain the reporting, investigation, and follow-up procedures that may follow, and address directly the risk of reprisal and the possible need for shelter.

Almost every state requires physicians to report suspected child and elder abuse and neglect to local protective services or law enforcement authorities.[40,41] It is not evident, however, that mandatory reporting of domestic violence would contribute to the safety of battered women or facilitate their access to appropriate resources. In fact, few states have mechanisms for reporting domestic violence to protective services. A more appropriate alternative to mandatory reporting for domestic violence would be to expand and increase funding for resource options for battered women and their children, including shelters and safe homes.

When a patient subjected to domestic violence is legally a minor, physicians are required in every state to report the abuse to their local child-abuse protective services. Similarly, depending on the particular state statute, if the victim is an elderly person or is disabled, physicians may be required to report the abuse under elder-abuse or abuse-of-the-disabled statutes.

Informed Consent

Informed consent for all nonemergency medical interventions must be obtained from competent adult victims of abuse, similar to any other adult patients. Interventions include taking photographs or roentgenograms of injuries or arranging referrals to the appropriate agency. It is important to encourage patients to consent to specific interventions and to give assurances of safety and confidentiality. However, no intervention should be forced on an unwilling patient. Overriding a patient's refusal violates the ethical principle of respect for patient autonomy. In the case of domestic violence, it also further disempowers the patient. Therefore, respecting the choices of persons who have been abused is also important for therapeutic reasons.

CONCLUSIONS

- Due to the prevalence and medical consequences of domestic violence, physicians should routinely inquire about abuse as part of the medical history. Physicians must also consider battering in the differential diagnosis for a number of medical complaints, particularly when treating women.
- Physicians who are likely to have the opportunity to detect abuse in the course of their work have an obligation to familiarize themselves with protocols for diagnosing and treating domestic violence and with community resources for battered women and their children.
- Physicians also have a duty to be aware of societal misconceptions about domestic violence and prevent these from affecting the diagnosis and management of abuse. Such misconceptions include the belief that abuse is a rare occurrence; that domestic violence does not occur in "normal" relationships; that domestic violence is a private problem best resolved without outside interference; and that victims are responsible for the abuse.
- The medical profession must demonstrate a greater commitment to ending domestic violence and helping its victims. Medical societies should work collaboratively with established services for those who are abused. Physicians must participate in community-wide efforts to establish and strengthen resources for victims and abusers. In particular, shelters and safe homes for battered women and their children must be expanded and better funded. Law enforcement reforms that would ensure greater enforcement of protection orders should be advocated. There should be more research into the effectiveness of rehabilitation and prevention programs for abusers.
- In order to improve physician knowledge of domestic violence, physicians must be better trained to identify domestic violence and to work cooperatively with the range of community services currently involved. Training on family violence should include education about the dynamics of abuse as well as presentations of diagnosis and management protocols. Hospitals should adopt protocols specific to domestic violence, and they should require additional training for those physicians who are likely

to see victims of abuse. Comprehensive training on domestic violence should be required in medical school curricula and in residency programs for specialties in which domestic violence is likely to be encountered.

- Informed consent for nonemergency interventions must be obtained from victims of domestic violence.
- Physicians must discuss the problem of domestic violence with patients in privacy and safety. For mentally competent adult victims, physicians must not disclose an abuse diagnosis to spouses or any other third party without the consent of the patient.

The Council thanks Anne Flitcraft, MD, for her critical review of this report.

References

1. Stark E, Flitcraft A, Zuckerman D, Grey A, Robison J, Frazier W. *Wife Abuse in the Medical Setting: An Introduction for Health Personnel.* Washington, DC: Office of Domestic Violence; 1981. Monograph 7.
2. Rosenberg ML, Stark E, Zahn MA. Interpersonal violence: homicide and spouse abuse. In: Last JM, ed. *Maxcy-Rosenau Public Health and Preventive Medicine.* 12th ed. East Norwalk, Conn: Appleton-Century-Crofts; 1986:1399-1426.
3. Council on Scientific Affairs, American Medical Association. Report B of the Council on Scientific Affairs: violence against women. In: *Proceedings of the House of Delegates of the American Medical Association.* Chicago, Ill: American Medical Association. In press.
4. Klaus PA, Rand MR. *Family Violence.* Washington, DC: Bureau of Justice Statistics, US Dept of Justice; 1984. Special report.
5. Walker LE. *The Battered Woman Syndrome.* New York, NY: Springer Publishing Co Inc; 1984.
6. Snyder DK. Differential patterns of wife abuse: a data-base typology. *J Clin Psychol.* 1981;49:878-885.
7. Langan PA, Innes CA. *Preventing Domestic Violence Against Women.* Washington, DC: Bureau of Justice Statistics, US Dept of Justice; 1986.
8. Bureau of Justice Statistics. *Report to the Nation on Crime and Justice: The Data.* Washington, DC: Office of Justice Programs, US Dept of Justice; October 1983.
9. McLeod M. Women against men: an examination of domestic violence based on an analysis of official data and national victimization data. *Justice Q.* 1984: 170-193.
10. Centers for Disease Control. Family and other intimate assaults—Atlanta, 1984. *MMWR.* 1990;39: 525-528.
11. Dobash RE, Dobash RP. Wives: the 'appropriate' victims of marital violence. *Victimology.* 1978; 2:426-442.
12. Straus MA, Gelles RJ, Steinmetz SK. *Behind Closed Doors: Violence in the American Family.* New York, NY: Doubleday & Co Inc; 1980.
13. Stark E, Flitcraft A. Violence among intimates: an epidemiological review. In: VanHasselt VB, Morrison RL, Bellack AS, Hersen M, eds. *Handbook of Family Violence.* New York, NY: Plenum Press; 1988:293-317.
14. Frieze IH, Browne A. Violence in marriage. In: Ohlin L, Tonry M, eds. *Family Violence.* Chicago, Ill: University of Chicago Press; 1989;2:163-218.
15. Yllo K. Political and methodological debates in wife abuse research. In: Yllo K, Bograd M, eds. *Feminist Perspectives on Wife Abuse.* Beverly Hills, Calif: Sage Publications; 1988:28-50.
16. Straus MA, Gelles RJ. Societal change and change in family violence from 1975 to 1985 as revealed by two national surveys. *J Marriage Fam.* 1986;48:465-479.
17. Stark E. *The Battering Syndrome: Social Knowledge, Social Therapy and the Abuse of Women.* Binghamton, NY: State University of New York–Binghamton; 1984. Dissertation.
18. McClear SV, Anwar RA. The role of the emergency physician in the prevention of domestic violence. *Ann Emerg Med.* 1987;16:1155-1161.
19. Geffner R, Pagelow MD. Victims of spouse abuse. In: Ammerman RT, Hersen M, eds. *Treatment of Family Violence.* New York, NY: John Wiley & Sons Inc; 1990:113-135.
20. Pellegrino ED, Thomasma DC. *For the Patient's Good: The Restoration of Beneficence in Health Care.* New York, NY: Oxford University Press; 1988.
21. Kurz D, Stark E. Not-so-benign neglect: the medical response to battering. In: Yllo K, Bograd M, eds. *Feminist Perspectives on Wife Abuse.* Beverly Hills, Calif: Sage Publications; 1988:249-266.
22. Margolin G, Sibner L, Gleberman L. Wife battering. In: VanHasselt VB, Morrison RL, Bellack AS, Hersen M, eds. *Handbook of Family Violence.* New York, NY: Plenum Press; 1988:89-117.
23. Stark E, Flitcraft A. Personal power and institutional victimization: treating the dual trauma of woman battering. In: Ochberg F, ed. *Post-traumatic Therapy.* New York, NY: Brunner/Mazel Inc; 1987.
24. Burge SK. Violence against women as a health care issue. *Fam Med.* 1989;21:368-373.
25. McLeer SV, Anwar RAH, Herman S, Maquiling K. Education is not enough: a systems failure in protecting battered women. *Ann Emerg Med.* 1989;18:651-653.
26. Jacobson A, Richardson B. Assault experiences of 100 psychiatric inpatients: evidence of the need for routine inquiry. *Am J Psychiatry.* 1987;144: 908-913.
27. Helton A, McFarlane J, Anderson E. Battered and pregnant: a prevalence study. *Am J Public Health.* 1987;77:166-174.
28. Warshaw C. Limitations of the medical model in the care of battered women. *Gender Soc.* 1989; 3:506-517.
29. Bowker LH, Maurer L. The medical treatment of battered wives. *Women Health.* 1987;12:25-45.
30. King MC, Ryan J. Abused women: dispelling myths and encouraging intervention. *Nurse Pract.* 1989;14:47-58.
31. Star B, Clark C, Goety K. Psychosocial aspects of wife battering. *Soc Casework.* October 1979.
32. Casanave NA, Straus MA. Race, class, network embeddedness and family violence: a search for potent support systems. *J Comp Fam Stud.* 1979; 10:281-299.
33. Schulman M. *Survey of Spousal Violence Against Women in Kentucky.* Washington, DC: Kentucky Commission on Women, Law Enforcement Assistance Administration, US Dept of Justice; 1979. Harris study 792701.
34. Bograd M. Family systems approaches to wife battering: a feminist critique. *Am J Orthopsychiatry.* 1984;54:558-568.
35. Rath G, Jarratt L. Battered wife syndrome: overview and presentation in the office setting. *South Dakota J Med.* 1990;43:19-25.
36. Sedlak A. Prevention of wife abuse. In: VanHasselt VB, Morrison RL, Bellack AS, Hersen M, eds. *Handbook of Family Violence.* New York, NY: Plenum Press; 1988:319-358.
37. *Hearings Before the Senate Subcommittee on Children, Families, Drugs, and Alcoholism,* 101st Cong, 2nd Sess (1990) (testimony of Jann Jackson, MS).
38. *Violence Against Women, July 1990.* Washington, DC: Congressional Caucus for Women's Issues; July 1990:7. Fact sheet.
39. Council on Ethical and Judicial Affairs, American Medical Association. Opinion 5.05: confidentiality. *Current Opinions of the Council on Ethical and Judicial Affairs.* Chicago, Ill: American Medical Association; 1989.
40. Faller K. Unanticipated problems in the United States child protection system. *Child Abuse Negl.* 1985;9:63-69.
41. Brewer R, Jones J. Reporting elder abuse: limitations of statutes. *Ann Emerg Med.* 1989;18:1217-1221.

Let's Be Clear

Violence Is a Public Health Problem

WE have worked for more than 10 years in the US Public Health Service to clarify the patterns of violence through surveillance and research and to identify and evaluate interventions to prevent and reduce the impact of violence. It is time to be clear about what we mean by violence and why we believe that violence is a public health problem. Violence is the intentional use of physical force against another person or against oneself, which either results in or has a high likelihood of resulting in injury or death. Violence includes suicidal acts as well as interpersonal violence such as rape, assault, child abuse, or elder abuse. Fatal violence results in suicides and homicides.

The term *violence* has been used to connote both a subset of behaviors (which produce injuries) and outcomes (ie, the injuries themselves). We use *violence* to refer to a particular class of behaviors that cause injuries. By convention, the public health community refers to injuries from violence as "intentional injuries." Although this description is not entirely satisfactory, it is meant to distinguish injuries due to violence from injuries due to unintended motor vehicle crashes, falls, drownings, and burns.

Having clarified what we mean by the term *violence*, we must still explain why violence is a public health problem. Three hard questions need to be answered.

Why Should Public Health Practitioners Concern Themselves With Violence?

The health consequences of violence are tremendous, but traditionally our society has turned to the criminal justice sector to protect us from such violence. Why involve public health practitioners? Why not just beef up our efforts in criminal justice?

In answering this question, we must first recognize that criminal justice has been and will continue to be an important component of our efforts to curb violence. We must also admit that the application of criminal justice measures alone is not enough.

Indeed, the incidence of injuries and deaths from violence has continued to increase in the face of ever greater resources devoted to criminal justice. In fact, the level of violence is so high that by any traditional measure of public health importance, fatal and nonfatal injuries resulting from interpersonal violence have become one of the most important public health problems facing our country.

The criminal justice system relies on arrests and incarcerations to deter, incapacitate, and rehabilitate convicted offenders. Criminal justice professionals themselves have stated for years that much of the problem of violence is a "social problem," beyond the purview of the police and the criminal justice system. For example, violence between family members and acquaintances accounts for more than half of all homicides. Most violent injuries do not stem immediately from criminal activities such as robbery. They occur as the result of violent arguments among people who know each other, and they generally do not occur in public.

Therefore, one reason that the public health community should become involved is that the problem is beyond the reach of the criminal justice system working alone. Another reason is that the public health community introduces a primary prevention focus to the problem of violence. The essence of public health is prevention, and it is that very essence that will enable the public health community to address the issues and problems in a manner that complements the efforts of the criminal justice system. By mobilizing the broad array of existing resources in medicine, mental health, social services, and substance abuse services toward the prevention of injuries and deaths from violence, considerable progress can be made.

Do We in Public Health Know How to Prevent Violence?

The short answer to that question is no. If we knew how to prevent violence, you would have heard about it before now. But a more accurate, complete answer to that question is no, we don't have the answers in hand, but we know how to get them! Public health brings to the table a time-tested, systematic approach to reducing the burden of illness, suffering, and premature death among human populations.

The public health approach consists of health-event surveillance, epidemiologic analysis, and intervention design and evaluation, focused unwaveringly on a single, clear outcome—the prevention of a particular illness or injury. This approach was originally developed to combat infectious diseases, when such diseases were the leading causes of death. It has been successfully applied, however, to many causes of premature death and preventable physical illness including lung cancer, coronary heart disease, and, more recently, motor vehicle crashes.

From the Division of Injury Control, National Center for Environmental Health and Injury Control, Centers for Disease Control, Public Health Service, US Department of Health and Human Services, Atlanta, Ga.

Reprint requests to Division of Injury Control, Mail Stop F-36, National Center for Environmental Health and Injury Control, Centers for Disease Control, Atlanta, GA 30333 (Dr Rosenberg).

The public health approach to violence faces several daunting challenges. Not only is violence a multifaceted problem, with each face requiring a separate approach, but violence is intimately intertwined with a variety of major social problems for which no easy solutions are apparent. Poverty, unemployment, racism, and other injustices contribute in complex ways to violent behavior. These social problems deserve attention on their own, and it seems clear that their remediation would substantially reduce the incidence of violent injuries and deaths.

Public health action to reduce the incidence and health consequences of violence faces other major impediments. Several distinctive characteristics of American society—characteristics highly valued by some—appear to be important determinants of violent behavior. The depiction of violence on television, in movies, and in other media, and ready access to firearms, are two examples. Exposure, especially of impressionable children and youths, to the creatively captivating scenes of aggression and violence depicted in the media fosters our acceptance and expectation of violence in America and probably contributes to the frequency of aggressive acts themselves. Firearms may or may not cause violent behavior, but there is increasingly compelling scientific evidence that they markedly elevate the severity of the health consequences of such behavior. The quarrelsome debate and the paralyzing ambivalence of American society about these issues has sometimes prevented, and still threatens to prevent, adequate research into the effect of media violence and access to firearms on violent behavior and associated injuries.

These social problems and issues are not synonymous with violence. However, they undoubtedly will continue to complicate and impede efforts by the public health community to reduce violent behavior and injuries. They will severely test the versatility of the public health model. We are just now beginning to apply public health methods to the prevention of injuries from violence. Will we be successful? Time alone will tell. But, given the track record of success for public health, we have every reason to be optimistic.

Is There a Commitment From the Public Health Sector to Address This Critical Public Health Problem?

This question we can answer quite definitively yes. The Centers for Disease Control has made the prevention of violence one of its highest priorities, and we now have a variety of projects under way that pertain, either directly or indirectly, to reducing the health consequences of violence.

First, we are developing a comprehensive National Plan for Injury Control. Seven panels of experts were commissioned to develop recommendations for specific parts of the injury control field. One panel was commissioned to develop recommendations for the prevention of injuries from violence.

A major recommendation of this panel was to develop a national system or infrastructure for preventing violence. Such a system would provide surveillance, direct resources for prevention to those at highest risk, empower communities to address the problem of violence at the community level, evaluate intervention activities, and train workers in the skills needed to accomplish the task. Accomplishing these various tasks will require not only federal commitment but the commitment and coordinated efforts of state and local governments and a wide range of private-sector organizations. Encouraging such involvement and coordinating these efforts are two aspects of the work that the Centers for Disease Control does.

Another major recommendation of the violence panel is that firearm injuries should be prevented. There is much debate on how to do this, but there is a growing consensus that immediate access to highly lethal weapons is one of the most critical elements in the causation of many homicides. As health officials concerned with stopping the bloodshed, we cannot ignore this issue. Just as we were able to save countless lives from motor vehicle injuries without banning cars, we can save many lives from firearm injuries without a total ban on firearms. There is no controversy in the area of children having unsupervised access to loaded guns. No one believes that children should have unsupervised access to guns, but few people are doing anything to prevent children from having such access. This, at least, is a place to start. Parents should be encouraged and assisted in every possible way to prevent their children from carrying guns or having unsupervised access to guns. Such efforts to empower families should begin now, while we in public health continue to explore the scientific issues associated with this question, through careful research and the evaluation of existing programs designed to reduce ready access to guns.

Second, we are developing guidelines for those who want to develop programs to prevent youth violence in their own communities. These guidelines are designed to prevent youth violence in general, but, in recognition of the disproportionate burden of violence borne by minority populations, we have sought extensive input on these guidelines from leaders of minority communities and those who have already implemented innovative programs in inner cities and urban centers.

Third, we will support the design, implementation, and evaluation of multifaceted community-based youth violence prevention programs. This fiscal year we plan to fund and work collaboratively with at least two communities to develop such programs and to scientifically evaluate their effectiveness. Multifaceted programs are needed because of the complex web of factors that cause violence and violence-related injuries. Community-based programs are needed to assure involvement in, ownership of, and responsibility for the activities by community residents. Successful prevention activities need to be identified, documented, and shared without delay to facilitate the most rapid progress possible in reducing violent injuries and deaths.

Fourth, James O. Mason, MD, assistant secretary for health, Department of Health and Human Services, has asked the Centers for Disease Control to lead the development of a new Public Health Service–wide activity to identify, develop, and implement effective, community-based interventions for the prevention of youth violence.

In summary, violence is a major cause of injuries and deaths. The prevention of these injuries and deaths is an appropriate, and indeed a necessary, public health focus. The problem of violence probably has no simple solution, but the public health method of health-event surveillance, epidemiologic analysis, and intervention design and evaluation can undoubtedly make important contributions to the solution.

Mark L. Rosenberg, MD, MPP
Patrick W. O'Carroll, MD, MPH
Kenneth E. Powell, MD, MPH

The Firearm Fatality Reporting System

A Proposal

RECOMMENDATION: [R]equire that firearm injuries, in addition to being reportable to the police, be reportable to health departments. Place greater emphasis on coding the type of firearm on the death certificate. Develop a national fatal firearm injury reporting system, comparable to FARS [Fatal Accident Reporting System], with sufficient data for documenting the firearm problem and designing prevention strategies.

—from *Cost of Injury in the United States*[1]

Firearms are the vehicle of death for approximately 34 000 people each year in the United States. The estimated lifetime costs for firearm injuries that occurred in 1985 will be $14.4 billion.[1] Firearm policy, as expressed most often through legislation, is in part health policy. For groups such as young African-American males, for whom almost half of all deaths are caused by gunfire,[2] gun policy may be more influential to their health status than any other form of health policy.

But gun policy has been driven more with an ear to rhetoric than with an eye toward health statistics. This is due in part to the inability of health professionals to provide data that will answer crucial policy questions.

For example: Are there temporal trends in the proportion of gun deaths from small, cheap handguns (Saturday night specials) vs more sophisticated weaponry? Do newly manufactured guns figure disproportionately in firearm homicides or suicides? How many deaths, and what percentage of all gun deaths, are attributable to paramilitary "assault" weapons? Are certain types of guns preferentially used for adolescent suicide, which has been increasing dramatically in recent decades?[3] Are there particular characteristics common to the guns that are involved in unintended, childhood shootings? Does the risk-to-benefit ratio for defensive handgun ownership vary among subsets of the population?

Questions such as these deserve answers based on reliable data, but these data are at present difficult or impossible to assemble. Vital statistics records for gun mortality are E-coded (using the external cause of death codes in the *International Statistical Classification of Diseases, Injuries, and Causes of Death, Ninth Revision*[4]), and the type of gun involved can be recorded by use of the code's fourth digit. But in about 80% of firearm homicides and 66% of firearm suicides and unintentional shootings, the type of gun is not specified on the death certificate.[5] Death certificates present only a crude assessment of intent—they do not distinguish among the types of homicides, for example. They contain little information on persons who die from gunshot wounds, less on the circumstances, and none at all on other involved persons.

Special studies that use medical examiner or coroner records or police reports can yield more information on gun deaths.[6,7] These studies, however, are expensive and fail to provide ongoing, timely information for most geographic areas. The ability of policymakers to respond to changing trends in gun deaths is thereby compromised.

The Uniform Crime Reporting System, maintained by the Federal Bureau of Investigation, provides information, at least for homicides. For example, it grossly specifies the type of gun used in murders. This reporting program is "a cooperative effort of approximately 16,000 city, county, and state law enforcement agencies voluntarily reporting data on crime brought to their attention."[8] Firearm suicides, which outnumber firearm homicides, and unintended gun deaths are not covered by the Uniform Crime Reports (UCR). Moreover, approximately 10% of homicides in the United States are not included in the UCR database.[9]

A Firearm Fatality Reporting System is needed. One can be patterned after the Fatal Accident Reporting System (FARS), which is maintained by the National Highway Traffic Safety Administration and which has reported on all motor vehicle–related fatalities since 1975. FARS collects uniform data from the states and reports on up to 90 different data elements characterizing each fatal crash and the vehicles and people involved in that crash. In 1989, FARS collected data on 45 555 fatalities involving 40 718 crashes. The annual budget for FARS is approximately $3.5 million.

The FARS data have been used, for example, to evaluate seatbelt laws,[10] child restraint laws,[11,12] and changes in speed limit laws[13]; to detect vehicles that are at high risk for injury involvement[14]; to monitor trends in motor vehicle safety[15]; and to monitor the role of alcohol in highway fatalities.[16] The existence of the FARS database has been crucial to the development of highway safety.

As is the case with highway fatalities, gun deaths are routinely investigated by medical examiners or coroners and

From the The Johns Hopkins Injury Prevention Center, The Johns Hopkins School of Hygiene and Public Health, Baltimore, Md (Mr Teret and Dr Beilenson); and the University of California, Davis, School of Medicine, Sacramento (Dr Wintemute).

Reprint requests to The Johns Hopkins Injury Prevention Center, 624 N Broadway, Hampton House 548, Baltimore, MD 21205 (Mr Teret).

by police. A good deal of information, therefore, is currently collected at the state and local levels, but this information is not uniform, nor are the medical data reported to a national repository. A Firearm Fatality Reporting System, which might best be located within the Centers for Disease Control, could rely on data currently collected at the state and local levels in much the same way FARS does. Information maintained at the federal level need not contain identifiers, so that the confidentiality interests of involved parties are protected.

At a minimum, data collected on firearm fatalities should include the following:

- Information on the gun itself, such as type, make, model, caliber, and serial number, which would allow researchers to determine other variables such as year of manufacture.
- Type of death—homicide, suicide, unintended, or undetermined.
- Information on the victim, such as age, race, sex, and drug/alcohol involvement.
- Information on the shooter, such as age, race, sex, relationship to the victim, and drug/alcohol involvement.
- Information on the circumstances of the shooting, such as date, time, type of location, and whether it occurred during commission of another crime.
- Involvement of emergency medical services.

In 1981, Wright and Rossi,[17] having reviewed the literature on weapons, crime and violence, wrote the following:

> The published literature is more noteworthy for what it does *not* show than for what it does. There is, it appears, scarcely a single finding in the literature that could be said to have been indisputably established. In part, this reflects the highly politicized nature of research in this area, but perhaps more importantly, it results from a near-total absence of sound and nationally generalizable data from which reliable information about weapons, crime, and violence might be extracted.

In the decade since that observation was written, there have been more than 300 000 additional firearm deaths in the United States, and we still do not systematically collect data.

Informed decisions must be made regarding gun risks and benefits, a topic that is emotionally and politically charged. The Firearm Fatality Reporting System would bring important, new, and needed information to help with the resolution of difficult issues.[18] The creation of such a system should be recognized as a national health priority.

Stephen P. Teret, JD, MPH
Garen J. Wintemute, MD, MPH
Peter L. Beilenson, MD, MPH

This work was supported in part by grant R49CCR302484-05 from the Division of Injury Control, Center for Environmental Health and Injury Control, Centers for Disease Control, Atlanta, Ga.

1. Rice DP, MacKenzie EJ, et al. *Cost of Injury in the United States: A Report to Congress.* Atlanta, Ga: Centers for Disease Control; 1989.
2. Fingerhut LA, Kleinman JC, Godfrey E, Rosenberg H. Firearm mortality among children, youth, and young adults 1-34 years of age: trends and current status, United States, 1979-88. *Monthly Vital Statistics Rep.* 1991;39:1-15.
3. Boyd JH, Moscicki EK. Firearms and youth suicide. *Am J Public Health.* 1986; 76:1240-1242.
4. *International Statistical Classification of Diseases, Injuries, and Causes of Death, Ninth Revision.* Geneva, Switzerland: World Health Organization; 1977.
5. Baker SP, O'Neill B, Ginsberg MJ, Li G. *The Injury Fact Book.* 2nd ed. New York, NY: Oxford University Press; 1991.
6. Wintemute GJ, Teret SP, Kraus JF, Wright MA, Bradfield G. When children shoot children: 88 unintended deaths in California. *JAMA.* 1987;257:3107-3109.
7. Kellermann AL, Reay DT. Protection or peril? an analysis of firearm-related deaths in the home. *N Engl J Med.* 1986;314:1557-1560.
8. Federal Bureau of Investigation. *Crime in the United States—1987.* Washington, DC: Federal Bureau of Investigation, US Dept of Justice; 1988.
9. Rokaw WM, Mercy JA, Smith JC. Comparing death certificate data with FBI crime reporting statistics on US homicides. *Public Health Rep.* 1990;105:447-455.
10. Wells JK, Williams AF, Fields M. Coverage gaps in seat belt use laws. *Am J Public Health.* 1989;79:332-333.
11. Teret SP, Jones AS, Williams AF, Wells JK. Child restraint laws: an analysis of gaps in coverage. *Am J Public Health.* 1986;76:31-34.
12. Wagenaar AC, Webster DW, Maybee RG. Effects of child restraint laws on traffic fatalities in eleven states. *J Trauma.* 1987;27:726-732.
13. Baum HM, Wells JK, Lund AK. Motor vehicle crash fatalities in the second year of 65 mph speed limits. *J Safety Res.* 1990;21:1-8.
14. Robertson LS. Risk of fatal rollover in utility vehicles relative to static stability. *Am J Public Health.* 1989;79:300-303.
15. Robertson LS. Automobile safety regulations and death reductions in the United States. *Am J Public Health.* 1981;71:818-822.
16. Fell JC, Klein T. The nature of the reduction in alcohol in US fatal crashes. Warrendale, Pa: Society of Automotive Engineers Inc; 1986. Technical paper series 860038.
17. Wright J, Rossi P. *Weapons, Crime and Violence in America: Executive Summary.* Washington, DC: National Institute of Justice, US Dept of Justice; 1981. Quoted in: National Committee on Injury Prevention and Control. *Injury Prevention: Meeting the Challenge.* New York, NY: Oxford University Press; 1989.
18. Kellermann AL, Lee RK, Mercy JA, Banton J. The epidemiologic basis for the prevention of firearm injuries. *Annu Rev Public Health.* 1991;12:17-40.

Abuse of Pregnant Women and Adverse Birth Outcome

Current Knowledge and Implications for Practice

ABUSE of pregnant women is not rare. The prevalence of physical assault of women during pregnancy has been estimated at 8% in a random sample drawn from public and private prenatal clinics,[1] and between 7% and 11% in nonrandom samples drawn from university obstetric clinic services.[2,3] Rates of overall violence against pregnant women gathered by the Second National Family Violence Survey[4] were as follows: 154 acts of violence per 1000 during the first 4 months of pregnancy and 170 acts of violence per 1000 women during the fifth through ninth months. (Pregnant women's risk of what was characterized as "abusive violence" was 60.6% greater than that of nonpregnant women in this national probability sample of 6002 households, but this was interpreted as an artifact of age because women under 25 years of age were more likely both to be pregnant and to be abused by husbands and partners.)

Nevertheless, the assault of women during pregnancy occurs with sufficient frequency to pose a significant concern for the possible threat to the health of the pregnant woman and her developing fetus.

Current Knowledge

There has been little study of or focused clinical effort on the risks to mother and fetus associated with physical or sexual abuse during pregnancy. Only a single, small study has addressed the issue of adverse birth outcome in association with abuse of pregnant women. The results of that study suggest an increased risk of low birth weight in women abused during pregnancy.[5]

An Institute of Medicine committee[6] examined the causes of low birth weight and pointed to the need for more systematic and rigorous examination of the risk of low birth weight. The report did not mention maternal injury, either intentional or unintentional, but did include a discussion of psychological factors that impinge on pregnant women.

Methodologic Problems.—The few clinical studies on abuse of pregnant women contain numerous methodologic problems that limit the extent to which these studies can inform clinical practice and guide future research. These methodologic problems include (1) small selected samples[7]; (2) limited descriptions of the timing, severity, locus, and treatment given for injuries[1,8]; (3) absence of corroboration with specific neonatal findings[5]; (4) confounded inferences of cause and effect with spurious variables[5]; (5) inability to generalize results of the findings to specific populations because of selected samples and study designs that do not use stratification on major social and demographic variables[1,9]; (6) possible recall biases both with regard to violence and to other risk exposures in pregnancy[1,7,8]; (7) poor validity and reliability due to underdeveloped study instruments[1,5,7,8,10,11]; and (8) statistical methods with little power to exclude type I and type II errors and to examine hypothesized effects of mediating variables.[1,7,8]

These methodologic difficulties result, implicitly, from the nature of the issue of family violence and the challenges it poses to investigators. Family violence is inherently multifactorial in nature. Practice and instrumentation in this area are far from standardized. Many risks and obstacles prevent accurate measurement of exposure and outcome. Rigorous study design involving large samples is needed but funding in this area has been limited.

Postulated Etiology.—While the association between abuse and adverse pregnancy outcome has not been extensively studied, several causal mechanisms can be postulated. The postulated relationship between victimization of battered pregnant women and their children's low birth weight can be understood as direct or indirect.

The direct causal pathway between physical and sexual victimization of a pregnant woman and adverse birth outcome could operate through a variety of biologic mechanisms. A physical or sexual assault involving abdominal trauma can cause abruptio placentae, which, depending on the gestational age of the fetus, could lead to fetal loss or early onset of labor and the delivery of a live, low-birth-weight or preterm infant.[12] Other consequences of abdominal trauma during pregnancy may include fetal fractures, rupture of the mother's uterus, liver, or spleen, pelvic fractures, and antepartum hemorrhage.[13] Additionally, trauma may cause uterine contractions, premature rupture of membranes, and infection leading to early onset of labor and possible fetal loss.[12] Finally, the victimization of a woman may lead to the exacerbation of chronic illnesses such as hypertension, diabetes, or asthma, which may have deleterious effects on the fetus.

An indirect causal pathway can be derived by considering the meaning of the victimization experience for a woman as realized in our and other research and clinical experiences. These experiences focus on the relationship between a woman and her victimizer, in which the victimizer uses a variety of strategies and methods to coerce and to exert control over the woman in the relationship. Victimization in this perspective

This article is one of a number of articles on violence that will appear in upcoming issues of THE JOURNAL. The reader is referred to the June 10, 1992, issue, which will be dedicated to studies of violence.

From the Department of Medicine, Children's Hospital, and the Department of Pediatrics, Harvard Medical School, Boston, Mass (Drs Newberger, Barkan, and McCormick and Mss Gary and Schechter); the Department of Obstetrics and Gynecology, Harvard Medical School, and the Department of Maternal and Child Health, Harvard School of Public Health, Boston, Mass (Dr Lieberman); and the Department of Sociology, Wheaton College, Norton, Mass (Dr Yllo).

Reprint requests to Children's Hospital, 300 Longwood Ave, Boston, MA 02115 (Dr Newberger).

may be defined in terms of particular assaultive acts,[14] by control techniques that include verbal intimidation, emotional abuse, and challenges to the woman's competency as a person, including, for example, her capacity to care for her children.[15]

Therefore, physical or sexual victimization might also lead to one or more of the following intermediate risks: (1) elevated physical and psychological stress; (2) isolation and inadequate access to prenatal care and other health care services; (3) behavioral risks such as cigarette smoking, alcohol use, and illegal drug use in reaction to the psychological distress of victimization; and (4) inadequate maternal nutrition as a consequence of financial privation or denial of nutrients as part of the victimization pattern.

The literature associating these indirect risks with diminished fetal growth and with the early onset of labor culminating in the delivery of a low-birth-weight and/or preterm infant is fairly extensive.

Although in general the literature linking stress and anxiety to obstetric outcome has been equivocal, there is a sound basis for the notion that maternal emotional distress may be linked to poor reproductive outcome. Animal research has demonstrated that exposing animals to stressors during gestation is associated with low birth weight, smaller litter size, and decreased neonatal survival.[16]

Maternal psychological stress has been associated with depression in both pregnant and nonpregnant women.[17,18] Stress and/or depression may have direct or indirect effects on the fetus. Direct effects have been hypothesized to involve the release of catecholamines resulting in precipitation of preterm delivery or placental hypoperfusion resulting in delayed fetal growth.[19] Stressful events and depression have been linked to pregnancy and birth complications.[20] Emotional distress may also increase the frequency of behavioral risks associated with neonatal or obstetric problems such as cigarette smoking, alcohol consumption, and decreased utilization of prenatal care.[16,19] A recent study confirmed the association between maternal depression and psychological stress, and between maternal depression and substance use and low weight gain during pregnancy.[17] Another study postulated that the relationship between maternal psychological stress and low birth weight may result from the effect of psychological stress on maternal weight gain.[21]

Current data suggest that the negative effects of maternal psychological stress and depression on neonatal outcome are ameliorated by social support.[22] Studies of work-related stress, both physical and psychological, suggest a link to low birth weight[23,24] and preterm delivery.[23-27]

Well-substantiated evidence links maternal alcohol consumption with miscarriage[28,29] and low birth weight.[30-32] The impact of marijuana use on decreased fetal growth has been suggested,[33-35] and the impact of cocaine use has been more convincingly documented.[33,36]

In the United States, maternal cigarette smoking is one of the most important risk factors for fetal growth retardation.[37-39] Smoking has been reported to slow fetal growth, double the risk of low birth weight, and increase the risk of stillbirth.[40,41]

Numerous studies have examined the relationship between adequacy of prenatal care and low birth weight and preterm delivery. These studies fairly consistently show that lack of or inadequate prenatal care is associated with an increased incidence of low birth weight even after controlling for important confounding variables.[42-46]

Impacts on Women.—The impact of abuse on women is extensive and embraces medical and psychological effects that may increase risks during pregnancy. The physical impacts can affect every organ system, and abuse may escalate in frequency and severity, especially during pregnancy.[7] In the absence of studies that systematically compare the risks and the nature of violence against pregnant women with those of other abused women, no clear patterns of vulnerability and trauma have been discerned. Apart from the substantial direct effects on pregnant women's physical safety (ie, abuse of the most vulnerable organ systems such as the central nervous system, integument, reproductive organs, facial organs, and abdominal viscera), such abuse by these women's partners appears to conform to a pattern of coercive control that includes restricting access to preventive and curative health care.[15]

The psychological effects of victimization include shame, fear, diminished self-esteem, self-blaming, and depression (in response to the continued sense of terror and need to mollify and contain the violence of the partner), and a sense of diminished personal instrumentality, because of few available resources to protect herself or to extricate herself from the relationship.[47] (Although this phenomenon has also been characterized as "learned helplessness," we, among other students of woman abuse, note that many women are indeed quite resourceful in protecting themselves and in seeking options, even in the face of continued threats and harmful actions and limited resources as part of the pattern of victimization.[48])

Psychological impacts may also be associated with a reluctance to disclose one's status as a victim to friends or to providers of health, social, and other services. They also appear to be associated with expressing psychosomatic and emotional complaints when seeking medical care, denying victimization when responding to direct questions about abuse, avoiding service contacts that might inflame the rage of their abusers, and exhibiting a vulnerability to use and abuse alcohol and illicit drugs.[3,47,49]

Implications for Practice

The burden of these posited associations for the clinical practice that considers the effect of the abuse of pregnant women on birth outcome is clear: direct and indirect causal relationships must be postulated and attention to multiple causal pathways must be considered. In the absence of a corpus of systematic research on the abuse of pregnant women and its consequences, clinicians should consider a range of possible physical and psychological consequences to a victimized woman and act to address them in a thoughtful and comprehensive fashion.

Interview Approach.—We believe that all women should have the opportunity to expand beyond the confines of the usual medical history to relate their life circumstances before and during the pregnancy and their experiences of victimization. Most women will not volunteer information about abuse experiences unless they are asked specifically about them. This interview effort should also try to gather insights into their relationships with the battering partners, the women's fears, and their perceptions of professional responses to their efforts to seek help and protection in the past, as well as the women's concerns about their pregnancies, deliveries, and the evolving condition of their babies. Interviewing must always be done apart from their male partners.

Sometimes women will deny to professional personnel that they are victimized, even when questions are posed to them directly. Victimized women appear more likely to disclose the circumstances of their victimizations to other women and to personnel who offer protection and who are sympathetic to the plight of battered women and can provide support and access to help.

Although the amount of time women spend in the hospital after delivering is decreasing, especially because of efforts to reduce the costs of hospitalization, aggressive efforts can be made in the obstetric service to identify and to protect battered women. This work has been pioneered by Prof McFarlane and her colleagues at the Texas Women's University School of Nursing, Houston. They have developed, in association with the Metropolitan Houston Chapter of the March of Dimes Birth Defects Foundation, a *Protocol of Care for the Battered Woman.*[50] They suggest the use of a schematic body map to guide interview questions on specific loci of trauma.

Linkages to Battered Women's Services.—Based on our experience at Children's Hospital, Boston, Mass, we propose that all medical and surgical services for women construct linkages to the battered women's service movement. Programs now exist in many communities. Such connection would provide access to protection, crisis intervention, and support for battered women. Ideally, after a disclosure of victimization to a physician, nurse, or social worker, the woman would be seen as quickly as possible by an advocate or the social worker, who would provide her with information about protection, legal rights, and when needed, shelter. In the course of the initial contact, an assessment would be made of the level of violence in the home, the availability of weapons, and the woman's previous experience with court and police interventions. A safety plan would be developed with the woman. There would be collaboration with medical and nursing staff to provide care for the woman and her children, including attending all case conferences and participating in hospital discharge planning. Services provided would include the following: (1) housing advocacy with shelter and emergency housing transfers; (2) court accompaniment; (3) referrals for legal and medical care; and (4) referrals to counseling support groups. The goals of such an effort are to empower women to better protect themselves and their children and to develop networks of support in the community.

Eli H. Newberger, MD
Susan E. Barkan, PhD
Ellice S. Lieberman, MD, DrPH
Marie C. McCormick, MD, ScD
Kersti Yllo, PhD
Lisa T. Gary, MSW
Susan Schechter, MSW

This work was supported in part by a grant from the Noonan Memorial Fund of the Medical Foundation, Boston, Mass, and grant MH18265-08 from the National Institute of Mental Health, Bethesda, Md.

1. Helton A, McFarlane J, Anderson E. Battered and pregnant: a prevalence study. *Am J Public Health.* 1987;77:1337-1339.
2. Hilliard P. Physical abuse in pregnancy. *Obstet Gyncecol.* 1985;66:185-190.
3. Amaro H, Fried L, Cabral H, Zuckerman B. Violence during pregnancy and substance abuse. *Am J Public Health.* 1990;80:575-579.
4. Gelles R. Violence and pregnancy: are pregnant women at greater risk of abuse? *J Marriage Fam.* August 1988:841-847.
5. Bullock L, McFarlane J. The birthweight/battering connection. *Am J Nurs.* 1989; 1153-1155.
6. Institute of Medicine. *Preventing Low Birthweight.* Washington, DC: National Academy Press; 1985:72.
7. Gelles R. Violence and pregnancy: a note on the extent of the problem and needed services. *Fam Coordinator.* 1975;24:81-86.
8. Helton A, Snodgrass F. Battering during pregnancy: intervention services. *Birth.* 1987;14:142-147.
9. Hawkins D. Devalued racial stereotypes: ideological barriers to the prevention of family violence among blacks. In: Hampton R, ed. *Violence in the Black Family: Correlates and Consequences.* Lexington, Mass: Lexington Books; 1987.
10. Sorenson S, Stein J, Seigal J, Golding J, Burnam A. The prevalence of adult sexual assault. *Am J Epidemiol.* 1987;126:1154-1163.
11. Russell DEH. The prevalence of wife rape. In: Russell D, ed. *Rape and Marriage.* New York, NY: Collier Books; 1982:57-72.
12. Pearlman MD, Tintinalli JE, Lorenz RP. Blunt trauma during pregnancy. *N Engl J Med.* 1990;323:1609-1613.
13. Sammons MN. Battered and pregnant. *Am J Maternal Child Nurs.* 1981;6:246-250.
14. Gary LT. Feminist practice and family violence. In: Bricker-Jenkins M, Hooyman NR, Gottlieb N, eds. *Feminist Social Work Practice in Clinical Settings.* Newbury Park, Calif: Sage Publications; 1991:19-32.
15. McKibben L, De Vos E, Newberger E. Victimization of mothers of abused children: a controlled study. *Pediatrics.* 1989;84:531-535.
16. Istvan J. Stress, anxiety, and birth outcomes: a critical review of the evidence. *Psychol Bull.* 1986;100:331-348.
17. Zuckerman B, Amaro H, Bauchner H, Cabral H. Depressive symptoms during pregnancy: relationship to poor health behaviors. *Am J Obstet Gynecol.* 1989;160: 1107-1111.
18. Brown GW, Harris TO. *Social Origins of Depression.* New York, NY: Free Press; 1978.
19. McAnarney ER, Stevens-Simon C. Maternal psychological stress/depression and low birth weight: is there a relationship? *AJDC.* 1990;144:789-792.
20. Norbeck JS, Tilden VP. Life stress, social support, and emotional disequilibrium in complications of pregnancy: a prospective, multivariate study. *J Health Soc Behav.* 1983;24:30-46.
21. Picone TA, Allen LH, Schramm MM, Olsen PN. Pregnancy outcome in North American women, I: effects of diet, cigarette smoking, and psychological stress on maternal weight gain. *Am J Clin Nutr.* 1989;6:1205-1213.
22. Boyce WT, Schaefer C, Vitti C. Permanence and change: psychological factors on the outcome of adolescent pregnancy. *Soc Sci Med.* 1985;11:1279-1287.
23. Homer CJ, James SA, Siegal E. Work-related psychological stress and risk of preterm, low birthweight delivery. *Am J Public Health.* 1990;80:173-177.
24. Homer CJ, Beresford SA, James SA, Siegal E, Wilcox S. Work related physical exertion and risk of preterm, low birthweight delivery. *Paediatr Perinat Epidemiol.* 1990;4:161-174.
25. Mammelle N, Laumon B, Lazar P. Prematurity and occupational activity during pregnancy. *Am J Epidemiol.* 1984;119:309-322.
26. Zuckerman BS, Frank D, Hingson R, et al. Impact of maternal work outside the home during pregnancy on neonatal outcome. *Pediatrics.* 1986;77:459-464.
27. Teitelman AM, Welch LS, Hellenbrand KG, Bracken MB. Effect of maternal work activity on preterm birth and low birth weight. *Am J Epidemiol.* 1990;131:104-114.
28. Harlap S, Shiono P. Alcohol, smoking, and incidence of spontaneous abortions in the first and second trimester. *Lancet.* 1980;2:173-176.
29. Kline J, Shrout P, Stein Z, Susser M, Warburton D. Drinking during pregnancy and spontaneous abortion. *Lancet.* 1980;2:176-180.
30. Ouellette EM, Rosett HL, Rosman NP, Weiner L. Adverse effects on offspring of maternal alcohol abuse during pregnancy. *N Engl J Med.* 1977;297:528-530.
31. Mills JL, Graubard BI, Harley EE, Rhoads GG, Berendes HW. Maternal alcohol consumption and birth weight: how much drinking during pregnancy is safe? *JAMA.* 1984;252:1875-1879.
32. Little RE. Moderate alcohol use during pregnancy and decreased infant birth weight. *Am J Public Health.* 1977;67:1154-1156.
33. Zuckerman B, Frank DA, Hingson R, et al. Effects of maternal marijuana and cocaine use on fetal growth. *N Engl J Med.* 1989;320:762-768.
34. Hatch EE, Bracken MB. Effect of marijuana use in pregnancy on fetal growth. *Am J Epidemiol.* 1986;124:986-993.
35. Linn S, Schoenbaum SC, Monson RR, Rosner R, Stubblefield PC, Ryan KJ. The association of marijuana use with outcome of pregnancy. *Am J Public Health.* 1983; 73:1161-1164.
36. Chasnoff IJ, Burns WJ, Schnoll SH, Burns KA. Cocaine use in pregnancy. *N Engl J Med.* 1985;313:666-669.
37. Simpson WJ. A preliminary report of cigarette smoking and the incidence of prematurity. *Am J Obstet Gynecol.* 1957;73:808-815.
38. Butler NR, Goldstein H, Ross EM. Cigarette smoking in pregnancy: its influence on birth weight and prenatal mortality. *BMJ.* 1972;2:127-130.
39. Abel EL. Smoking during pregnancy: a review of effects on growth and development of offspring. *Hum Biol.* 1980;52:593-625.
40. Public Health Service. *Healthy People: The Surgeon General's Report on Health Promotion and Disease Prevention.* Washington, DC: Public Health Service; 1979: 24-25. US Dept of Health, Education, and Welfare publication PHS 79-55071.
41. Stein Z, Kline J. Smoking, alcohol and reproduction. *Am J Public Health.* 1983; 73:1154-1156.
42. Gortmaker SL. The effects of prenatal care upon the health of the newborn. *Am J Public Health.* 1979;69:653-660.
43. Eisner V, Brazie JV, Pratt MW, Hexter AC. The risk of low birthweight. *Am J Public Health.* 1979;69:887-893.
44. Elster AB. The effect of maternal age, parity and prenatal care in perinatal outcome in adolescent mothers. *Am J Obstet Gynecol.* 1984;149:845-847.
45. Showstack JA, Budetti PP, Minkler D. Factors associated with birthweight: an exploration of the roles of prenatal care and length of gestation. *Am J Public Health.* 1984;74:1003-1008.
46. Donaldson DJ, Billy JOG. The impact of prenatal care on birthweight: evidence from an international data set. *Med Care.* 1984;22:177-188.
47. Walker L. *The Battered Woman Syndrome.* New York, NY: Springer Publishing Co Inc; 1984.
48. Gondolf E, Fisher E. *Battered Women as Survivors: An Alternative to Treating Learned Helplessness.* Lexington, Mass: Lexington Books; 1988.
49. Goldberg W, Tomlanovich M. Domestic violence in the emergency department new findings. *JAMA.* 1984;251:3259-3264.
50. Helton A, Anderson E, McFarlane J. *Protocol of Care for the Battered Woman.* Houston, Tex: Metropolitan Houston Chapter of the March of Dimes Birth Defects Foundation; 1986.

Violence in America: A Public Health Emergency

Time to Bite the Bullet Back

Violence, according to one dictionary, is defined as "(1) exertion of any physical force so as to injure or abuse, (2) injury by or as if by distortion, infringement, or profanation, (3) intense, turbulent and often destructive action, or force." In his book *Powershift* Alvin Toffler identifies violence or the threat of violence as one of the three fundamental sources of all human power, the other two being money and knowledge. Toffler convincingly argues that these power sources influence every person and all groups including government. Of the three, violence is the lowest form of power because it can only be used to punish. Knowledge and money are far more versatile and can be used in an infinite variety of positive as well as negative or manipulative ways.[1] The violence referred to in this issue of *JAMA* is the interpersonal kind rather than such types as war or that produced by forces of nature.

Response to *JAMA*'s Call for Papers

The response to a call for papers on any aspects of interpersonal violence, made last August on behalf of the editors of *JAMA* and all nine AMA specialty journals, was extraordinary.[2] *JAMA* alone received 131 topical papers for peer review and consideration. Of these, 12 appear in this issue; one relevant paper has been published in each *JAMA* since May 5, and another cluster of papers emphasizing domestic violence will appear in the June 17 issue. The specialty journals also received a great many manuscripts and published from one to 12 articles each in their June issues, in total 59. This outpouring of manuscripts not only confirms what we all know—that violence in the United States is a major issue—it underscores that violence is also a medical/public health issue, which is keenly felt by innumerable physicians and subject to medical/epidemiologic research.

The 1985 Surgeon General's Conference

One of us (C.E.K.) convened the Surgeon General's Workshop on Violence and Public Health at Leesburg, Va, in October 1985. The recommendations of the 150 assembled experts were reported by the Surgeon General to the Senate Committee on Children, Families, Drugs and Alcoholism.[3] Regional, state, and local workshops followed to create a new awareness of the possibilities for understanding and dealing with violence provided by multidisciplinary approaches. Pediatricians, psychiatrists, and other physicians, along with administrators and the public, were challenged to consider violence as a public health issue and to seek out its root causes and best treatments.

Seven years later, violence in our country has not diminished; instead, violence makes constant headlines. In fact, the incidence of violence has increased, especially among some groups.

- One million US inhabitants die prematurely each year as the result of intentional homicide or suicide.
- From 1960 to 1980 the population of the United States increased by 26%; the homicide rate due to guns increased 160%.
- The leading cause of death in both black and white teenage boys in America is gunshot wounds.
- The number of deaths due to firearms is seven times greater in the United States than in the United Kingdom.
- The death rate from trauma in France is 66% that of the US rate, and the rate in the Netherlands is only 39%.
- Armed assaults in California schools are on a sharp increase.
- One third of students in 31 Illinois high schools have brought some weapons to school for self-defense.
- Suicide is the third leading cause of death among children and adolescents in the United States, a rate that has doubled in the last 30 years, the increase almost solely due to firearms.
- Of the fatalities in the 1992 Los Angeles, Calif, riots, the vast majority occurred as a result of gunshot wounds.

New Research in Firearm Fatalities/Deaths by Gunshot Wounds

- In this issue of *JAMA*, Fingerhut and colleagues[4,5] document extraordinarily high firearm fatality rates in many core metropolitan counties, with rates for black male and female teenagers increasing sharply in recent years to reach alarming levels.

From the National Safe Kids Campaign, Washington, DC (Dr Koop), and the Scientific Publications Group, American Medical Association, Chicago, Ill (Dr Lundberg).

Reprint requests to Scientific Publications Group, American Medical Association, 515 N State St, Chicago, IL 60610 (Dr Lundberg).

• Saltzman et al[6] demonstrate that firearm-associated family and intimate assaults in Atlanta, Ga, are 12 times more likely to result in death than nonfirearm assaults.

• Weil and Hemenway[7] document in a national sample that large numbers of handgun owners keep their guns loaded in their homes and that many loaded weapons are not locked up, even if children are in the household. This dangerous behavior seemed not to be altered with training.

• Callahan and Rivara[8] show that one third of Seattle, Wash, high school students report easy access to handguns, 6% own a handgun and 6% of males have carried a handgun to school.

These research findings, together with other articles in these issues, and an array of related data paint a grotesque picture of a society steeped in violence, especially by firearms, and so numbed by the ubiquity and prevalence of violence as to seemingly accept it as inevitable. We do not agree. No society, including ours, need be permeated by firearm homicide. This is unacceptable. Prior solutions have not succeeded. New approaches are required. Two such are included in adjacent commentaries.[9,10]

What Now?

Regarding violence in our society as purely a sociologic matter, or one of law enforcement, has led to unmitigated failure. It is time to test further whether violence can be amenable to medical/public health interventions.

We believe violence in America to be a public health emergency, largely unresponsive to methods thus far used in its control. The solutions are very complex, but possible. We urge all persons in authority to take the following actions:

1. Support additional major research on the causes, prevention, and cures of violence.
2. Stimulate the education of all Americans about what is now known and what can now be done to address this emergency.
3. Demand legislation intended to reverse the upward trend of firearm injuries and deaths, the end result that is most out of control.

Proposed New Legislation

Automobiles, intended to be a means of transportation, when used inappropriately frequently become lethal weapons and kill human beings. Firearms are intended to be lethal weapons. When used inappropriately in peace time, they, too, frequently kill human beings.

In the state of Texas in 1990, deaths from firearms, for the first time in many decades, surpassed deaths from motor vehicles, 3443 to 3309, respectively, as the leading cause of injury mortality.[11] In the 1970s and 1980s, defining motor vehicle casualties as a public health issue and initiating intervention activity succeeded in reversing the upward trend of such fatalities, without banning or confiscating automobiles. We believe that comparable results can be anticipated by similarly treating gunshot wound casualties. But the decline in fatalities will not occur overnight and will require a major coordinated effort.

The right to own or operate a motor vehicle carries with it certain responsibilities. Among them are that the operator meet certain criteria:

• be a certain age and physical/mental condition;
• be identifiable as owner or operator;
• be able to demonstrate knowledge and skill in operating the motor vehicle safely;
• be subject to performance monitoring; and
• be willing to forfeit the right to operate or own a vehicle if these responsibilities are abrogated.

We propose that the right to own or operate a firearm carries with it the same prior conditions, namely, that the owner and operator of a firearm also meet specific criteria:

• be of a certain age and physical/mental condition;
• be required to demonstrate knowledge and skill in proper use of that firearm;
• be monitored in the firearm's use; and
• forfeit the right to own or operate the firearm if these conditions are abrogated.

These restrictions should apply uniformly to all firearms and to all US inhabitants across all states through a system of gun registration and licensing for gun owners and users. No grandfather clauses should be allowed.

Anticipated Resistance and Support

We recognize the enormous amount of change and expense necessary to effect any major proposal such as this having to do with guns. But we believe that anything short of this proposed registration and licensing for gun ownership and use would be too little action to recommend at this time. We also believe that there is great public sentiment in support of this proposal.

A vast lobby of special interests supports the utterly unfettered ownership and use of firearms. It is certain vigorously to oppose this proposal at any cost. One of us (G.D.L.) has met with representatives of the National Rifle Association in Washington, DC, to discuss ways to counter the acknowledged epidemic of firearm homicides. We invite that organization and any other dissenting persons and groups, to make their own rational proposals for countering this acute public health emergency of injuries and homicides, especially those occurring in young black men and women. We can wait no longer to act.

C. Everett Koop, MD
George D. Lundberg, MD

1. Toffler A. *Powershift.* New York, NY: Bantam Books Inc; 1990:2,17,38,467-469.
2. Lundberg GD, Koop CE. The AMA scientific journals—theme issues on violence: call for papers. *JAMA.* 1991;266:1126.
3. Surgeon General. *Surgeon General's Workshop on Violence and Public Health, Leesburg, Va, October 27-29, 1985.* Rockville, Md: Office of Maternal and Child Health, Bureau of Maternal and Child Health and Resources Development, Health Resources and Services Administration, US Public Health Service, US Dept of Health and Human Services; 1986. Report to the Senate Committee on Children, Families, Drugs and Alcoholism.
4. Fingerhut LA, Ingram DD, Feldman JJ. Firearm and nonfirearm homicide among persons 15 to 19 years of age: differences by level of urbanization, United States, 1979 to 1989. *JAMA.* 1992;267:3048-3053.
5. Fingerhut LA, Ingram DD, Feldman JJ. Firearm homicide among black teenage males in metropolitan counties, 1983 through 1985 to 1987 through 1989. *JAMA.* 1992;267:3054-3058.
6. Saltzman LE, Mercy JA, O'Carroll PW, Rosenberg ML, Rhodes PH. Weapon involvement and injury outcomes in family and intimate assaults. *JAMA.* 1992;267:3043-3047.
7. Weil DS, Hemenway D. Loaded guns in the home: an analysis of a national random survey of gun owners. *JAMA.* 1992;267:3033-3037.
8. Callahan CM, Rivara FP. Urban high school youth and handguns: a school-based survey. *JAMA.* 1992;267:3038-3042.
9. Rosenberg ML, O'Carroll PW, Powell KE. Let's be clear: violence is a public health problem. *JAMA.* 1992;267:3071-3072.
10. Teret SP, Wintemute GJ, Beilenson P. The Firearm Fatality Reporting System: a proposal. *JAMA.* 1992;267:3073-3074.
11. Zane DF, Preece MJ, Patterson PJ, Svenkerud EK. Firearm-related mortality in Texas (1985-1990). *Tex Med.* 1991;87:63-65.

Violence, Values, and Gender

"I want to do a study of battered women."
"Fine. There are data from the rape crisis team in the ED that need to be pulled together."
"No, not rape. I want to study battered women."
"What's a battered woman?"

Dialogue between medical student and adviser
New Haven, Conn, 1975

Violence epidemiology is still in its infancy. In our offices, clinics, and emergency departments we all see injury and its consequences, perhaps daily.

And yet, like a clinical Heisenberg's uncertainty principle, the more closely we focus on injuries, the less we seem to understand the violent relationships that culminate in these injuries. When we begin to make the connection between our patients' health problems and violence, we experience the same sort of epiphany that came with child abuse in the 1960s.

I was shocked into recognizing the complex interplay of poor health, injury, and violence during residency when I was called to the emergency department to admit a 35-year-old woman for yet another bout of acute pancreatitis. She was nearly blind, with wide scars over her left breast and shoulder, and multiple scars over her abdomen and flanks. Her several-volume medical record documented bilateral retinal detachments, burns over her torso from hot grease, a fractured jaw, multiple stab wounds to the abdomen, and a gunshot wound that required a partial hepatic resection. In the discharge summary for each hospitalization, house officers through the years had carefully noted "the patient is a 22-year-old . . . 25-year-old . . . 27-year-old . . . 31-year-old woman with a long and complicated history of trauma secondary to alcohol abuse."

The recurrent assaults were characterized as episodic injuries; alcoholism, not her violent relationship, became the prism through which we viewed this patient's life. In fact, of course, violence is more than the sum total of injuries, and optimal clinical intervention must address the social context in which violence occurs, not simply the pattern or severity of the resultant injuries.

Child abuse intervention programs initiated in the mid-1960s were the first to characterize violence within the context of ongoing social and familial relationships. Since then, we have extended the model to encompass protective services for abused elderly and handicapped individuals who are victims of abuse. With domestic violence—a major focus in this issue of THE JOURNAL—it is not age but gender that characterizes the experience of abuse.

When we[1] reported our findings that domestic violence was a leading cause of women's injuries, the initial response from the medical profession was to focus on emergency care. Yet a history of battering has proven important as a backdrop to many vexing issues in women's health care: alcoholism, suicide attempts, drug use and abuse, depression, and child abuse. It is now evident that ambulatory and primary care facilities, mental health and substance abuse programs must provide services to address the sequelae of abuse and the medical problems that arise from women's isolation in violent relationships.

From the Division of General Medicine, University of Connecticut Health Center, Farmington, Conn.
Reprint requests to Outpatient Services, University of Connecticut Health Center, 80 Coventry St, Farmington, CT 06112 (Dr Flitcraft).

Through the Prism of Gender: The Adult Trauma History

The report from the American Medical Association (AMA) Council on Scientific Affairs[2] reviews the epidemiology and clinical dimensions of rape, physical and sexual assaults in marital, cohabiting, and dating relationships, and the long-term effects of child sexual abuse—unveiling women's vulnerability to violence across the life span. The common denominator for women of all ages is that social partners—not strangers—pose the greatest threat of violence. In other words, the predominance of assaults on women occurs within ongoing familial, social, and domestic relationships. As a result, female victims of abuse present a distinct "adult trauma history" typified by recurrent injuries generally accompanied by sexual assault, threats, and verbal abuse.

The inescapable significance of women's vulnerability to violence is revealed in the article by Marzuk et al[3] on the epidemiology of murder-suicide. Their intent was to unify and classify data on homicide-suicide episodes, a unique class of violence. But they discovered that the most common type, representing fully one half to three fourths of all murder-suicides in the United States, typically involved a male between the ages of 18 and 60 years who physically abused his girlfriend or wife, feared her infidelity or estrangement, murdered her, and committed suicide, usually by a firearm. The importance of this work perhaps lies less in its typology of murder-suicide, than in its identification of possible predictors of lethal domestic violence and emphasis on the role of firearms in homicide and suicide.[4]

The Challenge in Clinical Practice

McFarlane and coworkers[5] demystify the problem of identifying women involved in abusive relationships. They highlight the importance of routine assessment for abuse in nonemergent settings, particularly prenatal care. Using three straightforward questions in a safe, confidential, and interpersonal encounter, they found that 17% of pregnant women in their public health clinic population were abused, 60% of whom reported recurrent episodes of violence within the index pregnancy. Abused women were twice as likely not to begin prenatal care until the third trimester, suggesting that domestic violence may limit women's utilization of early prenatal care.

These authors use a scale that gave a "severity of physical abuse" score according to the severity of the resultant injury. For instance, "threats of abuse, including use of a weapon" are ranked as the least violent of abusive acts. Consequently, black women appeared to experience fewer episodes of violence compared with their Hispanic and white counterparts. Homicide data suggest that this is not the case.[6] Is it intuitively obvious that the severity of abuse parallels the severity of injuries? Consider for a moment the woman who, when asked whether the violence is escalating, responds, "Yes, I mean no. No, I guess it's better. He doesn't hit me anymore, but he sleeps with a gun under his pillow." An alternative interpretation may be that severity of abuse differs little across ethnic groups and that threats with and access to a weapon should be ranked in a category with a high probability of significant injury, predictive of severe abuse. Thus, outright violence and coercive control, introduced by Jones and Schechter,[7] undermine a woman's capacity to design and implement proactive safety plans.

The report from the AMA Council on Ethical and Judicial Affairs[8] highlights beneficence and nonmaleficence as the principles to guide physicians' intervention in domestic violence. Importantly, our responsibilities extend to "participation in efforts to secure a safe place, including offering hospitalization if necessary for patients when there are no available shelters." But having emphasized safety, the report's distinction between child abuse and woman abuse becomes crucial. In the case of woman abuse, protective services (the basis of child abuse intervention) are replaced by informative and interpretive encounters that facilitate patient empowerment and autonomy.[9]

Consequently, "[s]pouses, partners, or other third parties, including the police, should not be notified of an abuse diagnosis without the expressed consent of the patient." Nor, I would add, should we contact these parties to confirm or substantiate a patient's report of abuse. Again, in contrast to policy in cases of suspected child abuse, "It is not evident, however, that mandatory reporting of domestic violence [by physicians] would contribute to the safety of battered women or would facilitate their access to appropriate resources." When we are addressing the abuse of competent adults, "[o]verriding a patient's refusal violates the ethical principle of respect for patient autonomy." The tenets of beneficence, nonmaleficence, confidentiality, and patient's autonomy provide a strong foundation for the development of an appropriate and empowering medical response to domestic violence. When women who have been abused are given the power to act, they are able to regain control of their lives and are more likely to make the decisions necessary to ensure a safe future.

As physicians organize to address domestic violence, we join forces with others who have been dedicated to eliminating this problem, forging relationships across institutional and disciplinary lines. The interagency child death review team described by Durfee et al[10] exemplifies a kind of institutional morbidity and mortality conference that can identify problems, gather data, and generate more effective intervention strategies. Adaptation of this model to review incidents of both fatal and nonfatal domestic assaults may facilitate cooperation between health care organizations, community-based services for battered women, and the complex array of legal, law enforcement, and social services vital to violence intervention and prevention efforts.

Personal and Professional Values

In medical practice, knowledge, skills, and attitudes are recognized as the necessary elements of clinical expertise. However, attitudes can be at odds with practice skills and knowledge. As discussed by Orentlicher,[11] corporal punishment remains legal in most states' public schools despite strong positions against it by the AMA, the American Academy of Pediatrics, the American Psychiatric Association, and American Public Health Association. Results from the study by McCormick[12] demonstrate the considerable confusion among physicians on the advisability of corporal punishment in the home. Widely differing definitions of corporal punishment prevent meaningful comparison of these two articles, but policymakers, physicians, and parents share the frustration that knowledge transforms behavior only when appropriate skills and values converge in the right political climate. Deep ambiguities persist on the societal and community levels regarding the difference between caretakers' legitimate authority and abusive behavior.

Fortunately, there is no longer legal ambiguity with respect to the use of force in intimate relationships between adults. State laws have established partner or spouse abuse as a criminal act. Legislative actions vary by state, but include mandated arrest when police are called to intervene in domestic violence cases. Policies developed in recent years urge judges to grant battered women child custody, mandate court-assigned treatment programs for batterers, and provide for more than a thousand community-based shelter and advocacy programs for victims of family violence. We have witnessed a profound change in the public response to domestic violence over the past 15 years.

Nevertheless, informal social norms and stereotypic gender roles still legitimate control of one partner over the other and may allow us to rationalize abuse in adult relationships. Sugg and Inui[13] in their survey of primary care physicians' attitudes about domestic violence conclude that "physicians found exploring domestic violence in the clinical setting analogous to 'opening Pandora's box.' " In the face of domestic violence, physicians experience fear and a sense of powerlessness and they perceive a loss of control, all of which parallel the feelings of the abused patient. But the physicians' strategies—denial, rationalization, and minimization—echo the voices of the abuser who neither identifies nor accepts responsibility for his violent behavior.

Interpersonal abuse was not foreign to the physicians interviewed by Sugg and Inui, nor is it foreign to many of us. Fourteen percent of male physicians and 31% of female physicians had been victims of abuse at some point in their lives. Yet only two physicians had been able to address violence with their patients; one of the physicians had sought counseling to cope with his own history of abusive behavior.

As the medical profession participates in violence prevention and intervention efforts, advances in knowledge, skills, and attitudes are bound to follow. This change will prompt a deeper understanding of the abuse of control and authority in our own professional—and personal—lives.

Anne H. Flitcraft, MD

1. Stark E, Flitcraft A, Frazier W. Medicine and patriarchal violence: the social construction of a private event. *Int J Health Serv.* 1979;9:461-493.
2. Council on Scientific Affairs, American Medical Association. Violence against women: relevance for medical practitioners. *JAMA.* 1992;267:3184-3189.
3. Marzuk PM, Tardiff K, Hirsch CS. The epidemiology of murder-suicide. *JAMA.* 1992;267:3179-3183.
4. Kellerman AL, Lee RK, Mercy JA, Banton J. The epidemiological basis for the prevention of firearm injuries. *Annu Rev Public Health.* 1991;12:17-40.
5. McFarlane J, Parker B, Soeken K, Bullock L. Assessing for abuse during pregnancy: severity and frequency of injuries and associated entry into prenatal care. *JAMA.* 1992;267:3176-3178.
6. Mercy JA, Saltzman L. Fatal violence among spouses in the United States, 1976-85. *Am J Public Health.* 1989;79:595-599.
7. Jones A, Schechter S. *When Love Goes Wrong.* New York, NY: Harper Collins Publishers; 1992.
8. Council on Ethical and Judicial Affairs, American Medical Association. Physicians and domestic violence: ethical considerations. *JAMA.* 1992;267:3190-3193.
9. Emanuel EJ, Emanuel LL. Four models of the physician-patient relationship. *JAMA.* 1992;267:2221-2226.
10. Durfee MJ, Gellert GA, Tilton-Durfee D. Origins and clinical relevance of child death review teams. *JAMA.* 1992;267:3172-3175.
11. Orentlicher D. Corporal punishment in the schools. *JAMA.* 1992;267:3205-3208.
12. McCormick KF. Attitudes of primary care physicians toward corporal punishment. *JAMA.* 1992;267:3161-3165.
13. Sugg NK, Inui T. Primary care physicians' response to domestic violence: opening Pandora's box. *JAMA.* 1992;267:3157-3160.

Knife and Gun Clubs of America

My friend Marie is 29 years old. Until she and a friend stopped to talk in a park in Pomona, California, last week, she was perfectly healthy. Palomares Park sits behind a stucco wall just off Arrow Highway, near its intersection with Orange Grove Avenue, less than half a mile from the large regional hospital where I work as a pathologist. If you are brave enough to drive into the park, you'll see the usual jungle gyms and slides and swings, basketball hoops and tennis courts, trees and flowers and nicely manicured grassy expanses. What Marie and her friend had not realized or noticed was the silence. No one was enjoying a family picnic, the swings were still; the enchanting screams and noise of children you expect to hear at a park were eerily absent. At 2:30 in the afternoon, the park was as quiet as a cemetery. Only when it was too late to respond did they understand. People were milling around, but in the shadows of the park.

It was a cool day, I remember, with a nice breeze, and the air was clear enough to see in the distance the snow-capped San Gabriel Mountains, which stand as silent, watchful sentinels over the troubles in this valley. Marie's friend told me later they were parked near the swings, under the full light of the sun, chatting, with the windows rolled down, when a young man in his early 20s lunged from the shadows and pointed a gun at Marie's friend, pressed it against his temple, and demanded his wallet. Of course her friend handed it over. When the gunman reached for Marie's wedding ring, her friend sensed the youth's finger begin to squeeze the trigger. Believing his death was imminent, the friend grabbed for the gun at the moment the bullet fired. It shot off the tip of his finger. Barely slowed in its trajectory, the bullet pierced Marie under her left arm, went through part of her stomach, severed the splenic artery, punctured the left kidney, and exited near her spine. An approaching vehicle scared off the criminal, and Marie's friend heroically drove her to our emergency department, a busy receptacle of violence in this once lovely part of southern California.

Marie works in our lab as a medical technologist. Because she is a friend, I went to the emergency department as soon as I heard what happened. Shootings and knifings happen every day, and the bloody, torn, and ripped bodies come and go through our ER as regularly as patients with any natural affliction, with any usual malady that requires transfusions, sutures, organ removal, or transfer to the undertaker. The stories are usually the same, only the faces change: gang shootings, a bad drug deal, innocent bystanders. The sad and beaten bodies end up either in the intensive care unit or in the morgue, waiting for the coroner to have another opening on the conveyor belt of carnage that is his practice in Los Angeles County.

Marie lost her spleen and has had 6 units of blood; her left kidney is still hemorrhaging, and it may have to be removed. She lies on a bed in the ICU under heavy morphine sedation, hooked up to chest tubes, central lines, IVs, heart monitors, catheters, all the things our technologically advanced society has invented to shield hospitalized patients from the grip of death. All because she expected a pretty little park to be a safe haven, a place to relax for a few minutes with a friend. Her ignorance of today's reality nearly killed her; she expected this park to be like the parks she used to visit as a child two decades ago.

Why should it take something like this, a friend in critical condition, to make me mad about violence? When you read every Monday morning in the *Los Angeles Times* about the 15 murders over the weekend, after a while that expectation becomes incorporated into your world view, as much a fact of life as the Lakers beating the Utah Jazz. You just turn the page and have another sip of coffee and look at your watch. It's negligence, desensitization to the pain in the world. It's like seeing pictures of people starving in Sudan: we lament for a moment, then turn back to our dinner. Or we believe homicides happen only in east Los Angeles; it's somebody else's problem; it can't happen in Beverly Hills or in our own neighborhoods. Perhaps it's an ethnic problem, we say; violence doesn't descend upon the privileged, the politicians, the wealthy. By remaining silent, we are accomplices in shoving our society toward an era of dyscivilization, of an impairment that permits pockets of mankind's primitive past to emerge, to spread like algae on a dead lake.

We have become complacent about violence. It's become just another common ailment we can suture together and make right with the phenomenal and ever-ready technomagic in the hospital. But the unfortunate thing is that we cannot alter our diet to prevent the squeezing of the trigger. We cannot exercise or lose weight and outrun the bullet. Safe sex, clean thoughts, and God will not dull the edge of the blade. Through our equanimity in regarding homicide as just another disease, we have allowed it to share that uneasy pedestal, with cancer and heart disease, as one of America's leading killers. We can no longer look the other way. Must we wait until this epidemic of violence drops a friend, a colleague, or oneself to admit its dark reality?

Laurence J. Purdy, MD
Pomona, Calif

Edited by Roxanne K. Young, Associate Editor.

First Encounter

For almost a year of my life, death meant cadavers. Between gross anatomy, neuroanatomy, and microanatomy, I spent four of five weekday afternoons last year in a cool laboratory full of cadavers. Despite my initial apprehension, I grew more and more comfortable with the bodies until I truly felt that I knew Death: what it looked like, smelled like, felt like against the back of my hand. I *knew* Death.

Death is dead bodies. Their skin is waxy, their organs are a uniform gray, they smell like preservative. Death is dead. But I realize now that in all the time I spent dissecting cadavers, I was distanced from Death. I have since seen Death, and that is not what it looked like.

The night I saw Death started pleasantly enough. I was to join my father in Boston for dinner and a Celtics game. We decided to meet near the Boston Garden and walk to the North End for our dinner. The North End of Boston is the Italian section. Its winding streets lined by three-story brownstones are commonly known as the safest in New England. The area is a throwback to the city neighborhoods of yesteryear where everyone knows everyone else, where people live their whole lives on the same street on which they were born. There is a real sense of community living there and, for an "inner" section of a large city, a conspicuous lack of street violence. We found one of the many quiet family restaurants on Hanover Street and went in.

We had just about finished dinner when a young couple burst through the restaurant door and dove into a corner, the man covering the woman.

"Everybody down on the floor!" screamed the owner. "They're shooting in the streets!" My father slid off his chair and I joined him on the floor. This can't be happening, I thought. This is the North End. There must be some kind of mistake.

Several long minutes passed. Then someone outside started screaming about blood. The owner peeked out the window. My dad, an emergency medical technician, shouted, "Does someone out there need medical help?"

"Oh God yes!" a girl screamed back. "He's covered with blood!"

We stood and cautiously made our way to the door. Inching it open, we stepped out to the sidewalk. As the door closed behind us, I looked up, and I saw Death–alive–for the first time.

It was sitting on the chest of a young man of my age who was 10 feet away, slumped on the passenger seat of a car its door open–at the curb. His head was tilted back as though he were resting. His desperate breathing was raspy. It seemed as if he were trying to speak, but with every effort, blood gushed from his mouth. A man–possibly a police officer–knelt next to him, pressing what looked like a sweatshirt against the young man's throat.

"He's finished," my dad said, shaking his head. "Poor kid."

"But he's alive!" The medical student in me protested. I *knew* he was alive. I knew he was young. And I knew all too well how resilient such a body was. I was the one who had studied it, taken it apart, admired its refined effectiveness. I knew that compression would minimize the bleeding until an ambulance arrived, that a transfusion would replace the lost blood. I knew that we were 20 blocks from one of the best hospitals in the world. There, physicians could easily arrest the probable hypovolemic shock. A few sutures, emergency surgery, surely he would make it. I knew it.

"He's gone," my dad said.

What did he know? I glared at him, then turned back to the young man. His chest heaved beneath the red wetness of his shirt. His stomach muscles contracted, then relaxed. He arched his back, coughed a bloody cough, then all was terribly still. More police arrived. The street began to fill with people while police tried to keep them away from the car. Sirens. Lights. An ambulance arrived, the crowd slowly moved aside, but my eyes never left the body.

"It happens fast," I mumbled.

"Yeah," my dad replied. "It's a fine line."

We turned and walked away, each absorbed in his own thoughts. Finally I stopped and said, "I think I just had my first look at the enemy. The one I'm training to fight the rest of my life."

"Death?" he asked.

"Yeah," I replied, and continued walking.

A few hours later we said our good-byes. Dad headed home, and I drove to school. A light drizzle had begun.

I stopped my car on top of a hill near school, got out, and stood looking out over the city, over the lights, over the buildings, looking over the living and the dead. I swore out loud at Death, and I cursed the violence in my country. I told Death that I knew it was going to win the war in the end but that I didn't care. I would be damned if I was going to let it win all the battles.

Daniel J. McCullough III
Worcester, Mass

At Large

With Dennis L. Breo

JFK's death—the plain truth from the MDs who did the autopsy

There are two and only two physicians who know exactly what happened—and didn't happen—during their autopsy of President John F. Kennedy on the night of November 22, 1963, at the Naval Medical Center in Bethesda, Md. The two, former US Navy pathologists James Joseph Humes, MD, and "J" Thornton Boswell, MD, convened last month in a Florida hotel for two days of extraordinary interviews with *JAMA* editor George D. Lundberg, MD, himself a former military pathologist, and this reporter about the events of that fateful night. It is the only time that Humes and Boswell have publicly discussed their famous case, and it was the result of seven years of efforts by Lundberg to persuade them to do so.

Bullets came from above and behind

The scientific evidence they documented during their autopsy provides irrefutable proof that President Kennedy was struck by only two bullets that came from above and behind from a high-velocity weapon that caused the fatal wounds. This autopsy proof, combined with the bullet and rifle evidence found at the scene of the crime, and the subsequent detailed documentation of a six-month investigation involving the enormous resources of the local, state, and federal law enforcement agencies, proves the 1964 Warren Commission conclusion that Kennedy was killed by a lone assassin, Lee Harvey Oswald.

Humes, who was in charge, calls it "probably the least secret autopsy in the history of the world." It was Humes and Boswell who opened the casket when the President's body was brought by ambulance from Andrews Air Force Base after the flight from Dallas. It was Humes and Boswell who lifted the former President from his casket and placed him on the examining table to begin a four-hour autopsy. (They were joined later at the autopsy table by Army Lt Col Pierre Finck, MC, who participated as an expert consultant; Finck, who now lives in Switzerland, declined to come to Florida for the joint interview.) Humes says he is breaking his 29-year silence "because I am tired of being beaten upon by people who are supremely ignorant of the scientific facts of the President's death."

Coincidentally, on the second day of the interviews, Boswell told the group that a Fort Worth physician, Charles Crenshaw, MD, had appeared on TV that very morning to argue the claim in his recent book, *JFK: Conspiracy of Silence*, that when he allegedly observed the dead President at Dallas' Parkland Hospital, he was positive that the bullets struck Kennedy from the front, not the back, "as the public has been led to believe." Crenshaw, who was a surgical resident in 1963, is not mentioned in the Warren Commission's 888-page summary report and his 203-page, generously spaced paperback was written with the aid of two assassination-conspiracy buffs. Crenshaw's book is only the latest in a long parade of conspiracy theories purporting to tell how Kennedy was really killed, including the 1991 release of Oliver Stone's film, *JFK*. Humes and Boswell had agreed to the *JAMA* interview without the slightest idea that Crenshaw's book had been published.

Now, his face incredulous with disbelief, Humes exploded with his summation. Pointing toward the window, the exasperated pathologist said, "If a bullet or a BB were fired through that window, it would leave a small hole where it entered and a beveled crater where it exited. That is what 'J' and I found when we examined the President's skull. There was a small elliptical entrance wound on the outside of the back of the skull, where the bullet entered, and a beveled larger wound on the inside of the back of the skull where the bullet tore through and exploded out the right side of the head. When we recovered the missing bone fragments and reconstructed this gaping wound where the bullet exited, we found this same pattern—a small wound where the bullet struck the inside of the skull and a beveled larger wound where it exited. This is *always* the pattern of a through-and-through wound of the cranium—the beveling or crater effect appears on the *inside* of the skull at the *entrance* wound and on the *outside* of the skull at the *exit* wound. The crater effect is produced when the bony tissue of the skull turns inside out where the bullet leaves."

'A foolproof finding'

He concludes, "In 1963, we proved at the autopsy table that President Kennedy was struck from above and behind by the fatal shot. The pattern of the entrance and exit wounds in the skull proves it, and if we stayed here until hell freezes over, nothing will change this proof. It happens 100 times out of 100, and I will defend it until I die. This is the essence of our autopsy, and it is supreme ignorance to argue any other scenario. This is a law of physics and it is foolproof—absolutely, unequivocally, and without question. The conspiracy buffs have totally ignored this central scientific fact, and everything else is hogwash. There was no interference with our autopsy, and there was no conspiracy to suppress the findings."

Though the evidence is less well defined, Humes emphasizes that his autopsy found that the other bullet that struck Kennedy, the so-called "magic bullet" that was the first to hit Kennedy and that also hit Texas Gov John Connally, was also fired from above and behind. He says, "There was an 'abrasion collar' where this bullet entered at the base of the President's neck, and this scorching and splitting of the skin from the heat and scraping generated by the entering bullet is proof that it entered from behind. Unfortunately, at the time of the autopsy, the tracheostomy performed on the President at Dallas in an attempt to save his life obliterated the exit wound through the front of his neck near the Adam's apple. Soft-tissue wounds are much more iffy than bone wounds, but there is no doubt from whence cometh those bullets—from rear to front from a high-velocity rifle."

Still, the other scenarios continue to be painted. "Recently," Humes notes, "there were about 300 people at a convention in Dallas, each hawking a different conspiracy theory about how the President was killed. I think this kind of general idiocy is a tragedy—it almost defies belief—but I guess it is the price we pay for living in a free country. I can only question the motives of those who propound these ridiculous theories for a price and who have turned the President's death into a profit-making industry."

Humes and Boswell had a long, long day 29 years ago, and, in many ways, it has never ended. The 6-foot, 4-inch, physically energetic Humes is a commanding presence, and he says, "I was in charge of the autopsy—period. Nobody tried to interfere—make that perfectly clear." The 5-foot, 9-inch, pipe-puffing Boswell is precise and methodical, and he says, "We documented our findings in spades. It's all there in the records. And Jim is not the kind of guy anybody pushes around." Their comments on the record are essential because polls show, in the wake of the film *JFK* and the glut of conspiracy-theorist authors, that many, if not most Americans disbelieve the Warren Commission finding that Oswald, "acting alone and without assistance," killed Kennedy. To set the record straight, they agreed to relive for *JAMA* their actions of Friday, November 22, 1963.

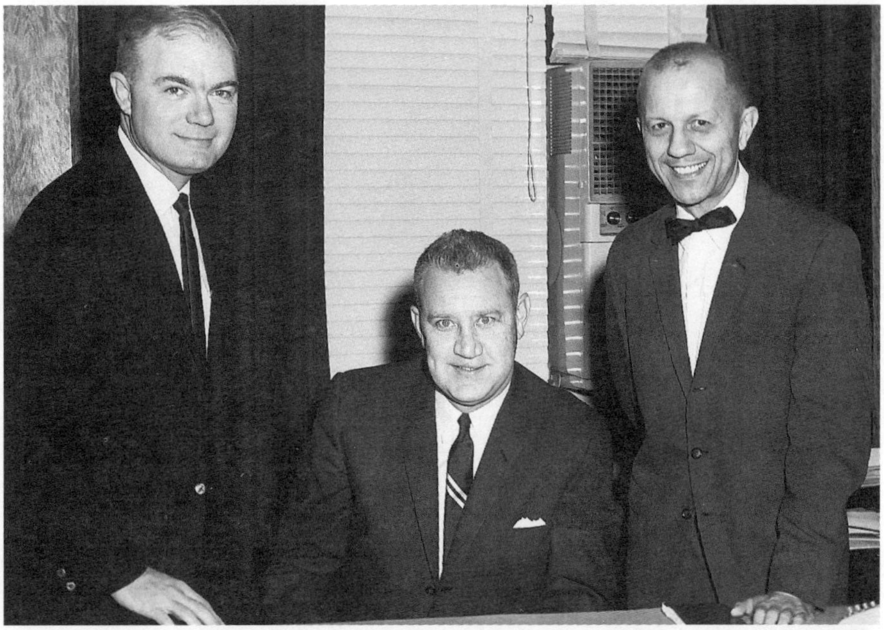

Photo: US Naval Medical School

The three pathologists who performed the autopsy on President John F. Kennedy on the night of November 22, 1963, were photographed days later (top photo, from left): US Navy Cmdr J. Thornton Boswell, MC; US Navy Cmdr James Joseph Humes, MC; and US Army Lt Col Pierre Finck, MC. Breaking their 29-year silence on this famous case, Drs Humes (left in bottom photo) and Boswell were interviewed by *JAMA* last April.

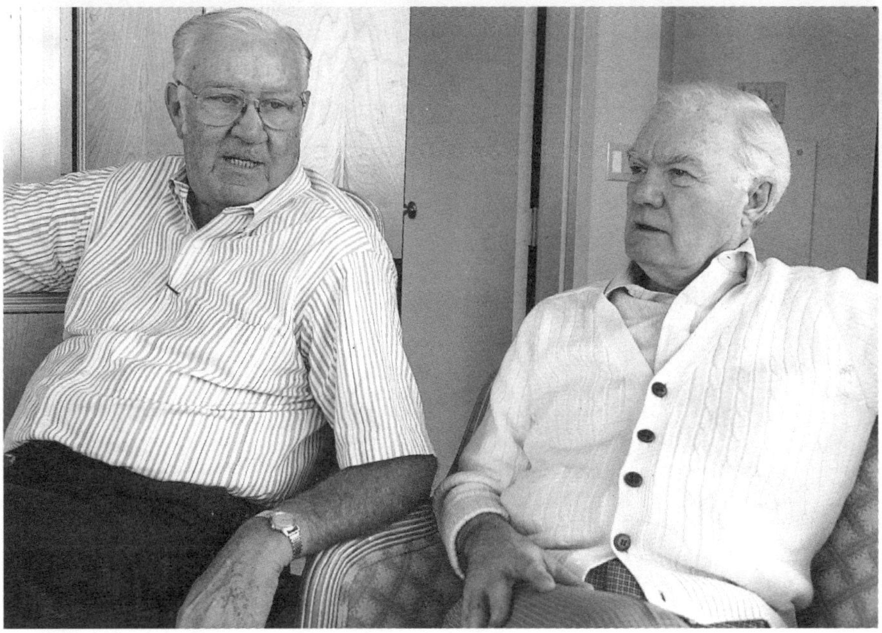

Photo: Dennis L. Breo

...

On the day the President was shot at 12:30 PM, while riding in an open motorcade through the sunny streets of Dallas, it was cold and gray in the Washington, DC, area. Commander Humes, then 39, was the director of labs of the Naval Medical School in Bethesda, Md. Commander Boswell, then 41, was chief of pathology at the naval hospital, which was part of the Bethesda National Naval Medical Center. Humes was Boswell's boss.

Humes had signed on with the US Navy in 1943 to complete his undergraduate work at Villanova University, Villanova, Pa, as part of the Navy's V-12 enlistment program. After earning his medical degree at Jefferson Medical College, Philadelphia, in 1948, he completed his internship and residency in anatomic and clinical pathology at the Bethesda medical center; the US Naval Hospital in Philadelphia; and the Armed Forces Institute of Pathology in Washington, DC. He was certified by the American Board of Pathology in anatomic and clinical pathology in 1955. His postings included military hospitals in the Canal Zone, Hawaii, and San Diego. He was appointed chief of pathology at the Naval Medical School in 1960 and promoted to director of labs for the medical school in 196l. By 1963, he had performed several autopsies on military personnel killed by gunshot wounds and he had also spent seven years at the Bethesda facility, which he "knew like the back of my hand." Boswell, a graduate of the Ohio State University Medical School, received his certification in anatomic pathology in 1957 and clinical pathology in 1959. He, too, had previously autopsied several gunshot wounds, and most of his military experience was at the naval hospital in Bethesda.

Ironically, shortly before President Kennedy was shot and pronounced dead at 1 PM at Dallas' Parkland Hospital, Humes left the medical center to go

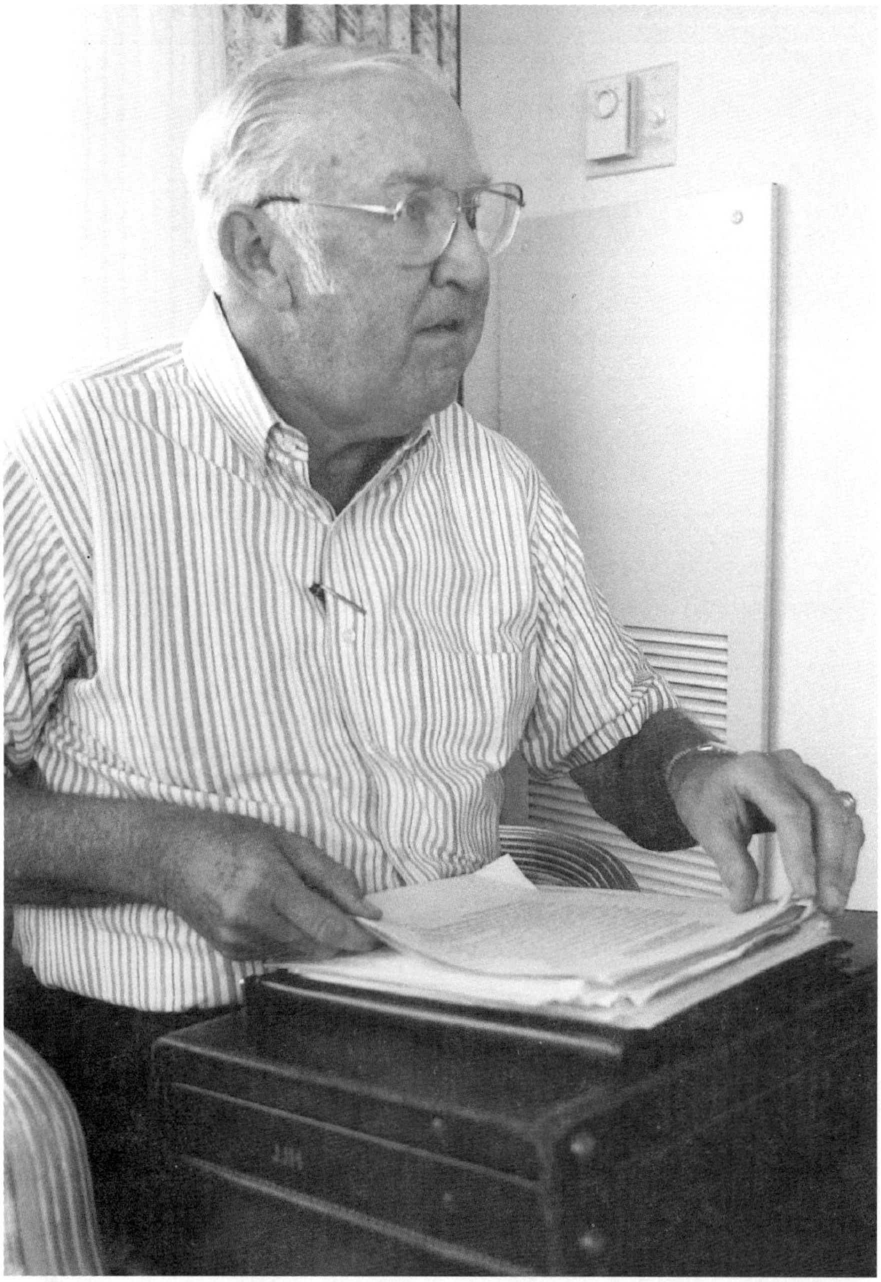
Photo: Dennis L. Breo

Dr Humes: 'This was the least secret autopsy in the world and the cause of death was blatantly obvious. There is no doubt from whence cometh those bullets—from rear to front from a high-velocity rifle.'

home. He had promised to help his wife, Ann, prepare for a dinner party for 24 that evening, almost all of them military personnel. Five of the Humeses' seven children were in school, with the youngest two at home. The radio and TV were off, and the couple did not learn of the tragic news until their older children returned on the school bus. He recalls, "The kids told Ann, 'The President's been shot,' and she was telling them, 'That's a terrible thing to say,' when we turned on the TV and learned for ourselves. My wife and I were both very upset, and we decided that a dinner party on this evening was out of the question." Washington phone circuits were jammed, and while Ann Humes tried to get a line to call her guests to cancel, Commander Humes took his son out for a haircut; his first communion was scheduled for the next morning. When father and son returned, they found that Ann Humes had finally found an open phone line, only to have the operator interrupt with an emergency call from the Surgeon General of the Navy, Admiral Edward Kenney. It was 5:15 PM and Admiral Kenney said, "Jim, you better hurry over to the hospital."

By the time he arrived at the hospital, Humes was "beginning to get the message that the President's body was en route. There was great commotion and a cordon of Marines and military police." Once inside, he was told by Admiral Kenney, the ranking military officer, " 'to be prepared to do an autopsy' on the late President."

'Find the cause of death'

"My orders were to find the cause of death and I was told to get anyone I thought necessary to help do the autopsy, but to limit it to only the help I needed. Hell, I could have called in people from Paris and Rome if I thought it necessary, but as it turned out, I didn't. About this time, I also received a phone call from Dr Bruce Smith, the deputy director of the Armed Forces Institute of Pathology [AFIP], offering me whatever help I might need. Bruce was a friend and I thanked him, saying I would call later if I needed help."

While Humes had been preparing for his dinner party, Boswell had been at the hospital going over autopsy slides with pathology residents. He recalls, "Early in the afternoon, we received a call from Dr Bruce Smith from AFIP, saying, 'The President's body is on its way to Bethesda for an autopsy.' I argued, 'That's stupid. The autopsy should be done at AFIP [which was located five miles away at the Walter Reed Army Medical Center].' After all, the AFIP was the apex of military pathology and, perhaps, world pathology. I was told, 'That's the way it is. Admiral [George] Burkley [the President's personal physician] wants Bethesda.' Apparently, Admiral Burkley had called the AFIP from Air Force One en route from Dallas. Later, I was told that Jackie Kennedy selected Bethesda because her husband had been a Navy man."

Humes was in total charge

By 7:30 PM, Humes was in his scrubs in the hospital's new morgue, built only four months earlier. He had selected Dr Boswell as his assistant. The morgue was at the back of the hospital, and, as Dr Humes stepped *outside* the morgue onto the loading dock, he noticed a crowd milling about and an unknown man carrying a large, old-fashioned "Speed Graphic" camera. Still outside the morgue, the pathologist told the unknown cameraman, "Get out!" Then, Humes asked, "Who's in charge here?"

The answer was only 2 feet away, as a man in full military dress answered, "I am. Who wants to know?" Humes explains, "The man who said he was in charge outside the morgue was some general representing the military section of the District of Columbia. I told him what my assignment was and asked him about the chap with the camera. Well, seconds later, this chap with the camera was sent away."

No generals in the morgue

As the general remained *outside* the morgue, Humes stepped back inside to prepare to receive the President's body. He emphasizes, "Nobody made any decision in the morgue except ME. Nobody distracted or influenced me in any way, shape, or form."

Jackie and Bobby Kennedy and a host of others accompanied the motorcade bringing the President's body from Andrews AFB to the Naval Medical Hospital morgue. While Jackie and Bobby Kennedy and the other VIPs were met at the front of the hospital and escorted to upstairs rooms, the casket was brought to the morgue at the rear of the hospital by Admiral Burkley. The bronze casket had one broken handle, and Humes and Boswell opened it. Humes says, "We found the unclothed body of President John F. Kennedy, wrapped in sheets in a swaddling manner, the massive head wound wrapped around and around with gauze and bandages." Together, they lifted the body onto an examining table, and Humes emphasizes, "There was no body bag anywhere near the scene. I cannot imagine how this talk about the President's body being delivered in a body bag got started, but it is absolutely false."

Opening the casket was a "shocking experience" for Humes, who was a Kennedy supporter. He recalls, "His identifying facial features were all intact and there he was, the President of the United States, now dead at age 46 with a terrible wound of the head. He wasn't that much older than me, and other than the head wound, he looked perfectly normal. He was a remarkable human specimen and looked as if he could have lived forever. It was very, very distressing." After the initial shock, however, Humes and Boswell got down to business. Humes notes, "This is what we are trained to do, and we got down to the task at hand."

As Admiral Burkley, the President's personal physician, stood by their side, a team of 10 "locked in" and proceeded to start what would turn out to be a thorough four-hour autopsy. Humes emphasizes, "I was in charge from start to finish and there was no interference—zero. It was myself, 'J' [Boswell], [Dr] Finck, two Navy enlisted men who served as autopsy technicians, three radiologists, including chief Jack Ebersole, MD, and two photographers, including the medical school's chief of photography, John Stringer. We took 14 x-rays of the body from head to toe and we took 52 photos from every possible angle."

He dispels the myth that no photos were allowed. "The medical school's director of photography was a civilian, John Stringer, and, in my opinion, he was one of the best medical photographers in the world. He took 25 black-and-white photos and 27 color photos, all with large 4-by-5-inch negatives. No significant aspect of the autopsy was left unphotographed." He adds, "The wounds were so obvious that there was no need to shave the hair before photographs were taken."

Responding to published reports that photo negatives were seized by the FBI and that the FBI took its own photo-

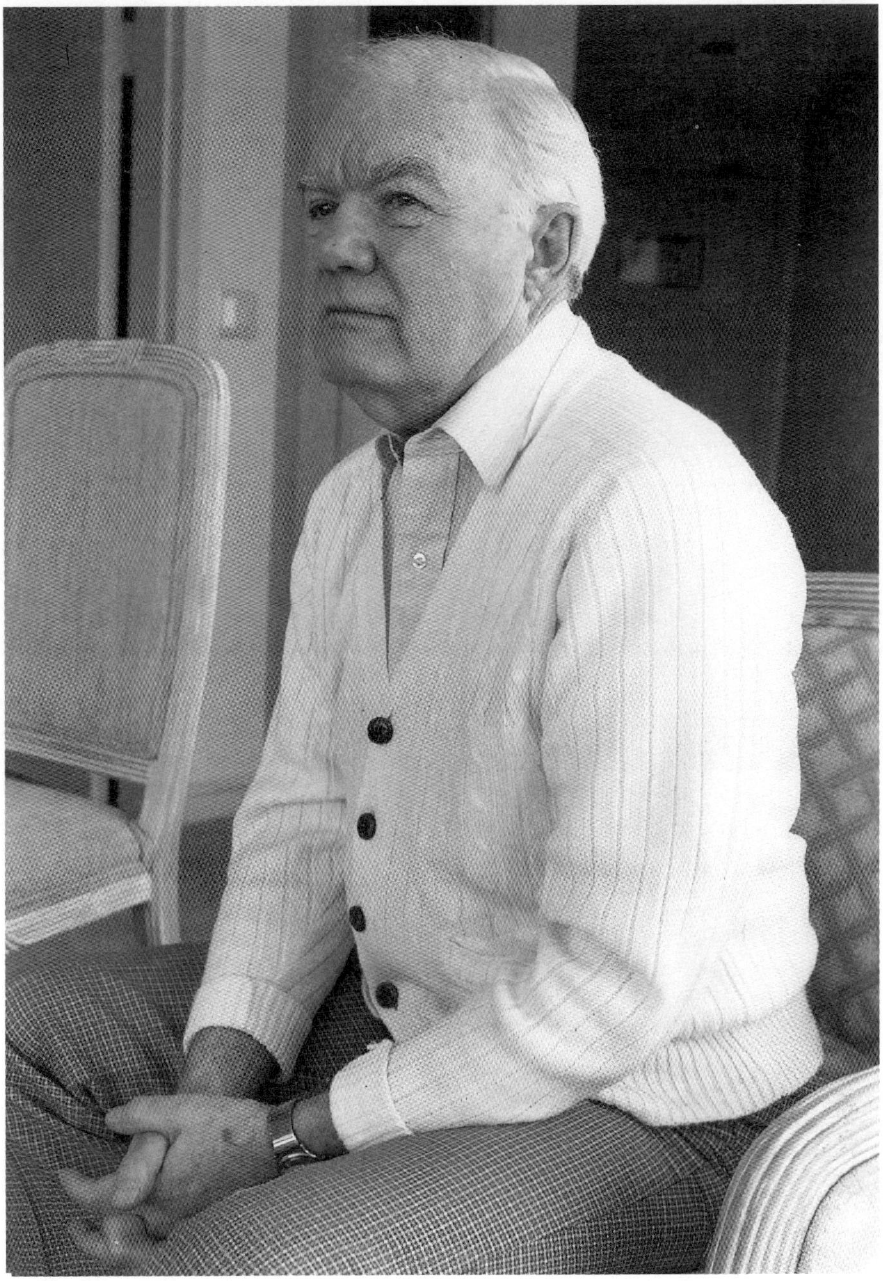

Photo: Dennis L. Breo

Dr Boswell: 'We documented our findings in spades. It's all there in the records.'

graphs, Humes is incredulous. He says, "Yes, there were FBI and Secret Service people milling about the room. And, at one point, there was an unauthorized Navy corpsman taking photos in the morgue and the FBI quite properly seized and destroyed that film, since the photographer did not have credentials. However, the official photos taken by John Stringer were never touched, and no one from the FBI even had a camera, let alone the intention to take autopsy photos. These reports are an incredible lie."

He dispels another myth—that the morgue was controlled by generals and other brass in uniform. "The President's military aides from the Air Force, Army, and Navy were all present," Humes says, "and they were all in dress uniforms, but they were not generals and their influence on the autopsy was zero. The only high-ranking officer was Admiral Burkley, and he left shortly after the autopsy began to join Jackie and Bobby Kennedy upstairs."

And a third myth—that he was not qualified to do a gunshot autopsy. "I'd done gunshot wounds before and this one was perfectly obvious—there was a huge hole on the right side of the President's head that only could have resulted from the exit of a high-velocity missile. Dr Bruce Smith [the deputy director of the Armed Forces Institute of Pathology] had initially thought that we might want a neuropathologist as a consultant, but once we opened the casket and saw the devastating nature of the President's head wound, we knew that there was no need for the skills of a neuropathologist. I called Dr Smith back and told him what we had found, and he decided to make available Dr Pierre A. Finck, who was one of the AFIP's experts in ballistics. I had never before met Dr Finck, who arrived at about 9:15 PM."

Finck, a shy, retiring man who had been trained in Europe, was an Army colonel, and he had trouble getting by all the Marines and sailors who were providing security outside the Navy hospital. Once inside, he completed the autopsy team.

Humes emphasizes, "There was a lot of commotion, but we are trained to focus on the task at hand, even under crowded conditions. Bethesda was a large teaching hospital. The morgue room contained an amphitheater which sat 30 to 40 people, and we were used to seeing authorized medical personnel come and go to observe autopsies." Still, he says that the scene in the autopsy room was "somewhat like trying to do delicate neurosurgery in a three-ring circus." The crowd did not influence the autopsy results, Humes says.

Boswell adds, "Sure, there were FBI and Secret Service people observing the autopsy and talking on their radios to people outside the room, and we could hear a play-by-play of what we were doing and talking about, but nobody tried to interfere and we were able to focus on the matter at hand." He adds, "The FBI and Secret Service told us that two fragments of the President's skull had been recovered in Dallas and were being rushed to Bethesda and that bullet fragments had also been recovered in Dallas."

Humes provides a poignant remembrance of the scene. "The people around the President were totally devastated," he says. "They were still in a state of shock and the reality of what had happened had not yet sunk in. Unless you live in Washington, it's hard to imagine the mind-boggling aura that surrounds the President of the United States. These people thought they had let the President down, and now their hero was gone." Boswell adds, "The people who accompanied the President's body to the morgue were the most disturbed and distressed people I have ever seen."

Humes continues, "We were unfazed by all the commotion and concentrated on getting our x-rays, which we read right at the table, and our photographs, which we relied upon for future documentation. 'J' and I both took down autopsy notes and diagrams."

Fatal wound 'blatantly obvious'

The pathologists found two wounds from a high-velocity missile that would later be matched to the military-jacketed bullets fired from above and behind the President by Lee Harvey Oswald. The fatal shot entered the back of the President's skull and exploded away almost a 6-inch section on the right side of his head; the second bullet entered at the base of his neck, but its exit track was not immediately apparent.

"The fatal wound was blatantly obvious," Humes recalls. "The entrance wound was elliptical, 15 millimeters long and 6 millimeters wide, and located 2.5 centimeters to the right and slightly above the external occipital protuberance. The inside of the skull displayed the characteristic beveled appearance. The x-rays disclosed fine dustlike metallic fragments from back to front where the bullet traversed the head before creating an explosive exit wound on the right temporal-parietal area. These fragments were not grossly visible. Two small fragments of bullet were recovered from inside the skull—measuring 3 by 1 millimeters and 7 by 2 millimeters.

"The head was so devastated by the exploding bullet and the gaping jagged stellate wound it created—it blew out 13 centimeters of skull bone and skin—that we did not even have to use a saw to remove the skullcap. We peeled the scalp back, and the calvarium crumbled in my hands from the fracture lines, which went off in all directions. We made an incision high in the spinal cord and removed the brain, which was preserved in formalin. Two thirds of the right cerebrum had been blown away.

"After the brain was removed, we looked more closely at the wound, and noted that the inside of the rear of the skull bone was absolutely intact and beveled and that there could be no question from whence cometh that bullet—from rear to front. When we received the two missing fragments of the President's skull and were able to piece together two thirds of the deficit at the right front of the head, we saw the same pattern on the outer table of the skull—a bullet that traveled from rear to front. Every theorist who says the bullet came from the front has ignored this critical irrefutable diagnostic fact. We did everything within the means of reasonable people to record with x-rays and photos what we saw."

The second bullet was more of a puzzle. "If we made a mistake," Humes says, "it was in not calling Dallas before we started the autopsy. Our information from Parkland Hospital in Dallas before we started the autopsy was zero. If only we had seen the President's clothes, tracking the second bullet would have been a piece of cake, but we didn't have the clothes. In hindsight, we could have saved ourselves a lot of trouble if we had known that the doctors at Parkland performed a tracheostomy in an attempt to save the President's life and that this procedure obliterated the exit wound of the bullet that entered at the base of the neck."

'Time to quit speculating'

"The tracheostomy was a gaping wound, about 3 to 4 centimeters around, and we didn't think of it as an exit wound. We also noticed that the Dallas doctors had tried to place chest tubes in the front of the President's chest, but the tubes had not gone in and we found no increase of blood or fluid in the pleural cavity. There was a contusion of the extreme apical portion of the right upper lobe of the lung but no laceration.

This article is one of a number of articles on violence that will appear in upcoming issues of THE JOURNAL. The reader is referred to the June 10, 1992, issue, which will be dedicated to studies of violence.

We also noted damage to the neck muscles, trachea, and pleura, but there was no bullet. It was bothering me very greatly, like nothing you can imagine, that we could find neither the second bullet nor its exit track. 'J' and I both knew that bullets can do funny things in the body, and we thought it might have been deflected down to the extremities. We x-rayed the entire body, but did not find a bullet." The autopsy was also criticized because the pathologists did not dissect the President's neck to track the second bullet. Humes says bluntly, "Dissecting the neck was totally unnecessary and would have been criminal.

"By midnight, we decided it was time to quit speculating about the second bullet, and I am very comfortable with this decision. It is true that we were influenced by the fact that we knew Jackie Kennedy was waiting upstairs to accompany the body to the White House and that Admiral Burkley wanted us to hurry as much as possible. By midnight, our task was done—it was perfectly obvious what had killed the man. The second bullet was important, but not of overriding importance. We knew we would find the explanation sooner or later."

The explanation came sooner, the next morning at 7:30 when Humes called Dallas to talk to Dr Malcolm Perry, the surgeon who had performed the tracheostomy. "The light came on when I talked to Dr Perry," Humes says. "Of course, the bullet had exited through the neck." Referring to Dr Crenshaw's contention that the wound in the front of the neck was small and round *after the tracheostomy was performed* and at the time the President was placed in a casket, Dr Humes says, "We found a gaping wound in the front of the neck where the tracheostomy had been performed, and if Dr Crenshaw was correct, the only possible explanation is that the neck wound was intentionally enlarged while the body was en route from Dallas, and the insinuation of this scenario does not deserve a response."

Humes and Boswell had remained at the morgue until 5 that morning, helping to embalm the President's body. Humes says, "We were able to almost perfectly restore the President's appearance, and a local funeral home brought out a beautiful mahogany casket to replace the bronze one from Dallas. When Admiral Burkley and Bobby and Jackie Kennedy left to take the body to the White House, 'J' and I finally went home." Boswell says, "The mood in Washington was so apprehensive that the commanding officer of the US Naval Medical School, Capt J. H. 'Smokey' Stover, asked me to drive behind Jim to make sure that he got home safely."

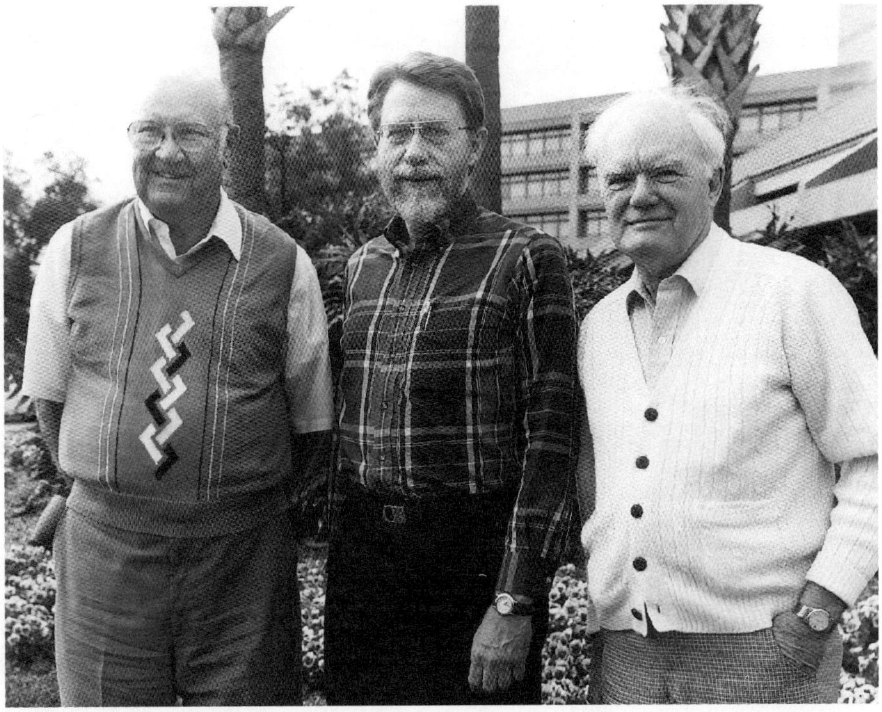

Photo: Dennis L. Breo

Thanks to seven years of pursuit by George Lundberg, MD (center), editor of *JAMA*, Drs Humes (left) and Boswell finally got together on a grassy knoll in Florida to discuss the 1963 autopsy of President John F. Kennedy. Later, Dr Lundberg said he 'completely believes' the autopsy report that Kennedy was killed 'by only two bullets that struck him from above and behind and caused fatal high-velocity wounds.'

Humes spent most of Saturday, November 23, drafting the autopsy report. In the process, he burned his autopsy notes, but not really. "This is the criticism I keep hearing over and over again," he says, "that I burned my notes and that this means there must have been a conspiracy. Well, it's true that I burned my original notes because they were stained with the President's blood, and I did not want them to become a collector's item, but I burned them *after* I had copied verbatim in my own handwriting the entire contents. I make no apology for this, but I will explain my reason:

"One of my assignments had been to escort foreign Navy officers around US bases. Along the way, we'd always try to show the foreign officers slices of Americana. On one of these trips, we saw an exhibit that purported to be the chair on which President Abraham Lincoln sat when he was shot at Ford's Theater. There were stains on the back of the chair that were reported to be from Lincoln's blood. I was appalled at this type of display, though I later learned that the stains were from macassar, a hair preparation of the day that inspired the antimacassar doily, and not from Lincoln's blood. In any event, when I saw that my own notes were stained with Kennedy's blood, I vowed that this type of revolting object would not fall into the wrong hands. I burned the notes that night in my fireplace."

Admiral Burkley wanted the autopsy report by midnight Sunday, November 24, and early Sunday morning Humes returned to the Naval medical school to go over his handwritten report with Drs Boswell and Finck. The three pathologists met in the office of Adm C. B. Galloway, the commanding officer of the National Naval Medical Center. While talking, they were called to watch a nearby TV set—Jack Ruby had just shot Lee Harvey Oswald in Dallas. Returning to their report, the three experts had no trouble agreeing on the facts of their autopsy. The report, "A63-272," was the 272nd autopsy performed that year at the hospital. The admiral's secretary typed the handwritten report into six pages. Humes says, "Our conclusions have stood the test of time." The cause of death is given as "gunshot wound, head." The summary, as published in the 1964 Warren Commission report, reads as follows:

The original 1963 autopsy report

"It is our opinion that the deceased died as a result of two perforating gunshot wounds inflicted by high-velocity projectiles fired by a person or persons unknown. The projectiles were fired from a point behind and somewhat above the level of the deceased. The observations and available information do not permit a satisfactory estimate as to the sequence of the two wounds.

"The fatal missile entered the skull above and to the right of the external occipital protuberance. A portion of the projectile traversed the cranial cavity in a posterior-anterior direction (see lateral skull roentgenograms), depositing minute particles along its path. A portion of the projectile made its exit through the parietal bone on the right, carrying with it portions of cerebrum, skull, and scalp. The two wounds of the skull combined with the force of the missile produced extensive fragmentation of the skull, laceration of the superior sagittal sinus, and of the right cerebral hemisphere.

"The other missile entered the right superior posterior thorax above the scapula and traversed the soft tissues of the supra-scapular and supra-clavicular portions of the base of the right side of the neck. This missile produced contusions of the right apical parietal pleura and of the apical portion of the right upper lobe of the lung. The missile contused the strap muscles of the right side of the neck, damaged the trachea, and made its exit through the anterior surface of the neck. As far as can be ascertained, this missile struck no bony structures in its path through the body.

"In addition, it is our opinion that the wound of the skull produced such extensive damage to the brain as to preclude the possibility of the deceased surviving this injury.

"A supplementary report will be submitted following more detailed examinations of the brain and of microscopic sections. However, it is not anticipated that these examinations will materially alter the findings."

That night, Humes hand-delivered the autopsy report, signed by Humes, Boswell, and Finck, to Admiral Burkley at the White House. On December 6, 1963, Humes alone submitted to Burkley his supplementary report, writing in the final summary: "This supplementary report covers in more detail the extensive degree of cerebral trauma in this case. However, neither this portion of the examination nor the microscopic examinations alter the previously submitted report or add significant details to the cause of death."

Shortly afterward, Humes turned over everything from the autopsy to Admiral Burkley—bullet fragments, microscopic slides, paraffin blocks of tissue, undeveloped film, x-rays—and the preserved, unsectioned President's brain. "Burkley said he wanted everything," Humes says, "and he came out to Bethesda to get it. I gave it to him all in one package. What was left at Bethesda? Zero. I didn't make a copy of anything. Frankly, I was glad to be out from under the responsibility. Admiral Burkley gave me a receipt for the autopsy materials, including the brain. It was my understanding that all the autopsy materials, except the brain, would be placed in the National Archives. He told me that the family wanted to inter the brain with the President's body. I don't know what happened to the brain, but I do know that Admiral Burkley was an honorable man."

The medical autopsy of President John F. Kennedy was concluded. The conspiracy autopsies had yet to begin.

...

Humes and Boswell concede that Kennedy's body was illegally moved from Dallas, in violation of Texas laws requiring that Texas homicides be autopsied in Texas, and that there would have been less confusion if the autopsy had been performed in Dallas, but Humes emphasizes:

"There was a very, very good reason why this happened. Lyndon Johnson did not know what was going on in Dallas on this day, and for all he knew a cabal could have been in the works. He wanted to get back to his base and his base was Washington, DC. He would not leave without Jackie Kennedy, and she would not leave without her husband's body. Johnson had to get back to Washington, and, ergo, the body had to be brought back. That's that, and I cannot believe that any reasonable person would disagree with this course of action."

He adds, "Several days after the autopsy, I got a call from someone in Dallas demanding that we return the bronze casket that had carried the President's body from Parkland Hospital to Bethesda. I told him I had no idea what had happened to that casket, and I didn't—it wasn't my responsibility. He was very insistent, but so was I."

Autopsy confirmed four times

The autopsy findings have been confirmed many times since 1963, a fact that has been largely ignored in the current hoopla over the film *JFK* and over Dr Crenshaw's new book and media appearances. The first time was the publication of the Warren Commission report in 1964, and Humes has brought to the interview a copy of his own Warren Commission report signed by Chief Justice Earl Warren. It was only during their interviews with Warren Commission investigators that Humes and Boswell saw for the first time the clothing worn by President Kennedy.

Humes says, "Once we saw the holes in the back of the President's suit jacket and shirt and the nicks on his shirt collar and the knot of his necktie, the path of the second bullet was confirmed. That bullet was traveling very fast and it had to go somewhere. I believe in the single-bullet theory that it struck Governor Connally immediately after exiting the President's throat."

Boswell adds, "Having seen the clothing, I now know that I created a terrible problem with my own autopsy drawings. My drawings of the bullet holes on the night of the autopsy did not precisely match up with the actual holes in the clothing, because we were not aware that the President's suit jacket had humped up on his back while he waved at the spectators. These errors were later exploited by the conspiracy crowd to fit their premises and purposes." The clothing was kept in the National Archives, along with the rest of the autopsy materials.

Photos not published

Both Humes and Boswell agreed to the commission's stipulation that the autopsy photos were not to be viewed. Humes explains, "I agreed with the commission's decision not to make the photos part of the official report. I had stated in the autopsy, 'The complexity of these fractures and the fragments thus produced tax satisfactory verbal description and are better appreciated in photos and roentgenograms which are prepared,' and I meant it. The head wound was devastating, and if the photos were made part of the commission report they would have become public. I did not think that these photos should appear on the front pages of newspapers, and I did not trust the ability of the commission to keep them secret. So, 'J' and I worked with an artist to reconstruct drawings of the President's wounds, based upon our original measurements. These drawings are very accurate and met the purposes of the Warren Commission. In 1964, there were no crazy conspiracy theories about the death of the President."

It was not until November 1, 1966, that the two pathologists saw the autopsy photos—when they were summoned to the National Archives to help categorize all autopsy materials.

The second confirmation of their autopsy came in 1968, as the result of a request made by Drs Humes and Boswell themselves. In 1968, there *were* crazy conspiracy theories coming out of the woodwork. On January 26, 1968, Boswell sent a letter to Ramsey Clark, then the US attorney general, in an attempt to put the issue to rest. The letter read:

"As you are aware, the autopsy findings in the case of the late President John F. Kennedy, including x-rays and photographs, have been the subject of continuing controversy and speculation. Dr Humes and I, as the pathologists concerned, have felt for some time that an impartial board of experts, including pathologists and radiologists, should examine the available material.

"If such a board were to be nominated in an attempt to resolve many of the allegations concerning the autopsy report, it might wish to question the autopsy participants before more time elapses and memory fades; therefore, it would be my hope that such a board would be convened at an early date. Dr Humes and I would make ourselves available at the request of such a board.

"I hope that this letter will not be considered presumptuous, but this matter is of great concern to us, and I believe to the country as well."

Four physicians were subsequently appointed to a blue-ribbon panel to evaluate the original autopsy. The four included:

- William H. Carnes, MD, professor of pathology at the University of Utah, Salt Lake City, and a member of Utah's Medical Examiner's Commission. He was nominated by J. E. Wallace Sterling, the president of Stanford University.
- Russell S. Fisher, MD, professor of forensic pathology at the University of Maryland and chief medical examiner of the state of Maryland. He was nominated by Dr Oscar B. Hunter, Jr, president of the College of American Pathologists.
- Russell H. Morgan, MD, professor of radiology at The Johns Hopkins University School of Medicine, Baltimore, Md. He was nominated by Dr Lincoln Gordon, president of The Johns Hopkins University.
- Alan R. Moritz, MD, professor of pathology at Case Western Reserve University, Cleveland, Ohio, and former professor of forensic medicine at Harvard University, Cambridge, Mass. He was nominated by Dr John A. Hannah, president of Michigan State University.

None of the four had any previous connection with prior investigations or reports on the President's assassination. After an exhaustive study of all relevant materials, the four members of the panel signed and submitted a 16-page report to Attorney General Clark in April 1968, unanimously concluding:

"Examination of the clothing and of the photographs and x-rays taken at autopsy reveal that President Kennedy was struck by two bullets fired from above and behind him, one of which traversed the base of the neck on the right side without striking bone and the other of which entered the skull from behind and exploded its right side. The photographs and x-rays discussed herein support the above-quoted portions [the conclusion] of the original Autopsy Report and the above-quoted medical conclusions of the Warren Commission Report."

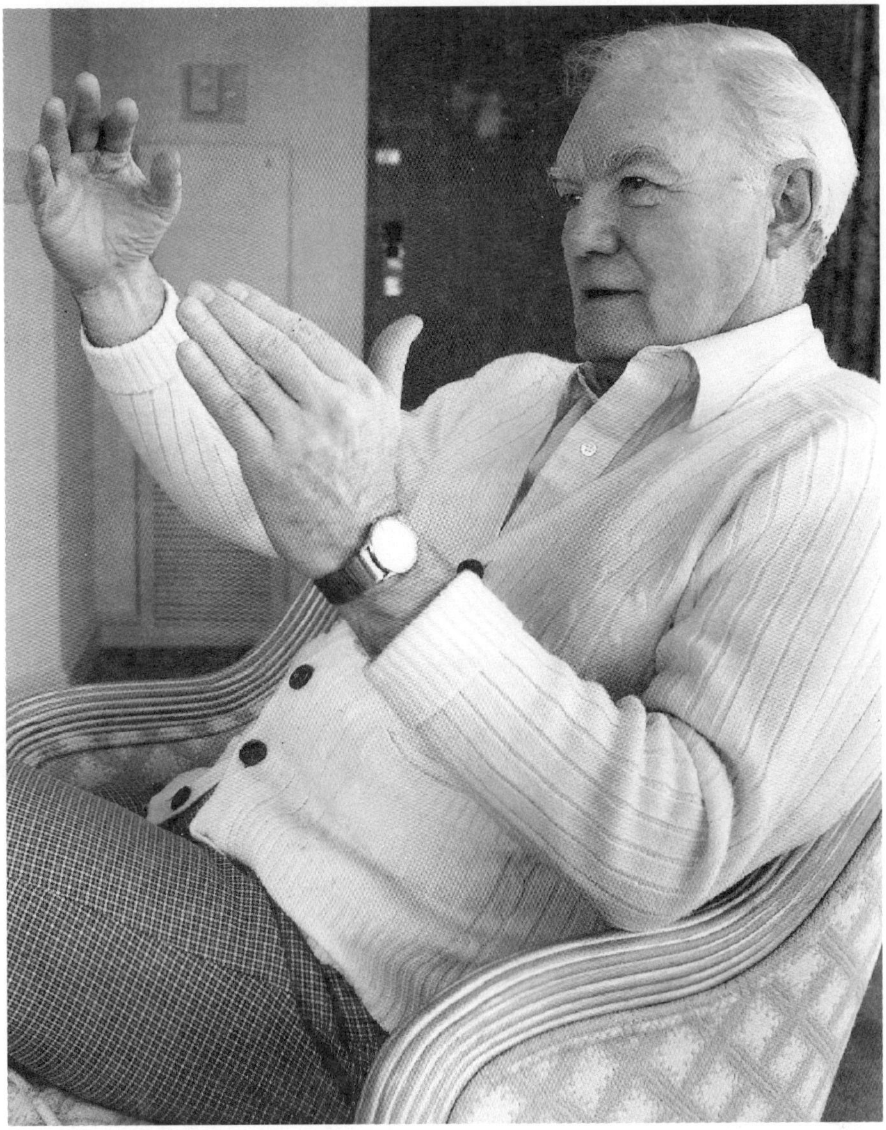

Photo: Dennis L. Breo

Dr Boswell: 'It appears that [filmmaker] Oliver Stone may have taken Dr Finck's mistaken perceptions about the alleged military presence in the morgue and used it as the sole mistaken basis for the autopsy scenes in his movie, *JFK*.'

The panel's report noted, "The possibility that the path of the bullet through the neck might have been more satisfactorily explored by the insertion of a finger or probe was considered. Obviously, the cutaneous wound in the back was too small to permit the insertion of a finger. The insertion of a metal probe would have carried the risk of creating a false passage—in part because of the changed relationship of muscles at the time of autopsy and in part because of the existence of postmortem rigidity. Although the precise path of the bullet could undoubtedly have been demonstrated by complete dissection of the soft tissue between the two cutaneous wounds, there is no reason to believe that the information disclosed thereby would alter significantly the conclusions expressed in this report."

The Garrison prosecution

The next confirmation came in 1969 in New Orleans when Pierre Finck was subpoenaed to testify at the trial of Clay Shaw, as part of District Attorney Jim Garrison's conspiracy prosecution. Shaw, of course, was acquitted, and, until the publication of this interview, Finck's testimony was the only *public* airing of the expert medical opinions on the assassination.

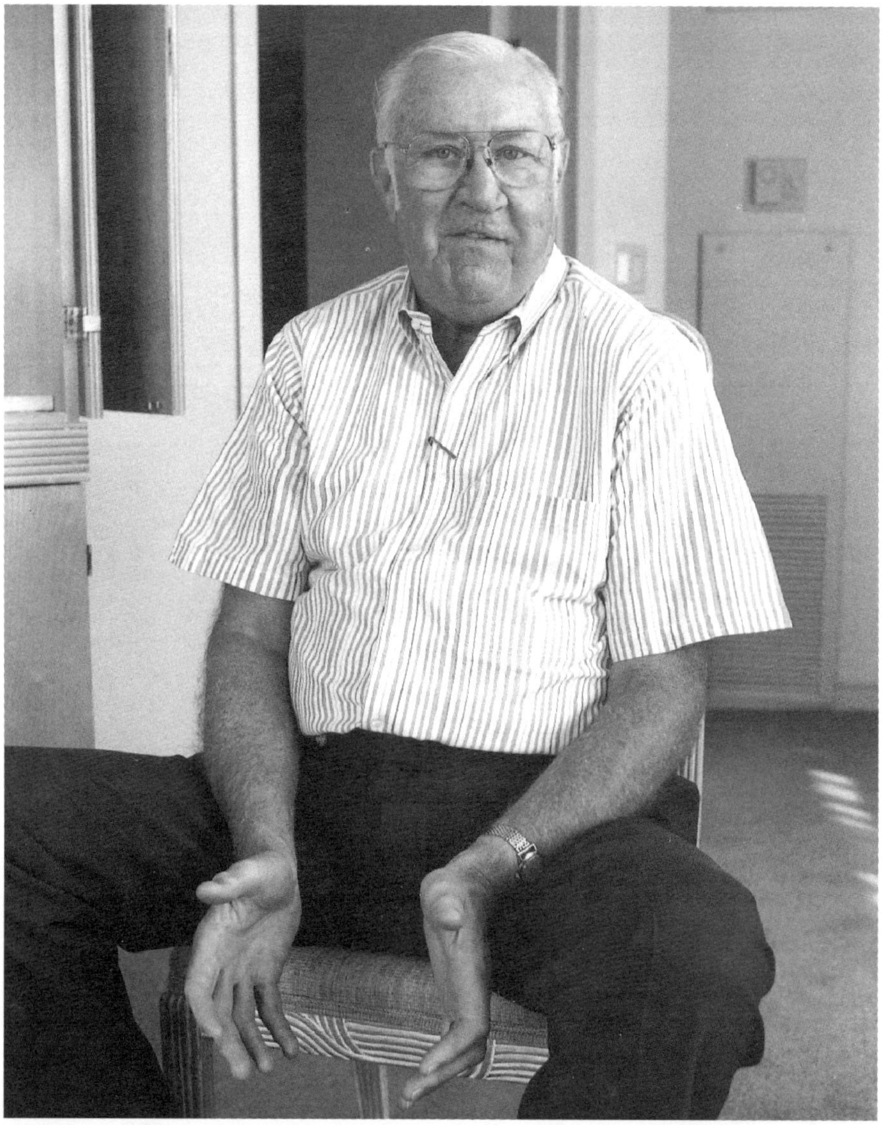

Photo: Dennis L. Breo

Dr Humes: 'There was no interference with our autopsy and nobody tried to suppress the findings.'

Boswell says, "A careful reading of the entire transcript of Dr Finck's testimony shows that he held tightly to the facts of our autopsy and supported its conclusions. However, Pierre was a meek and mild man who had been trained abroad, not in the United States. He was very 'brass conscious,' and he thought that generals were out of this world. At Bethesda, Finck was out of his element—an Army colonel in a Navy hospital—and he apparently mistook the President's military aides and other military personnel for generals. During the trial, Garrison was able to exploit Pierre's misperceptions about the scene to give the impression that it was controlled by generals. Jim [Humes] and I state categorically that there was no interference with our autopsy. The patient was extraordinary, the autopsy was ordinary, or at least as ordinary as it could be under the circumstances."

Boswell knows because he, too, was in New Orleans in 1969 at the request of the US Justice Department. "The Justice Department was so convinced that Garrison was on a fishing expedition in his prosecution of Clay Shaw," Boswell says, "that it summoned me to New Orleans to refute Finck's testimony, if necessary. It turned out that it wasn't necessary." It now appears, Boswell adds, that filmmaker Oliver Stone may have taken Finck's mistaken perceptions about the alleged military presence in the morgue, as detailed in the transcript of the trial, and used it as the sole basis for the mistaken autopsy scenes in his movie *JFK*. Humes calls the movie scenes "absolutely false and ridiculous," but we are getting ahead of the story.

The next confirmation of the President's autopsy came from the 1977 House Select Committee on Assassinations. Congress appointed a panel of nine experts chaired by forensic pathologist Michael Baden, MD, to investigate the medical findings. In his 1989 book, *Unnatural Death—Confessions of a Medical Examiner,* Baden agrees with the findings of Humes-Boswell-Finck but still terms Kennedy's autopsy the "exemplar" of the "bungled autopsy." He writes, "Despite all these errors and for the wrong reasons, Humes came to the right conclusions—that Kennedy had been shot by two bullets from behind, one in the head and one in the back. They [the wounds] were poorly tracked, but he got the two most important things right."

Humes says he has not read Baden's book and does not intend to. Mindful that this is a rare attack upon an autopsy that was solidly endorsed by an expert panel in 1968, he reacts to this quoted passage by saying, "Imagine that—we got it right, AS DUMB AS WE ARE! What possible purpose can be served by this kind of attack?"

Apprised of Baden's comment, "[Commander Humes] had never done one like it before," Humes incredulously exclaims, "Who had?" As Baden's written criticisms are read to him, Humes indignantly explodes, "False . . . false . . . false. My God, where does this stuff come from?" To cite but one example, Baden writes, "He [Humes] also knew that religious Catholics tend to be opposed to autopsies. And he was not in a position to press the issue." Humes replies, "Come on, now. I am a devout Catholic and for 19 years I was director of laboratories at St John Hospital, in Detroit, Mich, which is a Catholic hospital with a very active autopsy service. This autopsy was requested by the Kennedy family, who are Catholics."

JFK, the film, termed a 'hoax'

Then, there is the film, *JFK.* Jack Valenti, a former aide to President Lyndon Johnson and the current president of the Motion Picture Association of America, recently described *JFK* as based on the "hallucinatory bleatings of an author named Jim Garrison, a discredited former district attorney in New Orleans." He also calls it a "hoax," a "smear," and "pure fiction," rivaling the Nazi propaganda films of Leni Riefenstahl.

Syndicated columnist George Will says, "*JFK* is cartoon history by Stone, who is 45 going on 8. In his three-hour lie, Stone falsifies so much he may be an intellectual sociopath, indifferent to truth." *New York Times* columnist Anthony Stone says, "Oliver Stone used as his mouthpiece, Jim Garrison, the former New Orleans district attorney, who in real life bribed witnesses to prosecute an innocent man—and was laughed out of court. Stone alleges a conspiracy among the Army, the CIA, Lyndon Johnson, and countless others—without a shred of evidence." Stone has been quoted as saying his critics are motivated by a "fear of facts." *Chicago Tribune* reporter Paul Galloway responds, "Nope. They were angry with the way he disregarded the facts."

Humes does not disagree with these criticisms of Stone, which he finds mild. His son had recently persuaded him to see *JFK*, and now he tells his colleague, Boswell, "'J,' if you see this movie, believe me, you'll need heavy sedation. The autopsy scene bears no relation to reality, the man they have playing me looks older than I am now, and the triangulated shooting scene is preposterously impossible."

Conspiracy fanciers, including Stone, have tried to make much of the fact that the privately owned Zapruder film of the assassination shows Kennedy's head lurching *backward* after being hit. Humes and Boswell have both seen the Zapruder film "30 to 40 times," and they note that studies published two decades ago by surgeon John Lattimer demonstrated that an object struck in the rear by a high-velocity missile similar to the bullets that hit Kennedy *always falls backward* as a result of the jet-propulsion effect created by tissues exploding out the front.

JAMA's Lundberg, a stickler for detail, poses some questions that remain official mysteries:

Who ordered the autopsy?

Who ordered the autopsy?

"It must have been Jackie Kennedy," says Humes. "She made the request through Admiral Burkley." Boswell says, "It must have been Robert Kennedy. He was acting on behalf of the family." Lundberg counters, "Well, we have a lot of 'must haves,' but no answer." Humes says, "Well, George, I hope you're not saying that we shouldn't have done the autopsy! My orders came from Ed Kenney, the surgeon-general of the Navy. The President's personal physician, Admiral Burkley, was standing beside me at the autopsy table. Jackie Kennedy was waiting upstairs for the body with Robert Kennedy, and what greater authority can you have than the Attorney General of the United States [Robert Kennedy]?" Lundberg concludes, "OK, there were verbal OKs all over the place." Boswell adds, "Captain Stover [the medical center's commanding officer] was very thorough, and I'm sure he had someone complete the paperwork."

Who made the absolute identity?

Humes chuckles, "Well, the President's face was not exactly unknown. And the body was accompanied by the FBI, the Secret Service, military aides, and Kennedy family members. We saw no need for dental x-rays."

What happened to the brain?

Boswell says, "I believe that it was buried with the body." Humes says, "I don't know, but I do know that I personally handed it over to Admiral Burkley and that he told me that the family intended to bury it with the body. I believe Admiral Burkley."

What was the condition of Kennedy's adrenal glands?

Humes says, "I am not prepared to answer this question now, except to say that the President was *not* 'cushingoid' and did not have the appearance of a man with the odd fat deposits and facial puffiness associated with the cushingoid appearance. As his activities indicate, he was a very healthy and vigorous man. At some time in the near future, 'J' and I will have to sit down and write for history our report of the condition of the President's adrenal glands."

Should the body be exhumed for another autopsy to remove all doubts?

Humes is appalled. "That suggestion is ridiculous on the face of it. There is nothing further to be learned." Boswell adds, "The family would never permit it, anyway."

Boswell concludes, "In hindsight, we might have called in a civilian pathologist like Russell Fisher, who was right next door in Baltimore. We didn't need him to confirm our findings, but it might have removed the doubts about military control." Humes says, "Russell was a friend and we easily could have asked him to come in to help, but we had no problem in determining the cause of death."

'Irrefutable evidence'

Lundberg says, "I am extremely pleased that, finally, we are able to have published in the peer-reviewed literature the actual findings of what took place at the autopsy table on November 22, 1963. I completely believe that this information, as personally given by Jim [Humes] and 'J' [Boswell], is scientifically sound and, in my judgment, provides irrefutable evidence that President Kennedy was killed by only two bullets that struck him from above and behind and that caused fatal high-velocity wounds."

Humes concludes, "I really have not had much ongoing interest in the autopsy. We did what we had to do in 1963, and we did it right. And, I can't say that the criticism has hurt my career." Indeed, Humes retired from the Navy in 1967 with the rank of captain; worked 19 years at Detroit's St John Hospital as vice president for medical affairs and director of laboratories; and served from 1986 through 1989 as a field inspector for the Accreditation Council for Graduate Medical Education. In 1980, he was awarded the Distinguished Service Award presented jointly by the College of American Pathologists and the American Society of Clinical Pathologists (ASCP). He was president of ASCP from 1974 to 1975; president of the Michigan Society of Pathologists in 1974; the first president of the American Registry of Pathology from 1976 through 1978; and a member of the AMA House of Delegates from 1978 through 1988. Now semiretired, he is a clinical professor of pathology at the University of Florida School of Medicine, Jacksonville, and lives in nearby Ponte Vedra, Fla, where he has his choice of playing 105 golf holes, including the Tournament Players Championship course at Sawgrass. Boswell retired from the Navy in 1965, with the rank of commander, and worked in supervisory pathology positions at Suburban Hospital, Bethesda, Md, from 1965 through 1972; and with a large pathology group in Fairfax, Va, from 1972 to 1983. Now retired, he lives in Bethesda.

Humes stops the interview where he started. "The President was killed by a devastating gunshot wound to the head fired from above and behind by a high-velocity rifle. The second bullet that struck him in the back of the neck was also fired from above and behind. That's it. Everything else is adventitious."

It is an apt description. The adventitia, of course, are the external coatings of the blood vessels, giving rise to the adjective, "adventitious," for "added from another source and not inherent or innate . . . arising or occurring sporadically or in other than the usual location."

It is the perfect description for the growing industry of conspiracy theories from people who are ignorant of the essential facts and yet purport to know how President Kennedy must have been killed, at least in their minds. □

JFK's death, part II—Dallas MDs recall their memories

Only 90 minutes passed in Dallas from the time Lee Harvey Oswald raised his rifle at 12:30 PM until the slain body of President John F. Kennedy was escorted aboard Air Force One for the 1500-mile flight to Andrews Air Force Base in Maryland and the autopsy at the US Naval Medical Center in Bethesda. The medical team at Dallas' Parkland Memorial Hospital spent only 25 frenzied minutes in their futile effort to resuscitate Kennedy, but that whirlwind of events and emotions produced indelible personal memories.

In truth, though, there were no examinations, measurements, or photographs performed in Parkland's Trauma Room 1 that in any way, shape, or form allowed any of the physicians attending the President to make any meaningful evaluation of the entry and exit gunshot wounds and the forensic cicumstances of death. That assignment was left to the autopsy pathologists at the Naval Medical Center, and their comments in the preceding story stand as the definitive version that Kennedy was struck by only two bullets fired from behind and above from a high-velocity rifle.

This is the unanimous appraisal of four Dallas physicians who have broken their 29-year silence to speak with this reporter about their famous 1963 case. Malcolm Perry, MD, a surgeon, worked the hardest to try to save the patient and performed a tracheostomy in an attempt to create an airway for the dying Kennedy. Jim Carrico, MD, a first-year surgical resident, was the first physician to treat Kennedy, at 12:35 PM, and the first to notice the small bubbling wound in the front of the neck that necessitated the tracheostomy. M. T. "Pepper" Jenkins, MD, the hospital's longtime chief of anesthesiology, rushed to the scene to try to help ventilate the patient. Charles Baxter, MD, a surgeon, assisted in the resuscitation attempt. These were the four key players on the Parkland medical team of November 22, 1963.

Previously, the four have kept their memories private, but they agreed to be interviewed by *JAMA* in the wake of a new book written by one of their former Parkland Hospital colleagues, Charles Crenshaw, MD, that has bolstered conspiracy theorists because of Crenshaw's incredible 1992 claim that the bullets "struck Kennedy from the front" and that the autopsy photos must have been altered, proving "there was something rotten in America in 1963." Crenshaw attributes these statements and others to his alleged intense eyewitness observations of the dying President.

Although the other four Parkland physicians have some doubt about whether Dr Crenshaw wrote most of the sensationalistic book or deferred to his two coauthors, both of whom are conspiracy theorists, and although they are reluctant to publicly condemn Crenshaw's claims, they emphasize that they believe Crenshaw is wrong.

Since it is hard to prove a negative, no one can say with certainty what some suspect—that Crenshaw was *not* even in the trauma room; none of the four recalls ever seeing him at the scene.

'Dreams of notoriety'

Dr Perry says, "In 1963, Chuck Crenshaw was a junior resident and he absolutely did not participate in a meaningful way in the attempt to resuscitate the President and in the medical decision making. I do not remember even seeing him in the room." Dr Jenkins says, "He may have been in the room, but he was not among the inner circle attending to the patient." Dr Carrico says, "Charles has extended his conclusions far beyond his direct examinations. Everyone in that room was trying to save a life, not figure out forensics." Baxter adds, "Jim [Carrico] has just made a very astute observation."

Why, then, would Crenshaw make such claims and write a book representing himself as being in the forefront of the resuscitation effort?

Baxter says, "Charles and I grew up in Paris, Texas, and I've known him since he was three years old. His claims are ridiculous. The only motive I can see is a desire for personal recognition and monetary gain."

Thumbing rapidly through Crenshaw's slender paperback book, Carrico stops at page 15 and quotes Crenshaw's words, " 'Many of us have dreamed that history's grand scheme will involve us in some far-reaching role or experience thrusting us into notoriety and dramatically changing our lives.' " Carrico concludes, "There's your answer, in Charles's own words. I don't have those kind of dreams."

Jenkins says simply, "Crenshaw's conclusions are dead wrong."

Perry concludes, "When I first heard about Crenshaw's claims, I was considering a lawsuit, but after I saw Charles on TV one day all my anger melted. It was so pathetic to see him on TV saying this bogus stuff to reach out for his day in the sun that I ended up feeling sorry for him." He adds, "Crenshaw says that the rest of us are part of a conspiracy of silence and that he withheld his information for 29 years because of a fear his career would be ruined. Well, if he really felt he had valuable information and kept it secret for all those years, I find that despicable."

Crenshaw's book insinuates that the Bethesda autopsy pathologists altered Kennedy's wounds and it specifically charges that "the incision Perry had made in his [Kennedy's] throat at Parkland for the tracheostomy had been enlarged and mangled, as if someone had conducted another procedure. It looked to be the work of a butcher. No doubt, someone had gone to a great deal of trouble to show a different story than we had seen at Parkland."

Well, the physician who did that work at Parkland—Dr Perry—and three physicians who observed the tracheostomy—Drs Baxter, Carrico, and Jenkins—all say that the autopsy photos of the throat wound are "very compatible" with what they saw in Parkland Trauma Room 1. Dr Baxter says, "I was right there and the tracheostomy I observed and the autopsy photos look the same—very compatible." Dr Carrico says, "I've seen the autopsy photos and they are very compatible to the actual tracheostomy." Dr Jenkins adds, "They're the same." Dr Perry concludes, "Of course, tissues sag and stretch after death, but any suggestion that this wound was intentionally enlarged is wrong. When I talked to Commander Humes the morning after the assassination and told him we had done a tracheostomy, he said, 'That explains it—the bullet exited through the throat.' "

Drs Baxter, Carrico, Jenkins, and Perry emphasize that their experiences in the trauma room do not qualify them to reach conclusions about the direction from which the fatal missiles were fired. In fact, Dr Jenkins doubts if any of the Parkland physicians even had a good look at the President's head, explaining, "I was standing at the head of the table in the position the anesthesiologist most often assumes closest to the patient's head. My presence there and the President's great shock of hair and the location of the head wound were such that it was not visible to those standing down each side of the gurney where they were carrying out their resuscitative maneuvers." However, all four agree, in Carrico's words, that, "Nothing we observed contradicts the autopsy finding that the bullets were fired from above and behind by a high-velocity rifle."

As a result of Crenshaw's media allegations, the four other Dallas physicians have been besieged with calls from other members of the Parkland medical team that was on the scene on November 22, 1963. Baxter says, "I can assure you that these calls are uniformly in disagreement with Crenshaw's claims. Most of those who know the facts express disgust at Crenshaw's actions and question if he was involved in the care of the President at all. There has not been one call supporting his position."

Crenshaw also claims in his book to have received a telephone call from President Lyndon B. Johnson, asking him to extract a confession from the dying Lee Harvey Oswald. Baxter responds, "Did that happen? Heavens no ... imagine that, the President of the United States personally calls for Chuck Crenshaw." Another Crenshaw claim is that he was the last to view President Kennedy's body as he closed the casket and that it was at this point that he observed the head wound. Dr Jenkins responds, "It is highly unlikely that any physician would have closed that casket."

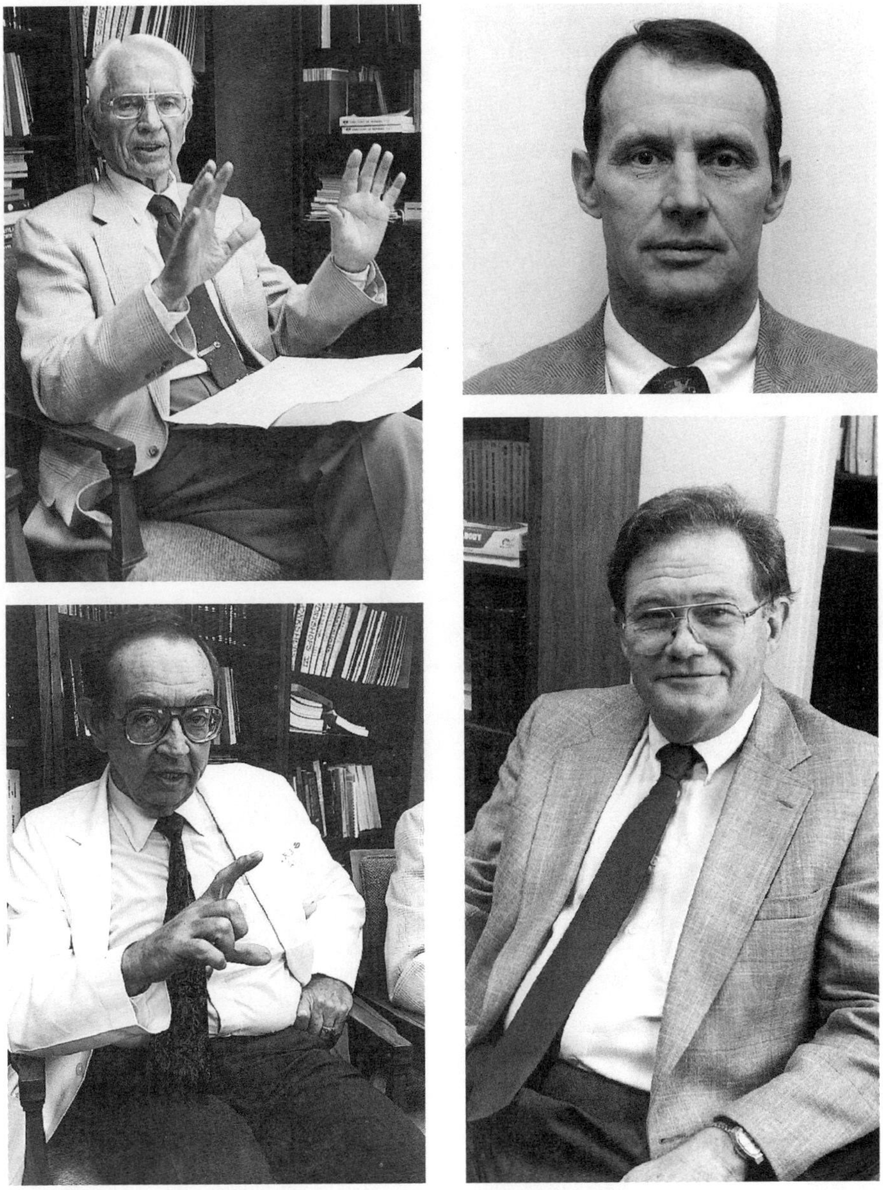

Photos: Dennis L. Breo

Parkland Hospital physicians who tried unsuccessfully to resuscitate President John F. Kennedy included (clockwise from top left) anesthesiologist Pepper Jenkins, surgeon Malcolm Perry, surgical resident Jim Carrico, and surgeon Charles Baxter.

Carrico emphasizes, "We were trying to save a life, not worrying about entry and exit wounds." Perry says, "The President's pupils were widely dilated, his face was a deep blue, and he was in agonal respiration, with his chin jerking. Jim [Carrico] was having trouble inserting the endotracheal tube because of the wound to the trachea and I didn't even wipe off the blood before doing the 'trach.' I grabbed a knife and made a quick and large incision; it only took two or three minutes." He adds, "So many people have theories about the assassination, but I have yet to meet one who has read the entire 26 volumes of the Warren Commission report."

The continuing controversy over the assassination and the refusal to believe the 26-volume, elephantinely documented Warren Commission report obscure the real human tragedy of the event. Pepper Jenkins recalls one poignant anecdote:

"The President was a bigger man than I recalled from seeing him on TV. He must have had really severe back pain, judging by the size of the back brace we cut off. He was tightly laced into this brace with wide Ace bandages making figure-of-eight loops around his trunk and around his thighs. His feet were sticking off one end of the gurney and his head was at the other end, cradled in my arms. I was standing with the front of my jacket against his head wound, an alignment that put me in the best position to carry out artificial ventilation.

I was getting gushes of blood down my jacket and onto my shoes.

"Jacqueline Kennedy was circling the room, walking behind my back. The Secret Service could not keep her out of the room. She looked shell-shocked. As she circled and circled, I noticed that her hands were cupped in front of her, as if she were cradling something. As she passed by, she nudged me with an elbow and handed me what she had been nursing in her hands—a large chunk of her husband's brain tissues. I quickly handed it to a nurse."

'It's too late, Mac'

It was Dr William Kemp Clark, a Parkland Hospital neurosurgeon, who most closely observed Kennedy's massive head wound. He told Dr Perry, "It's too late, Mac. There's nothing more to be done." It was Dr Clark who pronounced the President dead at 1 PM, only 25 minutes after he was wheeled into the emergency room.

By this time, the Secret Service had allowed a Catholic priest to enter the room to administer the last rites. Jenkins recalls, "All of the medical staff seemed to disappear, dissolve, fade from the room, except, I believe, for me and Dr Baxter. I was busy disconnecting the electrocardiographic leads, removing the IVs, and extracting the endotracheal tube. However, before I could finish these duties, Mrs Kennedy returned to the President's side and I retreated to a corner of the room. She kissed the President on the foot, on the leg, on the thigh, on the abdomen, on the chest, and then on the face. She still looked drawn, pale, shocked, and remote. I doubt if she remembers any part of this. Then the priest began the last rites in deliberate, resonant, and slow tones, and then it was over."

Jenkins recalls that Secret Service agents then "grabbed the President's gurney on each side and wheeled it out of the room, all but running over Dr Earl Rose, the Dallas medical examiner [whose office was right across the hall from the emergency room]."

Dr Rose, who is now retired in Iowa City, also gave *JAMA* a rare interview to pick up the narrative. "I was in their way," Rose recalls. "I was face to face with Secret Service Agent Roy H. Kellerman, and I was trying to explain to him that Texas law applied in the instant case of the death of the President and that the law required an autopsy to be performed in Texas.

"Agent Kellerman had experienced a tragedy on his watch and, although he had no legal authority, he believed that his primary responsibility was to transport the body back to Washington, DC.

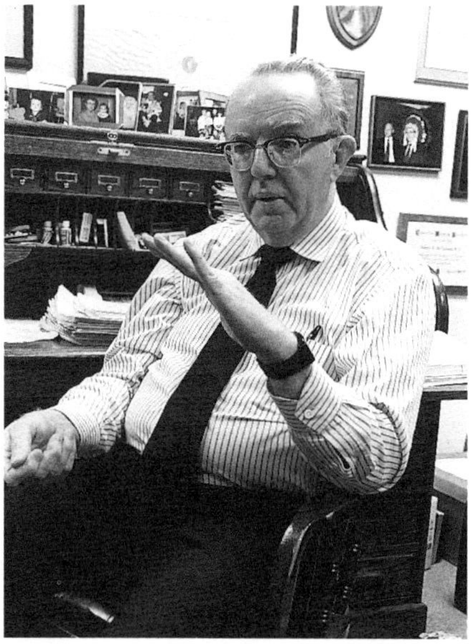

Photo: Dennis L. Breo

Ignoring the autopsy evidence, Dallas surgeon Robert McClelland maintains a "strong opinion" that the bullets that struck Kennedy came from the front. He bases this conclusion on his viewing of the Zapruder film of the assassination.

He was very distressed, apparently taking the death as a personal affront, and he and I were not communicating. It was not a hostile discussion, but he and I were expressing differing views on what was appropriate."

A standoff over removing the body

Theron Ward, a Dallas Justice of the Peace, was at the hospital to assert the applicable Texas law, but, in Rose's words, "he did nothing . . . he was frozen with fear. In effect, no one was in charge of the situation. Agent Kellerman tried three tactics to have his way—he asserted his identity as representing the Secret Service; he appealed for sympathy to Mrs Kennedy; and he used body language to attempt to bully, or, should I say, intimidate. I don't recall the exact words, but he and I exchanged firm and emotionally charged words. At no time did I feel I was in physical danger because he and the others were armed. I was not looking at Agent Kellerman's gun, I was looking at his eyes, and they were very intense. His eyes said that he meant to get the President's body back to Washington."

In 1963, Rose was 6-feet, 2-inches tall and solidly built. He was not the kind to back down from a fight if he believed he was right. "I was raised in western South Dakota," he said, "and I carried that baggage with me. People raised in western South Dakota may lose a fight, but they don't get bullied or intimidated." The standoff, however, was soon over. Rose says, "Finally, without saying any more, I simply stood aside. I felt that it was unwise to do anything more to accelerate or exacerbate the tension. There was nothing more I could do to keep the body in Dallas. I had no minions, no armies to enforce the will of the medical examiner."

Later that day, Rose autopsied patrolman J. D. Tippit, who was killed by Oswald; two days later, he autopsied Oswald himself, who was killed by Jack Ruby; a few years later, he autopsied Ruby.

It is 29 years later and Rose, who has a law degree as well as a medical degree, still feels strongly that the Kennedy autopsy should have been performed in Dallas. "The law was broken," Rose says, "and it is very disquieting to me to sacrifice the law as it exists for any individual, including the President. Having one set of rules for the rich and famous and another for the poor is antithetical to justice. There have been many arguments to try to justify the removal of the body, but to me they all seem like retrospective and self-serving theories. People are governed by rules and in a time of crisis it is even more important to uphold the rules, as this case amply demonstrates."

Rose believes that a Dallas autopsy, which he would have performed, "would have been free of any perceptions of outside influences to compromise the results. After all, if Oswald had lived, his trial would have been held in Texas and a Texas autopsy would have assured a tight chain of custody on all the evidence. In Dallas, we had access to the President's clothing and to the medical team who had treated him, and these are very important considerations."

Further, Rose believes that the removal of the body was the first step in creating disbelief about what had happened. "Silence and concealment are the mother's milk of conspiracy theories," he says. "If we have learned anything in the 29 years since the President was shot, it is that silence and concealment breed theories of conspiracy and the only answer is to open up the records, without self-serving rules of secrecy, and let the American people judge for themselves."

Rose, who is a board-certified forensic pathologist and who has personally examined Kennedy's autopsy materials and records, next turned his attention to the claims made by Dr Crenshaw, who is a surgeon. "I believe that Dr Crenshaw believes what he is saying when he argues that the shots came from the front," Rose says, "but he is mistaken." Pressed on his degree of confidence in this statement, Rose finally says, "I am absolutely sure that he is in error."

Rose was a member of the 1977 House

Select Committee on Assassinations that had access to the entire autopsy file of President Kennedy and that supported the autopsy conclusions. Though he thinks the Bethesda autopsy was "less than optimal," Rose has no argument with the central fact, saying, "I agree that the two wounds to the neck and head came from behind and above and that there is no room for doubt on this finding. The physical evidence corroborates this without question." He concludes, "Do not attribute to conspiracy what can be explained by distrust, inexperience, or ineptitude." Offering his own appraisal of who killed Kennedy, Rose says, "Oswald is the prime suspect and there is no credible evidence for any other suspect. However, there will always be reservations until all the evidence is disclosed. Only this morning the US Justice Department again opposed on the grounds of national security a Congressional resolution to open the Kennedy files."

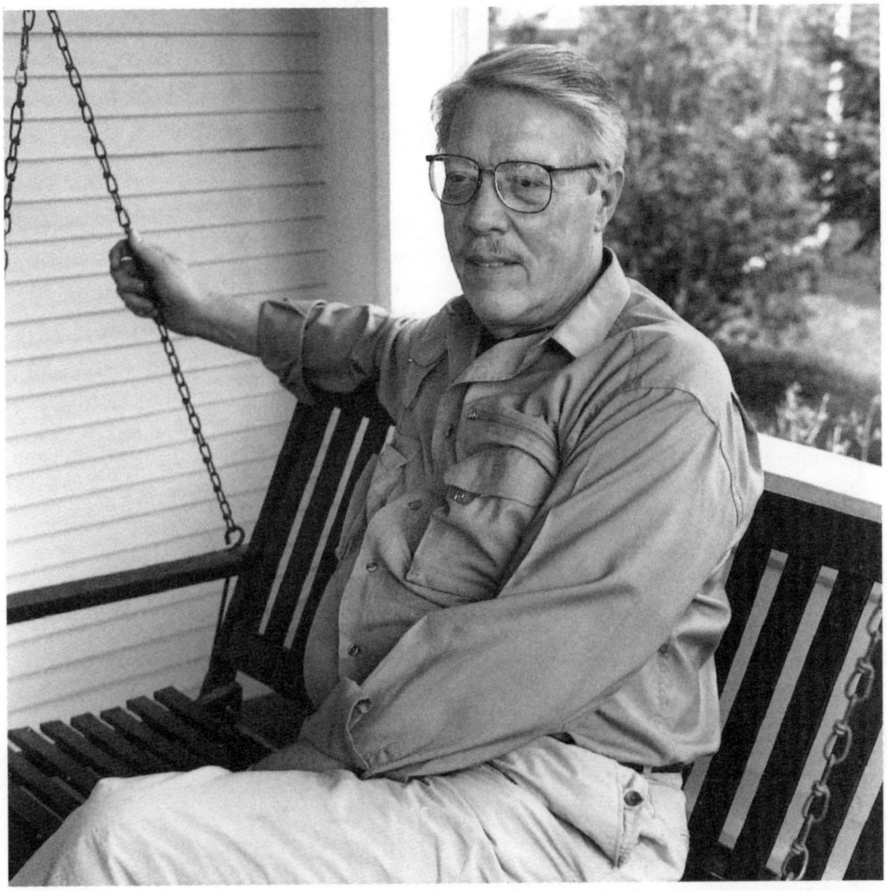

Photo: Dennis L. Breo

Dr Earl Rose: "The law was broken, but I had no minions, no armies to enforce the will of the medical examiner and perform the autopsy in Dallas."

Mistakes and conspiracies

One might think that all this demonstration of facts and expression of expert medical opinion would end the controversy over the President's autopsy, but one would probably be wrong. Even in that Parkland Hospital trauma room there was one other physician who still disbelieves the President's autopsy report. Robert McClelland, MD, is a respected surgeon who assisted in the last steps of the tracheostomy on President Kennedy. Interviewed in Dallas, he told this reporter that he maintains a "strong opinion" that the fatal head wound came from the front. Pressed on his reasons, he says, "After I saw the Zapruder film in 1969, I became convinced that the backward lurch of the head had to have come from a shot from the front. Unlike Crenshaw, I do not believe that one can tell the direction from which the bullet came simply by looking at the head wound, as I did, but the wound I observed did appear consistent with a shot from the front. That observation is secondary to my viewing of the Zapruder film, which convinced me that the shots were from the front." Reminded that at least 16 pathologists have also studied the Zapruder film and *also* examined the autopsy clothing, notes, photos, and x-rays and have concluded the opposite, McClelland remains unshaken. "I can't speak for them," he says, "and although I am not an expert in ballistics, pathology, or physics, I still have a strong opinion that the head shot came from the front."

So it goes. McClelland had originally mistakenly written in his hospital chart that the wound to Kennedy's head struck the *left* temple. This error, as published in the Warren report, later prompted a call from the office of New Orleans District Attorney Jim Garrison, who wanted to bring him to New Orleans in 1969 to testify in the conspiracy trial of Clay Shaw. McClelland recalls, "Well, when I told the investigator that I had made a mistake in 1963, there was a sudden silence at the other end of the line."

Mistakes do happen and contribute to conspiracy theories. Similarly, Dr Jenkins wrote in a 1963 report that Kennedy's "cerebellum" had been blown out, when he meant "cerebrum." Dr Perry appeared at a riotous press conference on the day of the assassination and said that the fatal shot "might have come" from the front. All have become grist for the rumor mill.

Jenkins was a technical consultant to the making of the film *JFK*, advising on the layout and equipment of the Parkland Hospital trauma room. Assured of director Oliver Stone's passion for authenticity, Jenkins was able to help re-create the 1963 room right down to the last detail and also to re-create the original Parkland emergency room entrance, which in subsequent decades has been engulfed by the complex of new buildings constructed at the parent University of Texas Southwestern Medical Center, Dallas. When Jenkins showed up at the set for a day of shooting, he noticed that the actors representing the medical team were all being issued blood-soaked scrub suits. Advising Stone that only he and Mrs Kennedy were splattered with blood, Jenkins was told by the director, "Oh, doc, people expect to see blood!" Jenkins notes, "So much for authenticity." Jenkins himself made a cameo appearance in the film, but says, "I was so bored with the film that I fell asleep and missed my two seconds on camera!"

People expect to read about conspiracy theories and this probably will not change. Earl Rose concludes, "The defamers of the truth can only be confronted and defeated by the truth."

This special report is our attempt to confront the defamers of the truth. □

Letter From Trincomalee

Innocence Abroad

Last July, I returned from working as a physician in Sri Lankan refugee camps. The 4-month experience was interesting medically—treating malaria, typhoid, and vitamin A deficiency. But I more easily learned the necessary pharmacology than I solved the ethical questions that arose.

Volunteering in War-torn Sri Lanka

I volunteered to work in Sri Lanka with the French medical assistance group Médecins Sans Frontières (MSF)—Doctors Without Borders. It was my first experience working in the Third World. In 1971, MSF began to provide medical assistance in Biafra and Bangladesh. The organization has grown rapidly and now operates some 80 missions in 27 countries.

Sri Lanka, formerly Ceylon, is an island off the southern tip of India. Since the 1950s, there have been intermittent clashes between the majority Sinhalese (predominantly Buddhist) and minority Tamils (predominantly Hindu) over the designation of Sinhalese as the official language and ethnic quotas on admission to university and government jobs for the Tamils.[1(pp41-56)] Civil war erupted in 1983, pitting the southern Sri Lankan army against various Tamil guerrilla groups, most prominently the Tamil Tigers (Liberation Tigers of Tamil Eelam) who seek a separate state (Eelam).[2]

The US government has full diplomatic relations with Sri Lanka, but recently has prohibited the sale of lethal weapons to the country because of human rights violations. Both Asia Watch and Amnesty International issue frequent bulletins describing human rights abuses, including widespread arrests, "disappearances," and civilian massacres.[3]

The general level of health of the population is quite good—in the top five of Asian countries. In 1988, infant mortality was estimated at 33 per 1000 live births.[1(p108)] Sri Lanka is rich in natural resources and had one of the better per-capita gross national products in developing Asian countries before the war.[4] It is blessed with rice paddies, fish, bananas, tea plantations, and fertile soil. The people are accustomed to vaccinating children and to the idea that it may sometimes be best to deliver babies in the hospital.

Due to the war and frequent nighttime raids by the army or the rebels, many civilians have fled. Some 210 000 have gone to southern India,[5] and others have chosen to stay in regional refugee camps believing themselves safer there.

Since the outbreak of the war, many professionals have left the country, including physicians. Even before 1983, apparently a considerable number of physicians left the country for higher salaries elsewhere. For a number of years, the government organized a system of field midwives, public health inspectors, and assistant medical officers who should be able to do the health work in peacetime, but many of these medical workers have left the north and others fear to travel. In 1986, MSF was asked to temporarily replace needed physicians and has been there ever since in four locations in the battle-scarred north and east. In addition to providing surgeons and anesthetists for the hospitals, MSF has fielded mobile teams of physicians and nurses who visit refugee camps and small villages. The organization also provides safe transport in its vehicles for vaccines, medical supplies, patients, and local medical personnel.

My job was to oversee the vaccine program the nurses and local personnel ran and to hold outpatient clinics, focusing on prenatal care and various acute complaints—colds, scabies, malaria, and pneumonias. Much time was spent in travel to and from these clinics—3 hours by boat across the Trincomalee Bay and another 2 hours by truck each day. The clinics were staffed by local volunteer health workers, who were a great help in draining abscesses and changing dressings for the innumerable skin infections that the tropics breed.

The Sri Lankan government's attitude toward MSF is ambivalent in the extreme. On one hand the government formally requested assistance from the French organization. On the other hand, MSF works in the north and east and most of the help goes to the Tamils, the very people who are rebelling against the government.

The philosophy of MSF is to treat anyone in need of care: civilian, rebel, or government soldier. This concept of neutrality in health care was naturally difficult for some state officials to grasp. Many government agents—police and army—were angry that we might be treating the Tigers or their families and would sometimes harass us, searching our vehicles and medical bags. We Westerners and the women and pediatric patients we brought with us were usually left alone. However, a young Tamil man would have difficulty getting through the military roadblocks and checkpoints even with us—he would be assumed to be a Tiger and might be detained for "questioning" and perhaps not be seen again.

Every week we had to go to the army headquarters to request a pass to visit villages held by the rebels. There were frequent military roadblocks along the rutted roads. In our white trucks with huge red and white crosses on the sides and roof, a flashing blue light, and mounted flags, we tried to ensure rapid identification of ourselves as neutral parties.

Ethical Dilemmas and the Rules of War

During my first month, I went to a rebel Tiger village and saw a man with an injured arm who had waited 6 days for our arrival. He said he had been shot by a soldier while working in his rice paddy. His ulna was obviously broken. As I brought him back with me to the hospital in our little boat, a navy cruiser stopped us and trained two machine guns on him. They wanted to know his name, what village he was from, and how he had been injured, and they appeared to want to take him with them. I said only that he had hurt his arm and now needed to go to the hospital. I realized I had no idea what the rules were in such matters, or if any even existed. Could they just haul him off the boat? Didn't that violate the Geneva convention or something? After I stood there nervously for a few seconds, they reluctantly shoved off.

Edited by Annette Flanagin, RN, MA, Assistant to the Editor.
Reprints not available.

Realizing that they might subsequently arrest him at the hospital, I went to the International Committee of the Red Cross. The Red Cross resident delegate explained to me that of course the army or police could arrest any patient at any time they wished on whatever charges they chose. I was obligated to tell them anything they wanted to know, except for items of medical confidentiality. And all I could do if a patient was arrested was strongly advise that he needed some medical care. If the government said that they would provide it at a prison hospital, that was sufficient. The Red Cross could attempt to visit the patient afterward, but there were no guarantees. This was my first lesson. I realized how little I understood about the rules in civil war.

The rebels would flag our truck down repeatedly to request medical supplies such as bandages, medications, and antibiotics. So did the army units stationed in outlying areas. I was afraid of jeopardizing our freedom to travel if I gave the Tigers medicines and the government found out. I imagined it must be difficult for the rebels to obtain medicine from their headquarters in the north, but they were obviously getting guns and ammunition, so couldn't they get medicine as well? I was confident that the army could obtain its own medical supplies, but if I gave them some, would that ingratiate us with them and make our travel easier? I decided that we would treat anyone from either side with an acute complaint, but that we would not give either party supplies for possible future use. I wasn't at all sure if this was the best solution.

On an almost daily basis, a Tamil woman at a clinic would tearfully tell of a husband or brother or son who had disappeared while in the paddy or had been taken in for questioning and had not been seen since, or worse yet, whose body had been found in a well. Compared with such tragedies, scabies and malaria seemed inconsequential. Indeed, the greatest single source of morbidity and mortality in Sri Lanka is the violence of the war, perpetuated by the army and the rebels. How could I address that? Despite the villagers' hope that as a foreigner I could help, all I could do was make an attempt at sympathy and take the name and details to add to the long lists handed in to the Red Cross. The United States is supplying foreign aid. Should I write to my US congressmen? In the long run, wouldn't it make more sense for me to agitate in Washington or at the United Nations for a settlement of the war than to lance abscesses and prescribe chloroquine?

In my fourth month of work, another event quickly personalized these heretofore more abstract ethical ruminations. The army attacked one of the MSF vehicles in a neighboring district on an authorized trip. A helicopter opened fire on the truck, destroying it and seriously injuring a nurse and driver, and slightly wounding another nurse and doctor. The truck's occupants used the radio to contact MSF headquarters. We all could hear their desperate pleas for someone to get the helicopter to stop attacking, interspersed with the sounds of gunfire. Suddenly, all the theoretical risks became real.

Immediately, all the teams were ordered to leave the field and come south to the capitol, Colombo. It was the fourth attack in 3 months on one of MSF's trucks—the other three had only been warning shots fired around a truck when the army alleged they could not identify it as an MSF vehicle, but this attack was clearly more than just a warning.

With all four teams present (some 20 health workers), many questions were raised: If we stay despite the attack, are we telling the army that it is open season on international humanitarian organizations (seen as "Tiger lovers" already by most of the rank-and-file military)? If we leave, will the adverse publicity cause the Western governments supporting the Sri Lanka government to push harder for a negotiated settlement and to stop the torture and human rights violations? Or is that hopelessly naive? Ultimately, is it worth risking our lives for this mission? What is my individual duty as a health worker to my patients? Obviously if I am dead, I won't be doing much health work. On the other hand, our departure would clearly hurt those people already suffering most from the war.

Initially, the government blamed the attack on MSF, stating that the team did not have permission to travel and that a rebel truck was behind the MSF truck, firing on the helicopter, neither of which was true. A government commission ultimately ruled that MSF had been at fault, straying into the midst of a battle, despite the fact that the army had given permission to travel on that route. It was decided that MSF would stay in Sri Lanka if better security could be negotiated, but this would not take place until I was scheduled to return home.

Taxi Driver, Witness, or Substitute Doctor?

I am left with a hazy impression of what I accomplished in Sri Lanka. Personally, even before the helicopter attack, I had been uncomfortable with MSF's style of assistance in Sri Lanka. I advocated more teaching of Sri Lankan locals, while my coworkers discounted this approach. I had been feeling that my major contribution during my stay was as an exalted taxi driver/security guard, giving safe transport to patients and vaccines. Was I replacing physicians who were political refugees or physicians choosing a better economic life? Or was I hung up on being a "doctor" and not recognizing that my very presence here as a witness, recording the injustices for the Red Cross or whomever, was more important than whatever suturing I might do or babies I delivered? How does one decide how much compromise is acceptable and at what point must one draw the line and say we can't continue to work here under these conditions? What exactly am I willing to risk my life for?

I can draw no grand conclusion from my experiences in Sri Lanka. I have gained an increased awareness of the complexity of ethical decisions in a war-torn country with a culture very different from my own, however unoriginal that may be. My experience is not unique. There have been similar war conditions in Sudan, El Salvador, Liberia, Croatia, and other countries. Many nongovernmental organizations are toiling away, doing much the same type of work and wrestling with many of these same issues.

Now that I'm back in America, my moral dilemmas consist of deciding where I stand on national health insurance and discussing code status with my patients. It's not the same as wondering what to do about murdered people on the side of the road, but I have come a long way from my medical-school conception of what ethical problems a physician might face.

Sean Stitham, MD
Alaska Native Medical Center
Anchorage

1. Ross RR, Savada, AM, eds. *Sri Lanka: A Country Study*. Washington, DC: Federal Research Division, Library of Congress; 1988.
2. Weaver MA. The gods and the stars. *New Yorker*. March 21, 1988:39-69.
3. Rathman R. *Sri Lanka: Human Rights Violations Escalation in the Northeast*. Los Angeles, Calif: Amnesty International; September 10, 1991. News release.
4. *Economic and Social Survey of Asia and the Pacific*. Bangkok, Thailand: United Nations; 1981:40.
5. West J. Passage to Jaffna. *Asiaweek*. March 8, 1991:13-22.

From the Office of the General Counsel

Corporal Punishment in the Schools

DESPITE broad opposition by professional organizations to corporal punishment in the schools, more than half of the states in this country still permit corporal punishment of students. As of May 1992, only 21 states (Alaska, Arizona, California, Connecticut, Hawaii, Iowa, Maine, Massachusetts, Minnesota, Montana, Nebraska, New Hampshire, New Jersey, New York, North Dakota, Oregon, Rhode Island, South Dakota, Vermont, Virginia, and Wisconsin) and the District of Columbia had bans on corporal punishment, either by statute or regulation (Nadine Block, MEd National Coalition to Abolish Corporal Punishment in Schools, Columbus, Ohio, oral communication, May 1992). In states that allow corporal punishment, most major cities have forbidden its use.[1(p23)] Typically, the prohibition applies only to public schools[2-4]; however, it may apply to both public and private schools.[5] In March 1992, Michigan became the first state to roll back its prohibition (*New York Times.* March 11, 1992:B8); 1 month later, Kentucky became the second state to do so. Corporal punishment in the schools has been challenged under the federal constitution, but courts have concluded that such punishment is acceptable, except when used excessively.

Corporal punishment of students has been defined by the American Medical Association as the "intentional infliction of pain or discomfort and/or use of physical force upon a student as punishment for an offense or behavior."[6] It does not include the use of physical force in self-defense or to protect other people or property. Corporal punishment takes many forms, including spanking, shaking, choking, excessive exercise, disrobement, and confinement in an uncomfortable space.[7(p48)] It has been imposed for violent acts, like fighting with another student, and nonviolent acts, like possessing cigarettes, talking in class, swearing, throwing food, and missing football practice.[7(p49)]

The abolition of corporal punishment in the schools has been advocated by the American Medical Association,[6] the American Academy of Pediatrics,[8] the American Psychiatric Association,[9] the American Public Health Association,[10] and other professional groups. Corporal punishment has already been banned in Great Britain, France, Germany, Spain, Greece, Italy, China, Russia, and many other countries (Nadine Block, MEd National Coalition to Abolish Corporal Punishment in Schools, Columbus, Ohio, written communication, March 1992). The opposition to corporal punishment reflects several concerns: the right of children to be free from physical assault, the lack of evidence showing a need for corporal punishment, the risk of serious harm to students, and the possibility that use of physical force on students will teach them that physical force is an appropriate method of resolving conflicts. The continued use of corporal punishment in most states in this country appears to reflect anachronistic views of children's rights and of the role of physical force in maintaining order in the schools.

The Legal Context

The schools are the only public institution in which corporal punishment is still permitted.[11] Corporal punishment was formerly employed in the prisons and the military, but it has since been outlawed in both settings.[6] Children are the only citizens who are regularly subjected to physical punishment. Ordinarily, any physical harm suffered at the hands of another person constitutes a battery, punishable by civil liability and criminal penalties.

Under federal court rulings, the legality of corporal punishment in the schools is largely governed by state law. The US Supreme Court considered the constitutionality of corporal punishment in *Ingraham v Wright.*[12] In that case, decided in 1977, the Court held that corporal punishment of students never violates the prohibition against cruel and unusual punishment found in the Eighth Amendment to the US Constitution, no matter how severe the force used. According to the Court, the Eighth Amendment was adopted to protect individuals convicted of crimes, not children paddled by their teachers.[12]

The Supreme Court did not decide in the *Ingraham* case, nor has it ever decided whether the Fourteenth Amendment's right of substantive due process applies to corporal punishment of students.[12(p659,n12)] The substantive due process question is whether the right to liberty limits the amount of force that may be used against schoolchildren. The lower federal courts have examined the applicability of the right to liberty; however, they have imposed few limitations on corporal punishment under that right. The US Court of Appeals for the Fifth Circuit (which includes Texas, Louisiana, and Mississippi) has held that corporal punishment of students never violates the right to liberty.[13] Other appellate courts have applied the same standard in corporal punishment cases as that developed for police brutality cases. For example, according to the Fourth Circuit Court of Appeal (which includes Maryland, Virginia, West Virginia, North Carolina, and South Carolina) and the Tenth Circuit Court of Appeal (which includes Kansas, Oklahoma, New Mexico, Colorado, Utah, and Wyoming), the question is

> whether the force applied caused injury so severe, was so disproportionate to the need presented, and was so inspired by malice or sadism rather than a merely careless or unwise excess of zeal that it amounted to a brutal and inhumane abuse of official power literally shocking to the conscience.[14(p613,n7),15(p655)]

The Third Circuit Court of Appeal (which includes Delaware, New Jersey, Pennsylvania, and the Virgin Islands) and the Eighth Circuit Court of Appeal (which includes Arkansas, Missouri, Iowa, Minnesota, Nebraska, South Dakota, and North Dakota) also have adopted their constitutional standards from police brutality cases, but their standards are somewhat more protective of students. These courts look at the need for corporal punishment, the relationship between the need and the amount of force used, the extent of injury caused by the punishment, and whether the punishment was administered "in a good faith effort to maintain discipline or maliciously and sadistically for the very purpose of causing harm."[16(p520),17(p564)]

The Supreme Court in *Ingraham* did hold that students are protected by the Fourteenth Amendment's requirement of procedural due process.[12] That is, students are entitled to procedural safeguards to prevent unjustified uses of corporal punishment. However, the Court did not require any kind of hearing or other opportunity for the student to challenge the imposition of corporal punishment before the punishment is administered. Thus, for example, the student need not be given a chance to correct any misimpressions that the teacher has about the student's behavior. As the Supreme Court observed in an earlier case, however,

> [d]isciplinarians, although proceeding in utmost good faith, frequently act on the reports and advice of others; and the controlling facts and the nature of the conduct under challenge are often disputed.[18]

Despite the concern about inaccuracy, the *Ingraham* Court concluded that adequate procedural protections are provided by state common law. According to traditional principles of the common law, which date back more than 200 years, teachers are permitted to employ a degree of force that is "reasonably necessary" for the "proper control" and education of school children.[12,19,20] If a teacher uses excessive force against a student, then the teacher will be liable under state law for civil damages and possibly criminal penalties.[12] The Supreme Court found that this risk of penalties for excessive force provides sufficient procedural safeguards for students and that therefore due process does not require any additional safeguards.

In deciding whether force is reasonable under the common law, courts look at a number of factors: the nature of the misbehavior, the teacher's motive for inflicting punishment, the likelihood that the force would cause serious or permanent injury, whether the force is proportionate to the misbehavior, the student's age, and the student's physical and mental health.[21-24]

A teacher has been found liable for damages for punching a student three or four times, causing bruises of the chest, arms, and back, after the student struck the teacher a light blow in the back and shot a rubber band into the teacher's face.[24] Liability has also been imposed for pushing a student against a chalkboard and a wall, fracturing the student's clavicle, after the student "improvised sounds in a song which the class was supposed to sing in unison."[25] A teacher has escaped liability after striking the palms of all the students in a class three or four times with a rubber strap because the students had been noisy while leaving class one day and while the teacher was away from the classroom on another day.[26] A teacher was also exonerated after paddling a student four times because of "disruptive behavior in the classroom."[27]

In sum, the law can be characterized as follows: In the absence of a state or local prohibition of corporal punishment, the common law permits school officials to impose force that is reasonably necessary for the proper control and education of children. Procedural due process is satisfied if states subject school officials to civil and/or criminal penalties when the force used exceeds the common law standard of reasonable necessity. Finally, the student generally has a claim for violation of the right to liberty, in addition to a common law claim, when the punishment is "so grossly excessive as to be shocking to the conscience."[15(p656)]

Under these legal rules, corporal punishment has been used liberally. According to data reported to the federal government, there were more than 1 million incidents of corporal punishment in the public schools during the 1986-1987 academic year.[28] Some commentators believe that these data underestimate the actual incidence of corporal punishment in the schools.[11]

If the common law standard were applied strictly, corporal punishment would never be permitted in the schools. As stated previously, the common law holds that teachers may use only force that is reasonably necessary for disciplinary and educational purposes. Research, however, has shown that alternative methods of managing student behavior are more effective than corporal punishment.[8,11,29] Consequently, there should be no need to use corporal punishment in the schools.

Alternative Approaches

Experts have developed a wide range of techniques that are more effective than corporal punishment for responding to the problem of student misbehavior. With these techniques, discipline can be maintained without resorting to physical punishment.

Praise for good behavior and role modeling of proper behavior are examples of effective positive reinforcement techniques.[11,30] In a study of London, England, schoolchildren, there was better student behavior in schools where teachers more frequently praised student work or otherwise showed appreciation for the efforts and accomplishments of the students.[31(p215)] Other studies have found that praise for good behavior is more likely than criticism of misbehavior to promote appropriate student conduct.[32(p374),33] Praise and other encouragement improve behavior by providing feedback to students on what constitutes desirable behavior. In addition, teacher approval improves behavior by enhancing student self-esteem and morale; the better students feel about themselves, the more likely they are to engage in productive activities.[31(p215)] Role modeling of proper behavior was also correlated with better student behavior in the London study. When children like and respect adults in positions of authority, they have a strong tendency to copy the adults' behavior and adopt their values and attitudes.[31(p217)] Discussions about values and student involvement in the development of disciplinary codes also are useful positive methods of behavioral modification.[11(p164)] When students are given greater responsibility at school, they may develop a greater commitment to their education.[31(p216)] As in other contexts, positive reinforcement in the school setting is more effective and longer lasting than negative reinforcement at building character and modifying behavior.[11(p163),30(p272)]

When punishment is necessary, a number of noncorporal alternatives are available, including verbal reprimands, separation of misbehavers by using "time out"[34(pp480-481)] or a "discipline room," loss of privileges, and after-school detention. These methods are effective both for enforcing rules and for helping students become more skillful at developing internal mechanisms of self-control.[11,35]

Often there may be a need to focus on the classroom skills of teachers. The use of corporal punishment appears to be more frequent by teachers who are less experienced, more subject to anxiety, and more likely to act impulsively.[36] Teacher training in communication strategies, educational psychology, and management of student misbehavior can improve the response of teachers to behavioral problems.[11,30] More importantly, better classroom skills can prevent disruptive behavior by students. Teachers who employ good educational techniques experience fewer behavioral problems; students are more engaged in their lessons and less prone to disruptive conduct.[37] In some cases, misbehavior may reflect problems at home or other underlying problems that can be helped by referral to social service agencies. There are also structural changes in the classroom environment that can reduce problems with student misbehavior. Smaller classes and greater use of teacher's aides are important modifications. Even modest changes that make for a more pleasant and comfortable environment can improve student behavior. For example, there is some evidence that good upkeep and attractive decoration of classrooms is associated with better behavior.[31(pp215-216)]

Experimental research on punishment may explain, at least in part, why corporal punishment is not as effective as alternative disciplinary measures. In particular, many of the characteristics of effective corporal punishment are not achievable or acceptable in the classroom setting. For example, corporal punishment is most successful when it is imposed with complete surprise and therefore without prior discussion or explanation, immediately after the occurrence of the misbehavior, and with each occurrence of the misbehavior.[38] In general, the severity of the punishment needs to be high to be effective.[38]

The effectiveness of alternative methods is reflected by the lack of problems in schools that no longer use corporal punishment. When schools have eliminated corporal punishment, there has not been a corresponding increase in disciplinary problems.[39(pp398-399)]

When physical force is used in other contexts without justification, society condemns the force as unacceptable violence. Society should do the same with corporal punishment in the schools.

Negative Consequences

Corporal punishment is not only less effective than alternative approaches to behavioral management, it can also be harmful. While the physical injury from corporal punishment in the schools is typically mild and transient, some students require medical evaluation and/or treatment for injuries, including abrasions, broken bones, nerve or muscle damage, and cerebral hemorrhage. In rare cases, students have died as a result of corporal punishment.[6,11]

Corporal punishment also may have detrimental psychological or counterproductive behavioral effects. Students who are physically punished may experience loss of self-esteem, increased anxiety and fear, and depression.[6,30,38(p364),40] In one study, a strong relationship was found between reports of unfair, harsh, and inconsistent childhood discipline in the home and the development of major depression and alcoholism during adulthood. The relationship was independent of parental psychiatric status and socioeconomic class.[41] Corporal punishment has also been linked to poor attention span and deficient academic performance;[6,11] children who are physically punished may view the teacher as an "aversive individual" who should be avoided.[30(p273),32(pp377-378)] In addi tion, because punishment tends to reinforce any behavior that is successful at preventing further punishment, students may respond to corporal punishment with tardiness or truancy.[38(pp364-365)]

By sending the message that physical aggression is an acceptable means of dealing with anger, corporal punishment may promote aggressive and destructive behavior by students.[11,29,38(p366)] In a three-country comparison of playground behavior, researchers found an association between aggressive behavior by adults and aggressive behavior by children.[42] Corporal punishment has been linked with aggression against teachers and other students and with vandalism against school property.[6(p90),30(p274)] Aggressive behavior against the teacher who imposed the punishment may be employed as a retaliatory mechanism; aggression toward other people or property in the environment appears to be a general response to physical punishment when the punishment occurs in the presence of others.[38(pp365-366)]

Physical punishment during childhood has also been linked to subsequent family violence and other antisocial behavior. Children who are physically punished at home are more likely to physically assault their siblings; adults who were physically punished during childhood are more likely to assault their spouses and children.[43(p142),44] The association between childhood punishment and delinquency has generally been shown for severe physical punishment; there is also evidence suggesting that moderate punishment may predispose to aggressive behavior by the child who is punished.[45] The focus on physical punishment should not obscure the fact that nonphysical punitive measures may be equally harmful if used in an abusive manner.[46(pp169-170)]

The problems with corporal punishment are compounded by an arbitrariness in its use. The administration of corporal punishment in the schools is often related to considerations that are not relevant to student misbehavior. Corporal punishment occurs more in the Southeast, in rural schools, and in smaller schools. Black students are twice as likely as white students to receive corporal punishment; in 1986-1987, a federal government survey found that black students accounted for 16.1% of elementary and secondary school enrollment and 31.4% of episodes of corporal punishment.[28] Students with learning disabilities are also more likely to be physically punished (*New York Times*. March 11, 1992:B8). Corporal punishment is often administered to a degree greatly disproportionate to the student's misbehavior. In one case in which a student used "foul language," a teacher wrapped his arm around the student's neck and applied sufficient pressure to render the student unconscious and cause him to fall face down. The fall resulted in a broken nose, fractured teeth, and other injuries requiring hospitalization.[16] In another case, a student was spanked more than 20 times with a wooden paddle because he was slow in leaving the stage of the school auditorium. As a result of the injuries suffered, the student missed 11 days of school.[47(pp2-3)]

Children's Rights

It is not clear that corporal punishment of students would be justified even if it were an effective method of behavioral control. Like adults, children are entitled to be treated with dignity and respect and to learn in an environment free of physical abuse or the threat of abuse. When society condones physical punishments of students that would not be permitted for any adult, it sends a troubling message about the moral worth of children, a message that is more consistent with the anachronistic view of children as chattel than with the contemporary view of children as human beings who are entitled to the same rights as adults unless there is a compelling reason to treat them differently.

It is particularly troubling that physical punishment is considered most acceptable for those individuals who should be most protected from the risk of physical abuse. Because of their physical and psychological immaturity, children are especially vulnerable to harm from corporal punishment. They are powerless to protect themselves or to lobby for changes in the law. Yet, in school (and at home), they are more susceptible than any other group to being physically punished. The case law on the constitutionality of corporal punishment has been especially unfortunate. It is difficult to understand why criminals should be entitled to more protection under the Eighth Amendment than students. It is also difficult to understand why the Fourteenth Amendment's standard for excessive punishment should be drawn from police brutality cases.

Need for Action

Considerable progress has been achieved in recent years in eliminating corporal punishment from the schools. Before 1984, only six states had abolished corporal punishment of students. Since 1984, 17 more states banned corporal punishment from the schools (*American Medical News*. March 9, 1992:53) before Michigan and Kentucky revoked their bans earlier this year. Utah recently enacted legislation prohibiting corporal punishment of a student unless the student's parent has given written permission for such punishment.[48] Currently, federal legislation is being considered that would deny federal funds to educational programs that permit corporal punishment of students.[49] Individually and through their professional societies, physicians can lobby for passage of this legislation, as well as for passage of legislation that would prohibit corporal punishment in states where corporal punishment is still permitted. While desirable, legislation is not necessary for the elimination of corporal punishment in the schools. Local school boards, or individual schools, can decide to forgo corporal punishment on their own, and they should be encouraged to do so.

The elimination of corporal punishment from all schools would not only enhance the educational process, it would also send a powerful message to society about the necessity of ending violence against children. The government cannot provide an effective leadership role in the effort to stop physical abuse of children when it sanctions corporal punishment of children in its own institutions.

David Orentlicher, MD, JD
Ethics and Health Policy Counsel
American Medical Association
Chicago, Ill

1. Block N, Fathman R. Convincing state legislatures to ban corporal punishment. *Child Leg Rights J.* 1988;9:21-24.
2. Cal Educ Code §49001.
3. Mont Code Ann §20-4-302.
4. Minn Stat §127.45.
5. NJ Rev Stat §18A:6-1.
6. Board of Trustees, American Medical Association. Corporal punishment in schools. In: *Proceedings of the House of Delegates, 134th Annual Meeting.* Chicago, Ill: American Medical Association; 1985:88-92.
7. Clarke J, Liberman-Lascoe R, Hyman IA. Corporal punishment in school as reported in nationwide newspapers. *Child Youth Serv.* 1982;4:47-55.
8. Committee on School Health, American Academy of Pediatrics. Corporal punishment in schools. *Pediatrics.* 1991;88:173.
9. Board of Trustees, American Psychiatric Association. *Corporal Punishment in Schools.* Position statement 890001; 1989.
10. Governing Council, American Public Health Association. Corporal punishment of children in schools and institutions. *Am J Public Health.* 1980;70:308.
11. Poole SR, Ushkow MC, Nader PR, et al. The role of the pediatrician in abolishing corporal punishment in schools. *Pediatrics.* 1991;88:162-167.
12. *Ingraham v Wright*, 430 US 651 (1977).
13. *Coleman v Franklin Parish School Board*, 702 F2d 74 (5th Cir 1983).
14. *Hall v Tawney*, 621 F2d 607 (4th Cir 1980).
15. *Garcia v Miera*, 817 F2d 650 (10th Cir 1987).
16. *Metzger v Osbeck*, 841 F2d 518 (3d Cir 1988).
17. *Wise v Pea Ridge School District*, 855 F2d 560 (8th Cir 1988).
18. *Goss v Lopez*, 419 US 565 (1975).
19. Harper FV, James F, Gray OS. *The Law of Torts.* 2nd ed. Boston, Mass: Little Brown & Co Inc; 1986:389.
20. American Law Institute. *Restatement of the Law Second: Torts 2d.* Rochester, Minn: American Law Institute Publishers; 1985:§147(2).
21. *Tinkham v Kole*, 252 Iowa 1303, 110 NW2d 258 (Iowa 1961).
22. *Willoughby v Lehrbass*, 150 Mich App 319, 388 NW2d 688 (Mich Ct App 1986).
23. *Gaspersohn v Harnett County Board of Education*, 75 NC App 23, 330 SE2d 489 (NC Ct App 1985).
24. *Thomas v Bedford*, 389 So2d 405 (La Ct App 1980).
25. *Sansone v Bechtel*, 180 Conn 96, 429 A2d 820 (1980).
26. *LeBoyd v Jenkins*, 381 So2d 1290 (La Ct App 1980).
27. *Maddox v Boutwell*, 176 Ga App 492, 336 SE2d 599 (Ga Ct App 1985).
28. *1986 Elementary and Secondary School Civil Rights Survey: National Summaries.* Washington, DC: Office for Civil Rights, US Dept of Education; 1987: Table 1.
29. Rudolph AM, Hoffman JI, Rudolph CD. *Rudolph's Pediatrics.* 19th ed. Norwalk, Conn: Appleton & Lange; 1991:30.
30. Dubanoski RA, Inaba M, Gerkewicz K. Corporal punishment in schools: myths, problems and alternatives. *Child Abuse Negl.* 1983;7:271-278.
31. Rutter M. School influences on children's behavior and development: the 1979 Kenneth Blackfan Lecture, Children's Hospital Medical Center, Boston. *Pediatrics.* 1980;65:208-220.
32. Wise JH. The carrot not the stick: comparing the use of reward to corporal punishment in promoting discipline, learning, and human relationships in the classroom. In: Hyman IA, Wise JH. *Corporal Punishment in American Education: Readings in History, Practice, and Alternatives.* Philadelphia, Pa: Temple University Press; 1979:373-383.
33. Lamberth J. The effects of punishment on academic achievement: a review of recent research. In: Hyman IA, Wise JH. *Corporal Punishment in American Education: Readings in History, Practice. and Alternatives.* Philadelphia, Pa: Templé University Press; 1979:384-393.
34. Radin N. Alternatives to suspension and corporal punishment. *Urban Educ.* 1988;22:476-495.
35. Behrman RE, Kliegman RM, Nelson WE, Vaughan VC. *Nelson Textbook of Pediatrics.* 14th ed. Philadelphia, Pa: WB Saunders Co; 1992:48.
36. Rust JO, Kinnard KQ. Personality characteristics of the users of corporal punishment in the schools. *J Sch Psychol.* 1983;21:91-105.
37. Jones VF, Jones LS. *Comprehensive Classroom Management: Motivating and Managing Students.* 3rd ed. Boston, Mass: Allyn and Bacon Inc; 1990:253-278.
38. Bongiovanni AF. An analysis of research on punishment and its relation to the use of corporal punishment in the schools. In: Hyman IA, Wise JH. *Corporal Punishment in American Education: Readings in History, Practice, and Alternatives.* Philadelphia, Pa: Temple University Press; 1979:351-372.
39. Hyman IA. A social science analysis of evidence cited in litigation on corporal punishment in the schools. In: Hyman IA, Wise JH. *Corporal Punishment in American Education: Readings in History, Practice, and Alternatives.* Philadelphia, Pa: Temple University Press; 1979:394-404.
40. Rohner RP, Kean KJ, Cournoyer DE. Effects of corporal punishment, perceived caretaker warmth, and cultural beliefs on the psychological adjustment of children in St. Kitts, West Indies. *J Marriage Fam.* 1991;53:681-693.
41. Holmes SJ, Robins LN. The role of parental disciplinary practices in the development of depresssion and alcoholism. *Psychiatry.* 1988;51:24-36.
42. Bellak L, Antell M. An intercultural study of aggressive behavior on children's playgrounds. *Am J Orthopsychiatry.* 1974;44:503-511.
43. Straus M. Discipline and deviance: physical punishment of children and violence and other crime in adulthood. *Soc Probl.* 1991;38:133-154.
44. Kaufman J, Zigler E. Do abused children become. abusive parents? *Am J Orthopsychiatry.* 1987;57:186-192.
45. Larzelere RE. Moderate spanking: model or deterrent of children's aggression in the family? *J Fam Violence.* 1986;1:27-36.
46. McCord J. Questioning the value of punishment. *Soc Probl.* 1991;38:167-179.
47. Piele PK. Neither corporal punishment cruel nor due process due: the United States Supreme Court's decision in *Ingraham v Wright. J Law Educ.* 1978;7:1-19.
48. Utah Code Ann §53A-11-702.
49. HR 1522, 102d Cong, 1st Sess (1991).

JAMA 100 Years Ago

March 26, 1892

Assaults Upon Medical Men

The profession is pretty well disciplined to expect to hear of assaults on medical men by insane persons or patients. But for them to be assailed by persons in normal mental condition is fortunately a decidedly rare occurrence. An incident of this latter kind, however, is said to have transpired at Chattanooga, Tennessee, February 24. A man and his wife took part in the onslaught, which was made in the public street, with a cowhide. The physician is spoken of as holding an important position in one of the colleges of the city and as a man of prominence in his calling. The assaulted party made a vigorous defense and succeeded in breaking away from these people and in subsequently having them brought in court. The explanation of the affair, as it came out at the hearing before the justice, was that these assailants had employed the doctor to treat a sick child who had died, and the parents thought the doctor had been responsible for the child's death. It appears that while the child was yet alive, the parents consulted another practitioner who told them that their child had been wrongly treated and would probably die. When, therefore, the death took place, the parents, moved by grief and rage, undertook to avenge themselves by publicly castigating the physician of their lost child. There is something so illogical about the accounts of this assault as conveyed to the newspapers over the telegraph wires, that we are inclined to the belief that the truth is not all told in those accounts. Persons who become frenzied by losses or affliction are capable of many inconsiderate acts, but it is exceedingly rare that that frenzy is vented against the profession devoted to healing the sick. But at the same time, no physician, however conscientious or careful, can tell what day or hour he may not be made the object of some undeserved attack, malicious accusation, blackmail, or suit for damages; "for sufferance is the badge of all our race."

Not long ago, an extraordinary incident in the lives of two physicians of Brooklyn, called attention to some of the risks incident to medical practice. It was brought to light in a suit at law of one of these physicians. These physicians were engaged in an instrumental obstetrical case, when word was taken to the husband of the patient that the life of the latter was being endangered by the use of instruments. At the critical point of the operation the husband suddenly appeared in the doorway with a shotgun and threatened the lives of the attendants if his wife should not survive the operation. Here was a conjunction of ignorance, wrath and gunpowder ripe for murder, if the work of the physicians had not ended in the recovery of the patient. In requital for their trouble and peril, these physicians were obliged to bring suit for payment for their services. All of which gives a glimpse of the possible conditions that may surprise the practitioner almost any day, and that will be encountered, as a rule, patiently and silently. Dignity, silence and patience are the lessons inculcated in the school of medical experience. *JAMA*. 1892;18:399-400

April 16, 1892

Castration Recommended as a Substitute for Capital Punishment

Dr. W.A. Hammond has addressed the New York Society of Medical Jurisprudence, at its last regular meeting, on the advantages of castration as a punishment for murder. As reported in the *Medical News*, April 2, Dr. Hammond restricts the scope of his suggestion to the male sex. "Women have become so accustomed to the removal of the ovaries, and these organs are so much less essential to womanhood than the testicles are to manhood, that it might be necessary to substitute imprisonment for life in their case." Female murderers are far less numerous than the males, so that this consideration is not of great moment.

Dr. Hammond seems to be serious in the matter, but he is not sanguine that the measure will be adopted in the lifetime of any of his hearers. For as it took many hundreds of years to abolish torture, and other inhumanities on the part of temporal and ecclesiastical powers, so it may take a long agitation before modern society can consent to his amendment. It is evident that neither capital punishment nor life-imprisonment have that amount of deterrent influence over the criminal class that could be desired, and Dr. Hammond argues that castration would be more effective than either of the older methods. He quotes a French writer who has said that the dignity of a man resides in his testicles, and also the three negroes, castrated in Missouri as punishment for rape, that capital punishment would have been their preference. Many a criminal has told Dr. Hammond, he says, that they would rather hang than lose the organs in question. Juries would feel less squeamish about decreeing guilt, in cases of doubtful testimony, if life-taking were not one of the consequences of finding a man guilty. The punishment would be continuous, and not momentary and intense, and in the continuance of a punitive award will be found its greatest effect. Castration changes the whole relations of the man; and while the brand upon him would be as bad as, or worse than, the mark upon Cain, he would be removed from many criminal tendencies. He cannot open his mouth without exposing what happened to him; his facial expression becomes altered; he becomes effeminate and cowardly. He loses his appetite for alcoholic drink. In the case of a man who mutilated himself while delirious from alcohol, this act was the means of his reformation.

Criminals thus changed might in many instances, be made useful to society much more so than dead men, even if it be the law that slays them. They could be made members of church-choirs, the vocal qualifications of eunuchs are well- known–safe typewriters, dry-nurses, laundry men, policemen, sailors, soldiers, legislators, reporters for mild society newspapers, and other places where originality and "dash" are not requisite.

The brutality of animal nature is reduced by emasculation, Dr. Hammond continues to argue. The fierce ram becomes mild, and the night-roving tom-cat ceases his pugnacious raids. The eunuchs of the Orient are described by travelers as a mild and obedient type of persons, generally trustworthy and fond of the care of young children.

As a means of stopping the propagation of criminals, this form of punishment would be no less effective than hanging. If it had been employed for the last few hundred years the number of criminal acts would have been many thousands less by this time, and the administration of justice would now have become much simpler and less expensive.

In the discussion following the paper, it was stated that more proof is needed to show that castrated males are not liable to commit acts of violence, and even murder. Many crimes are reported as having been perpetrated in the harems of the Orient, and it cannot always be shown that the eunuchs are guiltless. They have a not very enviable reputation in the matter of low cunning, conspiracy and greed, with their usual concomitant traits. Dr. Hammond has limited his present study or discourse to the crime of murder, incidentally referring to the minor blemishes of rape, wife-beating, alcoholism and suicidal proclivities. There is a class of despicable male creatures, in our cities, who prey upon and deprave women, and afterwards beat them, for whom this punitive measure would be admirably adapted to begin experiments with. If it worked well with them, it might be carried upwards into higher walks of vice. *JAMA* 1892;18:499-500

Resident Forum

Why Women Stay

By giving up my privacy and risking criticism by colleagues and friends, I will try to illustrate the painful and humiliating fact that domestic abuse penetrates even the "best" families and affects the "strongest" people. I know. I am a survivor of spouse abuse. One of the most difficult emotional decisions to understand is why, at the first sign of aggression or mistreatment, a woman does not or cannot leave a man who abuses her. It sounds straightforward and easy, but is it?

Let me begin by saying that abusive relationships do not start with violence. Women do not enter into a relationship saying, "It's okay to hurt me." Even abusive relationships usually start romantically, sharing love and trust, building dreams together, and often having children—just as in a normal relationship.

Often, the spouse's controlling behavior is not seen immediately, but develops slowly over time. When a woman realizes how damaging her relationship is, she often has already made an emotional commitment and developed a sense of loyalty to her partner. The bonds between the couple have been built over time and do not suddenly cease to exist. Once abuse enters the relationship, her emotional ties are a great source of turmoil. I know when I took my marriage vows, I meant "for better or for worse." But when "until death do us part" suddenly became a frightening reality, I was faced with some terrifying decisions.

There are myriad and complex reasons for staying in an abusive relationship. The simplest for society to grasp is the fact that many women have no other source of financial support or housing. We ask them to leave their homes behind, cloaked only by the temporary safety of darkness, to hide in community shelters (when there is room), or to live on the streets. Now add the responsibility of caring for several small children onto her shoulders. How many people would choose to take their children from their home, with no guarantee of food or shelter? How realistic are the options that we insist are the "obvious solutions" to this problem?

The fear of retaliation and further victimization by the abuser is another serious concern. The abused woman realizes that if the abuser catches her preparing to leave, or finds her once she has gone, his threats to harm her or her family may soon become a reality. Once, when I tried to leave my ex-husband, he took my dachshund puppy and beat him against the wall. He told me to remember those cries, because if I ever left him or tried to get help, those cries would haunt me, because they would be the cries of my young niece. At that moment, I knew he was capable of every horrible threat he had ever made, and my life was in grave danger.

Abuse by an intimate partner, either emotional or physical, is a commonly unrecognized cause of illness and injury among women. Recent estimates reveal that from 2 million to 4 million women are battered by their "significant other" each year. How long can we, the medical community, continue to ignore this horrifying crime? Physicians are on the front lines of dealing with victims of these acts of violence and have the ability to affect the prevalence of this form of aggression. We also have the responsibility to show compassion.

How can you help? First, educate yourselves, as well as your colleagues and community, about domestic violence. Try not to make value judgments. Your interaction with an abused patient has an incredible effect on her; she is searching for someone to believe her and, if possible, to offer an alternative. An attack by a loved one is an emotionally shattering experience. She needs compassion, not criticism or condescension.

Finally, realize that your actions, or lack of action, can have a huge impact on her life. Be aware that by not asking whether domestic abuse is the cause of your patient's injuries, you could be closing your eyes to the fact that this woman will most likely return home, only to be beaten again . . . and again.

G. L. Bundow, MD
Columbia, SC

Poetry and Medicine

The Man With a Hole in His Face

He has the lower part,
a crescent of face
on the right, and an eye

that sits precipitously
beside the moist hole
where the rest of his face was.

The hole is stuffed
with curls of gauze.

His nurse comes before dawn,
at the moment
the eye fears for its balance,

and fills the wound,
sculpting a tortured landscape
of pack ice.

The man's eye does not close
because any blink
is death,

nor does the eye rest
in mine
when I ask the questions
he is weary of answering.

While I wait here quietly
in arctic waste,
the pack ice cracks
with terrifying songs.

Over the moist hole
where the rest of his face was,
he rises.

This man is the man in the moon.

Jack Coulehan, MD
Setauket, NY

VIOLENCE

Articles published previously in *American Medical News*

The billion-dollar epidemic

By Harris Meyer

FAMILY VIOLENCE costs the nation billions of dollars, experts in the field agree. "It's not out of bounds to talk about $5 to $10 billion a year," says Richard Gelles, PhD, director of the family violence research program at the University of Rhode Island.

Researchers can only guess at precisely how many dollars this intimate plague drains from the economy and from other health care needs.

In 1987, Dr. Gelles and a colleague estimated that annual health care costs resulting from family violence were $44 million. That estimate was based on the low 1980 National Crime Survey estimate of 192,000 assaults within families. They estimated that domestic violence annually caused 21,000 hospitalizations, 99,800 hospitalization days, 28,700 emergency department visits and 39,900 physician visits.

But Dr. Gelles' $5 billion to $10 billion estimate takes into account newer, more accurate estimates of the incidence of family violence, and defines the social costs of the problem more broadly than just health care.

There is evidence to support the higher figure. Consider, for example, that just one hospital, Rush Presbyterian St. Luke's Medical Center in Chicago, ran up one-year charges of $1,156,408, for acute care only, for the 708 patients seen in its family violence program.

Experts agree that Gelles' ballpark estimate is not unreasonable. "It would be powerful to know that billions spent on health care is due to intimate violence," says Linda Saltzman, PhD, a criminologist in the Centers for Disease Control's Division of Injury Control. "There's no question we're spending inordinate amounts of money."

The most obvious component in estimating the cost of family violence is the direct expense of emergency department and doctors' office visits. In one recent year, Rush in Chicago found that the average charge for medical services provided to abused women, children, old people and the few abused men was $1,633. That did not include psychosocial or follow-up care. Elder abuse victims, because of their greater frailty, ran up a much higher average charge—$7,300.

The direct cost of injury treatment, however, may be the smallest part of the costs of battering to the health care system, says Evan Stark, PhD, an assistant professor at Rutgers University. A big item is investigative and protective services in child abuse cases, Dr. Gelles says. For instance, the American Assn. for Protecting Children says that the cost of these services just for children kept in their parents' homes, not out-of-home or foster placements, is $1.4 billion a year.

There are costs to the criminal justice system. For instance, the nation's police spend a third of their time responding to domestic violence calls. And abused children often become delinquent adolescents. Deborah Daro of the National Committee for Prevention of Child Abuse estimates it costs $15 million a year to incarcerate this group in juvenile facilities.

In addition, family violence victims lose productivity on the job. A conservative estimate of the adult earnings loss of children who suffered severe injuries from abuse is $658 million to $1.3 billion a year, Daro says.

But the big outlays, Dr. Stark argues, are associated with secondary psychosocial problems, such as alcoholism, attempted suicide, pregnancy problems and continuing medical utilization for related complaints. These aren't included in Dr. Gelles' larger cost estimate.

Finally, there are sizable social service and income support costs also not included in Dr. Gelles' number, such as welfare and disability payments, shelters and foster care. Foster care alone might consume an additional $5 billion to $10 billion a year, Dr. Gelles says. There's also the economic value of lives lost in family violence episodes.

When these direct and indirect costs of family violence are tallied, this elusive epidemic surely ranks as one of the nation's most expensive health problems. Productivity losses and other costs for family violence injuries are possibly far greater than for the other leading diseases because of the much younger average age of the victims.

Says Dr. Gelles: "If you move to reasonable extrapolations, you can get a figure so high it seems domestic violence is the No. 1 draw on the domestic economy. It might be, but I don't want to make the figure unbelievable."

Nation begins to see family violence as public health issue

By Rebecca Voelker

IN 1992, a family wracked by violence is likely to have more than its day in court.

Its members may spend the night in an emergency department. Or a morning in counseling at a community health clinic. Maybe an afternoon in a physician's office, describing a history of abuse.

After decades in the domain of criminal justice, family violence has arrived in the sphere of public health.

The shift has been gradual. Health and

medical experts say it began in the early 1960s, when the late C. Henry Kempe, MD, published his work on the "battered child syndrome."

For the first time, medical personnel were told they had a duty to inquire about the causes of children's bruises, broken limbs and deaths.

Dr. Kempe's work also came at a time when new social forces gripped the country. The focus was on the rights of the disadvantaged and those who could not lobby for themselves.

Given the political climate, experts say, it's no accident that child abuse surfaced at that time. And in a sense, children paved the way for women.

As the women's rights movement gained steam in the 1970s, public attention focused on wife battering and other crimes of violence directed primarily against women. Once again, the medical community was prompted to ask questions. Why did many women present with bruises, black eyes and broken limbs?

Public awareness of violence against women and children rose dramatically, but health and medical communities were characterized as slow to respond. By the late 1970s, however, the extent of the problem started to emerge.

At that time the U.S. Public Health Service began work on national health objectives for 1990. As researchers reviewed reams of statistics, the impact of violence was undeniable.

"People began to re-examine what the mortality data told us," recalls James Mercy, PhD, epidemiology chief in the injury control division at the Centers for Disease Control.

"It became very evident that if physicians were going to be responsive to major causes of mortality and morbidity, we couldn't ignore suicide and homicide. That was the first time there was an acknowledgment that these were legitimate areas for public health to address."

The resulting health goals included a section on stress and violent behavior. However, health officials remained somewhat removed from family violence until the mid-1980s. In 1983, CDC started its violence epidemiology unit. A year later, researchers there focused on family violence by working with the domestic violence unit of the Atlanta police.

Says Mark Rosenberg, MD, director of injury control at CDC, "It was clear that one type [of violence] of large proportion was domestic and family violence. The estimate is that 25% of violence is among people who are related."

As the interest in family violence grew, public health and medical experts say a turning point came in 1985. Former Surgeon General C. Everett Koop, MD, called for a Leesburg, Va., workshop on violence and health. A flurry of similar meetings followed, as did new research on homicide, suicide and unintentional injuries.

Public health professionals offered a perspective that went beyond arrests and incarceration. Dr. Rosenberg says, "The public health approach is broad-based. There is one thing that characterizes it–the focus on prevention. Public health is looking at prevention of the injury, treatment of the injury and rehabilitation of the individual."

Experts concede there is no pill or vaccine that will quell the devastation of family violence. However, thanks to smallpox, polio and a list of other infectious diseases, there is a systematic approach.

Through surveillance techniques, public health experts will gain a better understanding of who the victims of violence are, as well as who inflicts violence. Surveillance can also reveal circumstances that promote violent acts–alcohol use or poverty, for instance.

"We use these patterns to pick out individuals at greatest risk," Dr. Rosenberg explains. Supplemented with more in-depth research, surveillance may answer questions such as whether potential victims can be identified before violence occurs and how severe the long-term consequences of abuse really are.

In the hands of physicians, this information can lead to the next step in the public health approach against violence–intervention.

"It's critical that we work with health care professionals" to make sure that safe havens and treatment are accessible, says Dr. Rosenberg. "These are the lives of the physicians' patients. It's their patients who are at risk; it's their communities that are at risk."

Finally, public health brings a multidisciplinary approach to family violence. The issue is so complex and pervasive that it requires a broad coalition of caregivers–pediatricians, geriatricians, ob-gyns, psychiatrists, trauma surgeons and family physicians. With collaboration from these groups, Dr. Rosenberg believes the public health approach will beat the odds. "Smallpox was a fact of life, but now it doesn't exist on the face of the Earth. Violence is a fact of life, but we can have the same impact."

Is the rate of family violence increasing or decreasing?

By Beverly Merz

IS FAMILY violence increasing in the United States? Although it is difficult to obtain reliable data, many authorities contend that it probably is.

On the other hand, one set of landmark studies indicates that the rate of family violence may actually be declining. The studies conducted by Richard Gelles, PhD, professor of sociology and anthropology at the University of Rhode Island, and Murray Straus, PhD, of the University of New Hampshire, were the first in which data was collected from family members, rather than extrapolated from police reports.

The first national study, conducted in 1976, surveyed 2,146 individual family members, asking participants to identify how they, as well as their spouses and a referent child, responded to conflicts with family members. The participants were given a choice of 20 responses ranging from "discussed the issue calmly" to "used a knife or gun." The choice of responses encompassed the range of verbal and physical abuse; it did not include sexual abuse.

More than 3% of parents reported that they committed a potentially injurious act of violence against their children that year. More than 16% of women reported that they had been struck by their husbands at least once during their marriages. Almost 4% were victims of physically abusive violence each year. Approximately 0.2% were at some time threatened with weapons.

Nearly 5% of men surveyed reported they had been hit by their wives. However, the investigators determined that more than 75% had been hit because they initiated the violence.

A decade later, however, Drs. Gelles and Straus employed Louis Harris Associates to telephone 60,002 households, asking virtually the same questions interviewers had asked in 1976.

The Second National Family Violence Survey revealed that the rate of child abuse apparently had declined by 47%–from 3.6% to 1.9%–and that the rate of violent abuse to wives had dropped from 3.8% to 3.0%, a 27% decline. Only the rate of violence against husbands remained virtually unchanged.

"Quite frankly, we had expected to find no change in the rate of domestic violence. The rate of decline was more than we ever could have expected," Dr. Gelles said.

The second study might have contained methodological artifacts because the subjects were interviewed by telephone rather than in person, a feature that eliminated many of the lowest income households (those without phones), Dr. Gelles said. He and Dr. Straus also acknowledge that by 1985 publicity stigmatizing wife-beaters and child-abusers may have rendered people more reluctant to admit that they engaged in such behaviors. The researchers think, however, that reluctance among abusers might have been offset by an increased willingness of victims to speak up.

They speculate that several factors–an increase in childbearing age and decrease in numbers of unwanted children born, improvements in the economy, increasing alternatives for battered women, the development of treatment programs for abusers and the enactment of stronger legal measures against offenders–were responsible for the decline.

Giving comfort to the abused

By Janice Perrone

IN 1975, Courtney Esposito's boyfriend beat her. "I went to a clinic and was basically laughed at," she remembers. "People were amused that this had happened. The doctor gave me crutches and pain pills. But he didn't do a physical exam, didn't screen for broken bones or head injuries. He didn't take it seriously, and his attitude made me feel ashamed. My main purpose in going there was to get help. My main goal once I got there was just to leave."

In 1991 another woman's boyfriend beat her, severely, and she went to a hospital emergency department in Princeton, N.J. "The doctor said to her, 'Another one of you women. I'll patch you up and send you on your way and you'll go right back to him. I'm sure I'll see you again in a few weeks,' " said Esposito, who often makes presentations to health care professionals about domestic violence. "In 15 years there was no improvement in the attitude of the attending physician."

Experts agree that scenes such as these are still played out all too often in the offices and emergency departments to which abused women come seeking help. A physician's uncaring or judgmental attitude can compound the psychological damage done to a victim of abuse and discourage her from taking action to protect herself.

Said Carole Warshaw, MD, head of an AMA committee that helped to prepare guidelines to help physicians identify and counsel victims of domestic violence: "Only a small percentage of doctors have taken an active interest in these issues and deal with them appropriately."

Yet the physician's role can be crucial, said Dr. Warshaw. "Battered women are often reluctant to reveal they've been abused for a myriad of reasons, including shame, fear and humiliation. A physician may be the first and only person they reach out to for help. If the physician is blaming or judgmental, a woman who has been battered will probably try to protect herself from further abuse by withdrawing, and will be less likely to reach out [for help] again. But studies have shown that if battered women are asked about abuse directly, in a gentle, caring way, they do respond."

Identifying victims of domestic violence

First, say the experts, physicians must be alert to the possibility of domestic violence. "Often, physicians don't think about family violence," Esposito said. "One of the biggest problems in identifying victims is that doctors just don't ask any questions."

Esposito, Dr. Warshaw and others involved in the domestic violence field agree that it's critical for health care personnel to *routinely* assess female patients for abuse. "The thinking used to be–ask questions when you see clues for abuse. But the problem is so prevalent that now we feel doctors should ask every woman about abuse and violence in her life," said Dr. Warshaw, the director of behavioral science for the primary care internal medicine residency at Chicago's Cook County Hospital.

"Sometimes patients are afraid to tell you what happened in their own words, but if you ask them direct questions they may at least answer 'yes' or 'no' or give non-verbal responses. This makes it easier for women to reveal the abuse without feeling that they're telling on their partner."

Asking questions routinely also will identify women who are in danger but who have been hurt only once or who have been threatened but not yet hit, said Esposito.

"If you look only for black eyes, broken jaws and bruises, you're missing most victims. There will be many victims whose lives may be in imminent danger but who don't have a mark on them."

Esposito also advises physicians to hang posters from local domestic violence programs in their offices. "It helps patients realize that abuse is a health care issue and also may help them open up when you ask questions about it."

Doctors may need to practice asking sensitive questions before they feel comfortable doing it. Esposito suggests practicing in front of a mirror, into a tape recorder or with friends. "They should practice until they feel uncomfortable when they *don't* ask patients."

Dr. Warshaw said that not only is it often uncomfortable for physicians to ask the questions, but it's also often personally painful for them to hear the answers.

"Physicians need to begin to recognize that one reason they might not be routinely screening is because it is difficult to hear about violence. Having protocols is not enough. If MDs aren't able to work with the feelings that may be evoked by talking to women who've experienced violence, they may avoid asking the questions."

She suggests that physicians examine their reactions to patients' stories. They can discuss the situation with a colleague or have a consultant come in to talk with them about the issue.

"It's also possible to have someone else in the office, a nurse, for example, do the screening. The important thing is that someone ask."

It's abuse—now what?

Once a physician has determined that a woman has been abused, it is vitally important that he or she not inflict further injury by exhibiting an uncaring or judgmental attitude. "Don't ask the victim why she doesn't leave, or why she puts up with it. That makes her behavior the problem when the problem is *his* behavior," said Esposito. "We do it unwittingly, but all it does is isolate the victim further."

Dr. Warshaw acknowledged that it may be difficult for physicians to empathize with someone who seems to tolerate being treated badly, someone who feels helpless and overwhelmed. "As physicians, we're trained to be aggressive and in control."

But physicians also need to realize that abusers often try to humiliate their victims, she said. "So if physicians treat a patient in a objectifying and invalidating way, they are actually recreating an abusive experience."

Esposito pointed out that the abuser may have threatened the woman, her children or her relatives. The doctor also may not realize that divorce increases the likelihood that a violent incident will occur.

"Doctors think that, if you leave, the abuse will stop. But sometimes it escalates. The idea is not to tell her 'you should do this' but to be kind and open doors for her. That's a better intervention."

Esposito advised doctors to tell the patient that she's done the right thing by coming for medical help and by talking about the abuse. "Even if she says she's not being abused but you think she is, it's still important to let her know that you're a safe person to talk to about it. She'll talk when she's ready."

Patients may also be concerned that the doctor will think less of them if they admit to being abused, or that their physician will report the abuse to the police. "It's important to note that violence in the family is common and that the conversation is just between the two of you," Esposito noted.

"Just acknowledging the issue with a battered woman is a success. Let her know that you want to help. Tell her that you will treat her for her physical or emotional injuries and refer her to others who can help with day-to-day safety."

Domestic Violence: A Guide for Health Care Professionals, published by the Division on Women of the State of New Jersey's Dept. of Community Affairs, lists many other steps for health care professionals to take when their patient has been battered:

- A suspected victim should be treated with warmth and respect and as an adult. Refer to her as "Ms." or "Mrs." and not by her first name.
- If a patient feels guilty or ashamed, counter it by saying that a violent act is always the responsibility of the violent person. Stress that no one deserves to be beaten. If she becomes angry about her suffering, tell her you share her anger. It will make it easier for her to consider the next step in escaping a violent life.
- If time is available, allow the patient to talk herself out. But do not encourage her to talk if you don't have the time to listen; this will only add to feelings of rejection and isolation.
- Tell the patient that she is not alone, that other patients have come to you with similar problems. Tell her that battering is widespread and that education, race or religion make little difference in who batters.
- Don't get angry for the patient. You can't live a patient's life for her. Besides, a time of crisis may not be the right time for a patient to make a life-changing decision. Helping her become calm and composed will enable her to consider alternatives.
- Tell her that battering frequently leads to other problems such as alcohol or child abuse.
- Regardless of whether victims return to their homes, they should be encouraged to have a plan of action for the next episode of violence. This includes keeping important documents handy and having immediate access to an extra set of keys, emergency money, transportation, phone numbers for the police and rescue squad, the address of a safe house and the local domestic violence hot-line number.
- Resist the temptation to pressure the patient to accept help or to unnecessarily contact her at a later date. Such intervention not only constitutes a violation of privacy but may put victims in greater danger.

Perhaps one of the best responses is to stress that many patients, from all walks of life and in all conditions, have gotten help and gone on to make new lives for themselves.

"Doctors can empower patients by acquainting them with strategies that have worked for others and by supporting them in reaching their own conclusions," said Esposito, who helped write the New Jersey manual. "Give them options, not orders. Show concern for their safety, give reassurance, respect, information, referrals and, most importantly, hope for the future."

Doctors can help by serving as 'intimate friends'

By Flora Johnson Skelly

ROBERT E. MCAFEE, MD, vice chairman of the AMA Board of Trustees, tells a story about his first meeting with Kevin J. Fullin, MD. A Kenosha, Wis., cardiologist, Dr. Fullin has helped to develop a hospital-based advocacy program for victims of domestic violence, and in 1991 was chosen by the AMA to appear in a series of national advertisements recognizing the dedication of America's doctors.

Dr. McAfee, a surgeon, said to Dr. Fullin: "I understand you treat battered women."

Dr. Fullin replied: "And so do you." Although figures on family violence are hard to come by, there's little doubt that its victims are seen by almost all physicians in almost all specialties. "We see the victims of violence actually in larger numbers than the police," notes Deborah Prothrow-Stith, MD, assistant dean at the Harvard School of Public Health and a former Massachusetts Commissioner of Public Health.

Dr. McAfee acknowledges that he has certainly seen victims of family violence. He also acknowledges that he may not have recognized some of them.

"I recall patients who came to me with

relatively minor injuries, but great anxiety," he says. "Perhaps I didn't ask the right questions. If I had been more perceptive ... " Instead, he says with deep regret, he dismissed these patients' conditions as "non-surgical problems."

But Dr. McAfee will not make many such mistakes again; nor, if he has his way, will other physicians.

As a primary spokesman for the AMA's new Physicians' Campaign Against Family Violence, he is leading a national effort to raise physician awareness about this problem and engage the medical community in efforts to address it.

There are many reasons for physicians to get involved in such a campaign, Dr. McAfee says. The most obvious is that they are seeing these patients in large numbers. The tide will ebb only when physicians begin to treat the problems that cause these injuries and deaths.

Marshall Rosman, PhD, director of the AMA's Dept. of Mental Health, makes the point this way: "When you see a pregnant woman with a bruise to the abdomen and diagnose that as a bruise, that is an incorrect diagnosis. And an incorrect diagnosis will lead to incorrect treatment.

"She was kicked in the belly. The treatment for that is very different from the treatment you would order for a simple bruise." AMA officials also note that physicians enjoy a unique position of public trust, and with it unique responsibilities. An AMA survey found, for example, that more than 80% of Americans said that they could tell a physician if they had been either a victim or a perpetrator of family violence–significantly more than the 75% who would tell a police officer and about as many as would tell a priest, pastor or rabbi. A fourth said physicians could do a great deal, and another 44% said physicians could offer some help to control or reduce the amount of family violence.

There is also the not-inconsiderable factor of rising health care costs. Dr. McAfee said in a speech in February: "Violence affects physicians because we are criticized from so many quarters for the rising cost of health care when in truth one of the factors driving costs up is the reality that the United States is one of the most violent nations in the so-called civilized world."

And, finally, there are the obligations of citizenship. In an interview, Dr. McAfee said, "If you have any cognizance at all of the worsening problem of violence happening in this country, you have to ask, 'What can I do?' Part of the physician's code of ethics is to be a good citizen. You are obliged to do a bit more because you are a physician."

Do these emerging demands on physicians require a shift in their traditional roles? In some sense, yes, the experts say.

Physicians are being asked to play a greater role in prevention, and spend more time counseling patients. But that demand is being made of physicians in a number of contexts.

Addressing family violence requires physicians to go still further: In some cases, they may need to be aware of and make referrals to various social service agencies. They may need to help start programs, as Dr. Fullin did. Dr. McAfee says the AMA may even be asking its members to press for shifts in public policy affecting family violence. But in another sense, says Sandra Kaplan, MD, of the Division of Child and Adolescent Psychiatry of North Shore University Hospital in Manhasset, N.Y., physicians are really being asked only to return to their traditional roles.

"This problem demands that we again become very involved with our patients and their families," says Dr. Kaplan, a member of the AMA's advisory panel on family violence. "It's a return to the physician as an intimate friend of the family, to what medicine was once so honored and cherished for in our culture. That's the kind of medicine that this demands."

When the golden years are tarnished

By Flora Johnson Skelly

A PHYSICIAN treating elderly patients must always be on the lookout for abuse. "Regardless of the history being provided by person, family or caregiver, there's potential for abuse, neglect or exploitation of an elderly patient," said Kenneth Chelucci, MD, director of emergency services at Riverside Hospital in Toledo, Ohio.

How to identify an abused elder

"Guidelines for Physicians: Identification of Abuse Victims," a document prepared by the Elder Abuse Prevention Project, Community Care Organization of Milwaukee County Inc. and distributed by the Wisconsin Bureau on Aging, lists a number of signs in three categories:

- Physical indicators: Burns, bruises, contractures, decubitus, dehydration, diarrhea, impaction, lacerations, malnutrition, urine burns/excoriations, incontinence, poor hygiene, duplication of medication, alcohol/substance abuse, repetitive hospital admissions.
- Family/caregiver indicators: The elder may not be allowed to speak for himself/herself or be interviewed without the presence of the caregiver; obvious absence of assistance, or indifference or anger by the caregiver toward the elder person; family member or caregiver "blames" the elder (e.g., accusation that incontinence is a deliberate act); aggressive behavior toward the elder; previous history of abuse by family member/caregiver to others; unwillingness or reluctance of family member/caregiver to comply with service providers in planning for care and implementation; family history of alcohol/drug abuse or mental illness; conflicting accounts of incidents by the family, supporters and victim.
- Behavioral indicators: Agitation, anxiety, withdrawal, isolation, confusion, fear, depression, anger, disorientation, resignation, hesitation to talk openly, implausible stories, non-responsiveness.

The document notes that, although these behaviors "do not in themselves indicate abuse or neglect of an elder person," they suggest that the physician should take a closer look at the situation.

What to do

The best option for a physician who believes an elderly patient is being abused is usually to report the abuse to an agency that can offer a multidisciplinary intervention. That agency will usually be the state's Dept. of Human Services, said Julie Coyle, director of Catholic Charities for the Eastern Region of the Toledo (Ohio) Diocese.

Both she and Dr. Chelucci noted that the physician should also document the abuse. Their manual, *Elder Abuse: Acute Care Resource Manual*, gives detailed information on how to document abuse and on how to build a multidisciplinary team to handle cases of abuse. (It can be ordered for $19.95 plus $2.50 shipping and handling from Elder Abuse Specialists, 3826 Martha Ave., Toledo, Ohio 43612; (419) 476-4583, (419) 729-6128.)

In many states, physicians are legally

required to report instances of elder abuse. But in states where there are no reporting laws, or where reporting is voluntary, the physician's responsibility is not as clear-cut.

Experts note that elderly patients may be reluctant to have abuse reported to authorities; the reasons can include pride; fear of retaliation, isolation, institutionalization or abandonment, or a sense of guilt or responsibility toward the abusers. Although some experts believe that reporting is always desirable, others believe the patient's wishes should be respected.

But the experts also say that physicians can play a crucial role in determining whether patients seek or accept help. "If a physician says, 'I can see what's happening to you. I'm worried. This is what I want you to do,' that would more likely convince an older person that they would indeed want to receive services," said Jane Raymond, elder abuse specialist for Wisconsin Bureau on Aging.

Even if the physician cannot persuade the patient to allow reporting of the abuse, "the physician can at least affirm the patient's story and empower the patient to make decisions that could really make a difference."

'Red flags' offer clues in spotting domestic abuse

By Janice Perrone

"OVER THE years people in this field have determined what clues indicate that abuse is happening," said Carole Warshaw, MD, chair of an AMA committee that helped prepare guidelines to help physicians recognize and counsel victims of abuse.

Although many women who are being abused will show none of these signs, Dr. Warshaw noted, when the signs *are* present "physicians should see them as red flags."

- An abused woman may make appointments but not show up.
- The batterer may come with her and try to stay close at hand during the examination, in order to monitor what is said.
- She may have multiple injuries at a number of sites.

Sites favored by batterers include, initially, the face, and subsequently, the "bathing suit pattern"–the area that would be covered by a one-piece bathing suit. This is because abusers learn to injure their victims in areas that will be covered by clothing.

- She may also have sustained injuries on the neck from strangulation attempts and fractures to her upper extremities, which result from efforts to defend herself.
- If she is not being treated for severe trauma, her complaints may include headaches, insomnia, choking sensations and stomach, chest, pelvic and back pains.
- If she has medical disorders such as diabetes and hypertension, these may have been aggravated by the abuse, especially if the abuser refuses to allow her to take medication.
- She may be shy, frightened, embarrassed, evasive, anxious or passive.
- She may be hesitant to provide information about how she was injured, and her explanation may not fit the observed injuries.
- She may cry.
- She or her spouse may have a history of psychiatric problems–such as depression, anxiety, panic disorder or suicide attempts–or of alcohol or drug abuse.
- She may have a history of "accidents."

"But keep in mind that lack of an extensive history doesn't automatically mean there hasn't been abuse," warned Courtney Esposito, who lectures to health care professionals on domestic violence. "A victim may not return to the same physician after each beating or may be prevented from seeking treatment."

Finally, research shows that a significant number of women are beaten while pregnant.

"And abusers go for what represents the baby," said Esposito. "If a pregnant woman presents with injuries to her breasts, genitalia and abdomen, it is very likely the result of a beating."

Questions to ask women patients

Experts on family violence agree that physicians should routinely ask women patients about possible abuse. Many suggest that such questions should be asked even if the patient shows no signs of having been abused.

Domestic Violence: A Guide for Health Care Professionals, published by the Division on Women of the State of New Jersey's Dept. of Community Affairs, suggests several questions that will help elicit information about abuse:

- Have you ever experienced a relationship in which you were hit, punched, kicked, threatened or hurt in any way? . . . Are you in such a relationship now?
- You mentioned your partner uses drugs/alcohol. How does your partner act when drinking or on drugs? . . . Is he verbally or physically abusive?
- Has there been any time when you and your partner have physically fought?
- You mentioned that your partner loses his temper with the children. How are things between the two of you?
- You seem to have some special concern about your partner. Can you tell me more? . . . Are you fearful? . . . Has he ever hurt you?
- Do your verbal fights include physical contact?
- Many patients tell me that they had an argument with a partner and later state they were beaten. Could this be happening to you? . . . Are you being beaten?
- Sometimes when a partner is overprotective and as jealous as you describe, they react strongly and use physical force. Is this happening in your situation?
- I notice you have a number of bruises. Could you tell me how they happened? . . . Did someone hit you?

VIOLENCE

Articles published previously in the Specialty Journals of the American Medical Association

Trauma

The Motor End Plate of Violence

The editors of the American Medical Association scientific journals are devoting their June issues to the subject of violence in our society. The impact of violence on societal structures has produced medical, social, psychological, and economic effects which are quite staggering and increasing. The recent riots in Los Angeles resulting in more than 50 deaths triggered by a court decision are evidence of the volatility of violence in our society. Violence is inherently mediagenic. Several distinguished surgeon-traumatologists have been asked to participate in this issue of the ARCHIVES because of their interest, knowledge, and leadership in these areas. They have discussed the impact of violence on a discipline which has responded to injuries resulting from civil disorders, auto-pedestrian accidents, and the ever-increasing availability and use of guns.

Although the pathogenesis of violence is multifactorial, **trauma is the motor end plate of violence.** Civilian trauma in urban areas has made intense, costly demands on surgeons and hospitals during the last decade. A combination of drugs, crime, alcohol, gang warfare, and faster modes of transportation have contributed to the disturbing number of penetrating and blunt injuries admitted to hospitals. The American Board of Surgery states that trauma is one of its primary areas of responsibility which includes "the comprehensive management of trauma, including musculoskeletal, hand, and head injuries. The responsibility for all phases of care of the injured patient is an essential component of General Surgery."[1]

Our involvement in 20th century global wars provided fertile training ground for surgeons. The discipline of Traumatology evolved from these experiences. In more recent years war has been replaced by geometrically increasing violence in our urban areas. Some have observed that the surgical lessons of war have converted many surgeons from mediocrity to excellence. Trauma is an intensive part of training modern-day surgeons. Access to these experiences has become increasingly important to surgical postgraduate education. The improved care of the trauma patient resulting from military and civilian experiences has been chimerical for all phases of our society. Violence has reached suburban and rural America. Concerned individuals have begun to address communication and transportation needs as part of the overall trauma system to deal with an increasing number of injuries in rural areas.

In addition to improved patient care, Traumatology has (1) become a valuable educational tool, (2) opened up new vistas of research, and (3) become a multidisciplinary effort. The trauma center has enabled the salvage of cases previously thought not possible, identified curable lesions that could be lethal if left unrecognized, and played a vital role in the development of our intensive care units. Trauma care and the intensive care unit are inseparable. (See Moore et al in this issue.) It is difficult to imagine what effect violence would have had on our hospitals had trauma units not been available in urban areas.

The recent closure of trauma centers, mainly for financial reasons, is a matter of continuing national concern as addressed in this issue. These specialized units are considered by many as an **albatross** at budget time or moments of tranquility. This reaction rapidly escalates to that of institutional and metropolitan **treasures** in case of fire, earthquake, or other regional-local-national disasters. Despite being widely lauded during moments of crises, the public's memory and gratitude for the trauma unit is too often short-lived. Two perceptions regarding trauma centers continue to plague hospitals: (1) trauma centers siphon needed resources from the remainder of the hospital, and (2) the nontrauma patient does not have equal and immediate access to these same resources. However, the demands of traumatologists and society to meet high standards of care for the victims of violence have brought new resources and additional personnel previously unavailable to these institutions.

Surgery is addressing on a continual basis the participation of surgeons in the care of trauma patients. In a recent report by Richardson and Miller,[2] two thirds of the current general surgery residents completing their training believed that trauma was a rewarding field, but only 18% wanted it as a career or as a major part of their practice. Richardson and Miller further state that the interest of these residents in trauma fellowships was very low and that their primary reasons for these negative feelings were the large amount of nonoperative care rendered in treating blunt trauma patients and the unsavory type of patients encountered with most penetrating trauma injuries.

Esposito and colleagues[3] undertook a survey of the Washington State Chapter of the American College of Surgeons to document their opinions on trauma care issues and found that 39% of the total sample of surgeons who responded would prefer not to treat any trauma patients. Their conclusions were driven by the perception that trauma would have a negative impact on their practice and their perception of increased medical-legal risk. Reimbursement and location of practice were less influential factors.

The problems confronting surgery in a society with escalating violence will require sustained high-quality professional services for these victims, a reversal of the erosion of financial support for trauma centers, adequate funding for trauma-based biomedical research, and a renewed commitment from our surgical colleagues. **Traumatologists cannot do it alone!** In addition there is a spectrum of bioethical issues generated by trauma center clinical successes.

As surgeons we cannot isolate ourselves from societal trends that profoundly affect our professional activities. Because we do not live in a completed society, injustice will continue to be one of the root causes of violence. If we are to disrupt this cycle of violence, as citizens and surgeons too, we must be as concerned about the absence of justice as the mere presence of peace.

CLAUDE H. ORGAN, JR, MD
Editor
Oakland, Calif

References

1. *Booklet of Information (1991-1992).* Philadelphia, Pa: The American Board of Surgery Inc; p 9.

2. Richardson JD, Miller FB. Will future surgeons be interested in trauma call? Results of a resident survey. *J Trauma.* 1992;32:229-235.

3. Esposito TJ, Maier RV, Rivara FP, Carrico CJ. Why surgeons prefer not to care for trauma patients. *Arch Surg.* 1991;126:292-297.

Future Shock

Donald Trunkey, MD

The intent of this article is to give my vision for the future of trauma care. To do so, it is necessary to establish a very brief history of trauma systems and to describe the current status of trauma systems and trauma care.

According to Majno,[1] it was the Greeks who introduced the first rudimentary trauma system. The wounded were tended to in barracks (*klisiai*) or in nearby ships. The Romans expanded this concept and provided special quarters called *valetudinaria*. Most *valetudinaria* were built during the first and second centuries AD, and their primary purpose was as sites at which medical care was provided to the Roman legionaries. These *valetudinaria* were relatively sophisticated, and there was a ready regular medical corps. At least 85 army physicians have been noted from casualty records. Paradoxically, in Rome, there were no hospitals, and civilian trauma most likely was handled by private physicians.

The next effort to introduce a system of trauma care was by Dominique Larrey, the great French military surgeon. His contribution can best be appreciated by his efforts before the Russian campaign.[2] Larrey did not know which country Napolean was planning to attack, and there was even conjecture that there may be an invasion of England. He left Paris on February 24, 1812, and was ordered to Mentz, Germany. Shortly thereafter he went to Magdeburg and then on to Berlin, where he began preparations for the campaign, still not knowing precisely where the French army was headed. In his own words, "Previously to my departure from this capitol, I organized six divisions of flying ambulances, each one consisting of eight surgeons. The surgeons-major exercised their divisions daily, according to my instructions, in the performance of operations, and the application of bandages. The greatest degree of emulation, and the strictest discipline, were prevalent among all the surgeons"[3] Earlier in his preparation for the capture of Corfu, Greece, Larrey laid down three rules for his army surgeons.

> The first of these, which had for its object the prevention of disease and contagion, embodied some of my views on hygiene which I shall not repeat here as they have been given in my account of the campaign in America. They emphasize the supreme importance of seeing to the cleanliness and sanitation of the vessels and detail the means of preventing the ill effects of idleness by constant exercise. The second set of instructions laid down rules for the placing of medical officers in ships, their duties during a voyage and at the time of landing, and for the disbursal between the ships of surgical instruments, materials for dressing, medicaments and light foods. It is especially important to impress upon surgeons destined for far off expeditions that they should not assemble all their materials in one and the same place, on account of the dangers inherent in a voyage and the possibility of everything being lost should the vessel unhappily founder. Such things ought to be as widely distributed, which makes for easier transport and is infinitely more convenient, as we found by experience in Egypt.[3]

It is evident that Larrey had a clear grasp of the details for building a trauma system to support Napoleon. In 1976, the American College of Surgeons Committee on Trauma first developed a formal outline of injury care called *Optimal Criteria for Care of the Injured Patient*. Task forces of the Committee on Trauma have met approximately every 4 years and have updated the criteria, which are now used extensively in establishing regional and state trauma systems.

CURRENT STATUS

Although the American College of Surgeons Committee on Trauma has written extensively on the optimal criteria for trauma care, the current status of trauma care in the United States is less than optimal. It has been recently estimated that less than 25% of the entire geographic area of the United States is serviced by a trauma system.[4] The 75% of the country that is not serviced primarily comprises the Midwest, Rocky Mountain West, and other rural areas. In a report published in 1988,[5] only two states were found to have all eight recommended components of a trauma system. Nineteen states had one or more of the essential components, whereas 29 states had no formal trauma center designation. Since publication of that report, some states have initiated the process, but it should also be pointed out that at least 61 trauma centers have been closed for various reasons.[6] Paradoxically, there are nine studies in the surgical literature that support the efficacy of a trauma system once it has been established.[7-15]

The reasons for suboptimal trauma systems are complex and many, some of which I have previously addressed.[4,16-18] One of the more comprehensive reviews of trauma care in a single state has been conducted by Udell Reseach Associates, West Palm Beach, Fla (unpublished data, 1989). A summary of their findings shows

Accepted for publication March 24, 1992.
From the Oregon Health Sciences University, Portland.
Reprint requests to Oregon Health Sciences University, 3181 SW Sam Jackson Park Rd, L223, Portland, OR 97201 (Dr Trunkey).

that in 1989 114 800 persons in Texas suffered traumatic injury severe enough to require hospitalization. The cost of this care, which was provided by 403 hospitals, was almost $600 million. During the same year, the costs of care for 30 860 patients with trauma was uncompensated, resulting in a loss to hospitals of $157 million. One of the most interesting findings by Udell was that 34 hospitals, which is less than 10% of the hospitals in the state with emergency departments, provided 69.5% of this uncompensated trauma care. The same hospitals provided 76.5% of the uncompensated hospital care for patients with *major* trauma and 82% of the uncompensated care for severely injured patients with trauma.

The average hospital in Texas treating patients with major trauma provided $3 291 940 in uncompensated trauma care in 1989. There was a significant difference between government-owned teaching hospitals, which provided an average of $8 387 910 in uncompensated trauma care, and private teaching hospitals, which provided an average of $2 459 790 in uncompensated care.

Before the Texas study, many trauma surgeons assumed that most of the uncompensated care was for inner city populations. However, the Texas study showed that the estimated annual cost to rural hospitals for all injured patients who required transfer was $9 138 000. Thirty percent of these transferred patients were identified as unsponsored patients, resulting in uncompensated care costing rural hospitals $3 043 000. An additional loss of $14 144 000 was attributed to uncompensated care for injured patients admitted to the rural hospitals.

There are other reasons why trauma care is suboptimal, some of which relate to hospital administrators and surgeons. Results of a 1991 survey by Esposito et al[19] of Washington State surgeons showed that 39% of all responding surgeons preferred not to treat patients with trauma. Forty-three percent of general surgeons and neurosurgeons preferred not to treat patients with trauma compared with only 14% of orthopedic surgeons. Thirty percent of surgeons would not be on-call for trauma care if such coverage was not mandatory in their hospitals. The survey also documented some of the reasons why surgeons preferred not to care for patients with trauma. These included disruption of an elective surgery practice, labor-intensive level of care for patients with trauma, lower reimbursement rates, liability risk, and increased cost of malpractice premiums. Almost all of these concerns are myths and cannot be substantiated by studies in the literature.

In a related study, Dailey et al[6] surveyed 61 hospitals in the United States that had terminated their trauma services. Three were level 1 centers; 37, level 2 centers; and two, level 3 centers. The authors identified 26 factors that may have prompted or contributed to the closure of the trauma centers. The most important factor was the perceived cost of uncompensated care. The second reason for closure was high operating costs, specifically costs associated with trauma services. The third reason was inadequate reimbursement from medical assistance programs, and the fifth reason was reduced compensation for patients with trauma under the prospective payment system (involving diagnosis related groups). Significantly, the fourth reason for closure was unwillingness of physicians to be on call.

Another example of a suboptimal trauma system is the trauma system of the US military. In March 1986, *American Medical Association News* reported that only three in 10 casualties could be treated promptly under the current level of readiness.[20] This was due to a shortage of physicians, particularly anesthesiologists, general surgeons, and orthopedic surgeons; less than 30% of these positions were staffed. It is difficult for the military to recruit physicians because of low reimbursement compared with civilian-generated income. In addition, civilian surgeons and specialists are not supporting the military by belonging to the reserve forces as they had in previous generations. This is particularly true in academic centers. An associated problem is the lack of integration of military training programs into civilian trauma centers, where resident and military attending surgeons could keep up their skills in trauma management. Conversely, there has been no indication from the US Department of Defense that military hospitals can regularly care for civilian patients with trauma except in a few isolated instances.

This brief summary of the current status of trauma care in the United States shows that present trauma systems and trauma care are not optimal. It must be reemphasized that the surgical literature[7-15] strongly supports the efficacy of trauma systems once they are established. This is made even more poignant by two studies[21,22] showing that the patient with trauma who is transported to a trauma center and ultimately to a rehabilitation center has at least an 80% chance of returning to a productive life. Will this suboptimal trauma care continue? What will the future of trauma management be?

FUTURE

The American Heritage Dictionary defines *prognosticate* as "to predict, using present indications as a guide."[23] Based on the previous background information and other data, I would like to make prognoses in three areas: financing trauma care, trauma systems, and future trauma.

Trauma Finances

In 1990, Eastman and associates[24] reported at the annual meeting of the American Association for the Surgery of Trauma some of the reimbursement problems of trauma centers. They demonstrated in a nonrandomized survey that trauma care is underfunded. This study confirmed a perception held by many trauma center directors for some time. The causes of this underfunding include the following: more self-pay patients compared with other hospitalized patients, a reduced collection ratio for patients receiving Medicaid and Medicare, inability to cost shift all of the losses, and inappropriate assignment and poor definition of diagnosis related groups.

I believe it is safe to predict that if it remains in the hands of politicians, health care financing reform will be a slow process. Conceivably, if a democrat were elected president of the United States in 1992, there might be more rapid evolution to some type of national health insurance. However, neither the democrats nor the republicans currently have a plan that incorporates the positive aspects of the Canadian, German, and Japanese systems, and yet is uniquely American to solve some of our complex problems. However, results of an experiment currently being carried out in Oregon might address some of these financing problems.

In 1988, legislation was passed in Oregon that set in motion the Oregon Experiment. The purpose of this experiment was to give health care access to all Oregonians and, at the same time, rationalize this care based on rationing criteria determined by the health care community and the public. A health services commission was established consisting of five physicians, one public health nurse, one social worker, and four consumers of health care. Under the direction of the health services commission, diseases and injury were divided into diagnosis treatment pairs. Based on professional input of numerous subcommittees, these diagnosis treatment pairs were examined from the standpoint of outcome, cost benefit, quality of life, effective treatment, and other parameters of overall good. The commission developed 17 categories of health services and ranked these categories on the basis of value to society, value to an individual at risk of needing the service, and whether each category was an essential component of a basic health care package. One of the most important steps in the entire process was then to present these diagnosis treatment pairs to public groups for prioritization and commentary. Based on the commission's standards and public input, each of the 709 diagnosis treatment pairs was then given a priority ranking. In general, with few exceptions, injury was given a relatively high priority among the first 200 diagnosis treatment pairs listed. Ultimately, the state legislature recommended that the first 587 diagnostic treatment pairs on the list be funded.

Based on this Oregon Experience, I am very optimistic about the future of funding for trauma care. Thanks to numerous colleagues, there is a wealth of outcome studies in the surgical literature that document the efficacy of trauma care and the positive aspects of rehabilitation and returning patients to productive lives. It is inconceivable to me that any governmental group or lay group scrutinizing trauma as a health care problem would not assign it a high priority for appropriate funding.

Between now and the year 2000, major reform in health care delivery and financing is fairly certain. Part of this reform is being driven by the public at large, particularly older individuals who are now fearful of the costs of health care and whether or not they will be covered by entitlement programs. Interestingly, the data from most trauma studies show that older individuals have a higher mortality rate after trauma, and, although cancer and heart disease are the big killers in this age group, trauma is still a very significant problem. Another group pushing for health care reform is American business. It is inconceivable to me that business leaders will not recognize the importance of regionalized trauma care and appropriate funding for trauma care since such efforts may well return one of their workers to the work force. Thus, it would appear that the major impediments to health care reform will come from Congress, the executive branch of government, insurance companies, trial lawyers, and some health care providers. I do not believe the groups opposing health care reform will be able to stop the current populist revolt.

Trauma Systems

The American College of Surgeons Committee on Trauma has defined eight components of a trauma system.[25] The patient components are access to care, prehospitalization care, hospitalization care, and rehabilitation, while the societal components are prevention, disaster care, education, and research. Not all of these components have been developed at the same rate, and each has its own unique problems as state agencies operating emergency medical services try to develop a comprehensive system. What will the future be for these various components?

Access to trauma care will improve immensely from modern technology and particularly from advances in satellite communication. Satellites are already being used in Africa to improve access to trauma care. Some countries are experimenting with provision of global coverage for citizens who are injured in other countries. Switzerland, through a very extensive network and in conjunction with the airline, Swiss Air, already provides global coverage to all its citizens. Access to health care in rural areas could be markedly improved by simple technologic means. Radio transmitters in farm machinery or in vehicles could automatically start sending out a signal after an accident has occurred. This would activate the emergency medical service system, and rescue vehicles and personnel would be sent to the scene. Such devices have already been tested in Australia, with promising results.

Prehospitalization care will undergo major advances between now and the year 2000. A recent study[26] compared prehospitalization care in Germany with prehospitalization care in the United States at comparable trauma centers. Early outcome was significantly better in the German system and was attributed to the presence of a physician as part of the prehospitalization team. The implication was that lifesaving techniques such as intubation of the pleural cavity or the airway were better achieved when a physician was present. If results of this study can be confirmed, it might have far-reaching implications on the North American model for prehospitalization care.

It is very likely that some treatments currently delivered in the hospital will be removed to the prehospitalization setting. Definitive or prophylactic treatment of brain edema has to be initiated as soon as possible. Any positive results of the current multi-institutional lazaroid (21-aminosteroid) studies could obviously be extended into the prehospitalization setting. Similarly, if effective inhibiting agents to chloride movement into cells could be identified, these would also be best used in prehospitalization care. Monoclonal antibodies to cytokines or monokines would be most effective during the peak periods of activity of the cytokines or monokines, which are probably in the prehospitalization period. I am not as hopeful as some investigators for finding a substitute for blood. Experimental work with hemoglobin solution still reveals significant complications. In addition, results of preliminary studies from the Ben Taub Hospital in Houston, Tex, suggest that it might be better to withhold fluid resuscitation until definitive surgery is initiated.[27]

Hospital care of the patient with trauma will continue to be the area with the most exciting advances and applications as new information from research studies emerges. Brain injury still accounts for most deaths and morbidity after traumatic insult. Within the next 3 years, new, fast, computed tomographic scanners will be available that can be used in the resuscitation area. This will allow simultaneous resuscitation and diagnosis of head and torso injury even in the hemodynamically unstable patient. Multi-institutional trials using free-radical scavengers and other agents to specifically treat and prevent brain edema will be also used. Results of experiments with animals that show nerves to be capable of regeneration are just now showing promise and will probably be introduced for human protocols within the next 10 years.

The treatment of chest injuries will benefit from percutaneous techniques such as thoroscopy. Prototype computed tomographic scans now available will be extensively used to evaluate the mediastinum and to determine whether myocardial contusion is a significant problem. Patients with abdominal injuries will benefit from the same rapid diagnosis provided to patients with head injury. Selective management of penetrating and blunt injuries will be commonplace. There will be increased use of interventional radiology techniques to control hemorrhage and drain fluid collections. Laparoscopy will have a limited role.

Patients with orthopedic injuries and maxillofacial injuries will benefit from improvements in technology and the introduction of bone substitutes. There will be increased use of percutaneous fixation devices placed with either computed tomographic or ultrasonographic guidance. There will be increased emphasis on treating bony injuries as soon as possible after injury to reduce the inflammatory response and increase mobilization.

We should see conceptual improvements in anesthesia and analgesia. As soon as initial evaluation and resuscitation is achieved, anesthesia or analgesia will be initiated to reduce the catecholamine response and other counterregulatory hormones. "Intensive care" will be introduced in the emergency department and continued through the operation into the intensive care setting. Newer analgesic agents and methods of delivery will eliminate 90% of postinjury pain.

In the intensive care setting, I predict major debates on the efficacy of open- or closed-loop computer systems. Most surgeons will object to being removed from the decision loop. Noninvasive monitoring will be the gold standard. Infectious deaths will continue to decrease as nutrition and management of organ failure improves. Improved nursing care combined with the availability of medical personnel will force the concentration of patients into a few centers.

It is highly likely that between now and the year 2000 rehabilitation for the patient with trauma will finally become regionalized. With increasing outcome research, it will be impossible for third-party payers and the government to ignore the advantages of a rehabilitation system. There will be increased emphasis on linking these rehabilitation centers to the acute care centers in order to expedite care and improve communication. Legislators will become involved in increasing funding to rehabilitation units and addressing the disincentives that currently exist to prevent patients from returning to productive lives. Preventive-care activities will increase dramatically between now and the year 2000. I predict very little progress in modifying behavior, and, thus, predict increased use of passive restraints and new technology to minimize body injury after an accident. Gun control will finally be sensibly addressed by Congress, but inner city violence will continue unabated because of the underlying social problems.

Medical care for disaster victims will undergo minimal progress because of government and bureaucratic ineptness compounded by public apathy. The public will become increasingly aware of trauma as a health and social issue during the next decade. Because of changes in health care financing, young surgeons will be more interested in trauma care as a career. This will lead to more fellowships and eventually to some type of professional recognition. Providing trauma care in rural areas will continue to vex us.

The down side of the research component of a trauma system will be the decrease in basic science funding. This will be offset, in part, by an increase in outcome research and randomized clinical trials. A separate study section for trauma care in the National Institutes of Health will finally be approved. Basic research will continue, with a particular emphasis on the pathogenesis of brain edema. Monokines and cytokines will be extensively studied, and studies will be initiated to block or upregulate the effects of these compounds. Cell adhesion molecules will be shown to be important in the inflammatory cascade, particularly in leukocyte homing, cellular migration, and phagocytosis. Metabolic studies, including studies of organ flux and cell metabolism, will be extensively performed with humans as research with other animals decreases. There will be increased emphasis on studying target organs or tissue, such as the endothelial cell, after injury and sepsis. Fewer centers will be funded, thus concentrating bench research.

Future Trauma

As mentioned, urban violence is unlikely to abate. The underlying social causes are unlikely to be seriously addressed by Congress in the next 10 years. Similarly, it will be difficult to totally address the problem of access to trauma care in rural areas. It will be increasingly difficult to convince surgeons to pursue careers in rural areas. There will be increased efforts to incorporate the smaller rural hospitals into a regionalized trauma system, with communication and transportation markedly improving as a result. Mortality rates will decrease in rural communities that have been integrated into a trauma system.

Unfortunately, the risk of armed conflict between nations will not decrease in the next decade, even with the dissolution of the Soviet Union. Developing countries will continue to be sites of conflict because of despots or ethnic clashes. Many of these developing countries will have increased access to high-technology weapons. For example, Brazil, India, and North Korea all have the capability for intercontinental ballistic missiles. The addition of nuclear or biological chemical warheads is modestly easy. I predict that the United Nations will become increasingly involved in "police" actions in countries such as Yugoslavia and Libya.

There will be many changes in our armed forces as a consequence of the changes in the former Soviet Union. The number of armed forces personnel will decrease from 750 000 to 535 000, a reduction of about 29%. Staffing of the army medical department will decrease to about 52 000, an 18% reduction. This implies increased reliance on medical officers in the reserve forces, particularly surgeons and anesthesiologists. Maintenance of trauma skills will become a major issue. Conceivably, reserve units will be based near level 1 and 2 trauma centers. Thus, monthly weekend training could take place at these designated sites.

The final area of future trauma will be in space. The National Aeronautics and Space Administration (NASA) now predicts that the space station *Freedom* will have a permanent crew by the year 2000 or 2001, with a 20-year life span planned for this orbiting laboratory (Fig 1). A

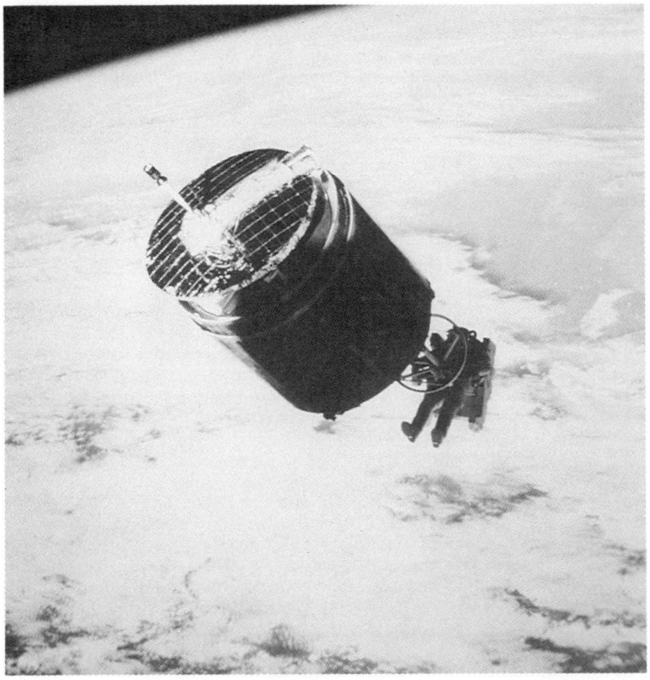

Fig 1.—*An early artist's depiction of the space station* Freedom. *Cutbacks in funding will most likely lead to design changes.*

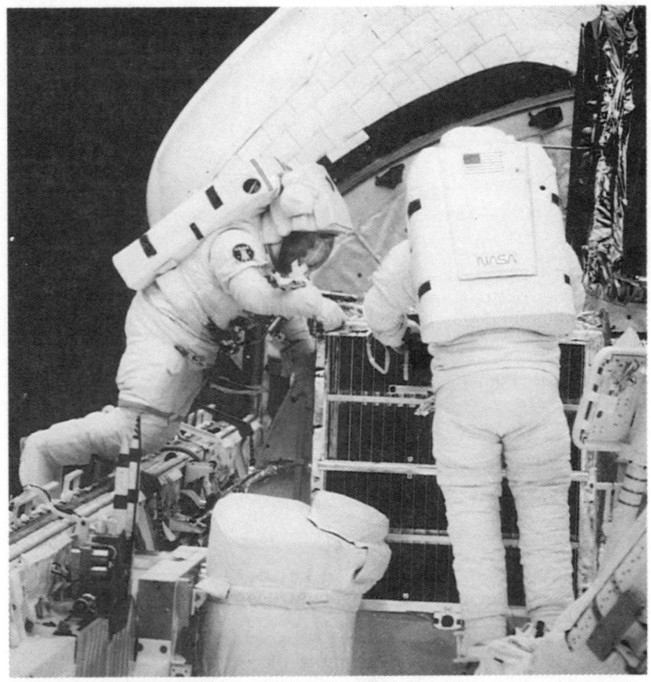

Fig 2.—*Two astronauts work in the cargo bay of a space shuttle. Exposure to sharp objects and the work itself make trauma a likely possibility. Trauma care is the obvious corollary.*

mission to Mars is beyond the early planning phases and will undoubtedly be an international effort.

Health care on *Freedom* will be an immediate problem. The health maintenance facility will be a part of the crew's health care system and will include an exercise countermeasure facility and an environmental health system. Several years ago, NASA considered the type of health care that should be provided, ranging from a first-aid kit and a scientist cross-trained as an emergency medical technician to care essentially equivalent to terrestrial care. Because of major funding cutbacks and other exigencies, a decision was made to initially provide only minimal health care facilities on *Freedom,* then phase in increases in the sophistication of equipment and personnel. The current plan includes an assured crew return vehicle that could bring an ill or injured patient back to Earth.

Trauma will undoubtedly be one of the major health hazards facing any crew on *Freedom,* a lunar mission, or a mission to Mars (Figs 2 and 3). Eventually, NASA will need a surgeon on-board *Freedom* and the vehicle involved in the mission to Mars. Diagnostic and therapeutic equipment will have to be miniaturized and capable of down-linking to consultants on Earth. It may be necessary to introduce a centrifuge either on the space station or on a space vehicle to mimic a partial-gravity or 1*g* environment to treat ill or injured crew members. The surgeon will have to be a true general surgeon who can provide intensive care. In addition, this individual would be invaluable in performing life science research projects.

Although trauma will be a major challenge, there will be other challenges, too, such as dealing with solar radiation particles and galactic cosmic radiation. Environmental hazards within the space station or any vehicle going to Mars will be a concern and must be identified and appropriately treated. Crew performance, including psychologic aspects, will have to be addressed by the on-board physician-surgeon. One of the more exciting aspects of being such a surgeon would be the opportunity to perform research to better understand the pathophysiologic effects of a microgravity environment. Any physician on-board *Freedom* would have to deal with the Controlled Ecological Life Support System with which *Freedom* would be equipped. Some of the mundane things that we take for granted on Earth in an operating room will have to be addressed, including the following: suctioning, patient fixation, and dealing with contaminated substances; blood and excrement can become major problems in a microgravity environment.

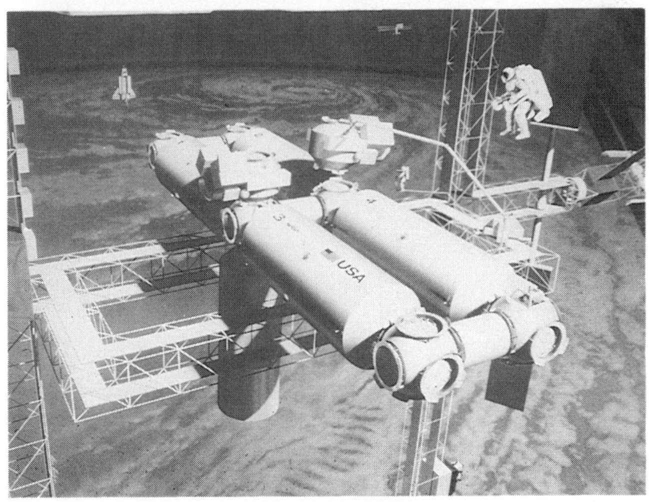

Fig 3.—*An astronaut "goes EVA" (extra vehicular activity) to rescue a damaged communications satellite. Although velocity is not nearly as important in a microgravity environment as on Earth in contributing to trauma forces, mass is and can cause significant crush injury.*

The provision of trauma care in space is an exciting challenge. It will require the development of new techniques, equipment, and methods not even considered in a terrestrial environment in 1992. The potential for research is unlimited, and any new knowledge will obviously have application even on Earth. I personally would welcome the opportunity to be on-call for trauma care on *Freedom*.

Photographs provided courtesy of NASA.

References

1. Majno G. *The Healing Hand: Man and Wound in the Ancient World.* Cambridge, Mass: Harvard University Press; 1975:339-422.
2. Larrey DJ. *Memoirs of Military Surgery.* Birmingham, Ala: Gryphon Editions; 1985. Classics of Surgery Library.
3. Dible JH. Napolean's Surgery. London, England: William Heinemann Medical; 1970.
4. Trunkey DD. What's wrong with trauma care? *Bull Am Coll Surg.* 1990;75:10-15.
5. West JG, Williams JJ, Trunkey DD, Wolferth CC. Trauma systems: current status-future challenges. *JAMA.* 1988;259:3597-3600.
6. Dailey JT, Teter A, Provenzano G, Cowley RA. Trauma center closures: a national assessment. *J Trauma.* In press.
7. Draaisma JMT, Haan AFG, Goris RJA. Preventable trauma deaths in the Netherlands: a prospective multicenter study. *J Trauma.* 1989;29:1552-1557.
8. Jacobs LM, Sinclair A, Beiser A, D'Agostino RB. Prehospital advanced life support: benefits in trauma. *J Trauma.* 1984;24:8-13.
9. Alexander RA, Pons PT, Krischer J, Hunt P. The effect of advanced life support in sophisticated hospital systems on motor vehicle mortality. *J Trauma.* 1984;24:486-490.
10. West JG, Cales RH, Gazzaniga AB. Impact of regionalization: the Orange County experience. *Arch Surg.* 1983;118:740-744.
11. West JG, Trunkey DD, Lim RC. Systems of trauma care: a study of two counties. *Arch Surg.* 1979;114:455-460.
12. Shackford SR, Hollingworth-Fridlund P, Cooper GF, et al. The effect of regionalization upon the quality of trauma care as assessed by concurrent audit before and after institution of a trauma system. *J Trauma.* 1986;26:812-820.
13. Ornato JP, Craren EJ, Nelson NM, Kimball KA. Impact of improved emergency medical services and emergency trauma care on the reduction and mortality from trauma. *J Trauma.* 1985;25:575-579.
14. Smith JM, Martin LM, Young WW, Macioce DP. Do trauma centers improve outcome over non-trauma centers: the evaluation of regional trauma care using discharge abstract data and patient management categories. *J Trauma.* 1990;30:1533-1538.
15. Smith RF, Frateschi L, Sloan EP, et al. The impact of volume on outcome in seriously injured trauma patients: two years experience of the Chicago trauma system. *J Trauma.* 1990;30:1066-1076.
16. Trunkey DD. Trauma care at mid-passage: a personal viewpoint. *J Trauma.* 1988;28:889-895.
17. Trunkey DD. Presidential address: on the nature of things that go bang in the night. *Surgery.* 1980;92:123-132.
18. Trunkey DD. Reflections on recent experiences. *J Trauma.* In press.
19. Esposito TJ, Maier RV, Rivara FP, Carrico CJ. Why surgeons prefer not to care for trauma patients. *Arch Surg.* 1991;126:292-297.
20. Krieger L. House bill would allow peacetime MD draft. *Am Med Assoc News.* 1986;29(11):15.
21. McKenzie CJ, Siegel JA, Shapiro S, Moody M, Smith RT. Functional recovery and medical costs of trauma: an analysis by type and severity of injury. *J Trauma.* 1988;28:281-297.
22. Rhodes M, Aronson J, Moerkirk G, Petrash E. Quality of life after the trauma center. *J Trauma.* 1988;28:931-938.
23. Morris W, ed. *The American Heritage Dictionary of the English Language.* Boston, Mass: Houghton Mifflin Co; 1981:1045.
24. Eastman AB, Rice CL, Bishop GF, Richardson JD. An analysis of the critical problem of trauma center reimbursement. *J Trauma.* 1991;31:920-926.
25. American College of Surgeons Committee on Trauma. *Resources for Optimal Care of the Injured Patient.* Chicago, Ill: American College of Surgeons; 1990.
26. Frame SB, Nerlich ML, Schmidt U, et al. On scene helicopter transport of the multitrauma patient: comparison of a German and an American system. *J Trauma.* In press.
27. Martin RR, Bickell W, Mattox KL, Burch M, Pepe PE. Prospective evaluation of preoperative volume resuscitation in hypotensive patients with penetrating truncal injuries: preliminary report. *J Trauma.* In press.

The gun and the sanctity of human life; or The bullet as pathogen

Lester Adelson, M.D.

Thoughtful clinicians and researchers are constantly on the alert for pathogens, whatever their nature, acting on the premise that identification of harmful environmental agents will lead to the introduction of measures to eliminate or control them.

In this presentation I discuss the bullet as a pathogen in our "peace-time" American society, a designation often considered a tragic joke by those of us who function professionally in metropolitan coroners' or medical examiners' offices, where we deal with violent death daily and, all too frequently, several times daily. I shall also mention briefly the epidemiology of gunshot incidents inasmuch as epidemiology may point to etiology.

Fatal and nonfatal gunshot incidents, whether they be attempted or successful homicides and suicides, accidents, or of undetermined origin, have multifaceted causations involving more than the presence of a potentially deadly firearm; but all too often a gun escalates the degree of violence to irreversible lethality. ("Wife, son 9, see man slain after minor car crash."[1] The victim was shot in the head.)

Human personality, intellectual capacity, emotional stability, our national historical heritage, community custom, popular entertainment (television, motion pictures, radio, and "comic" books), alcohol and other psychoactive drugs, and our legal system with its ramifications play roles in these tragedies. Although a gun is involved in most American homicides, it alone does not explain this blotch on our national face.

Discussion of firearms traumata possesses a relevance matched by comparatively few other remediable (an important qualification) life-and-death phenomena on the current American scene. The past decade witnessed a horrifying increase in homicidal and nonfatal gunshot crimes in our country. I do not call this a "wave" of homicides. Waves come, break, and recede. Rather, this dismal aspect of our society may be likened to a flood, with the water line (or blood line) constantly rising. ("Homicides are up 47% from '78's 1st quarter."[2])

This article, which appeared in *The Pharos* (Summer 1980), is reprinted here in its entirety.

The author (AOA, Tufts University, 1940) was formerly professor of forensic pathology at Case Western Reserve University School of Medicine, Cleveland, Ohio, and Chief Deputy Coroner at the Cuyahoga County (Ohio) Coroner's Office. The penetrating concepts embodied in this seminal contribution are as operative today as they were in 1980.—*The Editor.*

The Sanctity of Human Life

Before presenting some factual aspects of firearms incidents, I offer a few words about the moral aspect of this complicated subject.

The term, *sanctity of human life,* is not a trite phrase or a banal cliché. We physicians know it to be an article of deep professional and personal faith. All human life is sacred, and it is only the exigencies of war, excusable killings or justifiable homicides, and capital punishment (There, too, is an endlessly debatable subject.) that justify the deliberate termination of a human life.

Death is truly democratic, and we who deal with it in our autopsy and consulting rooms, and courtrooms know full well that regardless of race, religion, ethnic background, or life style of the homicide victim, the blood is always equally red, and the tears shed for the death of a loved one are equally salty.

Because most gunshot incidents arise from criminal acts with their sequelae of arrests and other steps of the law enforcement-judicial process, we must constantly bear in mind the thesis that justice exists only when those who have *not* been injured by a crime are as indignant as those who have been harmed by an unlawful act.

In a consideration of gunshot incidents, we deal with more than matters of life and death and more than simply medical or legal facts. We are concerned also with the quality of life. The news media inform the community about how many people have been done to death, whether by firearms, motor vehicles, or other traumatizing modalities. Unless the victim is a public figure such as Governor George Wallace, comparatively little attention is paid to nonfatal incidents, which range in gravity from minor to serious totally disabling injuries. Many nameless George Wallaces live out their shortened lives as paraplegics or worse because a missile transected their spinal cords. And there are those condemned to a vegetative existence as a consequence of a cerebral bullet injury.

Even when the gunshot victim recovers completely physically, how can one assess the degree of emotional trauma endured by the wounded subject, his family, and his friends? How in these days of double-digit inflation does one calculate the cost in dollars and cents of hospital care (operating room and what goes with it, blood bank, intensive care unit, special duty nurses, X rays), days lost from work by the human bullet target, police investigation, courtroom procedures, and all the rest? Where will this human and financial disaster end?

Gunshot fatalities are the visible tip of this iceberg of injury. Nonfatal wounds are more numerous and in many ways as or more important than those in which the victim was dead on or after arrival at the hospital. Thanks to advances in medical care made over the past several decades, many gunshot patients survive today who formerly would have succumbed quickly or slowly and agonizingly. A chilling thought presents itself: What would today's gunshot homicide toll be if we had our current assault rate combined with the medical skills and techniques that were available in the days before World War II and in the 1950s? What a mass disaster we would face if medical progress had *not* kept pace with the mounting level of violence!

The spectrum of physically and emotionally traumatic human behavior in contemporary American society is deeply disturbing. There is no humor in death, no happiness in disability, and no joy in suffering. These are the bitter fruits of the tree of violence, and the availability of handguns fertilizes the soil for the growth of this malignant phenomenon.

In all fairness we must acknowledge that firearms can be and indeed are used occasionally to protect the lives of innocent people, to safe-guard the privacy of one's home and the safety of one's belongings, over and above the fascination they hold for gun collectors and the fun they provide for hobby shooters.

Legally justifiable gunshot homicides are yet another aspect of the violence around us, whether the weapon was fired by a civilian or a police officer. Many law-abiding citizens are vociferous in their claim to their right (some consider it an obligation) to keep a loaded gun in their homes or on their persons to protect them from those who would harm or rob them. Their views, whether expressed individually or through such organizations as the National Rifle Association (NRA), must be kept in mind when we consider what can be done about firearms control.

Many of our fellow physicians, as learned and dedicated healers as the rest of us, I am sure, are quick to condemn any attempt at gun control. An editorial reprint entitled "Approved Therapy for Handgun Menace: 'Get the Bullet'" appeared in the *American Medical News*.[3] It evoked a spate of letters from physicians with communications headed by such phrases as "Get the criminal, not the bullet," "Passing a law is shooting from the hip," and "MD opposes handgun curbs."[4]

A Hard Look at Guns in Twentieth-Century U.S.A.

If we are to discuss the complex subject of gun control, we must do so on the basis of solid information, not emotion and prejudice. What are the *facts* about guns in our country today?

The Federal Bureau of Investigation (FBI) tells us that more than 20,000 homicides (culpable murders, manslaughters, and justifiable killings) occur annually in the United States. Put differently, every twenty-six minutes, a man, woman, or child is slaughtered in our nation by one means or another.[5] (These figures do *not* include fatal auto accidents classified as "vehicular homicides.") In 1976, homicide ranked as the twelfth most common "cause of death" in the United States, surpassing such serious "medical" entities as congenital anomalies, nephritis, nephrosis, and septicemia.[6] (Strictly speaking, homicide is not a *cause* but rather a *manner* of death. The *cause* of death is the responsible disease or injury. The *manner* of death is the fashion in which the *cause* arose.)

The weapon used most frequently with homicidal intent in America is a firearm, whether it be a handgun, shoulder gun, submachine gun, or some type of homemade lethal hardware, called a "zip" gun. Current national figures indicate that the number of homicides and attempted homicides perpetrated with firearms exceeds the number of homicides committed by all other forms of violence combined.[7] Handguns comprise the majority of firearms.

Firearms are used in three of four major crimes causing injury and death—homicide, aggravated assault, and armed robbery. They are the favorite weapon of the airplane hijacker. Since 1967, the number of firearms homicides in the United States has increased by 48 percent. During this same interval, homicides committed with other weapons increased by 10 percent.[8]

Of all weapons, firearms are the most deadly and the most versatile. They permit attacks at greater range and from positions of better concealment than do other lethal instrumentalities by persons physically or psychologically unable to overpower their intended victims through personal contact.

Since the start of this century, more than 850,000 American *civilians* have been killed by bullets. This number exceeds the total military casualties suffered by our armed forces in all the "big" and "little" wars we have fought from the War of Independence through Vietnam. This is a record no other industrialized nation can approach.[5] To make this matter more timely, more Americans were slain at home during the first four years of the 1970s than were killed in combat during the entire span of the Vietnam hostilities. This gruesome statistic supports the contention that our nation is in the midst of a murder "epidemic" unparalleled in our history. Indeed, murder now ranks as major "cause" of death in some age-race portions of our society.[9] The killers are "typical Americans," 70 percent of their victims are friends or relatives, and only 2 percent of the assailants are judged "criminally insane."[10]

Bullet Fatalities—A Personal Statement

My association with the Coroner's Office of Cuyahoga County, Ohio (Cleveland and its suburbs) spans three decades. Thus I am familiar with the urban handgun-homicide complex on the basis of almost daily personal experience. When I started to work in this governmental agency, the annual county homicide toll was less than 100, of which 50 to 60 percent involved guns. Starting in the mid-sixties, the homicide incidence and rate rose sharply. Now nearly 80 percent of these bloody episodes are gun-dependent. Of these, the weapons in approximately 80 percent of cases are handguns.

In my community, guns, especially handguns, account for roughly four times as many homicides as all other forms of lethal, criminal violence combined.[9,11]

If there were in excess of 200 deaths annually in my county from typhoid fever, as there are from criminally caused gunshot fatalities, there would be mass hysteria. Yet these murders and manslaughters are accepted by the majority of our citizens as a reasonable price to pay for living in "the best location in the nation."

A Brief Glance at Geography and History

Where strict gun control laws are enforced, homicides in general and assassinations occur infrequently. There were 189 murders in Tokyo in 1974 compared with more than 1500 in New York City. Only one in Tokyo involved a gun. During that same year there were 1708 murders in all of Japan of which only 72 (4 percent) were gun-caused, and firearms were utilized in less than 2 percent of armed robberies.[12]

Data from Western European nations are similar. Great Britain, with its population in excess of 50 million, has fewer annual killings than the borough of Manhattan with its 1.7 million inhabitants. In short, the United States averages *fifty* times as many gun homicides as the combined populations of England, Germany, and Japan.[13]

One author puts this aspect of our society in the following words:

> To foreign observers, nothing is more astonishing than our casual recourse to violence in personal disputes, unless it is our failure to restrain it by law—in particular, our failure to control the indiscriminate sale and use of guns, which in recent years has lain at the heart of the controversy and at the same time has made it politically insoluble.[14]

It is more than coincidence that all four American presidents killed in office in the century that elapsed between Lincoln's murder at Ford's theater in 1865 and Kennedy's assassination in Dealey Plaza in 1963 involved firearms. Lincoln, Garfield, and McKinley were shot with handguns. Kennedy was killed with an Italian military rifle. In this same context, attempted and, fortunately, unsuccessful assassinations of our nation's chief executives and of candidates for that high office all involved guns. (Recall the recent failed misdeeds of Sara Jane Moore and Lynette "Squeaky" Fromme.) Governor Wallace was crippled by Arthur Bremer in 1972, and Senator Robert Kennedy was killed in Los Angeles in 1968 during his campaign to win California's votes for the Democratic Party's nomination for president. Guns!! Guns!! Guns!! I recall no other industrialized North American or Western European nation that has had such a high, violent mortality in its top government leaders during the past century.

The Psychology and Psychopathology of the Shooter

The most reasonable explanation for the use of firearms in the majority of culpable homicides is that a gun, illegally used, is a coward's weapon. This is true whether the killing is committed in connection with a family argument, political terrorism, an armed robbery, a drunken quarrel between friends, or a skulking assassination. With its peculiar lethality, a gun converts a spat into a slaying and a quarrel into a killing. A handgun is effective at a distance of many feet, a shotgun kills or seriously injures at a muzzle-target distance of many yards, and a rifle is effective at hundreds of yards. (Remember what Lee Harvey Oswald, lurking in the Texas School Book Depository, did to his unsuspecting victim in a moving vehicle several hundred yards away, to comprehend the potential lethality of this weapon.)

The corollary of this unique firearms feature is that a slayer can kill with emotional impunity. Konrad Lorenz points out:

> The deep, emotional layers of our personality simply do not register the fact that the crooking of the forefinger to release a shot tears the entrails of another man. No sane man would even go rabbit hunting for pleasure if the necessity of killing his prey with his natural weapons brought home to him the full, emotional realization of what he is actually doing.[15]

Reams have been written about the psychiatric significance of the gun. Some observers consider the gun to be a sex symbol of male chauvinism with its ability to make the weakest man the peer of the strongest. ("God made man, but Colt made all men equal.") Some analysts state that the attitude of at least part of the masculine portion of the progun faction to the "threat" of gun control springs from a castration complex, or even worse. Certainly a gun can flatter the ego of a man who has nothing else to be vain about.

There appears to be a deep psychological drive motivating those who keep guns in their homes, stores, or auto glove compartments. For good or ill, man has always wanted to control his environment and the men around him. A gun gives him this "magical" power.

The gun (and the use of a gun) haunts American speech. Would it be going off half-cocked to suggest that, just as a shot in the dark, nothing penetrated the American idiom as deeply as the gun? The idea is not too wide off the mark. The gun has given the American tongue the big shot who is quick on the trigger, the straight shooter, the flash in the pan, and the dud.[16]

Guns create feelings of self-esteem, permitting even the least potent to join "The Superman Club." As part of its "magical" power, a firearm is "a key which can unlock any door."[17] With it, the misguided possessor believes that he can go anywhere and have everything he wants. No other weapon gives this feeling of mastery. On the basis of interviews with men convicted of armed robbery, a nationally syndicated psychiatrist concluded that in many instances the most important element in the crime was not the acquisition of money or jewels but rather the brief interval during which these armed individuals could force someone to do as they commanded. The firearm becomes a mechanism by which to compensate for feelings of inadequacy and represents a dangerous outlet for aggressive impulses.[17]

A gun is the favorite weapon of the political assassin. Other than for poisoning homicides, extremely rare today, the use of bombs (correctly termed "infernal machines"), and arson, practically every other attempt at man slaying requires that the assailant either come within arm's length or actual grips with his intended victim. Fatal injuries by knives thrown at rather than manually plunged into the victim are rare in the real world despite their comparative frequency in the "reel" world of Hollywood.

Facile access to firearms by their legal purchase, leaving aside for the moment their availability by their being borrowed or stolen, is an invitation to their wrongful use by the neurotic, the psychotic, and the socially maladjusted. Who can forget the multihomicides carried out by Charles Whitman in Austin, Texas (sixteen victims killed and thirty wounded, all but two by guns) and by Howard Unruh, who fatally shot thirteen neighbors and strangers within ten minutes in Camden, New Jersey?[5]

Shot and Killed on Duty

A firearm is the lethal instrumentality in virtually every homicide of a law enforcement officer killed in line of duty. During the past half-century, guns were responsible for over 90 percent of such fatalities, with pistols and revolvers constituting 95 percent of the fatal armament. Homicides involving "peace officers" occur throughout the United States at an average number of 100 yearly. In 1976, 110 law enforcement officers died as a consequence of criminal action, 93 by firearms.[18]

These sorry statistics become more impressive when they are compared with their counterparts in the British Isles. A recent study revealed that "over the past 10 years, *one* or *two* [emphasis added] British police officers have been killed on duty each year."[19]

Guns in America

The United States is the only industrialized nation that does not *effectively* regulate private ownership of firearms. The consequence of this sad fact is that our civilian population is the most heavily armed in history.[20] Approximately 100 million firearms of all types are in American civilian possession, and half of American homes have one or more firearms.[8] Sales of handguns and long guns have increased during the recent past, and we manufacture and sell more than 2.5 million handguns each year. Thus a new firearm is purchased every 13.5 seconds.[21]

Are we "hung up" on guns because of our frontier heritage? Canada, with the same frontier tradition as we, has only a fraction of our homicide rate.[5,22] Australia, historically much closed to a frontier tradition than we and with a similar melting-pot makeup, has one-seventh the proportionate private handgun ownership as we, thanks to an efficient system of law enforcement.[5]

Although only one-fourth of our firearms are handguns, they account for almost three-quarters of firearms homicides. The criminal's primary weapon is a handgun, and the ready availability of handguns makes it easy for extremist groups and misdirected individuals to obtain them. Put succinctly, where there are more firearms, there is more firearm violence. Conversely, where there are fewer firearms, there is a decrease in this modality of injury and death.

Accidental Firearms Casualties

The inevitable result of guns in the hands of those who misuse them is a depressing list of fatal and nonfatal *accidental* shootings. By accidental shootings, I mean incidents wherein persons are shot by mischance or misadventure, whether the responsible person was the victim "playing" with or cleaning a loaded gun, or some other person who unintentionally precipitated the traumatizing event. A typical group of such frightening events is made up of the following headlines: "3-year old boy shoots his mother to death";[23] "4-year old shot, killed by playmate";[24] "Boy 3, kills sister with parent's gun";[25] "6-year old is shot to death in 'find gun for $1' scheme."[26] It is evident that these tragedies would not have occurred had a loaded gun not been conveniently nearby.[27]

Approximately three thousand Americans die each year from accidental firearms injuries. Another twenty thousand are shot and survive.[8] Inasmuch as an accidental firearm death represents as premature a wastage of human life as that taken by a sadistic or psychotic killer, this facet of the gun problem deserves a moment's attention.

Like homicides, firearms accidents parallel the pattern of firearms ownership. The fallacy that a gun in the home represents protection for its residents is rebutted by data that prove that such household weapons are more likely to cause harm and death to those who own them, their children, and their friends than they prove to be an effective defense or reliable deterrent to those who would enter these homes, bent on robbery, burglary, or rape. Indeed, household weapons more often provide successful burglars and robbers with a ready arsenal than they prevent these marauders from carrying out their foul deeds.[28]

The Dispute

Any discussion of gun control requires that those who favor controlling firearms concede the inescapable fact that non-availability of guns will *not* eliminate homicide or nonfatal assaults. People killed each other and themselves long before the Chinese invented gunpowder.

The logic-destructive arguments of both sides in the current gun control debate are equally self-destructive.

> Every side has a sizable amount of good sense and logic to depend on; but instead of simply saying they want to have a good time with their guns—something not frowned on even in Puritan America—the hunters have concocted all sorts of weird Constitutional and conservation arguments to defend their position. Instead of saying that they want to make as much money as they possibly can—which has never been considered as a sin in America—the gun merchants also throw up great cloudbanks of patriotic fluff. And the antigun people, who could effectively restrict their arguments to showing that guns are not an absolute necessity for the American way of life, have instead clobbered the senses with distorted statistics, hysterically interpreted.[22]

Many concerned people believe that a substantial portion of our murders and manslaughters would not have occurred had a firearm not been readily at hand. The man who puts a Saturday Night Special into his pocket before he visits his neighborhood poolroom or the woman who puts a pistol into her purse before she goes shopping are not the same persons they would have been were they not "toting" these items.

A critical feature related to the number of firearms in the community is the life span of a gun. If a "shooting iron" is properly looked after (that is, cleaned and oiled regularly), its life expectancy is many years. Many firearms used to commit crimes in our country are several decades old.[8] If we manufacture, import, or assemble no additional guns in this country for the next twenty or thirty years, we have currently on hand (and *in* hand?) a sufficient number of these weapons to decimate the population. Firearms longevity provides a rebuttal to the slogan, "Guns don't kill people. People kill people." The response to this statement is "Guns don't die. People die."

A second sloganeering argument promulgated by our progun fellow-citizens is, "When guns are outlawed, only outlaws will have guns." Ergo, it follows logically that the law-obeying majority should have guns to protect themselves from the depredations of the habitual law breakers, who seemingly abound in our society.

There is no gainsaying the fact that the professional criminal is always able to get a gun, whether he buys, steals, borrows, or smuggles it across our international borders, and he will *not* register it, regardless of any law that requires public recording of gun possession. The majority of American homicides, however, are committed by law-abiding people who know and frequently "love" each other, and who express aggression in this explosive manner.

Said differently, although the confirmed criminal will

not register his gun, many people *become* criminals only after they have misused the weapon. The accessibility of a firearm permits the instantaneous metamorphosis of a law-abiding (hot-headed?) person into a murderer. The public has the misconception that most murders are perpetrated by criminals who kill to achieve profit and power, the Godfather image. Psychiatric studies reveal the opposite to be true. Most homicides are not associated with other felonies and are not perpetrated as the result of Mafia-type contracts.[28]

Consideration of the foregoing facts and arguments raises the question, How much longer must we wait and how many more lives must be lost to firearms before effective measures are forthcoming that will exert meaningful control over these presently all-too-readily accessible, death-dealing weapons? The current American approach to firearms—practically a laissez-faire attitude—is bankrupt.

One argument put forth by opponents of attempts at firearms control by state or federal legislative action is that it is their constitutional "right . . . to keep and bear arms." Taken out of context this phrase reverses the meaning of the constitutional intent, as has been demonstrated repeatedly by judicial interpretations.

The Second Amendment to the Constitution, which states, "A *well-regulated Militia* [emphasis added], being necessary to the security of a free State, the right of the people to keep and bear Arms, shall not be infringed," was enacted in the eighteenth century, when its provisions were essential for the survival of a struggling, infant nation, beset on all sides by actual and potential enemies. Moreover, the citizen did not then enjoy the protection we have today, when help is available at practically a moment's notice, thanks to modern communications and police mobility. Consequently, a citizen required some means to protect the privacy of his home and the personal safety of himself and his family.

These provisions are invoked today by many persons to justify their keeping a loaded firearm in their homes when the need for a "well-regulated Militia," in the sense intended by the Second Amendment, disappeared long ago. The "well-regulated Militia" of the eighteenth century is today's National Guard, and the "right to bear arms" is not synonymous with a citizen's putting a "piece" into his pocket or into her purse.

In talking about constitutional rights, we should recall that the Preamble to this governmental bulwark states that one of the purposes for its enactment it to "insure domestic Tranquility." Domestic tranquility means that one is safe in one's home, at one's place of work, and on the streets of one's community. The guns now used to kill and cripple make a mockery of these words.

Putting legalities aside for the moment, we must not overlook the right that supersedes and antedates all constitutional rights, and that is the right *not* to be killed by a fool, a maniac, or a robber who would use a gun with deadly purpose. No occupant of a premature grave who died as a result of the wrongful use of a firearm enjoys *any* constitutional rights.

The Legislative Approach to Firearms Control

Several contrasting concepts must be kept in mind when we come to grips with "passing a law" to reduce the slaughter by firearms. Enacting a law often does not guarantee an effective solution to a simple, let alone a complex, emotionally laden issue.[29] Bad laws are the worst form of tyranny, because they legalize governmental activities that are oppressive or unjust. A good law must be enforceable and enforced; otherwise the legislative process is a farce.

When legislation that could lead to a decrease in homicidal violence is discussed, we are confronted by doctrines of defeat and discouragement. Antigun control proponents iterate the proposition that firearms surveillance is a waste of time, money, and energy that could be more fruitfully expended for other purposes.[30]

There is no denying that an effective gun law, however one defines it, will not (repeat *not*) prevent gunshot incidents, fatal or nonfatal. But such a law should reduce their number. If the law does not cure, let it mitigate the multifold misery. The law need not prohibit. Let it regulate. If we can not eliminate the problem, let us attempt to control it.

Current American federal, state, and municipal gun laws fill a printed volume of 389 pages, which is a legislative crazy quilt.[31] A recent Associated Press dispatch carried the lead, "Guns across the line—Local firearms control laws don't halt crime, U.S. says."[32] This not surprising item tells us that a federal study concluded that *strict, local* gun control laws are not effective in keeping handguns away from lawbreakers. The study also established that many of the weapons were Saturday Night Specials, frequently obtained in lawful fashion.

Guns and what goes with them (ammunition, hunting gear, et cetera) are a multimillion dollar, legitimate business.[33] The progun lobby, financed primarily by arms manufacturers and spearheaded by the NRA, is a major objector to change in statutory approaches to firearms. Gun control advocates should proceed with respect for the concerns that motivate opposition to gun regulation.

The approach of gun confiscation is neither wise nor workable. What we need is a sound *federal* law that is clear, uniform, and precise. Such a law should regulate the sale and ownership of guns *and* ammunition, thus permitting the institution of some type of prophylaxis. We physicians are aware of the superiority of prevention over treatment of potentially fatal diseases.

A recent nation-wide poll of 1500 adults revealed that 84 percent favor regulation of newly purchased handguns, and 70 percent support an outright ban on Saturday Night Specials. (This label is a misnomer. These weapons, which "draw heavily on the emotions and lightly on the purse,"[22] are effective every day of the week, morning, noon, *and* night.) Moreover, 70 percent of those interviewed said that a stand on gun control could affect their votes for a specific candidate.[34] A recent Harris survey indicates that most Americans favor a law that requires that privately owned guns be registered with federal authorities.[35]

The need for a nationwide effort dedicated to this life-and-death matter is self-evident. In a democracy the populace gets the type of government it chooses. This is especially true if we elect a Congress shaking in mortal fear of the NRA, which threatens to ensure the defeat of any officeholder who votes for a federal gun-regulation law.[14] Despite the results of the polls cited earlier, a recent attempt to regulate handguns was defeated in the House of Representatives by a four-to-one margin, thus sustaining the potential criminal's right to "bear arms" (that is, to purchase, import, assemble, and ultimately to use arms unlawfully).[36] Dr. Milton Eisenhower, head of the National Commission on Violence, declared that the United States held "the distinction of being the clear leader in violent crime among modern, stable nations," as well as having the highest gun-to-population ratio in the world, other than for Switzerland. He said, further, "I continue to be perplexed by the blind, emotional resistance that greets any proposal to bring this senseless excess under control."[29]

We should be able to reduce the number of handguns used for malicious purposes without interfering with legitimate gun sports. A compromise should be worked out through wise leadership. But unless our public officials have the voters' support, they will not dare to incur the wrath of the NRA.

But any law, even a well-administered, "good" law, is too blunt an instrument to control the gun problem by itself. We need education and indoctrination in our schools, homes, and houses of worship, and we need constant reminding by the responsible segment of our news media that the basis of a decent society is respect and regard for the sanctity of all human life.

L'Envoi

Here are three summing-up statements.

By . . . our readiness to allow arms to be purchased at will and fired at whim; by allowing our movie and television screens to teach our children that the hero is one who masters the art of shooting and the technique of killing . . . we have created an atmosphere in which violence and hatred have become popular pastimes. —*Doctor Martin Luther King, Jr., November 1963.*[8, p.V] (Dr. King was fatally shot in Memphis, Tennessee on April 4, 1968.)

We have a responsibility to the victims of crime and violence . . . . It is a responsibility to put away childish things—to make the possession and use of firearms a matter undertaken only by serious people who will use them with the restraint and maturity that their dangerous nature deserves—and demands. —*Senator Robert F. Kennedy, July 11, 1967.*[8,p.V] (Senator Kennedy was fatally shot on June 5, 1968 in Los Angeles, California.)

The current banality is that, like the weather, violence is what everybody discusses and does nothing about. For the violated and for everybody else in danger of being violated, violence is not banal.

There is of course no single manifestation of this social disease, no single causative mechanism, no single cure. There are, however, "small steps" that can be taken by the federal government, steps capable of being administered and enforced, which can save no small number of lives and retard the frightening escalation of this evil: (1) the restriction of the manufacture, distribution and sale of cheap handguns (the so-called Saturday night specials), and (2) the registration of all handguns.

Implementation of legislation of these two measures, were it to save a single life, would warrant such action by the federal government.

How large a holocaust must we have to bestir us to act? —*Editor Naomi M. Kanof, 1975.*[37]

How many "shocks to the national conscience" do we need before we do something positive? The medical profession, charged with and sworn to the maintenance and restoration of health, the preservation of life, and the prevention of death, should speak out responsibly and responsively in the debate about this danger until effective measures for handgun control are properly implemented.

References

1. Plain Dealer (Cleveland, Ohio morning newspaper), Sept. 13, 1979.
2. Plain Dealer, October 7, 1979.
3. Editorial reprint of item by J. H. Felts in N.C. Med. J.: Approved therapy for hand gun menace: 'Get the bullet.' A.M.A. News, March 1, 1976.
4. Letters to the Editor. A.M.A. News, June 14, 1976.
5. Godwin, J.: Murder U.S.A.: The Ways We Kill Each Other. New York, Ballantine Books, 1978.
6. Monthly vital statistics report. Provisional statistics—Annual summary for the United States, 1976. D.H.E.W. Pub. No. (PHS) 78-1120, 25:3, 7, 26, 28, 1977.
7. Ray, M.W., Brenner, R.N., and Kravitz, M.: Firearm Use in Violent Crime. Washington, D.C., U.S. Government Printing Office, 1978.
8. Newton, G.D., Jr, and Zimring, F.F.: Firearms and Violence in American Life: A Staff Report Submitted to the National Commission on the Causes and Prevention of Violence. Washington, D.C., U.S. Government Printing Office, 1970.
9. Rushforth, N.B., Ford, A.B., Hirsch, C.S., Rushforth, N.M., and Adelson, L.: Violent death in a metropolitan community: Changing patterns in homicide (1958-1974). N. Engl. J. Med. 297:531-38, 1977.
10. U.S. in murder epidemic. Police Command (Official publication of the National Association of Chiefs of Police). August 16, 1979.
11. Hirsch, C.S., Rushforth, N.B., Ford, A.B., and Adelson, L.: Homicide and suicide in a metropolitan county: I. Long-term trends. J.A.M.A. 223:900-905, 1973.
12. Pearlstine, N.: A disarming people. Japanese assassins have a high failure rate, thanks to extremely strict gun-control law. Wall Street J. Sept. 12, 1975.
13. TRB: Crime fighting. New Republic. Nov. 16, 1978.
14. Harris, R.: Annals of Legislation: If you love your guns. New Yorker. April 20, 1968, p.56.
15. Lorenz, K.: On Aggression. New York, Harcourt, Brace & World, Inc., 1966, p. 242.
16. Loh, J.: Our sad love affair with guns. Associated Press Newsfeature in Plain Dealer, Nov. 12, 1967.
17. Menninger, W.: Having gun in hand triggers self-esteem. Column in Plain Dealer, July 1, 1976.
18. FBI Law Enforcement Bull. March 1977.
19. Stead, P.J.: Fewer police deaths in Great Britain. Quoted in Law Enforcement Assistance Administration Newsletter. 6:15, 1976.
20. Wright, J.D.: The demography of gun control. The Nation, Sept. 20, 1975, p. 241.
21. New gun sold in U.S. every 13.5 seconds. Police Times, October 1978.
22. Sherrill, R.: The Saturday Night Special. New York, Penguin Books, Inc., 1975, P. 74.
23. UPI dispatch. Plain Dealer, Aug. 10, 1974.
24. Plain Dealer, May 5, 1973.
25. Plain Dealer, Dec. 1, 1975.
26. Plain Dealer, Feb. 9, 1979.
27. Rushforth, N.B., Hirsch, C.S., Ford, A.B., and Adelson, L.: Accidental firearm fatalities in a metropolitan county (1958-1973). Am. J. Epidemiol. 100:499-505, 1974.
28. Pasternack, S.A.: The American connection: Handguns and homicide. Hospital Tribune, 8:2, 1978.
29. Bakal, C.: The failure of federal gun control. Saturday Review, July 3, 1977, p. 12.
30. Gardner, E.S.: Why gun registration can't cut crimes. American Rifleman, May 1971, p. 17.
31. Dept. of the Treasury: Bureau of Alcohol, Tobacco and Firearms: Firearms Regulations. Arlington, Virginia, 1977.
32. Plain Dealer, Feb.18, 1976.
33. Halverson, G.: Guns: $2 billion business—and thriving. Christian Science Monitor, Nov. 2, Nov. 13, and Nov. 14, 1975.
34. Law Enforcement Assistance Administration Newsletter: 7:5, 1978.
35. Harris Survey: Plain Dealer, Aug. 16, 1979.
36. Editorial: Whose right to arms? Plain Dealer, June 10, 1978.
37. Kanof, N.M.: Memo from the editor. J. Am. Med. Wom. Assoc. 30:470, 1975.

Surgical Critical Care

The Next Challenge in Regionalized Trauma Systems

Frederick A. Moore, MD, Ernest E. Moore, MD

Regionalized trauma centers were developed to provide optimal care for patients with high injury-severity and have, in fact, resulted in improved survival by ensuring early appropriate intervention.[1-3] However, to further reduce preventable deaths, these centers must now focus on the later phases of therapy that is delivered in the intensive care unit (ICU). Historically, trauma surgeons have been effective leaders in this arena, but now a variety of nonsurgeons (eg, anesthesiologists, pulmonologists, and pediatricians) with special interest in critical care believe they can best manage the severely injured.[4-10] They argue that trauma surgeons do not possess the necessary skills nor can devote the time needed to effectively care for the critically ill patient. Trauma surgeons, however, are best positioned to be critical care experts and have implicit responsibilities to comprehensively manage their patients. Abdicating ICU responsibilities to nonsurgeons will clearly fragment patient management and render this costly, advanced care substantially less efficient. Additionally, the ICU will not be optimally integrated into the trauma system. Finally, trauma surgeons will lose ongoing intellectual stimulation and an ideal clinical research environment. The purposes of this article are (*a*) to define a trauma surgeon, (*b*) to explain why critical care is an integral component of this unique profession, and (*c*) to characterize the important roles for trauma surgeons in the ICU.

DEFINITION OF A TRAUMA SURGEON

A trauma surgeon has special expertise and responsibility that spans from prehospitalization care and initial emergency department evaluation through operative intervention to critical care and rehabilitation. The American Board of Surgeons certifies that general surgeons possess the basic knowledge and technical skills to become trauma surgeons, but these surgeons must participate in sufficient clinical work and ongoing educational programs to confront the unique challenges of treating severely injured patients. The trauma surgeon should be (*a*) cognizant of diagnostic options and employ them at the right time in the right patient; (*b*) able to prioritize and coordinate treatment of patients with multiple injuries; (*c*) capable of operating on the neck, chest, abdomen, and extremities to definitively manage life-threatening vascular as well as visceral wounds, (*d*) responsible for the critical care of their patients, and (*e*) actively involved in injury prevention and rehabilitation programs.

While emergent operative intervention is imperative for the early survival of some patients, many high-acuity patients do not require these high-profile efforts. Both patient types, however, benefit from timely, state-of-the-art, high-quality critical care. There is a definable body of surgical expertise (eg, resuscitation, mechanical ventilation, optimal oxygen transport, antibiotic therapy, and nutritional repletion) that needs to be applied appropriately. While nonsurgeons may be capable of performing these tasks individually, they cannot integrate them as effectively in patients with multisystem injuries. The trauma surgeon who oversees resuscitation in the emergency department and interventions in the operating room uses the perspective gained from early contact with the patient to facilitate prompt decisions in the ICU as well as to institute appropriate surveillance for anticipated late complications. Late complications are often the result of the initial tissue trauma/ischemic event or technical imperfections in emergency trauma operation. These common surgical problems are not part of a nonsurgeon's training or subsequent experience. Additionally, trauma surgeons have the responsibility of caring for their patients from admission until discharge from the hospital and cannot be relegated to a "visiting observer" role during the pivotal phase of critical care. Continuity of care is essential, and the patient/surgeon relationship must be maintained. While the nonsurgeon who is an organ-specific specialist can play a valuable role in the care of patients with complex, preexisting disease, their role needs to be clearly defined as a consultant role.

TRAUMA CARE IS CRITICAL CARE

Recent trends in surgical practice and training render the qualified trauma surgeon increasingly scarce. Regionalized trauma systems, which rapidly triage patients with high injury-severity to designated centers, have grown

Accepted for publication March 23, 1992.

From the Surgical Critical Care Unit (Dr F. Moore) and the Department of Surgery (Dr E. Moore), Denver (Colo) General Hospital.

Reprint requests to Department of Surgery, Denver General Hospital, 777 Bannock St, Denver, CO 80204-4507 (Dr F. Moore).

out of the demonstration that survival is enhanced when such triage is performed. It is in these settings that the general surgeons have evolved into accomplished trauma surgeons. Ironically, in level 1 trauma centers, the demand for tertiary referral in academic surgery has caused general surgery to be partitioned into groups such as endocrine, breast, and tumor surgery; upper gastrointestinal tract, hepatobiliary, and pancreatic surgery; and colorectal surgery, and resident trainees are subliminally encouraged to pursue additional specialty fellowship training. Level 2 community surgeons are similarly preoccupied with maintaining a referral base and pragmatically adjust their practices to match financial realities. In both settings, an antiquated billing system has encouraged nonsurgeons to aggressively compete to provide nonoperative critical care.

The explosion in critical care knowledge and technology intimidates practicing surgeons. Consequently, surgeons have relied on other physicians to provide complex preoperative as well as postoperative care. The current medicolegal system unfortunately encourages this behavior. Collectively, these adverse factors discourage surgeons from sustaining a genuine interest in critical care and, thus, maintaining clinical expertise. Consequently, the traditionally dominant role of the surgeon in the clinical management and administration of the ICU has eroded. In academic centers, trauma surgeons have begun to reclaim this territory. A large portion of their practices are devoted to nonoperative critical care of patients with blunt injuries. Out of necessity, they have kept up with the ever increasing body of critical care knowledge and advances in technology. Intellectually, they enjoy the distinction of being critical care experts and have been reasonably well rewarded financially for these activities. Lastly, trauma surgeons have effectively used the ICU as their clinical laboratory and are increasingly being recognized academically for their accomplishments in the ICU. It is hoped that this trend extends more widely to reach level 2 community trauma centers.

THE TRAUMA SURGEON'S ROLES IN AN ICU

Critical Care Specialist

Management of life-threatening injuries is based on priority actions most necessary for survival. Resuscitation in the emergency department is generally initiated before a specific diagnosis is made. Life-threatening injuries are then addressed, often in the operating room. The prevailing focus is to maximize resuscitation; but, additionally, core hypothermia is reversed, coagulopathy corrected, and mechanical ventilation stabilized. Sophisticated monitoring tools and techniques are then used in the ICU to help ensure surgical success. Finally, non–life-threatening injuries are addressed systemically. This may require secondary transport to the radiology department as well as additional trips to the operating room for further intervention by a surgical specialist. Subsequent ICU care often requires extended mechanical ventilation, aggressive hemodynamic monitoring and intervention, metabolic assessment with tailored nutritional support, and administration of antibiotics. Appropriate surveillance and prompt treatment of septic complications is part of routine care. If multiple organ failure develops, acuity of care increases to an entirely different level. Postinjury multiple organ failure is extremely complex, and patients cannot afford fragmented care.

Historically, trauma surgeons have been the identified leaders in this arena. Nonsurgeons, however, argue that trauma surgeons do not possess the skills necessary to care for critically ill patients. Traditionally, general surgery residents, by virtue of daily exposure to a variety of patients, learned to manage patients with complex medical problems. More recently, the American Board of Surgery has increased the emphasis on critical care in both the written and oral examinations. Most training programs now have formal critical care rotations. Consequently, general surgeons are trained to be critical care specialists and, if they become trauma surgeons, they have sufficient clinical exposure to maintain these skills. Critical care is an integral component of the treatment of the severely injured patient, whether it is performed in the emergency department, operating room, or ICU. Moreover, most admissions to the ICU for treatment of blunt trauma are nonoperative cases, and these patients require high-acuity care.

A second argument levied against trauma surgeons is their lack of availability. This should not be a problem for the trauma surgeon who is active in critical care. The income generated from cognitive services delivered in the ICU relieves them of the need for daily schedules full of elective surgeries. On the other hand, the complete trauma surgeon must remain active in meeting the operative challenges of general surgery. Acknowledging that the individual trauma surgeon cannot be at the bedside 24 hours per day, systems must be developed to ensure that the immediate needs of critically injured patients are met. Such needs can be met by other trauma surgeons or a designated critical care team. In the latter case, however, these surrogate deputies must not forget that the attending trauma surgeon is ultimately responsible for the patient and must religiously maintain communication with the trauma surgeon.

ICU Director

Hospitals vary greatly in patient population and services rendered and, consequently, different systems and goals are in place for delivering critical care. However, institutions that have made the commitment to be part of a trauma system as a level 1 trauma center must involve a trauma surgeon in the administration of the ICU, preferably as the director. While this is a time-consuming job, it is a necessary one if the ICU is to be optimally integrated into the trauma system. The trauma surgeon understands how the various components (eg, emergency department, operating room, radiology department, social services department, and rehabilitation unit) function together. The trauma surgeon has the professional interest in and obligation to make the system work best for patients with trauma. Basic surgical training and ongoing clinical experience provide the foundation for determining how new monitoring techniques and therapies are best applied to critically injured patients. The ICU personnel (eg, nurses, respiratory therapists, pharmacists, and social workers) need to interact with a trauma specialist who has the authority to establish rational policies and procedures. The ICU director is responsible for developing an ICU environment where other surgical specialists can care for their patients, but the ICU director should not become every patient's intensivist. The ICU is an invaluable resource that needs to be used appropriately. Consequently, the ICU director should follow up all patients from the periphery and must have the professional recognition (ie, as a surgical colleague) as well as the authority (ie, as appointed by the chairperson of the surgery department) to intervene when (*a*) care deviates from established standards, (*b*) care is clearly futile, or (*c*) limited numbers of beds mandate difficult triage decisions. On a broader scale, the ICU director needs to be involved in an ongoing quality assessment and improvement program. This should identify real problems in the system. Data from such a program, if assessed in a constructive self-review process, can be used to devise a strategy to improve care.

Education and Research

The rapid growth of medical knowledge and technology employed in ICUs has created a need for physicians who have developed special skills in critical care medicine. This broad and complex body of knowledge crosses a variety of specialty interests. Consequently, no one specialty can claim critical care as its sovereign domain. Future intensive care physicians will come from the specialty groups (eg, surgery, anesthesiology, pulmonary medicine, and pediatrics) that provide essential training. The ICU has traditionally been an invaluable resource for surgical training programs. Continual exposure to patients with complex medical problems forces trainees to become physiologically oriented and to integrate multisystem problems into a unified problem list. They learn to be responsible for their patients and to use consultants to provide insight about specific issues. Diligent care is rewarded by successful outcomes. This commitment to patient care has gained professional respect for surgeons, and they are recognized as being much more than mere operating technicians. Systems, however, must be developed to sustain this heritage. Surgery residents and their attending staff members must determine ventilator orders, independent of nonsurgeons. If they do not, mechanical ventilation will become a bewildering therapy. Pulmonary artery catheter placement and intelligent use of available physiologic data must be routine. Infectious disease consultants should not be summoned to diagnose and treat routine surgical infections, nor should a nonsurgeon be allowed to dictate nutritional support. Bedside supervision and teaching by surgeons with a special interest in critical care is essential. Trauma surgeons are ideally suited to serve as role models in surgery training programs.

To maintain a dominant role in critical care, surgeons must preserve their scientific legitimacy by active involvement in clinical and basic research. Comparatively, trauma surgeons have contributed heavily to this evolving body of knowledge. Our current understanding of shock resuscitation, treatment of infection, metabolic stress assessment, nutrition support, pathogenesis of multiple organ failure, and many other topics is derived from careful clinical research performed by trauma surgeons. In part, success stems from the fact that trauma surgeons have access (as attending physicians) to a large number of high-risk patients. Moreover, they control the total ICU environment, thus facilitating clean dissection of clinical questions. Basic research is an important catalyst to an academic career in trauma care permitting new observations in the ICU to be explored promptly at the bench level. Moreover, experience and new knowledge in the basic arena prepares the trauma surgeon to design strategies for clinical research that are more driven by mechanisms and hypotheses.

COMMENT

Trauma surgeons have been instrumental in organizing regionalized trauma systems, and such systems have reduced mortality by ensuring early and appropriate interventions. The next challenge is to optimize the later phases of critical care. Trauma surgeons are acknowledged critical care specialists and need to exert leadership in this arena. Despite current trends, they cannot relinquish ICU management and administration to the nonsurgeon specializing in intense care. Patient care will suffer, the ICU will not be optimally integrated in the trauma system, and trauma surgery will lose credibility as a profession.

We thank Jacqueline Ward for her excellent preparation of the manuscript.

References

1. Cales RH, Trunkey DD. Preventable trauma deaths. *JAMA.* 1985;254:1059-1063.
2. Davis JW, Hoyt DB, McArdle MS, Mackersie RC, Shackford SR, Eastman AB. The significance of critical care errors in causing preventable death in trauma patients in a trauma system. *J Trauma.* 1991;31:813-818.
3. Hoyt DB, Fridlund P, Davis JW, Mackersie RC, Fortlage D. An evaluation of provider and disease related morbidity in a level I trauma service: directions for quality improvement. *J Trauma.* In press.
4. King EG, Sibbald WJ. The territorial imperative. *Chest.* 1988;93:1121-1122.
5. Kelley MA. Critical care medicine: a new specialty? *N Engl J Med.* 1988;318:1613-1617.
6. Gallagher TJ. Guidelines for care: the time has come. *Crit Care Med.* 1991;19:138-140.
7. Meyers AA, Fakhry SM, Sheldon GF. Critical care education in general surgery residencies. *Surgery.* 1989;106:392-399.
8. Holcroft JW. Who should be responsible for care of the critically ill surgical patient? *Arch Surg.* 1990;125:1103-1104.
9. Trash AL, Faber DR. The intensive care unit: who's in charge? *Arch Surg.* 1990;125:1105-1108.
10. Fakhry SM, Buehrer JL, Sheldon GF, Meyer AA. A comparison of intensive care unit care of surgical patients in teaching and nonteaching hospitals. *Ann Surg.* 1991;214:19-23.

Recidivism in an Urban Trauma Center

R. Stephen Smith, MD; William R. Fry, MD; Diane J. Morabito, RN, MPH; Claude H. Organ, Jr, MD

• The incidence of recurrent injury requiring evaluation and treatment at an urban trauma center was assessed by examination of data from the registry of an urban trauma unit. A subgroup of 342 recidivists sustained 711 traumatic injuries. This represented 6.4% of trauma service activations or consultations. The rates of recurrence in random groups of 100 patients with trauma and 50 patients with traumatic deaths were 5% and 12%, respectively. These rates of recurrent injury are lower than those of several previous reports. Comparison of patients with recurrent episodes of trauma with patients who experience a single episode of trauma revealed significant differences in age, sex distribution, mechanism of injury, and fatal outcomes. Recidivists averaged only 7.9 months between episodes of injury. In patients with recurrent trauma with fatal outcomes, the mean interval between initial injury and death was 18.8 months. Early identification of patients at high risk for recurrence may provide an opportunity for behavior modification.

(*Arch Surg.* 1992;127:668-670)

Many urban trauma systems are experiencing critical system strain. Justification for the expense and effort required to provide modern trauma systems is based on the concept that trauma robs our society of productive young people in the prime of life.[1] A serious injury (Abbreviated Injury Score>3) requiring evaluation and treatment in a trauma center is considered an isolated and unusual event. However, the public perception that a traumatic injury is a singular lifetime experience may be false.

Recently published data indicate that many individuals are injured repeatedly and frequently. Additionally, many patients with trauma are involved in illegal activity at the time of injury, are unemployed, and are uninsured.[2] Therefore, the benefit to our society of trauma centers and systems is called into question.

The purpose of this study was to determine the rate of recidivism in a busy urban trauma center and to identify those factors that may indicate that a patient with trauma has a high likelihood of recurrent injury. If such factors can be identified, efforts at behavioral modification of high-risk patients may be effective.

SUBJECTS, MATERIALS, AND METHODS

To determine the incidence of recurrent trauma, trauma registry data from Highland General Hospital were retrieved and examined. The 5-year study period was from September 1986 to October 1991. Highland General Hospital is an urban trauma unit in Oakland, Calif, that primarily serves an adult population. All patients who required activation of the hospital trauma team or consultation by the trauma service were included in the registry. Patients admitted to the hospital and patients treated and released from the emergency department were included. Registry data were evaluated in three ways: (1) the entire registry of 10 894 patient contacts was examined for repetitive users of the trauma system, (2) the medical records of 100 random patients with trauma treated during 1991 were reviewed for history of previous episodes of trauma, and (3) the medical records of 50 random patients who died secondary to trauma were reviewed for evidence of previous injury.

Medical records were examined for evidence of previous trauma, age, sex, mechanism of injury, and intervals between different episodes of trauma. Statistical comparison of these groups was performed with χ^2 analysis or Student's *t* test. Statistical significance was defined as $P<.05$.

RESULTS

During this study period 10 894 patient contacts were entered in the Highland General Hospital trauma registry. The mechanism of injury was blunt trauma in 63% of cases and penetrating trauma in 37% of cases. Seventy-six percent of the contacts were male and 24% were female (3:1 ratio).

A subset of 342 recidivists used our trauma service for 711 activations (mean activations, 2.07 per patient; range, two to seven activations) or consultations. This subset accounted for 6.5% of the total activity of the trauma service. Two hundred ninety-seven (87%) of the recidivists were male. During the study period, 580 deaths occurred as a result of trauma; 42 (7.5%) of these deaths were of patients with recurrent trauma. Unlike the total population with trauma, the patients with recurrent trauma were more likely to have been injured with a penetrating mechanism (435 [61%] of 711 cases) than with a blunt mechanism (276 [39%] of 711 cases). Death in the recurrent group was caused by penetrating trauma in 80% cases compared with 60% for all patients with trauma.

Patients with recurrent trauma were more predominantly male (87%) than the general trauma population (76%). The mean age of the patients with recurrent trauma

Accepted for publication March 26, 1992.

From the Department of Surgery, Division of Trauma, University of California–Davis, East Bay, Oakland.

Reprint requests to the Department of Surgery, University of California–Davis, East Bay, 1411 E 31st St, Oakland, CA 94602 (Dr Smith).

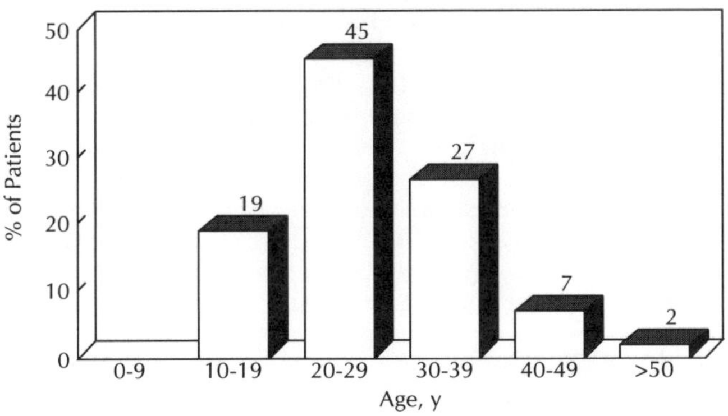

Fig 1.—*Age of recidivist at first traumatic injury.*

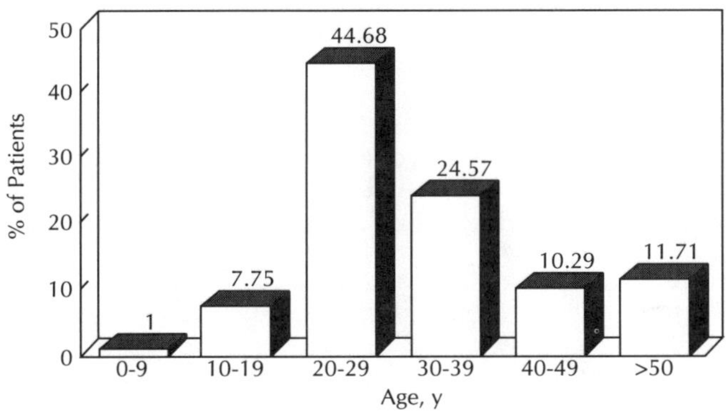

Fig 2.—*Distribution of all patients with trauma by age.*

Table 1.—Comparison of Patients With Single Episodes of Trauma With Patients With Multiple Episodes

	No. of Patients	Mean Age, y	No. (%) of Male Patients*	Penetrating Trauma, No. (%) of Patients*	Mortality, No. (%) of Patients*
Single episode	10 552	33.0	8020 (76)	3904 (37)	538 (5.1)
Multiple episodes	342	27.7	298 (87)	209 (61)	42 (12.3)

*$P<.001$.

was 27.7 years (range, 16 to 68 years), while the mean age of all patients with trauma was 33.0 years. Ninety-three percent of patients with recurrent trauma were younger than age 40 years at the time of initial injury (Fig 1). In the nonrecurrent population, 78% of patients were younger than age 40 years (Fig 2).

Among the recidivists, the mean interval between trauma incidents was 7.9 months (range, 0 to 54 months). In the 42 patients with recurrent trauma (12%) who sustained a fatal outcome, the mean interval between the initial incident and death was 18.8 months (range, 2 to 46 months). Five patients were readmitted to the trauma service within 24 hours of their initial injury. Differences in population groups that achieved statistical significance are listed in Table 1.

The medical records of 100 patients with presumed nonrecurrent trauma in 1991 were examined for comparison with those of the patients with recurrent trauma. Data obtained from the review of these records closely approximated the characteristics of the entire registry. Blunt trauma was the mechanism of injury in 67% of cases. The mean age of patients was 33.0 years (range, 16 to 97 years). Five of these randomly chosen patients had a history of previous significant trauma that had been treated at another trauma center or at our hospital before the establishment of the trauma registry.

The medical records of 50 randomly chosen patients with traumatic deaths were examined. Six (12%) of these patients had evidence of previous significant trauma. Penetrating trauma was the cause of death in 32 (64%) of these patients. The mean age of this group was 32.9 years (range, 15 to 87 years). Analysis of this group of patients with random deaths showed the population to be very similar to the general population with trauma. A comparison with study groups is presented in Table 2.

COMMENT

Trauma was once "the neglected disease of modern society." It is now known that trauma is the leading cause of death in Americans younger than age 44 years and the third leading cause of death when all age groups are considered. Because of the predominantly younger patient population that it affects, trauma is the leading cause of

Table 2.—Comparison of Study Groups*

Characteristic	All Trauma	Recurrent Trauma	Random Trauma	Deaths in Patients With Recurrent Trauma	Random Deaths
No. of patients	10 894	342	100	43	50
Sex					
Male	8279 (76)	298 (87)	82 (82)	40 (93)	40 (80)
Female	2615 (24)	44 (13)	18 (18)	3 (7)	10 (20)
Mean age, y	33.0	27.7	33.0	27.0	32.9
Age <40 y	8497 (78)	318 (93)	80 (80)	41 (95)	39 (78)
Penetrating injuries	4031 (37)	209 (61)	33 (33)	34 (80)	32 (64)
Blunt injuries	6863 (63)	133 (39)	67 (67)	9 (20)	18 (36)
Recidivism	711 (6.4)	342 (100)	5 (5)	43 (100)	6 (12)
Mean interval, mo	. . .	7.9†	. . .	18.8‡	. . .

*Unless otherwise indicated, data are numbers (%) of patients.
†Interval between episodes of trauma.
‡Interval between initial trauma service activation and the episode of fatal trauma.

years of life lost in the United States.[3] Because this age group is commonly involved in accidents, it has been generally expected that many successfully treated patients with trauma would return to a productive role in society. This opinion has been one of the factors that has led legislative bodies and public opinion to support the improvement of trauma care despite the significant expenditures required.

In the previous 2 decades, Trunkey[1] and others[4-8] have documented that improved outcome after injury can be achieved in hospitals with a significant commitment to trauma care. These studies paved the way for the development of trauma systems and centers in many areas of the United States. However, recent reports have described urban trauma as a chronic recurrent disease peculiar to unemployed, uninsured law breakers.[2,9] It is unlikely that popular support of trauma systems and centers can be maintained if this is indeed the case. The widespread closure of trauma centers in urban areas, such as Los Angeles, Calif, may be the harbinger of a national trend partially based on this perception of patients with trauma. The reluctance of many general surgeons to actively participate in trauma care in their communities may also be a result of this perception.[10]

The trauma unit from which these data were retrieved is located in an urban area that set a record for homicides in 1991 for the third consecutive year and is presently on a course predicted to surpass that record. Statistics confirm that violent crime is becoming more common in areas that have traditionally been spared (*San Francisco Examiner*. January 12, 1992:B-1). Penetrating injuries are present in 37% of the patients with trauma who are brought to our trauma center.

Before initiating this review, we anticipated finding a high rate of recidivism, as has been reported from other urban centers.[2,9] Our analysis identified 342 patients with more than one incident of trauma treated by our trauma service. This represents only 6.4% of the activations or consultations of our trauma service, significantly less than those in the recent reports by Sims et al[9] and Morrisey et al,[2] with recurrence rates of 44% and 32.6%, respectively. These reports concentrated on penetrating injuries or assaults, while we included all patients with trauma in our study. We believe that our analysis places the recidivism rate in a more balanced perspective. Other reasons for this difference are difficult to assess.

Patients injured prior to 1986 are not in the Highland General Hospital trauma registry. Highland General Hospital is in a geographic area that is served by multiple trauma centers and it is possible that some of our patients may have been taken to other trauma centers for subsequent episodes of trauma. Potential patients with recurrent trauma may have relocated to another area. However, our evaluation of the medical records of 100 random patients with trauma (5% with recurrent trauma) and 50 random patients with traumatic deaths (12% with recurrent trauma) failed to show rates of recidivism comparable with those of other reports.

Among our patients with recurrent trauma, penetrating injuries were much more common than in the total population with trauma (61% vs 37%). The cause of death among the recidivist group was also much more likely to be penetrating trauma when compared with the entire registry (80% vs 60%). Patients with recurrent trauma were also more likely to be male (87% vs 76%) and younger (mean age, 27.7 vs 33.0 years) than the other groups of patients in the study. The mean interval between episodes of trauma was short (7.9 months) and the mean time from initial presentation to the trauma service to the time of death in the 42 patients with recurrent trauma was 18.8 months. The brief period between initial injury and subsequent injury or death seems to indicate a high-risk environment and life-style in recidivists. If intervention and behavior modification are to be successful it appears necessary to initiate such programs as soon as possible after injury. These efforts should probably be initiated immediately after contact with the trauma service. Male patients younger than age 30 years admitted with penetrating injuries are the group most likely to benefit from such posttrauma psychosocial counseling.

Analysis of these data suggests that for a subgroup of patients with trauma recidivism is a significant problem. This group is more likely to have been injured with a penetrating mechanism, to be young and male, and to subsequently have a fatal outcome following trauma. Our information does not provide definitive criteria that may be used to identify patients at higher risk for recurrent episodes of trauma since the so-called average trauma patient is a young male. Further study of socioeconomic, cultural, and psychological factors, such as drug or alcohol abuse, gang membership, employment status, home situation, and education, may reveal risk criteria that can be applied to the clinical environment. Early identification of this group of patients could provide an opportunity to initiate a program of counseling and behavior modification with the goal of altering life-styles to avoid trauma recidivism.

While a small percentage of our patient population with trauma represents a group of patients with chronic recurrent trauma, the majority of our patients do not fall into this category. We believe that the goal of returning patients to productive, useful roles in society is not inconsistent with our clinical experience and that continued support for trauma systems is both justified and desirable. Programs for behavior modification directed at teenagers, such as "Youth Alive" and "Teens On Target," may hold an important position in the rehabilitation phase of trauma care for high-risk groups.

References

1. Trunkey DD. Trauma. *Sci Am*. 1983;246:28-35.
2. Morrisey MC, Byrd RC, Deitch EA. The incidence of recurrent penetrating trauma in an urban trauma center. *J Trauma*. 1991;31:1536-1538.
3. Committee on Trauma Research, Commission of Life Sciences, National Research Council and Institute of Medicine. *Injury in America: A Continuing Public Health Problem*. Washington DC: National Academy Press; 1985:13-36.
4. Trunkey DD, Lim RC. Analysis of 425 consecutive trauma fatalities: an autopsy study. *J Am Coll Emerg Phys*. 1974;3:368-371.
5. Trunkey DD. Bay area trauma care. *San Francisco Med*. 1982;55:22-25.
6. West JG, Trunkey DD, Lim RC. Systems of trauma care: a study of two counties. *Arch Surg*. 1979;114:455-460.
7. West JG, Cales RH, Gazziniga AB. Impact of regionalization: the Orange County experience. *Arch Surg*. 1983;118:740-744.
8. Cales RH. Trauma mortality in Orange County: the effect of implementation of a regional trauma system. *Ann Emerg Med*. 1984;13:1-10.
9. Sims DW, Bivins BA, Obeid FN, et al. Urban trauma: a chronic recurrent disease. *J Trauma*. 1989;29:940.
10. Trunkey DD. What's wrong with trauma care? *Bull Am Coll Surg*. 1990;75:10-15.

Injury and Violence in Los Angeles

Impact on Access to Health Care and Surgical Education

Arthur W. Fleming, MD; Rosalyn P. Sterling-Scott, MD; Gabriel Carabello, MD; Imani Imari-Williams, PA-C; Brenda Allmond, RN; Randall S. Foster, MHA; Frank Kennedy, MD; William C. Shoemaker, MD

• The Los Angeles County (California) Trauma Hospital System was designed to ensure that all patients requiring specialized trauma care would be transported directly to a trauma center using established trauma triage criteria. The designation and implementation of all level 1, 2, and 3 (rural) trauma centers were completed between October 1983 and July 1985. However, by February 1, 1985, one level 2 trauma center withdrew, and nine other level 2 and 3 trauma centers followed suit over the next few months and years. The reasons for closure of these 10 trauma centers were almost exclusively related to economic factors. The major impact of trauma center closure on surgical educational programs at the Drew University of Medicine and Science and the Martin Luther King, Jr/Charles R. Drew Medical Center have been additive and cumulative. The high volume of patients with trauma has been cited, sometimes correctly and sometimes incorrectly, as the primary reason for a lack of access to health care for patients without trauma. We have developed a blueprint for survival that, when fully implemented, will improve access to health care for all residents in our catchment area and optimize surgical education. While the Los Angeles County Trauma Hospital System has had many difficulties during the last 9 years, the population it serves is greater than that in 42 states in the United States. The experiences gained in Los Angeles County may be beneficial to statewide systems in the United States and in countries of comparable size.

(*Arch Surg.* 1992;127:671-676)

Injury is the principal public health problem in the United States today. Injury causes almost half the deaths in children aged 1 to 4 years, more than half the deaths in children aged 5 to 14 years, and nearly four fifths of the deaths of persons aged 15 to 24 years.[1] Two people are injured every second; every 15 seconds, one person is injured severely enough to be hospitalized; one person dies of injury-related conditions every 4 minutes; and one person is severely or permanently disabled because of injury every 7 minutes.[1,2]

Whether measured in dollar costs, physician contacts, premature deaths, or years of productive life lost, injuries are the most serious health problem facing this country. The aggregate cost for the 57 million persons injured in 1985 was $158 billion, with nearly 75% of that sum ($116 billion) being the cost for care delivered in the year after injury and approximately 25% ($41 billion) being the estimated cost for care delivered in later years.[2,3]

Numerous studies have shown that a large percentage of deaths due to injury are preventable. Accurate matching of patients with available treatment resources should logically result in reduced mortality and morbidity. To this end, California's Los Angeles County (LAC) sought to develop a comprehensive emergency care system. The purpose of this article is to review the evolution of trauma centers in the largest trauma system in the United States and to describe its impact on both access to care in our underserved community and the development of our surgery education program.

UNIQUENESS OF LAC

Los Angeles is a sprawling city of 465 square miles in an expansive county covering 4000 square miles. The county's emergency medical system serves a population estimated at more than 9 million documented and 2 million undocumented people. The total population of LAC is greater than the population of 42 states in the United States. This is also the largest population in the United States served by a single emergency medical service system.

Formal planning for a trauma system in LAC began in September 1979 when the Board of Supervisors of LAC instructed the Department of Health Services to study and make recommendations on the need for a trauma hospital system in LAC.

In 1981, a trauma questionnaire was distributed to the 97 hospitals in LAC with licensed basic emergency medical services to determine the trauma caseload. Based on survey results from the 88 responding hospitals (91%), an estimated 8100 cases of severe trauma occurred in LAC in 1980. At the time of the survey, patients with trauma were

Accepted for publication March 26, 1992.

From the Departments of Surgery (Drs Fleming, Sterling-Scott, Carabello, and Kennedy; Ms Imari-Williams; and Ms Allmond) and Emergency Medicine (Mr Foster and Dr Shoemaker), Charles R. Drew University of Medicine and Science, Martin Luther King, Jr/Charles R. Drew Medical Center, Los Angeles, Calif.

Reprint requests to Department of Surgery, Charles R. Drew University of Medicine and Science, Martin Luther King, Jr/Charles R. Drew Medical Center, 12021 S Wilmington Ave, Los Angeles, CA 90059 (Dr Fleming).

Table 1.—Reasons for Hospitals Withdrawing From the Los Angeles County (California) Trauma System*

Inadequate financial reimbursement
High volume of indigent care
Unmet surgeon expectations and needs
Unavailability of neurosurgeons
Difficult timing of trauma events; often high volume of trauma patients
Potentially violent and dangerous visitors
Disruptive impact on private practice of hospitals
Perception that trauma victims are not from local communities

*From *Planning Retreat Final Report 1990,* Los Angeles, Calif, Los Angeles County Trauma System Blue Ribbon Advisory Committee, Department of Health Services, 1990, page 16.

routinely taken to the nearest hospital for care. Thus, the average number of patients with trauma per institution per year was 92, with many hospitals treating fewer patients and an occasional hospital treating several hundred patients.

After 4 years of planning, discussion, public hearings, and deliberations by the Board of Supervisors, a number of difficult issues were resolved and the salient characteristics of the Trauma Hospital System were finally adopted by the Board on January 25, 1983. The plan to implement a trauma care network included a process for the selection and designation of level 1 trauma centers first, and, second, a process for the selection and designation of level 2 trauma centers in the areas not covered by level 1 facilities.

Request for proposals were distributed on February 4, 1983, with a May 5, 1983, submission deadline. Key criteria for trauma center designation included the following:

1. Commitment by the hospital and its medical staff to treat and care for any patient presenting
2. Demonstrated capacity and ability to care for 750 patients with trauma annually, including surgical and intensive care unit capacities/capabilities
3. A helipad (with appropriate licenses), and
4. Graduate medical education programs in surgery and surgical specialties accredited by the Accreditation Council for Graduate Medical Education.

Considerable enthusiasm for designation as a level 1 trauma center was exhibited by many hospitals. Activities included (but were not limited to) hiring consultants from the East Coast to assist in proposal preparation; major construction and remodeling of emergency departments; building of heliports; and documentation of rotations of surgical residents to certain hospitals to satisfy criteria for designation as a level 1 trauma center. Based on a review of the proposals and surveys conducted by out-of-state reviewers on May 23 to 24, 1983, the Department of Health Services identified nine hospitals that satisfied the criteria for level 1 trauma centers. The Board of Supervisors approved the Department's recommendations to designate nine hospitals as level 1 trauma centers on October 11, 1983. On December 15, 1983, the Martin Luther King, Jr/Charles R. Drew (King-Drew) Medical Center (KDMC), seven other adult facilities, and one pediatric center were implemented as level 1 trauma centers.

The next step was to designate level 2 trauma centers

Table 2.—Characteristics of Los Angeles County (California) Trauma Centers

Center	Average No. of Patients Per Year	No. of Beds Licensed for Use	Catchment Population
Level 1 Trauma Centers			
King-Drew Medical Center	2520	480	995 600
University of Southern California Medical Center	3180	2045	1 209 915
Harbor UCLA Medical Center	1200	553	709 250
Cedars-Sinai Medical Center	936	1119	354 891
Childrens Hospital of Los Angeles	336	331	Unknown
Huntington Memorial Hospital	636	606	540 972
Long Beach Memorial Medical Center	960	998	486 759
St Mary Medical Center	600	556	199 610
UCLA Medical Center	756	711	541 330
Level 2 Trauma Centers			
Holy Cross Hospital	588	264	466 002
Northridge Hospital Medical Center	552	349	445 388
Level 3 Trauma Centers			
Henry Mayo Newhall Memorial Hospital	264	133	99 999
Westlake Community Hospital	60	126	58 108

for patients with trauma who were not near level 1 trauma centers. In turn, rural trauma centers were designated to provide service to areas not covered by level 1 and level 2 trauma centers. A total of 23 hospitals were designated as trauma centers. Before completion of the designation process for all trauma centers, one level 2 trauma center, California Hospital Medical Center, withdrew from the trauma system. By 1989, only 13 trauma centers remained in the system. Reasons for hospital withdrawal are summarized in Table 1. The difficulties encountered in maintaining physician commitment to caring for patients with trauma in LAC are reflected nationwide, especially by residents as they plan their careers.[4]

There currently are nine level 1 trauma centers (including three public, county-run hospitals), two level 2 trauma centers, and two level 3 trauma centers in LAC that care for an estimated 12 600 patients with trauma admitted annually (Table 2). Fifty-five percent of these patients are treated in the public hospitals. The geographic distribution of the original and current trauma centers is illustrated in Fig 1.

Two factors that contribute to injury in LAC are gang activity and alcohol and drug abuse. The number of reported gang members in LAC has doubled since 1985 to at least 100 000 members in 1000 cliques. This is in stark contrast to the 10 000 to 15 000 gang members in Chicago, Ill, and New York City. Gang violence has claimed the

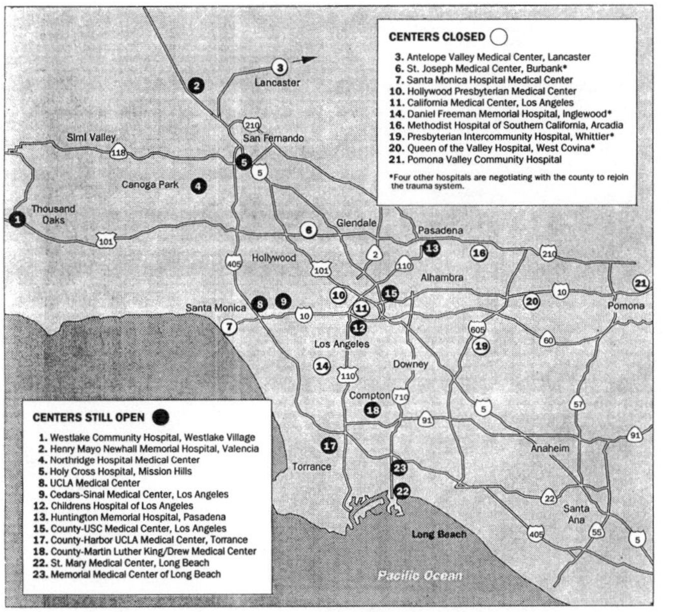

Fig 1.—*Map of all existing and closed trauma centers in Los Angeles County, Calif. Copyright, 1990,* Los Angeles Times. *Reprinted by permission.*

lives of more than 700 people in LAC in 1991, continuing a wave of bloodshed that has been rising for a decade (*Daily Breeze*. December 9, 1991:A1).

The relationship between alcohol use and homicide was characterized using data from the Los Angeles City Police Department and the Los Angeles Medical Examiner's Office regarding 4950 victims of criminal homicides in Los Angeles from 1970 through 1979. Alcohol was detected in the blood of 1883 (46%) of the 4092 homicide victims who were tested.[5]

Subsequent homicide and autopsy reviews revealed that south central Los Angeles (the KDMC catchment area) contained 17% of the county's population and was the site of 51% of the county's homicides. In addition, 51% of the victims found in this area had detectable levels of alcohol, cocaine, or alcohol and cocaine in their blood.

Violence has also increased in the pediatric population. Between 1989 and 1991, 547 children younger than age 17 years suffered gunshot wounds. Seventy-three of these children were aged 12 years or younger. Caring for infants and children brought to the hospital in traumatic, full cardiac arrest because of gunshot wounds and seeing infants and children who are dead-on-arrival because of gunshot wounds to the head has been particularly stressful not only for young surgical residents, but also for the whole health care team involved with such patients.

UNIQUENESS OF THE CHARLES R. DREW UNIVERSITY OF MEDICINE AND SCIENCE AND THE LAC–MARTIN LUTHER KING, JR/CHARLES R. DREW MEDICAL CENTER

The founding of the Charles R. Drew University of Medicine and Science (originally the Charles R. Drew Postgraduate Medical School) and KDMC (originally the LAC-Martin Luther King, Jr, General Hospital) was one of several contemporaneous events that signaled the turning point of the American conscience.[6] The report of the Governor's Commission, chaired by John A. McCone, after the Watts revolt in August 1965 recognized that the residents of Watts and surrounding areas had significant health problems that were not met by existing health facilities and services.[7] Based on statewide formulas, the Department of Public Health determined that only 21% of the residents of Watts were receiving the hospital care they needed and concluded that a 394-bed, acute general hospital was needed.[8] King-Drew Medical Center opened its doors in March 1972 on the site of a former public housing project purchased in 1966 for $100 000.[6] The Charles R. Drew Postgraduate Medical School was incorporated as a private, nonprofit institution in August 1966 and as the academic arm of the hospital. The mission of the school was and continues to be "to conduct medical education and research in the context of service to a defined population and to train persons to provide care with competence and compassion to this and other underserved populations."[9] In 1978, an affiliation agreement was signed between the Charles R. Drew Postgraduate Medical School and UCLA, initiating the Drew/UCLA Medical Education Program. The first class of 21 students was admitted in fall 1981. Students complete their first 2 years at UCLA School of Medicine and their third and fourth years at KDMC. The Drew/UCLA Medical Education Program is fully accredited by the Liaison Council on Medical Education as a program of the UCLA School of Medicine. In recognition of the graduate medical education program and the School of Allied Health, the Charles R. Drew Postgraduate Medical School gained designation as a university in 1987.

King-Drew Medical Center has a catchment area of a little more than 1 million documented residents and an unknown number of undocumented residents. Only 10 cities in the United States have a population greater than 1 million. By 1976, an ad hoc committee appointed by the dean of Drew University and charged with evaluating the Department of Surgery recognized that "The hospital, beautiful in concept and appearance, was quickly found to be inadequate in design and available space."[10]

IMPACT ON ACCESS TO HEALTH CARE

Between March 1983 and December 1983, an average of 22 patients with major trauma (excluding isolated head injuries) were treated each month at KDMC, or approximately 264 annually. It was anticipated that after implementing a level 1 trauma center at KDMC the number of patients with major trauma presenting annually would increase threefold to 792.

In its first month as a trauma center (December 15, 1983, to January 14, 1984), the number of patients evaluated increased threefold. To accommodate this increase, the following changes were made: (1) placement of interns and residents on every-other-night on-call duty, resulting in average work weeks of 110 hours (for 6 months); (2) discontinuation of interns' rotations to internal medicine, pediatrics, anesthesiology, and emergency medicine units; (3) alteration or discontinuation of rotations to all surgical subspecialty units (orthopedics, neurosurgery, plastic surgery, and urology); and (4) implementation of a rule requiring that faculty stay in-house when on-call.[11]

By 1985, the total number of patients with trauma treated at KDMC was 3325. Table 3 details the activity of our trauma center by mechanism of patient injury from 1985 to 1991. Before closure of the third largest designated trauma center in LAC (Daniel Freeman Memorial Hospital, the trauma center closest to KDMC) in 1987, we were faced with an inability to adequately handle the routine

Table 3.—Patients With Trauma Presenting to King-Drew Medical Center From 1985 to 1991

	1985 (N=3325)	1986 (N=3233)	1987 (N=4093)	1988 (N=3473)	1989 (N=3764)	1990 (N=3518)	1991 (N=3788)	Total (N=25 144)
Total No. of patients discharged from the emergency department	**133**	**136**	**750**	**683**	**905**	**900**	**976**	**4483**
Total No. of patients admitted	**3192**	**3097**	**3343**	**2790**	**2859**	**2618**	**2762**	**20 661**
Patients with gunshot wounds	606	794	1472	1044	1308	1259	1408	**7891**
Patients with stab wounds	415	423	550	347	378	343	351	**2807**
Patients who were assaulted	682	570	632	495	494	405	336	**3614**
Patients who were victims of other types of violence	1489	1310	689	904	679	611	667	**6349**

caseload. The reasons for this inability were as follows: (1) Patients frequently had to be kept in the operating room for recovery because the postanesthesia recovery room and the surgical intensive care unit (SICU) were full. (2) Patients requiring SICU beds were triaged prematurely to the ward. (3) Elective surgeries had to be canceled because of patients with trauma who needed emergency surgery or lack of nurses to staff the operating room. (4) Chronic, unrelenting, nursing shortages resulted from inadequate compensation and extremely stressful working conditions. As a result, beds in surgery wards became filled only with patients with or without trauma who needed emergency or urgent care. The severity of illnesses of the other patients in-house increased, further exacerbating the stressful working conditions.

The closure of trauma care facilities at Daniel Freeman Memorial Hospital contributed to an increase in the number of patients with trauma treated at KDMC of 500% more than the original projections. The volume of patients treated represented more than a 1000% increase in the volume treated before trauma center designation. Because of trauma center closures, the KDMC catchment area was expanded in easterly and westerly directions in 1987 and 1989, respectively. These boundary changes intensified the problem of managing the acutely ill. In 1989, the State Department of Health Services' Licensing and Certification Division concluded that patient overcrowding and nursing staff shortages in both the emergency department and inpatient wards at KDMC violated state codes. Balancing the patient-nurse ratio became a critical objective for KDMC because such a balance was necessary for KDMC to remain open as a tertiary care center. Thus, in November 1989, 33 beds in each the surgery and general medicine units and 27 beds in the pediatrics unit were no longer allowed to be used in an attempt to relieve this untenable situation. These reductions represented approximately one third of the beds on each of the units. The pediatrics unit was again licensed to use these beds in August 1990. The general medicine unit was again licensed to use 15 of the 33 beds in November 1991. Likewise, the surgery unit was licensed to use 15 of the 33 beds in February 1992.

An increased number of patients with gunshot wounds were treated from 1985 to 1991, as illustrated in Table 3. The number of injuries resulting from large-caliber/high-velocity missiles has also escalated during the last 6 years. It should be noted that 27% of patients with gunshot wounds were treated as outpatients. The numbers of victims of motor vehicle accidents, stabbings, and assaults treated has remained relatively constant.

The magnitude of the impact on health care access at KDMC might be better understood by reviewing a comparison of the number of beds the facility was licensed to use with the number of patients with trauma admitted during 1990 in LAC trauma centers (Fig 2). During the last 8 years, all of our hospital beds have been occupied with "the sickest of the sick," with an additional 5% of patients requring admission to the hospital staying in the emergency department because no hospital beds were available. Approximately 40% of the adjusted daily admissions (total admissions excluding newborns and their mothers) are admissions to the surgical services, and of these, approximately 60% are admissions related to trauma. In addition, 60% of the patients with trauma are victims of violence. Based on these data, trauma accounts for 24% of adjusted daily admissions.

The hospital evaluated 14 929 acutely ill medical and surgical patients in 1990 whose conditions were reported in telephone calls to 911. An equivalent number of such patients were treated at LAC/University of Southern California Medical Center, a facility with three times the number of operating beds as KDMC. The volume of patients at KDMC whose conditions were reported via 911 telephone calls surpassed that of LAC-Harbor/UCLA Medical Center by 9269 patients, or 264%, despite having 19% fewer operating beds (Fig 3). A contributory factor to the high level of activity at KDMC was the closing of 15 of the 20 hospitals in operation in south central Los Angeles at the time of the Watts riots.

The large number of patients with trauma significantly interfered with the timely care of other diseases requiring surgical intervention. For example, in July 1991, 159 scheduled operations were canceled. The most common reasons for cancellation were as follows: prioritization of urgent cases (39 cases [25%]); postanesthesia recovery room/SICU overload (33 cases [21%]); staffing shortages (15 cases [9%]); and overbooked operating rooms (14 cases [9%]). Attempts to divert paramedic ambulances to other facilities were not uniformly successful. When all three public trauma centers were closed, we basically still received patients with trauma for whom ours was the

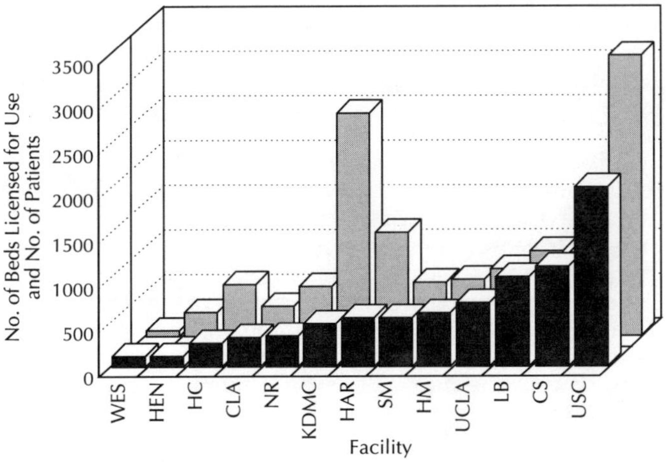

Fig 2.—*The number of beds facilities are licensed to use (dark bars) and the number of patients with trauma (light bars) admitted to Los Angeles County (California) trauma centers in 1990. WES indicates Westlake Community Hospital; HUN, Huntington Memorial Hospital; HC, Holy Cross Hospital; CLA, Children's Hospital of Los Angeles; NR, Northridge Hospital Medical Center; KDMC, Martin Luther King, Jr/Charles R. Drew Medical Center; HAR, Harbor UCLA Medical Center; SM, St Mary Medical Center; HM, Henry Mayo Newhall Memorial Hospital; LB, Memorial Medical Center of Long Beach; CS, Cedars-Sinai Medical Center; and USC, University of Southern California Medical Center.*

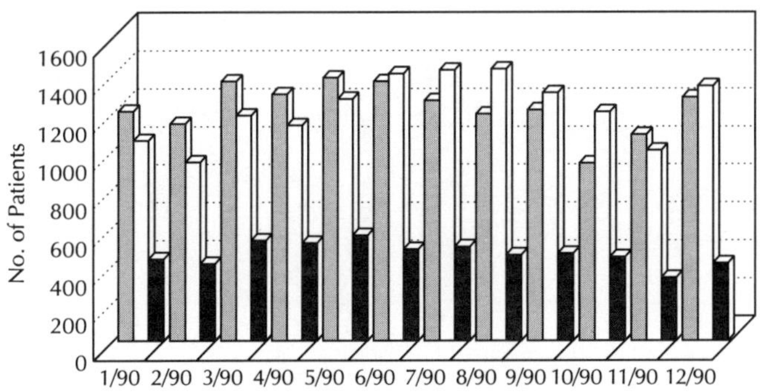

Fig 3.—*Distribution of patients with trauma among emergency departments of the three public level 1 trauma centers in Los Angeles County (California) in 1990. Light bars indicate the University of Southern California; open bars, Martin Luther King, Jr/Charles R. Drew Medical Center; and dark bars, Harbor/UCLA.*

closest hospital because there were no suitable alternatives. For instance, in June 1991 we were closed 19% of the month, but still received 51 patients during the closed periods. On one occasion, eight patients were brought to KDMC during a 12-hour closed period.

IMPACT ON GENERAL SURGERY RESIDENCY EDUCATION

When KDMC opened in March 1972, it was notified by the Residency Review Committee (RRC) that provisional approval was given for a 4-year surgical residency program to begin on July 1, 1972. In 1975, a request was made for a 5-year program, which gained full approval. At that time the number of residents had increased to 23. Between 1978 and 1982, the program was on probation. It subsequently lost its accreditation in October 1982. After reconsideration, the decision to withdraw accreditation was sustained. One of the primary concerns of the Residency Review Committee was an inadequate exposure of residents to a sufficiently broad spectrum and volume of surgical experience.

An application for a new general surgery residency program with rotations to other hospitals, which offered additional exposure to elective surgery, was submitted and approved in 1983. In 1984, the program was expanded to 6 years and 24 residents, and in 1989, to 34 residents. Our General Surgery Residency Program currently has full accreditation. The 34 residency positions are filled at the following levels: postgraduate year 1, 12 residents; 2, six residents; and 3 through 6, four residents each.[6]

Despite the negative impact on recruitment caused by being on probation between 1978 and 1982, 93% of all graduates have taken the Qualifying Examination of the American Board of Surgery. Thirty (77%) of the 39 residents taking the Qualifying Examination and 23 (88%) of the 26 graduates taking the Certifying Examination passed the tests. The four June 1991 graduates have passed the Qualifying Examination and will be taking the Certifying Examination this year.

Numerous innovative approaches have been and are being developed to maintain a balance of exposure for residency training, while increasing surgical care in a county with decreasing resources. These approaches include the following: (1) integrating our residency program with the California Medical Center, a 321-bed community hospital near downtown Los Angeles; (2) affiliation (with plans to integrate) our residency program with the Long Beach Memorial Medical Center, a 998-bed volunteer hospital in Long Beach; (3) initiation of the first Physician's Assistant Postgraduate Surgical Residency Program west of the Mississippi River; (4) establishment of a Trauma/Critical Care Fellowship; and (5) institution of a trauma rotation for two of the eight surgical training programs of the United States Army (begun in July 1989). We are in the process of developing the Drew University Surgical Service at California Medical Center and establishing a freestanding trauma center on the KDMC campus.

FREESTANDING TRAUMA CENTER ON THE KDMC CAMPUS

In May 1988, the LAC Board of Supervisors recognized the continued and growing need to provide emergency and trauma care services at KDMC and authorized plans for a self-contained, freestanding trauma center complete with diagnostic radiology and intensive care services as well as operating rooms. The center is now undergoing mechanical and structural development. The space allocation review was completed in August 1989, followed by completion of the schematic design in December 1989. Construction costs for the project have been projected to be $65 400 000. Funding has been planned through revenue bonds and bond anticipation notes. The anticipated ground-breaking will take place in September 1992. The new trauma center is expected to be completed in 1995.

The new trauma center will increase our operating room capability by 33% and our SICU capacity by 100%. An intermediate care area, which currently does not exist, will also be established. We anticipate that the current operating room will be used exclusively for treatment of patients without trauma.

COMMENT

F. William Blaisdell, MD, in his 1991 presidential address to the American Association for Surgery of Trauma, stated that, "Whether or not national health insurance is passed, the last 25 years have demonstrated that there will always be those who have problems with access to mainstream health care and that there is a need for hospitals that will provide for the neglected patients and neglected diseases."[12] King-Drew Medical Center, with 480 beds licensed for use, 80 of which are for psychiatric patients, and 36 of which are temporarily not licensed for use, can truthfully say that it has offered care under extraordinary circumstances. Like many of the present and previous public hospitals, KDMC experiences a myriad of adversities in the daily management of too many patients.

The academic consequences of the failure of a trauma system were explored by Fischer et al[13] based on their experience in Houston, Tex. The University of Texas Medical School at Houston suffered a severe decrease in variety of clinical experience provided to surgical residents and medical students as well as a severe reduction in faculty-generated billing at its private hospital, Hermann Hospital, under conditions very similar to those in Los Angeles. A severe shortage of SICU nurses also played a major role in compounding the problems.

Despite a nursing shortage and the unavailability of 33% of surgical beds at KDMC because of licensing restrictions throughout 1990 and 1991, the annual census of patients with trauma for both years exceeded the figures from the 1988 census. Unlike the Texas medical school, we did not have the luxury of diverting patients to another facility. The potential benefits to our surgical training program of having residents in the 90th to 98th percentile for trauma experience may not be fully appreciated. In fact, one level 1 trauma center in LAC has expounded on the benefits of nonoperative trauma management in postgraduate surgical training.[14] Despite our heavy load of operative cases, our chief residents each manage, nonoperatively, more than 100 cases of blunt trauma. As the number of endoscopic surgeries increases, the number of elective open procedures will decrease. An oral presentation by the American Board of Surgery in March 1992 suggested that treatment of patients with trauma as part of a residency training program may be used to fulfill several important operative categories for completion of surgical residency training (eg, criteria regarding training in head and neck, liver, pancreas, and vascular injuries) provided that more than the minimal number of trauma cases have been managed.

The value of institutionally shared trauma rotations as viable solutions to deficiencies in trauma training has been discussed by Richardson et al.[15] Likewise, we have enjoyed a successful relationship with two military surgical residency programs.

The caseload of patients with trauma at KDMC has undoubtedly been a challenge not only to the surgery, emergency medicine, anesthesiology, radiology, pathology, and nursing departments, but also to all the ancillary support staff. Several innovative approaches have been implemented to cope with the difficulties encountered.

Injury in the United States is the most important public health problem we face. We see the advancement of trauma management as crucial to our survival as a struggling public institution in the largest county in the United States. Three quarters of a century ago, Charles Mayo indicated that the objects of medical education are to heal the sick and advance medical science. By today's standards, we might add this object: to prepare medical students and residents as physicians and specialists of tomorrow. If the management of trauma is reviewed in the context of these three objectives, perhaps more young surgeons would share our commitment to treating the most common cause of premature death in the United States.

References

1. Committee to Review the Status and Progress of the Injury Control Program at the Centers for Disease Control. *Injury Control.* Washington, DC: National Academy Press; 1988:9.
2. Rice DP, MacKenzie EJ, et al. *Cost of Injury in the United States: A Report to Congress.* San Francisco, Calif: Institute for Health & Aging, University of California, and Injury Prevention Center, The Johns Hopkins University; 1989.
3. Committee on Trauma Research, Commission of Life Sciences, National Research Council, Institute of Medicine. *Injury in America: A Continuing Public Health Problem.* Washington, DC: National Academy Press; 1985.
4. Richardson JD, Miller FB. Will future surgeons be interested in trauma care? *J Trauma.* 1992;32:229-235.
5. Goodman RA, Mercy JA, Loya F, et al. Alcohol use and interpersonal violence: alcohol detected in homicide victims. *Am J Public Health.* 1986;76:144-149.
6. Fleming AW. Martin Luther King, Jr, General Hospital and the Charles R. Drew Postgraduate Medical School. In: Organ CH Jr, Kosiba MM, eds. *A Century of Black Surgeons: The USA Experience.* Norman, Okla: Transcript Press; 1987:377-425.
7. Governor's Commission of Los Angeles Riots. *Violence in the City: An End or a Beginning?* Los Angeles, Calif: State of California's Governor's Commission of Los Angeles Riots; 1965:1-101.
8. *Recommendation to the State Advisory Hospital Council.* Los Angeles, Calif: State Department of Public Health; 1965.
9. Haynes MA. Charles R. Drew Postgraduate Medical School (Medical Schools of the West). *West J Med.* 1984;140:308-310.
10. *Report of the Ad Hoc Review Committee for Renewal of Surgery Chairmanship to M. Alfred Haynes, MD, Acting Executive Dean.* Los Angeles, Calif: Drew University; 1976:1-5.
11. Fleming AW, Olivier M. Crisis in trauma management. *Drew Med Soc J.* 1987;3:1-2.
12. Blaisdell FW. 1991 AAST presidential address: the pre-medicare role of city/county hospitals in education and health care. *J Trauma.* 1992;32:217-228.
13. Fischer RP, Pepe PE, Reed RL II, Parks DH, Prentice FD, Mattox KL. Academic consequences of a trauma system failure. *J Trauma.* 1990;30:784-791.
14. Hiatt JR, Tompkins RK. The importance of nonoperative trauma in postgraduate surgical education. *J Trauma.* 1987;27:769-773.
15. Richardson JD, Freeark RJ, Miller FB, Baker WH, Polk HC Jr. Institutionally shared trauma rotations are viable solutions to deficiencies in trauma training. *J Trauma.* 1989;29:1211-1216.

Blood in Our Streets

The Status and Evolution of Trauma Care Systems

A. Brent Eastman, MD

• Injury is our nation's leading public health problem. Victims of violence need expert and immediate medical attention. A model exists for optimal care of the injured patient—the trauma care system. This article outlines the history of trauma care, the components of the ideal, inclusive trauma care system, its efficacy, and the challenges and opportunities facing those who advocate such systems.
(*Arch Surg.* 1992;127:677-681)

In late 20th-century America, injury is the leading cause of years of potential life lost and often maims and disables when it does not kill. Every year, more than 140 000 people die of injuries. Another 70 million sustain nonfatal injuries and 340 000 become permanently disabled. Injury accounts for more years of potential life lost than cancer and heart disease combined (Fig 1). Injury is this nation's leading public health problem as stated in the 1985 report of the National Academy of Sciences.[1]

The cost of injury to this nation was estimated to be $180 billion in 1988. This exceeds all other disease categories including cancer and heart disease.[2] The victims of violence, whether intentional or unintentional, need expert and immediate medical attention. The failure to develop an organized system of care only adds to the devastation of serious injury. The phrase "victim of violence" pertains as much to the victim of drunk driving as to the victim of gunshot wounds.

Our first goal should be to prevent the violence but, failing that, we must provide a system for optimal care of the injured patient. In fact, an organized community-based system of trauma care may be a highly effective tool in preventing injury.

HISTORY

Man's earliest writings, including Homer's *Iliad*, allude to the care of the injured patient.[3] Many of the advances of such care have derived from the experience of military conflicts. Hippocrates himself believed war to be the proper school for surgeons. Perhaps the earliest documentation of a rudimentary "Trauma Care System" is the description of medical care for the Roman Legions about 100 AD. They had 24 surgeons, well-organized first aid, and field ambulances, and hospitals were maintained near every important encampment.[4]

Historically, "trauma centers" in this country were city/county hospitals. As stated by Blaisdell[5] in his presidential address to the American Association for the Surgery of Trauma in 1991, "They (the great city/county hospitals) were the primary institutions for care of trauma during most of our country's history, and the vast majority of advances in trauma care arose from these hospitals."

Other than these de facto trauma centers, injured patients typically were taken to "the nearest hospital." It is only in the last 25 years that trauma care systems have evolved as the optimal way to care for injured patients. Trauma centers are a critical component, but only one part, of a trauma care system.

SYSTEM AND COMPONENTS

Trauma care system is a term for the coordinated effort to provide care to the injured patient from the time of injury (before admission to the hospital) through definitive treatment in the hospital, and afterward in rehabilitation. The delivery of care is *regionalized* to match the severity of injury to the available resources in a given geographic area.

The components of a trauma care system must provide a continuum of care and allow for the measurement of success. The components and their relationship to one another are shown in Fig 2.[6,7]

In addition to these component parts of the system, there are a variety of providers[8] such as (1) system management personnel; (2) prehospital providers; (3) acute care facilities; and (4) rehabilitation services. The planning and development of trauma care systems have been well described. The following sequence of events is necessary to develop a trauma care system[9]: (1) determine need; (2) establish authority; (3) develop trauma criteria; (4) democratize the process; (5) obtain outside review and verification; (6) formalize designation; and (7) ensure viability through assessment of ongoing needs and quality assurance.

West et al[10] also described a step-by-step process for the development, management, and analysis of a compre-

Accepted for publication March 26, 1992.
From the Trauma Center, Scripps Memorial Hospital, La Jolla, Calif, and the Department of Surgery, University of California, San Diego.
Reprint requests to Trauma Center, Scripps Memorial Hospital, PO Box 28, La Jolla, CA 92038-0028 (Dr Eastman).

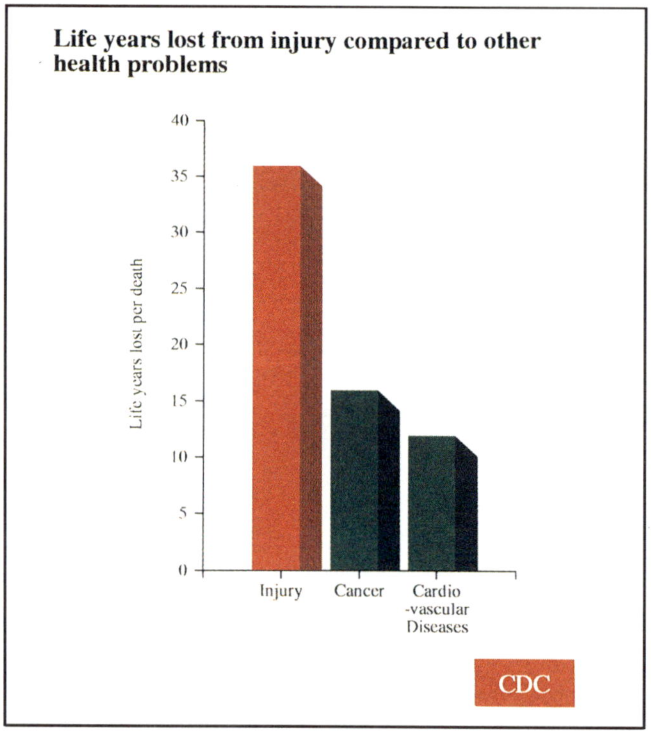

Figure 1.

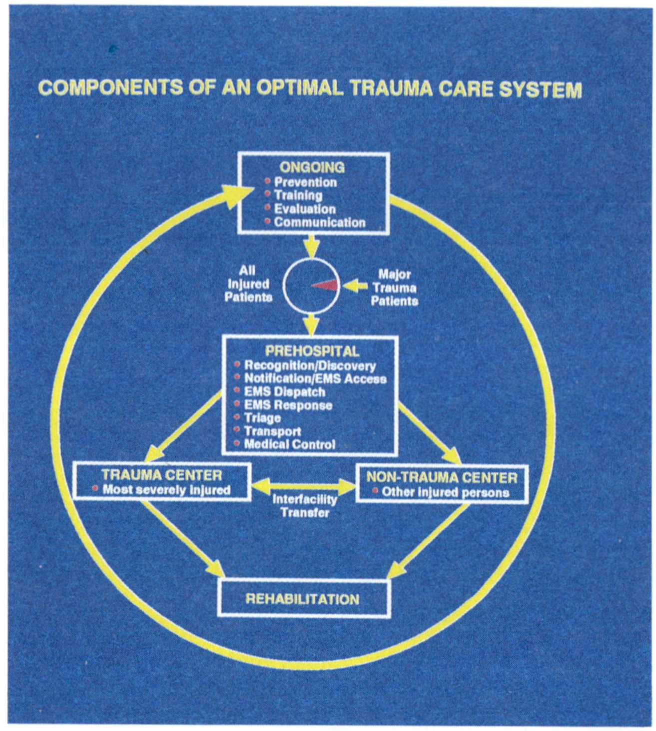

Figure 2.

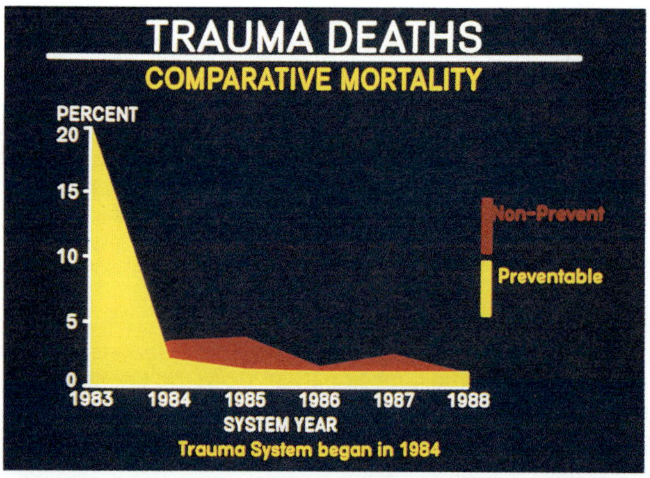

Figure 3.

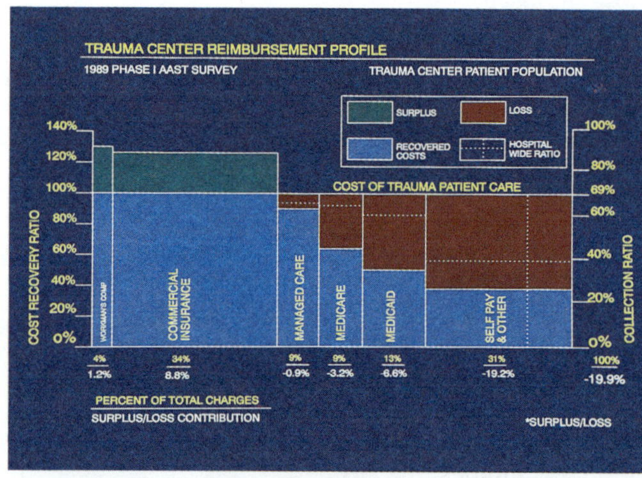

Figure 4.

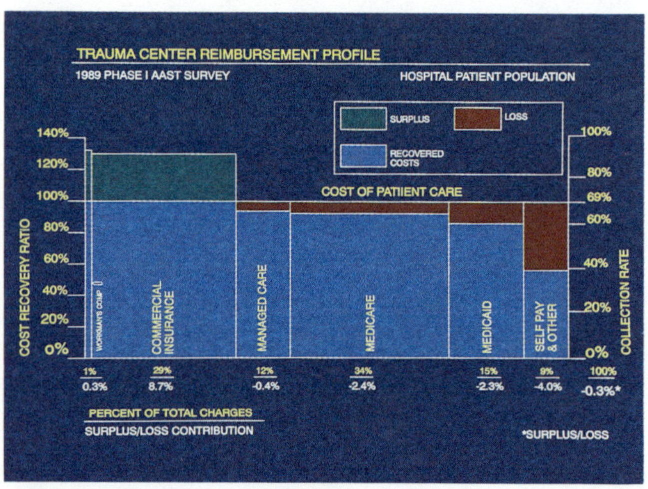

Figure 5.

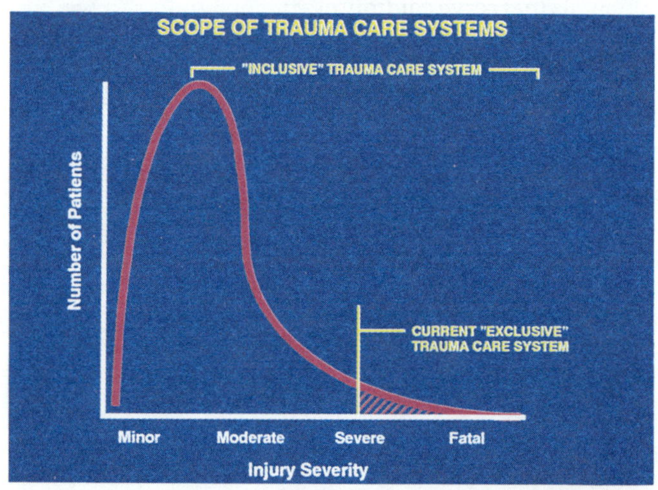

Figure 6.

Fig 1.—*Years of potential life lost. From Rice et al.*[2]

Fig 2.—*Components of an optimal trauma care system. From Eastman et al.*[7]

Fig 3.—*Preventable death rate in San Diego County, Calif.*[16]

Fig 4.—*Reimbursement profile for the trauma center patient population: 19% overall loss.*[23]

Fig 5.—*Reimbursement profile for the general hospital patient population: 0.1% overall loss.*[23]

Fig 6.—*Scope of inclusive trauma care system.*[7]

hensive system of trauma care. The most widely recognized system guidelines are those presented by the American College of Emergency Physicians[8] and American College of Surgeons Committee on Trauma (ACS/COT).[9] The National Highway Traffic Safety Administration has used these guidelines and developed a "how-to" manual for states and counties.[11] It is, therefore, not necessary to "reinvent the wheel" as new communities embark on the development of trauma care systems.

The use of aeromedical transportation in the Vietnam conflict established the principle that rapid transport to definitive care facilities saves lives.[12] A seminal study comparing preventable deaths in a trauma center with those in hospitals without trauma centers was a catalyst for the development of trauma care systems in 1979.[13] From the late 1970s through the 1980s, there was a flurry of activity designating trauma centers and establishing trauma care systems. The ACS/COT established a verification process whereby hospitals could request a site visit to determine whether they met the following ACS/COT criteria for level I, II, or III centers.[9]

Level I.—Regional Resource Trauma Centers. These include the primary hospital in the trauma care system with the capability of providing total care for every aspect of injury. Education and research programs are also essential.

Level II.—Community Trauma Centers. These centers are also expected to provide total care for injured patients but do not have the same educational and research requirements. These will be the most prevalent facility in most communities.

Level III.—Rural Trauma Hospitals. These include hospitals that serve communities without all the resources associated with a level I or II institution; provide optimal care with available resources; and often imply stabilization and transfer.[9]

A recent study showed a total of 457 state-designated or ACS-verified trauma centers in this country. This study estimated another 20 hospitals that function as trauma centers but are neither designated by a state nor verified by the ACS/COT, as well as 23 states in which the trauma center designation process is in place.[14]

There are now some states (Maryland, Virginia, Pennsylvania, Washington, and Oregon) with statewide trauma care systems. There are also systems established in individual counties such as the San Diego Trauma Care System in California. We have clearly entered a new era of trauma care systems, not just trauma centers. This movement has been given added impetus by enactment of the Federal Trauma Care Systems Planning and Development Act (PL101-590) in 1990 to provide assistance to states to plan, implement, and monitor organized trauma care systems.

EFFICACY OF TRAUMA CARE SYSTEMS

There have now been multiple studies verifying as much as a 50% reduction in preventable deaths (ie, deaths that would not have occurred with prompt and appropriate care) after implementation of regionalized trauma care.[14-19] San Diego County documented a countywide preventable death rate of 22% before the implementation of the trauma care system in 1984 (unpublished data, Hospital Council of San Diego and Imperial Counties. *Trauma Needs Assessment Study*. San Diego, Calif: Amherst Associates Inc; 1982). This rate fell to less than 2% and has remained at that level through 1991 (Fig 3).[16] Although less well documented than decreased mortality, there is also evidence of lower morbidity rates with organized trauma care. Mackenzie et al[20] evaluated rehabilitation following trauma in two level I trauma centers in an urban area. They analyzed 487 injured patients 1 year after trauma and found that 83% of the total had returned to full- or part-time work, school, or housekeeping. When injured patients are rehabilitated rapidly, the economic consequences are immense.

CHALLENGES

Despite the proven efficacy of trauma care systems in reducing death and disability, less than 25% of this country is served by such systems. Not only have most areas not developed such systems, but a number of those that were implemented have subsequently failed. Many of the designated trauma centers have closed their doors.[21] A study initiated by the Eastern Association for the Surgery of Trauma identified 95 hospitals that had dropped their trauma center designation in the past 5 to 6 years.[14]

The General Accounting Office recently reported a study that examined the reasons for trauma center closures in major urban areas. They found that " . . . primarily closures were due to financial losses sustained from treating the uninsured and patients covered by Medicaid and other government-assisted programs."[22] The survey by Dailey et al[21] showed similar causes for trauma center closures. They found that economic concerns were listed as four of the five most important factors: (1) cost of uncompensated care delivered to the uninsured or inadequately insured; (2) high operating costs associated with trauma services; (3) inadequate reimbursement for medical assistance programs; (4) unwillingness of physicians to be on call; (5) reduced compensation for trauma patient care under the prospective payment system (diagnosis related groups).

A study of 25 trauma centers indicated that underfunding results from a combination of the following.

1. Adverse selection, that is, attracting patients who incur above-average costs. It is estimated that the cost of admission of the average patient with trauma is two to three times greater than other hospital admissions of patients with acute conditions.

2. Disproportionate share, that is, attracting a higher proportion of indigent patients.[23]

The reimbursement profile compared the patient population with trauma with the general hospital population in those hospitals surveyed (Figs 4 and 5). The left y-axis reflects the cost recovery ratio. The x-axis displays proportionate contribution of payer's sources. The aggregate data revealed a 19.9% loss in the patient population with trauma compared with −0.3% in the general hospital population.

It is a paradox that the very object of a trauma care system, namely, of concentrating the most critically injured patients in a limited number of designated trauma centers, has proved to be the primary cause of center closures and system failure. The problem is compounded by increasing numbers of uninsured persons in this country. The number of uninsured was estimated to be 37 million in 1986.[24] It has been estimated that unsponsored trauma care totaled approximately $1 billion in 1988 and represented approximately 10% to 12% of the total $8.3 billion in unsponsored care provided by the nation's acute care hospitals that year.[25]

Parallel to the hospital reimbursement crisis is inadequate reimbursement for physicians. Provision of trauma care is difficult at best, as violent injury is a nocturnal disease, disruptive of regular schedules, exposing physicians and other health care providers to increased risk of AIDS, hepatitis, and possibly medicolegal problems. These factors, along with poor reimbursement for their efforts, have caused a general reluctance of many surgeons to provide trauma care. Esposito et al[26] reported in a survey of the Washington chapter of the ACS that only 39% of those surveyed were willing to participate in the care of patients with trauma. Reasons cited for nonparticipation were negative impact on practice and perception of increased medicolegal risk. This attitude was also reflected in a survey of surgical residents conducted by Richardson and Miller.[27] They found that only 21% of residents were interested in trauma care as a career or major part of their surgical practice.

The root problem with closure of many trauma centers is the lack of surgical commitment to the trauma program. This is not so much lack of surgical altruism as a lack of society's willingness to pay the bill. The state of California last year soundly defeated an alcohol tax initiative ("a nickel a drink"). This surcharge on alcohol would have made a significant contribution to funding the state's trauma programs. It seemed appropriate given the high correlation between alcohol and motor vehicle crashes.

Another major challenge is the development of rural trauma care systems. The problems of trauma care are quite different in urban and in rural areas. The urban areas are characterized by large populations contained within limited geographic spaces. This setting is associated with violent crimes, drug-related crime, gang warfare, and large indigent populations. The sheer number of seriously injured patients may overwhelm both prehospital providers and acute care facilities. Since indigent populations tend to be concentrated in urban areas, economic problems are magnified. However, the basic resources for regionalized trauma care exist in cities and, therefore, most systems have been developed in the urban setting.

Rural areas face unique problems in developing trauma care systems. These areas encompass the greater land mass but contain a minority of the population. This creates different logistic problems, including long travel times, difficult access, sparse populations, small hospitals, and limited financial and human resources. It should be emphasized that these are limited but not inferior human resources. Baker et al[28] reported geographic variations in mortality rates associated with motor vehicle crashes. Their study showed that the mortality rate was highest in counties of low population density. This inverse correlation between death rate per 100 000 in motor vehicle crashes and population density was partially attributed to poor access to trauma care in the rural areas. The development of rural trauma care systems must be based on realistic assessment of available resources. The grave mistake thus far has been the attempt to impose the "urban model" on the rural area. This has led to a sense of defeatism and has impeded the development of rural trauma care systems.

THE OPPORTUNITIES

Perhaps nowhere in modern medicine is the challenge and the opportunity greater than in the attempt to decrease the rates of death and disability from injury by implementing regionalized trauma care systems. Financial problems faced by trauma centers reflect the economic turmoil confronting our nation's health care system. We are in the midst of a national health care reform debate. Effective reform will lay the foundation for financially troubled trauma care systems. The opportunity exists to establish equitable payment programs for verified hospitals and qualified physicians who provide this sophisticated trauma care.

There are also opportunities to generate supplemental financial support for trauma centers and regional systems. These options are well outlined by Champion and Mabee[25] and include the following: (1) sin taxes, ie, cigarette tax and alcohol tax; (2) surcharges on driver's license fees, traffic violation penalties, 911 telephone numbers, and motor vehicle registrations; (3) trauma financing pool—a federal/state/private sector financing pool developed to reimburse qualified centers for documented uncompensated care; (4) adjustment of diagnosis related group–based reimbursement; and (5) increased reimbursement in return for managed regional trauma care.

The current health care reform debate is being driven by the demand for more cost-effective health care. The efficiencies and efficacy of regionalized trauma care systems could serve as a model for cost-effective medical care, and this might be expected to generate support from a nation that is currently spending approximately 12% of its gross national product on health care.

Rural trauma care provides one of our greatest opportunities for improvement. Since the urban model is not applicable, we must design a system that addresses the specific needs of rural America. The critical feature will be the linkage between existing systems and sharing of resources. This will demand sophisticated communication and transportation systems. The Optimal Resources Document produced by the ACS/COT is currently undergoing revision. An important addition will be the establishment of criteria for level IV trauma centers. These are facilities that lack the resources to be a level I, II, or III center, and yet are the only facilities in their rural areas available to provide initial care to severely injured patients. It is important to acknowledge the role that such facilities play and provide them with standards of care that are commensurate with resources available. An exchange of personnel, both physicians and nurses, between level I and level III and IV facilities could result in a better understanding of the special problems in rural America. Such exchanges should facilitate more expeditious transfers of injured patients when their needs outstrip the resources of the rural facility.

Another program being considered by the ACS/COT is a Trauma Advisory Panel. This is a 31-person panel made up of trauma experts. These trauma surgeons have committed to be available 24 hours a day via a toll-free number to be coordinated through the Chicago, Ill, office of the ACS. One of these experts will be available every day to consult with and advise physicians regarding trauma care issues in the more isolated areas of this country. This program is another attempt at establishing linkage between level I and II trauma centers and rural America.

As trauma care systems have evolved, it is clear that they have been "exclusive" in nature. They have focused only on the most critically injured patients who require the resources of a trauma center. This approach, however, has largely ignored the other 85% of injured patients who still need care in facilities other than designated trauma centers. If we are to truly establish injury as a national health priority, we must develop "inclusive" systems (Fig 6). The scope of a trauma care system needs to be expanded to include *all* hospitals that provide care to persons who are injured in the geographic region served by the system. This inclusive approach has the potential to minimize morbidity and disability following a person's injury, whether that injury is minor, major, or critical. The goals of the inclusive trauma care system are to match each hospital's trauma care resources with the needs of the injured persons, ensure flexibility within the system so that patients with different needs have access to the appropriate hospital, and continuously strive to provide optimal care to the population it serves.[7] The inclusive system will be the most cost-effective system in that it uses the resources of all facilities and personnel within a given region.

The opportunity to provide universal access to optimal care given available resources is an attainable goal. It is also an imperative goal in our violent society. Violence in this context refers not only to "crimes of violence" but the equally violent nature of death and disability caused by drunk drivers.

In a message to the ACS/COT in October 1991, William Roper, MD, MPH, Director of the Centers for Disease Control, Atlanta, Ga, announced his recommendation to the Secretary of Health and Human Services, to establish a National Center for Injury Control. When established, this center will add clear focus as well as increased funding for research in trauma care.

Another promising opportunity for a trauma care system is to serve as a community focal point for injury prevention and confront violence where it occurs. This is the greatest challenge as well as solution to the costly problem of injury. The ultimate goal of any trauma care system should be to put itself out of business. However, failing that, we must strive to establish trauma care systems across this country. Until the violence of our roadways and streets is extinguished, there will be blood in our streets and the need for regionalized trauma care.

References

1. Committee on Trauma Research. *Injury in America: A Continuing Public Health Problem.* Washington, DC: National Academy Press; 1985.
2. Rice DP, Mackenzie EJ. *Cost of Injury in the United States: A Report to Congress.* Atlanta, Ga: Centers for Disease Control; 1989.
3. Homer; Murray AT, trans. *The Iliad.* Cambridge, Mass: Harvard University Press; 1967.
4. Durant W. *The Story of Civilization: Caesar and Christ.* New York, NY: Simon & Schuster; 1944;3:312.
5. Blaisdell WF. The pre-Medicare role of city/county hospitals in education and health care. *J Trauma.* 1991;32:217-228.
6. Eastman AB, Lewis FR, Champion HR, Mattox KL. Regional trauma care systems design: critical concepts. *Am J Surg.* 1987;154:79-87.
7. Eastman AB, Schwab WC, Annest JL.Trauma care systems. Presented at the Third National Injury Control Conference; April 22-25, 1991; Denver, Colo.
8. American College of Emergency Physicians. Guidelines for trauma care systems. *Ann Emerg Med.* 1987;16:459-463.
9. American College of Surgeons Committee on Trauma. *Resources for Optimal Care of the Injured Patient.* Chicago, Ill: American College of Surgeons; 1990.
10. West JG, Williams MJ, Trunkey DO, Wolferth CC. Trauma systems current status: future challenges. *JAMA.* 1988;259:3597-3600.
11. US Dept of Transportation, National Highway Traffic Safety Administration. *Development of Trauma Systems: A State and Community Guide.* Washington, DC: Office of Enforcement and Emergency Medicine; 1989.
12. Haacker LP. Time and its effect on casualties in WWII and Vietnam. *Arch Surg.* 1969;98:39-40.
13. West JG, Trunkey DO, Lim RC. Systems of trauma care: a study of two counties. *Arch Surg.* 1979;114:455-460.
14. Eastern Association for the Surgery of Trauma. *Preliminary Survey of US Trauma Centers and State-by-State Analysis of Trauma System Development.* Reston, Va: Timothy Bell & Co; 1991.
15. Cales RH. Trauma mortality in Orange County: the effect of implementation of a regional trauma system. *Ann Emerg Med.* 1984;13:1-10.
16. San Diego County Division of Emergency Medical Services. *Trauma System Reports.* San Diego, Calif: Dept of Health Services, Division of Emergency Medical Services; 1991.
17. US Dept of Transportation, National Highway Traffic Safety Administration. *Medical Services Program and Its Relationship to Highway Safety.* Washington, DC: Office of Enforcement and Emergency Medical Services; 1985. Technical Report DOT HS 806832.
18. Champion HR, Teter H. Trauma care systems: the federal role. *J Trauma.* 1988;28:877-879.
19. Shacksford SR, Hollingsworth-Fridlund P, Cooper GF, Eastman AB. The effect of regionalization upon quality of trauma care as assessed by concurrent audit before and after institution of a trauma system: a preliminary report. *J Trauma.* 1986;26:812-820.
20. Mackenzie EJ, Siegel JH, Shapiro S, Moody M, Smith RT. Function, recovery and medical costs of trauma: an analysis by type and severity of injury. *J Trauma.* 1988;28:281-297.
21. Dailey JT, Teter H, Provenzano G, Cowley AR. Trauma center closures: a national assessment. Presented at the 51st Annual Meeting of the American Association for the Surgery of Trauma; September 13, 1991; Philadelphia, Pa.
22. United States General Accounting Office. *Trauma Care Lifesaving System Threatened by Unreimbursed Costs and Other Factors.* Washington, DC: General Accounting Office; 1991.
23. Eastman AB, Rice CL, Bishop GS, et al. An analysis of the critical problem of trauma center reimbursement. *J Trauma.* 1991;31:920-926.
24. US Congressional Research Service. Health Insurance and the Uninsured: Background Data and Analysis GPO. Washington, DC: Congressional Research Service; 1988.
25. Champion HR, Mabee MS. *An American Crisis in Trauma Care Reimbursement.* Washington, DC: Washington Hospital Surgical Critical Care Services; 1990.
26. Esposito PJ, Maier RV, Rivara FP, Carrico CJ. Why surgeons prefer not to care for trauma patients. *Arch Surg.* 1991;126:292-297.
27. Richardson DJ, Miller FB. Will future surgeons be interested in trauma care? results of a resident survey. Presented at the 51st Annual Meeting of the American Association for the Surgery of Trauma. September 12, 1991; Philadelphia, Pa.
28. Baker SP, Whitfield MA, O'Neill B. Geographic variation in mortality from motor vehicle crashes. *N Engl J Med.* 1987;316:1384-1387.

Visceral Injuries

David H. Wisner, MD, F. William Blaisdell, MD

• Abdominal visceral injuries are encountered by every surgeon who deals with trauma. It is simple and useful to divide abdominal visceral injuries into those caused by penetrating mechanisms of injury and those due to blunt mechanisms. Determination of the need for operative intervention is generally easier after penetrating trauma. Gunshot wounds to the abdomen should be explored, as should stab wounds to the anterior abdomen that penetrate the fascia. A midline incision is the standard approach to abdominal visceral injuries because of its ease and versatility. Abdominal exploration should be consistent and systemic so as not to miss significant injuries. Hollow viscus injury is most common after penetrating injury, while blunt injury most often results in injury to solid viscera. Diagnostic and operative aspects of the treatment of specific visceral injuries are reviewed.

(*Arch Surg.* 1992;127:687-693)

Abdominal visceral trauma is best dichotomized by mechanism of injury. The major mechanism of injury categories are those caused by blunt force and those caused by penetration of the abdomen. With both mechanisms, there are challenges with diagnosis and treatment.

Diagnosis after penetrating injury is more straightforward than after blunt injury. Gunshot wounds in and about the abdomen have an 80% to 90% incidence of serious associated visceral injury.[1] For this reason, we believe that gunshot wounds to the abdomen merit laparotomy in almost all instances. Rare exceptions are patients in whom it is apparent that the wound is clearly superficial and probably did not penetrate the peritoneal cavity. Selective exploration of patients with gunshot wounds to the abdomen has been proposed.[2,3] Given the high incidence of visceral disruption with such a mechanism of injury, we consider this policy unwise.

Treatment of stab wounds to the abdomen is more controversial than treatment of abdominal gunshot wounds.[4-6] Associated visceral injury from stab wounds is less common than after gunshot wounds, and if all abdomens are explored, the incidence of nontherapeutic laparotomy can be as high as 30% to 50%. For this reason, indirect assessment is often used to determine the need for operation. If the patient has generalized tenderness after a stab wound to the abdomen, a decision for operative intervention is easy. If the tenderness is limited to the periwound area only, however, the decision is not as straightforward. For stab wounds anterior to the midaxillary line, we favor local wound exploration to determine if the wound has penetrated the abdominal wall fascia. If there has been fascial penetration or the local exploration is indeterminate, abdominal exploration is done. If the wound has not penetrated the fascia, the patient is only observed. Because of the thick musculature of the back and flanks, wounds posterior to the posterior axillary line in stable and minimally symptomatic patients are treated with observation, urinalysis, serial abdominal examinations, and serial determinations of the hematocrit level and white blood cell count.[7,8] Progressive findings suggestive of intra-abdominal injury result in laparotomy.

Less aggressive approaches to stab wounds to the abdomen have been suggested.[9,10] Peritoneal lavage can be used with criteria for positivity ranging from the blunt trauma standard red blood cell count of 0.1×10^{12}/L down to a count for positivity of as low as 0.001×10^{12}/L. As would be expected, lower criteria for positivity result in fewer false-negative results at the expense of an increased false-positive rate.

A final approach to abdominal stab wounds in stable minimally symptomatic patients, even those with wounds to the anterior abdomen, is observation. Operative intervention is reserved for those who develop increasing signs or symptoms with time.[5,11]

When blunt trauma is confined to the abdomen or lower ribs, clinical assessment is the best initial indicator for laparotomy. Diffuse tenderness and hemodynamic instability that is resistant to initial volume resuscitation are indications for exploration. With prolonged observation, increasing tenderness or elevations in the white blood cell count or serum amylase concentration can also be indications for exploration. A falling hematocrit concentration in a stable patient under observation can be another indication for abdominal exploration. An alternative to exploration in such situations is to obtain a computed tomogram (CT) of the abdomen. Computed tomography, although it may miss bowel, pancreatic, and other visceral injuries in the early postinjury period, is a good test for large amounts of intraperitoneal blood, and the sensitivity increases with time.[12,13]

If, when a patient presents in the emergency department, there are associated injuries that make evaluation

Accepted for publication March 23, 1992.

From the Department of Surgery, University of California, Davis, Medical Center, Sacramento.

Reprint requests to Department of Surgery, University of California, Davis, Medical Center, 4301 X St, Room 2310, Sacramento, CA 95817 (Dr Wisner).

of the vital signs and abdomen difficult or unreliable, indirect means of assessment are appropriate. This is particularly true for patients with an altered level of consciousness. In the acute setting, when possible central nervous system injuries require immediate diagnosis or treatment, peritoneal lavage should be done. The advantages of peritoneal lavage over CT in such a setting is that it can be done more rapidly and with the patient under direct observation.[14] In the absence of gross blood on insertion of the lavage catheter, the full lavage procedure can be performed concurrent with other diagnostic and therapeutic maneuvers. For example, in a patient with multisystem injury and a decreased level of consciousness, diagnostic peritoneal lavage should be done shortly after arrival in the emergency department. A grossly positive result should prompt immediate abdominal exploration in most instances. If the result is grossly negative, the patient can be sent for a CT of the head with the lavage catheter still in place and the lavage fluid infusing.

Peritoneal lavage and CT of the abdomen have an appreciable false-negative rate, probably approximately 2% to 5% in each instance.[15-17] This emphasizes the importance of paying attention to the patient's clinical condition. If there are clear clinical indications for abdominal exploration, an operation should be done regardless of whether the peritoneal lavage or CT of the abdomen was negative.

Following penetrating trauma, the most likely injury is to a hollow viscus, small bowel, or colon because they occupy most of the volume of the abdominal cavity. The most important initial problem is contamination. With contamination, each hour that goes by before recognition results in increased morbidity. Following blunt trauma, solid organs, such as the spleen, liver, kidney, and pancreas, are most often injured. The mesentery of the small or large bowel can also be injured from a blunt mechanism. In the assessment of blunt trauma, the most important initial priority is to monitor bleeding. Blunt trauma can be safely observed if blood loss is negligible and the patient is adequately resuscitated. If shock is prevented, the patient is in good condition for the later surgery.

CONDUCT OF THE OPERATION

A midline incision should be used for abdominal exploration after trauma. This provides the best exposure of the entire abdomen and can be easily extended, if necessary, into the chest. Because most injuries from blunt trauma that require treatment are in the upper abdomen, the initial incision for exploration should be in the epigastrium. Extension in an inferior direction can be done easily as needed. In patients with penetrating injury, the approach should still be midline, but the location and extent of the initial incision should be tailored to the site of the wound.

In all instances where there is an abdominal injury, exposure is of paramount importance. To allow for vigorous retraction, the falciform ligament should be divided early after entry into the abdomen. Exposure of the liver and spleen requires a sufficiently long incision so that the abdominal musculature can be retracted laterally. This will often require extension to below the umbilicus, particularly in obese patients and those with a narrow costal margin. The addition of paraxiphoid extension can increase the exposure when a liver or splenic injury is encountered. If the injury is to the spleen, the paraxiphoid extension should be to the left; if the injury is to the liver, the extension should be to the right of the xiphoid. On rare occasion, median sternotomy is helpful for exposure of the dome of the liver. While exposure is improved, packing the liver injury to control bleeding can be more difficult if a sternotomy has been done.

When blood is encountered on entering the abdomen, all four quadrants should be quickly packed. The object of packing is to temporarily control bleeding until a quick survey of the abdomen can be done. A clot will often localize the source of bleeding, and when it is encountered in a quadrant during packing, that quadrant should be the first to be inspected later in further detail. If possible, each quadrant should undergo a brief inspection before embarking on definitive treatment of any specific injury. There is nothing worse than to select a relatively minor injury for initial treatment, only to have the patient exsanguinate from another unrecognized site. This is the reason for a complete initial survey of the abdomen. Liver and spleen injuries are often associated with one another and priorities for treatment should be based on the threat of exsanguination, ease of temporary control with packing, and relative ease of definitive treatment.

Initial four-quadrant packing, followed by more definitive inspection and control of injuries, should also generally be done after penetrating trauma, although a more directed approach can be taken if the path of the knife or bullet is known or is obvious.

After packing, the quadrants should be examined in a serial fashion. The precise means by which the viscera are inspected is not as important as making sure that the inspection is done in a systematic manner and is complete. We prefer to begin in the left upper quadrant. The left hemidiaphragm should be inspected and palpated. Small injuries are easily missed. The lateral segment of the left lobe of the liver should be bimanually palpated. The anterior surface of the left kidney should be visualized for the presence of a hematoma in Gerota's fascia and the kidney palpated. The greater curvature of the stomach is then inspected. The spleen should be visualized by gentle retraction toward the midline as much as attachments will allow. Inspection of the spleen and perisplenic area for injury or blood is important. Because of its consistency, splenic injuries can be missed if exploration is limited to palpation.

Attention is next directed to the right upper quadrant. The liver should be inspected and palpated. Bimanual palpation is particularly helpful in detecting injuries to the undersurface of the right lobe and injuries on the dome of the liver. The gallbladder should be inspected and palpated for the presence of gallstones. The right kidney can be inspected and palpated and at the same time the duodenal sweep visualized. Blood or bile staining of the periduodenal area mandates mobilization of the duodenum using the Kocher maneuver.

The lower quadrants are then inspected. This is facilitated by eviscerating the small bowel. This will reveal any gross mesenteric disruption or injuries to the colon, although definitive inspection is reserved for later. The lower quadrants should also be checked for the presence and size of retroperitoneal or pelvic hematomas. The pelvis should be inspected, with particular attention paid to the bladder. Bladder injury is particularly likely if gross hematuria is present. The tip and balloon of the bladder catheter can be palpated and the peritoneal surface of the dome of the bladder visualized.

After inspection of the lower quadrants and pelvis, visualization of the pancreas should be carried out. In thin patients, this can be done by pulling the stomach in an inferior direction and looking through the gastrohepatic ligament. If the presence of fat precludes an adequate view of the anterior surface of the pancreas via this route, the lesser sac should be entered via the gastrocolic ligament. The stomach can be retracted superiorly and the pancreas seen. This maneuver should be done in all cases where injury to the stomach is suspected, as it allows for inspection of the posterior wall of the stomach and the pancreas. This is facilitated by grasping the greater curvature and stretching the stomach so that its entire anterior and posterior surfaces are visible.

The small bowel is then eviscerated and run from the ligament of Treitz to the ileocecal valve. The duodenal-jejunal junction should be inspected. Hematomas in this area may be associated with either bowel injury or injuries to the body of the pancreas. The mesentery for each segment of the bowel should be stretched and inspected. A laparotomy pad should be used to wipe the surface of the bowel where necessary to avoid small injuries. If large holes in the bowel are encountered, they can be controlled temporarily with an atraumatic clamp or a temporizing figure-of-eight suture. When hematoma, discoloration, or the path of a missile or knife suggest injury to the mesenteric side of the bowel, the mesenteric surface in that location should be visualized by further opening the mesentery as necessary. When the ileocecal valve has been reached, inspection of the bowel should continue with the cecum and the rest of the colon. The same principles that apply to examination of the small bowel apply to the large bowel. When injury to the ascending or descending colon is suspected, that portion of the bowel should be mobilized on its mesentery.

TREATMENT OF SPECIFIC VISCERAL INJURIES

Bleeding takes precedence over contamination; therefore, the lesions that require initial treatment are those that are or have been bleeding.

Spleen

The spleen is inspected by gently retracting it medially. Adhesions to the diaphragm should be divided sharply. The fingers of the nondominant hand should enter the avascular plane posterior to the spleen and the tail of the pancreas. This is facilitated by dividing the splenophrenic ligament. The correct plane can best be identified by making sure that the back of the hand is right next to the surface of the left kidney. This ensures that the plane deep to the tail of the pancreas is entered instead of the plane between the tail of the pancreas and the splenic hilum. Traction on the splenic hilum and the spleen may result in tears of the splenic capsule, whereas traction exerted upward when the fingers are passed under the tail of the pancreas will not. Entering the plane behind the tail of the pancreas also allows for much greater mobilization of the spleen and, in many instances, it can be delivered completely into the wound. After mobilization of the tail of the pancreas, further mobility of the spleen can be accomplished by division of the splenocolic ligament and short gastric vessels as needed. Once the spleen is brought medially, packs can be placed behind it to keep it elevated.

If there are major associated injuries that require therapy or the patient is at any risk for the development of coagulopathy, the spleen should be removed.[18-20] Small lacerations that are not bleeding may be treated conservatively and do not require splenectomy unless the risk of coagulopathy is extreme.

Whenever the splenic salvage is contemplated, it should be borne in mind that the risk for subsequent development of overwhelming postsplenectomy sepsis is exceedingly low in adult trauma victims. Undue attempts at salvage should be abandoned if they significantly increase transfusion requirements or there is any risk of subsequent hemorrhage.[21] The length of the operative procedure should also not be excessively prolonged by attempts at salvage. Because of these considerations, we have a low threshold for splenectomy in adult patients. The risks are somewhat higher in children but are still low enough that common sense should be used in deciding when to attempt salvage and how long to persist in the attempt.[22,23]

If splenorrhaphy is to be attempted, the spleen must first be fully mobilized and visualized and bleeding controlled. After division of short gastric vessels, a vascular clamp can be placed across the splenic hilar vessels for temporary control. A dry field is created and further blood loss avoided while decisions are made regarding salvage.

Hilar injuries, if severe, preclude splenic salvage. If, however, the injury is peripheral and bleeding can be controlled by suture without compromising splenic viability, salvage may be possible. For major lacerations, we use absorbable sutures tied over bolsters of polytef felt. Alternatively, a sling of collagen mesh may be used to compress lacerations for hemostasis. On rare occasions, a hemisplenectomy can be done using vascular isolation and hilar clamping as described above for hemostasis during the resection.

We do not drain the splenic bed after splenectomy or splenorrhaphy. At the time of discharge, pneumococcal polysaccharide vaccine is administered and the patient is provided information about subsequent infection management. Definitive proof of the effectiveness of pneumococcal vaccine in preventing a disease as rare as overwhelming postsplenectomy sepsis is statistically impossible and emphasizes the rarity of this complication. Although there is no absolute clinical evidence that the vaccine is effective, enough theory and experimental evidence has been collected about the vaccine to have made it the standard of care.[18,24]

Liver

Because spontaneous hemostasis of the liver is common, many liver injuries are not significant clinically and are never recognized. Indirect assessment of the abdomen with peritoneal lavage and CT reveals a number of injuries for which no therapeutic intervention is required. Indications for operation are evidence of major blood loss on clinical assessment, increasing abdominal tenderness suggesting the presence of associated intra-abdominal injury, or a major parenchymal disruption seen on CT. An additional indication is a grossly positive peritoneal lavage result in a patient who is unstable or cannot be followed up clinically.

Penetrating liver injuries can be quite benign. As indicated previously, the liver is an excellent hemostatic organ, and secondary hemorrhage from liver injuries is rare. Therefore, if the lesion is not bleeding at the time of abdominal exploration, further treatment is usually meddlesome. If blood loss from the liver has been less than 500 mL and the liver is not actively bleeding, no specific treatment other than evacuation of the free blood is indicated. If blood loss has been greater than 500 mL and the liver is not actively bleeding, we usually place drains. Large wounds or the suggestion of a bile leak are other indications for drainage. Drainage permits monitoring for secondary hemorrhage and the egress of leaking bile. We use open-dependent drainage with a posterior incision placed just below the 12th rib and a two- to three-fingerbreadth incision in the muscle and fascial layers. Multiple soft Penrose drains are placed in the area of injury.

For penetrating liver injuries that are bleeding, the first maneuver that should be done is the Pringle maneuver, placement of a clamp across the portal triad. If this controls the hemorrhage, the laceration can be opened deep into the liver substance, inspected, and definitive control of bleeding points obtained with sutures. If a profusely bleeding laceration is controlled by placement of a clamp on the portal triad, but control of the bleeding site deep in the substance of the liver is difficult, the bleeding may respond to selective lobar artery ligation.[25,26] The proper hepatic artery should be dissected and vascular clamps applied in succession to the right and left lobar arteries. Whichever application controls the bleeding dictates the appropriate lobar artery to ligate. Lobar artery ligation is especially helpful and important for deep, centrally located liver injuries when opening the laceration fully and individually ligating bleeding points is difficult.

In blunt trauma, the lacerations and cracks in the liver are usually quite wide and direct visualization of bleeding points is easier than with penetrating injury. Portal triad clamping should be done and is sometimes successful in substantially decreasing the amount of bleeding. If this occurs, individual suture ligation of bleeding points should be undertaken. Sometimes, the magnitude of the liver injury and disrupted parenchymal surface is so great that individual suture ligation of bleeding points is not possible. This is particularly true if the patient develops coagulopathy. In such instances, the liver should be packed and the abdomen closed with the packs left in place. We believe that resection of liver tissue, especially formal anatomic resection, should rarely be done, and then primarily when a major segment is nonviable. Such resections create an even greater surface of bleeding liver parenchyma.

Hepatic venous and vena caval injuries are another circumstance in which liver packing can be employed. Portal clamping has minimal effect on the rate of bleeding from such injuries, a fact that can be a helpful clue in making the diagnosis. If portal clamping is not helpful, the liver should be mobilized from its ligamentous attachments. This allows not only for better visualization, but also for better manual compression of the liver parenchyma and temporary control of bleeding. If bleeding is massive, packing should be done without delay and the operation terminated.

Occasionally, particularly with large hepatic venous or caval injuries, packing does not successfully control bleeding, even temporarily. We have the most experience in this situation with atriocaval bypass.[27] This involves cannulation of the right atrium with a large-bore tube passed inferiorly to below the level of the renal veins. Tapes or clamps passed around the suprahepatic and infrahepatic vena cava and side holes cut in the tube in the right atrium result in shunting of blood past the area of injury. Coupling this with a Pringle maneuver produces vascular isolation of the liver and permits definitive repair of large venous injuries.

An alternative to atriocaval shunting now being used in liver transplantation is to place one end of a cannula in the iliac or femoral vein and the other end in the axillary or jugular vein. A nonocclusive pump is used to keep blood moving in the bypass circuit.[28,29]

Simple clamping of the vena cava above and below the liver without any form of shunting has also been suggested.[30,31] If the patient is normovolemic, this may be tolerated. If the patient is in hypovolemic shock, however, caval occlusion traps enough blood to precipitate immediate cardiac arrest. This technique is therefore rarely successful in trauma patients.

When the liver has been packed, timing of return to the operating room is important.[32,33] Optimally, the packs should be removed about 24 hours after their placement. They can be left in longer, however, if more time is needed to reverse the patient's coagulopathy, hypothermia, electrolyte abnormalities, and blood volume depletion. Packs should usually be changed before 48 hours have elapsed and sometimes may need to be replaced one or two times with repeated trips to the operating room.

All major liver injuries should be drained dependently as described above.

Kidney

When a patient has suffered penetrating trauma in the vicinity of a kidney or its blood supply, it is important to document an adequately functioning kidney on the contralateral side. This can be done preoperatively with an abbreviated intravenous pyelogram, but undue time should not be spent on this study in unstable or worrisome patients. The pyelogram can be done instead in the operating room and, although of poor quality, will usually demonstrate nephrograms. One alternative to pyelography that can be done in the operating room is to administer an intravenous dye such as indigo carmine or methylene blue. If the ureter on the injured side is clamped, excretion of dye in the urine implies a functioning kidney on the uninjured side. Another quick alternative in the operating room is to occlude the ureter on the contralateral side and look for proximal ureteral distention.

Penetrating injuries of the kidney should be explored. With blunt injuries, the approach should be more selective. Most perinephric hematomas in patients with blunt injury do not require intervention, but they should be explored if they are expanding or pulsatile because these characteristics suggest arterial injury.[34]

If a kidney is to be explored, vascular control should be obtained.[34,35] This can be done either before exploration of the perinephric hematoma or as part of the exploration.[34] If control is to be obtained before exploration, the retroperitoneum should be entered at the base of the mesentery at the ligament of Treitz. Dissection of the aorta and vena cava allows for control of the appropriate renal artery and vein. Because it is so short, the right renal vein requires independent exposure just above and lateral to the duodenum after a Kocher maneuver.

If vascular control is done as part of the renal exploration, Gerota's fascia should be incised and the kidney mobilized. The renal vessels are then easily identified and controlled from behind. This maneuver is particularly helpful if the kidney is massively injured and likely to require removal or if the patient is unstable owing to massive bleeding or associated injuries.[35]

If the patient's renal function is known to have been good and the opposite kidney is functional, most renal injuries associated with major bleeding or pelvic disruption are best treated with nephrectomy. When there is any question about the function of the opposite kidney, attempts to salvage the kidney are in order. This is particularly true if the patient is older, hypertensive, or has a history of renal disease. Renal pelvis injuries can be directly repaired. Injuries to the parenchyma usually respond to suture ligation of bleeding points, incorporation of absorbable hemostatic sponge into the repair, and drainage of the kidney. Heminephrectomy is also occasionally possible.

All major renal injuries should be drained unless a nephrectomy has been done. Because urine is the primary drainage fluid of concern, closed suction drains are appropriate. They should be placed in proximity to the kidney, but not abutting the repair.

Pancreas

The most challenging visceral injuries, other than major liver injuries, are to the pancreas.[36,37] When there is hemorrhage in the substance of the pancreas seen at laparotomy, the pancreas should be mobilized sufficiently to permit palpation of the area of injury. A Kocher maneuver should be done to permit bimanual palpation of injured areas in the head of the pancreas. Simple inspection is not adequate because the hematoma may smooth out the contour of the pancreas, and even large disruptions of pancreatic parenchyma may be missed.

The basic approach to penetrating and blunt injuries of the pancreas is the same.[36,38] Minor contusions and hematomas of the pancreas do not require any treatment. Minor lacerations of any portion of the pancreas should be drained. We favor open drainage using Penrose drains brought out through the left flank for injuries to the body and tail and through the right flank for injuries to the pancreatic head. Treatment of deep lacerations of the pancreas depends on their location and whether an associated ductal injury is unlikely. A distal pancreatectomy should be done if ductal injury is present or suspected.[39,40] Splenic salvage is possible when distal pancreatectomy is performed and requires division of the pancreatic branches of the splenic artery and vein. This is reasonable in stable patients with minimal associated injuries, but the additional operative time is not justified if there is any question about the patient's stability. Both the endocrine and exocrine morbidity of distal pancreatectomy for trauma are minimal, and internal drainage procedures to salvage pancreatic tissue should not be done. Such procedures expose the patient to the risks of a tenuous pancreaticoenteric anastomosis.

Severe injuries to the head of the pancreas, particularly if there is an associated duodenal injury, are challenging. Some can be treated with distal pancreatic resection, as up to 80% pancreatectomy can be performed with relative ease, particularly if the pancreas was normal before the injury and there is minimal surrounding inflammation. In almost all other injuries, simple drainage should be done. Pancreaticoduodenectomy in the patient with trauma has a high mortality rate and should be avoided unless the injury is so massive that débridement of dead and devitalized tissue results in a de facto pancreaticoduodenal resection. Reconstruction after pancreaticoduodenectomy is difficult because the common bile duct and pancreatic duct are small in patients with trauma, most of whom do not have preexisting disease and chronic ductal dilatation.

When the head of the pancreas has been severely injured or when there is an associated duodenal injury, the pancreatic injury and duodenal repair can be temporarily protected from secretion and activation of pancreatic juice and digestive enzymes by performance of a pyloric exclusion procedure.[41] A gastrotomy is done on the greater curvature of the stomach and the pylorus oversewn from inside with an absorbable collagen suture. A gastrojejunostomy is then constructed to restore gastrointestinal continuity. The head of the pancreas and duodenum are protected until the pyloric closure breaks down and normal gastrointestinal continuity restored. Should a duodenal fistula develop, the absence of gastric secretions ensures a more benign process.

Gastric and Duodenal Injury

Penetrating injuries to the stomach are relatively simple and usually lend themselves to direct repair. The stomach has a good blood supply and heals well. Blunt traumatic rupture of the stomach is rare, but can usually be treated with direct repair after débridement of overtly damaged tissue. Gross blood from a nasogastric tube is a helpful sign in the diagnosis of gastric injury, but is not always present even with severe injuries.

Most penetrating duodenal injuries can be treated with simple repair and will heal nicely. Severe injuries may sometimes require resection of a short segment of duodenum and primary anastomosis. An alternative is internal drainage or use of serosal patch of jejunum. For complex or tenuous duodenal repairs, pyloric exclusion should be done.

Blunt duodenal injuries with perforation should be repaired using the same principles as for penetrating injuries. An unusual form of blunt duodenal injury is the development of submucosal or subserosal hematomas with luminal compromise but no perforation.[42] Sometimes these injuries are noticed in nonoperated patients on upper gastrointestinal series obtained because of unexplained obstruction. In such instances, the patient should be treated conservatively and the hematoma usually gradually resorbs and resolves. When such hematomas do not resolve or are noticed at laparotomy, they should be incised and drained.

Duodenal injuries should be drained dependently using open drains and a large drain site.

Small Intestine

Small-bowel injury is common after penetrating trauma because the small bowel fills much of the volume of the peritoneal cavity. High-speed motor vehicle accidents and the widespread use of seat belts have resulted in an increasing number of blunt intestinal injuries as well.[43,44] The small intestine has an excellent blood supply and small perforations are easily treated with primary repair or resection and primary anastomosis if there are multiple injuries in one segment. When there is compromise of the circulation to the bowel or more than half of the circumference has been damaged, resection is indicated. We routinely perform side-to-side, functional end-to-end stapled anastomoses because they can be done rapidly and the resultant anastomotic lumen is large.[45]

Operative treatment of penetrating and blunt small intestine injuries is similar, although blunt intestinal injury tends more often to involve long sections of bowel and mesentery and more often requires resection. For both mechanisms of injury, if there is any question of bowel viability, reexploration of the abdomen 24 hours following initial treatment is indicated to verify bowel viability and the integrity of the anastomosis or repair.

Colon and Rectum

Most colon injuries are the result of penetrating trauma, but, on occasion, blunt trauma will also lead to perforation or devascularization of the large bowel.[43,44] We treat a majority of colon injuries with either primary repair alone or with resection and end colostomy formed from the proximal margin of resection. We do not perform exteriorization of colonic repairs or proximal diversion to protect more distal repairs.[46,47]

Minor isolated penetrating trauma of the colon is treated at most centers, including our own, with primary closure when it is recognized within 6 to 8 hours of injury, regardless of whether it involves the right or left colon. Stab wounds, in particular, lend themselves to primary repair. When dealing with gunshot wounds, the decision may be more difficult and depends on the extent of damage. Primary repair is clearly a good risk when the colonic injury is not massive, the patient is stable, there are no severe associated injuries, the injury has been recognized within 6 to 8 hours of injury, and there has not been massive peritoneal contamination.[48] When there is doubt about appropriate treatment, resection and proximal colostomy is the most conservative and safest approach. Resection and colostomy are also the most appropriate methods of treatment if there is an associated mesenteric injury and vascular compromise.

Blunt colonic injuries usually involve a segment of colon and have associated compromise of the colonic blood supply. Resection and colostomy are indicated in these patients.

Rectal injuries may result from penetrating trauma or may occur in association with pelvic fracture. These are best treated with proximal sigmoid colostomy and mucous fistula. This should be followed by dilation of the anal sphincter and gentle irrigation and washout of the rectal segment through the mucous fistula. Large perineal lacerations, often seen in conjunction with compound or open pelvic fractures, should also be treated with proximal diversion and rectal washout.

Bladder

Gross hematuria, regardless of the mechanism of injury, mandates performance of a cystogram because of the relatively high incidence of bladder injury associated with this finding. Penetrating retroperitoneal injuries to the bladder can be treated with simple catheter drainage, but associated rectal or major vascular injury must be ruled out. Retroperitoneal injuries can also be repaired directly by incising the bladder and performing the repair from inside. Intraperitoneal injuries from penetrating trauma should be primarily repaired and a suprapubic catheter placed.

Most blunt bladder injuries occur in association with pelvic fracture. When the rupture is retroperitoneal, it can be treated with simple urethral catheter drainage. Intraperitoneal ruptures are treated with primary repair and suprapubic cystostomy.[49]

References

1. Feliciano DV, Burch JM, Spjut-Patrinely V, Mattox KL, Jordan GL Jr. Abdominal gunshot wounds: an urban trauma center's experience with 300 consecutive patients. *Ann Surg.* 1988;208:362-370.
2. Nance FC. Abdominal trauma at the Southern Surgical Association, 1888-1987. *Ann Surg.* 1988;207:742-753.
3. Lowe RJ, Saletta JD, Read R, Radhakrishnan J, Moss GS. Should laparotomy be mandatory or selective in gunshot wounds of the abdomen? *J Trauma.* 1977;17:903-907.
4. Sirinek KR, Page CP, Root HD, Levine BA. Is exploratory celiotomy necessary for all patients with truncal stab wounds? *Arch Surg.* 1990;125:844-848.
5. Demetriades D, Rabinowitz B. Indications for operation in abdominal stab wounds: a prospective study of 651 patients. *Ann Surg.* 1987;205:129-132.
6. Holcroft JW, Blaisdell FW. Trauma to the torso. In: Wilmore DW, Brennan MF, Harken AH, Holcroft JW, Meakins JL, eds. *American College of Surgeons: Care of the Surgical Patient.* New York, NY: Scientific American Inc; 1989;1:1-56.
7. Jackson GL, Thal ER. Management of stab wounds of the back and flank. *J Trauma.* 1979;19:660-664.
8. Blaisdell FW. General assessment, resuscitation and exploration of penetrating and blunt abdominal trauma. In: Blaisdell FW, Trunkey DD, eds. *Trauma Management.* New York, NY: Thieme-Stratton Inc; 1982:1-18.
9. Oreskovich MR, Carrico CJ. Stab wounds of the anterior abdomen: analysis of a management plan using local wound exploration and quantitative peritoneal lavage. *Ann Surg.* 1983;198:411-419.
10. Thal ER. Evaluation of peritoneal lavage and local exploration in lower chest and abdominal stab wounds. *J Trauma.* 1977;17:642-648.
11. Mariadason JG, Parsa MH, Ayuyao A, Freeman HP. Management of stab wounds to the thoracoabdominal region: a clinical approach. *Ann Surg.* 1988;207:335-340.
12. Grumbach K, Mechlin MB, Mintz MC. Computed tomography and ultrasound of the traumatized and acutely ill patient. *Emerg Med Clin North Am.* 1985;3:607-624.
13. Federle MP, Jeffrey RB Jr. Hemoperitoneum studied by computed tomography. *Radiology.* 1983;148:187-192.
14. Pevec WC, Peitzman AB, Udekwu AO, McCoy B, Straub W. Computed tomography in the evaluation of blunt abdominal trauma. *Surg Gynecol Obstet.* 1991;173:262-267.
15. Sorkey AJ, Farnell MB, Williams HJ Jr, Mucha P Jr, Ilstrup DM. The complementary roles of diagnostic peritoneal lavage and computed tomography in the evaluation of blunt abdominal trauma. *Surgery.* 1989;106:794-801.
16. Marx JA, Moore EE, Jorden RC, Eule J Jr. Limitations of computed tomography in the evaluation of acute abdominal trauma: a prospective comparison with diagnostic peritoneal lavage. *J Trauma.* 1985;25:933-937.
17. Henneman PL, Marx JA, Moore EE, Cantrill SV, Ammons LA. Diagnostic peritoneal lavage: accuracy in predicting necessary laparotomy following blunt and penetrating trauma. *J Trauma.* 1990;30:1345-1355.
18. Lucas CE. Splenic trauma: choice of management. *Ann Surg.* 1991;213:98-112.
19. Rappaport W, McIntyre KE Jr, Carmona R. The management of splenic trauma in the adult patient with blunt multiple injuries. *Surg Gynecol Obstet.* 1990;170:204-208.
20. Buckman RF Jr, Piano G, Dunham CM, Soutter I, Ramzy A, Militello PR. Major bowel and diaphragmatic injuries associated with blunt spleen or liver rupture. *J Trauma.* 1988;28:1317-1321.
21. Beal SL, Spisso JM. The risk of splenorrhaphy. *Arch Surg.* 1988;123:1158-1163.
22. Wisner DH, Blaisdell FW. When to save the ruptured spleen. *Surgery.* 1992;3:121-122.
23. Pearl RH, Wesson DE, Spence LJ, et al. Splenic injury: a 5-year update with improved results and changing criteria for conservative management. *J Pediatr Surg.* 1989;24:121-125.
24. Immunization Practices Advisory Committee, Centers for Disease Control. Update: pneumococcal polysaccharide vaccine usage—United States. *Ann Intern Med.* 1984;101:348-350.
25. Cogbill TH, Moore EE, Jurkovich GJ, Feliciano DV, Morris JA, Mucha P. Severe hepatic trauma: a multi-center experience with 1,335 liver injuries. *J Trauma.* 1988;28:1433-1438.
26. Lewis FR, Lim RC Jr. Blaisdell FW. Hepatic artery ligation: adjunct in the management of massive hemorrhage from the liver. *J Trauma.* 1974;14:743-755.
27. Schrock T, Blaisdell FW, Mathewson C. Management of blunt

trauma to the liver and hepatic veins. *Arch Surg.* 1968;96:698-704.

28. Griffith BP, Shaw BW, Hardesty RL, Iwatsuki S, Bahnson HT, Starzl TE. Venovenous bypass without systemic anticoagulation for transplantation of the human liver. *Surg Gynecol Obstet.* 1985;160:271-272.

29. Diebel LN, Wilson FR, Bender J, Paules B. A comparison of passive and active shunting for bypass of the retrohepatic IVC. *J Trauma.* 1991;31:987-990.

30. Heaney JP, Stanton WK, Habert DS, et al. An improved technique for vascular isolation of the liver: experimental study and case reports. *Ann Surg.* 1966;163:237-241.

31. Stain SC, Yellin AE, Donovan AJ. Hepatic trauma. *Arch Surg.* 1988;123:1251-1255.

32. Cué JI, Cryer HG, Miller FB, Richardson JD, Polk HC Jr. Packing and planned reexploration for hepatic and retroperitoneal hemorrhage: critical refinements of a useful technique. *J Trauma.* 1990;30:1007-1013.

33. Feliciano DV, Mattox KL, Burch JM, Bitondo CG, Jordan GL Jr. Packing for control of hepatic hemorrhage. *J Trauma.* 1986;26:738-743.

34. McAninch JW, Carroll PR. Renal exploration after trauma: indications and reconstructive techniques. *Urol Clin North Am.* 1989;16:203-212.

35. Corriere JN Jr, McAndrew JD, Benson GS. Intraoperative decision-making in renal trauma surgery. *J Trauma.* 1991;31:1390-1392.

36. Wisner DH, Wold RL, Frey CF. Diagnosis and treatment of pancreatic injuries: an analysis of management principles. *Arch Surg.* 1990;125:1109-1113.

37. Cogbill TH, Moore EE, Kashuk JL. Changing trends in the management of pancreatic trauma. *Arch Surg.* 1982;117:722-728.

38. Wynn M, Hill DM, Miller DR, Waxman K, Eisner ME, Gazzaniga AB. Management of pancreatic and duodenal trauma. *Am J Surg.* 1985;150:327-332.

39. Yellin AE, Vecchione TR, Donovan AJ. Distal pancreatectomy for pancreatic trauma. *Am J Surg.* 1972;124:135-142.

40. Balasegaram M. Surgical management of pancreatic trauma. *Curr Probl Surg.* 1979;16:5-59.

41. Vaughan GD, Frazier OH, Graham DY, Mattox KL, Petmecky FF, Jordan GL Jr. The use of pyloric exclusion in the management of severe duodenal injuries. *Am J Surg.* 1977;134:785-790.

42. Jones WR, Hardin WJ, Davis JT. Intramural hematoma of the duodenum: a review of the literature and case report. *Ann Surg.* 1971;173:534-544.

43. Wisner DH, Chun Y, Blaisdell FW. Blunt intestinal injury: keys to diagnosis and management. *Arch Surg.* 1990;125:1319-1323.

44. Dauterive AH, Flancbaum L, Cox EF. Blunt intestinal trauma: a modern-day review. *Ann Surg.* 1985;201:198-203.

45. Wisner DH. Surgical management of traumatic intestinal injuries. In: Sabiston DC Jr, ed. *Textbook of Surgery.* Philadelphia, Pa: WB Saunders Co; 1991:129-148.

46. Lou MA, Johnson AP, Atik M, Mandal AK, Alexander JL, Schlater TL. Exteriorized repair in the management of colon injuries. *Arch Surg.* 1981;116:926-929.

47. Mulherin JL Jr, Sawyers JL. Evaluation of three methods for managing penetrating colon injuries. *J Trauma.* 1975;15:580-587.

48. Stone HH, Fabian TC. Management of perforating colon trauma: randomization between primary closure and exteriorization. *Ann Surg.* 1979;190:430-436.

49. Corriere JN Jr, Sandler CM. Management of the ruptured bladder: seven years of experience with 111 cases. *J Trauma.* 1986;26:830-833.

Epidemiologic Changes in Gunshot Wounds in Washington, DC, 1983-1990

Daniel W. Webster, ScD, MPH; Howard R. Champion, FRCS(Edin); Patricia S. Gainer, JD, MPA; Leon Sykes, MD

• The purpose of this study was to examine temporal patterns in gunshot wound admission rates and wound profiles from 1983 through 1990 at a level I trauma center in Washington, DC. Data on trauma admissions were collected at the time of admission. Records were reviewed to identify patients admitted for gunshot wounds from assaults. Data on the number and location of entrance gunshot wounds, survival, complications, length of stay in the intensive care unit, and total inpatient days were recorded. Admissions due to gunshot wounds grew at an exponential rate beginning in 1987 and reached a level from 1989 through 1990 three times higher than the preepidemic rate. The mean number of entrance gunshot wounds per patient grew from 1.44 before the epidemic to 2.04 from 1988 through 1990. Multiple thoracic wounds became relatively more common from 1988 through 1990. This increase was partially responsible for reversing a downward trend in patient mortality. Temporal changes in admission rates and wound profiles were consistent with the city's epidemic of drug-related violence and with a shift in weaponry toward high-capacity, semiautomatic handguns.

(*Arch Surg.* 1992;127:694-698)

Interpersonal violence has grown to epidemic proportions in many US cities. Homicide is the 12th leading cause of death in the United States overall, and is the leading cause of death among black males aged 15 to 34 years.[1] Homicide rates for black males aged 15 to 24 years have nearly doubled between 1984 and 1988, and virtually all of the increase was attributable to gun-related homicides.[2] In 1985, even before the incidence of gun-related violence began to soar, direct medical care costs for treating patients with firearm injuries were estimated to be $863 million nationally.[3] Recent escalations in violence have placed considerable financial strain on urban trauma centers and have forced some to close.[4]

The increase in violence during the late 1980s in many US cities has been perhaps most dramatic in the nation's capital. The homicide rate in Washington, DC, per 100 000 population increased threefold, from 24 in 1985 to 78 in 1990,[5] during which time the city earned the appellation "murder capital of the nation" for having the highest rate of homicide of any US city. This dramatic increase has been largely attributed to violence surrounding the trade of crack-cocaine and has been most pronounced for gun homicides of young black males.[5]

Data collected by hospitals on fatal and nonfatal gunshot wounds (GSWs) can provide a more complete picture of gun violence than homicide statistics alone. Every firearm death represents an estimated 7.5 nonfatal shootings, 28% of which require hospitalization.[3] Hospital surveillance of injuries owing to firearm assaults indicate that many of these injuries do not show up in police statistics.[6]

Using medical records data, it is possible to study temporal changes in GSW profiles (ie, the number and location of entrance GSWs), which may be indicative of shifts in the prominence of particular types of gun attacks, the type of guns used, and the lethality of these attacks. For example, a study of violent crime in New York City revealed that homicide rates changed over time due to changes in the lethality of gun attacks, the lethality of attacks being largely determined by an assailant's intent to kill during assaults.[7] Drug-related assaults characteristically had a higher degree of intent to kill than assaults resulting from spontaneous arguments. Execution-style GSWs to the head or high numbers of GSWs to the chest are wound profiles indicative of a clear intent to kill.

MATERIALS AND METHODS

Data Collection

We used data collected at the Washington (DC) Hospital Center, a level I trauma center located in the north central part of Washington. The hospital treats 30% to 40% of all adult patients with GSWs who are treated at trauma centers in the city. Most of these patients are transported from high-crime sections of Washington.

Data collected for each GSW victim admitted included external cause of injuries, nature and severity of injuries, treatments and procedures, length of stay, complications, and patient discharge status. These data are reviewed and edited monthly for every trauma inpatient.

Patients admitted for GSWs were identified through a retrospective review of trauma admission records from January 1983 through December 1990. Cases were excluded if the GSWs were noted to be self-inflicted or unintentional. These exclusions left 1781 patients eligible for the study. For analyses of length of in-

Accepted for publication March 24, 1992.

From the Trauma, Surgical Critical Care, and Emergency Services, Washington (DC) Hospital Center. Dr Webster is now affiliated with The Johns Hopkins University Injury Prevention Center, Baltimore, Md.

Reprint requests to Trauma, Surgical Critical Care, and Emergency Services, Washington Hospital Center, Room 4B-46, 110 Irving St NW, Washington, DC 20010 (Dr Champion).

Description of Population of Patients Admitted for Gunshot Wounds From January 1983 Through December 1990								
		Age, y						
	Total	**<20**	**20-24**	**25-29**	**30-34**	**35-39**	**40**	**Unknown**
Admissions, No.	**1781**	273	492	401	253	141	166	55
Deaths in hospital, No. (%)	**379** (21)	58 (21)	87 (18)	77 (19)	55 (22)	25 (18)	37 (22)	40 (73)
Treated in intensive care unit, No. (%)	504 (28)	72 (26)	138 (28)	137 (34)	89 (35)	51 (36)	59 (36)	8 (15)

patient stay and number of days in the intensive care unit (ICU), the following categories of patients were excluded: patients who died in the hospital, patients who were discharged to another acute care facility, and patients who had significant injuries other than GSWs (eg, injuries associated with a motor vehicle crash that occurred after the shooting).

Data Analysis

Based on published homicide statistics, news reports of increased drug-related violence, and data from the firearms identification unit of the DC Metropolitan Police Department, we anticipated that there would be differences in GSW patterns between 1983 and 1986 and 1988 and 1990, with 1987 being the year of transition. Trends in GSW patterns were described using plots of monthly, quarterly, and annual time-series data. Five-month moving averages were calculated and plotted to smooth monthly plots. When appropriate, patients admitted for stab wounds due to assaults were used as a comparison group. For mortality and morbidity analyses, patients were assigned to one of four categories based on the location of wounds: (1) any head wound, (2) thoracic wound with no head wound, (3) wound to the face, neck, abdomen, or pelvic region and no head or thoracic wound, or (4) wounds confined to extremities.

Most of the analyses were descriptive in nature, and in some instances, statistical tests were unnecessary to determine that a temporal shift had occurred. The statistical significance of differences in proportions was assessed using Pearson's χ^2 analysis with Yates' correction. Annual medians were calculated to examine changes in length of inpatient stays since means are highly affected by extreme values.

Annual population estimates for the hospital's catchment area for trauma admissions were not available. Therefore, trends in the number of GSW admissions were analyzed without the benefit of data on the population located in the catchment area. It is unlikely that shifts in the population would have a substantial effect on GSW admission during the 8-year observation period. Neither the estimated 3.3% decline in the city's population from 1983 to 1990 nor the District of Columbia's emergency medical services system procedures for transporting patients to trauma centers are believed to have had a substantial effect on the volume of patients transported to any specific trauma center.

RESULTS

Description of Study Population

From January 1983 through December 1990, 1781 patients were admitted to Washington Hospital Center's level I trauma center for GSWs that were not believed to be self-inflicted or unintentional (Table). Overall, 21.3% (379 of 1781) died in the hospital and 28.3% (n = 504) were admitted to the ICU. Patients aged 20 to 24 years had the highest number of admissions (27.6%), and patients older than age 40 years had the highest risk of in-hospital mortality (22.3%). Only 8.5% (150 of 1755) of the patients were female (data not shown).

Gunshot Wound Admission Trends

Figure 1 shows a sharp increase in the number of GSW assault admissions that began during the last half of 1987.

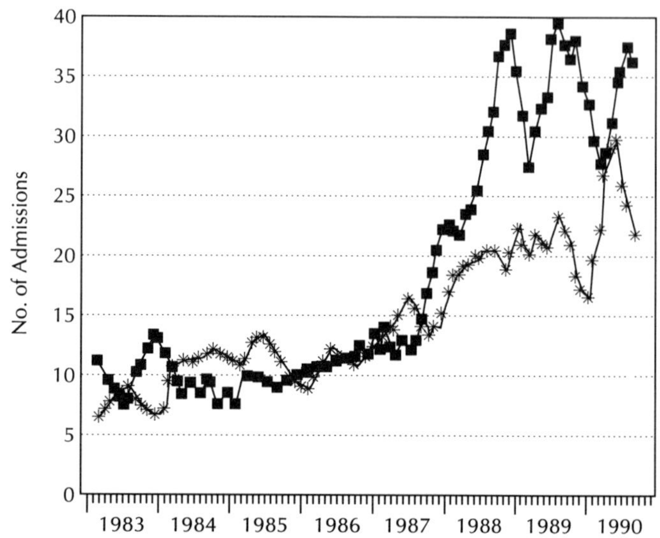

Fig 1.—*Five-month moving average of monthly admissions for gunshot wounds (squares) and stab wounds (asterisks) from 1983 through 1990 (calculated using monthly, quarterly, and annual time-series data).*

From January 1983 through June 1987, the mean±SD number of GSW assault admissions was 10.2±3.4 per month, with no apparent trend. Despite some normal monthly fluctuations, GSW admissions rose steadily from the last half of 1987 through January 1989. After having 46 admissions in January 1989, monthly GSW admission dropped off to 33.2±8.2 for the remainder of the study period, with considerable month-to-month variation.

Monthly admissions for stab wounds also began to increase in 1987, and from 1988 through 1990 (20.6±4.8) levels were double those from 1983 through 1986 (9.9±3.0). The less dramatic increase in admissions for stab wounds compared with GSWs altered the ratio of GSW to stab wound admissions from 1:1 from 1983 through 1986 to 1.5:1 from 1988 through 1990.

Consistent with the pattern of homicide increases in Washington, DC,[5] increases in GSW admissions were most pronounced among males younger than age 20 years. Admissions of teenagers for GSW assaults increased from an annual average of 7.5 admissions (6.4%) in 1983 and 1984 beginning in 1985 before leveling out to 76 admissions (19.3%) per year in 1989 and 1990. (Most serious injuries to children and adolescents younger than 18 years are treated at nearby Children's Hospital National Medical Center.) With the exception of those younger than 20 years, the general temporal pattern in GSW admissions did not vary substantially among age groups. The proportion of patients with GSWs who were female ranged from 5.0% in 1988 to 11.8% in 1990; however, no clear temporal pattern in the gender of patients with GSWs was evident.

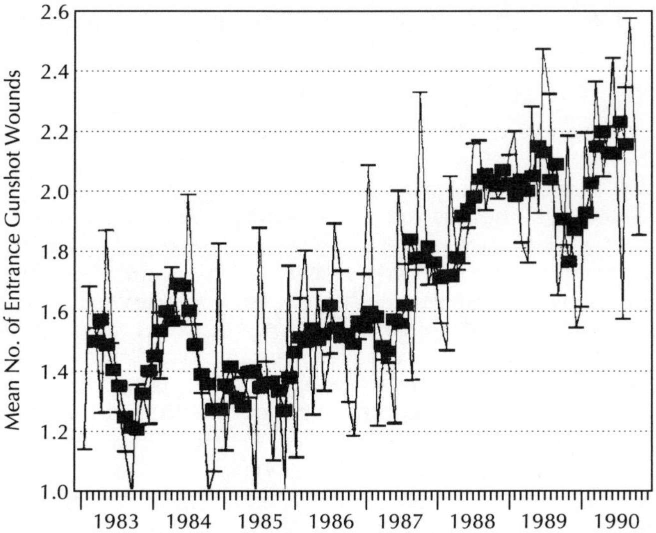

Fig 2.—*Mean number of entrance gunshot wounds per patient by month from 1983 through 1990. Squares indicate moving average; bars, observed value.*

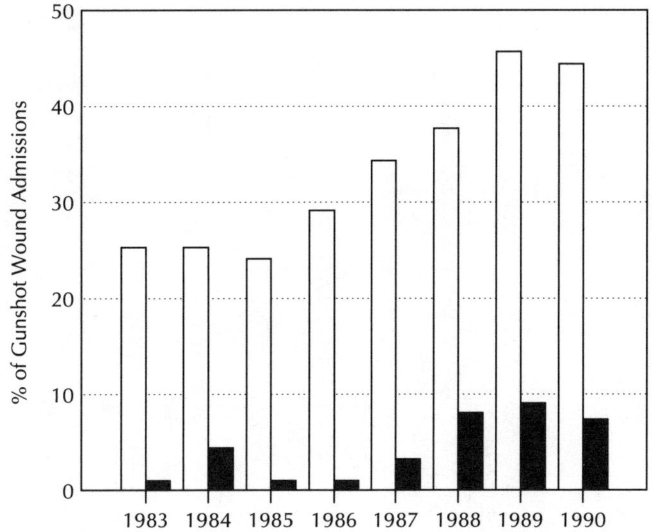

Fig 3.—*Percentage of all admissions for patients with two or more entrance gunshot wounds (shaded bars) and percentage of those with five or more entrance wounds (solid bars) from 1983 through 1990.*

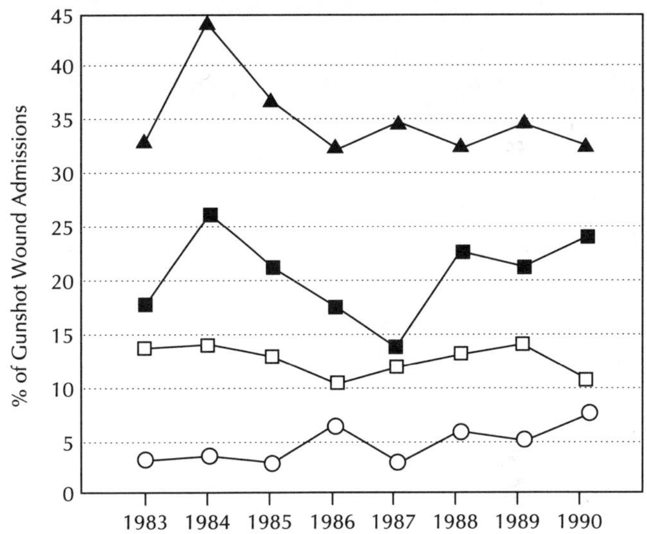

Fig 4.—*Patient mortality and the percentage of patients with gunshot wounds who have the most lethal wound profiles from 1983 through 1990. Triangles indicate one or more thoracic wound(s); solid squares, mortality; open squares, head wound(s); and open circles, multiple thoracic wound(s).*

Number of Wounds per Patient

The mean number of entrance GSWs per patient is displayed by month in Fig 2. From January 1983 through June 1987, the mean number of entrance GSWs per patient fluctuated around 1.44 ± 0.28. After a 13-month ascent that leveled off in August 1988, the mean number of GSWs per patient fell off somewhat to 2.04 ± 0.28 for the remaining study period.

Figure 3 depicts the temporal change in the percentage of patients with multiple entrance wounds. The proportion of patients with two or more entrance wounds grew from 25.9% (123 of 475) before 1987 to 43.0% (487 of 1132) from 1988 through 1990 (χ^2, 40.95; *df*, 1; $P<.001$). After 1987, the large number of entrance wounds also became more common. The proportion of patients with five or more entrance GSWs nearly quadrupled from 1.7% (eight of 475) from 1983 through 1986 to 7.9% (89 of 1132) from 1988 through 1990 (χ^2, 21.44; *df*, 1; $P<.001$).

Body Region and Patient Mortality

Patients with GSWs to the head and/or thorax made up 85.2% (323 of 379) of in-hospital deaths. As expected, patient mortality trends from 1983 through 1986 mirrored changes in the percentage of patients with head or thoracic wounds (Fig 4). The 1984 peak in mortality rate coincided with proportionate annual highs in patients with head wounds and/or thoracic wounds (58.3%, 67 of 115). The mortality rate declined from 1984 to 1986 as fewer patients presented with head or thoracic wounds. Patient mortality continued to decrease from 1986 to 13.6% (23 of 169) in 1987, even though the percentage of patients with head or chest wounds increased slightly between the two years.

Patient mortality increased from 1987 through 1990, even though the percentage of patients with head or chest wounds remained relatively constant until the percentage of admissions due to head wounds fell to 10.8% (42 of 390) in 1990. The increase in patient mortality during the last 3 years of the study was partially attributable to increases in the proportion of patients with multiple thoracic wounds, from 3.0% in 1987 to 7.6% in 1990. In-hospital mortality was 49.0% (48 of 98) among patients with multiple thoracic wounds compared with 30.5% (164 of 538) among patients with a single thoracic wound (χ^2, 11.94; *df*, 1; $P=.0005$).

The temporal pattern for GSW patient mortality was also a function of shifts in mortality from wounds to body regions with vital organs (Fig 5). For example, the rise in overall mortality from 1987 to 1988 and 1990 was driven by increases in mortality among patients with head wounds, from 45.0% (nine of 20) in 1987 to 62.0% (88 of 142) from 1988 through 1990 (χ^2, 1.45; *df*, 1; $P=.23$). Mortality among patients with thoracic wounds and no head wounds also grew from 15.3% (nine of 59) in 1987 to 35.1% (133 of 379) from 1988 through 1990 (χ^2, 8.29; *df*, 1; $P=.004$).

Morbidity

Annual median length of inpatient stay for patients with GSWs dropped from 5.5 days in 1985 to 3 days in 1987, then increased to 6 days in 1989 and 1990 (Fig 6).

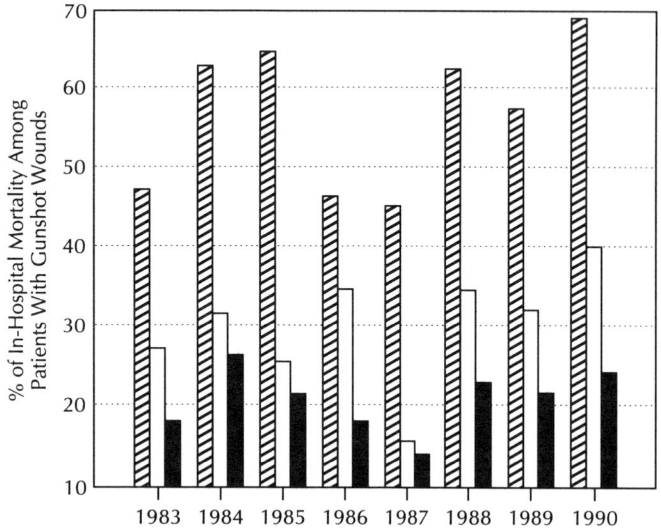

Fig 5.—*Percentage of patients with gunshot wounds who died in the hospital by body region of entrance wound(s) from 1983 through 1990. Hatched bars indicate head wound(s); shaded bars, thoracic wound(s); and solid bars, total of all gunshot wounds.*

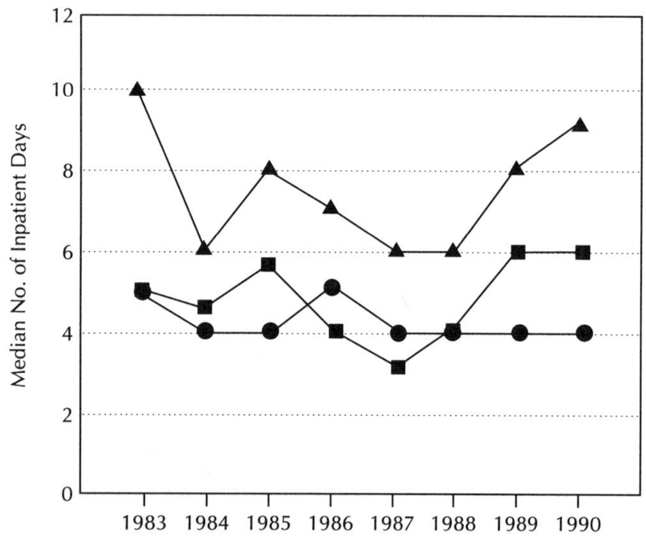

Fig 6.—*Median number of inpatient days for all patients with GSWs (squares), patients with GSWs to the thorax (triangles), and patients with stab wounds (circles) from 1983 through 1990.*

Although the temporal pattern of inpatient stay was partly attributable to proportional changes in the body regions wounded, the V-shaped pattern for median length of stay for all patients with GSWs from 1985 to 1990 follows the same pattern as trends for patients with thoracic wounds. Temporal patterns in median length of inpatient stay were similar for patients with wounds to the abdomen, face, or neck (data not shown). Trends in length of stay were not studied for patients with GSWs to the head who survived because such cases were relatively rare in the early and mid-1980s. Length of stay for patients with stab wounds varied little during the study period, suggesting that discharge practices for patients with penetrating trauma were unlikely to have affected the observed changes for patients with GSWs.

Temporal changes in average ICU stays for patients with GSWs followed virtually the same pattern as that of total inpatient stays (data not shown). Aggregate ICU stay averages were also propelled by dramatic increases for patients with thoracic wounds, as the mean number of ICU days went from 0.44 in 1987 to 2.22 in 1990.

COMMENT

The threefold increase in GSW admissions to Washington Hospital Center beginning with the last quarter of 1987 was consistent with the rate at which homicides increased in the District of Columbia.[5] Gunshot wounds also became more severe, which may have been partially responsible for the city's increase in homicides. The in-hospital mortality rate had declined steadily from 1984 to 1987, before shifting markedly upward from 1988 through 1990. This reversal in mortality trend was a function of higher mortality within body regions and an increase in the proportion of patients with multiple thoracic wounds. Trends in inpatient length of stay also suggest that GSWs became more severe.

Assessments of temporal changes in the lethality of gunshot injuries may be biased when relying solely on hospital data if the proportion of homicides in which the victim dies at the scene changes over time. Unfortunately, data on the site of death for homicides were not available from the city medical examiner. Police data indicating a 51% increase in the ratio of gun-related homicides to assaults between 1983 through 1987 and 1988 through 1990 support the hypothesis that gun attacks in Washington, DC, have become more lethal.[5]

The epidemic of gun violence in our nation's capital has led to substantial increases in medical care costs that have been borne primarily by taxpayers and trauma centers. Hospital costs associated with treating victims of criminal violence in the District of Columbia were estimated to be $20.4 million in 1989.[8] Washington Hospital Center's costs of treating patients with GSWs were not available throughout the study period; however, increases in patient volume alone resulted in a dramatic rise in costs. Using financial data from patients with GSWs in fiscal 1990 (July 1, 1989 through June 30, 1990), the mean cost for hospital care per patient with GSWs was estimated to be $14 757, excluding physician fees. (This estimate is based on an estimated Medicare cost-to-charge ratio of 0.57.) During the preepidemic period, admissions for GSW assaults averaged 10.24 per month or 123 per year. The 385 GSW admissions in fiscal 1990, therefore, represent 262 more than would have been expected if the epidemic of gun violence had not occurred. This increase in GSW admissions translates into an additional $3.9 million in hospital costs for fiscal 1990; however, the increased financial burden of treating patients with GSWs is likely to have been greater because the severity of wounds increased concomitantly with patient volume. Only half of the hospital's costs for treating patients with GSWs were reimbursed in fiscal 1990 because 37% of patients with GSWs were uninsured and 35% were covered by government programs that do not reimburse payments for the full cost of care.

Despite the unfortunate consequences for the victim, the increasing number and severity of GSWs treated at Washington Hospital Center has made for excellent training opportunities for surgeons, especially military surgeons who rotate through the trauma service. Although differences between GSWs of civilian and military patients have been documented,[9,10] the increasing incidence of multiple GSWs from military-style street weapons is closing this gap (*Am Med News*. April 14, 1989:3).

Despite differences in surgical treatment of many wounds of civilian and military patients, skills in basic assessment and resuscitation are largely transferrable.

Police data on homicide motives suggest that the violence associated with the trade of crack-cocaine played a key role in the onset of the city's epidemic of gun-related homicides and assaults. Drug-related homicides grew from 14% in 1986 to 53% in 1988, and accounted for 80% of the increase in homicides during that period.[5] Although the proportion of homicides considered to be drug-related declined in 1990, and other indexes suggest that the relative importance of drugs in violent crime has begun to diminish in Washington, DC, the legacy of sophisticated weaponry is very much in evidence.[11]

More and more assailants have switched from revolvers to high-capacity semiautomatic pistols. In 1987, revolvers outnumbered semiautomatic pistols by a ratio of 2:1 among the handguns seized by the DC Metropolitan Police Department. From 1987 to 1990, the number of semiautomatic pistols confiscated doubled, while the number of revolvers seized did not change. By 1991, semiautomatic pistols outnumbered revolvers 1011 to 799 among guns confiscated by the police (*The Washington Post*. February 2, 1992:A1). Earlier research indicated that the types of guns confiscated by police are likely to be representative of those used in all assaults and homicides.[12] Data collected by the Federal Bureau of Alcohol, Tobacco, and Firearms indicate that the shift toward semiautomatic pistols during the late 1980s was not unique to the nation's capital (*Atlanta Journal and Constitution*. May 21, 1989).

Although little research has been done in this area, the increased popularity of high-capacity semiautomatic pistols could have significant effect on public safety. High-capacity semiautomatic handguns enable assailants to fire more bullets at their victims more quickly than do revolvers, both increasing the likelihood of hitting one or more victims and increasing the number of wounds to any particular victim. Our data do not allow us to assess any increase in the likelihood of one or more victims being wounded in gun assaults. Trauma surgeons in Los Angeles (Calif) have noted an increase in multiple-victim incidents involving assault-style weapons (*Am Med News*. April 14, 1989:3). Although it is difficult to quantify such incidents, using existing medical or police data, we observed increases in the percentage of patients with two or more GSWs, the mean number of entrance wounds per patient, and the proportion of patients with five or more entrance wounds.

The available data preclude us from directly attributing changes in the number of wounds per patient to changes in gun type. Information about the type of weapon used in an attack usually is not available from medical records, and even if such information was available, correlations between the type of gun and the number of wounds may be confounded by the degree of the assailant's intent to kill. That is, assailants who are more deliberate in their attempts to kill their victims by shooting them multiple times (eg, drug enforcers) may be more likely to use high-capacity, rapid-fire guns. If that is the case, the observed increase in the number of wounds per patient may be partly attributable to a disproportionate increase in gun attacks that were very deliberate attempts to kill the victims.

Although there has most likely been some increase in the intent to kill during gun attacks due to the increasing prominence of drug-related violence, the observed increase in wounds per victim is likely to have been facilitated by the availability of semiautomatic guns with high-capacity ammunition clips. Uzis and Tech-9s, originally designed for military use, can hold more than 30 rounds and can fire up to eight rounds per second.

Epidemiologic studies that provide good estimates of the harm attributable to high-capacity semiautomatic weapons, while taking into account confounding effects related to assailant intentions, would be important contributions to the policy debate concerning the banning or regulation of the sale of this class of weapon. While well-controlled epidemiologic studies could provide more precise estimates of the degree to which high-capacity semiautomatic guns are more harmful than other handguns, the design of these guns may be so inherently dangerous to public safety that immediate legislative action is warranted. The American Medical Association and the American College of Surgeons have called for legislative efforts to restrict civilian access to high-capacity, high-rate-of-fire automatic or semiautomatic firearms.[13,14] The enactment and enforcement of such restrictions should reduce the number and the severity of firearm injuries.

References

1. National Center for Health Statistics. *Vital Statistics of the United States, 1987, II: Mortality: part A*. Hyattsville, Md: US Dept of Health and Human Services, Public Health Service, Centers for Disease Control; 1989.
2. Fingerhut LA, Kleinman JC, Godfrey E, Rosenberg H. *Firearm Mortality Among Children, Youth, and Young Adults 1-34 Years of Age: Trends and Current Status: United States, 1979-1988*. Hyattsville, Md: National Center for Health Statistics; 1991;39(suppl):1-6. Monthly Vital Statistics Report.
3. Rice DP, MacKenzie EJ, et al. *Cost of Injury in the United States: Report to Congress*. San Francisco, Calif: University of California, Institute for Health and Aging and The Johns Hopkins University, Injury Prevention Center; 1989.
4. US General Accounting Office. *Trauma Care: Lifesaving System Threatened by Unreimbursed Costs and Other Factors*. Washington, DC: General Accounting Office; 1991. Publication GAO/HRD-91-57.
5. Office of Criminal Justice Plans and Analysis. *Crime and Justice Report: 1990*. Washington, DC: Government of the District of Columbia; 1991.
6. Barancik JI, Chatterjee BF, Greene YC, Michenzi EM, Fife D. Northeastern Ohio trauma study, I: magnitude of the problem. *Am J Public Health*. 1983;73:744-751.
7. Swersey AJ. *Patterns of Criminal Homicide in Harlem and New York City*. New Haven, Conn: Yale School of Organization and Management; 1981.
8. Billings J, Teicholz N. *The Costs of Criminal Violence in the District of Columbia Hospitals*. Washington, DC: District of Columbia Hospital Association; October 1991.
9. Smith AM, Hazen SJ. What makes war surgery different? *Mil Med*. 1991;156:33-35.
10. Rignault DP. Is war surgery a specialty? *Mil Med*. 1990;155(pt 1):91-97.
11. Office of Criminal Justice Plans and Analysis. *Drug Abuse Indicators Trend Report for the District of Columbia*. Washington, DC: Government of the District of Columbia; 1991.
12. Zimring F. The medium is the message: firearm calibre as a determinant of death from assaults. *J Leg Stud*. 1972;1:97-124.
13. American Medical Association. *Substitute Resolution 264*. June 1989;A-89:385.
14. Statement on gun control. *Am Coll Surg Bull*. 1991;76:2.

Trauma in the Geriatric Patient

C. William Schwab, MD, Donald R. Kauder, MD

• **Elderly individuals are living longer, healthier, and more active lives, and, in the process, they are continually exposed to the risk of injury. Trauma is now the fifth most common cause of death in people over the age of 65 years, and the elderly suffer disproportionately high injury-related mortality rates compared with younger adults. They consume a vast portion of health care resources and their care precipitates some of the most difficult ethical and sociologic questions in modern medicine. Physiologically, the elderly present a unique and complex picture that requires an understanding of the process of aging and the concomitant effects of acquired diseases. As surgeons involved in the care of the injured, we find ourselves becoming more frequently involved with this national dilemma. This review provides some insights and guidelines for the care of the injured elderly, with the hope of improving our understanding and their outcome.**

(*Arch Surg.* 1992;127:701-706)

There is increasing awareness in the United States regarding the rapid growth of the elderly population. The 1980 US census counted almost 26.5 million people over the age of 65 years, 11.3% of the populace. The most recent census, completed in 1990, has yielded continued striking growth in America's elderly population. People 65 years of age and older now number 30.9 million, representing a 21.3% increase in this segment of the population and accounting for 12.5% of the total.[1] According to US Census Bureau projections, those over the age of 65 years will number 52 million by the year 2020 and will increase to 68 million by 2040, at which point they will exceed 20% of our population. Furthermore, the subset of persons 85 years of age and older is growing at an even faster rate. The Census Bureau forecasts 6.7 million Americans in this age group by 2020 and 12.2 million by 2040.[2]

Although the population is aging, this does not necessarily imply that the elderly are becoming less mobile and confined. In fact, more and more people are approaching their later years in excellent health and are maintaining that health for a much longer period of time. Advances in the diagnosis and treatment of cardiovascular disease, diabetes, and arthritis have delayed and, in some cases, reduced the complications of these conditions, allowing a more active life-style. Since the elderly continue to engage in many of the same activities as younger individuals, albeit at a less intense level, they are exposed to similar risks of injury. There is, however, a large discrepancy in rates of injury and mortality secondary to injury compared with younger individuals. Persons aged 65 years and older account for 27.9% of deaths due to accidental causes and have higher population-based accident mortality rates than any other age group.[3]

Apart from their unique medical and surgical problems, many geriatric patients have additional social and ethical issues that complicate their care. Although surgeons are in the unique position of having the potential to improve outcome in the injured elderly, unfortunately, there is little available in the literature to guide us through the intricacies of these more complex cases. Only recently have trauma surgeons focused on studies aimed at identifying the problems of trauma in the elderly.

MECHANISMS OF INJURY

The elderly experience the same types of injuries as younger people. However, there are distinct differences in injury pattern, effect, postinjury course, and outcome that occur with advancing age. These relate to changes in life-style, preexisting disease states, and the natural process of aging. Motor vehicle crashes are the most common type of fatal incident in the elderly through age 80 years, and falls are the second most common type. After age 80 years, the situation reverses, and falls become the predominant mechanism, probably because of changes in life-style and activity level. In fact, 70% of all deaths due to falls occur in the geriatric population.[4]

Falls are the most frequent cause of accidental injury in those over 75 years old and are the second most common injury sustained by people 65 to 74 years of age. Many of those who fall do so from a level surface and sustain an isolated orthopedic injury, such as a fractured wrist or hip. The individual who suffers this mechanism of injury is characteristically older and may fall for any number of reasons.

Falls may occur simply due to the vagaries of aging. Age-related changes in postural stability, balance, motor strength, and coordination can make the elderly more prone to tripping and, furthermore, can reduce the ability to counteract a fall after tripping. Changes in visual

Accepted for publication March 23, 1992.

From the Division of Traumatology and Surgical Critical Care, Department of Surgery, University of Pennsylvania Medical Center, Philadelphia.

Reprint requests to Division of Traumatology and Surgical Critical Care, Hospital of the University of Pennsylvania, 3400 Spruce St, Philadelphia, PA 19104 (Dr Schwab).

acuity, diminution in hearing, and progressive memory loss can lead to the inability to recognize and avoid environmental hazards. Acute or preexisting chronic disease states can also lead to a fall. Syncope is commonly implicated. A sudden diminution in cerebral blood flow (due to cardiac dysrhythmia, venous pooling, autonomic insufficiency) or a metabolic derangement (hypoglycemia, hypoxia, anemia) is often the cause. Drop attacks, defined as sudden unexplained weakness of the lower extremities, are also common. For these reasons, all patients presenting with a fall-related injury require a thorough search for an inciting event and a concentrated effort to delineate any underlying problems, both medical and environmental.

A fall from a level surface does not involve a great deal of energy transfer. Nonetheless, the morbidity and mortality from this type of incident are high. The incidence of fractures following this type of fall is reported to be between 8% and 40%.[5] Of those who are hospitalized following a fall, only 50% will be alive 1 year later.[6] This probably is due to their limited physiologic reserve and relatively fragile status at the time of the fall.

The kinds of patients just described are commonly seen only by an orthopedic surgeon. Those who require the services of a general surgeon have usually suffered a different falling mechanism. These patients tend to be healthier and more active, and, like their younger counterparts, they are injured while at work, while engaged in home repair, or while performing some other activity that places them at a greater height. Besides fractures, these fall victims have significant rates of severe injury to the head and face, chest, abdomen, and axial skeleton. An Injury Severity Score (ISS) over 15 is common.[7] As a result of the multiplicity of injuries, physiologic derangements are common. Although it is usually the severity of injury and not an underlying disease that brings this population to our attention, as with the older fall group, one must delineate the events leading to the fall to be sure that a new or occult medical problem is not missed.

The exposure of the elderly to motor vehicle trauma is a consequence of the increasing growth of the elderly population and of the growing number of elderly drivers and occupants of motor vehicles. There are 21.8 million licensed drivers aged 65 years and older in the United States, accounting for about 13% of all licensed drivers.[3] Those over 75 years of age number 6.6 million, or about 4% of those behind the wheel. Unfortunately, the elderly suffer an alarmingly high motor vehicle crash rate. The over-75 age group has the highest rate of fatal crashes of any age group and a crash rate second only to that of "new" drivers aged 16 through 25 years.[3] Motor vehicle–related injury ranks first as the mechanism of injury that brings the injured elderly to a trauma center.[7] In contrast to younger drivers, the elderly are more likely to be involved in crashes closer to home, in good weather, and during daylight hours. Alcohol plays less of a role in crashes involving the elderly, as only 6.6% of fatally injured drivers over 65 years have blood alcohol levels greater than 0.10%, compared with 23% for all other age categories.[8]

Hard scientific data explaining these crash statistics are not readily available, but, as in falls, these accidents probably follow the cause-and-effect phenomena of preexisting medical conditions, physiologic diminution of cerebral and motor skills, and increased exposure by continued use of the automobile as primary source of transportation. Cognitive deficits in memory and judgment can compound the problem when a potentially dangerous situation is encountered. Alterations in visual and auditory acuity may make it more difficult to recognize and avoid dangerous traffic situations. New medications or unanticipated drug interactions may also cause mental aberrations that can interfere with safe driving. Deterioration in strength and slower reaction times may also contribute and make the elderly driver more prone to a road crash. Certainly, exacerbations of acute or chronic medical conditions, such as coronary and cerebrovascular diseases, are known to be precipitating events in traffic crashes.

The third and most devastating mechanism of injury in the elderly occurs when an older person is struck by a moving vehicle. The population over 65 years accounts for more than 22% of automobile-pedestrian fatalities in the United States and has the highest population-based fatality rate of any age group (4.7 per 100 000 population).[8] Even if an elderly individual exercises caution when approaching a roadway, the process of aging may expose that person to an increased risk of injury. Postural changes secondary to musculoskeletal decline lead to progressive kyphosis. The resultant stooped posture makes it more difficult to lift the head to see traffic signals. Additionally, alterations in gait and strength may lead to a slow shuffling walk. Most traffic signals are set to allow a crossing rate of 4 feet per second. This rate may not give the elderly person time to clear the intersection and may explain why those over the age of 65 years account for 46% of all fatalities that occur in crosswalks.[8] Diminution in peripheral vision and progressive hearing loss also limit access to important information needed to make rational decisions regarding crossing the street. As with motor vehicle crashes, age-related alterations in memory, cognitive skills, and judgment also play a large part in these incidents.

While falls and vehicular trauma account for the majority of serious injuries in our geriatric population, the elderly are all too frequently involved as victims of violent crime. Although the literature specifically addressing this issue is sparse, violent assaults account for 4% to 14% of trauma admissions in this population.[7,9-13] Poor vision, decreased strength and coordination, improper balance, and cognitive changes leading to poor judgment combine to make the elderly particularly vulnerable. Assaults with blunt instruments are the most frequent crimes reported, but assaults with firearms and knives are becoming more common. The problems of elder and parental abuse have attracted recent focus, and, as with potential victims of child abuse, one must maintain a high index of suspicion when an elderly individual appears bruised, battered, poorly nourished, or unkempt. These cases often require hospitalization and involvement of and investigation by social services personnel.

OUTCOME

The outcome of elderly trauma patients can be assessed using a variety of measures. Perhaps the most visible acute measure is the overall rate of deaths occurring among hospitalized geriatric trauma victims. This has been reported to be in the range of 15% to 30%, far in excess of the 4% to 8% mortality rate expected in younger individuals.[14] Other measures include the complication rate, length of stay, disposition at discharge, and, perhaps most important, long-term functional status. Several authors have attempted to delineate predictors of outcome, but, again, good scientific literature is scant.

The trauma outcome "gold standards" have been applied to the geriatric subgroup with only variable results. Oreskovich et al,[15] reviewing 100 trauma victims over 70 years old, found that the ISS had little correlation with mortality. Horst et al[16] reported on trauma patients over the age of 60 years admitted to an intensive care unit and also found that the ISS was a poor predictor of mortality. Several studies, however, have shown that the ISS is a reasonable predictor of mortality. Finelli et al[13] in 1989 reviewed over 46 000 patients entered in the Multiple Trauma Outcome Study and confirmed the original work with ISS by Baker et al[17] in 1974, in which persons older than 50 years had a higher mortality rate than younger patients for any given level of ISS. van Aalst et al[11] found the ISS as well as the Glasgow Coma Score, the Revised Trauma Score, and the TRISS probability of survival to be predictive. Our own work has shown that, overall, geriatric trauma patients die with less severe injuries than their younger counterparts. Additionally, while the mortality rates from severe head injuries and exsanguination are similar among the young and the old, the elderly die of multiple organ failure and sepsis at a higher rate than younger patients, and with less severe injuries.[7]

Attempts have been made to correlate physiologic parameters with survival. While Horst et al[16] found no relationship between the Trauma Score and mortality rate, Oreskovich et al[15] and Finelli et al[13] reported good predictive value for patients with altered physiologic characteristics. Specifically, they found that the Glasgow Coma Score and the presence of shock were both correlated with poor outcome. Some interesting work addressing these contradictions was recently reported by Scalea and coworkers.[18] Using invasive monitoring to assess the cardiovascular status of all elderly patients at high risk for mortality, they found that some patients who were "hemodynamically stable" had derangements in cardiac performance, vascular tone, and oxygen metabolism. By improving oxygen consumption using fairly simple measures, such as accurate volume loading and inotropic support, survival was improved. We believe that these observations explain why some physiologic scoring tools may be inaccurate in predicting outcome.

More important, this observation highlights the concept of "limited physiologic reserve" in the elderly trauma victim and spotlights a key difference between the average younger trauma patient with normal physiologic characteristics and the elderly patient with outwardly normal "numbers" but with underlying physiologic derangements. This poorly quantified concept is consistent with the known physiologic alterations that occur in virtually every organ system as people undergo the normal aging process. The extent of underlying abnormal physiologic characteristics is widely variable among people and even between any individual's separate organ systems. The "limited reserve" concept has yet to be specifically studied in relation to injury outcome and remains a subjective component that most physicians understand and accept but seem unable to quantify. Our impression is that, after age 55 years and especially by age 65 years, each individual is unique, with widely variable responses to injury. Injury-related physiologic alterations take a different toll on each organ system and each person. Finally, outcome is difficult to predict except in extreme cases.

Intuitively, it seems logical that people with multiple medical problems would do poorly after sustaining multiple severe injuries. However, successful attempts to link the relationship between preexisting disease and mortality are scarce. In a recent case-control study, Morris et al[19] focused primarily on preexisting disease and its relationship to mortality in trauma patients. They found that cirrhosis, congenital coagulopathy, ischemic heart disease, chronic obstructive pulmonary disease, and diabetes all significantly increased the risk of dying. It is no coincidence that these disease states all increase in frequency and severity with advancing age. In related work, these authors also found that trauma victims with one or more preexisting conditions stayed in the hospital significantly longer than those without a preexisting condition.[20] However, this effect was most marked among younger patients and among those with less severe injuries. The implications for increased hospital costs and patient outcome are sobering.

Although mortality rates are the most visible means of measuring outcome, functional status at the time of discharge and over the long term is of far greater importance to the elderly survivors of severe injury and their families. Oreskovich et al[15] reported a dismal functional outcome in their study, in which 85% of elderly trauma victims survived but only 8% returned to their previous level of independence. The remainder required some form of assistance at home or in a nursing facility. One year after discharge, 72% were still in a nursing home. This work prompted a study by DeMaria et al[10] to delineate factors that determine the potential for long-term recovery in elderly trauma victims. They found that, at discharge, one third of survivors were independent, one third were dependent but living at home, and one third required a nursing care facility. Eventually, 89% of patients returned home and 57% were fully independent. van Aalst et al[11] reported on factors influencing function and independence following severe injuries in the geriatric population. Shock on admission, the presence of a severe head injury, age greater than 75 years, and the development of infectious complications were all found to be harbingers of poor outcome. The work of van Aalst et al supported that of DeMaria et al and showed that the majority of survivors of severe injury (67%) returned to a level of independence. Unfortunately, in all of these studies, variability in the measures of functional outcome makes comparisons somewhat difficult. This is an area in which there is little good science and one that will clearly benefit from further investigation.

Despite the shortcomings in the literature, the potential for achieving a favorable outcome in seriously injured geriatric patients warrants aggressive therapy and support, at least at the initial phase of contact. To this end, some basic principles of treatment of the severely injured geriatric patient will be reviewed.

TREATMENT CONSIDERATIONS

In a young person, one can safely assume a predictable normal physiologic response to trauma and a rare history of significant preexisting disease. These same assumptions cannot be made in an elderly individual.

The Advanced Trauma Life Support course serves as a good framework for the evaluation and resuscitation of geriatric trauma victims. During the initial assessment phase, one must take every opportunity to obtain a complete medical history and guard against a false sense of security in the patient with no "apparent" life-threatening injury. A relatively minor injury may be life-threatening in an individual with limited physiologic reserve. The window of opportunity to collect this type of data can thus be unexpectedly small, for the condition of a seemingly stable geriatric patient can deteriorate rapidly and with few warning signs. Attempts to glean this information can be overshadowed by the frenetic nature of the resuscitation process. Simply making a telephone call to a reliable relative or personal physician can provide invaluable information about the patient's baseline status that can completely change one's approach to diagnosis and treatment. The evaluation and support of the cardiovascular system can be especially challenging, as the work of Scalea et al[18] has illustrated. Of 15 patients entered into their original protocol, all of whom were initially considered "stable," eight had a cardiac output less than 3.5 L/min, and none of these patients had an adequate response to volume loading. Of the seven patients with a normal cardiac output, five had inadequate oxygen delivery.

Age-related changes in the cardiovascular system lead to progressive stiffening of the myocardium, resulting in a less effective pumping mechanism. One can expect an 80-year-old to have half the cardiac output of a 20-year-old, even in the absence of significant atherosclerotic cardiovascular disease.[14] There is a concomitant decrease in cardiac reserve. The myocardium becomes less sensitive to exogenous and endogenous catecholamines, and electrical conduction abnormalities can be exacerbated by the physiologic stress of the patient's injuries. As a result, the normal compensatory tachycardia in response to hypovolemia, pain, and anxiety expected in a younger individual may be blunted or absent. Ingestion of commonly prescribed β-blockers can also muddy an already confusing and complicated picture by altering the normal chronotropic response. A "normal" heart rate in this setting should be viewed with suspicion. When the clinical situation warrants, prudent administration of crystalloid is indicated, but early use of red blood cell transfusion to augment oxygen delivery should be considered, especially in any shock state or with a low hemoglobin level. If the patient's response to standard therapy is inappropriate or inadequate, the use of early invasive monitoring with an oximetric pulmonary artery catheter, as suggested by Scalea et al,[18] is indicated. The margin of error for guesswork is slim, especially when one suspects the presence of underlying ischemic cardiovascular disease. The elderly are as intolerant of overresuscitation as they are of hypovolemia.[21]

Perhaps as important as the cardiovascular status is the patient's pulmonary condition. Progressive changes in the elasticity of the lungs and chest wall lead to decreased pulmonary compliance and reduced ability to mount an effective cough. Alveolar and small airway support diminishes with advancing age, resulting in an overall diminution in total lung surface area. Age-related changes in lung defense mechanisms also occur. Pseudociliated bronchial mucosa atrophies, resulting in decreased mucociliary clearance of foreign material and bacteria. In addition, the oropharynx of elderly individuals tends to be colonized with gram-negative organisms.[22] In this milieu, even a "minor" injury to the chest can compromise the elderly trauma victim. Therapy in this setting must be directed at maintaining adequate oxygenation and controlling the pain associated with chest wall injury. Frequently, addressing the pain will go far toward ensuring satisfactory pulmonary toilet. Systemic analgesic therapy must be used with caution in this setting to avoid any respiratory depression, but, at the same time, pain must be relieved. Regional anesthetic therapy, such as epidural anesthesia, intrapleural catheters, and intercostal nerve blocks, are therefore attractive and are our mainstays of care. In patients presenting with respiratory distress or in whom conservative means of pulmonary support fail, early mechanical ventilation must be considered. While recognizing that this may lead to a higher incidence of pulmonary infectious complications,[22] allowing the patient to become hypoxic or to markedly increase the work of breathing can be disastrous.

Similar caution must be taken in the evaluation of the geriatric patient with the potential for an intracranial injury. With increasing age, the brain undergoes progressive atrophy. All other things being equal, the brain can be expected to decrease in size by 10% between the ages of 30 and 70 years.[14] As aging proceeds, functional changes accompany the structural alterations. Subtle changes in cognitive ability, memory, and data acquisition are common and may confound the evaluation of the patient's mental status. It is an error, however, to ascribe alterations in mental status to the changes of senility, for these structural changes in the brain can mask significant intracranial pathologic conditions. As the brain's mass decreases, the space between the brain surface and the skull increases. The bridging veins are stretched. As a result, a relatively minor blow to the head can cause significant bleeding or swelling that will not be immediately apparent due to the increased "dead space" within the skull. Liberal, aggressive use of computed tomography is essential.

The diagnosis of abdominal injury is also difficult, since the physical examination of the abdomen in the elderly is frequently unreliable. While diagnostic peritoneal lavage is the "gold standard," many elderly patients are at a stage in life where they have had previous abdominal surgery. In this population, double-contrast computed tomography is a reasonable alternative. Care must be taken, however, to ensure adequate hydration. Elderly patients tend to be volume contracted, especially those taking diuretic agents. Add to this even a modest degree of blood loss, and the stage is set for renal failure induced by the administration of the intravenous contrast medium needed to do an adequate computed tomography study. A "dry" scan, done without the aid of intravenous contrast, can be a useful alternative.

Renal mass declines progressively with age, so that, by the age of 65 years, there is a 30% to 40% loss of the glomeruli.[4] The functional nephrons that remain frequently show degenerative changes in the tubules and thickening of the basement membrane. The result is that the glomerular filtration rate diminishes. It is an error to assume that a normal serum creatinine level represents normal renal function in this setting. Calculation of the creatinine clearance can be an important guide prior to the administration of dye or a potentially nephrotoxic drug. Adequate and accurate volume resuscitation must be assured.

The treatment considerations just reviewed serve as a

background for care. Unfortunately, there is not sufficient space to discuss the management of specific injuries. The principles of diagnosis and management for individual injuries should be the same irrespective of age. It is the increasing incidence of physiologic changes and antecedent disease states that mandates a different overall approach to the geriatric trauma population. For ease of consideration, we think in terms of three age subsets: 55 through 64 years, 65 through 74 years, and 75 years or older. Each subset warrants a slightly different approach, integrating the above principles and heightening one's awareness that, with increasing age, although the signs and symptoms may be minimal, the eventual outcome is frequently in doubt and commonly is poor, as seen in the following.

Treatment Axioms, 55 Through 64 Years

1. Assume some mild decrease in physiologic reserve
2. Suspect the presence of some common diseases of middle age (diabetes, arteriosclerotic cardiovascular disease, hypertension, previous surgery, previous transfusion)
3. Suspect the use of prescription or over-the-counter medications
4. Assume the patient is competent to provide an accurate medical history
5. Look for subtle signs of organ dysfunction, especially cardiovascular and respiratory systems; arterial blood gas measurements and electrocardiograms are crucial
6. In the presence of a history of loss of consciousness or abnormalities in cognitive function or personality, assume there is a serious brain injury until proven otherwise; computed tomographic scan is invaluable; magnetic resonance imaging may be a helpful adjunct
7. Proceed with standard diagnostic and management schemes, unless contraindicated by information collected during history taking

Treatment Axioms, 65 Through 74 Years

1. Accept the presence of age-related and acquired disease-induced physiologic alterations of organ systems
2. Accept the presence of acquired diseases and medications to correct or control them; assume a higher incidence of previous surgery and transfusion
3. Decide whether the patient is competent to give a reliable medical history; review the history as soon as possible with the patient's relatives or personal physician
4. Aggressively monitor the patient and control the physiologic characteristics to optimize cardiac performance and oxygen metabolism
5. Assume that any alteration in mental status or cognitive or sensory function indicates the presence of a brain injury; imaging of the brain is mandatory
6. Proceed with standard diagnostic and management schemes, including early, aggressive operative management
7. Be aware of poor outcome, especially with severe injury to the central nervous system or marked physiologic deterioration secondary to injury; check for advance directives

Treatment Axioms, 75 Years or Older

1. Proceed as in items 1 through 5 for patients 65 through 74 years of age
2. Assume a poor outcome with moderately severe injury, especially in the central nervous system or for any injury causing physiologic dysfunction
3. After aggressive initial resuscitation and diagnostic maneuvers, examine item 2 and discuss appropriateness of care with the patient (if competent) and family members
4. Attempt to be humane, and recognize the legal and ethical controversies involved; consider early consultation of experts in ethics and social services to help the family and medical team with difficult decisions

These guidelines must be viewed only as the framework around which individualized care should be built. They should also be linked to the social and ethical issues unique to each geriatric patient who has a life-threatening or permanently disabling injury.

SOCIOECONOMIC ISSUES

The cost of trauma care in the United States is huge, accounting for more than $87 billion per year in direct medical expenses and lost productivity.[23] The issue of cost must be viewed hand in hand with that of reimbursement, which has been shown to be inadequate to cover hospital costs.[24] The problem is magnified in the population over age 65 years, which accounts for nearly one third of these expenses.[15] Many of these people have the diagnosis related group (DRG)-based Medicare system as their primary health care coverage. In 1988, Schwab et al[25] addressed the issue of DRG-based reimbursement for trauma care in New Jersey, a state that uses an all DRG-based system. They concluded that the DRG-based prospective payment system was not capable of supporting trauma care. DeMaria et al[26] addressed this issue in a study that projected DRG reimbursement specifically for trauma patients over 65 years old. No correlation was found between hospital costs and reimbursement. Furthermore, the DRG system grossly underestimated costs in patients with severe injury, in those with one or more complications, and in those more than 80 years old. Clearly, efforts need to be directed toward modifying the Medicare system to adjust it to the reality of health care costs.

On the other hand, health care providers must be aware of the strong and direct association between costs, complications, and the length of stay. This is true through all age groups, but, in the elderly, postdischarge placement is another variable that profoundly affects length of stay and cost. In almost all cases, this relates to social and family issues. The eventual disposition of an elderly trauma victim often depends on the extent of the family support structure. Financial assistance as well as help in the home may have to come from either the extended family or some governmental agency. It is common for the children of an 85-year-old to be elderly themselves and potentially in poor health and thus unable or unwilling to take responsibility for a parent's postdischarge care and rehabilitation. The lack of private or commercial insurance coverage can similarly make it difficult to obtain resources for providing extended care, and the length of stay while discharge planning arrangements are made is likely to increase. In some cases, there is no family at all, and the patient essentially becomes a ward of the hospital.

The appropriate allocation of limited resources is another highly sensitive issue, especially regarding the decision to withhold or withdraw therapy. Recent Congressional legislation has mandated that patients admitted to hospitals must have the opportunity to place an advance directive in the medical record. Unfortunately, the sudden nature of trauma does not allow for such foresight. There are instances in which it is immediately apparent that meaningful survival is impossible. A patient sustaining trauma who presents in cardiac arrest is a good example of such a situation. A decision to withhold futile care is not difficult in that setting. Unfortunately, most circumstances are not so clear-cut, and early, frank discussions with the patient (if possible) and the family are paramount. In one recent report, 12% of deaths in elderly trauma victims occurred at the request of the patient, the family, and the physicians.[12]

The many issues involved in the care of the injured elderly are complex. What should be clear from this report is that the scope of the problem is growing by leaps and bounds. To date, however, few objective data are available to help the surgeon cope with the severely injured geriatric patient. This review provides a background that is intended to highlight several areas in which the care of the injured elderly is different from that of the young adult. What is needed is continual study and definition of physiologic response, good outcome data, an attempt to define what is lethal injury at the far end of life, and a dignified and human approach to this unique population.

References

1. *Projections of the Population of the United States, by Age, Sex, and Race: 1983 to 2080.* Washington, DC: US Bureau of the Census; 1990. US Census Statistics, ser P-25, No. 952.
2. Spencer G. *Projections of the Population of the United States by Age, Sex and Race: 1988 to 2080.* Washington, DC: US Bureau of the Census; 1989. Current Population Reports, ser P-25, No. 1018.
3. *Accident Facts: 1991 Edition.* Chicago, Ill: National Safety Council; 1991.
4. Schwab CW, Kauder DR. Geriatric trauma. In: Moore EE, Ducker TB, Edlich FR, et al, eds. *Early Care of the Injured Patient.* Toronto, Ontario: BC Decker Inc; 1990:328-334.
5. Perry BC. Falls among the elderly: a review of the methods and conclusions of epidemiologic studies. *J Am Geriatr Soc.* 1982;30:367-371.
6. Rubenstein LZ. Falls in the elderly: a clinical approach. *West J Med.* 1983;138:273-275.
7. Kauder DR, Civil ID, Schwab CW. Trauma in the elderly: a regional center's experience. Presented at the First Scientific Assembly for the Eastern Association for the Surgery of Trauma; 1988; Longboat Key, Fla.
8. *A Decade of Progress: Fatal Accident Reporting System, 1989.* Washington, DC: National Highway Traffic Safety Administration; 1991. US Dept of Transportation publication HS 807071.
9. Smith PC, Enderson BL, Maull KI. Trauma in the elderly: determinants of outcome. *South Med J.* 1990;78:171-177.
10. DeMaria EJ, Kenney PR, Merriam MA, Casanova LA, Gann DS. Aggressive trauma care benefits the elderly. *J Trauma.* 1987;27:1200-1206.
11. van Aalst JA, Morris JA Jr, Yates HK, Miller RS, Bass SM. Severely injured geriatric patients return to independent living: a study of factors influencing function and independence. *J Trauma.* 1991;31:1096-1102.
12. Osler T, Hales K, Baack B, et al. Trauma in the elderly. *Am J Surg.* 1988;156:537-543.
13. Finelli FC, Jonsson J, Champion GR, Morelli S, Fouty WJ. A case control study for major trauma in geriatric patients. *J Trauma.* 1989;29:541-548.
14. Kauder DR, Schwab CW. Comorbidity in geriatric patients. In: Maull K, Cleveland H, Strauch G, Wolferth C, eds. *Advances in Trauma.* St Louis, Mo: Mosby-Year Book Inc; 1990:215-230.
15. Oreskovich MR, Howard JD, Copass JK, Carrico JC. Geriatric trauma: injury patterns and outcome. *J Trauma.* 1984;24:565-572.
16. Horst HM, Obeid FN, Sorensen VJ, Bivins BA. Factors influencing survival of elderly trauma patients. *Crit Care Med.* 1986;14:681-684.
17. Baker SP, O'Neill B, Haddon E, Long WB. The injury severity score: a method for describing patients with multiple injuries and evaluating emergency care. *J Trauma.* 1974;14:187-196.
18. Scalea TM, Simon HM, Duncan AO, et al. Geriatric blunt multiple trauma: improved survival with early invasive monitoring. *J Trauma.* 1990;30:129-136.
19. Morris JA Jr, MacKenzie EJ, Edelstein SL. The effect of preexisting conditions on mortality in trauma patients. *JAMA.* 1990;263:1942-1946.
20. MacKenzie EF, Morris JA Jr, Edelstein SL. Effect of pre-existing disease on length of hospital stay in trauma patients. *J Trauma.* 1989;29:757-765.
21. Demarest GB, Osler TM, Clevenger FW. Injuries in the elderly: evaluation and initial response. *Geriatrics.* 1990;45:36-42.
22. Allen JE, Schwab CW. Blunt chest trauma in the elderly. *Am Surg.* 1985;51:697-700.
23. Weingarten MS, Wainwright ST, Saccheti AD. Trauma and aging effects on hospital costs and length of stay. *Ann Emerg Med.* 1988;17:10-14.
24. Jacobs LM. The effect of prospective reimbursement on trauma patients. *Am Coll Surg Bull.* 1985;70:17-28.
25. Schwab CW, Young G, Civil ID, et al. DRG reimbursement for trauma: the demise of the trauma center (the use of ISS grouping as an early predictor of total hospital cost). *J Trauma.* 1988;28:939-946.
26. DeMaria EJ, Merriam MA, Casanova LA, Gann DS, Kenney PR. Do DRG payments adequately reimburse the costs of trauma care in geriatric patients? *J Trauma.* 1988;28:1244-1249.

This month, the 10 scientific journals of the American Medical Association are concurrently publishing multiple articles on the medical, social, and economic effects of violence. Although our awareness of the consequences of this virulent societal problem has been heightened by the recent catastrophe that occurred in Los Angeles, Calif, the reality is that violence exists as a part of life in the world of the 1990s. Some manifestations of this problem that are pertinent to dermatology are described and discussed in several articles in this month's issue of the ARCHIVES.

Kenneth A. Arndt, MD
Editor

Skin Manifestations of Mustard Gas

A Clinical Study of 535 Patients Exposed to Mustard Gas

Ali-Z Momeni, MD; Shahla Enshaeih, MD; Montaza Meghdadi, MD; Maliheh Amindjavaheri, MD

• ***Background.***—**During the Iraq-Iran war (1980-1988), 535 patients who were exposed to mustard gas (one of the chemical warfare agents used by Iraq) were referred to our dermatology department. In this article, we have tried to review the skin manifestations of these patients.**

Observations.—**The skin lesions were of early or late onset. The early onset lesions consisted of erythema (76%), bulla (55%), and purpura (1.1%). These lesions were mostly found on the face and skin folds. The late-onset manifestations were pigmentation (20.4%) and desquamation (11.2%). Other complications were ophthalmic (85%), pulmonary (15%), and gastrointestinal (10%). Lymphopenia (7%) was the most serious laboratory disorder reported. Biopsy specimens of the lesions showed subepidermal bullae with mild dermal and epidermal necrosis.**

Conclusions.—**All patients were treated as for burns using sulfadiazine and furacine. All patients were cured in a period of 15 to 45 days. During a 6-month follow-up, no mortality was observed.**

(*Arch Dermatol.* 1992;128:775-780)

Mustard gas was synthesized in 1854. However, the vesicant properties of sulfur mustard (dichlorodiethylsulfide) were not described until 1887. During World War I, medical attention was first focused on the vesicant action of sulfur mustard on the skin, eyes, and respiratory tract.[1,2] This gas was first employed by the German army in July 1917.[3] Since serious systemic intoxication also followed after exposure, more attention was paid to these problems.

Although the use of chemical warfare was banned by the 1925 Geneva Protocol, it was used in the Iraq-Iran conflict (1980-1988). During the war, several Iranian soldiers and civilians were exposed to chemical warfare agents. Most of the toxic effects were found in the eyes, skin, and respiratory tract.[4] Those who had skin lesions were referred to our dermatology ward. The toxicologic analysis performed at that time revealed that most of the victims had been exposed to dichlorodiethylsulfide or mustard gas (Yperite), which has been reported as the most extensively used gas.[4-7]

PATIENTS AND METHODS

In total, 535 patients who had been exposed to mustard gas were admitted to our dermatology ward. A questionnaire and a special examination chart were designed, and routine examination tests, including complete blood cell count, hemoglobin, hematocrit, erythrocyte sedimentation rate, routine urinalysis, chest roentgenogram, and electrocardiogram, were performed for all patients. Toxicologic analysis was done in a limited group of these patients. Skin biopsy specimens were obtained in more than 80 patients in different clinical stages. Other special examinations, such as liver and renal function tests, electroencephalogram, blood gases, and protein electrophoresis, were performed whenever clinically required.

RESULTS

Toxicologic analysis performed locally and at other centers[4,5] revealed that the only gas used was mustard gas, even though in our ward this analysis was performed for only 60 patients.

The time interval between exposure and admission was between 24 and 48 hours. Most patients were young combatants, but there were also civilians, including women and children, who lived at the border near the war front and who were exposed to the gases. Ninety-five percent of the patients were male (508) and 5% were female (27). Most of the patients were young, with an average age of 22 years; however, there were

Accepted for publication March 2, 1992.
From the Department of Dermatology, Isfahan (Iran) University of Medical Sciences.
Reprint requests to PO Box 1191, Isfahan, Iran (Dr Momeni).

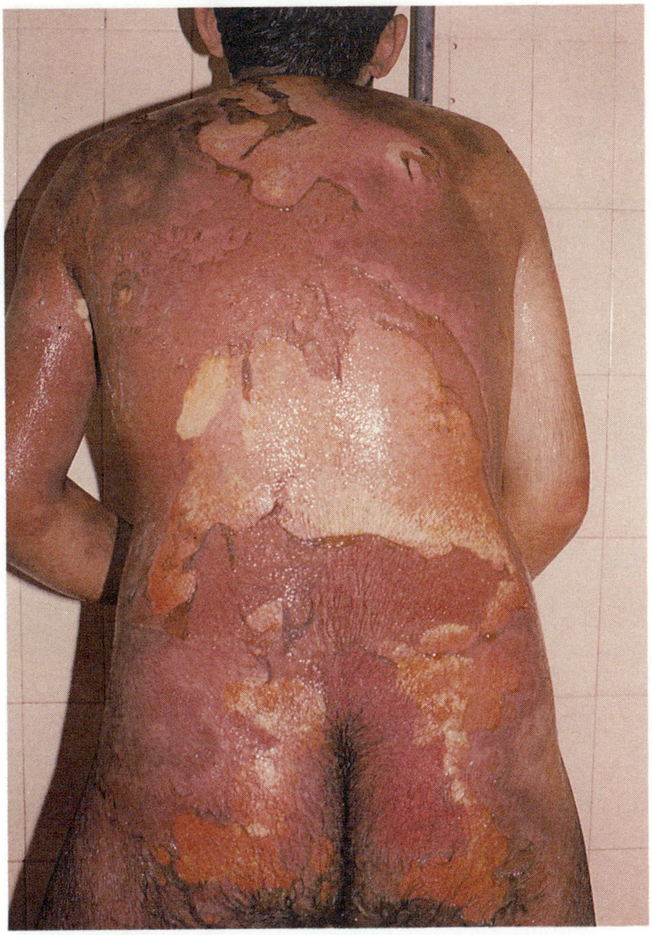

Fig 1.—Diffuse erythema and ulcerating lesions over the back.

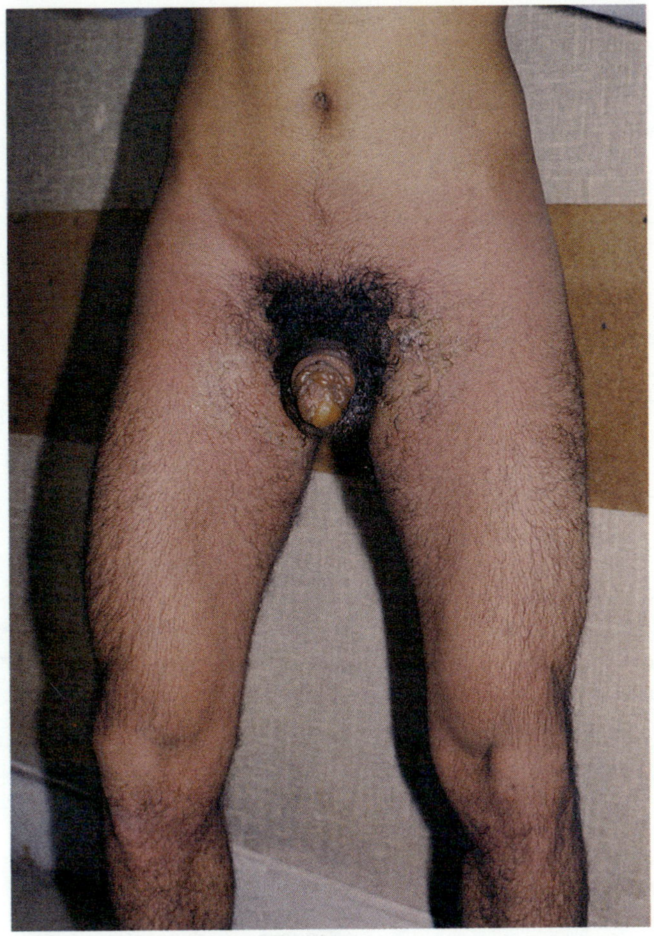

Fig 3.—Diffuse erythematous lesion over the genital area.

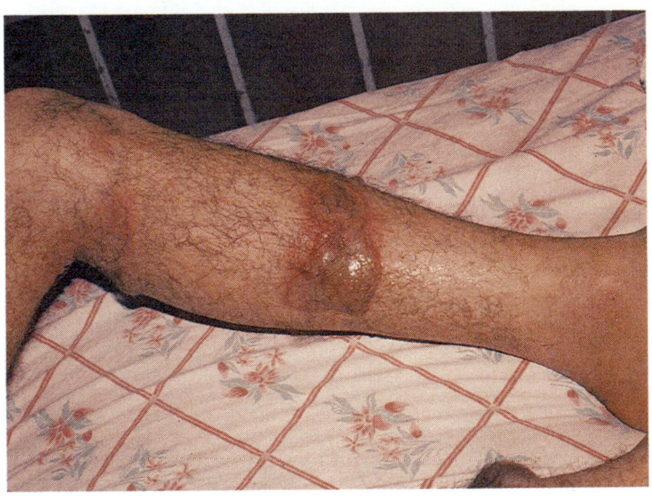

Fig 2.—Multiple bullae over the leg and thigh.

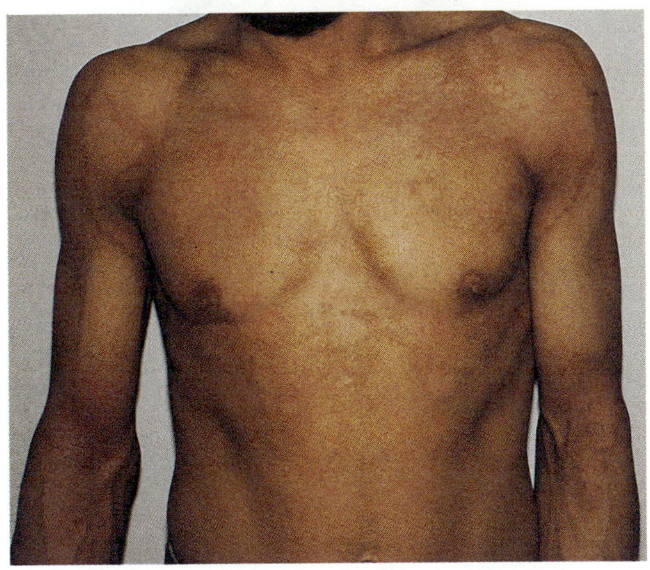

Fig 4.—Generalized hypopigmented and hyperpigmented macules over the trunk.

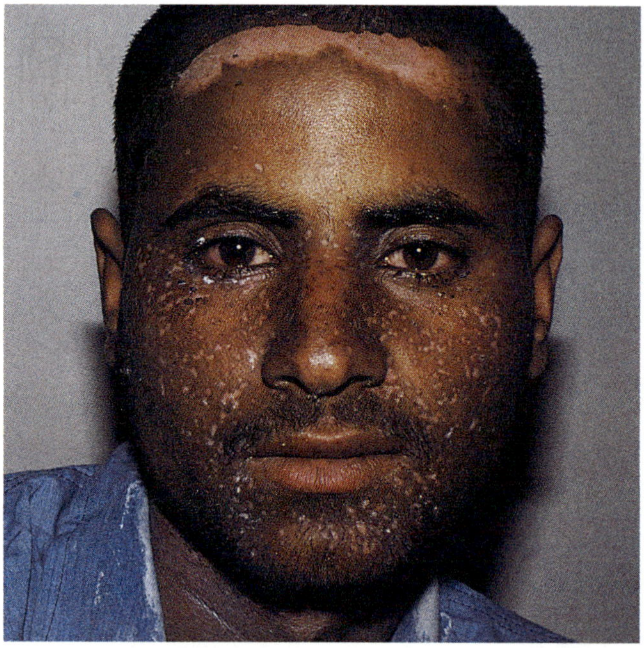

Fig 5.—Postinflammatory hypopigmented and hyperpigmented lesions over the site of the previous skin lesions.

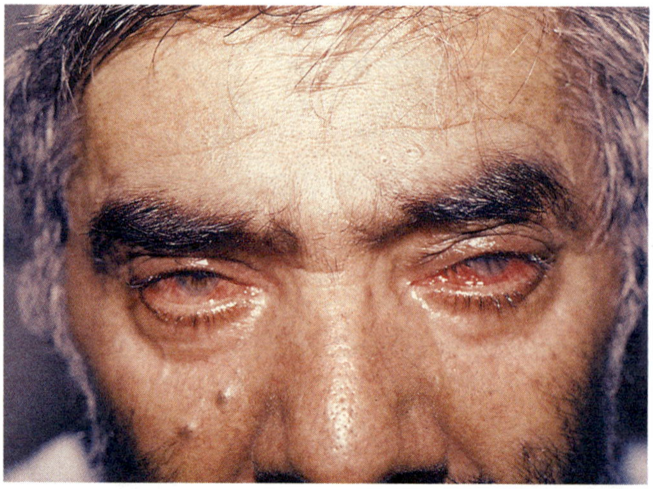

Fig 7.—Blepharokeratoconjunctivitis was one of the ophthalmic problems.

Table 1.—Skin Manifestations of Mustard(Yperite) Gas*

Clinical Manifestations	No. of Patients	%
Erythema	423	79.06
Bulla	295	55.14
Pigmentation	109	20.37
Scale	60	11.21
Urticaria	26	4.85
Purpura	6	1.12
Mucosal lesion	6	1.12

*Five hundred thirty-five patients were exposed to mustard gas.

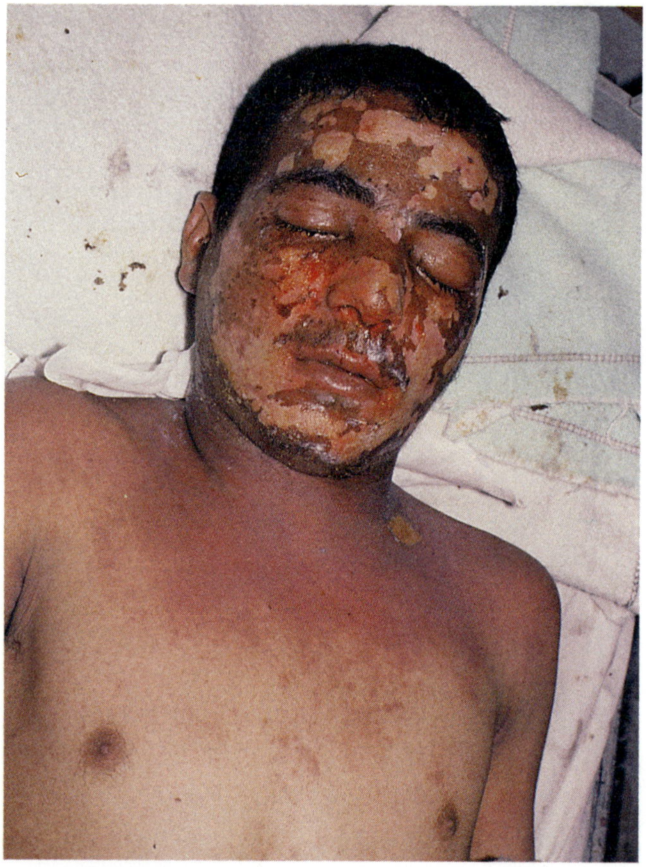

Fig 6.—Erythematous lesion over the chest with ulceration of the face.

15 children, including a 9-month-old infant, and a 70-year-old man. According to the history obtained from these patients, the main source of chemical agents were air bombs. At first, all patients had noticed a garlic smell, and, after an interval of 3 to 4 hours, eye irritation had started. These symptoms were followed by photophobia and conjunctivitis. Skin lesions started 8 to 24 hours after exposure. The first symptoms were itching and a burning sensation in most parts of the body, especially in the armpits, genital areas, and at the base of the neck. At first, the patients developed erythema and, gradually, after 2 to 3 days, blisters had appeared.

At the time of admission, 85% (455) of our patients had conjunctivitis and 92% (492) had skin lesions. Skin lesions in 30% (160) of the patients were not severe; therefore, these patients were discharged after 1 day but were followed up in the outpatient clinic.

Skin Lesions

As mentioned above, 92% (492) of patients had skin lesions (Table 1). These lesions started as erythema and bullae. Ulcers and necrosis appeared later and, finally, hypopigmentation and hyperpigmentation developed.

Erythema

Seventy-six percent (423) of our patients had erythematous lesions. These lesions were mostly found over

Table 2.—Location of Bullous Lesions of Mustard (Yperite) Gas*

Location	No. of Patients	%
Axillary	266	90.16
Genital	213	72.20
Face	104	35.25
Chest	89	30.16
Trunk	36	12.20
Other parts of the body	18	6.10

*Two hundred ninety-five patients had bullae.

Table 3.—Ophthalmic Manifestations of Mustard (Yperite) Gas*

Clinical Manifestations	No. of Patients	%
Conjunctivitis	455	85.04
Photophobia	332	62.05
Eyelid edema	64	11.96
Corneal abrasion	43	8.03

*Five hundred thirty-five patients were exposed to mustard gas.

the axillary area, neck, chest, face, and genital areas. A few of these patients had generalized erythrodermatous rashes. Erythematous areas were hypersensitive and the patients complained of a mild burning sensation over the affected areas. Erythema was followed by bulla formation or gradually disappeared after a few days or even after 2 to 3 weeks. Mild scaly areas and, very rarely, hypopigmentation and hyperpigmentation appeared over the previous erythematous areas. Hyperpigmentation was seen mostly over the sites that were under pressure, eg, areas covered by a belt or close-fitting socks.

Bulla

Blister and bulla lesions were present in 55% (295) of patients. Bullae appeared over previously erythematous lesions or on sites without any previous lesion, with mild erythema around them (Figs 1 through 6). A hyperpigmented area was seen around some of the blisters. The bullae were variable in size, from small vesicles to large bullae (15 cm). Sometimes large flaccid bullae developed that became confluent, and the epidermis came off in large sheets, leaving a raw, red exposed dermis making the skin surface look scalded. A positive Nikolsky's sign was usually present in these patients. Bullae were present mostly over the axillary region, genital areas, face, and chest; however, sometimes the bullae were so severe that they involved 60% to 80% of the whole body surface.

Bullous Lesions

Ninety percent (266 patients) of the lesions were found on the axilla; in 72% (213 patients), on the genital area; in 35% (104 patients), on the chest and back; and in 12% (36 patients), on the trunk and extremities. In 6% (18 patients), the severity of exposure was such that the lesions appeared on almost all parts of the body. However, the bullae were never seen on the palms and soles (Table 2).

During the first 2 days of admission, the patients did not complain of pain, although they had mild itching and burning sensations. Later on, pain appeared, and, in some cases, it was so unbearable that it necessitated the use of powerful sedatives. Bullae contained a yellowish fluid that clotted after 24 hours. At this time, drainage of the bullae was difficult, since this clotted material adhered to the floor of the bullae. However, if the bullae were opened and drained during the first 24 hours, recovery was good and the ulcers healed in 1 or 2 weeks. If the bullae were drained after 24 hours, then healing was difficult and could take 4 to 6 weeks. We did not test this phenomenon on individual patients; rather, we observed it among different patients receiving the same treatments.

Sometimes after a few days or weeks, new bullous lesions appeared over skin that formerly appeared normal. This presentation was rare and only 6% (33) of our patients had late-onset bullae.

In most patients, the ulcers healed, leaving no scars. True scars developed in only 4% (21) of our patients. Moreover, a pattern similar to scar formation was seen in 51.2% (274) of our patients.

Pigmentation

Pigmentation was seen in 20.4% (109) of our patients. These included the following: (1) postinflammatory hypopigmentation and hyperpigmentation over the site of the previous skin lesions (Fig 5); (2) prefollicular hypopigmentation and hyperpigmentation, which might have been due to mild prefollicular inflammation without any specific lesion; (3) generalized hyperpigmentation, which, in a few cases, was so severe that the formerly white-skinned patient turned black; (4) generalized hypopigmented and hyperpigmented macules and patches on the trunk, resembling tinea versicolor lesions (Fig 5); and (5) hyperpigmented patches over sites of previous pressure, such as under the belt, over the legs, and under close-fitting socks.

Purpuric Lesions

Purpura and ecchymosis were rare and only 1.1% (6) of our patients had this lesion, even though it was not specific.

Scales and Exfoliation

A few days or weeks after exposure, 11.2% (60) of patients developed scaling. This was mostly seen over the site of the previous erythematous rash. Generalized scaling and exfoliative erythroderma were rare, and only 1.6% (8) of patients showed this manifestation.

Urticaria

Urticaria developed in 4.9% (26) of patients. This was one of the latest manifestations, and the patients complained of urticaria a few weeks after admission or during the follow-up period. We think it might have occurred due to hypersensitivity or in response to a psychological factor, but it needs further investigation.

Mucosal Lesions

Mouth ulcers were very rare, and only 1.1% (6) of patients showed ulcerating lesions over the oral mucosa.

Other Manifestations

As mentioned before, those patients with skin lesions were referred to our dermatology ward; others with mostly pulmonary, ophthalmic, or gastrointestinal problems were sent to other wards. However, among our patients we had some with involvement of other organs.

Ophthalmic complications included conjunctivitis, blepharokeratoconjunctivitis, a burning sensation, and lacrimation. These findings were observed in 85% (455) of patients. Moreover, there was photophobia in 62% (332 patients), corneal edema and abrasion in 8% (43 patients), and edema of the eyelids in 12% (64 patients) (Table 3). Most patients had blurred vision, and a few of them complained of temporary blindness (Fig 7).

Since most of our patients were in good general condition, respiratory problems were less severe than reported.[6] In our group, only 15% (80) of patients had these manifestations. Respiratory symptoms included upper respiratory tract symptoms, such as a burning sensation in the mouth, pharyngodysphonia, and cough. Symptoms of the lower respiratory tract were less frequent and included cough, shortness of breath, tachypnea, and tachycardia.

Gastrointestinal symptoms were less frequent and were found in only 10% (53) of patients. The symptoms included nausea and vomiting. Gastrointestinal bleeding was rather rare and only four patients had this problem.

Neuropsychiatric Problems

There was no focal neurological abnormality in our patients. Psychiatric problems, however, were somewhat frequent and presented in 12% (64) of our patients. These included agitation, insomnia, depression, and muscle weakness.

Laboratory Findings

Hematologic disorders were the most serious complications among our patients. During the first 3 days of admission, complete blood cell counts were within normal limits and only 16 of our patients, who had secondary infections, showed leukocytosis. Later on, most patients developed lymphopenia with mild leukocytosis (ie, while the total number of leukocytes increased, the percentage of lymphocytes decreased), and in 6% (18 patients), pancytopenia occurred. Thrombocytopenia and anemia were the most prevalent findings. In those patients with leukopenia, skin lesions became infected. The most common organisms were *Staphylococcus*, *Streptococcus*, and *Pseudomonas*.[8]

Fortunately, leukopenia and anemia were rare in our patients, and other laboratory findings were within normal limits; only a few patients showed mild elevation of their transaminase levels, even though this was not significant.

Pathologic Findings

Biopsy specimens of the lesion in the erythematous stage showed intercellular and intracellular edema and nuclear pyknosis of the epidermis with mild edema at the upper dermis and perivascular lymphocytic infiltration in the dermis. The bullous lesion showed subepidermal bullae with infiltration of leukocytes in the upper dermis and perivascular infiltration of leukocytes and lymphocytes. In the ulcerating lesion, the epidermis showed mild necrosis with severe inflammatory cell response, including leukocytes and lymphocytes in the upper dermis. The hyperpigmented lesions showed hyperactivity of the melanocytes with increased melanin in the dermis.

Treatment

Those patients who were referred to our department had received first aid in local emergency clinics immediately after exposure. We treated them as follows: (1) daily bathing with permanganate (1/10 000) or tap water; (2) intravenous solutions were used for all patients during the first 24 hours, which was continued for those who had severe lesions, and their electrolyte levels were measured daily; (3) skin was left open (the patients were kept on sterile sheets while the skin was left open); (4) all patients were receiving high-energy diets including frequent nutritious liquids; (5) blisters were aspirated immediately and bullae bigger than 2×2 cm were opened as soon as possible; (6) patients were cared for as if they were burn patients by means of different ointments, such as 1% silver-sulfadiazine, constituents of an O/W ointment (polysorbate 60, polysorbate 80, glycerine, monostearate, methyl alcohol, liquid paraffin, propyleneglycol, and water), or furacine (0.2% nitrofurazone), with corticosteroid ointments (ie, 1% hydrocortisone) being used only for those with severe erythematous rashes; (7) if the patients had severe pain while dressing, morphine sulfate was administered; (8) in a few patients with infected lesions, antibiotics were used; (9) in patients with ophthalmic problems, eyes were irrigated with Ringer's solution and, when they had photophobia, the eyes were kept closed at least for 24 to 48 hours and 1% cyclopenolat or 15% sulfacetamide in hydroxypropylmethylcellulose or chlortetracycline was used daily as an eye ointment (corticosteroid ointments for ophthalmic problems were never used); (10) a urinary catheter was used for those patients with severe genital skin damage; (11) gastrointestinal problems were not severe in our patients and were treated symptomatically; (12) the 15% (80) of patients with respiratory problems received antibiotics, bromohexin, codeine compounds, and moist oxygen, but those who had severe problems (10 patients) were sent, under special care, to chest wards; and (13) those with bone marrow depression received fresh blood (18 patients).

Fortunately, all of our patients (except for those 10 patients about whom we have no information) recovered in 15 to 40 days. We followed up a group of these patients (250) for a period of 6 months, during which we observed no mortality, and all patients were in good condition.

COMMENT

We herein report the clinical presentations of sulfur mustard gas on 535 patients who were referred to our dermatology department. Although a brief toxicologic test performed on a limited number of patients (60) revealed the toxin used to be dichlorodiethylsulfide, our recognition of this gas was based on the reported clinical presentations.

It has been reported that the toxicologic effects of dichlorodiethylsulfide increases with higher temperatures and in humid atmospheres.[4,9,10] It is of great interest to know that most of our patients were exposed to the gas in humid tropical areas. The eye, skin, and respiratory tract are the most reported target organs,[6,11] among which the eye has been mentioned as be the most sensitive.[9,11] However, in our patients, skin lesions were more prevalent than eye lesions, with a ratio of 492 to 455. Although most of these patients were not using protective equipment, it is not clear why their eyes, which are normally more exposed, had fewer lesions than their skin. Other complications of dichlorodiethylsulfide gas are gastrointestinal,[4,12] psychological,[6,10] and hematologic.[13,14]

Skin lesions are reported as beginning 1 to 2 hours after exposure[9]; however, in our patients they appeared 8 to 24 hours after exposure. It may be that the gas used was diluted by the wind, or the duration of exposure was short. Thinner skin, such as the skin of the neck, axillae, and groin, is much more sensitive.[4] Our finding coincided with these reports, although we did not notice any palmoplantar lesions. It is that the absorbed agent disappears rapidly,[9] and the reported detection of intact sulfur mustard in tissues of casualties is difficult to accept.[15] However, 30 patients had late bullae formation over skin that previously appeared normal. Since all of our patients had been exposed to mustard gas for the first time, late bullae formation cannot be accounted for as hypersensitivity.[16] We think it might have developed due to the residue of gas in adipose tissues, or the lack of completely synchronous vesiccation might be attributable to the spread of the agent to new areas before the skin had been decontaminated.[4] Blister fluids are reported to be nontoxic.[6] We have noticed the same thing, as the fluids of ruptured bullae when in contact with healthy skin did not cause bullae formation.

As far as our treatments are concerned, we should mention that washing with 0.5% household bleach is the standard of treatment in many military systems.[17] However, in our patients we used pure water and, although it is reported to spread the toxin, we found out that heavy washing with pure water can be effective and satisfactory. We should add that all of our patients had been decontaminated in the war zone using pure water and that their clothes had been changed as well. Therefore, we emphasize that heavy washing is an effective means of decontamination.

Age had no important role in recovery. The only common factor involved was the severity of exposure. Unfortunately, nothing has been reported for other factors. Mortality rates have been reported to be 1% to 5%[17,18]; fortunately, in our patients there was no mortality. Sulfur mustard has been shown to be carcinogenic[19]; therefore, a much longer follow-up period is needed to study this effect.

References

1. Gliman A, Philops FS. The biological actions and therapeutic applications of the B-chloroethyl amines and sulfides. *Science.* 1946; 103:409-415.
2. Karnofsky DA, Graef I, Smith HW. Studies on the mechanism of nitrogen and sulfur mustards. *Am J Pathol.* 1984;24:275-292.
3. Atkinson WS. Delayed keratitis due to mustard gas. *Arch Ophthalmol.* 1948;38:291-301.
4. Sohrabpour H. Clinical manifestations of chemical agents on Iranian combatants. In: *First World Congress: New Compounds in Biological and Chemical Warfare: Toxicological Evaluation.* Ghent, Belgium, May 21-23, 1984.
5. Heyndrickx A, Heyndrickx B. Comparison of toxicological investigations in men in Southeast Asia, Afghanistan and Iran, concerning gas warfare. In: *First World Congress: New Compounds in Biological and Chemical Warfare: Toxicological Evaluation.* Ghent, Belgium, May 21-23, 1984.
6. Balali M. Clinical and laboratory finding in Iranian fighters with chemical gas poisonings. In: *First World Congress: New Compounds in Biological and Chemical Warfare: Toxicological Evaluation.* Ghent, Belgium, May 21-23, 1984.
7. Report of the United Nations Security Council, March 26th, 1984. New York, NY: United Nations Security Council publication SCOR 16433.
8. Mrozowsky B. Bacteriological determination of samples collected in gas warfare of Iran. In: *First World Congress: New Compounds in Biological and Chemical Warfare: Toxicological Evaluation.* Ghent, Belgium, May 21-23, 1984.
9. Smith JW, Dunn CMA. Medical defense against blistering chemical warfare agents. *Arch Dermatol.* 1991;127:1207-1213.
10. Colardyn F, Debersaques J. Clinical observation and therapy on injuries with vesicants. In: *First World Congress: New Compounds in Biological and Chemical Warfare: Toxicological Evaluation.* Ghent, Belgium, May 21-23, 1984.
11. Scholz RO, Woods AC. Relapsing and chronic ocular lesions following mustard gas burns. *Arch Pathol.* 1947;37:137-142.
12. Dhalliun F, Roels H. Autopsy observations in an Iranian soldier exposed to war gas. In: *First World Congress: New Compounds in Biological and Chemical Warfare: Toxicological Evaluation.* Ghent, Belgium, May 21-23, 1984.
13. Heyndrickx A, Van Steenberg EM. Methemoglobinemia in patients attacked by chemical and microbiological warfare agents. In: *First World Congress: New Compounds in Biological and Chemical Warfare: Toxicological Evaluation.* Ghent, Belgium, May 21-23, 1984.
14. Pauser G, Aloy A, Carvana M, Mutz N. Lethal intoxication by war gases on Iranian soldiers: therapeutic interventions on survivors of mustard gas and mycotoxin immersion. In: *First World Congress: New Compounds in Biological and Chemical Warfare: Toxicological Evaluation.* Ghent, Belgium, May 21-23, 1984.
15. Drasch G, Kretschmer E, Kauert G, Von Mayer L. Concentrations of mustard gas *bis*(2-chloroethyl) sulfide in the tissues of a victim of a vesicant exposure. *J Forensic Sci.* 1987;32:1788-1793.
16. More AM, Rockman JBA. Study of human hypersensitivity to compounds of the mustard gas type. *Can J Res.* 1950;28:169-176.
17. Heyndrickx A, Heyndrickx B. Treatment of Iranian soldiers attacked by chemical and microbiological war gases. In: *First World Congress: New Compounds in Biological and Chemical Warfare: Toxicological Evaluation.* Ghent, Belgium, May 21-23, 1984.
18. Willems, JL. Clinical management of mustard gas causalities. *Ann Med Milit Belg.* 1989;3(suppl):1-61.
19. Brookes P, Lawley PD. Effects of alkylating agent on T2 and T4 bacteriophages. *Biochem J.* 1963;89:138-144.

The Cutaneous Manifestations of Violence and Poverty

Janet A. Moy, MD, Miguel R. Sanchez, MD

• ***Background.***—**Violence is a public health issue that disproportionately affects the poor. Homelessness, drug abuse, and physical violence are seen with increasing frequency in poor communities. This article reviews the cutaneous manifestations of violence and the dermatologic problems commonly seen in the homeless. Particular emphasis is placed on the experience of municipal hospitals serving the urban poor.**

Observations.—**Dermatologic diseases are common in the homeless, and foot-related problems such as cellulitis and pyodermas are frequent causes of hospitalization. Unusual patterns of scarring and bruises in different stages of healing are seen in victims of physical violence. Trauma and sexually transmitted diseases result from sexual abuse. Serious skin infection and self-mutilating scarring are seen in intravenous drug abusers.**

Conclusions.—**Dermatologists are able to diagnose and treat the many skin problems seen in the poor and to identify the physical manifestations of abuse during routine skin examination. Findings of violence should be documented and reported to the appropriate investigational agencies.**

(*Arch Dermatol.* 1992;128:829-839)

Disease creates poverty and poverty disease, the vicious circle is closed.[1]

It is estimated that 25 to 30 million people live below the poverty level in the United States, and that another 25 to 30 million live marginally above the poverty level.[2] "The poor remain unhealthy as long as they remain poor,"[3] and, with few choices, depend on municipal hospitals for their medical care. These hospitals are facing problems that reflect the social dilemmas of our society. Issues such as drug abuse, homelessness, lack of universal access to health care, high health care costs, and acquired immunodeficiency syndrome (AIDS) disproportionally affect the poor. Violence permeates their lives, and increased levels of poverty lead to increased homicidal rates.[4] Thirty-eight percent of those patients admitted to a San Francisco (Calif) hospital for gunshots, stab wounds, or physical assault had incomes below the federal poverty level, and 56% were unemployed.[5]

In New York, NY, the care of the underclasses is largely provided by municipal hospitals of the Health and Hospitals Corporation, such as Bellevue Hospital Medical Center.

Bellevue hospital's expertise in treating trauma is renown. For this reason, it is the hospital of choice for policemen who are seriously injured, and, in such situations, police cars have been known to block the highways to transport a slain officer from outer boroughs.

Due to the large number of immigrants and persons who seek medical care late in their illnesses, the variety of diseases and range of clinical presentations is impressive. Providing health care to this population can be challenging. It is not enough to diagnose a disease and write prescriptions, but we have to intervene on their behalf with social service agencies, family members, and employers. In case after case, social problems have to be solved if the therapeutic plan is going to succeed.

Human immunodeficiency virus (HIV)–infected patients with severe skin problems, but without opportunistic infections, do not qualify for many benefits such as housing subsidies. Without a place to live, they are discharged to shelters where they are often assaulted when other residents learn of their HIV status.

Physicians have to understand the needs of the patient. A drug addict will try to manipulate the medical and nursing staff through a variety of clever and irritating drug-seeking behaviors. However, with good communication and clearly defined treatment goals and plans, the patient often accepts the medications identifed by his care providers as appropriate. A homeless person may press a health care provider for hospitalization when the severity of the skin disease may not seem to warrant inpatient care. Yet the patient's condition will worsen without hospitalization, because the patient will be unable to care for the disease while living in a shelter. Physicians become frustrated as patients whose skin conditions improve while hospitalized relapse within weeks of discharge.

Issues such as lack of compliance must be viewed as problems of both patients and caregivers. We have seen Hispanic and Chinese people incorrectly diagnosed, sometimes with tragic results, because they were unable to communicate their complaints. Patients

Accepted for publication March 4, 1992.

From the The Ronald O. Perelman Department of Dermatology, New York University (NY) Medical Center.

Reprint requests to The Ronald O. Perelman Department of Dermatology, New York University (NY) Medical Center, 550 First Ave, New York, NY 10016.

Table 1.—Racial Population at Bellevue Hospital Compared With the New York Metropolitan Area*

	Outpatients, %	Inpatients, %	New York, NY, %
Hispanic	45	36	15
African American	32	31	18
White	19	26	60
Asian	3	3	5
Other	1	2	2

*Adapted from the *National Data Book.*[7]

may take their medications incorrectly because they cannot read the directions on a medicine bottle.

Even when speaking the same language, communication is important. In the early years of the AIDS epidemic, we found that several men who had been counseled about safe sex continued to acquire sexually transmitted diseases (STDs). Some of these men had used condoms but, unable to read the instructions, had used them incorrectly and even washed and reused them.[6]

Health care providers may not understand the cultural significance of illness in foreign patients. For example, counseling Chinese patients with tuberculosis or Hansen's disease is essential. We have to guarantee them privacy since these diseases are stigmatized in their communities.

The hospital's designated catchment area is the lower half of Manhattan County, New York, but 40% of the hospital's patients come from the outer boroughs of New York and 4% come from upstate New York or adjacent states.

The lack of access to specialized health care for the poor and uninsured creates a critical demand for services such as dermatology in these facilities. With over 20 000 outpatient visits per year, the dermatology clinics, which include general dermatology, dermatologic surgery, pediatric dermatology, STDs, phototherapy, and special cutaneous diseases, are the busiest clinics next only to medicine, pediatrics, and obstetrics and gynecology.

In our hospital, 40% of dermatology clinic visits are funded by state programs (Medicaid), 20% by federal programs (Medicare), and 35% by "self-payers," the patients themselves. Self-payers include people who are marginally poor yet earn too much money to qualify for Medicaid benefits and those whose employers are unable to provide health care benefits. A graduated payment scale enables uninsured patients to be evaluated by a dermatologist, undergo diagnostic procedures, and receive medications for total fees that range from $14 to $130.

Minorities constitute a higher percentage of patients in the dermatology service compared with the population in the New York metropolitan area (Table 1).[7]

The inpatient dermatology service includes a 16-bed ward and a consultation service for the 1200-bed hospital. In contrast with the nationwide statistics for hospitalized patients, the majority of inpatients in our hospital are young. Fifty-six percent of inpatients on the medical service are between the ages of 18 and 44 years, and only 14% are 65 years or older.

Municipal hospitals have had disproportionately higher numbers of AIDS cases, as HIV infection has spread among uninsured homosexuals and intravenous drug abusers (IVDAs).

At any given time, approximately 15% of dermatology inpatients at our hospital are HIV infected and, in some medical wards, up to 60% of hospitalized patients suffer from AIDS. From 1987 through 1991, the average daily number of AIDS cases in New York has doubled to 2200 patients per day. Common reasons for admission include STDs, tuberculosis, measles, drug abuse–related illnesses, and HIV-associated infections.

The hospital maintains a 50-bed forensic psychiatry unit and a 40-bed inpatient ward for prisoners from New York corrections facilities such as Riker's Island prison and the Manhattan House of Detention. Prisoners are also seen in the outpatient clinics and constitute 7% of some medical clinic visits. In 1987, approximately 20% of all New York inmates and 44% of IVDAs were HIV seropositive.[8] We are sometimes asked to treat prisoners involved in highly publicized cases. We recently evaluated penile erosions in an HIV-seropositive prisoner arrested for sodomizing a school-aged child. The lesions were due to herpes simplex, placing the child at risk not only for HIV infection but also for anal herpes simplex. When dealing with emotionally charged cases such as this, it is essential that we put aside our personal feelings.

Homelessness

The term *homeless* refers to persons who lack "customary or regular access to a conventional dwelling or residence."[2] Based on psychologic and sociologic criteria, they can be divided into four groups: the chronically mentally ill, the undomiciled due to eviction or unemployment, the "skid row" alcoholic, and long-term "street people."[9]

Estimates of the numbers of homeless in the United States range from 250 000 to 3 million. New York has approximately 80 000 undomiciled individuals and has sheltered up to 4000 families.[10] In some US communities, families with children represent more than a third of the homeless population.[11]

Homelessness is bad for health.[12] When compared with indigent, but housed, counterparts, homeless men had significantly higher rates of hospitalization for psychiatric problems, twice the rate of hospitalization for physical problems, and a higher incidence of trauma.[9] In studies of homeless children, half had developmental delays, learning disabilities, anxiety or depressive disorders, and a variety of acute and chronic health problems for which they are more frequently hospitalized.[13]

Dermatologic disease is the most common health problem found in the homeless. Studies have found that the number of clinic visits and hospitalizations related to skin disease is substantially higher in the homeless than in poor undomiciled counterparts.[14] Also, with limited access to health care and a high prevalence of untreated psychiatric illness, homeless patients tend to

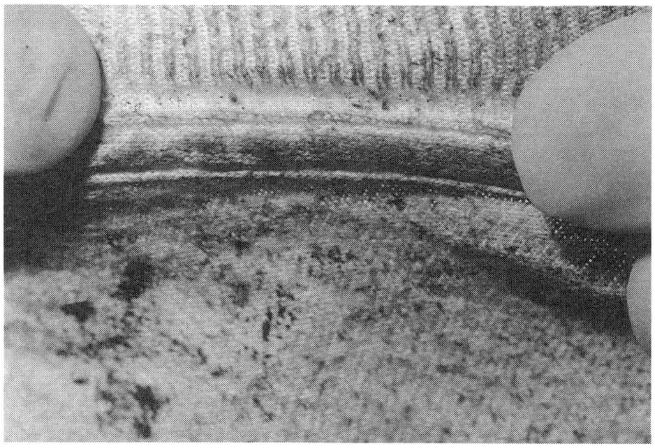

Fig 1.—Infestation with pediculosis corporis (var corporis) disproportionally affects the homeless. Body lice can be identified on clothing.

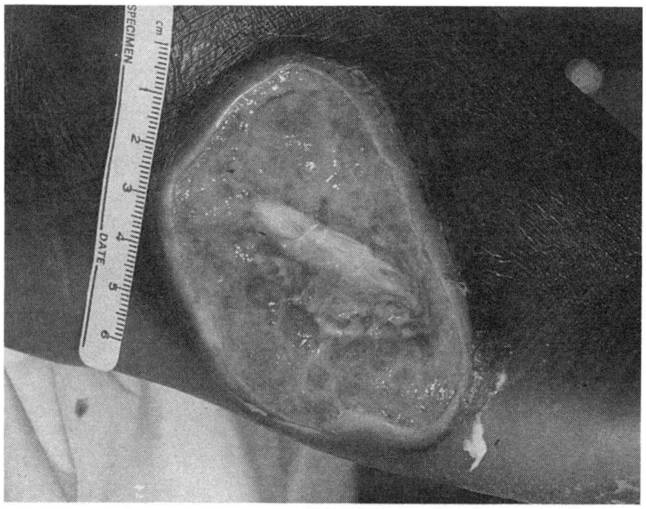

Fig 2.—Ulceration of the foot with exposed tendon from ill-fitting shoes in an undomiciled person.

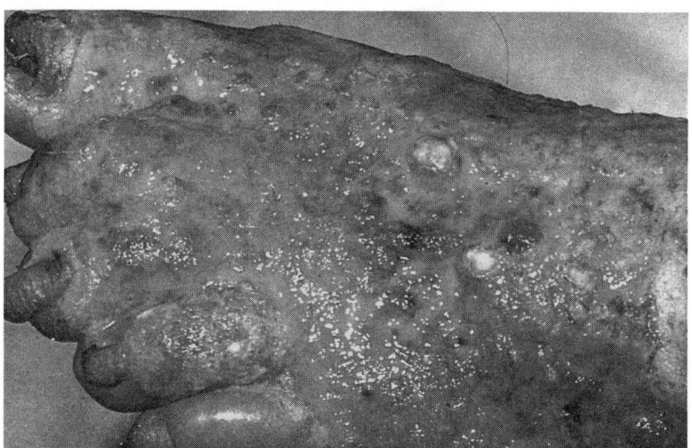

Fig 3.—Extensive ulceration of the foot overlying chronic osteomyelitis in an undomiciled person.

neglect their skin until cutaneous problems become serious and disabling.[15]

A survey of admissions to our inpatient dermatology ward over a 3-month period showed that 46% of patients admitted were homeless, either living on the street or in shelters, and 48% were admitted for cellulitis or other skin infections. Conversely, 81% of all patients admitted for cellulitis or other pyodermas were homeless.

Other frequently observed skin diseases in the homeless include impetigo, tinea infections, warts, leg ulcers, immersion foot, frostbite, erythromelalgia, scabies, pediculosis, seborrheic dermatitis, acne rosacea, eczematoid eruptions, xerosis, and pruritus (Fig 1).

Foot problems, a major source of morbidity in the homeless, are caused by cold injury, repeated trauma, prolonged standing, water exposure, and, as a result of alcohol and drug use, altered mental status and sensation.[16] Foot-related skin diseases, which include lymphedema, venous stasis disease, and tinea pedis infection, are predisposing factors for cellulitis, skin ulcers, gangrene, chronic nonhealing wounds, osteomyelitis, and squamous cell carcinoma (Fig 2). Recently, a 70-year-old undomiciled man was brought to the emergency department by a social worker because of leg pain. Physical examination showed a malodorous extensive skin ulcer extending into the fascia (Fig 3). The ulcer had been present for over 10 years, and the patient had refused all medical and social service interventions in the past. The patient was admitted and ultimately required amputation for nonhealing osteomyelitis.

Shelter dwellers tend to hide their skin problems due to fear of ridicule or ostracism by other residents, who mistake the rash for a contagious disease. Those who do manage to receive medical attention may have no place to clean their skin, apply medicines, or take prescribed drugs on a regular schedule. Frequently, homeless psoriatic patients require admission for exfoliative erythroderma or evaluation for septicemia that could have been prevented with routine topical therapy.

Although increasing pressure is being placed on the hospital to discharge patients as quickly as possible, it is difficult to discharge homeless patients because they have no suitable place to go. Commonly, patients refuse shelter placement, where they may not feel safe, and prefer to return to the streets. Shelters have a relatively large proportion of violent residents who have been classified as sociopathic, antisocial, or typical batterers.[17]

Once discharged from the hospital, the homeless are inadequately prepared to recuperate and are likely to deteriorate.[18] In one study, only a third of the patients attending a mission clinic had Medicaid insurance that enabled them to pay for outpatient care and medications, and only 4% were enrolled in Medicare.[9] Most homeless persons rely on emergency departments for health care, and many require rehospitalization. In our service, 17% of hospitalized patients had been admitted within the past year for treatment of the same problem.

When homeless persons acquire communicable diseases such as measles, varicella-zoster infection, or tu-

Table 2.—Comparison of Inpatient Drug and Alcohol Use at a Municipal and Neighboring Voluntary Hospital*

	Bellevue, %	Voluntary, %	Nationwide, %
Drug	30	. . .	2
Alcohol	20	. . .	8
Drug and/or alcohol	50	20	10

*Robert Maslansky, MD, oral communication, November 21, 1991. Bellevue indicates Bellevue Hospital Medical Center, New York, NY.

berculosis, hospitalization is required because they pose a public health problem. Tuberculosis is spreading rapidly among the homeless, prisoners, HIV-infected persons, and the poor. In a New York shelter-based clinic, 6% of patients had active tuberculosis and 27% had a positive tuberculin skin test result.[19]

Drug Abuse

Over the last 5 years, rates of drug abuse in the general population, particularly among casual users and the young, have decreased. However, there has been an increase in the numbers of heavy users of cocaine or alcohol.[20] The poor may be inclined to use drugs to alleviate the stresses and frustrations of economic adversity by maintaining a state of pleasure.[21] No accurate data are available on IVDAs, but it is estimated that there are between 1 and 1.5 million IVDAs in the United States. The number of deaths reported to the Drug Abuse Warning Network, commonly known as DAWN, from cocaine use tripled from 1984 through 1988, and the majority of drug related deaths reported in 1988 were due to cocaine (49%) and heroin (37%).[22]

The effects of drug abuse on families is devastating. Annually, over 300 000 infants are born to mothers who use "crack" cocaine, and 10 000 infants are born to chronic opiate users. Up to 10 million children in this country are raised by addicted parents,[23] and female drug users are more inclined to mistreat their children.

Compounding the drug abuse problem is the rising rate of HIV infection among IVDAs, their sexual partners, and offspring. Over 300 000 IVDAs nationwide may be infected with HIV. The New York State Department of Substance Abuse Services, Albany, has estimated that 8% of HIV seronegative IVDAs become infected each year.[24] The mortality due to infectious diseases in drug users deaths dramatically increased in New York from 1981 to 1986, which suggests that the addicts were also HIV infected.[25] When HIV-associated mortality was adjusted to accommodate these statistics, over 50% of AIDS-related deaths were associated with intravenous drug use.[24]

Astonishingly high rates of alcohol and nonmedical drug use can be found in the population served by city hospitals (Table 2).

Drug abuse is associated with a variety of criminal activities. In a recent US Justice Department study, between 54% and 80% of arrested men and women had evidence of illicit drug use by urine toxicology screening.[26] The violent environments associated with drug dealing, drug possession, robbery, and prostitution result in trauma, including gunshot injuries, knife

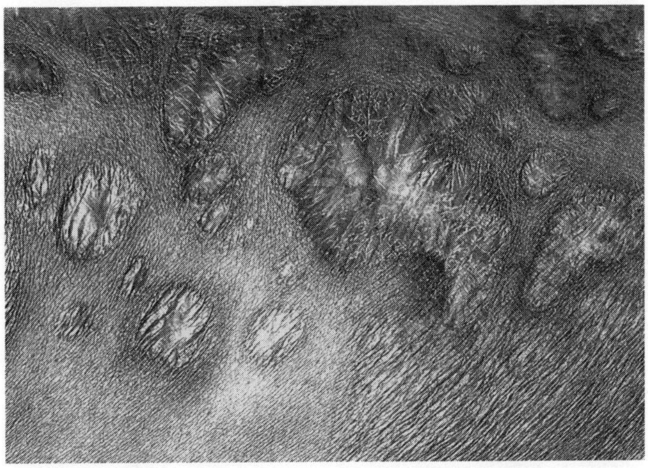

Fig 4.—"Punched-out," atrophic scars as a result of "skin popping" cocaine.

wounds, and beatings. Also, certain drugs, such as cocaine, predispose to heightened suspiciousness and violent behavior.

While personality and behavior changes are valuable indicators of drug abuse, skin signs can alert the clinician to nonmedical drug use. Burns, bullae, frostbite, and gangrene due to prolonged immobility and decreased sensation result from intoxication with drugs and alcohol. The most common precipitating factor in burn cases from one rehabilitation unit study was the use of alcohol and drugs.[27]

Specific skin findings of drug abuse depend on the route of drug administration.[28,29] Scarring, "track marks," or linear pigmentation along veins, bruising, and cellulitis are commonly seen with intravenous injection. Circular, atrophic, punched-out lesions result from "skin popping" or subcutaneous drug injection (Fig 4). Foreign-body granulomas form by the injection of various adulterants such as talc and sugar and from particulate material such as plastic or glass that is inadvertently injected. Tattoos may be placed to camouflage scars or may result from the deposition of carbon and other materials during drug injection.

Serious infection is the most common skin manifestation of drug abuse. Abscesses, cellulitis, and gangrene are the result of reusing needles and syringes and poor hygiene. Intra-arterial injection can cause a syndrome of vasospasm and widespread skin necrosis that results in limb amputation.[30]

The use of cocaine and the development of its inexpensive, freebase form, "crack," has devastated low-income communities. This drug is a stimulant, producing alertness and well-being in low doses and euphoria in high doses. Cocaine is highly addictive, and repeated use increases craving for the drug. When given free access to cocaine, monkeys will self administer the drug until they die of starvation, skin infection, or cardiovascular collapse.[31]

There are a number of skin findings associated with cocaine use. Nasal mucosa erythema and even nasal septum perforation can develop when the drug is inhaled. Madarosis, the loss of the eyebrows and eye-

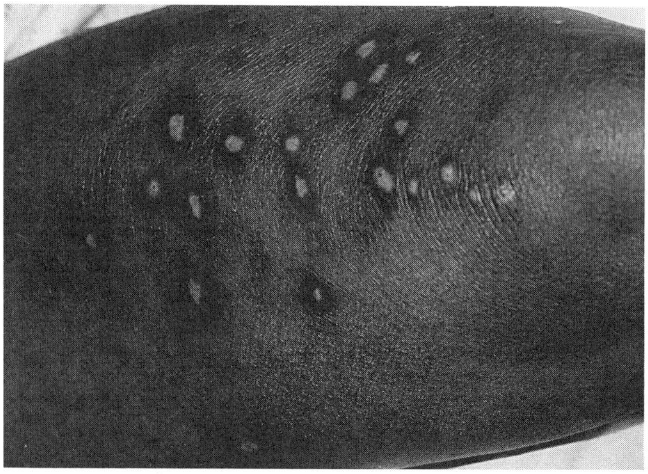

Fig 5.—Hypopigmented and hyperpigmented scars on the thigh representing self-induced excoriations in a cocaine addict.

lashes from hot vapors, has been reported with "freebasing," the smoking of cocaine.[32] Skin and muscle infarction has been seen as a result of vasoconstriction.[33] Widespread excoriations occur from delusional formication and other cocaine-induced behavioral abnormalities, such as self-mutilation and stereotypical repetitious skin picking (Fig 5).[31]

Cocaine users often report heightened sexual interest but delayed orgasm.[34] It has been suggested that this sexual dysfunction and the selling of sex for money to buy crack have been the reasons for the current syphilis epidemic.[35] In New York, the number of primary and secondary syphilis cases has more than doubled from 6465 in 1986 to 13 748 cases in 1989. Even more alarming, the reports of congenital syphilis have also risen from 33 cases in 1986 to 1017 in 1989 and continue to climb.[35,36]

The drug of choice among intravenous drug users remains heroin or diacetyl morphine. This opiate, illegal in the United States, produces central nervous system analgesia, drowsiness, and euphoria. The skin manifestations of heroin include "pseudo" acanthosis nigricans, cheilitis, thrombophlebitis, and vasculitis.[37] Cases of fixed drug eruptions and systemic amyloidosis have been reported.[38,39] Thrombosis and tissue necrosis from concentrated diluents and adulterants such as quinine have been reported.[40]

Child Abuse

During 1986, the most recent year for which figures are available, 360 000 cases of child abuse were reported in this country, with 1100 deaths and 6000 incidents of brain damage.[23] Since many cases are not identified or reported, the actual incidence could be 15 to 20 times higher.[23]

The strongest predictor of physical or sexual abuse against children in a community is the number of families with incomes significantly below the poverty level.[41] A study in a small-sized community found that one of every 130 children was treated each year for an intentional injury involving fights, rape, or child battery.[42] The rate of intentional injury is directly correlated with poverty and urbanization. Among the poor, child abuse has been reported at a rate of two to three cases per 1000 children. In homeless children, the prevalence is even higher, with a rate of 8.8 cases per 1000 children.

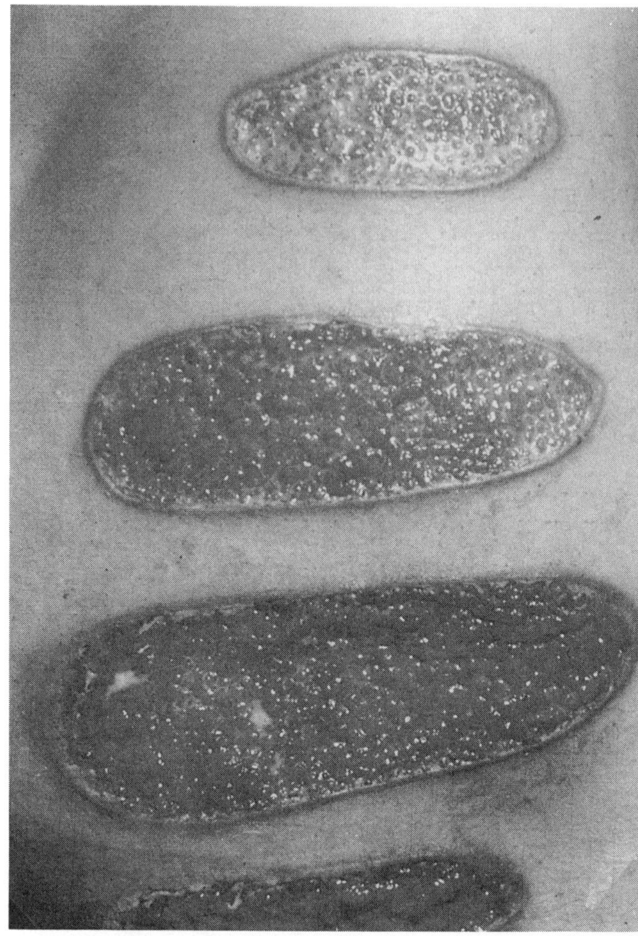

Fig 6.—Unexplained lesions with geometric patterns such as these thermal burns should be evaluated for abuse.

Factors that predispose to child abuse include psychologic instability of the parents, acute and chronic life stresses, social factors such as unemployment and substance abuse, behavioral and medical problems in the child, and a lack of family support systems. The abuser is often a parent or a person well known to the child, such as the mother's fiancee, babysitter, or stepfather.[43] Abused children tend to acquire deviant patterns of processing social information, which leads to the development of aggressive behavior,[44] and a cycle of abusive behavior is perpetuated. Poor single mothers are more likely to inflict physical punishment on their children. In one study, 89% of homeless or housed poor mothers had experienced either sexual or physical abuse.[45]

Child abuse, an emotional issue, requires the involvement of experienced health professionals. Dermatologists must be able to recognize the unmistakable stigmata of physical violence and report these findings to the appropriate investigational agency, or, at least, to the child's pediatrician.[46] Skin findings can be found in

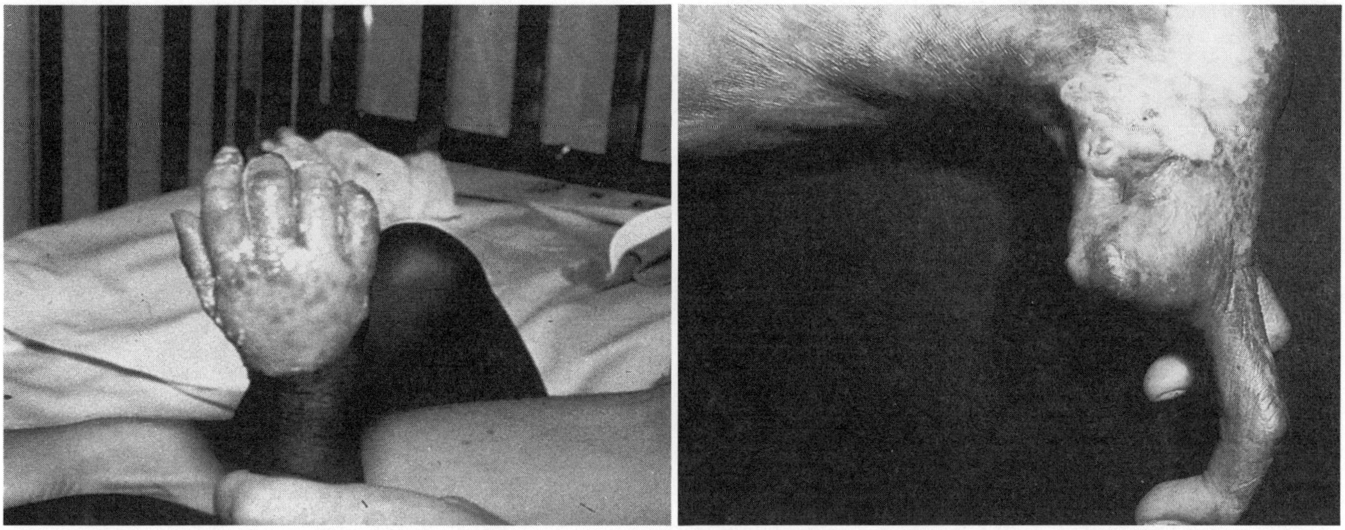

Fig 7.—Left, Sharply demarcated third-degree burn in a child caused by emersion of the hand into hot liquid. Right, The consequences of such trauma may be death or permanent physical deformity.

the vast majority of abused children. Injuries can occur in any child; however, multiple injuries over many body sites in different stages of healing should alert the physician. Unusual patterns and increased numbers of scars, keloids, and suspicious pigmentary changes must be investigated and well documented, preferably with photographs (Fig 6).

Injuries usually follow the caretaker's uncontrolled reaction to the child's unwanted behavior. They may be inflicted with a number of objects, including belts, paddles and boards, switches, and sticks or cords. The child may be slapped, choked, pinched or grabbed, punched, burned, or, less often, dropped, pushed, shaken, propelled, bitten, or kicked. The results include ecchymoses, lacerations, abrasions, or scratches and other signs of trauma that can appear alone or with fractures and rupture of viscera.[43]

Close observation of the skin can provide clues as to how the violence was inflicted. For instance, a small rectangular or square mark with a clear center can be made with a belt buckle, while a larger rectangle develops from a whack with a spatula or fly swatter. Symmetrical bruises occurring over areas of soft tissue rather than bony prominences may be marks caused by pressure from the thumb and forefinger while grabbing. Looplike bruises are often produced by striking with a rope or cord.

Intentional burns can be inflicted with an assortment of appliances including hot plates, irons, stoves, radiators, boiling liquids, electromagnetic batteries,[47] cigarettes, matches,[48] and even hair dryers[49] or microwave ovens.[50] Deliberate immersion into hot water more commonly involves the feet in a specific bootlike distribution not seen when a toddler accidentally falls into a hot bathtub.[23] (Fig 7).

An abused child is not necessarily neglected and may appear well groomed and well nourished. Neglected toddlers tend to have a disheveled appearance and can be malnourished.[46] Repeated episodes of infestation with scabies or lice, bites from rats or dogs, and injuries from accidental trauma such as burns and frostbite can be observed.

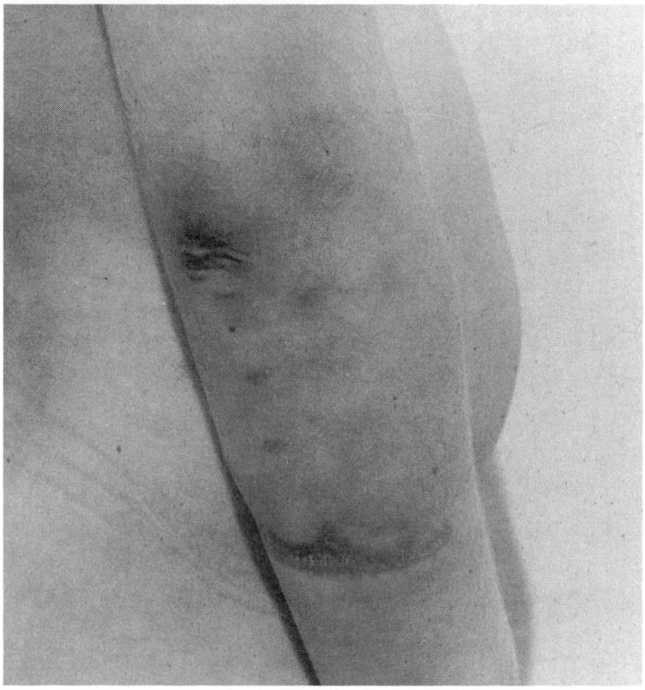

Fig 8.—Broad scars and ecchymosis in Ehlers-Danlos syndrome can simulate the signs of child abuse.

Once child abuse is suspected, the investigation must be thorough and thoughtful. It should be remembered that dermatologic diseases such as the Ehlers-Danlos syndrome,[51] bullous diseases, and staphylococcal scalded skin syndrome have been misdiagnosed as symptoms of child abuse.[52] For example, a social worker brought an 8-year-old Vietnamese girl to our pediatric clinic for evaluation of possible child abuse. Despite the resolute denial by parents and child that physical abuse had occurred, proceedings to move the child to a foster care home had been initiated. Physical examination revealed broad linear atrophic scars and bruises (Fig 8) in addition to hypermotility of hand joints. A skin biopsy specimen showed thin collagen fibers consistent with the diagnosis of Ehlers-Danlos syndrome.

Cultural practices must also be considered. The folk remedy *cupping* consists of extinguishing a lit candle under a cup on the skin, leaving circular patches of petechiae. The Southeast Asian practice of *cia gao*, which consists of vigorously rubbing a coin on the oiled skin of a sick child, results in skin markings which resemble flogging.[53]

Sexual abuse in children will be discussed below.

Spouse Abuse

Once considered rare, domestic violence is now identified as a national phenomenon arising from multiple social, cultural, and psychologic factors. The estimated incidence ranges from 1.5 million cases per year to half of all wed or unwed relationships.[54] In a study of 492 male and female patients attending a general hospital emergency department, 22% identified themselves as victims of domestic violence.[54] Of these, 62% were women, and 38% were men. Violent behavior may start when a wife becomes pregnant. In a study of 501 pregnant women attending a public prenatal clinic, 20% reported episodes of physical abuse during their marriage and, of these, 29% said that the abuse occurred during pregnancy.[55] White non-Hispanic women admit to abuse more frequently than their African-American or Hispanic counterparts.[55] Women are more likely to be the victims of domestic violence if they are poor and unmarried.[56]

Violent behavior includes being threatened with murder, being hit or punched, kicked, struck by an object, whipped, or stabbed. These victims suffer serious emotional trauma, and evidence of repeated skin and soft-tissue injuries, such as ecchymoses, hematomas, lacerations, abrasions, and burns, is common.[57,58] In a 5-year retrospective study, 20% of burn patients were victims of assault. The assailant was known to the victim in two thirds of cases and was usually a wife or girlfriend. Ten percent of burns were inflicted with chemicals such as lye, hot water, hot soup, or grease and often resulted in severe facial disfigurement. Another 16% were doused with gasoline and ignited.[27]

Recently, we saw a 48-year-old Hispanic woman who sought our help for a nonhealing, enlarging, aphthous ulcer of the tongue. Disfiguring burn scars on her face and neck from lye had been inflicted by her husband. There was a long history of physical abuse, and subsequent medical evaluation revealed that he had also infected her with HIV.

Dermatologists may identify spouse abuse during routine physical examination. A battered woman characteristically seeks medical care more often than her nonabused counterpart. Her complaints are often psychosomatic or unrelated to sustained injuries.[58] With adequate detection and screening methods for spouse abuse, the identification of battered women increased from 6% to 30% of female trauma cases in one emergency department study.[59]

Sexual Abuse

Sexual assault, defined as being pressured or forced to have sexual contact, is a violent crime. In one study of 491 rape victims, 82% had general traumatic injuries while only 39% sustained genital injury.[60] The lifetime prevalence of sexual assault in adults was 10% in a study of more than 3000 people.[61] In young white women with some college education, the prevalence was even higher, at 26%.[61] Rape statistics, however, are inaccurate, and it is estimated that 80% to 90% are never reported.[62]

The physical signs of sexual abuse include ecchymoses, hematomas, skin and soft-tissue trauma, and STDs. Traumatic injuries such as lacerations and abrasions may be confused with STDs.

Sexual assault also occurs in men. Mucosal injuries as a result of penetrating anal intercourse have been described in most male victims.[63] Most rapists are acquainted with, but not related to, their victims. Instances of threats of HIV transmission by attackers have also been reported.[63]

In our STD clinic, a man was referred to us with painful, infected anal fissures as a result of sexual assault. He had seen several proctologists and infectious disease specialists who had treated him for herpes, syphilis, gonorrhea, and chancroid despite a negative evaluation. The fissures healed with treatment, which included appropriate antibiotics, analgesics, stool softeners, and topical gentian violet.

The National Center on Child Abuse and Neglect, Washington, DC, estimates that 100 000 cases of abuse occur each year, with only 20% to 50% of incidents ever reported.[64] Most assaults occur around 10 years of age. Physical signs of sexual abuse in children are not usually obvious. The presence of genital or anal tags, ecchymoses, edema, erythema, lacerations, abrasions, fissures, and petechiae should be reported.[65] Genital ulcers must be evaluated for syphilis, herpes, and chancroid, and cases of condyloma must be thoroughly investigated.[66] The dermatologist's expertise enables the differentiation of child abuse from lichen sclerosus, vitiligo, bullous disease, and nonvenereal infections.[52]

Young prostitutes are often victims of sexual and/or physical abuse as children.[67] Prostitution, whether organized or entrepreneurial, is associated with a high incidence of HIV infection, alcoholism, drug addiction, police arrests, physical violence, and STDs.[68]

In our STD clinic, we were recently puzzled by a high rate of gonorrhea relapses until we learned that one of our female patients with psoriasis was using a hospital bathroom to supplement her income through prostitution while waiting for her phototherapy treatment.

Prostitutes are particularly vulnerable to physical violence. A prostitute diagnosed with secondary syphilis still managed to support her common law husband and 2-year-old child despite being 8 months pregnant. With considerable effort, she was persuaded to discontinue prostitution but returned to the clinic with numerous abrasions and ecchymoses. She had been forced to return to prostitution by her husband after beatings and homicidal threats. After counseling, she was able to flee from him.

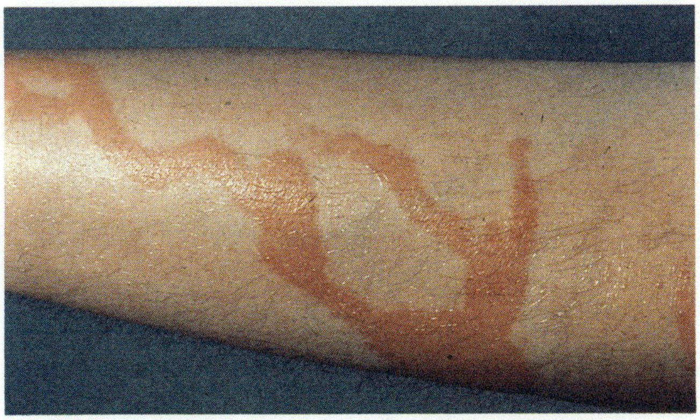

Fig 9.—Chemical burns have streak patterns such as this burn from phenol.

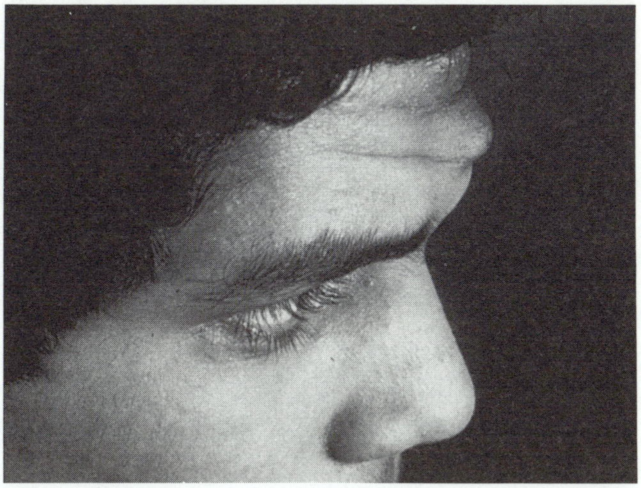

Fig 10.—Hamartomas developed in a patient secondary to head-banging.

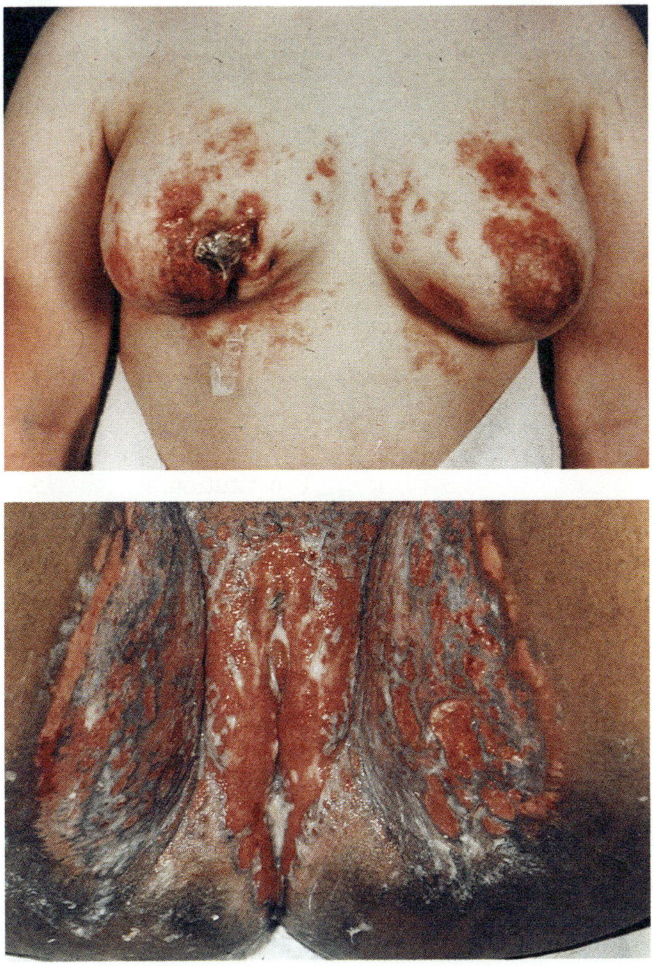

Fig 11.—Disfiguring injuries of the breasts (top) and external genitals (bottom) in two patients as a result of self-mutilation.

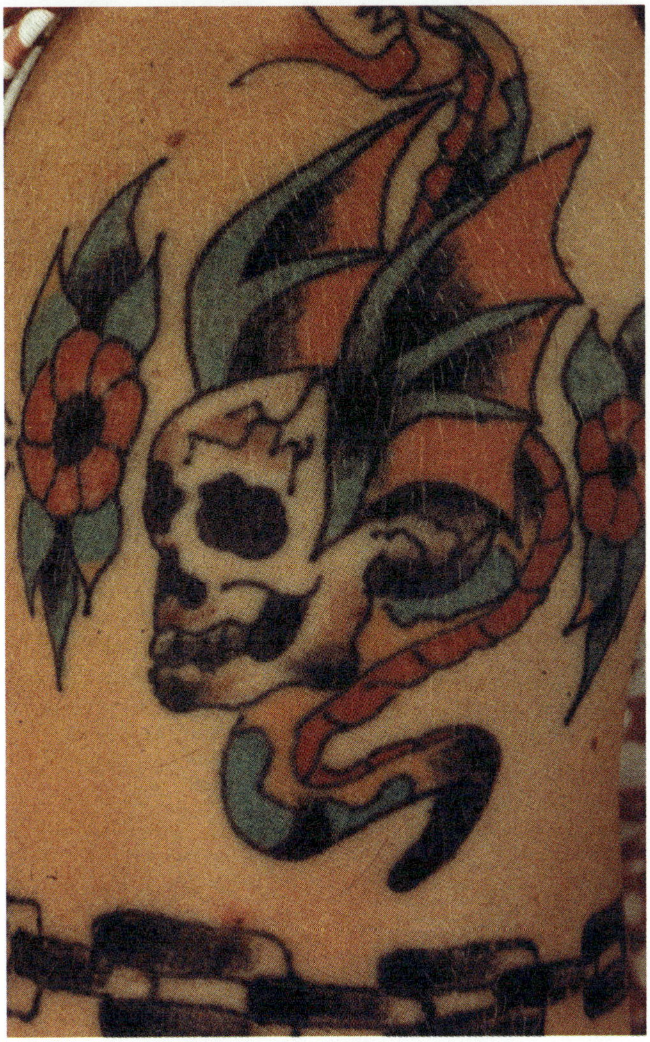

Fig 12.—Tattoos, sometimes sinister and bizarre, may be a means of group identification among prisoners.

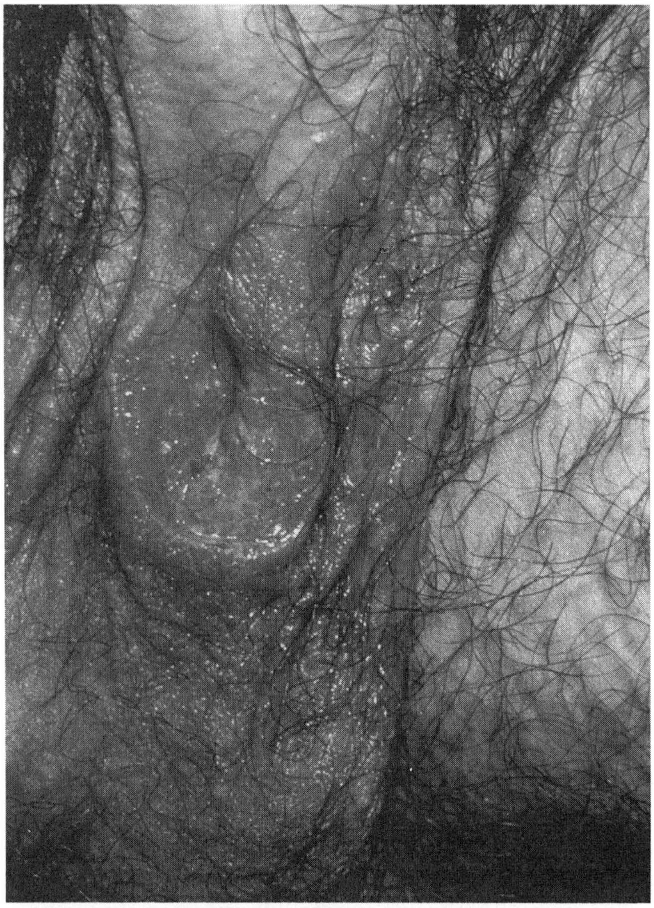

Fig 13.—A 32-year-old man with erythema ab igne and unusual ulcers at the base of his penis admitted after a negative medical evaluation to sadomasochistic practices that included drenching with boiling water.

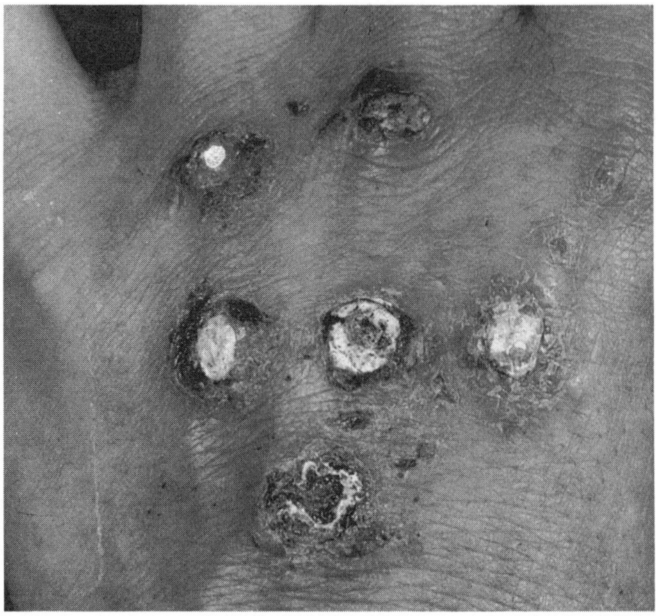

Fig 14.—Multiple intentional cigarette burns on the dorsal aspect of the hand.

Elder Abuse

Approximately 13% of the US population is now over 65 years of age, and it is estimated that by the year 2020 this number will rise to 17%.[69] Skin diseases are common in the geriatric population. Some problems that disproportionately affect the elderly poor are skin ulcers, cellulitis, fungal infections, pyodermas, nutritional deficiencies, xeroses, eczemas, and large or metastatic basal and squamous cell carcinomas.

The leading cause of morbidity and mortality among elderly Americans, however, is injury.[70] Every year in this country, between 500 000 and 1.4 million elderly persons become victims of neglect, physical abuse, verbal intimidation, exploitation, or abandonment by a caretaker.[71] In a recent study, 5% of an inner city, geriatric population required emergency department treatment or died of injury over a 1-year period. The rate of injuries was 48 per 1000 persons and, of these, 54% resulted from falls, 13% from motor vehicle accidents, and 7% from intentional violence.[71]

Identification of elderly people who are at high risk for serious injury is essential. Mistreatment is usually inflicted on a characteristically dependent and infirmed elderly person. The victim of elder abuse is often socially isolated, having lost most friends and relatives.[72] Senility and/or physical handicaps create dependency and burden on the caretaker. Studies, however, emphasize that the preponderance of personality disorders is found in the abuser.[73] The perpetrator is often a relative or aide who, facing situational and financial stresses, is increasingly dependent on the elder and more prone to abuse alcohol and drugs.

The signs of neglect, physical violence, and sexual abuse in the elderly are similar to those described in the sections on child abuse and sexual abuse above. Geometrically shaped bruises, burns, poor hygiene, urine burns, neglected decubiti, freeze injuries, and unexplained malnutrition, especially when recurrent, should raise suspicion (Fig 9).

Once elder abuse is identified, the dermatologist should discuss the problem with the patient's primary care physician and social worker and contact the appropriate investigational agency.

Self-Injury

Self-injurious behavior may be observed in some mentally handicapped or autistic persons, drug addicts, prisoners, patients with certain metabolic disorders, and psychotic or emotionally dysfunctional individuals.[74]

Self-injury associated with mental retardation is repetitive and stereotypic.[74] Destructive lip and finger biting is found in patients with Lesch-Nyhan syndrome, and repetitive skin picking and self-slugging can be a component of the Brachman-de Lange syndrome. Behaviors such as head-banging may be due to frontal lobe seizures in the mentally retarded.[75] (Fig 10). Self-mutilating behavior associated with psychoses tends to be sporadic.[74] Genital mutilation is almost always related to psychosis[74] in men but less frequently in women.[76]

Nonpsychotic people with normal intelligence who

produce factitial wounds usually have abnormal impulse control or borderline personality disorders. Self-mutilation may temporarily relieve the symptoms of racing thoughts, depersonalization, or marked anxiety in these patients[77] or may be an appeal for help.[78] The cause may be related to dysfunction of the serotonergic, dopaminergic, or opiate neurotransmitter pathways.[74]

The skin manifestations of self-injury include neurotic excoriations, trichotillomania, disfiguring tattoos, skin ulcers with geometric or bizarre patterns, burns, edematous purpuric plaques (Secretan's syndrome or l'oedema bleu), and panniculitis due to the injection of milk, feces, saliva, contaminated materials, and drugs[79] (Fig 11).

Prisoners and drug addicts carve or tattoo words and symbolic figures as means of group identification (Fig 12).[74] Self-mutilation can be a way to leave prison for a more comfortable infirmary.

Ornamental mutilation as practiced in certain cultures (African tribes) and social groups (punkers) or sadomasochistic sexual practices such as the piercing of nipples and genitals for sexual gratification should be distinguished from factitial dermatitis (Fig 13). These behaviors do not usually result in injury requiring medical treatment unless one of the participants has a serious psychiatric disorder. However, infected wounds, lacerations, handcuff chafes, puncture wounds, and cigarette burns can occur.

Self-inflicted thermal burns are rare and almost always associated with severe depression and chronic paranoid schizophrenia (Fig 14).[80] Fewer than half of patients who require hospitalization actually intend to kill themselves.

The behavioral and psychotherapeutic treatment of self-injurious behavior may be enhanced by the use of psycho-pharmacologic agents such as serotonin reuptake inhibitors and opiate and dopaminergic antagonists.[74,81]

COMMENT

Dermatologists must be aware of the many difficulties faced by the poor. These problems include homelessness, drug abuse, and injuries from violent behavior. The physician's task is challenging, yet we can deliver better medical care to the poor through an understanding of their psychosocial problems and economic frustrations. Dermatologists can be sensitive to these issues and can educate their staff and communities about the severity of these problems. Active participation in government is essential, since homelessness, drugs, and crime are also national health problems. Finally, dermatologists are in a unique position to identify manifestations of physical violence during routine skin examination. We may be called on to be advocates for patients, especially in cases of physical abuse and need to document our clinical findings and report them to the appropriate investigational agencies.

References

1. Siegerest HE. *Civilization and Disease.* Chicago, Ill: University of Chicago Press; 1962:241.
2. Rossi PH, Wright JD, Fisher, GA, Willis G. The urban homeless: estimating composition and size. *Science.* 1987;235:1336-1341.
3. Smith T. Poverty and health in the 90s. *BMJ.* 1990;301:349-350.
4. McDowall D. Poverty and homicide in Detroit, 1926-1978. *Violence Vict.* 1986;1:23-34.
5. Sumner BB, Mintz ER, Brown PL. Injuries caused by personal violence. *Injury.* 1987;1:258-260.
6. Marmor M, Krisenski K, Sanchez M, et al. Sex, drugs and HIV infection in New York City hospital outpatient population. *J Acq Immune Defec Syndr.* 1990;3:307-318.
7. Statistical abstract of the United States, year 1991. In: *The National Data Book.* 111th ed. Washington, DC: US Dept of Commerce, Economics and Statistics Administration, Bureau of the Census; 1991:27-34.
8. Smith P, Mikel J, Truman BI. HIV infection among women entering the New York State Correctional System. *Am J Public Health.* 1991;81:35.
9. Fischer PJ, Shapiro S, Breakey WR, Anthony JC, Kramer M. Mental health and social characteristics of the homeless: a survey of mission users. *Am J Public Health.* 1986;76:519-524.
10. Bassuk EL, Rubin L, Lauriat AS. Characteristics of sheltered homeless families. *Am J Public Health.* 1986;76:1097-1101.
11. American Academy of Pediatrics Committee on Child Abuse and Neglect. American Academy of Pediatrics guidelines for the evaluation of sexual abuse of children. *Pediatrics.* 1991;82:254-260.
12. Lowry S. Housing and health: health and homelessness. *BMJ.* 1990;300:32-34.
13. Wood DL, Burciaga Valdez R, Hayashi T, Shen A. Health of homeless children and housed, poor children. *Pediatrics.* 1990;86: 858-866.
14. Gelberg L, Linn LS, Usatine RP, Smith MH. Health, homelessness, and poverty: a study of clinic users. *Arch Intern Med.* 1990; 150:2325-2330.
15. Robertson MJ, Cousineau MR. Health status and access to health services among the urban homeless. *Am J Public Health.* 1986;76:561-563.
16. Wrenn K. Foot problems in homeless persons. *Ann Intern Med.* 1990;113:567-568.
17. Gondolf EW. Who are those guys? toward a behavioral typology of batterers. *Violence Vict.* 1988;3:187-203.
18. Tyler A. Hospitals spurn homeless. *Time Out.* 1985;5:12-15.
19. McAdam JM, Brickner PW, Scharer LL, Crocco JA, Duff AE. The spectrum of tuberculosis in a New York City men's shelter clinic (1982-1988). *Chest.* 1990;97:798-805.
20. The Third Triennial Report to Congress from the Secretary, Department of Health and Human Services. In: *Drug Abuse and Drug Abuse Research.* Rockville, Md: National Institute on Drug Abuse; 1991;13-31.
21. Serban G. Social stress and drug abuse. In: Serban G, ed. *Social and Medical Aspects of Drug Abuse.* New York, NY: SP Medical and Scientific Books; 1984:125-133.
22. National Institute on Drug Abuse. *Data From the Drug Abuse Warning Network (DAWN): Annual Data 1988, Statistical Series, Report I:8.* Washington, DC: US Dept of Health and Human Services; 1989. Publication ADM 89-1634.
23. Bays J. Substance abuse and child abuse: impact of addiction on the child. *Pediatr Clin North Am.* 1990;37:881-904.
24. Joseph SC. Current issues concerning AIDS in New York City. *N Y State J Med.* 1988;88:253-258.
25. Stoneburner RL DesJarlais DL, Benezra D, et al. A larger spectrum of severe HIV-1–related disease in intravenous drug users in New York City. *Science.* 1988;242:216-219.
26. Wish ED, Klumpp DA, Moorer AH, Brady E, Williams KM. *Analysis of Drugs and Crime Among Arrestees in the District of Columbia: Final Report.* Washington, DC: US Dept of Justice; 1988.
27. Brodzka W, Thornhill HL, Howard S. Burns: causes and risk factors. *Arch Phys Med Rehabil.* 1985;66:746-752.
28. Vollum DI. Skin lesions in drug addicts. *BMJ.* 1970;2:647-650.
29. Moy JA. Cutaneous manifestation of drug abuse. In: Fitzpatrick T, Eisen A, Wolff K, et al, eds. *Dermatology in General Medicine.* New York, NY: McGraw-Hill Internationl Book Co. In press.

30. Smith DJ Jr, Busuito MJ, Velanovich V, Spotts J, Heggers JP, Robson MC. Drug injection injuries of the upper extremity. *Ann Plast Surg.* 1989;22:19-24.

31. Aigner TG, Balster RL. Choice behavior in rhesus monkeys: cocaine versus food. *Science.* 1978;201:534-535.

32. Tames SM, Goldenring JM. Madarosis from cocaine use. *N Engl J Med.* 1986;314:1324.

33. Zamora-Quezeda JC, Dinerman H, Stadecker MJ, Kelly JJ. Muscle and skin infarction after free-basing cocaine (crack). *Ann Intern Med.* 1988;108:564-565.

34. Jaffe JH. Drug addiction and drug abuse. In: Goodman-Gilman A, Rall TW, Niew AS, et al, eds. *Goodman and Gilman's The Pharmacological Basis of Therapeutics.* 8th ed. New York, NY: Pergamon Press; 1990:541.

35. Rolfs RT, Goldberg M, Sharrar RB. Risk factors for syphilis: cocaine use and prostitution. *Am J Public Health.* 1990;80:853-857.

36. Zwerg-Greenberg MS, Singh T, Hoo M, et al. The association between congenital syphilis and cocaine/crack use in New York City: a case control study. *Am J Public Health.* 1991;81:1216-1318.

37. Young AW, Rosenberg FR. Cutaneous stigmas of heroin addiction. *Arch Dermatol.* 1971;104:80-86.

38. Derbes VJ. The fixed drug eruption. *JAMA.* 1964;190:765-766.

39. Neugarten J, Gallo GR, Buxbaum J, Katz LA, Rubenstein J, Baldwin DS. Amyloidosis in subcutaneous heroin abusers ('skin poppers' amyloidosis). *Am J Med.* 1986;81:635-640.

40. Dunne JH, Johnson WC. Necrotizing skin lesions in heroin addicts. *Arch Dermatol.* 1972;105:544-547.

41. Zuravin SJ. The epidemiology of child abuse and neglect: review of the literature and presentation of data. *Violence Vict.* 1989; 4:101-20.

42. Guyer B, Lescohier I, Gallagher SS, Hausman A, Azzara CV. Intentional injuries among children and adolescents in Massachusetts. *N Engl J Med.* 1989;321:1584-1589.

43. Johnson CF. Inflicted injury versus accidental injury in child abuse. *Pediatr Clin North Am.* 1990;37:791.

44. Dodge KA, Bates JE, Pettit GS. Mechanisms in the cycle of violence. *Science.* 1990;250:1678-1683.

45. Goodman LA. The prevalence of abuse among homeless and housed poor mothers: a comparison study. *Am J Orthopsychiatry.* 1991;61:489-500.

46. Council on Scientific Affairs. AMA diagnostic and treatment guidelines concerning child abuse and neglect. *JAMA.* 1985;254:796-800.

47. Mecrow IK. Burn to toddler's penis from an electrochemical battery. *BMJ.* 1988;297:1315.

48. Prescott PR. Hair dryer burns in children. *Pediatrics.* 1990; 86:692-697.

49. Montrey JA, Barcia PJ. Nonaccidental burns in child abuse. *South Med J.* 1985;78:1324-1326.

50. Reece RM. Unusual manifestations of child abuse. *Pediatr Clin North Am.* 1990;37:905-921.

51. McNamara J, Baler R, Lynch E. Ehlers-Danlos syndrome reported as child abuse. *Clin Pediatr.* 1985;24:317.

52. Levine V, Sanchez M, Nestor M. Localized vulvar pemphigoid in a child misdiagnosed as sexual abuse. *Arch Dermatol.* 1992;128: 804-806.

53. Feldman KW. Pseudoabusive burns in Asian refugees. *AJDC.* 1984;138:768-769.

54. Goldberg WG, Tomlanovich MC. Domestic violence victims in the emergency department: new findings. *JAMA.* 1984;251:3259-3264.

55. Berenson AB, Stiglich NJ, Wilkinson GS, Anderson GD. Drug abuse and other risk factors for physical abuse in pregnancy among white non-Hispanic, black, and Hispanic women. *Am J Obstet Gynecol.* 1991;164:1491-1496.

56. Gin NE, Rucker L, Frayne S, Cygan R, Hubbell FA. Prevalency of domestic violence among patients in three ambulatory care internal medicine clinics. *J Gen Intern Med.* 1991;6:317-322.

57. Frazer M. Domestic violence: a medicolegal review. *J Forensic Sci.* 1986;31:1409-1419.

58. Bergman B, Brismar B. A 5-year follow-up study of 117 battered women. *Am J Public Health.* 1991;81:1486-1489.

59. McLeer SV, Anwar RA, Herman S, Maquiling K. Education is not enough: a systems failure in protecting battered women. *Ann Emerg Med.* 1989;18:651-653.

60. Wupe ER. Genital injuries in assault victims. *Can Med Assoc J.* 1991;144:644-647.

61. Sorenson SB, Stein JA, Siegel JM, Golding JM, Burnam, MA. The prevalence of adult sexual assault: the LA epidemiologic catchment area project. *Am J Epidemiol.* 1987;126:1154-1164.

62. Hicks DJ. Sexual battery: management of the rape victim. In: Sciarra J, ed. *Gynecology and Obstetrics.* New York, NY: Harper & Row Publishers Inc; 1983;6:96.

63. Hillman R, O'Mara N, Tomlinson D, Harris JR. Adult male victims of sexual assault: an underdiagnosed condition. *Int J STD AIDS.* 1991;2:22-24.

64. Bachmann GA, Moeller TP, Benett J. Childhood sexual abuse and the consequences in adult women. *Obstet Gynecol.* 1988;71:632-642.

65. Muram D. Anal and perianal abnormalities in prepubertal victims of sexual abuse. *Am J Obstet Gynecol.* 1989;161:278-281.

66. Oriel JD. Anogenital papillomavirus infection in children. *BMJ.* 1988;296:1484-1485.

67. Seng MP. Child sexual abuse and adolescent prostitution: a cooperative analysis. *Adolescence.* 1989;24:665-675.

68. Caukins SE. The psychodynamics of male prostitution. *Am J Psychother.* 1976;30:44-51.

69. Fulmer TT, O'Malley TA. *Inadequate Care of the Elderly: A Health Care Perspective on Abuse and Neglect.* New York, NY: Springer Publishing Co Inc; 1987:180.

70. Grisso JA, Schwarz DF, Wishner AR, Weene B, Holmes JH, Sutton RL. Injuries in an elderly inner-city population. *J Am Geriatr Soc.* 1990;38:1326-1331.

71. Carlson MJ. Evidence of elderly abuse growing. *Ohio Med.* 1989;85:346-349.

72. Godkin MA, Wolfs RS, Pillemer KA. A case-comparison analysis of elder abuse and neglect. *Int J Aging Hum Dev.* 1989;28:207-225.

73. Pillemer K, Finkelhor D. Causes of elder abuse: caregiver stress versus problem relatives. *Am J Orthopsychiatry.* 1989;59: 179-187.

74. Winchel RM, Stanley M. Self-injurious behavior: a review of the behavior and biology of self-mutilation. *Am J Psychiatry.* 1991; 148:306-317.

75. Gedye A. Extreme self-injury attributed to frontal lobe seizures. *Am J Ment Retard.* 1989;94:20-26.

76. French AP, Nelson HL. Genital self mutilation in women. *Arch Gen Psychiatry.* 1972;27:618-620.

77. Favazza AR, Conterio K. Female habitual self-mutilators. *Acta Psychiatr Scand.* 1989;79:283-289.

78. Spraker MK. Cutaneous artifactual disease: an appeal for help. *Pediatr Clin North Am.* 1983;30:659-668.

79. Winkelmann RK, Barker SM. Factitial traumatic panniculitis. *J Am Acad Dermatol.* 1985;13:988-994.

80. Daniels SM, Fenley JD, Powers PS, Cruse CW. Self-inflicted burns: a ten-year retrospective study. *J Burn Care Rehabil.* 1991; 12:144-147.

81. Van-Moffaert MM. Self-mutilation: diagnosis and practical treatment. *Int J Psychiatry Med.* 1990;20:373-382.

Localized Vulvar Pemphigoid in a Child Misdiagnosed as Sexual Abuse

Victoria Levine, MD; Miguel Sanchez, MD; Mark Nestor, MD, PhD

• *Background.*—Various primary dermatoses can affect the vulva of children and be misdiagnosed as child abuse, with devastating social consequences.

Observation.—A 3-year-old girl with vulvar erosions was removed from her parent's care after a pediatrician and gynecologist diagnosed child abuse. Histopathologic and immunofluorescence studies were consistent with vulvar pemphigoid.

Conclusion.—Localized pemphigoid should be added to the differential diagnosis of vulvar lesions. Dermatologists, pediatricians, and gynecologists should be familiar with nonvenereal diseases that can exclusively affect this area. The dermatologist's expertise is particularly valuable in differentiating between primary diseases and sexual abuse.

(*Arch Dermatol.* 1992;128:804-806)

Increased publicity and professional awareness has led to a dramatic rise in the number of children evaluated for sexual abuse in recent years.[1,2] Between 30% and 64% of abused children present with evidence of anogenital trauma.[3,4] In cases that resulted in felony convictions, physical evidence was present in only 23%.[5] Because some cutaneous diseases can resemble lesions of child abuse in general,[6-8] and sexual abuse in particular,[9-11] it is critical that physicians recognize these conditions and prevent the stigma and suffering of erroneous accusations and investigations. We describe a 3-year-old girl with localized vulvar pemphigoid that was misdiagnosed as sexual abuse.

Accepted for publication March 13, 1992.

From the The Ronald O. Perelman Department of Dermatology, New York (NY) University Medical Center.

Reprint requests to Ronald O. Perelman Department of Dermatology, New York University Medical Center, 550 First Ave, New York, NY 10016 (Dr Sanchez).

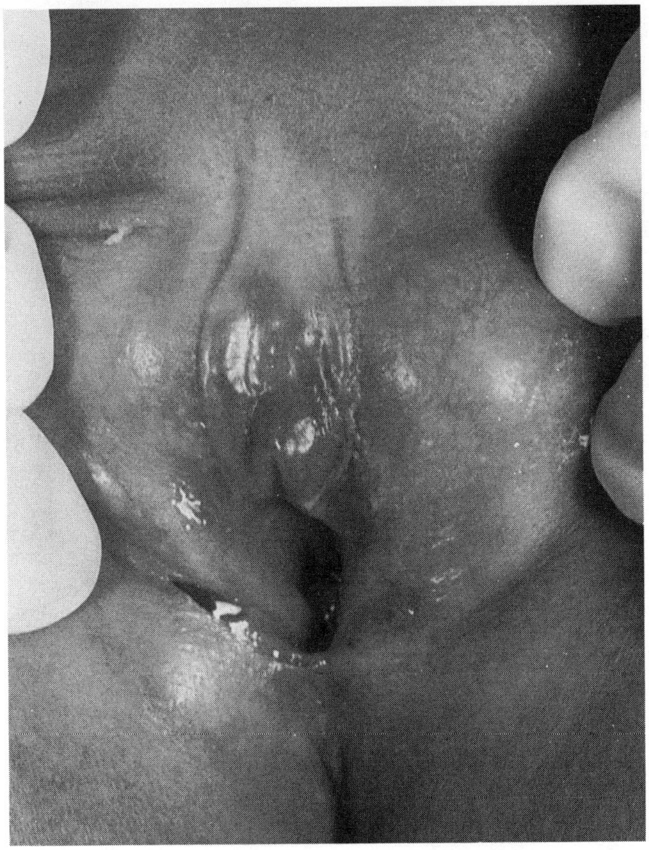

Fig 1.—Shallow vulvar ulcerations at 1, 4, 8, and 11 o'clock.

REPORT OF A CASE

A previously healthy 3-year-old girl developed slightly pruritic ulcers on the inner aspects of her labia and vestibule. Her mother noticed the lesions and brought her to a pediatrician, who concluded that the lesions were caused by exter-

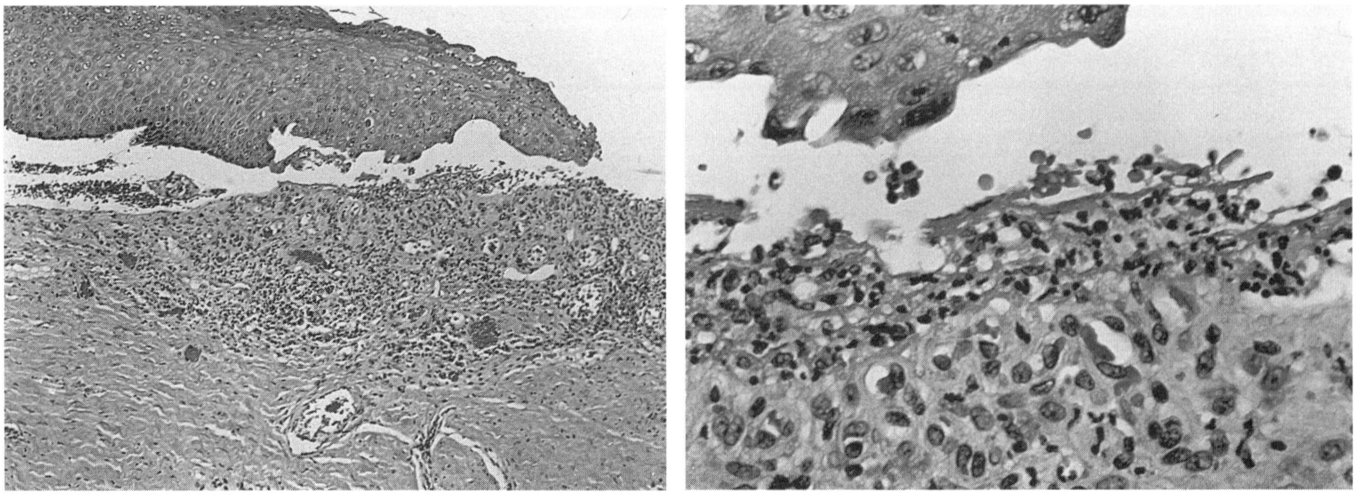

Fig 2.—Left, Subepidermal blister with a dermal mixed inflammatory cell infiltrate. Right, High-power magnification showing the presence of eosinophils.

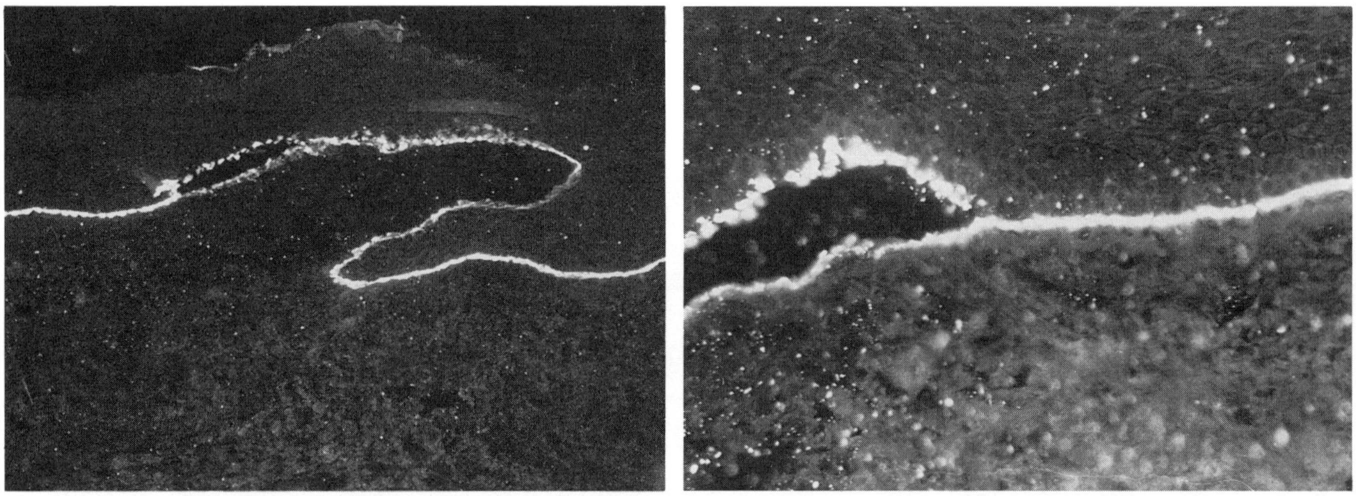

Fig 3.—Left, Linear deposition of IgG and C3 along the dermoepidermal junction, which is concentrated on the epidermal side of the vesicle. Right, High-power magnification of figure on the left.

nal trauma. The child was immediately hospitalized with a diagnosis of sexual abuse. A gynecologist reported a "stretched" hymen and microscopic tubular structures "resembling" adult hairs. Serologic tests for syphilis were nonreactive. Cultures for gonorrhea, chancroid, chlamydia, and yeast yielded no organisms, and smears for trichomonas and monilia were negative. Based on a diagnosis of sexual abuse, the child welfare agency began prosecuting the parents, who vehemently denied any sexual molestation. Pending final litigation, the child was returned to the mother's custody with the stipulation that the father move and have no contact with the child. The father continued to deny wrongdoing but complied.

Approximately 11 months later, the patient was examined by a dermatologist. Physical examination revealed four shallow, oval, well-demarcated ulcerations measuring 0.5 to 0.8 mm, which were slightly tender to the touch on the inferior inner aspect of the labia (Fig 1). No scarring, fissures, or milia were present. There were no additional cutaneous, ocular, or oral findings. A perilesional skin biopsy specimen stained with hematoxylin-eosin revealed a subepidermal blister with fibrosis of the lamina propria and a mixed inflammatory cell infiltrate containing eosinophils (Fig 2). Immunofluorescent stains on two separate skin biopsy specimens showed a subepidermal vesicle and linear deposits of IgG and C3 at the dermoepidermal junction with the majority of the stain on the epidermal aspect of the vesicle (Fig 3). Indirect immunofluorescence tests for pemphigoid and epidermolysis bullosa antigens were negative. The ulcers healed with application of fluocinolone ointment (0.025%).

COMMENT

The history of persistent vulvar ulcerations despite removal of the patient from the home environment as well as the physical appearance of the lesions, together with the histopathologic and immunofluorescence findings, support the diagnosis of localized pemphigoid of the vulva. Re-evaluation of the data presented in court lead to the conclusion that the "hairs" were cotton fibers and that the hymen was intact and normal. Of the previously reported cases of localized pemphigoid of the vulva, the youngest was in an 11-year-old girl.[12]

Other possible diagnoses, based on the histologic and immunofluorescence findings, include cicatricial pemphigoid and epidermolysis bullosa acquisita. Unfortunately, a saline split-skin immunofluorescence examination, to differentiate between pemphigoid and epidermolysis bullosa, was refused.

Despite persistent denial by the parents, normal psychologic testing of the child, and failure of the lesions to heal during a prolonged hospitalization, the physicians, faced with physical findings with which they had no experience, did not consider dermatologic disease and attributed the ulcers to sexual abuse. Incorrect descriptions of hair and hymen seemed to strengthen the case.

Based on the findings and testimony of dermatologists, the charges of child abuse were dropped and the family was reunited. However, by then the father had been forced to live away from home for over a year with the almost-certain prospect of incarceration, and the family had accumulated considerable legal expenses, experienced enormous psychologic stress, and endured public humiliation. Even the parents' attorneys had admitted that due to the medical evidence presented they had been convinced of the father's guilt and could not provide an adequate defense. The far-reaching consequences of the misdiagnosis of child sexual abuse in this case stress the importance of recognizing dermatologic diseases when considering the diagnosis of sexual abuse.

A number of dermatologic conditions, including mongolian spots,[6] phytophotodermatitis,[7] and Ehlers-Danlos syndrome[8] as well as chronic bullous dermatosis of childhood, linear IgA dermatosis, Crohn's disease, varicella, allergic contact dermatitis, and nonsexually transmitted vulvovaginal infections[11] can simulate child abuse. In lichen sclerosus et atrophicus, the vulva and perianal area may show purpura, excoriations, blistering, erosion, and bleeding. Several cases of lichen sclerosus misdiagnosed as sexual abuse in children have been reported.[9] Concern has been expressed that certain types of genital hygiene practices may either mimic or be considered a type of sexual abuse.[13]

Recently, efforts have been made to define and even standardize assessment and examination of children suspected of being sexually abused.[14] We feel that this case emphasizes that it is vital that any assessment include a specific examination by a dermatologist when any question arises regarding dermatologic manifestations of disease.

Health professionals must be made aware of the signs and symptoms of child abuse and sexual abuse to prevent continued suffering and its ultimate physical and psychologic sequelae. The recent Cleveland, England, child sexual abuse frenzy, when scores of diagnoses of sexual abuse were made without adequate evidence,[15] points to the necessity of both vigilance and care when diagnosing child sexual abuse to prevent the tremendous suffering that both the patient and family experience when a misdiagnosis is made.

References

1. Wild NJ. Sexual abuse of children in Leeds. *BMJ.* 1986;292: 1113-1116.
2. Mrazek PJ, Lynch MA, Bentovim A. Sexual abuse of children in the United Kingdom. *Child Abuse Negl.* 1983;7:147-153.
3. Tilelli JA, Turek D, Jaffe AC. Sexual abuse in children: clinical findings and implications for management. *N Engl J Med.* 1980;302: 319-323.
4. Claytor RN, Barth KL, Shubin CI. Evaluating child sexual abuse: observations regarding ano-genital injury. *Clin Pediatr.* 1989;28:419-422.
5. De Jong AR, Rose M. Frequency and significance of physical evidence in legally proven cases of child sexual abuse. *Pediatrics.* 1989;84:1022-1026.
6. Saulsbury FT, Hayden GF. Skin conditions simulating child abuse. *Pediatr Emerg Care.* 1985;1:147-150.
7. Owen SM, Durst RD. Ehlers-Danlos syndrome simulating child abuse. *Arch Dermatol.* 1984;120:97-101.
8. Coffman K, Boyce WT, Hansen RC. Phytophotodermatitis simulating child abuse. *AJDC.* 1985;139:239-240.
9. Handfield-Jones SE, Hinde FR, Kennedy CTC. Lichen sclerosus et atrophicus in children misdiagnosed as sexual abuse. *BMJ.* 1987;294:1404-1405.
10. Priestly BL, Bleehen SS. Lichen sclerosus et atrophicus in children misdiagnosed as sexual abuse. *BMJ.* 1987;295:211.
11. Herman-Giddens ME, Berson NL. Dermatologic conditions misdiagnosed as evidence of child abuse. *JAMA.* 1989;261:3548-3547.
12. DeCastro P, Jorizzo JL, Rajaraman S, Solomon AR, Briggaman RA, Raimer SS. Localized vulvar pemphigoid in a child. *Pediatr Dermatol.* 1985;2:302-307.
13. Herman-Giddens ME, Berson NL. Harmful genital care practices in children: a type of child abuse. *JAMA.* 1989;261:577-579.
14. Strickland SL. Sexual abuse assessment. *Pediatr Annu.* 1989; 18:498-500.
15. Fulginiti V, Krugman R. Cleveland, England: child abuse in the public eye. *AJDC.* 1989;143:651-652.

Family Violence, Child Abuse, and Anogenital Warts

Violence within the family is a problem that has reached epidemic proportions in the United States. According to "Family Violence: An Overview," published in January 1990 by the US Department of Health and Human Services, 1100 children are known to have died as a result of abuse or neglect in 1986 (the actual number is probably much larger). A 1979 Federal Bureau of Investigation report stated that 40% of murdered women and 10% of murdered men were killed by partners. Each year an estimated 2 to 4 million children suffer abuse or neglect at the hand of a parent, and 1.5 to 2 million women are battered by their partners. For many unfortunate Americans, home is anything but a sanctuary.

In addition to possible death or permanent physical impairment, child victims of family violence may suffer long-term psychological consequences. Some children withdraw and develop feelings of worthlessness, helplessness, hopelessness, and depression. Others exhibit aggressive and impulsive behavior and are at risk for delinquency, substance abuse, absenteeism from school or work, adolescent pregnancy, and prostitution. Abused children are more likely as adults to be abusive to their own children and to their spouses. All physicians are being called on to help interrupt this cycle of human suffering.

Child abuse encompasses physical abuse, physical and/or emotional neglect, and sexual abuse. Physical abuse frequently leaves cutaneous signs indicative of such abuse.[1] These signs include loop or curvilinear marks from small ropes and cords; linear bruising; ecchymoses from blunt trauma; binding injuries; traumatic alopecia; human bite marks; and thermal burns, such as cigarette burns, branding injuries, and immersion-type scald injuries. Abuse is more common in families with poor social support systems, and stress may precipitate an episode of abuse. Children who were premature infants, are handicapped, or who have other medical or behavioral problems are at increased risk for physical abuse. Since 1967, all 50 states have required physicians to report suspected cases of child abuse and neglect. The laws offer immunity from liability as long as the report is made without malice.

Although physical abuse frequently leaves cutaneous signs, physically abused children (at least those with acute injuries recognizable as abuse) are rarely seen by the dermatologist. A much more common problem to face our specialty is the evaluation of the child with anogenital warts. Are anogenital warts in a child indicative of sexual abuse?

Reports of anogenital warts in children are increasing and appear to reflect an increased incidence of infection in the adult population. In adults, almost all anogenital warts result from sexual transmission. For children, however, several routes of acquisition of anogenital human papillomavirus (HPV) infection seem possible.[2] These include transmission from an abusing adult, from an adult who is not abusing, from the mother either transplacentally or by passage through an infected birth canal, or, in the case of skin-type warts, from the child's own hands or those of other children or adults who have warts.

Great variation exists in the incidence of documented or strongly suspected child abuse reported in recent studies of children with anogenital warts,[2-5] ranging from a low of 11%[3] to a high of 91%.[5] Gutman et al[6] have recently reminded us that adequate assessment for child abuse should be done in all anogenital HPV-infected children. The evaluation should include: (1) assessment of medical and behavioral indicators of abuse; (2) a medical examination to identify physical indications of abuse (ie, signs of previous trauma; measurement of the transverse vaginal opening, which should be less than 4 mm in prepubertal girls[7]; and evaluation of anal sphincter tone); (3) assessment for infection with other sexually transmitted diseases (infection with gonorrhea or serologic evidence of syphilis is very suggestive of abuse and frequently indicates multiple abusers[5]; natal infections with *Chlamydia trachomatis* have recently been documented to persist as long as 28 months[8]; therefore, concomitant infection with this organism in the young child is not conclusive evidence of abuse); and (4) age-appropriate interviews of the child and caretakers by skilled personnel. Hopefully, future reports will document the extent to which children in studies have been examined, and only children with negative findings after full evaluation will be considered not to have been abused.

The appearance of anogenital warts is not helpful in determining whether or not they were sexually acquired.[4,8] Condyloma in children are seen more frequently on the skin than on the mucous membranes[8] and are frequently papillomalike, hyperkeratotic, and sharply demarcated. Typing of warts may be helpful;

however, such typing is not routinely available to the practitioner and, when performed, must still be correlated with physical and historical evidence of abuse.

In recent studies of 123 children with anogenital warts in which a known HPV type was detected in 109,[2-4,9] 74% were found to have HPV types 6 or 11 (those commonly associated with genital warts of adults), 4.6% had HPV 16 or 18 (also associated with adult genital warts and suspected to be oncogenic), and 18% had HPV types 2 or 3 (commonly found in skin warts). The vertical transmission from mother to infant of HPV types commonly associated with adult genital lesions is likely one source of genital warts as well as the source of laryngeal and conjunctival papillomatosis in young children. These viruses have been found in newborns with no apparent infection. One study demonstrated the presence of anogenital HPV types in 4% of the foreskins from infants undergoing routine circumcisions.[10] Warts acquired congenitally probably manifest themselves early in life, generally by age 3 years.

It is probable that HPV can also be transmitted during the routine care of young children or through benign contact with an infected adult (eg, bathing with the infant). In a recent study by Cohen et al[3] of 73 children with genital warts, 55 (75%) were under 3 years of age and abuse was suspected or documented in only two children under the age of 3 years. Even though anogenital warts may be acquired in benign ways in the young child, young children are frequently sexually abused and such abuse should be excluded. The probability of anogenital HPV infection being acquired because of sexual abuse appears to increase with the increasing age of the child.

Dermatologists are rarely trained to adequately examine the genital area of children for signs of abuse or to properly interview children or caretakers. Unless the dermatologist has these skills, children with anogenital warts should be referred to a local pediatrician experienced in evaluating children for possible abuse, or, if available, to a child abuse team often composed of a cooperating group of medical personnel, including physicians, psychologists, nurses, and social workers. Referrals should be made in a very nonaccusatory fashion. It is important for the dermatologist to maintain good rapport with the family so that they will return for adequate treatment and follow-up of the child. Occasionally, dermatologists may have difficulty finding an experienced primary care physician in their area to evaluate children with anogenital warts. Physicians may feel inadequately trained or occasionally are reluctant to undertake such an evaluation because of the time required to prepare a detailed written report for child protective services (CPS) agencies and potential time out of the office to testify in court should a case be brought to trial. Local medical and pediatric societies or local chapters of the American Academy of Pediatrics may be helpful in locating an appropriate physician for referrals. When the dermatologist must decide without consultation whether or not notification of CPS in warranted, Schachner and Hankin's article[11] on assessing sexual abuse in childhood condyloma accuminatum may be helpful in making this decision.

An argument could be made for reporting all children with anogenital warts directly to local CPS agencies. One problem with this approach is that the number of child abuse cases reported within the last 10 years has risen dramatically, while funding for personnel to properly investigate such cases has not grown proportionately. There is a danger, therefore, of overburdening an already stressed system, particularly if the incidence of anogenital warts in children continues to increase. Inexperienced and, at times, poorly trained case workers may be less capable of evaluating a child than an experienced physician or child abuse team. Some states have no specific degree requirements or licensure for CPS case workers and may offer as little as 40 hours of formal training (far less than is required to become a cosmetologist or law enforcement officer) before placing workers in the field to make what may be life or death decisions for children. Child Protective Services may require adult males in the family to move out of the home pending completion of an investigation. This can cause emotional trauma to family members, may result in unwarranted distrust, and may wreak financial havoc for the family. It seems most appropriate for experienced medical personnel to make the decision of whether or not referral to CPS is warranted.

If child abuse is proven, it generally results in punishment for the offender. Treatment programs for sex offenders are increasing in number, but it is difficult at this point in time to evaluate their effectiveness. When it becomes necessary to remove a child from the home, options for care are far less than ideal. Children are frequently "warehoused" in shelters or placed in less than adequate foster homes, which are part of an underfunded foster care program. It is probably safe to assume that abused and neglected children have no highly paid lobbyists working for them in state capitals to influence legislation on their behalf. As physicians, we should not only adequately treat the immediate physical problems of abused children but also be an advocate at the local and state levels for services, and moneys for these services, designed to protect the physical and mental health of young Americans who, through no fault of their own, are unable to protect and care for themselves.

Sharon S. Raimer, MD
Department of Dermatology and Pediatrics
Ben G. Raimer, MD
Department of Pediatrics
University of Texas Medical Branch
Galveston, TX 77555-0783

References

1. Raimer BG, Raimer SS, Hebeler JR. Cutaneous signs of child abuse. *J Am Acad Dermatol.* 1981;5:203-212.

2. Gibson PE, Gardner SD, Best SJ. Human papillomavirus types in anogenital warts of children. *J Med Virol.* 1990;30:142-145.

3. Cohen BA, Honig P, Androphy E. Anogenital warts in children: clinical and virologic evaluation for sexual abuse. *Arch Dermatol.* 1990;126:1575-1580.

4. Hanson RM, Glasson M, McCrossin I, Rogers M. Anogenital warts in childhood. *Child Abuse Neglect.* 1989;13:225-233.

5. Herman-Giddens ME, Gutman LT, Berson NL, The Duke Child Protection Team. Association of coexisting vaginal infections and

multiple abusers in female children with genital warts. *Sex Transm Dis.* 1988;15:63-67.
6. Gutman L, Herman-Giddens M, Prose N. Diagnosis of child sexual abuse in children with genital warts. *AJDC.* 1991;145:126.
7. Goff CW, Burke KR, Rickenback C, Buebendorf DP. Vaginal opening measurement in prepubertal girls. *AJDC.* 1989;143:1366-1368.
8. Bell TA, Stamm WE, Wag S, Kuo C, Holmes KK, Grayston JT. Chronic *Chlamydia trachomatis* infections in infants. *JAMA.* 1992;267:400-402.
9. Obalek S, Jablonska S, Favre M, Walezak L, Orth G. Condylomata acuminata in children: frequent association with human papillomaviruses responsible for cutaneous warts. *J Am Acad Dermatol.* 1990;23:205-213.
10. Roman A, Fife K. Human papillomavirus DNA associated with foreskins of normal newborns. *J Infect Dis.* 1986;153:855-861.
11. Schachner L, Hankin DE. Assessing child abuse in childhood condyloma accuminatum. *J Am Acad Dermatol.* 12:157-160, 1985.

Diagnosing Child Abuse

The Cost of Getting It Wrong

In this issue of the ARCHIVES, Levine et al[1] describe the situation of a 3-year-old girl with lesions on her vulva, removed from her parents' care on suspicion of sexual abuse diagnosed by both a pediatrician and a gynecologist. Only after a dermatologist performed a biopsy 11 months later and diagnosed the lesions as localized vulvar pemphigoid was custody returned to the parents.

This case is nót a bizarre aberration. Indeed, the footnotes to the article by Levine et al[1] indicate many instances in which skin conditions have simulated child abuse, including sexual abuse.

Publicity surrounding child abuse in recent years has created a concern, even a hysteria, about the harm being done to children. But there is another side to the problem that rarely receives much public attention—the injustices and injuries inflicted on children and families caught up in the child protection system.[2]

Other examples abound:

The New York Times Magazine (September 15, 1991:52) reported the story of a New Jersey family whose 1-month-old baby accidentally fell to the floor, sustaining two skull fractures. Maintaining the two injuries could not happen in one accident, the doctor in the emergency department accused the parents of child abuse and, although the baby recovered, the hospital kept the boy for a week until he was placed with his grandparents. Only supervised visits by the parents were allowed until 4 months later, when the court determined there had been no child abuse.

Similar accounts exist in the realm of sexual abuse. For example, a woman in upstate New York lost custody of her daughter for a period after she had asked a volunteer center if it was normal to become aroused while nursing. The volunteer associated the question, and the fact that the child was 2 years old, with sexual abuse. In another situation, parents were accused of sexual abuse by a technician who had developed photographs of the couple's naked children in normal postures.

I do not mean to belittle the problem of child abuse, which is serious and real. Child sexual abuse, in particular, has serious and lasting psychological consequences for many victims. But, as one commentator put it, "a visceral reaction may impair objectivity with the result that truth becomes a second victim."[3]

As greater awareness of child abuse has increased, reports from professionals and the community at large have increased—reports that have serious consequences for children and their families who are subjected to investigation, court appearances, medical and psychological examinations, and often short-term or long-term separation of family members while the case is being investigated. The family's privacy is violated, family relations are disrupted, and the child's caretakers are stigmatized.

The well-meaning efforts of doctors, social workers, teachers, and others have gone terribly wrong. On any given day, nearly 500 000 children in this country are living apart from their biological parents. Over half of the children will be kept away from their homes for a year or more; three of five will be placed in more than one setting during their stay; some will have 15 or more "homes" in their childhood; and some will never again live with any permanent family.[4]

It is not clear from the article on which I am commenting how long the 3-year-old remained away from her parents' home. At some point during the 11 months before the correct diagnosis, the father, accused of criminal sexual molestation, agreed to move and have no contact with the child. How can we judge the harm to this 3-year-old deprived of her mother's care for even a few days and her father's presence for 11 months?

There is a myth that child abuse crosses class lines, that it is an "all-American problem." Perhaps children whose parents are accused of abuse and neglect exist in well-off homes in the same proportion as in poor homes, but I doubt it. The child protection system is fraught with economic, ethnic, and cultural biases. Although the article does not let us know the background of the 3-year-old victim, one cannot help but wonder whether her family was poor, perhaps black or Hispanic, possibly non–English speaking.

Several studies in recent years have attempted to analyze how race and family income affect child abuse reporting. Among the findings of which the medical profession should be aware is that, compared with other agencies, hospitals identified a disproportionate number of black families. Similarly, a study found that medical personnel disproportionately reported child abuse among blacks. As the commentator reporting on these studies suggests, "the apparent bias may be attributable to the difference between seeing an injured child in an emergency room compared to a private office. Alternatively, it may represent an attempt by doctors to overlook abuse in affluent, white families."[5] Hospitals have been found to be especially biased in this regard.

Take the case of the black baby who died at age 8 weeks from "positional asphyxia"; the baby was unable to breathe after shifting in his cradle. It was a battery-powered swinging cradle that was later recalled under an order from the US Consumers Product Safety Commission. As a result of the tragedy, the four remaining children were taken from the baby's mother and placed in foster care. But the middle-class parents of a 6-week old baby who also suffocated, by a beanbag pillow that also was recalled, got tremendous sympathy and community support after their tragedy.

In 1962, child abuse was formally identified as a medical condition,[6] and the concept of a child abuse reporting statute was discussed at a conference called by the Children's Bureau of the-then US Department of Health, Education, and Welfare. By 1967, all 50 states had some form of legislation mandating specified professionals to report suspected cases of child abuse.

The enactment of broad and vague reporting laws in the 50 states and the creation of "mandatory reporters" have created a dangerous potential for overreporting. Most states' laws include a criminal penalty for failure to report and immunity from both criminal and civil liability to persons making reports in "good faith." Thus, it is clear why doctors, social workers, and other mandated reporters weight their decisions in favor of reporting despite the lasting damage experienced by children and their families as a result of investigative errors.

But mandatory reporting should bring responsibilities as well as prestige. (I use the word "prestige" deliberately. Last year, when dental hygienists in the state of New York realized they were not designated mandated reporters, their association lobbied to have them included in the legislation.) Professionals must have thorough training as to what is and *what is not* child abuse. Most medical students receive little or no training, and even some pediatric residencies have an inadequate focus on child abuse.[7] And information on the characteristics of child abuse should be kept current and disseminated. For example, in the early 1980s a group of California doctors established what they believed was a medical standard for detecting sexual abuse. Yet, in recent years new studies have shown that certain of these same physical characteristics considered to be signs of sexual abuse are normal in a large percentage of children (*The Wall Street Journal*. April 15, 1991:B1). It is important to be aware of the potential of overintervention and its consequences; it would indeed be tragic and ironic if parents, especially poor parents and racial- and linguistic-minority parents, hesitated to take their children for medical care because they were afraid of the consequences.

There is already evidence that some mandated reporters do not report in certain instances, but not for lack of knowledge and experience.[8] In a survey, these reporters stated that they do not comply with their mandate because they are attempting to protect children in the context of overloaded child protective systems and because they believe that reports often have negative consequences for the children involved. One pediatrician working with impoverished families stated she broke the law because, based on her experiences, families often failed to return for essential health services after a report was filed. Other doctors said they failed to report because a family had already accepted treatment. Others believed they could help the child better themselves. (The study also revealed a small group of consistent nonreporters who worked exclusively in private practice and failed to report because of personal consequences, lost time, and lost patients.)

It should be obvious that responsible professionals do not want to break the law. Finkelhor and Zellman[8] propose a plan for flexible reporting options for certain groups of well-trained reporters under certain conditions. Very briefly, their plan calls for a special status for certain professionals who could document formal child abuse training and experience. These professionals could apply for special status not currently available under the mandated reporting laws. For example, they could defer mandated reports until a later time, or they could make the report in confidence, deferring an investigation until later, or indefinitely.[8] Proposals like these recognize the risk of unwarranted and harmful intervention, such as the case described in this issue of the ARCHIVES.

There are many unanswered questions in the article: Is this child from a poor family? How does she receive her health care? Why was a dermatologist not consulted sooner? However, the biggest question remains: What would have happened to this little girl if a dermatologist had not seen her at all?

Elizabeth Vorenberg
National Coalition for
Child Protection Reform
9 Willard St
Cambridge, MA 02138

References

1. Levine V, Sanchez M, Nestor MS. Localized vulvar pemphigoid in a child misdiagnosed as sexual abuse. *Arch Dermatol.* 1992;128:804-806.

2. Wexler R. *Wounded Innocents: The Real Victims of the War Against Child Abuse.* Buffalo, NY: Prometheus Books; 1990.

3. Myers JEB. The child sexual abuse literature: a call for greater objectivity. *Mich Law Rev.* 1990;88:1709-1733.

4. Lost in the system: the problem in context. In: *Keeping Families Together: Facts on Family Preservation Services* [information packet]. New York, NY: The Edna McConnell Clark Foundation; 1991.

5. Meriweather MH. Child abuse reporting laws: time for a change. *Fam Law Q.* Summer 1986;20:141-171.

6. Kempe CH, Silverman FN, Steele BF, Droegemueller W, Silver HK. The battered-child syndrome. *JAMA.* 1962;181:17-24.

7. Hechler D. *The Battle and the Backlash: The Child Sexual Abuse War.* Lexington, Mass: Lexington Books; 1988:24-2

8. Finkelhor D, Zellman GL. Flexible reporting options for skille-child abuse professionals. *Child Abuse Negl.* 1991; 15:335-341.

Silent Violence

Poverty, greed, too many people, the right to bear arms (anyone *and* everyone), addiction, hopelessness, mental illness, genetic propensity, media bombardment. We're on the bullet train to Entropy!

Violence plagues our nation. Society suffers. The *Journal of the American Medical Association* is devoting its June 10th issue to the subject of violence. In the pages that follow you will find commentaries by Maryland Governor William Donald Schaefer, Baltimore Mayor Kurt L. Schmoke, *Baltimore Sun* reporter and author David Simon, American Academy of Otolaryngology–Head and Neck Surgery President Richard Holt, MD, and several articles by our colleagues addressing this most pressing and disturbing issue.

Violence takes many forms. The murderer, the rapist, the robber attack the individual. Another kind of violence, one not so obvious, attacks the whole of humankind. Air and water, the essential elements for existence, are being polluted at a staggering rate. What we dump into our land and water and air we eventually eat and drink and breathe. Everyone is affected. Environmental pollution is violence to the earth—trauma to all living things.

I am appalled at what I read and hear. Numbers like: 100 million metric tons of air pollutants in a single year; millions of pounds of pesticides being plowed into our agricultural fields; even more toxic wastes being dumped into our waterways. For every man, woman, and child in this country, more than a ton of toxic waste is produced. Millions. Billions. Tons. This is almost beyond comprehension. Is that why we discount their meaning—we seem to be ignoring what is happening all around us? This is the air we run in, picnic in, exist in!

The smoking issue was easy (especially for otolaryngologists). We saw, firsthand, in the larynx and oral cavity, the destruction caused by tobacco. Now the residual effects of smoking are becoming more apparent. Even if you do not smoke, you can get cancer by being around people who do. Airlines, hospitals, and many offices have responded accordingly and banned smoking. And, fortunately, tobacco use is down among adults in the United States. But what about the young, the blacks—the new targets for cigarette advertising? What about the rest of the world? Do we export tobacco and disease for profit? Does anyone care? And eventually the question becomes: with limited resources, whom do we treat? What about the person who knowingly chooses to smoke? Obviously, moral issues abound.

We can do something about smoking and smokers and the immediate space around us. But what about the air we breathe every time we go outside? Or the recycled inside? The huge volume of air pollutants is eating away our ozone layer protection—that layer of gas that filters out the sun's hazardous ultraviolet rays. The main culprit is the chlorofluorocarbons—chemicals used in air conditioning and refrigeration, foam packaging, aerosol sprays, and dry-cleaning solvents. We now know about their effects and the world has responded quite rapidly. But the total phaseout deadline by the year 2000 appears to be too slow. Scientists predict ozone depletions in some areas to be as much as 40%. This increased amount of radiation exposure to the earth kills the plankton and krill, the root of the ocean food chain; it raises temperatures; it decreases crop yields; it affects the immune system; it causes cataracts and cancers. The ramifications are enormous. Are we prepared to deal with them? Could we have prevented this?

Chlorofluorocarbons are not the only offenders. Did you know that of the more than 50 000 chemicals registered with the Environmental Protection Agency, 90% have had little or no testing for health risks? With all that we pour into our air, land, and water (eventually filtering back to the human body), shouldn't there be a Food and Drug Administration of chemicals? No Human Use Committee would approve such uncontrolled experimentation. Again, we *react* rather than *act*. We ban after we find there is a toxic effect. Why don't we find the effects first? Who dreams up these compounds? Where is accountability? No academic institution would permit such negligence. Where is conscience?

Words like acid rain, mutagens, polychlorinated biphenyls, global warming, leachate, desertification, aquifer permeate the pages of the papers. We are bombarded. Even nature seems against us. It is estimated that 20 000 lung cancer deaths occur each year due to exposure to radon gas—a naturally occurring substance in rocks and soil that leaks into our living space.

Many wrongs and their repercussions are obvious: overdevelopment of land, overconsumption and waste of fossil fuel by developed nations, toxic landfills and seepage, massive deforestation. If we do not kill one another individually, it seems we will collectively.

Physicians, as purveyors of health, must not only treat the havoc man heaps on man, but we must also try to prevent that which threatens our mass destruction. We cannot barricade and hide, we must act. We must serve as examples. We must educate ourselves and those around us. We must be willing to speak up. How can we accept less when we expect so much from ourselves. Difficult choices may have to be made. Sacrifice is in order. Are we willing to pay for what is right? Individually? As a society?

Only through the efforts of us all, can change for the better actually happen. Awareness, courage, action, change. It is possible.

MICHAEL E. JOHNS, MD
Baltimore, Md

Time to Take Back Our Streets—and Our Homes

Every time I pick up a newspaper I see a new headline, informing us of another senseless tragedy: a child killed playing with a loaded gun, a drive-by shooting that claims an innocent life, a drug-related killing. Crime and violence continue to escalate, in the cities, and across the state. As one homicide officer told me: the police have lost the streets to crime.

We hear of weapons—most of them guns—being recovered in schools, on street corners, and in homes. Violence on the streets poses a huge problem. We continue to spend more and more money every year on police protection, and on sophisticated computers and equipment to keep track of the criminals. Our prisons are jammed with inmates serving time for violent crimes, most of them involving a gun of some kind. Our hospital emergency departments are busy tending to the latest shooting victim. In 15 years as mayor of Baltimore, and while I served on the City Council before that, I saw what one police officer recently described as a "domestic arms race" between the police and the criminals. Every so often, the police would need upgraded equipment: stronger body armor or more powerful guns, to keep up with what the criminals on the streets were carrying. Now, more and more, police are confiscating more powerful weapons at crime scenes, in some cases, the rapid-fire assault-style weapons that have one purpose: to kill people.

There is violence in our homes that is unspeakable. There is domestic violence and child abuse, which both trouble me, and then there are loving parents who think nothing of leaving a dangerous piece of equipment within reach of a child. Since April 1991, when the Maryland General Assembly rejected a bill that would require people to keep guns locked away from youngsters, at least 14 children all over the state have been killed or injured because of the careless handling of a weapon. That is violence that occurs not on the street, but in the home. It is but a fraction of the shooting incidents that occur in Maryland, but a situation that could be avoided altogether.

What can we do about violence? Is it too much for us to overcome? We can try to protect the citizens through thoughtful laws intended to put a stop to careless storage of firearms that can injure young people, that restrict the availability of concealable Saturday Night Specials, and that ban the sale of powerful assault weapons. We can try to educate people, to explain that it is in their best interest to lock up a gun away from a child's reach, or stop easy access to weapons capable of firing dozens of rounds in seconds.

We can encourage families to stay together to prevent youngsters from falling into lives of crime. We can work with communities to take back the streets. We can call on all Maryland jurisdictions to pool their information about drugs, so often the reason for violence, to band together to fight the spread of violence that spills over county lines. We can look for new ways to rehabilitate prison inmates to discourage them from returning to lives of crime. We can hope a fraction of our combined efforts will make a difference, that doctors, legislators, police, and our citizens will continue to lobby for safer streets—and homes.

WILLIAM DONALD SCHAEFER
Governor, State of Maryland

A Public Health Solution to Violent Crime

On December 15, 1991, the United States celebrated the 200th anniversary of the Bill of Rights. On December 25, 1991, the Soviet Union officially turned off the lights, shut the door, and declared itself out of business. These two stunning successes—one demonstrating the staying power of democratic principles, the other the triumph of hope over conventional wisdom—showed America in its best light. Unfortunately at no time during either day, or during the 9 days separating them, was there so much as a pause in the grinding violence that grips our nation.

That violence shows America in its worst light and contrasts sharply with the international movement toward peace, democracy, and disarmament. Although communities throughout the United States are facing an alarming increase in violent crime, the problem is especially acute in cities, where state and local budgets for police and public safety are being frozen or cut because of the recession. That has left millions of city dwellers, in particular the poor, feeling even more fearful of being crime victims.

How violent have we become? The percentage of people committing violent crimes is actually quite small. Nevertheless, the numbers are shocking. Nationwide in 1990, there were 23 438 deaths from nonnegligent homicide. That's one every 22 minutes. At least half of those murders were committed with handguns.

Baltimore, Md, has not been immune to this epidemic of violent crime. There were 305 murders in Baltimore in 1990. That was the highest number since 1972 and a 16% increase over 1989. Similar increases were seen in other "index" crimes. The numbers of rape, robbery, and aggravated assault all rose during 1990 and are likely to do the same in 1991 and 1992.

But numbers and trends tell only a very small part of the story about violence and cities. They do not, for example, explain the impact of violence on America's cities. Even more important, they do not explain the cause or offer a solution. I will try to do both in this commentary.

The impact of violent crime on cities is pervasive and frequently devastating. Crime shatters families; it raises the cost of doing business; it erodes the tax base by driving the middle class to the suburbs; it disrupts learning; it takes resources away from other essential services; and, all too often, it steals our future by ending the lives of our children.

Several times in 1990 and 1991, the people of Baltimore watched in horror as a murdered child was first discovered, then eulogized, and then buried. These senseless and dispiriting killings, coming on top of many others, sap what the people of every city need most: the self-confidence not only to walk the streets, but also to make a long-term financial and spiritual investment in the neighborhoods bounded by those streets. Thus, the impact of the violence that is swirling through cities extends beyond the loss of life, property, and economic potential. Hope, too, is in jeopardy. And without hope, cities cannot survive.

Who or what is responsible for most of the violent crime that is rending America's urban communities? Easy access to firearms is part of the problem. In Baltimore, handguns were involved in more than 7000 violent crimes in 1990; and 68% of all homicides were committed with handguns. Guns also frequently show up in cases of suicide, domestic violence, and accidental death.

But weak firearm laws are only one piece of a much larger problem. The incessant violence that has become so much a part of American life is caused primarily by our national drug policies. For more than 75 years—longer, it turns out, than the life of communism in what was the Soviet Union—it has been the policy of the federal government to control substance abuse with the heavy hand of the criminal law. This policy has not only failed to stem drug abuse, which according to the government's most recent report rose 18% in 1991, it has created an epidemic of violence.

Why? First, because the profits available from illegal drugs are so large that traffickers and street dealers will go to any lengths, no matter how violent, to maintain those profits. And second, the lack of treatment and maintenance programs leads addicts to commit crimes in order to pay for illegal drugs. This pattern has not changed throughout the long history of the war on drugs, and will not change until responsibility for fighting substance abuse is transferred from the Attorney General to the Surgeon General.

For several years, I have advocated treating substance abuse as a public health problem. This is consistent with the stated view of the American Medical Association (AMA) that addiction is a disease. It is also common sense and offers the best chance of substantially reducing violent crime, especially in cities.

That lesson has already been learned with alcohol prohibition. We tried to engineer an alcohol-free society and ended up with huge criminal enterprises, government corruption, children lured into organized crime, and random violence that took the lives of countless innocent people. So we ended Prohibition and began treating alcoholism as a disease. We have also used social pressure and public education to reduce alcohol, as well as cigarette, consumption. Obviously, much more needs to be done to further reduce both drinking and smoking. However, as a nation we made a sound policy choice when we decided to approach alcohol abuse primarily as a health problem rather than as a crime problem.

We now need to change course with respect to drug abuse. Instead of spending billions of dollars trying to arrest and incarcerate America's large addict population—a policy that leaves our prisons overcrowded and violent offenders subject to early release—we should transfer that money to the public health system, where medical professionals could use it for treatment, prevention, and education. This policy would have the added benefit of slowing the spread of human immunodeficiency virus infection, which in cities is being transmitted primarily by intravenous drug use.

Better care for addicts and far less crime are not the only reasons for taking a public health approach to substance abuse. These changes in national policy are also tied to a broader concept of justice. For example, there are more African-American men under the supervision of the criminal justice system than there are in college. This is a national tragedy. Moreover, a huge majority of urban crime victims are minorities. (In 1990, 92% of Baltimore's murder victims were nonwhite.)

These statistics cry out for a new, more just, and humane strategy in the war on drugs—a war that even the federal government reluctantly admits it is currently losing. That new strategy could be modeled after the approach now used in the Netherlands. There have also been numerous public health strategies proposed by academics and policy analysts. I have suggested that a national commission be set up to study how all drugs, legal and illegal, should be regulated—an idea that I hope will eventually earn the support of the AMA and the entire medical community.

Several weeks ago I reminded a rally in Washington, DC, that an American had a better chance of being shot in an American city than in the Persian Gulf. That sad truth deserves to be relegated to history, and will be once substance abuse is viewed as a disease to be treated, not a crime to be punished.

MAYOR KURT L. SCHMOKE
Baltimore, Md

A Journalist's Eye View of the Trauma Physician's Dilemma

This one yours?" asks the nursing supervisor.

"Does he have a bullet in him?"

"Yes, indeed."

"Then he's ours," says Garvey, bored.

Across the corridor, two doctors and a six-pack of nurses are expending their collective talent on the prone body of a West Baltimore drug trafficker. The electrocardiogram is irregular, and blood is pouring down the gurney and onto a white tile floor.

"He's not doing real well," the supervisor adds, turning back toward the nursing station in University of Maryland Hospital's emergency room. "They're cracking the chest."

And to that, Richard Garvey can't hold his tongue.

After all, as a veteran detective in the Baltimore Police Department's homicide unit, Garvey has seen this sort of thing before. Night after night, his clients arrive as bleeders at his city's best trauma units—Johns Hopkins, Sinai, University of Maryland Hospital—where the vanguard of emergency medicine attempts to prolong the lives of the narcotics addicts, street dealers, and belligerent barroom drunks who comprise more than half of Baltimore's assault victims. To what ultimate purpose, Rich Garvey has no way of knowing.

"Crack his chest? Why do that?" Garvey asks the nurse, deadpan. "We've got a suspect on this one."

The nurse smiles and shakes her head. It's an old joke with homicide detectives: When you've got a stone whodunit, your victim is certain to die. When you've got a suspect in custody, the victim will surely survive. Emergency room veterans maintain a similar postulate: If the victim is a law-abiding taxpayer with medical insurance, he will surely die. If he's an addict, stick-up artist, or drug trafficker, he'll live to fight another day. Each profession finds itself lost in the flood of urban violence, each is rightly granted its share of cynicism. In this particular instance, however, which happens to fall on an overnight shift in April 1988, Rich Garvey feels reasonably assured that he will be able to chalk up a murder clearance.

"When they get to cracking the chest, they're as good as dead," the detective tells his partner, Donald Kincaid, in the emergency room's waiting room.

"Aw yeah," drawls Kincaid, a 22-year veteran. "I only seen one guy who lived after they cracked him. That was at Hopkins."

True enough, the victim in question is dead by morning, despite the best efforts of the university surgeons. A small-time narcotics peddler from west Baltimore, he was murdered because a junior partner had been snorting up too much profit and felt obliged to shoot his boss rather than make the money right. The victim and his assailant had lengthy criminal records, as did the lone witness to the murder—an addict who was firing heroin inside the Harlem Avenue stash-house when the shooting began.

And on the following night, when word reached Rich Garvey that his victim had rolled a seven in University's intensive care unit, he responded in a fashion that most cops would find entirely excusable: he grabbed hold of Donald Kincaid and danced a brief, awkward jig around the homicide unit.

"Hey, Donald. He's gonna die," joked Garvey. "He's gonna die and we know who did it!"

The reaction of those who labor in University Hospital's emergency room is unrecorded, but given the ethics of modern medicine, it's probably safe to assume that veteran doctors and nurses managed a little more restraint.

And yet if Baltimore's trauma teams are less visceral than police detectives in their overt response to the senselessness of urban mayhem, they, nevertheless, share the same frustration. Both professions are being asked to cope with an inner-city drug culture that has grown far beyond the sanctions of our society. Both professions are expending precious money and manpower trying to cope with a small but increasingly violent population of drug offenders that exists at society's margins. The philosophical cul-de-sac for an inner-city surgeon is the same as that for an inner-city detective: If a drug dealer falls in west Baltimore and there's no one there to hear him, does he make a sound?

A crime reporter with the *Baltimore Sun,* I spent 1988 with the Baltimore Police Department's homicide unit to write a book about inner-city violence and death investigation. Granted police department identification and assigned to a shift of detectives, I followed Baltimore's best criminal investigators to crime scenes, autopsies, courtrooms, and, of course, the hospital emergency rooms that cope with much of the city's violence.

Not only did I witness the response of my city's emergency medical system to the ravages of the drug war, I was afforded the view of veteran homicide detectives—truly outsiders to the medical sphere. These are men who are unrepentant in their opinions of society, unbeholden to any sympathetic or therapeutic view of the men and women they police. And from that perspective, what they witness in places like Johns Hopkins or the University of Maryland Hospital is little less than amazing. Night after night, Baltimore's detectives watch some of their nation's best and most expensive medicine practiced on people who for the most part played a role in their own victimization, men and women who rarely, if ever, have health insurance, who will not pay for the medical interventions that keep them alive, and who, after recovery, will promptly return to the drug trade that left them shot, stabbed, or bludgeoned.

A little less than half of Baltimore's homicides in 1988 were directly related to narcotics trafficking; arguments were responsible for another 25% of the slayings, and a good many of those arguments occur between people under the influence of alcohol or narcotics. Stranger-to-stranger murders—those involving robbery, rape, or burglary—accounted for only 16% of the total. Given those statistics, it is safe to estimate that about seven of every 10 assault victims who arrive at a Baltimore hospital are in some way culpable in the violence that has incapacitated them. And yet, to the never-ending amazement of homicide detectives, a drug trafficker who arrives in the Johns Hopkins trauma unit to be treated for gunshot wounds for the third time in 2 years is assured the same quality of care as a truly innocent victim—a Real Victim, as a detective might say—unfortunate enough to be critically wounded in a downtown mugging.

Burdened by a spiraling caseload, homicide detectives in Baltimore are, of course, delighted with the fact that this medical intervention produces fewer murders. In 1988, almost as many people were seriously assaulted in Baltimore as in Washington, DC, which had the worst per capita murder rate in the nation that year. The telling difference between the two cities is that in Baltimore, aggravated assault victims survived their wounds far more often than victims in the District of Columbia, only 35 miles to the south. Low ambulance response time and citywide access to state-of-the-art emergency care has artificially reduced Baltimore's murder rate, so much so that if assault victims in Maryland's largest city had been subjected to Washington's mortality, it would have recorded 414 murders in 1988, rather than 234.

With a lesser emergency medical system, Baltimore would no doubt be competing with Washington for the dubious distinction of leading the nation in murder—a theory further proved by the fact that the city recorded its all-time record number of slayings in the early 1970s, before the citywide trauma system came on line. And yet, despite the best efforts of police and health care professionals alike, the murder rate in my city continues to rise. Last year, the police department recorded 305 murders; this year, the toll is running slightly ahead of that count.

But while the homicide detectives might be grateful to be dealing with fewer slayings, they are, nevertheless, confounded by a high quality of care for any and all trauma victims. This is a noble ethic, true—the Hippocratic oath defined, perhaps—and yet for the police officers who stand in the corridors of Baltimore's hospitals every night, it all seems profoundly absurd.

After all, the police department in which they serve began long ago to prioritize and categorize its growing workload. In Baltimore, where law enforcement can bring only limited resources to its investigations, most drug-related slayings will get the attention of a detective for a few days at most—only long enough to work the most obvious leads before a fresh homicide requires that detective's attention. In contrast, the robbery and murder of a truly innocent victim is likely to get the attention of two or more detectives for weeks or even months. In 1988, the rape-murder of an 11-year-old girl—as true a victim as an American detective might find—received the attention of an investigator for the entire year. Instinctively, homicide detectives—and by extension police officials, prosecutors, and judges—know which incidents will produce genuine concern in the community and therefore require the greatest resources and most intense effort. As a result, practical politics and institutional rationalizations in law enforcement produce Hobson's choices on a daily basis.

In emergency medicine, however, our cultural values, our very ideals, argue against qualitative judgments about many of the men and women who arrive in our nation's trauma centers every night. Law and ethics guarantee even the most unrepentant drug trafficker the absolute right to medicine's best efforts. And even if that guarantee was somehow voided, there is no practical way for hospital officials to discern, at the moment that ambulances arrive at the emergency room door, which of the wounded are truly victims in every sense of the word.

The result is, of course, known to the entire medical community. At least 80 inner-city hospitals have abandoned their emergency rooms in recent years as the costs of drug violence involving uninsured patients become unmanageable. In other hospitals, those costs are simply passed on to paying patients when government subsidies for uninsured care prove woefully inadequate. Meanwhile, with more and more patients arriving at the emergency rooms that remain operational, the quality of trauma care—for drug traffickers, innocent victims, those involved in common accidents—is at risk.

For 1 full year, I saw the dilemma defined in a thousand ways. I met addicts who staggered into the same emergency rooms twice a week to save themselves from overdoses, then staggered back to a shooting gallery—a migration so frequent that nurses and interns came to regard some of them as old acquaintances. I saw people shot dead after returning to the drug trade within days of being released from hospitals after prolonged, costly treatment for earlier assaults. Once, in October of that year, I saw a Johns Hopkins intern working on the chest of a young east Baltimore shooting victim when he suddenly recognized scars from a previous medical adventure.

"Wait a sec. Were you here before?" the surgeon asked the kid. "I remember you. I remember you being here for a shooting before."

Wincing beneath an oxygen mask, the kid nodded in agreement. Last year, he told the intern. It was surgery followed by months at a north Baltimore rehabilitation hospital.

"Who shot you the first time?" the intern asked.

The kid shook his head.

"Who shot you this time?"

The kid shook his head again.

"How long before you get shot again?" asked the intern, now irritated.

The kid shrugged. "It happens," he muttered.

Is there a solution? Probably not.

There is no back-door escape for emergency medicine as exists in law enforcement. When the police are overwhelmed, they simply work those cases that matter most and drop the drug-related incidents after an investigative shake or two. When our courts are overwhelmed, they plea bargain. When the prisons are overcrowded, the parole board simply changes its guidelines to free a few more of the less dangerous inmates and increase the available bed space.

One detective I followed mustered enough cynicism to suggest something similar at the trauma units:

"You hook up a police computer at the admitting station," he offered over a dinner of domestic beer one evening. "And if a guy comes in with gunshot wounds, you run his sheet and see what kind of priors he has. Then you run him through the hospital computer and see how many times he's been treated there. If you have three confirmed drug-related episodes, you kick his ass out the emergency room door. I'm serious. Let him bleed to death."

An unlikely solution, but then again, police detectives are a unique breed. Cops become cops for a variety of reasons, but most of them share an ability to view the world in pure black-and-white; gray areas need not apply. Still, it would be hard to find an emergency room in Baltimore where some beleaguered resident or charge nurse has not on occasion entertained similar fantasies about a few particular patients.

No, there won't be any back doors for our urban hospitals, particularly given the federal prohibitions regarding patient transfers. By definition, our emergency rooms are all prisoners of 911.

And yet it seems to me that medicine has something to learn from the detectives who stand on its fringe. Blunt and uncompromising, most cops have little problem saying exactly what they think, exactly when they think it. In contrast, it seems that the medical profession has been talking around the edges of its dilemma for years now, bemoaning the high costs of violence, urging higher government subsidy, and quietly burying the remaining red ink in the bills of paying patients.

Perhaps we've reached that point where it pays to be blunt, even rude. Perhaps every itemized hospital bill should make it unequivocally clear to the consumer that he or she is payingdirectly some of the costs of our national drug policy, our high-end economic priorities, our failure to rebuild the cities. What response would there be—from individuals, from government—if every hospital bill identified graphically not only the costs of servicing the individual patient, but the amount of subsidy required to service not only the indigent and uninsured—as is appropriate—but those men and women who have given their lives over to drugs and brutality?

Perhaps such an honest assessment would lead to more practical solutions, perhaps not. But the drug epidemic is not going to disappear, and either way, a detective might say, it's going to have to get ugly. To speak out on this issue is to place on the bargaining table some of our oldest and dearest medical ethics. To remain silent is to place all of our urban medical systems and their standard of care at great risk. To a detective, at least, the choice seems obvious.

David Simon*
Baltimore, Md

*David Simon, a reporter for the *Baltimore Sun,* is the author of *Homicide: A Year on the Killing Streets,* published by Houghton Mifflin Co.

A Commentary on Violence

Twenty years ago, trauma to the face, head, and neck regions was primarily due to motor vehicle accidents, occupational and sports injuries, and the occasional altercation. Over the past two decades there has been an alarming escalation in domestic and interpersonal violence that now appears to be the main cause of maxillofacial trauma. Much of the trauma is alcohol or drug related and will often involve members of the same family, whether related by blood or by marriage. Such an observation reflects poorly on the strength and stability of the family unit and directs our attention to the proper target of our rehabilitation efforts—the improvement of the family unit integrity.

As the availability of drugs increases in our society, coupled with the generally depressed economy and high unemployment, drug-related violence, whether it is associated with the sale of drugs or the use of drugs, has developed as an outward sign of this pollution in our society. While most Americans, including those of us in the medical profession, would probably not feel too compassionate about drug dealers committing violent crimes against themselves (since it is a form of self-destruction), all are concerned about the near-innocent or innocent victims of these crimes. How often have we seen family members or innocent bystanders caught in the crossfire or fallout of a drug deal gone sour or injured as a result of a drug-induced craze?

Beatings, gunshot wounds, and stabbings all occur in the world of drug- and alcohol-related events. And, of more sobering influence, is the knowledge that it is not only the "criminal element" of the society who is involved in the incidents but also those people who engage in the daily productive machinery of America—lawyers, physicians, teachers. While violence is not as common in the latter groups, the fact that some utilize drugs perpetuates the need for the more unsavory elements.

Thus, it is a problem from which there is no escaping by the physician, particularly for those who treat the victims, both innocent and presumed guilty, and for those with a strong social conscience. Caring for the trauma victim is not the real challenge for us—we are competent professionally to handle any type of maxillofacial and head and neck trauma, whether by single practitioners or by a team effort. We have the skills and technology. *What is the difficult challenge* is the involvement by the physician in the process of rehabilitating the broken segment of society that is the origin of the problem itself—the inadequate family unit!

Gang-related violence is on the upswing. In large urban centers across the country, we are seeing more drive-by shootings, more beatings of innocent young people, and more attacks on brothers and sisters of suspected rival gang members. The weapons of this violence vary from knives and guns to boots and baseball bats. The head, face, and neck are particularly vulnerable targets. The attacks are cowardly and driven by peer pressure of other gang members to conform to their "rituals of initiation." Such acts result from a basic weakness in the development of strong personal and societal integrity and moral standards and in the failure to instill a sense of responsibility and honor in these young people. To many of them, "honor" lies in the act of violence and in going to jail as a "Badge of Courage." This mentality must be changed and basic human values and a respect for life must be reinstilled in today's youth.

The third significant problem we as physicians face today is the rising incidence of child and spousal abuse. These heinous acts of violence are seen across the entire spectrum of society, not just in lower-class, urban families. Who has not been personally outraged and angered when called in to the hospital to care for a child or a wife who has sustained blows to the head and face as a result of a parental or spousal beating? It almost makes one want to inflict the same damage on the perpetrator. However, our personal feelings notwithstanding, we must objectively understand the causes of the violent acts and develop a professional plan to improve the situation at the very heart of the problem—the family unit. Although there may be extenuating circumstances or confounding factors present, such as pressures at work, financial woes, infidelity, drugs and alcohol, the *basic* problem is the failure of the family unit to work together to help the member through the difficult times and to continue to face tribulations together. We, as facial surgeons, can piece the injuries back together quite well, in most circumstances. However, unless we take action to heal the underlying emotional injuries, we have done only part of our job. We must be cognizant of the psychosocial dynamics of the trauma victims' lives and involve ourselves and other professionals in their improvement. It is simply not enough to repair the facial injuries and discharge the patient. Violence within families tends to repeat itself unless some positive intervention occurs. It is the responsibility of the otolaryngologist–head and neck surgeon, as with all other physicians caring for victims of violence, to make an effort to do whatever can be done to improve the conditions in the family that led to the violent act. To *not* do so is to fail to completely care for our patients.

What else can be done by the physician in the cases of alcohol-, drug-, and gang-related violence? In addition to improving the family dynamics of the individual patient, the physician *must* become involved in community affairs, working with the schools, churches, support groups, and even the police, to provide a more positive community action and opportunities for rehabilitation of wayward individuals. The physician must become a recognized leader in, and contributor to, the return of the values of honesty, integrity, and respect to the family unit. For only with the teaching of the proper moral values to the youth today by the family, school, and other societal units can we hope to eventually curb and reverse the trend toward violence in America today.

G. Richard Holt, MD, MSE, MPH
President, The American Academy of Otolaryngology–Head and Neck Surgery Inc

Reprint requests to Suite 206, 12709 Toepperwein Rd, San Antonio, TX 78233 (Dr Holt).

Editorial Introduction

Otolaryngologists are well aware of the underrecognition that exists with regard to physical and acoustic trauma to the ear and surrounding temporal bone. By virtue of the important sensory, neural, and vascular structures housed within the temporal bone, trauma to this region can produce a broad constellation of symptoms, many of which bear heavily on an individual's ability to conduct everyday activities and effectively communicate. Temporal bone trauma frequently compromises the quality of life, cancels human productivity, and may be associated with loss of life. This form of violence causes injury that carries immeasurable costs to society at large, and considerable psychosocial impact on the victim.

Awareness of the problem of noise exposure in young adult populations has been slow to evolve. While the notion of staying "forever young" is prevalent in our society, young adults as a whole have only recently recognized that noise exposure accelerates the process of sensorineural degeneration. Initiatives by organizations such as the American Academy of Otolaryngology–Head and Neck Surgery appear to be succeeding in bringing about this awareness.

In many ways, trauma to the ear and surrounding temporal bone symbolizes the implications of violence in general. As otolaryngologists, we are confronted with patients who suffer hearing loss, vertigo, tinnitus, facial paralysis, cerebrospinal fluid leaks, and other indicators of acoustic and physical trauma to the temporal bone and its neural elements. In this commentary Dr Kinney surveys the vast array of mechanisms by which the temporal bone and inner ear can be traumatized. The true costs of such trauma, although incalculable, are readily apparent, as is the need for innovative solutions to the problem of violence in our society.

John Niparko, MD
Baltimore, Md

Violence and the Ear and Temporal Bone

Violence in our society frequently is directed toward our ability to hear as well as other functions related to the temporal bone. Important sensory and motor nerves as well as vascular structures traverse the temporal bone. Trauma to the temporal bone may impair the person's ability to perform everyday functions, also limiting the ability to communicate. The result of temporal bone trauma may have a significant effect on the victim's socioeconomic status.

Violence is defined by *Webster's Third New International Dictionary* as "exertion of any physical force so as to injure or abuse."[1] The purpose of this commentary will be to apply this definition of violence to the ear and temporal bone.

The physical forces that affect the ear and temporal bone may be separated into two categories. The first category is direct trauma to the ear or temporal bone, and the second category is acoustic trauma to the ear.

The temporal bone is located in the midposterior portion of the skull base. It contains otic capsule bone, the most dense bone of the human skeleton. The anatomy of the temporal bone involves numerous structures and functions other than hearing that may be involved with a violent act. The major vascular structures to the brain and head, the carotid artery and jugular vein, course through the temporal bone. The lower cranial nerves VI through XI have direct relationships to the temporal bone. The most frequent cranial nerve to be affected by violence to the temporal bone is the facial nerve.

Violent acts are usually perpetrated by one human against another. The most common of these occurs in the domestic situation. Not infrequently an open hand is used to strike the side of a person's head. This act may have a direct effect on the ear. There may be soft-tissue injury to the pinna; however, the most physical injury occurs if the hand causes a compression injury to the ear canal. The compression force may be sufficient to rupture the tympanic membrane. The tear most often occurs in the anterior or posterior inferior quadrant of the membrane. Most often there is a linear tear, but the tear may be triangular. The injury is painful and may be associated with bleeding and hearing loss. The physician should examine the ear carefully and remove any blood clots.

The opening in the tympanic membrane is examined carefully. If a straight edge is seen in the opening, this may represent a folded piece of the membrane. If possible, this folded piece of membrane should be teased back to its anatomic position. The injury may be stented by a circle of fine-grain paper to assist healing. Dry perforations should not be treated with drops. Ninety percent of traumatic perforations of the tympanic membrane will heal spontaneously. However, it may take 3 to 4 months for healing to be complete.

In addition to injury to the tympanic membrane from an open hand injury, there may be an effect on the inner ear. The compression may be sufficiently great to cause injury to the round window membrane, the annulus of the oval window, or the ossicular chain. When first examined, the patient should be questioned about a sensation of vertigo. The patient's eyes should be examined carefully for the presence of nystagmus. A patient who has been exposed to tympanic membrane trauma and has nystagmus has a true otologic emergency. This patient needs the attention of an otolaryngology–head and neck surgeon capable of exploration of the middle ear.

An audiogram should be performed to assess injury to the ossicles and inner ear. This does not need to be performed as an emergency. A conductive hearing loss greater than 20 dB may indicate an ossicular injury. Because of the acute nature of a middle ear injury surgery to correct an ossicular problem is best delayed until hemorrhage and mucosal reactivity has resolved, usually after 6 weeks.

The presence of a sensorineural hearing loss may be the result of an inner ear concussion. However, it may be the result of a tear in the round window membrane or oval window annulus. The otolaryngology–head and neck surgeon must make a judgment using the history, physical findings, and test results to determine the advisability of middle ear exploration for fistula.

The next level of violence to affect the ear and temporal bone is a mechanical force sufficiently great to fracture some portion of the temporal bone or even the otic capsule bone itself. A useful reference for consideration of a fracture of the otic capsule is an automobile accident at 65 mph. This reference is helpful when considering trauma to the head and the possibility of an otic capsule fracture.

Trauma sufficient to fracture the temporal bone is seen in two general categories. In the first category the head is thrown against an unmovable object such as in an automobile accident. The second is a missile directed toward the head such as a bullet from a gun. Although the first category is more common, the category of a missile directed toward the head is most often seen in a situation of violence.

When the skull is directed toward an immobile object, a number of injuries may occur. There may be soft-tissue injuries as well as injuries to the brain contents of the skull. In this type of injury rarely is there direct trauma to the temporal bone; rather, the point of contact would be the frontal bone, parietal bone, or occipital bone. There may be an effect on the temporal bone from a fracture that begins in one of these areas.

The fracture begins at a point of impact and travels toward the temporal bone. There it takes a course of least resistance. The most likely course will involve the carotid artery and the foramen lacerum. This course takes the fracture very close or through the geniculate ganglion.

The patient sustaining skull trauma should be examined carefully. Particular attention should be paid to the ear and temporal bone. Bleeding from the ear or blood in the middle ear is clinical evidence of a skull base fracture. A bony defect in the ear canal is also evidence of a temporal bone fracture. An attempt must be made to assess and record facial nerve function at the time of the initial examination. The physician must try to observe voluntary movement of the facial nerve. A patient lying supine in bed will have complete eye closure for upward of 48 hours after complete transection of the facial nerve. Therefore, a closed eye does not mean there is no injury to the facial nerve.

Temporal bone fractures are generally classified into longitudinal or transverse fractures. In reality the fractures can occur in most any imaginable direction of the skull base. Fractures that cross the internal auditory canal or otic capsule result in loss of auditory and vestibular function as well as a facial nerve injury.

Routine skull roentgenograms are no longer adequate to look for skull base fractures. A high-resolution computed tomographic scan with a bone algorithm should be obtained to identify a temporal bone fracture. The computed tomographic scan may be valuable to assess a fracture seen months or years after an injury. Dense otic capsule bone has a relatively poor blood supply and fractures often do not heal and may be seen years after the injury.

Treatment of temporal bone fractures begins with the stabilization of the intracranial injury, which is almost always present. Facial nerve injuries are managed after the risk of intracranial injury has passed.

A partial facial nerve paralysis is treated expectantly with an excellent prognosis for complete recovery. A total facial nerve paralysis must be evaluated by the history of onset and the computed tomographic scan. Traumatic facial nerve paralysis recovery is often benefited by surgical exploration and decompression and/or repair. The surgery to be performed is determined by the status of the inner ear function. The operating surgeon must remember that the facial nerve is often injured in more than one location. It courses the temporal bone, and the surgeon must be prepared to explore the entire nerve, including the labyrinthine portion to the internal auditory canal.

The most common trauma to the temporal bone by a missile is from a gunshot. In a close violent confrontation the assailant frequently points the gun to the side of the head or at the temporal bone. Even self-inflicted violence from a gunshot is directed toward the temporal bone.

A gunshot wound to the temporal bone most often results in instant death. However, because of the density of the temporal bone and the ballistic characteristics of the bullet, death may not be instant, and considerable injury may result to the temporal bone and adjacent structures. High-velocity copper-coated bullets tend to shatter the temporal bone. However, low-velocity lead bullets may only imbed into the skull base.

The patient sustaining a gunshot to the skull base needs to be stabilized intracranially. When possible a complete otolaryngology–head and neck examination is performed. Particular attention is paid to the cranial nerve function. Any cranial nerve deficit demands close attention to the status of adjacent structures. Particular attention is paid to the function of the IX, X, and XI cranial nerves because of their location within the neural compartment of the jugular bulb adjacent to the carotid artery. Studies of the vascular structures with digital subtraction angiography or conventional angiography must be performed.

Unfortunately, most of the cranial nerve injuries to the skull base from a gunshot wound will not recover, although the facial nerve can be repaired with good return of function. The most common skull base surgery to be performed following a gunshot to the ear and temporal bone will be to repair a major vascular injury.

Spinal fluid leaks following temporal bone trauma are common. The leak may exit the ear canal or pass through the eustachian tube to the nasopharynx. The risk of intracranial infection from a spinal fluid leak is apparent. Most leaks will close spontaneously. However, if the leak persists and surgical intervention is deemed necessary, consideration should be given to exploration of the ear and mastoid to identify the point of the leak with major intracranial exploration performed after the point of the leak has been identified.

Acoustic trauma to the ear presents a different type of physical force than noted in the previous sections of this commentary. It is here that the last word of the *Webster's* definition of violence is important. Although violence is a major social concern, it is sometimes difficult to determine when a physical force, such as an acoustic force, becomes abusive.

There is no doubt that extensive acoustic forces can injure or destroy inner ear function. Fortunately, the industrial complex is aware of this problem, and governmental agencies are attempting to regulate the noise exposure of a person in the workplace.

Unfortunately, there has been and still exists a pop culture of self-inflicted acoustic trauma in the younger generation. This group of young adults is just beginning to recognize that noise may prematurely produce degeneration of the sensorineural component of the auditory system. This is a form of self-inflicted violence. Public service programs to warn people of the effect of too-loud music are growing and are necessary.

Freedom and the rights of individuals are two of the most precious of all human experiences. However, society must decide when the rights of one individual infringe on the rights of another individual.

To this end, the question of acoustic violence must be addressed. The excessively loud playing of powerful personal radios in public can be abusive and considered an act of violence. Of greater concern is the excessive intensity of sound surrounding an individual operating a moving vehicle. The masking effect of too-loud sound renders the operator of the vehicle unable to react to the warning of an outside sound that might prevent an accident. There have been reports of massive sound systems in private vehicles causing violent injury or death to children in neighborhoods.

Violence in its many forms can have a major effect on the ear and the temporal bone. The socioeconomic and psychosocial effects of trauma to the temporal bone are significant. When thinking about violence and its effect on the ear and temporal bone, physicians and patients must remember the definition of violence: "exertion of any physical force so as to injure or abuse."

SAM E. KINNEY, MD
Section of Otology and Neurotology
Department of Otolaryngology and Communicative Disorders
The Cleveland Clinic Foundation
9500 Euclid Ave
Cleveland, OH 44195-5034

Reference

1. Gove PE, ed. *Webster's Third New International Dictionary*. Springfield, Mass: A & C Merriam Co Publishers; 1966:2554.

Physical Abuse of Children

A Retrospective Review and an Otolaryngology Perspective

Jay P. Willging, MD; Charles M. Bower, MD; Robin T. Cotton, MD

• Child abuse is a common problem seen by practicing physicians. To further define the incidence and the type of head and neck injury in children referred for evaluation of child abuse, a 5-year retrospective study of 4340 patients was undertaken. Of these patients, 2950 (68%) were victims of sexual abuse, while 1390 (32%) were victims of physical abuse. Forty-nine percent of patients abused physically had evidence of injury to the head and neck region, while only 1% of the sexually abused children had injuries in the head and neck area. The age of the patients ranged from 1 day to 17 years, with a mean of 5.6 years. More than 150 of these children were under the age of 1 year; 180 patients were admitted. The average age of the admitted patients was 2.1 years. The alleged perpetrator, mechanism of injury, and location of injury were tabulated. There were 11 deaths in the series (1.6%). Child abuse has been defined in our institution as *any injury inflicted* on a child. Identification and reporting of suspected child abuse is required by law and essential for the well-being of the abused child. Recommendations are made concerning the evaluation of these children, their management, and the physician's legal responsibility to report suspected cases of child abuse.

(*Arch Otolaryngol Head Neck Surg.* 1992;118:584-590)

The typical otolaryngologist's practice is composed of a large proportion of children. Because of the volume of children that are treated annually in any given office, the potential for encountering a child who is the victim of child abuse is high. It is mandatory that all physicians having contact with children be familiar with the common signs of, and risk factors for child abuse. In the United States, more than 2 million abuse cases involving children were reported in 1984.[1] Most of these cases occurred at the hands of one of the parents. Homicide is one of the top five causes of childhood death, accounting for 5% of all childhood deaths to the age of 18 years. Child abuse is the number one cause of death in the age group 6 to 12 months.[2]

Accepted for publication February 28, 1992.

From the Department of Pediatric Otolaryngology and Maxillofacial Surgery, Children's Hospital Medical Center, Cincinnati, Ohio.

Reprint requests to Department of Pediatric Otolaryngology and Maxillofacial Surgery, Children's Hospital Medical Center, Elland and Bethesda avenues, Cincinnati, OH 45229-2899 (Dr Willging).

The American Society to Prevent Cruelty to Children was founded in 1875. Awareness of this national problem remained low until Kempe et al[3] published the landmark article in 1962 describing child abuse as a medically recognizable condition, the battered child syndrome.[3] In 1974, the National Center for Child Abuse and Neglect was founded to promote research and public understanding of the problem of child abuse. The number of reported cases of child abuse continues to rise.

In our series, 1% of all children seen in the Children's Hospital Medical Center (Cincinnati, Ohio) emergency department had nonaccidental injuries. The risk of continued harm to the child is real and potentially lethal. Most childhood deaths from abuse have come after a pattern of abuse has developed. It is paramount that all cases of suspected abuse be reported to proper authorities for the welfare of the child as well as for the legal protection of the physician.

The number of victims of child abuse seen by practicing otolaryngologists has not been well defined nor has the role of the otolaryngologist been adequately established. The purpose of this article is to more accurately reflect the demographics of patients with abuse and to further define the spectrum of otolaryngologic injury of these patients. A retrospective review of 5 years' experience was therefore undertaken.

MATERIALS AND METHODS

We reviewed the records of all patients referred to the social service department for evaluation of suspected child abuse or neglect or suspected sexual abuse from January 1, 1986, through December 31, 1989, a period of 5 years. This group of patients initially was selected from emergency department encounters. Over the 5-year period, 379 348 children were seen in the emergency department at Children's Hospital Medical Center. Of these patients, 4340 (1.14%) were referred to the social services department for evaluation of suspected physical or sexual abuse; 1390 patients (32%) were victims of physical abuse, while 2950 (68%) were victims of sexual abuse. Children were referred to social services when there was documented evidence of injury, including neglect type of injuries, inflicted on a child. Referral was at the discretion of the attending physician in the emergency department at the time the child was seen. An attempt was not made to select children as victims of abuse based on the motive or intent of the perpetrator. This is a relatively broad definition of abuse; however, it is very justifiable as all of these children manifested injury at the hand of another person.

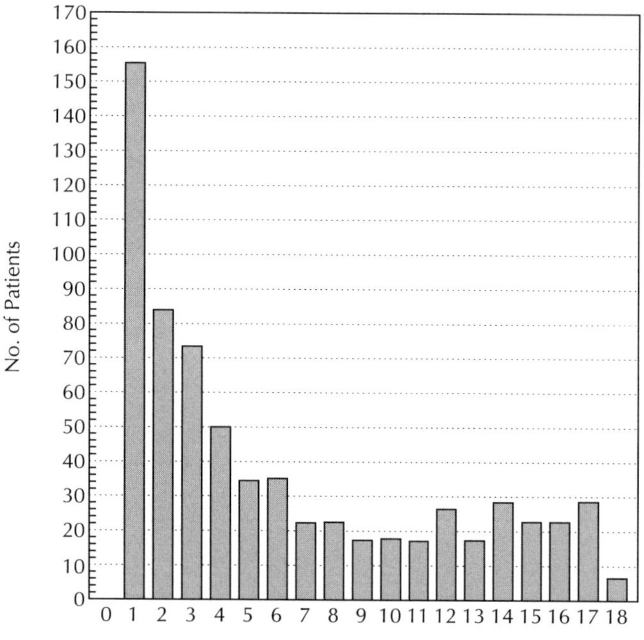

Age (in years) of victims on date of examination.

Once a referral to social services was made, all patients and families were evaluated by a social worker and a physician. The history surrounding the incident, alleged perpetrator, physical evaluation of the child, any supporting laboratory or roentgenographic evidence of injury, and disposition of the child was documented on a social services form. The data involved in this article were generated by review of the social services' forms over this 5-year period. A record was made for any child with manifestations of injury or abuse in the head and neck region. An attempt was made to decide whether this injury was a primary otolaryngologic process bringing the child to the emergency department for evaluation or an associated problem. The area and type of injury in the head and neck as well as associated regions was documented. The mechanism of injury, where delineated, was also documented. Operative procedures performed by an otolaryngologist were also tabulated.

The subsequent data were collected on DataEase 4.2 (DataEase International Inc, Trumbull, Conn) and analyzed by routine statistical methods.

RESULTS

Of the 379 348 patients evaluated in the emergency department over the 5-year period of the study, 4340 patients (1.14%) were referred for evaluation by social services for suspected abuse; 1390 patients (32%) were victims of physical abuse, while 2950 (68%) were referred for evaluation of sexual abuse. Of the 1390 physical abuse patients, 641 (49%) had evidence of injury to the head and neck, and 38 (1%) of the sexually abused children had head and neck injuries. The age of patients ranged from 1 day to 17.9 years with a mean of 5.6 years of age (Figure); 364 (54%) of these patients were male while 312 (46%) were female; and 49% of the patients were black, 49% of the patients were white, while less than 1% were Hispanic, or other race or nationality. The primary complaint and injury compelling referral to social services was located in the head and neck region in 555 (82%) of these patients, while the head and neck injury was associated with another more significant injury in 18%. Only 180 patients (27%) were admitted to the hospital for further evaluation, while 490 (72%) were treated as outpatients.

Table 1.—Alleged Perpetrator of Child Abuse

Perpetrator	No. (%)
Mother	175 (26)
Father	127 (19)
Parents	39 (6)
Mother's boyfriend	61 (9)
Father's girlfriend	3 (1)
Stepmother	10 (2)
Stepfather	36 (5)
Aunt	6 (1)
Uncle	15 (2)
Sibling	14 (2)
Neighbor	
Adult	5 (1)
Child	8 (1)
Babysitter	39 (6)
Related to sitter	5 (1)
Paid caregiver	4 (1)
Friend	15 (2)
Cousin	4 (1)
Grandparent	8 (1)
School personnel	4 (1)
Unknown	99 (15)

As might be expected, when the average age was calculated in the subgroups of inpatients vs outpatients, those patients admitted to the hospital were much younger. The average age of those admitted to the hospital was 2.1 years, while the average age of the remainder of the patients was 6.9 years. The reason that abuse was suspected and accidental injury excluded was provided by the history of the parents or caregivers in 73% of the cases. A significant discrepancy between the history and the sustained injury resulted in a suspicion of child abuse in 161 patients (24%). In 3% of patients, suspicions of abuse were raised because the mechanism of the injury was unclear, or there was inappropriate activity between the child and parents. In the majority of cases, the mother was the alleged perpetrator of the injury. This was followed in frequency by the father, the mother's boyfriend, parents, babysitters, stepfather, and a variety of other persons (Table 1).

The mechanism of the injury was a blow by a hand in 40% of these children, followed in frequency by a blow with an object (22%) and falls (19%). Shaken baby syndrome was noted in 38 patients (6%). Injury caused by burns, neglect, kicking, endangerment, falls, and asphyxia were less common (Table 2). The mechanism of injury was not apparent in 131 patients (19%).

Injury to the face and scalp predominated the type of abuse noted (89% of children). Ocular and periorbital injury (27%) and neck injury (11%) were noted less commonly, followed by trauma to the lips, central nervous system, ears, nose, and oral cavity (Table 3). When divided into types of injuries, the majority were ecchymoses or abrasions, accounting for 62% and 15% of injuries, respectively. Lacerations, fractures, hematomas or hemorrhages, and burns or blunt trauma were encoun-

Table 2.—Mechanism of Child Abuse*

Mechanism	Patients, No. (%)
Blow	
Hand	271 (40)
Foot	16 (2)
Object	150 (22)
Fall	93 (14)
Burn	31 (5)
Neglect	26 (4)
Endangerment	12 (2)
Bite	
Human	8 (1)
Animal	1 (. . .)
Hair pull	4 (1)
Sexual assault	38 (6)
Shaken baby syndrome	36 (6)
Asphyxia/hypoxia	8 (1)
Unknown	131 (19)
Munchausen's by proxy	0 (0)

*Children (679) with injuries to the head and neck area.

Table 3.—Location of Head and Neck Injury

Area	Injuries, No. (%)
Eyes	66 (10)
Periorbital	79 (12)
Ears	42 (6)
Nose	37 (5)
Lips	59 (9)
Face	435 (64)
Cranium	166 (25)
Neck	105 (16)
Oral cavity	15 (2)
Nasopharynx	3 (. . .)
Central nervous system	51 (8)

tered less frequently (Table 4). The majority of lacerations occurred on the lips and face; however, when an injury was noted in the oral cavity, oropharynx, and nasopharynx, the majority of these injuries were lacerations. Of the 57 fractures, the majority (81%) were skull fractures. Only four nasal fractures, three periorbital fractures, two other facial fractures, and two neck fractures were identified in this series. Thirty-three burns were encountered and the majority occurred on the face (48%). Other burns were noted to be distributed on the neck, the cranium, the lips and nose, and around the eyes.

In patients with head and neck injuries, a significant number of injuries were noted throughout the rest of the body. Associated injuries to the upper and lower extremities occurred in 160 and 154 children, respectively. This was followed in frequency by injury to the back in 121 children, to the chest in 92 children, to the buttocks in 86 children, and to the abdomen in 64 children. Oxygen deprivation was noted in eight children. Forced use or excess use of drugs was noted in eight children, while alcohol use was noted in two children with head and neck injuries.

An attempt was made to differentiate between inpatient and outpatient demographics and injury; 180 children were admitted vs 490 outpatients; and 55% of admitted patients were male, while 45% were female. Of those patients admitted, the average age was 2.1 years as opposed to an age of 6.9 years for the outpatient population; 45% of the admitted patients were black while 55% were white. In the outpatient population, these numbers were 51% and 49%, respectively. Evidence of significant central nervous system injury was present more commonly in the admitted patients. Ten children admitted to the hospital had evidence of central nervous system injury, including intracranial hemorrhage in 10 and hypoxia in three. Only one patient had any evidence of central nervous system injury treated as an outpatient.

Although the follow-up on these children was somewhat limited, the majority did not require significant intervention by an otolaryngologist. Closure of lacerations and cleaning of wounds were the main treatment provided on an outpatient basis. As mentioned previously, admission to the hospital for evaluation and treatment was required in 180 children. At least five of these children required intensive care unit observation for a period of time. Three children were pronounced dead on arrival at the emergency department.

Eleven deaths were identified during the study period from injuries associated with head and neck trauma (1.6%). One child was the victim of a rape, the remaining 10 sustained injuries by the direct action of a parent, or secondary to parental neglect. The range of ages of fatalities from abuse was 3 months to 8 years, with a median age of 1.5 years. Seven (64%) of these 11 patients were male, while 36% were female.

Head trauma significant enough to cause intracranial hemorrhage, brain edema, and herniation occurred in nine patients. Severe abdominal injuries associated with head trauma occurred in five patients. Asphyxiation occurred in two cases.

Two of the 11 families had contact with Children's Protective Services at least once in the past. One family was in counseling for previous abuse against the deceased child. One family had the children placed in foster care for several years until domestic problems were resolved, at which point the children were returned to parental custody. Significant family disorganization and a history of previous abuse must be viewed as significant risk factors for continued abuse, possibly leading to fatality.

COMMENT

Child abuse is an increasingly common problem seen by practicing physicians. More than 1% of patients seen in a busy emergency department in this series were referred to social services for evaluation of suspected child abuse (physical or sexual). Of these patients, 15% had injuries noted within the head and neck region. Otolaryngologists, therefore, must be aware of the typical signs and symptoms of child abuse, be able to recognize this disorder, be prepared to treat patients with significant injuries from child abuse, and know the appropriate evaluation and referral mechanisms available in their local area to care for children who are victims of child abuse.

Fortunately from the otolaryngologist's perspective, the majority of injuries to the head and neck region are benign; 62% of the injuries noted were ecchymoses, while 15% were abrasions, which required little more than rou-

Table 4.—Number of Injuries by Site and Type*

Site	Total	Ecchymosis	Abrasion	Lacerations	Burn	Hemorrhage	Foreign Body	Fracture	Blunt Trauma
Eyes	66	21 (37)	10 (15)	3 (0.5)	1 . . .	36 (55)	0 0	0 . . .	0 . . .
Periorbital	79	70 (89)	6 (8)	6 (8)	0 . . .	0 . . .	0 . . .	3 (0.4)	0 . . .
Ears	42	32 (76)	6 (14)	2 (5)	1 2	0 . . .	0 . . .	0 . . .	37 (88)
Nose	37	27 (73)	5 (14)	3 (8)	3 8	0 . . .	0 . . .	4 (11)	0 . . .
Lips	59	29 (49)	18 (31)	17 (29)	3 (51)	0 . . .	0 . . .	0 . . .	0 . . .
Face	435	375 (86)	77 (17)	23 (5)	15 (3)	0 . . .	0 . . .	2 (0.5)	1 . . .
Cranium	166	103 (62)	15 (9)	16 (10)	5 (3)	14 (8)	0 . . .	46 (28)	2 (1)
Neck	105	74 (70)	34 (32)	5 (5)	5 (5)	0 . . .	0 . . .	2 (2)	0 . . .
Oral cavity	15	3 (20)	2 (13)	7 (46)	0 . . .	0 . . .	0 . . .	0 . . .	0 . . .
Nasopharynx	3	0 . . .	0 . . .	2 (67)	0 . . .	0 . . .	0 . . .	0 . . .	0 . . .
Central nervous system	51	0 . . .	0 . . .	0 . . .	0 . . .	11 (21)	0 . . .	0 . . .	0 . . .
Total	**1058**	**734** (62)	**173** (15)	**84** (7)	**33** (3)	**61** (5)	**0** (0)	**57** (5)	**40** (3)

*Numbers in parentheses indicate percent. Percentages do not add up correctly due to unclassified injuries and multiple injuries per patient. More than one injury may occur per site. The total number of injuries was 1182; the total number of patients was 679.

tine wound care. Eighty-four lacerations were noted. Many of these required simple wound care only or closure in the emergency department. More significantly, however, 57 patients were seen with fractures in the head and neck region. Burns to the head and neck region were also reasonably common and were identified in 33 patients. Eleven fatalities were noted in this series, resulting from severe abdominal and closed head trauma in the majority of cases. The potential for escalation of the severity of abuse necessitates prompt intervention to stop the cycle of abuse.

An association of head and neck injuries with other injuries of the trunk and extremities was quite common in these children suspected of child abuse. The importance of a good general physical evaluation in any patient presenting with head and neck trauma, especially of unclear or inconsistent cause, cannot be overemphasized.

Definition of Abuse

It is very difficult to define child abuse. Approximately 90% of families in the United States use physical punishment as a method of discipline.[4] The right of parents to discipline their children is rooted deeply in our culture. Religious beliefs continue to complicate the matter of child abuse. For example, faith healing remains a common practice in many areas, with the refusal of routine medical care and often lifesaving medical intervention for the children. Cultural practices must also be evaluated in proper context. The piercing of earlobes is one such common practice that may be viewed as a form of unnecessary mutilation and, therefore, child abuse.

Where do parental rights, religious freedoms, and cultural norms stop and child abuse or child neglect begin? There is no consensus. One end of the spectrum abhors any type of physical violence directed toward a child. The other end of the spectrum condones graduated physical discipline that increases in intensity with the behavioral transgression. The adopted definition of child abuse must be sufficiently vague as to allow interpretation by local standards, yet be exclusive enough to define behavior that clearly is detrimental to the child's well-being. The definition of abuse used at the Children's Hospital Medical Center emergency department is *any injury inflicted* on a child. This very broad definition misses very few abuses but requires a large number of social service evaluations.

Interpretation will vary as to whether an individual act can be construed as child abuse. The physician is currently caught in this dilemma. Although any particular physician may feel a mode of punishment is inappropriate as a disciplinary means, he or she may not go so far as to feel it is actually abuse.[5] Every physician will need to determine in advance how to deal with a given situation, where the line of delineation exists between discipline and abuse. It is important that parental intention not be considered when looking at a given action, as it is inappropriate for a child to be abused "for his own good." It is noteworthy that the bulk of abuse cases reported by physicians are from younger physicians. The addition of child abuse to the medical student and residency training programs appears to have set some norms against which cases can be compared. It is imperative that continuing education courses address this important issue such that uniformity of reporting can be obtained.

While children are certainly prone to accidents, and presentation to emergency department with injuries sustained in these "accidents" is common, child abuse is a cause that should always be considered during the evaluation of an injured child. Certain injuries and certain patterns of injuries, furthermore, are often consistent with child abuse necessitating evaluation for this abuse.[4] Signs of child abuse can be plainly evident or very subtle. It is important to look for signs of past injury, regardless of the primary reason for the child presenting to the physician for examination.

A physician should examine a given injury and attempt to determine if it is an accidental or an inflicted injury. There is no specific test or questionnaire available to differentiate these two conditions.[6] A detailed history both from the parent and the child is vital to any assessment of child abuse. Seventy-three percent of patients in our series gave a history consistent with an abusive act. The caregivers may give fabricated histories because of embarrassment or fear of punishment. The injury must then be evaluated in the context of the obtained history. Otolaryngologists receive adequate training in trauma to accurately determine whether a given injury could develop in accordance with the given history. If any discrepancy exists between the history and the observed injury, child abuse should be highly suspected. In our series, nearly 25% of cases were identified on the basis of this discrepancy. For example, a child presents to the emergency department with a subcondylar fracture and a history of falling off his bike onto the pavement. On examination, there is a bruise in the contralateral parasymphyseal area and no abrasions anywhere on the face, mandible, or extremities. Because of the lack of expected associated injuries, the likelihood of child abuse is very high.

Physicians should learn to recognize the pattern and distribution of ecchymosis and erythema secondary to injuries sustained from common objects.[4,7] For example, a slap from an open hand to the face commonly shows multiple parallel marks. Marks resulting from belts and looped cords will have single or multiple apparently random marks depending on the direction of the blows at the time of contact. Any mark that has a regular geometric design is almost always the result of child abuse. Burns will also leave very characteristic lesions that must be explained.

Any time the suspicion of child abuse is entertained, the children must undergo a complete physical examination.[1,7] The entire body must be examined for other signs of child abuse. Multiple bruises of various ages are classic for an abused child. Skeletal roentgenograms of the extremities and chest may be indicated in the young child to document previous fractures in various states of healing.[8]

The child's behavior can suggest a potential problem and should be noted on entering the examination room.[1,9] Although behavior is an unreliable sign as an isolated indicator of abuse, when taken in context with the remainder of the history and physical examination, it may suggest a problem.

Infants are susceptible to severe intracranial injury when shaken vigorously. Due to poor head control and relative fragility of the intracranial bridging vessels, bilateral subdural hematomas and hemorrhagic retinopathy occur as a result of this acceleration injury.[10] Thirty-six cases of shaken babies were identified in our series over the 5-year study period. There is usually no sign of external trauma. When the triad of subdural hematoma, hemorrhagic retinopathy, and auricular ecchymosis exists (tin ear),[10,11] the cause appears to be a blow to the side of the head, causing angular acceleration with shearing of the ipsilateral bridging subdural veins. Severe cerebral swelling can occur with tentorial herniation and subsequent death.

Children who present as "life-threatening events" (near-miss sudden infant death syndrome) should be closely examined for signs of suffocation.[7] Two children with asphyxia were identified in our series. The nose should be closely examined for signs of pinching, the eyes checked for conjunctival hemorrhages, and the gums and oral cavity closely examined for bruising.

Pharyngeal lacerations may occur due to foreign bodies or subsequent to removal of the foreign body from the throat. Fifteen cases of oropharyngeal trauma, including lacerations, ecchymoses, and abrasions, have been treated at Children's Hospital Medical Center. Although not noted in our series, subcutaneous emphysema and mediastinitis are potential complications. Pharyngeal lacerations and foreign-body ingestions should always be viewed in the context of potential abuse. A torn frenulum is also highly suspicious of abuse in a young child and referral is always warranted.[12]

Medical neglect is a much more difficult area to define. Children with chronic problems, such as recurrent laryngeal papillomatosis, often require close follow-up and repeated endoscopic laser procedures to keep their disease under control. Multiple missed appointments are clearly detrimental to the child and would fall into the definition of child abuse by means of medical neglect.

Munchausen's by Proxy Syndrome

Munchausen's disease is a psychiatric illness characterized by Asher[13] in 1951, to describe fictitious injuries in patients. Meadow[14] in 1977 adapted the term *Munchausen's syndrome by proxy* for children who are the victims of the parents developing fictitious symptoms and complaints in the child, and seeking medical care by unknowing physicians. Multiple reports exist in the literature describing specific cases of Munchausen's syndrome by proxy.[15-18] The most common age group affected by this type of abuse are those under 6 years of age. The most common presenting complaints in many series are seizures.[16] However, other common symptoms, including apnea, ataxia, nystagmus, and headache[19-21] are complaints where otolaryngologists would commonly see the patients on a consultant basis.

The most frequent perpetrator is the mother.[19] She is frequently well educated and commonly has substantial medical background. The child presents with symptoms and physical findings that elude diagnosis. Often a very rare disorder is entertained. The child is subjected to a variety of uncomfortable and potentially hazardous examinations to arrive at an elusive diagnosis.[22]

It is not possible to diagnose Munchausen's syndrome by proxy on the first encounter with the patient. A pattern will develop with continued care that can be further substantiated by reviewing the entire medical record of the patient, including those treatments administered by other physicians. A pattern of repeated visits to the physician for evaluation of symptom exacerbations, frequently only occurring in the presence of the mother, may be seen. Descriptions of symptoms relayed by the mother may not correlate with objective physical examinations or test results. Failure of multiple treatment modalities that normally will control a given problem are often seen in Munchausen's syndrome by proxy. Diagnostic for this disorder are symptoms in the child that resolve in the absence of the suspected caregiver.[11,21,22]

All children suffering the Munchausen's syndrome by proxy suffer the morbidity of many unnecessary tests, but there is also an estimated 9% mortality rate associated with this syndrome.[15] Although not within the study period, one patient was encountered in our institution who was receiving toxic doses of ipecac [23,24] and who underwent an endoscopic procedure under general anesthesia by our service and multiple other invasive procedures by other services. The child later died of cardiac complications, and the true cause was not determined until autopsy results were released. Because of this, it is essential to diagnose this most difficult variant of child abuse, and remove the child from this environment. The parent must be confronted, but sufficient support personnel must be present to care for both the child and for the mentally ill parent.

Caustic Ingestions

Many children present to the emergency department with foreign-body aspirations and caustic ingestions. These combined account for a third of the pediatric accidental deaths, with 8% of these children having a previous history of caustic ingestion.[25] Seventy-eight percent of caustic ingestions occur while the child is being supervised.[26] The most significant factor that indicates risk of accidental poisoning is the family unit. Disorganized families, and families with internal strife and high stress levels, are predictors of accidental poisoning.[27] It must be borne in mind that a caustic ingestion may be a sign of other difficulties in the home and demonstrate a risk for child abuse. Determination of accidental injury vs neglect (failure to adequately protect the child from potential danger) vs child abuse is very difficult. Any hesitation as to which category a given case would fall in requires reporting as potential child abuse or neglect.

Risk Factors

Certain factors have been identified as being associated with child abuse, conditions that produce an environment where abusive behavior is more likely to be exhibited. Some of these factors are intrinsic to the child, others are environmental. Child abuse crosses all cultural, religious, and socioeconomic groups. It is important to recognize conditions that have an increased risk of leading to child abuse.

Low-birth-weight children requiring admission to a newborn intensive care unit or any condition that requires prolonged hospitalization affects parental-infant bonding.[9] Children with multiple handicaps or mental retardation are also at increased risk of abuse because of the demands placed on the parents.[28] Children with a defiant personality or who are hyperactive are similarly at risk for abuse.

Stressors in the home environment are closely linked to the development of child abuse. Examples of these stressors are financial problems, loss of a job, alcoholism, drug addiction, and marital problems.[29] Families where the parents utilize violence against each other to settle disagreements frequently turn their violent behavior on their children.[30]

Teenage mothers are also at higher risks for abusing their children than women who are older at the time of delivery.[8] The coping skills of these young women are frequently poor, and the social support they receive from family and government agencies is usually limited.

Physically handicapped and hearing-impaired children are at risk of abuse.[9,28,31] These children often are unable to express their problems to others. These children require a large amount of attention from their parents. It is recommended that all deaf children and children with handicaps undergo annual physical examinations, specifically looking for signs of physical and sexual abuse.[7]

In the history obtained when entertaining the possibility of abuse, it is always prudent to explore the personal characteristics of the parents and attempt to determine the degree of stress within which the family operates.[32] An assessment of the relative isolation of the family as well as the availability of financial resources may point out potential problems that place children at higher risk of being abused.

Reporting

All 50 states have statutes requiring the reporting of suspected child abuse. The Ohio Revised Code 2151.421 was enacted in 1970. The law applies to all children under the age of 18 years and any mentally retarded or physically handicapped child until the age of 21 years. The report must be made immediately in person or by telephone to appropriate authorities. This could include county welfare departments, child protective services, or local police departments. A written report is generally required within 72 hours of the verbal report. Any individual reporting suspected child abuse is granted absolute immunity from criminal and civil liability resulting from the reported incident. The statute continues in defining failure to report suspected cases of child abuse as a fourth-degree misdemeanor. A separate statute, however, child endangerment, may also apply to an individual failing to report child abuse. State medical boards may also sanction the physician for the conviction of a misdemeanor committed in the course of his or her practice.[33]

Physicians report fewer than 10% of the cases of child abuse.[7,34] It is important to realize that patient confidentiality in the doctor-patient relationship does not release a physician from reporting child abuse. The most common problem seems to be an inability to adequately define what is abuse. Eighty-six percent of physicians in a study by Morris et al[5] felt that spanking that leaves a bruise could be considered child abuse. Only 25% of these same physicians, however, would report this to the officials. It is important to know what the local standards are for abuse in a given region. Local hospitals are the best source of reference material. The failure to report child abuse, for any reason, can further endanger the child and bring criminal liability on the physician. Additionally, there have been multiple civil lawsuits brought to the courts on the child's behalf, suing for compensation for all injuries sustained after the diagnosis of child abuse was missed or therefore not reported to the proper authorities. These civil lawsuits leave the individuals who failed to make the report liable for potential multimillion-dollar settlements.

Professionals who deal with children have both a moral and a legal obligation to report cases of child abuse. It is certainly in the best interest of the child, because child abuse is a recurrent and usually escalating problem that exposes the child to substantial risk. Social agencies are best equipped to follow-up on cases of child abuse. A growing number of district attorneys view the enforcement of criminal laws prohibiting child abuse as an important part of their responsibilities.[35] The statute of limitations for child abuse has been extended to allow the prosecution of appropriate cases years after the infraction was committed. Disclosure of the event by children may not occur for months to years after the abuse due to the age of the victims, fear of reprisal, and general confusion. Because of this, discovery of cases of physical or sexual child abuse even years after the fact should still be reported to the proper authorities.

Goals of Identifying Child Abuse

The purpose of identifying victims of child abuse is not the punishment of the abuser but the protection of the child. Court-sanctioned separation of the child from the parent may be required in some circumstances to protect the child. Most of the time, however, psychosocial intervention can begin, leaving the child in the family environment. The main focus is on the development of improved parenting skills for the parents as well as the improvement of interpersonal relationships as a method to reduce child abuse.

Child abuse must be diagnosed so that the child can be helped. Organized multidisciplinary child abuse teams are best equipped to handle the multifaceted social aspects of child abuse, and physicians should take an active role when appropriate.[36] The physician should act as the child advocate and obtain a clear history and document the injuries with diagrams and photographs when possible. The physician should be willing to testify on behalf of the child should such circumstances arise.[2,35] Any physician having contact with children must be familiar with the common signs of child abuse, and most importantly, always view each injury in light of possible nonaccidental injury. There is no substitute for a proper diagnosis in cases of child abuse and there are moral and legal responsibilities to the child.

In conclusion, 15% of 4340 patients suspected of physical or sexual child abuse had evidence of injury in the head and neck region; 49% of the 1390 physically abused children had head and neck injuries. Most injuries were caused by blows with hands (40%) or an object (22%); 89% of injuries were to the face and scalp. There was a 1% incidence of death from abuse and/or neglect in our series. One child had been diagnosed and reported as being abused in the past. Ecchymoses and abrasions accounted for 62% and 15% of injuries, respectively. More serious injuries such as fractures or burns can occur. Younger patients (<2.1 years) and patients with more severe injuries require admission more frequently. Recognition of child abuse requires a good history and physical examination and an index of suspicion of abuse, especially in patients with inconsistent findings on examination relative to the reported mechanism of injury. Certain injuries require investigation for abuse and include "shaken baby syndrome," tin ear, near-miss sudden infant death syndrome with associated injuries, torn lingual frenulum, or persistent medical neglect. Reporting suspected cases of child abuse is required by law in all 50 states, however, only 10% of cases are reported by physicians. Increased recognition and reporting by physicians is an important step in the care of the victims of child abuse. Child abuse frequently escalates in intensity with time. It is essential to diagnose this disorder to prevent further injury. Parents often take their children to multiple treatment facilities, so the pattern of abuse is difficult to identify.

We are indebted to David O'Connor for his assistance in data management and Shirley Walston for transcription.

References

1. Fontana VJ. The maltreatment syndrome of children. *Pediatr Ann.* 1984;13:736-744.
2. Peters JM. Criminal prosecution of child abuse: recent trends. *Pediatr Ann.* 1989;18:505-509.
3. Kempe CH, Silverman FN, Steele BF, Droegenmueller W, Silver HK. The battered-child syndrome. *JAMA.* 1962;181:17-24.
4. Johnson CF. Inflicted injury versus accidental injury. *Pediatr Clin North Am.* 1990;37:791-814.
5. Morris JL, Johnson CF, Clasen M. To report or not to report: physicians' attitudes toward discipline and child abuse. *AJDC.* 1985; 139:194-197.
6. Newberger EH. Pediatric interview assessment of child abuse. *Pediatr Clin North Am.* 1990;37:943-954.
7. Manning SC, Casselbrant M, Lammers D. Otolaryngologic manifestations of child abuse. *Int J Pediatr Otolaryngol.* 1990;20:7-16.
8. Ozonoff MB. Emergency radiology in childhood. *Emerg Med Clin North Am* 1985;3:563-584.
9. Brookhouser PE, Sullivan P, Scanlon JM, Gabbarino J. Identifying the sexually abused deaf child: the otolaryngologist role. *Laryngoscope.* 1986;96:152-158.
10. Hanigan WC, Peterson RA, Njus G. Tin ear syndrome: rotational acceleration in pediatric head injuries. *Pediatrics.* 1987;80:618-622.
11. Reece RM. Unusual manifestations of child abuse. *Pediatr Clin North Am.* 1990;37:905-921.
12. Grace A, Grace S. Child abuse within the ear, nose and throat. *J Otolaryngol.* 1987;15:108-111.
13. Asher R. Munchausen's syndrome. *Lancet.* 1951;1:339-341.
14. Meadow R. Munchausen syndrome by proxy: the hinterland of child abuse. *Lancet.* 1977;57:92-98.
15. Sullivan SCA, Francis GL, Bain MW, Hartz J. Munchausen syndrome by proxy: 1990: a patent for problems? *Clin Pediatr.* 1991;30:112-116.
16. Mehl AL, Coble L, Johnson S. Munchausen syndrome by proxy: a family affair. *Child Abuse Neglect.* 1990;14:577-585.
17. Alexander R, Smith W, Stevenson R. Serial Munchausen syndrome by proxy. *Pediatrics.* 1990;86:581-585.
18. Mills RW, Burke S. Gastro-intestinal bleeding in a 15 month old male: a presentation of Munchausen's syndrome by proxy. *Clin Pediatr.* 1990;29:474-477.
19. Meadow R. Neurological and developmental variants of Munchausen syndrome by proxy. *Develop Med Child Neurol.* 1991;33:267-272.
20. Kravitz RM, Wilmott RW. Munchausen syndrome by proxy presenting as factitious apnea. *Clin Pediatr.* 1990;29:587-592.
21. Light MJ, Sheridan MS. Munchausen syndrome by proxy and apnea (MBPA): a survey of apnea programs. *Clin Pediatr.* 1990;29:162-168.
22. Meadow R. Munchausen syndrome by proxy. *Arch Dis Child.* 1982;57:92-98.
23. Feldman KW, Christopher DM, Opheim KB. Munchausen syndrome/bulimea by proxy: ipecac as a toxin in child abuse. *Child Abuse Neglect.* 1989;13:257-261.
24. Sutphen JL, Saulsburg FT. Intentional ipecac poisoning: Munchausen syndrome by proxy. *Pediatrics.* 1988;82:453-456.
25. Friedman EM. Caustic ingestions and foreign body aspiration: an overlooked form of child abuse. *Ann Otol Rhinol Laryngol.* 1987;96:710-712.
26. Jensen GD, Wilson WW. Preventative implications of a study of 100 poisonings in children. *Arch Dis Child.* 1980;55:643-647.
27. Sibert R. Stress in families of children who have ingested poisons. *BMJ.* 1975;3:87-89.
28. Benedict MI, White RB, Wulff LM, Hall BS. Reported maltreatment in children with multiple disabilities. *Child Abuse Neglect.* 1990;14:207-217.
29. Helfer RE. Epidemiology of child abuse and neglect. *Pediatr Ann.* 1984;13:748-751.
30. Council on Scientific Affairs, Council Report. AMA Diagnostic and Treatment Guidelines concerning child abuse and neglect. *JAMA.* 1985;254:796-800.
31. Brookhouser PE. Ensuring the safety of deaf children in residential schools. *Otolaryngol Head Neck Surg.* 1987;97:361-368.
32. Wolfe D. Child abuse prevention and intervention. *Pediatr Ann.* 1984;13:766-770.
33. Grey L. Physicians liability in child abuse reporting cases. *OSMA.* 1985;51:492-497.
34. Saulsburg FT, Campbell RE. Evaluation of child abuse reporting by physicians. *AJDC.* 1985;139:393-395.
35. Chadwick DL. Preparation for court testimony in child abuse cases. *Pediatr Clin North Am.* 1990;37:955-970.
36. Mundie GE. Team management of the maltreated child in the emergency room. *Pediatr Ann.* 1984;13:771-776.

Editorial Introduction

Society seems to tolerate a certain level of trauma. We have the technology to drastically reduce accidental injuries, but we do not enforce such safety rules until the level of education about a risk reaches some critical proportion, thus becoming the expected norm. Society has a hard time legislating safety. For instance, the reduction in highway speed limits that occurred in the early 1980s, purportedly to conserve fuel, was very unpopular despite the accident rate being lowered below a level we put up with through the 1970s.

The major cause of blunt laryngeal trauma that results in a need for surgical care has been high-speed motor vehicle accidents. Annually, we still kill nearly as many people on our highways as died in combat during the Vietnam conflict, but for some reason, society tolerates this level of personal injury. Recent efforts to increase seat belt use and newer air bag installations may further reduce the injury sustained in an accident. This type of safety equipment is important, but it does not deal with the problem of dangerous roads, dangerous cars, and dangerous drivers. As surgeons we tend to focus on the acute problem requiring intervention—intervention by us, naturally. More importantly, however, society needs to be involved in prevention of such trauma. The type of personal suffering described in this article on laryngeal trauma is an example of the information the public requires to assess the cost of such injuries.

In this discussion and in the article by Stiernberg et al on gunshot wounds, the recognition of increasing penetrating head and neck trauma is well identified. Crimes involving bodily threat or personal injury have increased to such a point that we hear about them on the news nightly. We have all come to know someone's family that is touched by it, if not experiencing it ourselves. In this light, it is astonishing to note that we have organizations committed to the preservation of the societal framework that perpetuates the mechanisms of much of the trauma.

Americans have many tough decisions to face in the next few years: decisions that may limit personal freedoms to protect society, decisions on how to deal with the cost (monetarily and personally) of the drug habit that our society keeps, and decisions on how to provide affordable, high-quality health care. Knowing how to fix an injury, as presented here, is important because the injuries will happen through a variety of means and someone needs to know how to deal with them expertly. Work spent on prevention of the injury is even more important, yet such work remains poorly rewarded. Prevention of these injuries will mean that society has educated itself and learned from its mistakes. The ability to learn is sure to be taken as the sign of a viable organism of high order.

WILLIAM J. RICHTSMEIER, MD, PHD
Baltimore, Md

Gunshot Wounds to the Head and Neck

Charles M. Stiernberg, MD; Robert A. Jahrsdoerfer, MD; Ann Gillenwater, MD; Stephanie A. Joe; Socorro V. Alcalen

• Gunshot wounds to the head and neck contribute to substantial medical, economic, and social problems in the United States today. The treatment of these patients requires the contemporary head and neck surgeon to be precisely informed in anatomy, wound ballistics, resuscitation, and surgical decision making. Ninety recent cases at the University of Texas Health Science Center affiliated hospitals in Houston were reviewed and are reported. Data show substantial trends in patient demographics and corroborate other reports in the trauma literature. Controversies in patient management continue, but current evidence favors a protocol of selective surgical exploration.

(*Arch Otolaryngol Head Neck Surg.* 1992;118:592-597)

Trauma by firearms in the United States remains a significant public health problem, with an estimated 33 000 gun-related deaths per year and many more nonfatal shootings per year.[1] As a subgroup of this large population, patients with gunshot wounds to the head and neck pose a wide range of medical and surgical challenges to the contemporary head and neck surgeon. The treatment of such cases requires a thorough knowledge base in wound ballistics, anatomy, resuscitation, and surgical decision making.

The objectives of this study were twofold: first, to review the most current demographic data and incidence of gunshot wounds to the head and neck at the authors' institute; and second, to review current concepts in wound ballistics and treatment of patients who sustain gunshot wounds to the head and neck.

SUBJECTS AND METHODS

All emergency department admissions to the University of Texas Health Science Center affiliated hospitals in Houston between January 1, 1991, and October 31, 1991, were screened for the diagnosis of gunshot wounds to the head or neck. Ninety cases were identified and retrospectively reviewed for data on age, sex, race, site of injury, and outcome. Information on the type of weapon used, the cause or motive of the injury, the number of hospital days, and whether the patient was taken to the operating room was also collected and analyzed.

Accepted for publication January 2, 1992.

From the Department of Otolaryngology—Head and Neck Surgery, The University of Texas Health Science Center at Houston.

Reprint requests to Department of Otolaryngology—Head and Neck Surgery, The University of Texas Health Science Center at Houston, 6431 Fannin St, Suite 6.132, Houston, TX 77030 (Dr Stiernberg).

RESULTS

Seventy-three males and seventeen females sustained gunshot wounds to the head or neck. Figures 1 through 4 depict the population in terms of age, race, site of injury, and patient outcome. Sixty-seven (74%) of 90 patients had wounds to the face (39) or head (28). Twenty-two (79%) of 28 head wounds were intracranial, and 14 of these were suicide attempts; all of these patients died within 1 day. Seventy-five charts documented which side of the head or neck had the entrance wound. There were 33 right-sided, 34 left-sided, four midline, and three bilateral wounds. Neck injuries were further categorized by zone, with three in zone 1, 17 in zone 2, and three in zone 3. Six patients had a combination of neck and face wounds. Most patients either spent only 1 day in the hospital (33) or were not admitted (27). Of the 27 patients not admitted, 10 had pellet wounds and were treated as outpatients. The average hospital stay for patients with shotgun wounds was 9.3 days, for those with handgun wounds, 6.3 days, and for those with rifle wounds, 1 day. Only 11 patients stayed longer than 10 days. Twenty-four patients required either diagnostic or therapeutic procedures in the operating room. Figure 5 shows the type of weapon used, the most common being a handgun, which was also the most deadly, with 24 deaths (46%) from 52 wounds. Shotguns accounted for only one death (7%) of 15 wounds, and rifles caused three deaths (43%) of seven wounds. The motive of the shooting is shown in Fig 6. All self-inflicted wounds were from suicide attempts.

Wound Ballistics

Ballistics is the study of the characteristics of projectiles in flight. The term *missile* is used herein to refer to the projectile shot from any firearm. Bullets pertain to the ammunition for handguns and rifles, while their projectiles are sometimes called "slugs." Shotguns can also fire single slugs, but their projectiles are more often called "pellets" or "shot."

The equation $KE = mv^2/2$ (KE indicating kinetic energy; m, mass; and v, velocity) is a fundamental law of physics for determining the kinetic energy of any mass that is moving. The wounding capability of a firearm is directly proportional to the kinetic energy of its missile on impact and how much kinetic energy is dissipated into the tissues. The critical variable is missile velocity. Doubling it quadruples kinetic energy, while doubling mass only doubles kinetic energy. There is a wide range of weapon

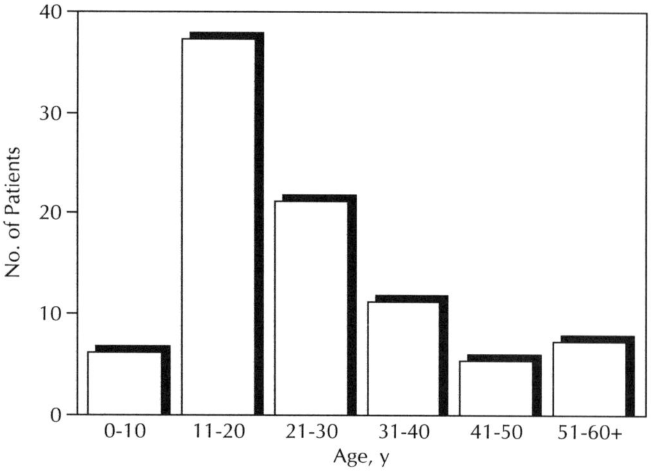

Fig 1.—*Distribution of patient ages.*

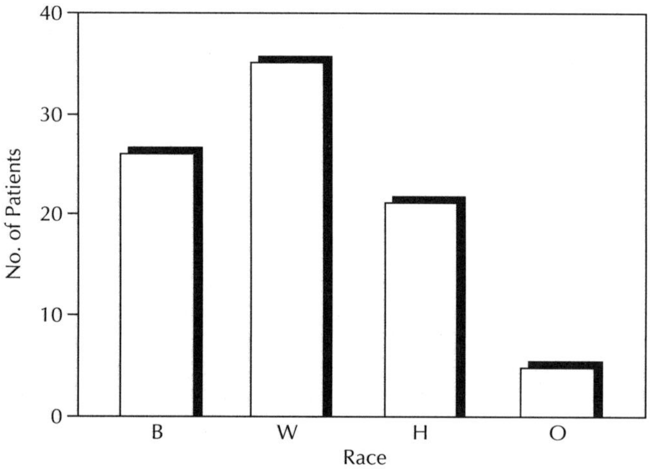

Fig 2.—*Distribution of races. H indicates Hispanic; O, other.*

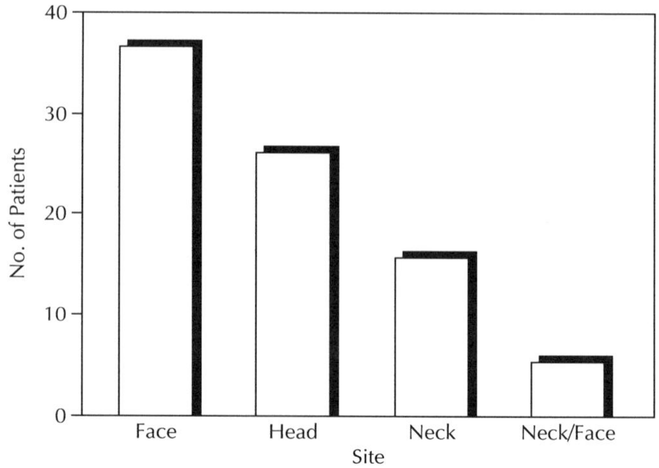

Fig 3.—*Distribution of sites of injury.*

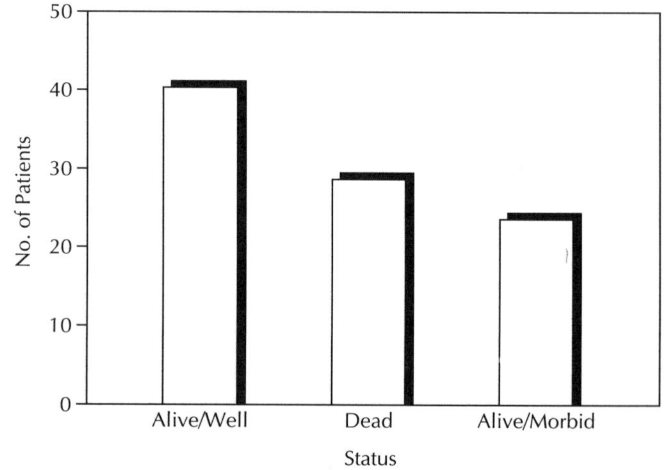

Fig 4.—*Distribution of patient status. Alive/well means the patient had no permanent sequelae. Dead refers to death as a direct or indirect result of the gunshot wound. Alive/morbid indicates the patient lived but not without some form of lasting disability, such as a cranial nerve palsy.*

velocities. The .22- and .25-caliber pistols fire bullets with slug velocities of about 91.4 m/s (300 ft/s). They cause much less tissue destruction than rifles, such as a .270-caliber hunting rifle, which has a missile velocity of about 670.6 m/s (2200 ft/s). The slow-velocity missiles also tend to be deflected by such structures as vessels, nerves, and fascial planes. The path of these slowly moving projectiles will therefore be much more erratic, sometimes having no relation to entrance and exit wounds. In contrast, high-velocity missiles cut straight through soft tissues and fracture bones with relative ease. Trauma surgeons therefore classify firearms into low-, medium-, and high-velocity weapons. This type of information in an individual case can provide insight into the severity of the injury.

Guns are most often referred to by caliber, which is a measure of the diameter of the gun's bore. If considered alone, caliber can be misleading. For example, a magnum handgun, which can use ammunition with more powder than an equivalent-caliber nonmagnum handgun, produces 20% to 60% more energy in the projectile. Holt and Kostohryz[2] explain this clearly in terms of foot-pounds of energy that a weapon can produce. A slug fired from a .22-caliber rifle may have as little kinetic energy as 135.6 J (100 ft-lb), while a .460-caliber rifle may yield 4068 J (3000 ft-lb).

Several other factors also influence the wounding capability of firearms. Flight stability and the angle that a bullet strikes its target greatly affect its path through human tissue. A projectile with a stable flight path, hitting the skin at 90°, traverses the neck quickly and dissipates energy over a greater distance than one of equal size and velocity striking the skin at an oblique angle and tumbling through the tissue.

The design of a bullet is another important factor to gunshot wound injuries. Figure 7 graphically depicts two types of high-velocity bullet designs and their effects on tissue. The military full-jacketed type is designed to pass sharply through tissues, leaving a cylinder-shaped permanent cavity. The sporting type, designed for hunting rifles, mushrooms on impact and consequently imparts far more energy to the surrounding tissue. It leaves a cone-shaped permanent cavity and a large exit wound.[3] Although the fully jacketed military design is theoretically supposed to cause less tissue damage, the missile from an M16 military rifle tumbles end-over-end easily, thereby causing significantly more destruction.[4]

As a missile passes through the head and neck, tissue is destroyed and either ejected out the entrance and exit wounds or compressed into the walls of the missile's tract. This creates a permanent cavity that is three to four times larger than the missile diameter, depending on the

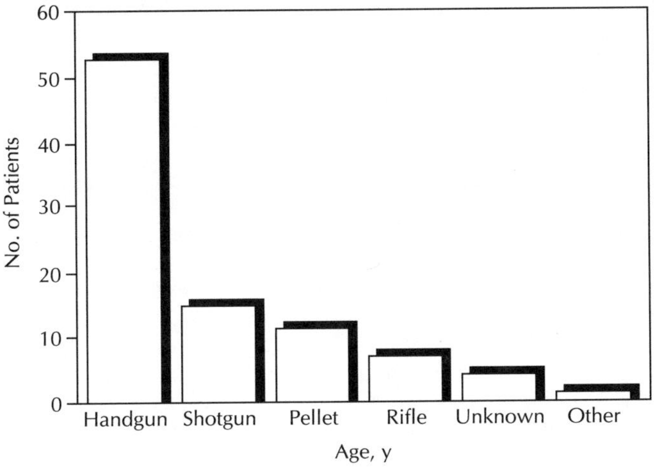

Fig 5.—*Distribution of the type of weapons used in gunshot wounds.*

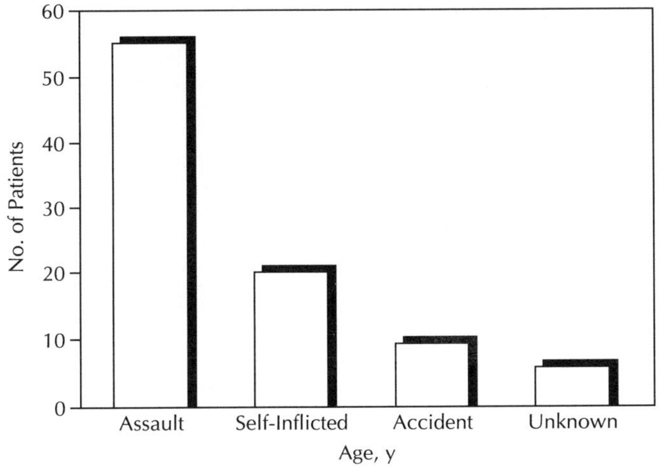

Fig 6.—*Distribution of mechanisms of injury. Assault refers to the gunshot wound being inflicted intentionally by another person. Self-inflicted refers to suicide attempt.*

amount of energy dissipated. In addition to this permanent cavity, the missile causes a pulsating temporary cavity that expands outward around the tract and can be 30 times larger than the missile's diameter. The duration of a temporary cavity is only 5 to 10 milliseconds. Higher-velocity weapons create wider temporary cavities that tend to injure structures a considerable distance from the actual missile tract.

The ballistic characteristics of shotguns are different from those of handguns and rifles. The ammunition of different shotguns varies in size, in amount of gun powder, and in number and size of pellets. The most important factor in the wounding capability of a shotgun, however, is distance of the weapon from the victim. Wounds from a shotgun fired from over 20 ft are similar to those of multiple slow-velocity weapons. On the other hand, shotgun blasts at a close range are more like high-velocity weapons. As the range decreases, the pattern of pellets striking the target will have a smaller diameter. At very close range, the size of the pellets makes little difference, since they act as one large mass traveling at a high velocity. It is also important for the surgeon to realize that a shotgun's wadding acts as a separate missile and may escape detection since it is radiolucent. If it remains deep

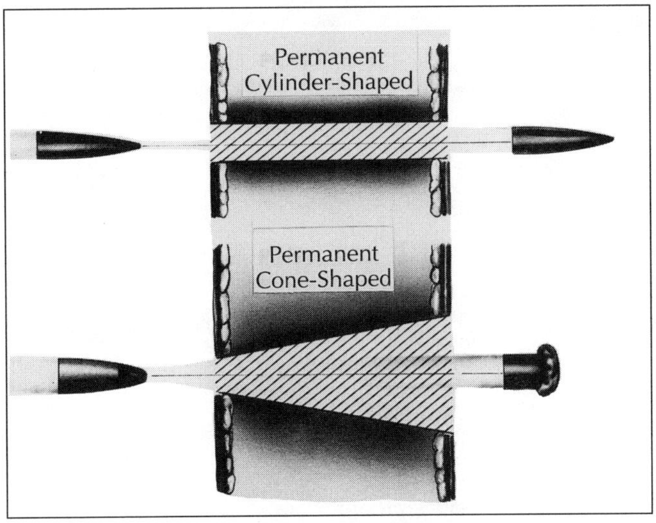

Fig 7.—*Types of permanent cavities produced by high velocity missiles. Top, Cylinder-shaped cavities are typically produced by military-type fully jacketed missiles. Bottom, Cone-shaped cavities are characteristic of missiles fired from sporting weapons (from Jahrsdoerfer et al[3]).*

within the tissues, wadding can be a significant nidus of infection.[5]

Patient Management

Fortunately, most patients who sustain gunshot wounds to the head and neck live long enough to arrive at an emergency department. Though initial stabilization begins in the field, it is continued in a systematic fashion on arrival at the hospital. With some special attention to particular areas, the steps for resuscitating a patient with a gunshot wound to the head and neck are basically the same as those taught in Advanced Trauma Life Support sponsored by the Committee on Trauma of the American College of Surgeons.[6]

Resuscitation begins with the airway. Signs and symptoms of airway injury or obstruction are listed in Table 1. Subcutaneous emphysema can result from a tear in the mucosa anywhere in the upper aerodigestive tract. Tracheal deviation can result from pneumothorax or hematoma in the neck. If massive swelling or distorted anatomy precludes endotracheal intubation, then cricothyrotomy or tracheostomy must be performed. Care should be taken, however, to avoid cutting in the region of a hematoma because of the possibility of major hemorrhage from an underlying vascular injury. Once the upper airway is secure, if the patient continues to show signs of hypoxia, a pneumothorax must be suspected. Roentgenograms of the chest and neck are indicated to look for pneumothorax, pneumomediastinum, and air in the soft tissues of the neck.

Active bleeding from a vascular injury must be controlled either simultaneously or immediately after securing the airway. When possible, direct pressure is the best method to control bleeding temporarily. Indiscriminate or blind clamping of such wounds is contraindicated. Occasionally, gunshot wounds have significant hemorrhage from an entrance or exit wound in the pharynx. Since direct pressure is difficult or impossible at this site, cricothyrotomy or tracheostomy should be done first, followed by pharyngeal packing.[7] Likewise, packing the nose for severe epistaxis from a gunshot wound may be necessary,

Table 1.—Signs and Symptoms of Penetrating Neck Trauma

- Airway
  - Respiratory distress
  - Stridor
  - Cyanosis
  - Hemoptysis
  - Hoarseness
  - Tracheal deviation
  - Subcutaneous emphysema
  - Sucking wound
- Vascular system
  - Hematoma
  - Persistent bleeding
  - Neurological deficit
  - Absent pulse
  - Hypovolemic shock
  - Bruit
  - Thrill
  - Change of sensorium
- Nervous system
  - Hemiplegia
  - Quadriplegia
  - Coma
  - Cranial nerve deficit
  - Change of sensorium
  - Hoarseness
- Esophagus/hypopharynx
  - Subcutaneous emphysema
  - Dysphagia
  - Odynophagia
  - Hematemesis
  - Hemoptysis
  - Tachycardia
  - Fever

but the surgeon must remain aware of the possibility that the cribriform plate has also been disrupted by the trauma.

Since clinical presentations and management of penetrating vascular wounds in the neck differ according to the anatomical level of injury, trauma surgeons divide the neck into three zones (Table 2). The contents of each zone include the following: zone 1, subclavian arteries and veins, the domes of the pleura, esophagus, great vessels of the neck, recurrent nerves, and trachea; zone 2, larynx, pharynx, base of tongue, carotid artery, jugular vein, phrenic nerve, and cranial nerves X and XII; zone 3, internal and external carotid arteries, vertebral artery, and cranial nerves IX, X, XI, and XII. Each zone has unique clinical characteristics. With major intrathoracic structures behind the clavicles and sternum, zone 1 penetrating trauma has the highest mortality.[8] Also, hemorrhage in this zone is often occult. In a study by Markflint et al,[9] 32% of surgically proved vascular injuries in zone 1 had no sign on preoperative clinical evaluation. When bleeding in this zone is diagnosed, an anterolateral or median thoracotomy may be necessary to control it. Zone 2 is the most common site of carotid artery injuries. Fortunately, hemorrhage is usually controlled by pressure, and surgical access is much easier in zone 2 than in the other two zones. Zone 3 poses the greatest problems for surgical exposure, particularly for distal control or repair of the carotid arteries.

Restoration of circulation in gunshot wound victims, who often present in hypovolemic shock, requires rapid replacement of the lost vascular volume. At least two large-bore intravenous lines should be started, with one of them in the lower extremity. Care should be taken to avoid putting a line in an arm on the same side as a subclavian injury, which could result in filling the chest cavity with intravenous fluid.

Table 2.—Anatomical Zones of the Neck

Zone	Superior Border	Inferior Border
1	Cricoid cartilage	Clavicles and sternum
2	Angle of mandible	Cricoid cartilage
3	Base of skull	Angle of mandible

Once a patient has been stabilized, a more thorough diagnostic workup can be initiated. Conscious patients who can communicate may have symptoms that reflect which organs and structures of the head and neck are injured. In addition to the airway, Table 1 lists signs and symptoms of injuries to the upper digestive, vascular, and nervous systems. Many of the signs overlap. For example, hemoptysis, hematemesis, and subcutaneous emphysema can present in patients with pharyngeal or esophageal injury as well as airway injuries.

Any wound in the midline of the neck or one that crosses the midline must be carefully evaluated for esophageal perforation. These patients may complain of dysphagia or odynophagia, or they may not have any symptoms. If the injury is older than 12 hours, an early neck abscess or mediastinitis may be present. Signs include tachycardia, fever, and radiographic evidence of a widened mediastinum or retropharyngeal space. Key diagnostic procedures are barium swallow and esophagoscopy. Both tests have false-negative rates that range widely among clinical studies, but most authorities agree that the combination can bring the sensitivity to above 90%.

A multitude of neurological injuries can occur from gunshot wounds to the head and neck. In addition to injuries to cranial nerves, phrenic nerves, and the brachial plexus, quadriplegia or paraplegia are often the outcome of gunshot wounds to the spinal cord. Radiographic evaluation of the vertebral column is therefore an important part of the early evaluation of these patients. A hematoma in the posterior triangle can indicate fracture of a transverse process, while a widened retropharyngeal space can mean edema or hemorrhage into this space from a cervical spine fracture. The clinician needs also to remember that hoarseness can signify either recurrent laryngeal or vagus nerve injury.

A thorough head and neck examination includes auscultation with a stethoscope to search for bruits in the neck and inspection of the patient's back to look for additional wounds. Care must be taken, however, to stabilize the cervical spine when rolling the patient over. Fiberoptic or indirect laryngoscopy are also important to uncover any laryngeal or hypopharyngeal injuries. If an abnormality is noted, further assessment should be done by direct laryngoscopy and esophagoscopy in the operating room.

Radiography is an invaluable tool in the evaluation of gunshot wounds to the head and neck. As previously mentioned, chest, cervical spine, and soft-tissue roentgenograms are routine in nearly all cases. Frequently, slow-velocity missiles from handguns break up and leave small metal particles in the projectile's path. Higher-velocity missiles can shatter bones, so films of the mandible or face may also be necessary to assess fractures.

Perhaps the most important radiographic study is arteriography. Indications for an arteriogram include any of those signs or symptoms listed under the vascular system in Table 1. In addition, patients in a coma or who are hemiplegic require arteriography, since these signs may be a result of vascular compromise to the central nervous system.

Arteriography is especially helpful in zones 1 and 3, where clinical assessment is much more difficult in comparison with zone II. Since significant morbidity is associated with exploring zone 1 for vascular injuries, arteriography is particularly useful here for reducing the number of negative explorations. In zone 3, arteriography is diagnostically beneficial for delineating the site of an injury and therapeutically beneficial for determining surgical accessibility. In those cases where surgical exposure would be difficult, embolization is often a practical option.[10] Indications for embolization of vessels in the neck include surgically inaccessible vessels, expendable vessels (ie, vertebral artery), and internal carotid artery injuries in comatose patients who are not candidates for revascularization.

Before World War II, watchful waiting was standard medical practice for stable patients who sustained gunshot wounds to the neck. This was associated with mortalities of about 15%. During World War II, mandatory exploration of all penetrating neck wounds led to decreased mortalities but a high rate of negative explorations, in the range of 60%. Today, most experts have adopted a policy of selective exploration, which has led to a decrease in the number of negative explorations, a decrease in medical costs, and no increase in morbidity or mortality.

Selective exploration of gunshot wounds is based on specific clinical variables identified in clinical studies over the past 15 to 20 years. In a study of 1000 patients who sustained penetrating trauma to the neck, May et al[11] reported that only 210 (21%) patients required exploration, and of these, 88% had significant injuries. They evaluated patients by angiography when there was no direct evidence of a vascular injury but a strong suspicion and when the wound was in zone 1 or 3. Their overall mortality was 3%. In another study by Ordog et al,[12] 31 of 110 patients underwent selective exploration for gunshot wounds to the neck. Twelve of the 31 surgical patients were taken to the operating room for unequivocal signs, while the other 19 patients underwent investigational studies before a decision was made for an exploration. In the latter group, only three patients had negative explorations despite positive findings during the workup. These investigators, as well as others, do not advocate selective exploration for all institutions. They stress the need for frequent physical examinations and 24-hour availability of radiological and endoscopic procedures for patients who are triaged to be observed.

A protocol for the management of gunshot wounds to the head and neck should certainly consider the principles of wound ballistics. All wounds resulting from high-velocity missiles should be surgically explored. These will require débridement and careful scrutiny of all structures in the area surrounding the missile's path. Another factor to weigh is which zone of the neck is injured. In clinically stable patients who have sustained a zone 2 gunshot wound, serial examination is highly reliable for detecting any adverse changes. Patients under observation should be admitted to an intensive care unit. For zone 3 wounds, surgical techniques are available to expose the base of skull for repair of vascular injuries, but there is a significant rate of cranial nerve injury in such cases.[13] The alternatives to repair are surgical ligation or radiologically guided embolization. With regard to the larynx, unless it is totally shattered, fractures and mucosal lacerations are the typical injuries. Exploration is usually performed through a laryngofissure. When the pharynx or esophagus are explored for repair of perforations, esophagoscopy will help to identify the level of injury.

COMMENT

The medical, economic, and social problems precipitated by gunshot wounds to the head and neck merely contribute to the much larger national problem of trauma by firearms. From epidemiological and medical perspectives, there is no comprehensive national database of trauma that includes site of injury and outcome. Nearly all reports that address management come from locally generated data. In scrutinizing the data in this review, however, trends that corroborate other reports can be identified. Specifically, males and blacks have the highest rate of gunshot wounds to the head and neck. This correlates well with statistics reported by Lee et al,[14] who found that males and blacks have the highest firearm mortality in Texas. The age group 11 to 20 years had more gunshot wounds than any other group in this study. Again, this supports data that relate the alarmingly high rate of death by trauma among young people.[15] Handguns were the most often used firearm causing wounds in this study, which confirms findings by Nelson et al.[16] Assault was the most common motive, and zone 2 of the neck was the most common neck zone injured.

Despite the predominance of current literature supporting selective surgical exploration, controversy continues over the best management for gunshot wounds to the head and neck. The two areas debated most often are the indications for arteriography and selective vs mandatory surgical exploration.[17,18] The chief proponents of using angiography in nearly all cases of gunshot wounds to the head and neck are surgeons who believe in selective exploration.[19] Some radiology colleagues, however, argue that angiography also has risks, and its use should therefore be selective as well. In a retrospective review by North et al,[20] 78 of 139 clinically stable patients presented with only a wound and no other sign or symptom. All patients underwent angiography, and only two of the 78 had radiographic evidence of a vascular injury. This study is biased, however, by the fact that only 62 of the patients had gunshot wounds, and the remainder had stab wounds. A new modality that is far less invasive and yet may prove to be of significant value in assessing vascular trauma is magnetic resonance imaging angiography.

Based on current literature and on data uncovered in this retrospective review, we advocate a protocol utilizing selective angiography and selective surgical exploration. It is acceptable, however, for this approach to differ from one institution to the next, depending on experience of the surgeons and nursing personnel, as well as other hospital resources.

References

1. Zane DF, Preece MJ, Patterson PJ, Svenkerud EK. Firearm related mortality. *Tex Med.* 1991;87:63-65.
2. Holt GR, Kostohryz G. Wound ballistics of gunshot injuries to the

head and neck. *Arch Otolaryngol Head Neck Surg.* 1983;109:313-318.
3. Jahrsdoerfer RA, Johns ME, Cantrell RW. Penetrating wounds of the head and neck. *Arch Otolaryngol Head Neck Surg.* 1979;105:721-725.
4. Lowry LD. Trauma. In: Schuller DE, ed. *Otolaryngology—Head and Neck Surgery.* St Louis, Mo: Mosby–Year Book; 1986;2:1621-1630.
5. Calhoun KH, Li S, Clark WD, Stiernberg CM, Quinn FB. Surgical care of submental gunshot wounds. *Arch Otolaryngol Head Neck Surg.* 1988;114:513-519.
6. Ramenofsky ML, Ali J, Aprahamian C, et al. *Advanced Trauma Life Support Course.* Chicago, Ill: The American College of Surgeons; 1989.
7. Crumley R. Soft tissue injuries of the neck. In: English GM, ed. *Otolaryngology.* Philadelphia, Pa: JB Lippincott; 1991;4:1-9.
8. Carducci B, Lowe RA, Dalsey W. Penetrating neck trauma: consensus and controversies. *Ann Emerg Med.* 1986;15:208-215.
9. Markflint LM, Snyder WH, Perry MO, Shires GT. Injuries in the base of the neck. *Arch Surg.* 1973;106:407-413.
10. Panetta T, Sclafani S, Goldstein AS. Percutaneous transcatheter embolization for arterial trauma. *J Vasc Surg.* 1985;2:54-64.
11. May M, Tucker HM, Dillard BM. Penetrating wounds of the neck in civilians. *Otolaryngol Clin North Am.* 1976;9:361-391.
12. Ordog GJ, Albin D, Wasserberger J, Schlater TL, Balasubramaniam S. 110 bullet wounds to the neck. *J Trauma.* 1985;25:238-246.
13. Fry RE, Fry WJ. Extracranial carotid artery injuries. *Surgery.* 1980;88:581-587.
14. Lee RK, Burau K, Clanton S. Firearm mortality in Texas, 1976-1985: how far is Fort Smith? *Tex Med.* 1991;87:78-83.
15. Martin WS, Gussack GS. Pediatric penetrating head and neck trauma. *Laryngoscope.* 1990;100:1288-1291.
16. Nelson CL, Puskarich CL, Marks A. Gunshot wounds: incidence, cost, and concepts of prevention. *Clin Orthop.* 1987;222:114-121.
17. Saleta JD, Lowe RJ, Lim LT, Thornton J, Delk S, Moss GS. Penetrating trauma of the neck. *J Trauma.* 1976;16:579-587.
18. Wood J, Fabian TC, Mangiante EC. Penetrating neck injuries: recommendations for selective management. *J Trauma.* 1989;29:602-605.
19. Livingstone AS. Vascular injuries of the head and neck. *Otolaryngol Clin North Am.* 1983;16:671-678.
20. North CM, Ahmadi J, Segall HD, Zee CS. Penetrating vascular injuries of the face and neck: clinical and angiographic correlation. *AJR Am J Roentgenol.* 1986;147:995-999.

The Acute Management of External Laryngeal Trauma

A 27-Year Experience

Steven D. Schaefer, MD

• The acute care of 139 consecutive patients with external laryngeal trauma over a 27-year period is reported. This article represents an effort to periodically reevaluate our care of this relatively infrequent injury and to share our changes and refinements in treatment. This series provides the means to test and establish basic principles in the acute care of external laryngeal trauma because (1) the number of years encompassed by the article, (2) most patients were managed by one physician, (3) the relative consistency of management principles throughout the series, and (4) the delivery of trauma care in Dallas County, Texas, reflects a broad sampling of this injury within the geographic area.

(*Arch Otolaryngol Head Neck Surg.* 1992;118:598-604)

External trauma to the larynx threatens both the quality and maintenance of life.[1] Essential to the vocal and airway sphincteric functions of the larynx is restoration of the skeletal framework and epithelial lining of this organ.[2] Essential to such preservation is the early recognition, accurate evaluation, and proper treatment of such injuries. Although external laryngeal trauma is infrequent, we have held for the past decade that sufficient knowledge now exists to permit more standardization of the immediate care of both blunt and penetrating laryngeal trauma.[3]

To learn from and to refine our acute treatment of external laryngeal trauma, we have periodically reviewed our experience with this injury at approximately 5-year intervals.[1,3-5] This process has focused on the specific areas of (1) incidence and changing mechanisms of external trauma, (2) improving diagnostic strategies, (3) clarifying criteria for surgical vs medical management, (4) addressing the benefit of immediate rather than delayed surgical treatment, (5) establishing principles for conservation of laryngeal anatomy, and (6) developing guidelines for laryngeal stenting. In this article, we have the unusual opportunity to reexamine the above areas from the perspective of a major trauma center, to revisit and test previous concepts expressed by the author and others, and to evaluate new patients and reevaluate previously described patients.[1,3-13]

Accepted for publication February 4, 1992.

From the Department of Otolaryngology, The University of Texas Southwestern Medical Center, Dallas. Dr Schaefer is now with the Department of Otolaryngology, New York (NY) Eye and Ear Infirmary, and Affiliated Hospitals of the New York Medical College.

Reprint requests to Department of Otolaryngology, New York Eye and Ear Infirmary, Second Ave at 14th St, New York, NY 10003 (Dr Schaefer).

MATERIALS

This is the fourth report in a current series of 139 patients managed between January 1965 and August 1991 at the University of Texas Southwestern Medical Center, Dallas, and affiliated hospitals (Parkland Memorial Medical Center, Veterans Administration Medical Center, Presbyterian Hospital, and John Peter Smith Hospital, all in Dallas). This series is composed of two patient groups. The first group consists of 52 patients acutely treated for external laryngeal trauma between 1965 and 1977. The retrospective analysis of these patients lead to the principles by which the subsequent group of 87 patients were managed, data were collected and evaluated, and results were reported (Table 1).[1,5] These aspects of the methodology have remained the same throughout the entire series. Since the long-term results of this series are important as a measure of outcome of such injuries, changes in the state of the airway or voice following our last report were sought during the current review, within the limitations of the review method and the mobility of the population.[5] Limited information was available as to the patterns of subsequent trauma in this population. However, many of the patients have been followed up for years and the trauma hospital network in Dallas County, Texas, is such that the series broadly reflects the various socioeconomic groups in the region.

Three changes that have occurred over the duration of this series are (1) patients reported after 1982 are confined to those treated at Parkland Memorial Medical Center, (2) treatment between 1977 and 1989 was primarily performed by, or at the direction of, the author, while care thereafter was given by the author or other faculty members using the principles previously reported by the author, and (3) retrieval of charts at Parkland Memorial Hospital for patients managed medically only (classified as group 1 patients) was incomplete after 1989 due to partial coding of records.[5] The latter change did not affect analysis of other patient groups because the same methodology for review of operating room logs, use of a computer search of operating room records, and the examination of personal records was conducted in the same manner by the author.

Inclusion in this report was limited to patients (1) treated within 24 hours of injury, with the exception of two patients treated within 36 hours after injury, (2) managed at the above institutions, and (3) sustaining external trauma to the larynx. These criteria were necessary to maintain the original intent of this series; ie, early management of external laryngeal injuries, rather than secondary management of the late sequelae of various forms of laryngeal trauma.

Duration of observation in the patients treated before 1978 ranged from 1 month to 20 years, and from less than 1 month to 5 years in those managed after 1978. The change in length of follow-up in the first group from previous reports reflects one patient having been recently examined for consideration of further treatment.[5]

MANAGEMENT

The diagnosis of external laryngeal injury was based on the history and physical examination (Table 2). Emergent measures included preservation of the airway, cardiac resuscitation, control of hemorrhage, and stabilization of neural and spinal inju-

Table 1.—Treatment Groups*

Management Group	1965-1977	1978-1982	1983-1988	1988-1991	Total
1	7	7	4	2	**20**
2	5	17	11	11	**51**
3	14	4	8	3	**29**
4	26	7	3	3	**39**

*N=139 patients.

Table 2.—Population Profile After 1977*

	Presenting Symptoms							Type of Injury		
Group	Hoarseness	Pain/ Tenderness	Hemoptysis	Dysphagia	Subcutaneous Emphysema	Impaired Respiration	Hematoma	MVA	Blunt	Penetrating
1	9	7	1	1	1	1	0	7	4	2
2	14	5	3	3	8	21	3	9	11	27
3	4	4	1	1	6	9	1	3	2	10
4	3	4	0	1	3	8	0	4	2	7

*N=87. MVA indicates motor vehicle accident.

ries, followed by a systematic search for other organ system trauma.[5] Throughout this series, tracheotomy was the preferred method of management of the unstable airway rather than endotracheal intubation. Our treatment protocol has been refined over the past decade and is as illustrated in Fig 1. In the past 8 years, computed tomographic scanning was selectively employed in patients with lesser injuries to aid in the determination of those individuals who would benefit from surgical management.[14] Over the entire 27 years of this series, management classification was divided into four groups reflecting the severity of the injury.[4] Informed consent for treatment was obtained throughout this series consistent with the regulations of The University of Texas Southwestern Medical Center and affiliated hospitals.

Group 1

Findings included minor endolaryngeal hematomas or lacerations, absence of a detectable laryngeal skeletal fracture, and minimal, if any, airway compromise. Computed tomography was used to investigate the integrity of the laryngeal cartilages in questionable cases (Fig 2). Patients were medically managed by employing a minimum of 24 hours of close observation, head-of-bed elevation, and humidification of inspired air and laryngoscopy. Flexible fiberoptic laryngoscopy has completely replaced indirect laryngoscopy over the past 10 years as the primary diagnostic procedure in this patient group.[3] Close observation was utilized because some patients initially presenting within an hour of injury developed significant endolaryngeal edema hours later, which compromised their airway. The classification of these patients was based on their final form of treatment. Steroids were prescribed inconsistently, both in this group and in group 2.

Group 2

Findings included edema, hematomas, minor mucosal disruption without exposed cartilage, and varying degrees of airway compromise. Patients were initially managed by tracheotomy under local anesthesia to preserve the airway, to avoid further trauma to the larynx, and to permit administration of general anesthesia. Endotracheal intubation was only used when (1) the laryngeal injury was minor and the patients were undergoing general anesthesia for other reasons or (2) the laryngeal injury was not suspected prior to administration of general anesthesia, and thus the department of otolaryngology was not consulted prior to intubation. Airway management was followed by direct laryngoscopy and rigid esophagoscopy to evaluate the extent of injury.[15] As these injuries were judged as likely to spontaneously resolve, no further operative intervention was performed. Beginning in years 16 and 17, computed tomographic scanning was used initially to confirm laryngeal fractures in patients who were difficult to examine by either indirect or direct laryngoscopy because of massive endolaryngeal edema or hematomas.[14] Before these years, such patients might have undergone open exploration of the larynx to determine the extent of injury. With subsequent experience and given specific theoretical considerations to be discussed later, open exploration of the larynx was considered unnecessary in this group if there were no fractures or if there were single nondisplaced fractures.

Groups 3 and 4

Findings included massive edema, large mucosal lacerations, exposed cartilage, displaced fractures, vocal fold immobility, and varying degrees of airway compromise. Following tracheotomy and endoscopy, the larynx was explored either through a midline thyrotomy or through a laryngofissure at the site of the paramedian fracture (Fig 3). All mucosal injuries were identified and carefully approximated with 5-0 or 6-0 absorbable sutures. The anterior margin of each true vocal fold was sutured to the thyroid cartilage or its external perichondrium at the thyroidotomy site to reconstitute the normal scaphoid configuration of the anterior commissure. Based on the experience in the patient group treated prior to 1978, this reconstruction technique proved valuable in minimizing the use of stents. Computed tomography was omitted in these patients because these injuries were so significant that it was apparent restorative surgery was required.

Group 4 patients differed from group 3 patients in that their injuries tended to be more severe, leaving the anterior larynx (true and/or false vocal fold) disrupted or the cartilaginous skeleton unstable. Therefore, to avoid potential adhesions in the anterior larynx or collapse or overriding of fragments of cartilage, a lumen-keeping stent was employed. In the initial patient group, stenting was performed with commercially available stents, a finger of a surgical glove filled with sponge rubber, or a modified endotracheal tube stent (Portex). Between 1975 and 1988, the endotracheal tube stent (Portex) was used exclusively.[16] After 1988, a Montgomery stent was used in one of three patients requiring stenting. These "lumen-keepers" were fixated with 2-0 polypropylene (Prolene) sutures passed externally through the laryngeal ventricle and cricothyroid membrane (Figs 4 and 5). Before 1975, stents were held in place by wire, which thereafter was abandoned because of breakage in three patients. Stents were removed at direct laryngoscopy under general anesthesia

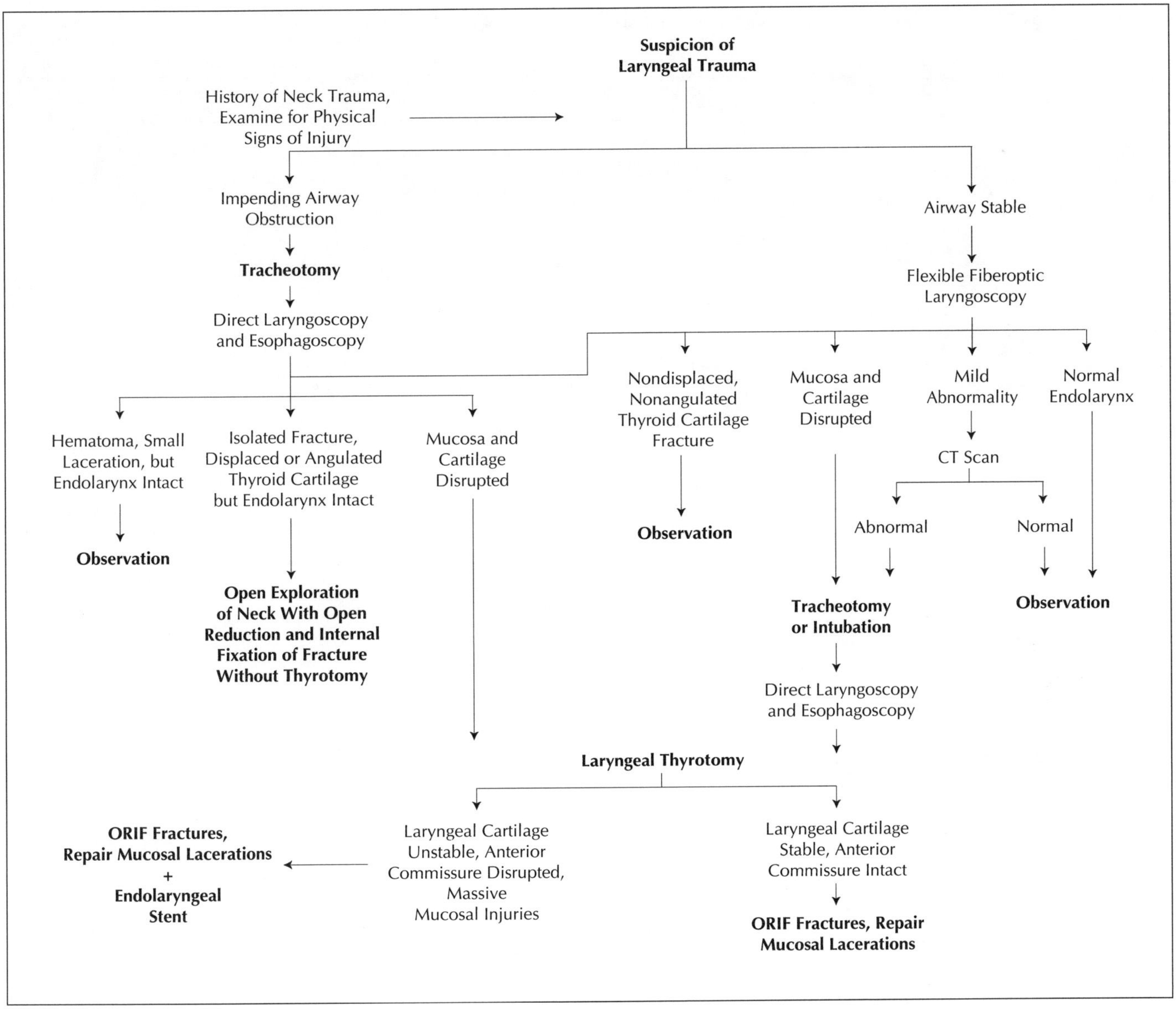

Fig 1.—*Algorithm of treatment protocol for acute management of external laryngeal trauma. ORIF indicates open reduction and internal fixation; CT, computed tomography.*

at approximately 4 weeks after injury until 1983, when the author realized that 2 weeks would suffice to stabilize the larynx and avoid the complications of prolonged stenting. During the 27 years of this report no skin grafts were used. One buccal mucosal graft was employed to cover a gunshot avulsion of the posterior cricoid ring. All fractured cartilage was repaired with either wire or nonabsorbable suture, with the latter primarily used after 1978. Removal or débridement of the laryngeal skeleton was limited to fragments that were totally avulsed from their blood supply. Arytenoid cartilages were preserved and mucosal sutures were used to position the arytenoid on the cricoid. Despite the severity of many of the injuries, the goal of the operations remained restoration of normal anatomic relationships in the hope of best preserving airway and vocal function.[5]

RESULTS

Consistent with earlier reports regarding this series, results are given in terms of incidence of laryngeal trauma and mechanism of injury over time, initial airway management, presenting symptoms, diagnostic improvements, restoration of airway and voice, and complications.

Incidence and Mechanism of Injury

The changing patterns of external laryngeal trauma are well illustrated by examining these patterns at Parkland Memorial Medical Center over the past 27 years. Parkland Memorial Medical Center is a level 1 trauma center for Dallas County, treating 139 466 emergency patients in 1990, 26 119 of whom were trauma patients. This large number of emergency visits reflects the extensive trauma network in Dallas County, which recently has included two other major hospitals. During the first 13 years of this series, 48 patients were identified at Parkland Memorial Medical Center as having sustained either acute blunt or penetrating trauma. During this period, emergency department visits averaged 155 780 per year. In the subsequent 10 years, 68 patients were treated for external laryngeal injuries while the emergency visits averaged 157 000 per year. In the following 4 years, 19 patients with this injury were cared for at Parkland Memorial Medical Center. Emergency department visits during this last period averaged 141 084 per year. During the last two peri-

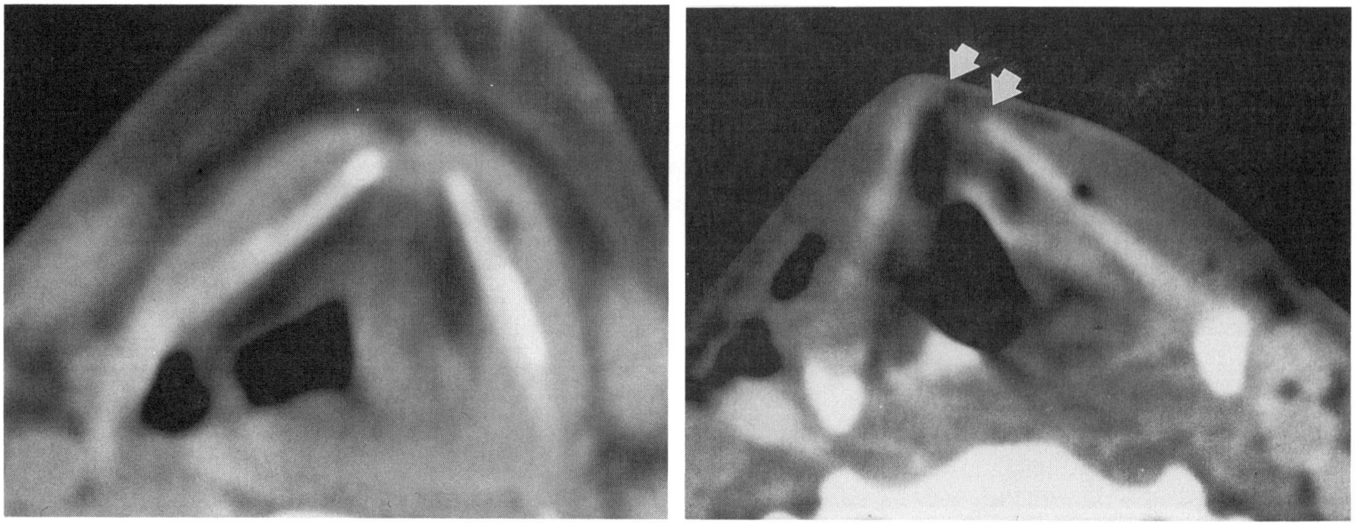

Fig 2.—*Laryngeal computed tomographic scans of two young men who have both sustained blunt trauma to the anterior aspect of the neck. Although the scans appear similar, the patient on the left has only edema and a hematoma of the left vocal fold. The other patient (right) has a paramedian thyroid cartilage fracture (arrows). Further computed tomographic sections of both patients clearly show the actual pathologic findings and illustrate the need for evaluation of the entire scan.*

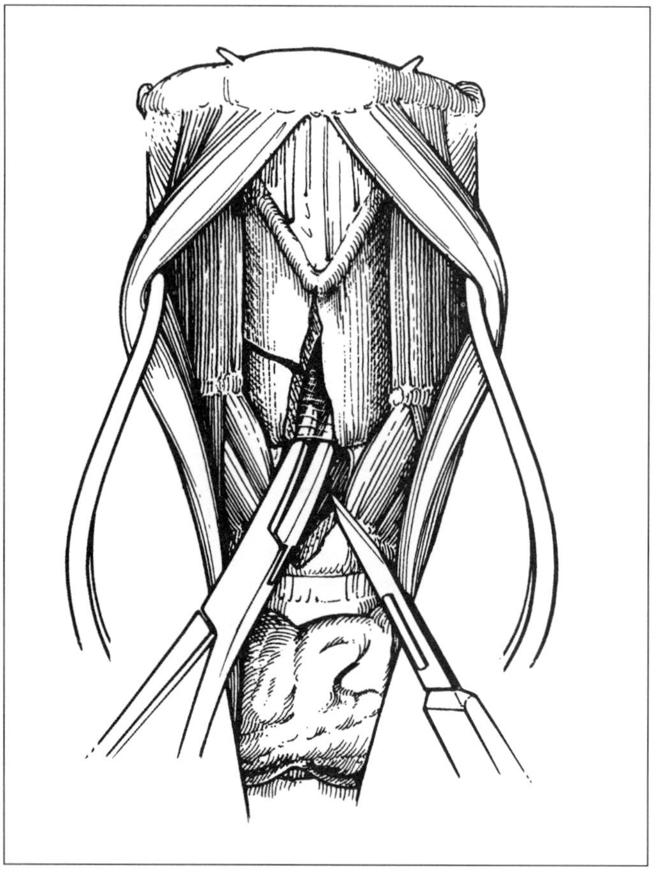

Fig 3.—*The larynx is entered in the midline using a curved hemostat to retract the thyroid cartilage as the scalpel divides the laryngeal mucosa at the anterior commissure.*

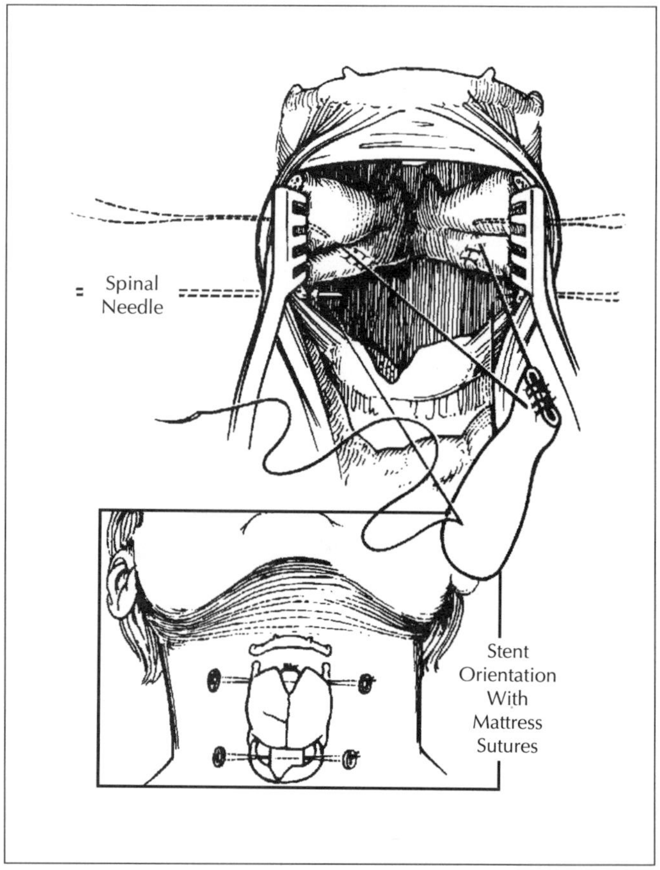

Fig 4.—*Top, Stent fixated in laryngeal lumen using polypropylene (Prolene) suture placed through the laryngeal ventricle and cricothyroid membrane. Bottom, Enlargement shows fixation sutures attached to buttons.*

ods of this series, there was a continued trend toward penetrating trauma due to acts of violence. To better assess the incidence of such trauma in Dallas County, all deaths recorded by the medical examiners office due to neck injuries were reviewed for the first 11 months of 1991. Of the 173 such deaths, 94 were from homicide, 24 from suicide, and 55 from accidents. Within these groups of individuals dying from neck trauma, the distribution of those suffering external laryngeal injuries was 15% (14/94), 75% (18/24), and 23% (12/55), respectively. Also

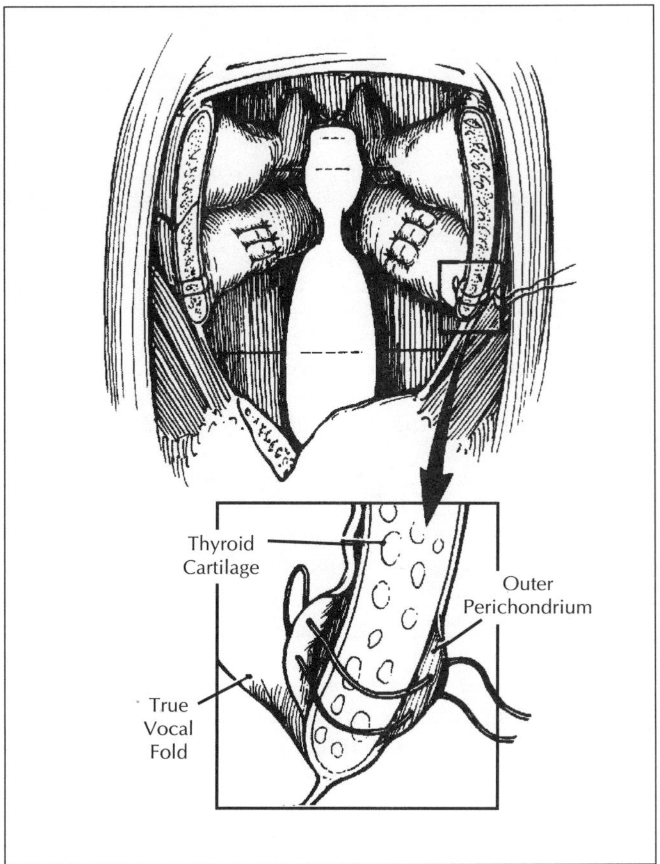

Fig 5.—*Enlargement shows reconstitution of anterior commissure by suturing anterior margin of true vocal fold to outer perichondrium of thyroid cartilage.*

within each of these groups, the most frequent respective mechanism of injury was penetrating trauma (gunshots and stab wounds), blunt trauma (hangings), and blunt trauma (multiple causes).

Initial Airway Management

As has been previously reported, before 1978 there was little agreement between the trauma and otolaryngology services at the University of Texas Southwestern Medical Center as to the best way to manage the potentially unstable airway following external laryngeal trauma. In the period before 1978, four patients did require emergent tracheotomy due to attempted orotracheal intubation. Since 1978 there has been a consensus to avoid intubation in the potentially injured airway and to employ tracheotomy under local anesthesia. Exceptions to this management protocol have been those patients (1) with a history of potential airway trauma and a normal-appearing larynx on direct fiberoptic laryngoscopy who are undergoing general anesthesia for other reasons and (2) with unrecognized laryngeal injuries. The latter group have become increasingly rare but often share the common history of a difficult intubation and further injury to the larynx by the endotracheal tube.

Presenting Symptoms

Presenting symptoms and method of injury for patients treated after 1977 are summarized in Table 2. No apparent correlation was noted between severity of injury and a particular symptom, with one exception. This exception is patients first presenting to the emergency department with difficulty in breathing tended to have more severe injuries.

Diagnostic Improvements

Two important diagnostic modalities have influenced the treatment of laryngeal trauma over the past decade. The first improvement is the routine use of fiberoptic direct laryngoscopy to identify patients with laryngeal trauma and to evaluate the extent of injury. The second modality is computed tomographic scanning in selected patients. Using the previously reported criteria of multiple or displaced fractures as an indication for open exploration, patients with only massive edema continue to be regarded as not benefiting from extensive surgery. In these patients, management is limited to tracheotomy, direct laryngoscopy, and esophagoscopy.[5] Others have had questionable findings on physical examination, and computed tomographic scanning has clearly identified those with displaced laryngeal fractures (Fig 2).

Restoration of Airway and Voice and Complications

The results by management group are summarized in Table 3. For consistency, the same measures of outcome are employed as used in our previous reports.[3,5] A good voice was one that was close to normal or comparable to the patient's preinjury voice. Moderate-to-marked hoarseness was described as a fair voice, and phonation just above a whisper was classified as poor. Airway quality was judged good if the patient denied restriction, fair if mild-to-moderate restriction persisted, and poor if permanent tracheotomy was required.

In group 1, 20 of 20 patients obtained a good airway and a good voice. In group 2, 43 of 51 patients were considered evaluable. Two of the nonevaluable patients died of their injuries, one from a concurrent crushed chest, and the other from a cervical spine gunshot wound. Two nonevaluable patients achieved a good voice, but never returned for removal of their tracheotomy tubes. The other nonevaluable patients did not return for follow-up care. Included with these nonevaluable patients is a 3-year-old child who sustained penetrating trauma to the neck from an assault. This individual was the only pediatric patient in the entire series. The results of these 43 patients are summarized in Table 3. The two patients with a fair voice reflect a recurrent laryngeal nerve injury and an unrepaired laceration of the free margin of the anterior third of the vocal fold in the other patient. In retrospect, the latter patient would have probably benefited from closure of the laceration, and our protocol now reflects this experience. In the patients managed after 1977, 20 underwent concurrent neck exploration without thyrotomy for vascular, pharyngeal, and esophageal injuries. Seven of these patients had minor fracture dislocations or angulated nondisplaced fractures of the thyroid or cricoid cartilages, which were reduced and fixated without entry into the larynx. Five of these 20 patients avoided tracheotomy through the use of fiberoptic endoscopy to identify airways acceptable for intubation. Complications included prolonged hospitalization due to pharyngocutaneous fistula and temporary loss of airway due to attempted orotracheal intubation in an unrecognized laryngeal injury. Follow-up in both groups 1 and 2 tended to be limited because patients often did not return once they were well and/or decannulated (range, 1 week to 5 years).

Table 3.—Results of Treatment of Evaluable Patients*

Group	Voice: Good	Voice: Fair	Voice: Poor	Airway: Good	Airway: Fair	Airway: Poor
1	20	0	0	20	0	0
2	38	3	0	40	1	0
3	18†	3	0	21	0	0
4‡	22	10	0	31	0	2

*N = 115.

†One patient achieved good voice after Teflon injection of true vocal fold following recurrent laryngeal nerve injury.

‡One patient was not evaluated for voice because of prolonged coma. Another patient required removal of a polyp and then developed a fair voice.

In group 3, 21 of the 29 patients were available for follow-up ranging from 1 month to 5 years. Reasons for nonevaluability varied from complications from other injuries to failure to return after decannulation. All evaluable patients underwent removal of their tracheotomy tube within 5 to 35 days after injury. Two patients had significant fracture dislocations of the thyroid cartilage without endolaryngeal lacerations. These two patients were treated by open reduction and suture fixation of the external perichondrium without entry into the larynx. Six months after injury, one patient underwent left true vocal fold Teflon injection for recurrent laryngeal nerve paralysis. Following this procedure the patient achieved a good voice.

Thirty-three of the 39 group 4 patients were evaluable, with follow-up ranging from 2 months to 20 years after injury. Tragically, reasons for nonevaluability included homicide in two patients while they were still tracheotomy dependent, with most patients simply not returning after completing treatment. Decannulation varied from 27 to 100 days after injury, with two patients in the group before 1978 requiring permanent tracheotomy. In one of these patients, tracheotomy was required for pulmonary toilet necessary for anoxic brain damage following cardiac arrest. The other patient was an elderly woman who preferred to use a small-diameter tracheotomy tube with a fair voice and a fair airway clinically (classified as a poor airway in this series because of the persistent tracheotomy tube). Voice and airway results are summarized in Table 3. No observable difference in outcome was seen between the various forms of stenting. Complications in group 4 included (1) avulsion of the mucous membrane of the hemilarynx from attempted intubation in one patient, (2) slippage or expulsion of the stent due to wire breakage in three patients treated before 1978, (3) total airway obstruction following attempted endotracheal intubation in four patients, and (4) removal of an anterior commissure polyp resulting in a fair voice in one patient. An additional patient previously reported as developing perichondritis 9 years after injury was later found to have carcinoma of the larynx.[1] Antibiotics, primarily cephalosporins after 1977, were given for 5 to 10 days after injury in group 3 and 4 patients. Steroids were not used in group 3 and 4 patients.

COMMENT

The results of 27 years of acute management of external laryngeal trauma at primarily one institution are reported. This series provides the means to reappraise and refine previous principles in the acute management of laryngeal injuries reported by the author and other investigators.[1-15,17]

Demographics of Laryngeal Trauma

The changing patterns and increasing incidence of violence in the United States is evident in this series. In this regard, the mandatory use of safety belts and a lower speed limits is felt to be the most likely cause for a reduction in blunt injuries in this series. However, our review of the county medical examiner's files demonstrates that too many individuals are still dying from automobile accidents that potentially are preventable if safety and speed limit laws are observed. Personal assaults continue to increase, relative to motor vehicle accidents. The actual number of assaults causing laryngeal trauma has decreased on a yearly basis for our population since our last report.[5] However, we believe this change probably reflects additional hospitals being more actively involved in the trauma network and reasons that we cannot account for, rather than a real decrease in such injuries given the rise in violent crimes in Dallas County.

Acute Management of the Airway

Over the past decade, we have had the opportunity to refine our views on intubation of the injured larynx. Specifically, the experience of the last 4 years suggests that patients with injuries not involving the lumen of the larynx can safely undergo intubation when performed by a skilled physician.[6] In contrast, significant persistent edema and potential further injury was seen even in our patients with minor intraluminal lacerations or hematoma who underwent intubation. In these patients and in those with greater injuries, tracheotomy performed under local anesthesia is strongly recommended for an emergent or elective airway.

Diagnostic Strategies

Flexible fiberoptic laryngoscopy and computed tomographic scanning have significantly influenced the care of the patients in this series. Flexible fiberoptic endoscopy has permitted evaluation and often correct assessment of the extent of endolaryngeal injury. This procedure has proven particularly useful in identifying those patients who can be managed without surgery vs those requiring repair of endolaryngeal lacerations. Computed tomographic scanning continues to be employed on a selective basis. The selection of patients for scanning has been recently summarized by us as follows: Patients with obvious fractures or large endolaryngeal lacerations on physical examination will require open exploration of the larynx, and, thus, computed tomographic findings are unlikely to influence the treatment decision to manage the patient surgically. Conversely, patients who have a history of minimal trauma to the anterior part of the neck, no laryngeal tenderness or subcutaneous emphysema, and normal fiberoptic endoscopy probably do not benefit from scanning. All other patients should be scanned to evaluate the integrity of the laryngeal skeleton, assess the condition of the cricoarytenoid joints, and examine endolaryngeal soft tissue not seen on fiberoptic endoscopy.[3] Although few patients with blunt trauma have been identified as having pharyngoesophageal injuries, rigid esophagoscopy continues to be employed in both blunt and penetrating trauma in patients undergoing direct laryngoscopy.[15] We recommend rigid over flexible esophagoscopy because previous investigations at our institution have shown the former to be much more sensitive in evaluating injuries of the pharyngoesophageal region.[17]

Operative Intervention

Beyond the need to establish an airway by tracheotomy or evaluate the injury by rigid endoscopy, surgical management should be considered when spontaneous resolution of the laryngeal injury is unlikely.[1] The results in groups 1 and 2 remain consistent throughout this series and suggest a full recovery without operative intervention is likely with laryngeal edema, hematomas without mucosal disruption, small lacerations of the endolarynx not involving the anterior commissure or free margin of the vocal fold, and small lacerations of the supraglottic larynx that do not disrupt the integrity of this site.[1,5] Single nondisplaced thyroid cartilage fractures have been historically treated in this series by observation. However, we have in the last 3 years managed angulated thyroid fractures as per the recommendations of Stanley et al[13] by open reduction and internal fixation. Such fractures have been reduced and fixated without performing a thyrotomy. This treatment is reflected in the inclusion of such patients in group 2.

Open vs Closed Reduction

Closed reduction has been suggested as an alternative to thyrotomy in patients with displaced or comminuted fractures of the laryngeal skeleton. We have no experience with such management. However, we feel these injuries are intrinsically unstable due to the muscular forces on the larynx and continue to recommend open reduction and internal fixation. During the evolution of this series, we observed simple lacerations of the anterior commissure or free margin of the vocal fold lead to impaired vocal function and now recommend these injuries, and those involving large endolaryngeal mucosal lacerations or displaced arytenoids, undergo open treatment via a thyrotomy.

Conservation of Anatomy

Until 1991, no patient in this series had undergone any form of mucous membrane or skin grafting. One patient with a gunshot shattering the posterior cricoid arch has since been treated using a buccal mucosal graft. Despite numerous significant blunt and gunshot wounds in this series, our efforts continue to focus on conservation of laryngeal tissue rather than employing total laryngectomy for severe injuries.[18] At times this has resulted in (1) a foreshortening of the anteroposterior dimension of the larynx due to loss of the anterior thyroid cartilage, (2) use of muscle flaps to replace loss of the anterior cricoid cartilage, or (3) mucosal advancement to cover mucous membrane denuded areas.

Operative Timing

Early treatment of external laryngeal injuries is not novel. The importance of early treatment was well demonstrated by Harris and Tobin[10] and Harris and Ainsworth[11] and has remained an important element of our series. To achieve optimal reduction of fractures and restoration of endolaryngeal anatomy, we believe early recognition and treatment are essential. Since we have little experience in delayed treatment of external laryngeal injuries, no comparison can be made with an alternatively treated population.

Indications for Stenting

A stent may be viewed as having three potential functions. First, such an appliance is used to compliment the fixation of the laryngeal skeleton by providing internal stenting. Second, the stent maintains the lumen of the larynx and, in performing this lumen-keeper function, prevents the formation of adhesions between lacerations or denuded mucous membrane. Finally, the stent serves as a keel to maintain the scaphoid shape of the anterior commissure, which is essential to normal vocalization. Given these functions, we have used stents only when (1) numerous cartilaginous fractures preclude stabilizing the laryngeal skeleton by open reduction and internal fixation, (2) massive endolaryngeal lacerations are likely to result in adhesions or stenosis, or (3) extensive lacerations or avulsion injury prevent restoration of a normal anterior commissure from probable web formation or blunting of this site. The length of stenting depends on the type of stent and the goals of the procedure. Our experience suggests 10 to 14 days is long enough to promote mechanical stability of the larynx without furthering significant mucosal injury.

We would like to express our appreciation to Bill Lene, Chief Field Agent of the Dallas County (Texas) Medical Examiners Office, and his staff for providing us with the information regarding incidence and mechanism of death in Dallas County.

References

1. Schaefer SD. Primary management of laryngeal trauma. *Ann Otol Rhinol Laryngol.* 1982;91:399-402.
2. Cohn AM, Larson DL. Laryngeal injury. *Arch Otolaryngol.* 1976;102:166-170.
3. Schaefer SD. State of the art: the acute treatment of external laryngeal injuries. *Arch Otolaryngol Head Neck Surg.* 1991;117:35-39.
4. Trone TH, Schaefer SD, Carder HM. Blunt and penetrating laryngeal trauma: a 13-year review. *Otolaryngol Head Neck Surg.* 1980;88:257-261.
5. Schaefer SD, Close LG. The acute management of laryngeal trauma: an update. *Ann Otol Rhinol Laryngol.* 1989;98:98-104.
6. Gussack GS, Jurkovich GJ, Luterman A, Mobile A. Laryngotracheal trauma: a protocol approach to a rare injury. *Laryngoscope.* 1986;96:660-665.
7. Olson NR, Miles WK. Treatment of acute blunt laryngeal injuries. *Ann Otol Rhinol Laryngol.* 1971;80:704-709.
8. Olson NR. Surgical treatment of acute blunt laryngeal injuries. *Ann Otol Rhinol Laryngol.* 1978;87:716-721.
9. Pennington CL. External trauma of the larynx and trachea: immediate treatment and management. *Ann Otol Rhinol Laryngol.* 1972;81:546-554.
10. Harris HH, Tobin HA. Acute injuries of the larynx and trachea in 49 patients. *Laryngoscope.* 1970;80:1376-1384.
11. Harris HH, Ainsworth JZ. Immediate management of laryngeal and tracheal injuries. *Laryngoscope.* 1965;75:1103-1115.
12. Fitz-Hugh GS, Wallenborn WM, McGovern F. Injuries of the larynx and cervical trauma. *Ann Otol Rhinol Laryngol.* 1962;71:419-442.
13. Stanley RB Jr, Cooper DS, Florman SH. Phonatory effects of thyroid cartilage fractures. *Ann Otol Rhinol Laryngol.* 1987;96:493-496.
14. Schaefer SD, Brown OE. Selective application of CT in the management of laryngeal trauma. *Laryngoscope.* 1983;93:1473-1475.
15. Krekorian EA. Laryngopharyngeal injuries. *Laryngoscope.* 1975;85:2069-2086.
16. Schaefer SD, Carder HM. 'How I do it'—head and neck: a targeted problem and its solution: fabrication of a simple laryngeal stent. *Laryngoscope.* 1980;90:1561-1563.
17. Weigelt JA, Thal ER, Snyder WH, et al. Diagnosis of penetrating cervical esophageal injuries. *Am J Surg.* 1987;154:619-622.
18. Harrison DFN. Bullet wounds of the larynx and trachea. *Arch Otolaryngol.* 1984;110:203-205.

Management of Combined Frontonaso-Orbital/Skull Base Fractures and Telecanthus in 355 Cases

Joram Raveh, MD, DMD; Kurt Laedrach, MD, DMD; Thiery Vuillemin, MD, DMD; Markus Zingg, MD, DMD

• In regard to the multiple problems of reconstruction concerning this fracture pattern, we developed various methods to achieve optimal results. As various vital regions, apart from the nasoethmoidal fractures and aesthetics, are involved, the proposed classification has direct implication for the surgical procedure. Even in intracranial fragment dislocations, cerebral contusion, and elevated intracranial pressure, the subcranial approach, in contrast with the transfrontal access, enables early definitive management of the skull base and the external facial frame in a one-stage procedure. Another method, the symmetrical centripetal compression of the canthal ligaments and naso-orbital bone fragments, enables correct reduction of the telecanthus. The significant reduction of morbidity and complication rate to a minimum confirms the efficiency of our treatment modalities.

(*Arch Otolaryngol Head Neck Surg.* 1992;118:605-614)

Of 5017 surgically treated facial fractures in our department, 475 cases showed concomitant severe skull base and frontal bone involvement, of which 355 had frontonaso-orbital disruption along with marked telecanthus. As shown in our series, the concomitant involvement of the skull base and frontal region in this fracture pattern is significantly common to high-velocity trauma cases. In such severe cases, the vast disruption includes intracranial dislocation of bone fragments along the anterior and middle skull base planes as well as multiple vast dural tears and optic nerve compression. This implies that multiple regions and very specific aspects must be appraised to enable optimal evaluation and planning. These may be summarized as follows: (1) concomitant involvement of the skull base and ethmoidal frontal sinuses in association with brain contusion, elevated intracranial pressure, multiple vast dural tears, cerebrospinal fluid leaks, and frequent herniation of devitalized brain tissue into the paranasal spaces and orbits; (2) direct compression of the optic nerve in the canal by bone fragments or as a result of pressure development and orbital apex syndrome; (3) concomitant lesions to the sagittal or cavernous sinuses, hypophysis, or major intracranial blood vessels; and (4) aesthetic and functional derangement as a result of the disrupted frontonaso-orbital rim frame, inward telescoped nasal buttress, and telecanthus.

The linkage of the various regions involved is obvious and should be considered accordingly as one entity. To date, the conventional treatment consists of a neurosurgical, transfrontal management of the skull base planes, while leaving the reduction of the facial frame to be performed by others in the same or in a separate session. The disadvantages directly related to the craniotomy and transfrontal procedure are the relatively high morbidity and complication rate. Furthermore, as adequate frontal lobe retraction is mandatory for the management of extensive skull base lesions, concomitant cerebral contusion, edema, and elevated intracranial pressure often preclude intracranial surgery. Apart from a local, limited, primary neurosurgical repair, the surgical definitive management must often be deferred for 10 days or even 2 to 3 weeks.[1-5] This implies that the reduction of the concomitant multiple fractures of the facial skeleton must also be postponed. The disadvantages directly related to such a deferral should be emphasized as follows: (1) the multiple dislocated facial frame fragments and, particularly, the disrupted frontonaso-ethmoidal and orbital skeleton hematoma and coagula often lead to obstruction of the sinus pathways and lymphatic drainage; edema and swelling of the soft tissues, as a result of insufficient drainage, develop within the first 24 to 48 hours, and, if surgery is deferred, often increase grotesquely; (2) the risk of acute or chronic infection is higher as the pressure and expansion of the soft tissues lead to further damage and promote unfavorable scar formation later on; (3) granulation tissue and osteoid interposition often make optimal reduction of the fragments difficult or even impossible; (4) optic nerve decompression, only effective within the first 8 hours, cannot be performed; and (5) deferral implies prolonged intensive care.

The longer the deferral, the less optimal the result will be, and we regard the initial 24 to 48 hours following trauma as the "golden period." Accordingly, we developed the subcranial approach[6-8] to enable an early one-stage definitive surgical management of these complex

Accepted for publication December 21, 1991.
From the Department of Craniomaxillofacial Surgery, University of Bern (Switzerland).
Presented at the American Association of Facial Plastic and Reconstructive Surgery Fall Meeting, Kansas City, Mo, September 28, 1991.
Reprint requests to Department of Craniomaxillofacial Surgery, Clinic of Otolaryngology–Head and Neck Surgery, University of Bern, 3010 Bern, Switzerland (Dr Raveh).

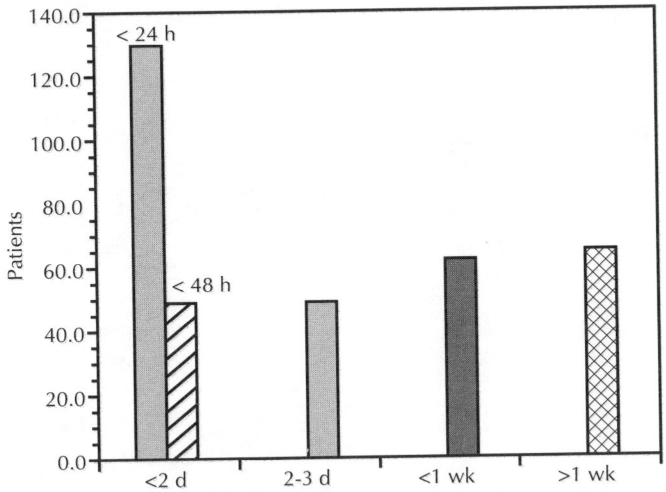

Fig 1.—*Time elapsed between trauma and surgical treatment in 355 patients with combined frontonaso-orbital and skull base fractures.*

injuries, in spite of major involvement of the neurocranium.

Furthermore, the subcranial approach made the development of a further technique possible: the symmetrical, centripetal compression of the naso-orbital frame fractures and canthal ligaments.[8] The reproduction of pretraumatic relations of this anatomically subtile and aesthetically delicate area still represents a challenge.[9-12] The purpose of this article is to highlight the advantages rendered by the subcranial approach and the techniques for reduction of the disrupted frontonaso-orbital complex.

MATERIALS AND METHODS

Facial fractures (5017) were surgically treated in our department during the years 1978 through 1989. Of these, 475 had combined frontal skull base and midface fractures, of which only 355 cases with major disruption of the nasal buttress, lateral displacement of the medial and inferior orbital rim frame, and marked telecanthus were evaluated in this series. As indicated in Fig 1, definitive one-stage management was feasible in 51% of cases in less than 48 hours. The deferral of 1 week or more was unavoidable in regard to involvement of further systems or late referrals from rural regions. In the preoperative evaluation, the neurosurgeon as well as the ophthalmologist were always involved.

Anatomic Considerations in Regard to the Fracture Pattern

The frontal, maxillary, and ethmoidal sinuses, in conjunction with the orbital cavity and the nasal buttress, may be regarded as shock absorbers. The fracture pattern in high-velocity trauma of the complex region may be classified in two separate cardinal categories as follows:

Type 1. Frontonaso-Ethmoidal and Medial Orbital Frame Fractures Without Skull Base Involvement.—The external facial frame and buttresses give way (Fig 2) and absorb and neutralize the entire force impact. In this type of fracture, the posterior walls of the frontal sinuses, the frontal skull base planes, and the optic nerve canal are left intact. Accordingly, the brain tissue and the dura are also left undamaged. This type of fracture only demands the reduction of the external frame fractures and telecanthus as well as the management of the frontal and ethmoidal sinuses. Exact clinical and radiologic evaluation are essential to exclude skull base and optic nerve involvement.

Type 1a. Additional Optic Nerve Involvement.—Same pattern as in type 1, except that the fracture along the medial orbital wall (Fig 2, top) involves the orbital apex and the medial wall of the optic canal with concomitant nerve compression. This seldom occurs, as most cases with involvement of the optic nerve canal correspond to type 2 injuries, dependent on the force impact.

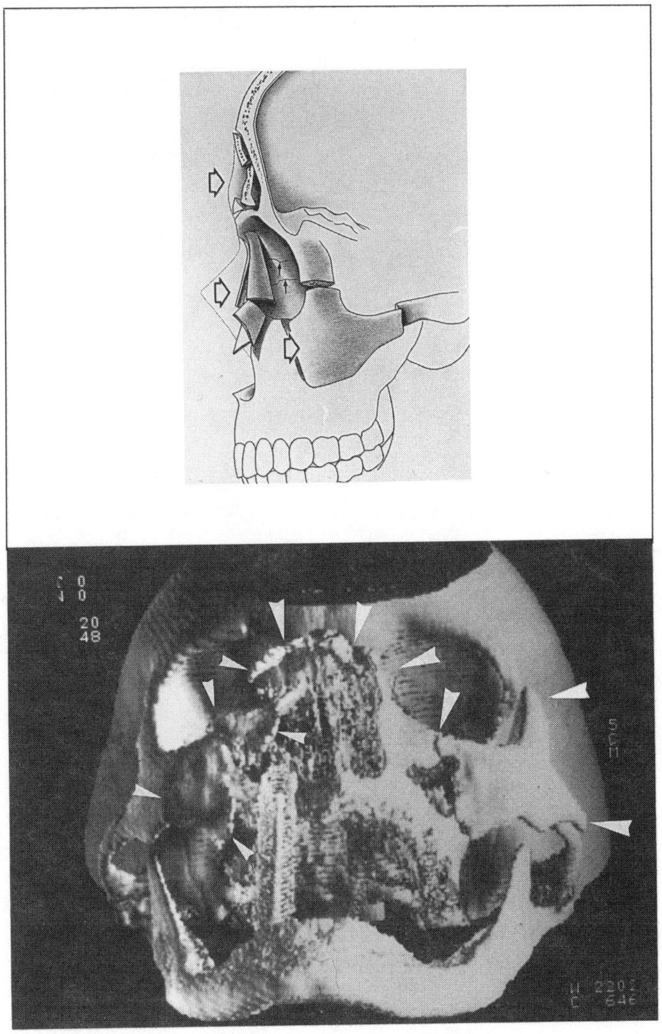

Fig 2.—*Frontonaso-orbital frame fracture pattern, type 1. Top, Schematic illustration of the type 1 fracture pattern: no concomitant skull base lesions. Type 1a: occasional involvement of the medial orbital wall may lead to optic nerve compression along the canal (arrows). Bottom, Preoperative three-dimensional computed tomographic scan demonstrating frontonaso-orbital frame (arrowheads) fractures, resulting in telecanthus.*

Type 2. Combined Skull Base, Frontonaso-Ethmoidal, and Medial Orbital Frame Fractures: Frequent Optic Nerve Compression.—The force impact is of such intensity that the pattern described in type 1 is insufficient to absorb and neutralize all of the force components. Thus, not only the external but also the internal palisades and buttresses give way and fracture (Fig 3, left). This includes intracranial dislocation of the posterior frontal sinus walls (Fig 3, center); inward telescoping of the fractured nasal buttress underneath the skull base, leading to further fractures; and intracranial dislocations along the anterior skull base planes (Fig 3, center and right). These include the ethmoidal and orbital roofs up to the temporal bone as well as the sphenoidal-parasellar areas. The dura, particularly at the anterior part of the skull base, is extremely adherent to the bone. Accordingly, multiple dural tears, pneumocranium, cerebrospinal fluid leaks, and brain tissue herniation into the comminuted ethmoidal, orbital, and frontal sinus compartments are extremely frequent. Lateral and inward displacement of the nasal walls and medial orbital rim frame fragments results in a telecanthus and flattening of the interorbital area. The force of impact often leads to further fractures and dislocations along the

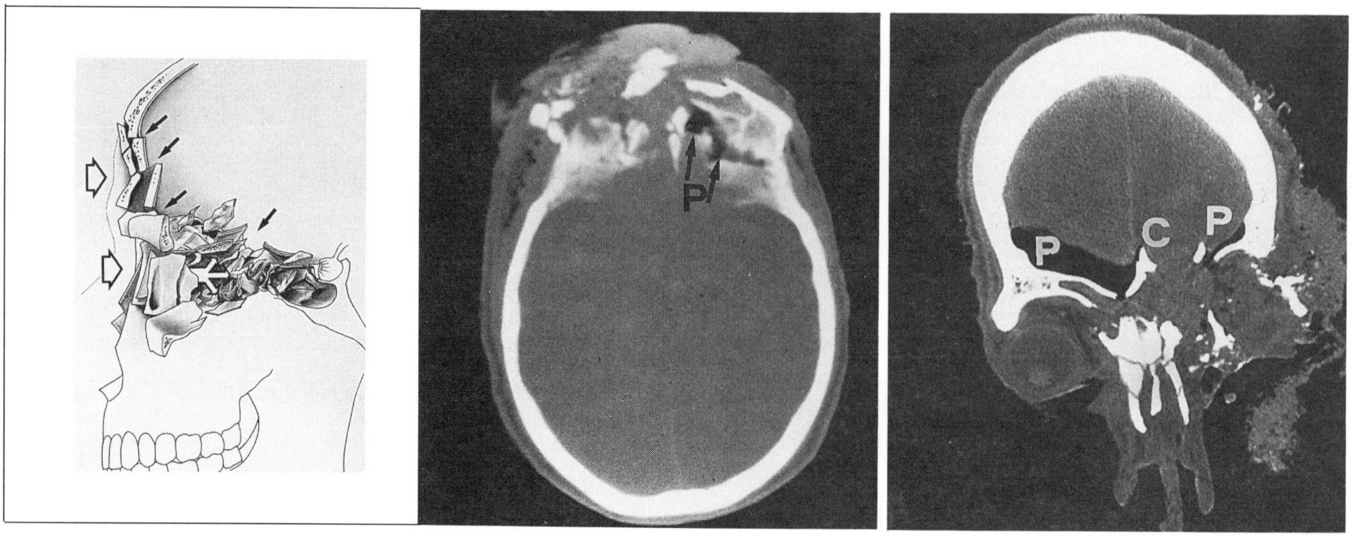

Fig 3.—*Frontonaso-ethmoidal and orbital fracture pattern, type 2. Left, Schematic illustration of the force components leading to concomitant intracranial fragment dislocation along the skull base and sphenoidal planes. Note frequent involvement of the medial orbital wall and optic nerve compression along the canal (arrows). Center, Axial computed tomographic scan illustrating major intracranial fragment dislocation involving all frontobasal skull base planes. P indicates pneumocranium. Right, Same case, coronal computed tomographic scan. Disattached and multifragment nasal bone/orbital frame fracture. P indicates pneumocranium; C, dislocated crista galli.*

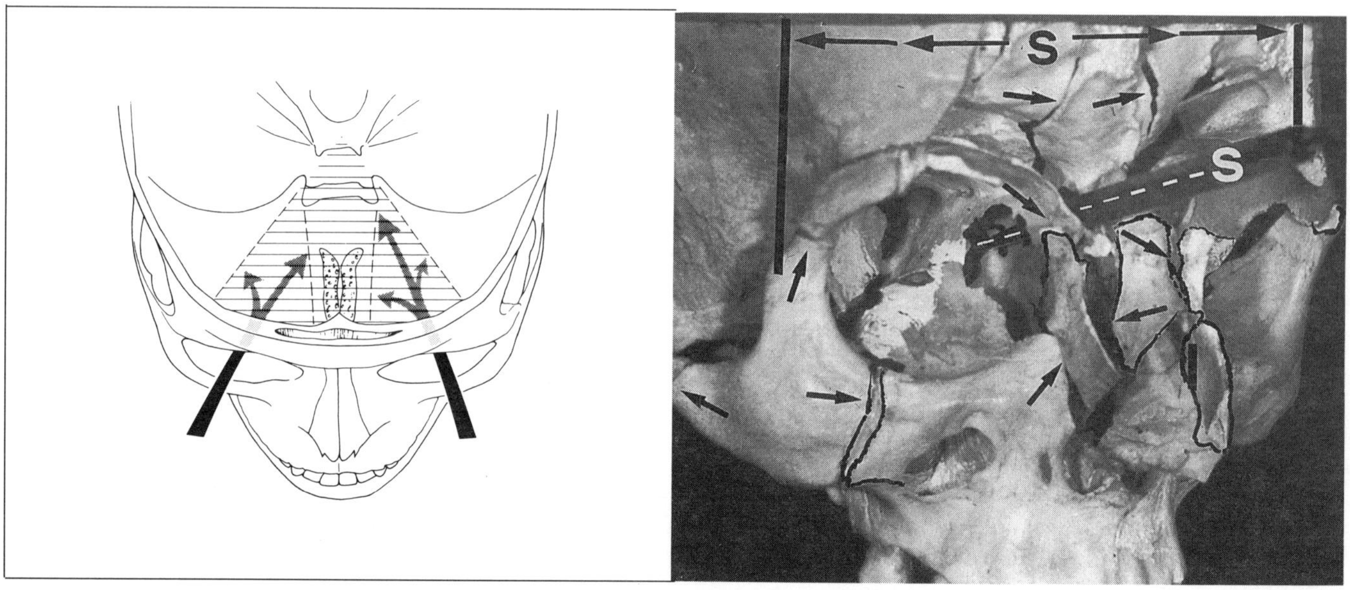

Fig 4.—*Left, Schematic illustration of the subcranial exposure avoiding the neurosurgical-transfrontal approach. In contrast with the classic limited transethmoidal exposure, the orbital roof and lateral walls are included. Right, Reproduced combined skull base–midface fractures (arrows) following removal of the frontal sinus walls. Extent of the subcranial exposure (S). Access to the sphenoid and optic canal wall is marked by a sonde.*

optic nerve canal with concomitant compression of the nerve. Even more often than direct nerve compression by the bone fragments is the development of an orbital apex syndrome due to hematoma and edema. This is the result of displaced medial orbital and lateral ethmoidal wall fragments into the orbital cavity, damaging the periorbital tissue.

Treatment Modalities and Methods

In all cases, clinical and radiologic examination, in regard to possible concomitant involvement of the skull base and optic nerve, is inevitable. This cannot be emphasized often enough.

Type 1, 1a. Frontonaso-Ethmoidal and Medial Orbital Frame: Fractures Without Skull Base Involvement.—As only the external facial frame is fractured and no skull base involvement is manifest, initial posttraumatic surgical management is usually feasible in all cases. As such cases are less complicated, in comparison with the severe fracture pattern in type 2, these were not included in this series. In the presence of a type 1a injury with optic nerve compression, urgent surgical treatment within the first 8 hours is indicated. The surgical management of the external skeletal frame is the same as in type 2.

Type 2. Combined Skull Base, Frontonaso-Ethmoidal, and Medial Orbital Frame Fractures: Frequent Optic Nerve Involvement.—In contrast with type 1, with fractures limited to the external frame, concomitant intracranial fragment dislocations, brain contusion, and edema as well as optic nerve compression are typical for this fracture pattern (Fig 3). The subcranial approach developed by us (Fig 4) enables an extensive exposure, thus making early definitive one-stage management of all skull base planes, including reduction of the frontonaso-orbital fractures, possible. This is particularly crucial if optic nerve decompression within the first 8 hours is indicated.

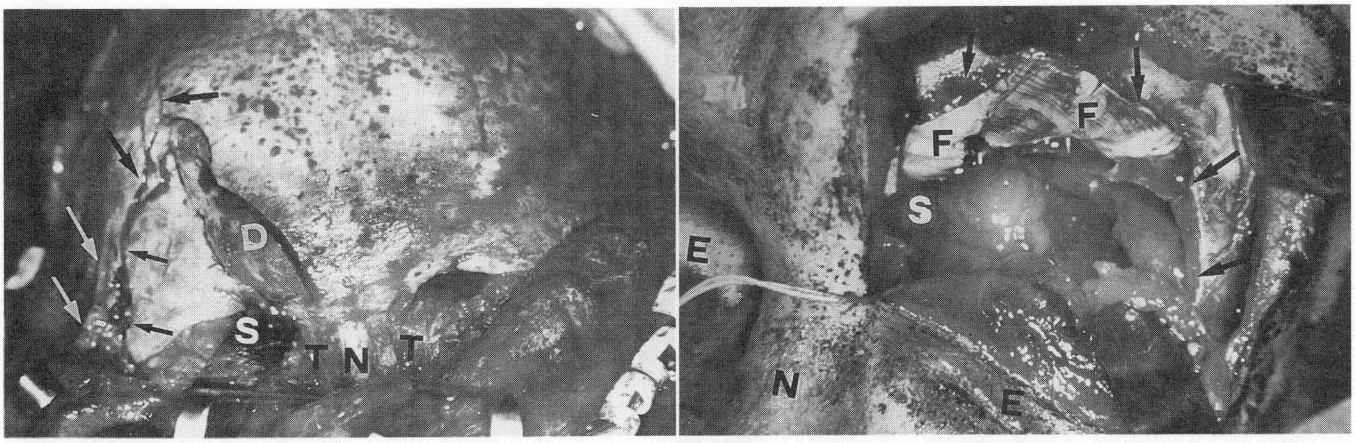

Fig 5.—*Incisions for the subcranial exposure. Left, Bicoronal flap. Frontoparietal dislocation (arrows). D indicates lacerated exposed dura; S, double-sided subcranial exposure of the orbital and ethmoidal roof, including the transethmoidal (T) access up to the sphenoid; and N, nasal bone. Right, Eyebrow incision, limited to the hair borders. E indicates retracted globe; arrows, fracture borders following temporary removal of the anteroposterior sinus walls/orbital roof; F, fascia lata layers aligning frontal lobe and sutured dura; N, nasal bone; and S, subcranial exposure of ethmoidal-orbital roof, sphenoid, and optic nerve decompression.*

Management of the Skull Base Planes and Optic Nerve Decompression.—The subcranial exposure of the skull base is performed by the coronal flap or eyebrow incision (Fig 5). The dural tears are sutured and aligned with fascia lata (Fig 5, right) and adapted with fibrin glue. Accessory alignment of the entire subcranial undersurface with fascia lata provides further optimal isolation from the paranasal spaces. In contrast, a pedicled transfrontally applied pericranial flap often turns out to be insufficient for the closure of multiple major dural tears along the posterior orbital-ethmoidal roof and parasellar-sphenoidal planes.

The frontal sinuses are never obliterated—on the contrary, these are meticulously reconstructed to regain correct physiologic function. A Portex tube is inserted into the subcranial compartment and frontal sinus and externalized into the nasal lumen to establish adequate drainage. The tube is left in situ for not less than 6 months to avoid obliteration of the pathways. Following this, the frontal bone fragments are reduced.

The broad subcranial exposure facilitates optic nerve decompression. Removal of the medial optic canal wall (Fig 6) enables the expansion of the nerve medially toward the subcranial compartment created by the removal of the comminuted ethmoidal cells. This, and the tube drainage of the subcranial compartment externalized into the nasal lumen, prevents postoperative development of pressure at the apical orbital cone and along the optic nerve.

Reduction of the Telecanthus: The Symmetrical Centripetal Cross-sided Compression Method.—This method is schematically illustrated in Fig 7 and includes both sides. Reduction of the nasal and medial orbital frame should only be undertaken after reconstruction of the frontal area for the achievement of a correct three-dimensional configuration. Two burr holes are then drilled into the lateral nasal wall fragments on both sides, where the canthal ligament should be adapted. An unresorbable thread is guided through the canthal ligament, and both ends are inserted through the burr holes and underneath the already exposed anterior skull base, through the perpendicular lamina, over to the contralateral frontal sinus lumen (Fig 7, right). Both ends are then guided through two further burr holes applied to the anterior frontal sinus wall. Tightening of both ends on each side results in a symmetrical centripetal compression of the reduced fragments and canthal ligaments.

If the lateral nasal walls are comminuted and practically pulverized, bone grafting is indicated. In the absence of osseous support beneath the canthal ligament, it will tend to be displaced laterally and upward. Later on, as a result of granulation tissue formation, displacement worsens. If this aspect is left unconsidered, postoperative telecanthus can be a complication. The bone grafts are usually harvested from the external calvarial table into which two burr holes are applied. Fixation of the canthal ligament is then performed in the manner already described. The major advantages of this procedure are as follows: (1) the canthal ligaments as well as the lateral nasal wall fragments are compressed and symmetrically pulled toward the midline; (2) the canthal ligament is not only adapted medially at the correct horizontal and vertical level but, as the thread is guided underneath the skull base, the ligament is also pulled simultaneously down and inward to guarantee the correct relation in the sagittal level; and (3) even if, during the remodeling period, resorption of the reduced nasal buttress bone fragments or bone grafts occur, the canthal ligaments will still remain in the correctly set position.

The following cases illustrate particular details and aspects concerning these techniques.

REPORT OF CASES

CASE 1.—As shown in Fig 8, the high-velocity force impact resulted in the disruption of the frontonaso-ethmoidal and medial orbital rim frame as well as intracranial fragment dislocation. Cerebrospinal fluid leaks, multiple dural tears, and devitalized brain tissue herniation along the orbital and ethmoidal compartments were manifest. Bilateral optic nerve compression was confirmed, making immediate surgery necessary. Immediate definitive management by the craniotomy transfrontal approach along with adequate frontal lobe retraction would have, in this case, not been feasible.

In contrast, immediate initial decompression and surgical management of all further regions by the subcranial approach was performed. The frontal and naso-orbital region was reconstructed using miniplates (AO-Synthes, Stratec Medical, Waldenburg, Switzerland). The zygomatic fractures in the orbital floor were reduced by the transconjunctival approach,[8] using lyophilized cartilage. Reduction of the telecanthus was performed as shown in Fig 7. Intensive care was limited to only 24 hours, and the patient was discharged after 11 days of hospitalization. Postoperative results are shown in Fig 8, panels g and h.

CASE 2.—This patient sustained a major disruption of the frontonaso-ethmoidal region (Fig 9). The telecanthus, along with inward telescoped nasal buttress and involvement of the skull and brain tissue, were even more marked than in patient 1. Six hours following trauma, one-stage definitive management was undertaken. Closure of the dural tears and reconstruction of the frontal region as well as reduction of the frontonaso-orbital fractures and telecanthus were performed by the bicoronal flap and subcranial approach. The postoperative roentgenogram (Fig 9, center right) illustrates the advantage of the centripetal com-

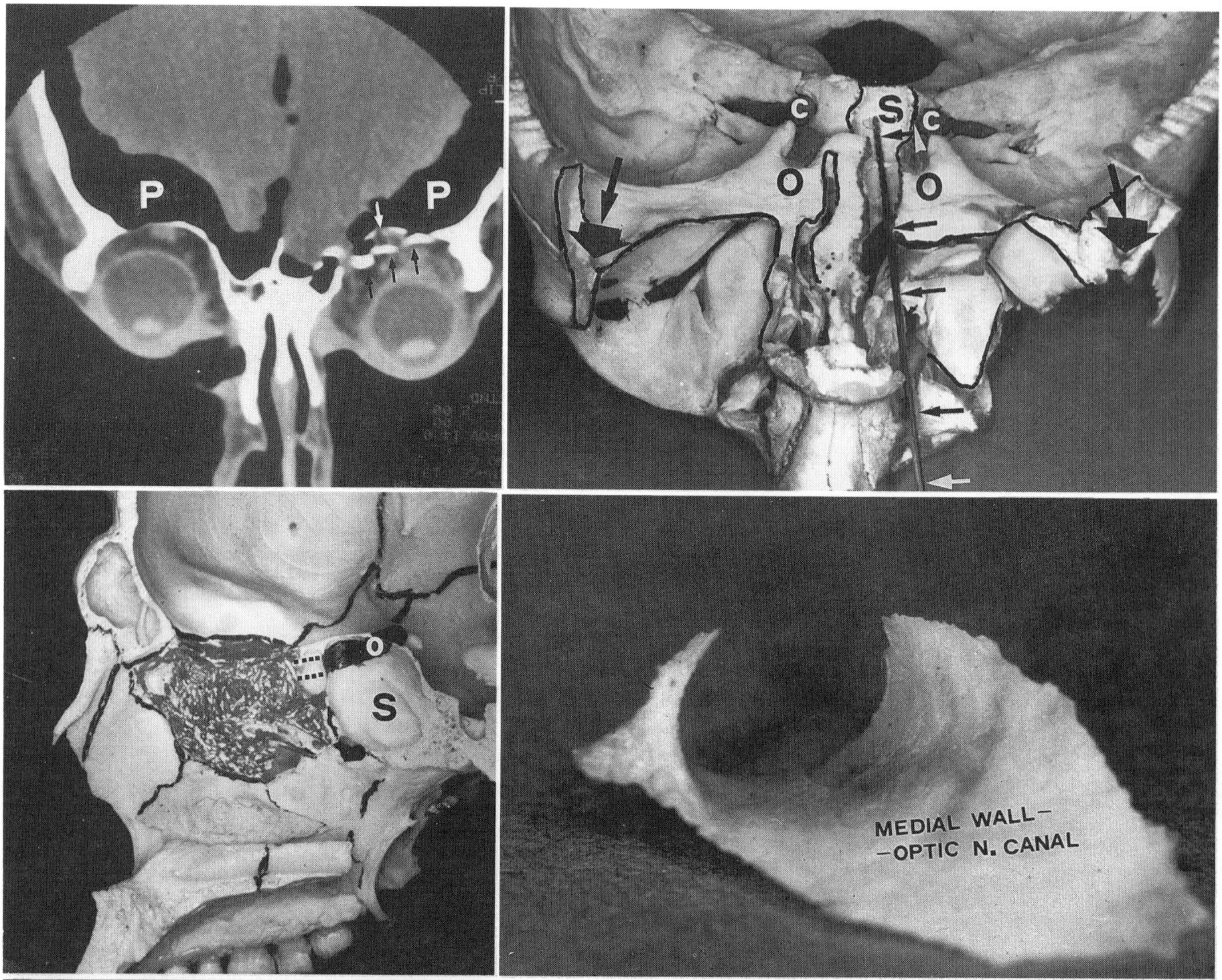

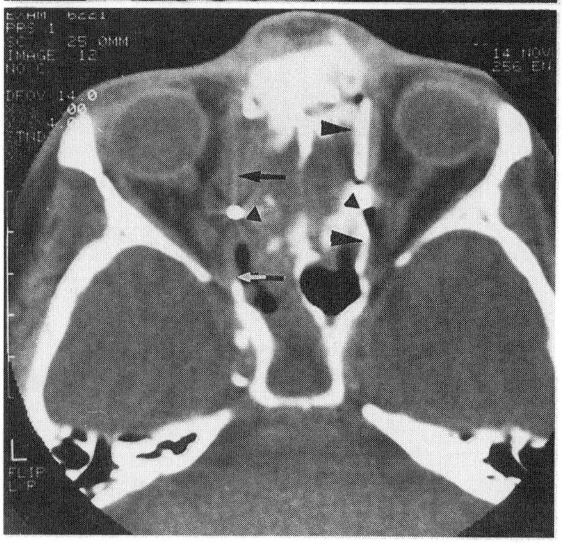

Fig 6.—*Top left, Coronal computed tomographic scan illustrating vast pneumocranium (P) and dislocated ethmoidal and orbital roof fractures (arrows) leading to optic nerve compression. Top right, Subcranial optic nerve decompression. Subcranial exposure including the lateral orbital walls (large arrows) and sphenoid (S) marked by a sonde (arrows). Removal of the medial nerve canal wall is facilitated. O indicates optic nerve; C, the immediate adjacency of the carotid artery to the sphenoid. Center left, Broken line indicates projection of the osteotomy line for removal of the medial optic nerve canal wall (O), enabling the subcranial expansion and decompression of the nerve. S indicates sphenoid. Center right, Removed medial optic nerve canal wall compressing the nerve in a trauma case. Bottom, Postoperative axial computed tomographic scan, same case (center right) after doubled-sided skull base repair by the subcranial exposure. Triangles indicate ethmoidal artery clips on both sides; arrows (left side), removed partial medial orbital and total medial optic nerve canal wall; arrowheads (right side), in contrast, preserved medial orbital and nerve canal walls.*

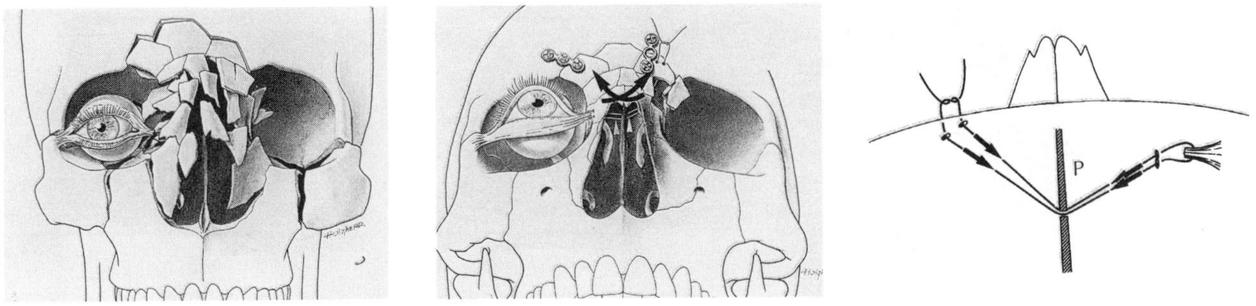

Fig 7.—*Left, Schematic illustration of the frontonaso-orbital fracture pattern and telecantus in type 2. Center and right, Centripetal-subcranial cross-sided compression for reduction of the telecanthus. P indicates lamina perpendicularis. Both thread ends guided through the canthal ligament underneath the skull base to the frontal wall: tightening provides symmetrical compression of the fragments and ligaments toward the midline pulled medially and downward (see text).*

pression of the naso-orbital fractures, limiting the application of miniplates to the load-bearing buttresses. Postoperative views (Fig 9, bottom left and right) confirm the efficiency of this method.

RESULTS

The minimum follow-up period in this series was 1 year. The maximum follow-up period of 5 years and more included 49.8% of patients. The remaining 41.9% of patients had a follow-up period of 2 to 5 years. The departments of ophthalmology and neurosurgery and the dental school were involved in the evaluation. In regard to the insurance system in Switzerland, enabling and even implying such intensive recall activities, the compliance was exceptionally favorable. It should be emphasized that, in spite of severe involvement of the neurocranium, most patients were discharged from intensive care after 1 to 2 days. Swelling subsided rapidly 1 to 2 days postoperatively, in contrast with deferred cases. If no other systems were involved, hospitalizations were limited to 10 to 11 days.

Evaluation of the Reduced Intercanthal Distance and Frontonaso-Orbital Fractures

The examination was specifically related to the results concerning the skull base and reduction of the frontal, nasoethmoidal, and medial-orbital frame as well as the intercanthal distance. Further aspects, such as symmetry of the zygomas, reconstruction of the orbital walls, diplopia, enophthalmos, strabismus, and globe position would have been beyond the scope of this article and are the subject of further articles. The anthropometric measurements (Table 1) were performed according to the study of Farkas[13] in a normal population to allow for an adequate comparative evaluation. This series of 355 cases included 302 males and 53 females. Thus, in regard to the values described in the study by Farkas concerning only male subjects, we did not integrate the female subjects. The distances were even slightly less than in the male subjects, and the success rate was the same. The measurements were within the normal limits. The width and inclination of the palpebral fissure, in relation to the canthal line, were calculated and found to be normal in most patients. Accordingly, as shown in Table 2, the indication for secondary correction was reduced to only a few cases. As a postoperative intercanthal distance may be within the normal limits, a significant aberration in the individual pretraumatic width may yet manifest. Thus, the criteria for evaluation should not only include the measurements but, furthermore, the comparison of pretraumatic photographs, including the opinion of relatives. Accordingly, the criteria for insufficient reduction were particularly strict. Only in 1.9% of patients (Table 2) was insufficient reduction observed. In regard to the symmetrical, centripetal compression method, as described in this article, asymmetrical displacement of the medial canthal ligament of 1 to 2 mm above and 3 to 3.5 mm below the canthal line was observed in only eight patients.

Cerebrospinal Fluid Leaks

The incidence of postoperative cerebrospinal fluid leaks was only 2.8%, which compares favorably with that reported in the literature. Further, 1.1% of the recurrent cerebrospinal fluid leaks occurred postoperatively in those patients still confused, restless, and not fully awake, which removed the ethmoidal roof packing that extruded into the nasal lumen. Further, cerebrospinal fluid leaks were a result of insufficient closure of the dural tears and revision was indicated.

Meningitis

Postoperative meningitis was observed in 1.1% of patients. This included mostly late referrals in whom persisting meningitis and even abscess formation were already manifest.

Mortality

Four patients died 6 days to 3 weeks postoperatively. One patient presented with meningitis and intracranial abscess formation preoperatively, while the remaining patients succumbed to causes not directly related to surgery.

Frontal Sinus Infection

Acute frontal sinusitis was observed in 1.7% of patients due to insufficient drainage, which was a result of loss or accidental removal of the Portex or its obliteration. In those patients resistant to antibiotics, revision was performed.

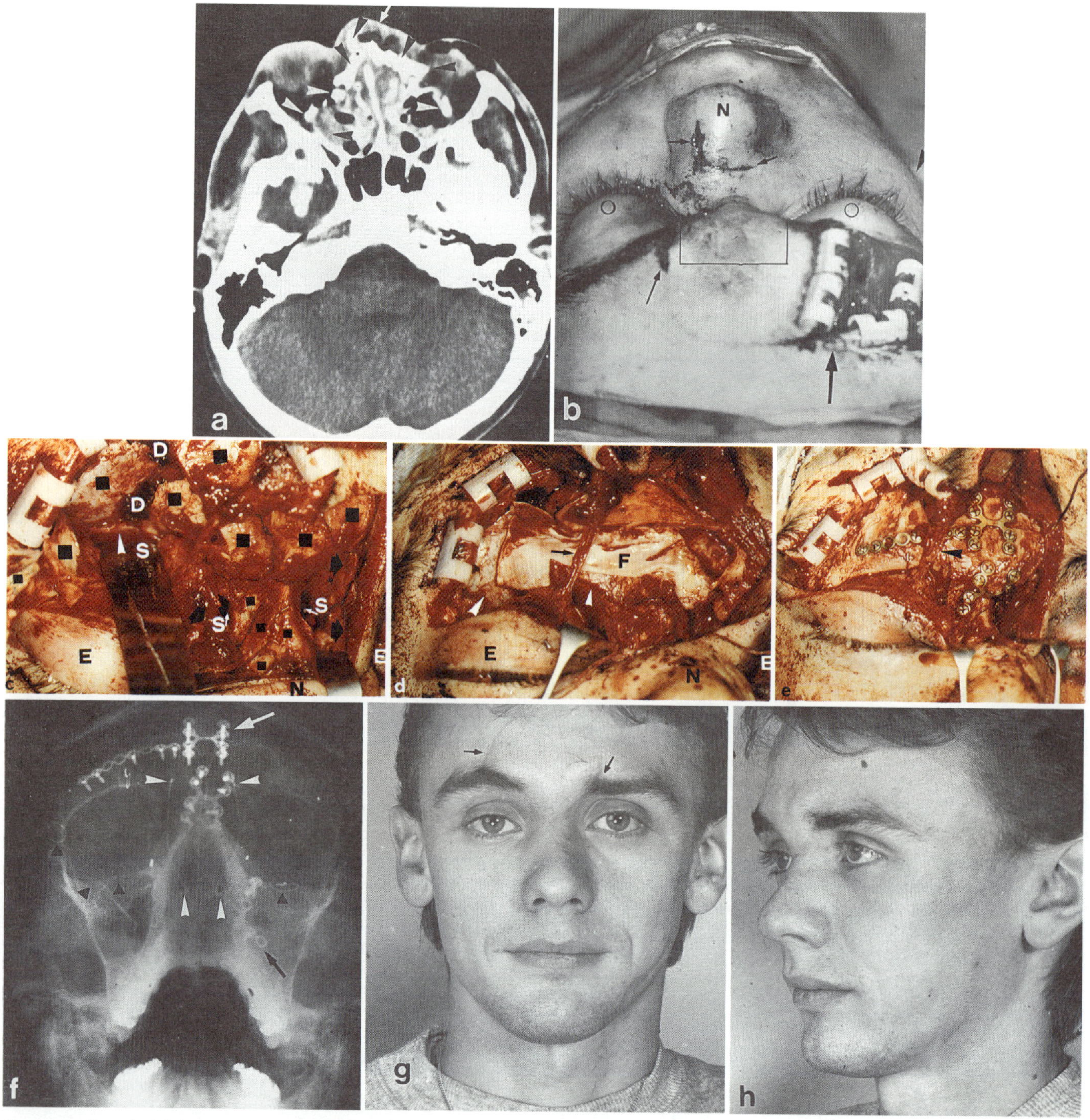

Fig 8.—*a, Case 1. Axial computed tomographic scan. Type 2 pattern-inward telescoped nasal buttress (arrow) and lateral displacement of the impacted lateral nasal walls and ethmoidal compartment (arrowheads). Severe amaurotic optic nerve compression on both sides. Multiple dural laceration and cerebrospinal fluid leaks. b, Same patient. Open laceration wounds (arrows). Note the asymmetry of the front, zygoma (arrowhead), and orbitae (circles). The nasal buttress is telescoped inward; only the tip of the nose is emerged (N). Telecanthus is indicated by the bar. c, Same patient, following removal of devitalized brain tissue herniated into the orbital cavity and frontal sinus. D indicates lacerated dura. Intracranially dislocated bone fragments (squares); arrowhead, distal part of the orbital roof after removal of the intracranially dislocated segments; nasal frame already repositioned. Laterally displaced nasal wall fragments (large arrow). E indicates eyes. d, Temporary removal of intracranially dislocated frontal bone, oribtal, and ethmoidal roof fragments. Double-sided optic nerve decompression. F indicates frontal lobes and dural tears along all skull base planes aligned with fascia; E, eyes; arrows, preserved supraorbital nerve. e, Titanium miniplate osteosynthesis. Reduction and centripetal compression of the nasal bone fragments and canthal ligaments, as in Fig 9, center right and bottom left. Arrowhead, preserved supraorbital nerve. f, Postoperative roentgenogram. The centripetal compression method enables reduction of miniplate application to a minimum (arrows). Infraorbital rim and orbital floor reduction (triangles) by the transconjunctival approach avoiding miniplates. Portex tube drainage of the skull base (arrowheads). g and h, Postoperative view of the same patient. Arrows indicate visible traumatically induced laceration scars.*

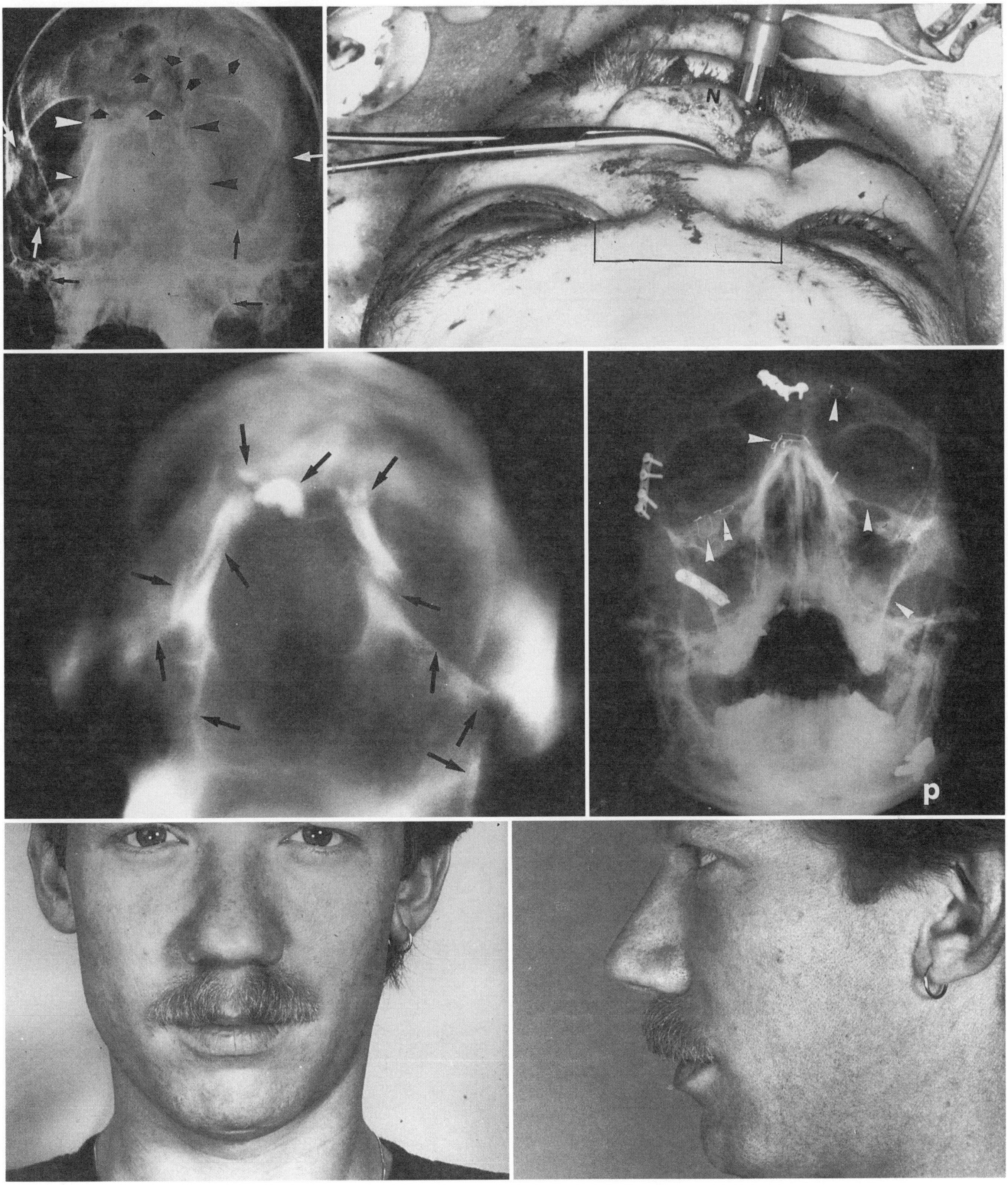

Fig 9.—*Top left, Preoperative roentgenogram revealing the extent of the frontobasal skull base (large arrows) and naso-orbital, Le Fort I through III and zygoma fractures (arrows). Lateral displacement of the multifragmentary fractured nasal walls (arrowheads). Note the right-sided displacement of the Le Fort I palate fracture. Top right, Preoperative view, same patient. The inward telescoped and laterally displaced nasal skeleton have led to a marked telecanthus (bar). Only the tip of the nose is emerged (N). Center left, Same patient's tomogram illustrating the multiple laterally dislocated fractures (arrows) and the enlargement of the intercanthal distance in the nasal cavity. Center right, Patient's roentgenogram 1 year postoperatively. Application of miniplates and ligatures (arrowheads) was limited to the necessary minimum. Reduction of the medial orbital rim frame, nasal skeleton, and telecanthus by the centripetal compression method. P indicates plate osteosynthesis of the lower jaw. No intermaxillary fixation. Bottom left and right, Same patient's frontal and lateral view 6 months postoperatively.*

Table 1.—Postoperative Measurements in 302 Men With Combined Frontonaso-Orbital and Skull Base Fractures: Comparison With Anthropometric Values in a Normal White Population

Distance	Postoperative Anthropometric Values in 302 Men		Anthropometric Values in Normal White Men*	
	Mean, mm	SD	Mean, mm	SD
Intercanthal	32.8	2.2	32.0	3.0
Interpupilary	62.3	3.7	63.0	3.0
Lateral intercanthal	91.2	5.8	90.0	4.0
Bizygomatic	129.7	11.6	144.0	6.0

*From Farkas.[13]

Table 2.—Postoperative Complications in 355 Patients With Combined Frontonaso-Orbital and Skull Base Fractures

Complication	%
Insufficient reduction	
Medial canthal ligament	1.9
Nasal frame	2.5
Cerebrospinal fluid leak	2.8 (1.1*)
Meningitis	1.1
Mortality	1.1
Frontal sinus mucocele	3.0
Frontal sinus infection	1.7
Orbital apex syndrome	0.8

*The 1.1% is due to accidental packing removal by the patient.

Frontal Sinus Mucocele

Chronic infection, along with formation of a mucocele, was observed in 3.0% of patients. The reasons are the same as mentioned above. In regard to long-term follow-up, this represents a significant reduction of the complication rate. This is the reason for our policy since 1978 not to obliterate but to reconstruct meticulously the sinus and its pathways. However, an observation period of only 5 to 13 years is not sufficient for definitive conclusions.

Orbital Apex Syndrome

Postoperative development of pressure at the apical area of the orbital cone, leading to optic nerve compression and dysfunction, was observed in 1.2% of patients. The reason was obliteration of the Portex tube drainage and excessive packing of the skull base. After immediate partial removal of the packing (extruded into the nasal lumen) and cleaning of the tube, two patients regained normal optic nerve function.

COMMENT

The goal of this article is to highlight the major advantages of the subcranial exposure of the skull base planes, representing the key for successful management of severe disruption of the frontonaso-ethmoidal and medial orbital frame. Concomitant intracranial impaction of the median-paramedian skull base plane, including the sellar-sphenoidal area, vertical rotation, and intracranial dislocation of the orbital roof and distal part of the greater wings, is common. A well-known access route is the transethmoidal approach. The relatively poor exposure limited to the median skull base plane is insufficient for the visualization and repair of extensive vast multiple dural tears and intracranial fragment dislocation. This explains the high recurrence rate of cerebrospinal fluid leaks,[14-19] up to 20% to 25% of the patients managed by this approach, or meningitis later on, in even less severe cases. Thus, in the absence of an adequate alternative, the neurosurgical, transfrontal approach remained the method of choice for the management of such severe involvement of the neurocranium and skull base. As reduction of the facial frame is performed by others mainly referring to the reduction of the fractures and aesthetics,[9-12,20] these major aspects are left insufficiently described and evaluated.

In the presence of concomitant brain contusion, edema, and elevated intracranial pressure as well as brain tissue herniation, adequate frontal lobe retraction is often contraindicated. A deferral, until the brain edema and the elevated pressure have subsided, is in such cases often unavoidable.[1-4] The deferral of such complex fractures presents a cardinal disadvantage. As a rule, the longer the deferral, the lesser the results will be. Particularly if optic nerve compression manifests, a posttraumatic deferral of more than 8 hours may lead to irreversible damage. Extracranial decompression of the optic nerve by the transorbital,[21] transethmoidal,[22] and transantral[23] approaches are well-known methods. Yet, these studies mainly include a relatively limited number of trauma cases and refer mainly to selected, less extensive injuries. Admittedly, the craniotomy and frontal lobe retraction provide generous exposure of the skull base and frontal region. By comparison, the price, in regard to the disadvantages alluded to, is much too high. Thus, the subcranial approach is an adequate alternative to the transfrontal access to the skull base.

The subcranial approach renders the following advantages: (1) in spite of concomitant severe skull base involvement, intracranial fragment dislocation, brain contusion, and elevated intracranial pressure, or even brain tissue herniation, the majority of the cases can be managed in an early one-stage procedure; (2) performance of the symmetrical cross-sided centripetal compression for reduction of the naso-orbital walls and telecanthus; (3) the subcranial compartment, created after radical removal of the comminuted ethmoidal cells, facilitates optic nerve decompression and expansion toward the midline, reducing significantly postoperative development of pressure along the apical orbital cone and optic nerve (apex syndrome); (4) watertight closure of multiple and vast dural tears and optimal alignment of the skull base toward the paranasal spaces; and (5) the drainage of the subcranial compartment and frontal sinus externalized into the nasal lumen for 6 months reduces dysfunction, infection, empyema, or mucus retention of the frontal sinuses to a minimum.

Comments that this method has no advantages in comparison with the conventional procedure[24] are particularly counterproductive in the absence of a comparative study in regard to the extent of trauma and achieved results, including long-term follow-up.

In our opinion, there is no justification to declare a case successful only in regard to the reduction of the facial frame leaving other complications, such as recurrent cerebrospinal fluid leaks, meningitis, optic nerve damage, or recurrent functional disorders of the frontal and paranasal spaces, unconsidered. This implies a long-term follow-up and, in regard to credibility, interdisciplinary evaluation is unambiguous.

We would like to thank the Stanley Thomas Johnson Foundation, Bern, Switzerland, for the generous support of the scientific programs, and Hans Holzherr for the high quality of the schematic drawings.

References

1. Arendall RE, Meirowsky AM. Air sinus wounds: an analysis of 163 consecutive cases incurred in the Korean War, 1950-1952. *Neurosurgery.* 1983;13:377-380.

2. Loew F, Pertuiset B, Chaumier EE, et al. Traumatic spontaneous and postoperative CSF rhinorrhea. *Adv Tech Stand Neurosurg.* 1984;11:169-207.

3. Probst C. Neurochirurgische Aspekte bei fronto-basalen Verletzungen mit Liquorfisteln: Erfahrungen bei 205 operierten Patienten. *Aktuel Traumatol.* 1986;16:43-49.

4. Gruss JS. Fronto-naso-orbital trauma. *Clin Plast Surg.* 1982;9:577-589.

5. Manson PN, Crawley WA, Hoopes JE. Frontal cranioplasty: risk factors and choice of cranial vault reconstructive material. *Plast Reconstr Surg.* 1986;77:888-900.

6. Raveh J. Schwere Gesichtsschädelverletzungen: Eigene Erfahrungen und Modifikationen. *Aktuel Probl Otorhinolarnygol.* 1979;3:145-154.

7. Raveh J, Neiger M. Die Wiederherstellung bei schweren Gesichtsschädelverletzungen. *Schweiz Monatsschr Zahn Med.* 1981;91:206-217.

8. Raveh J, Vuillemin T. Subcranial management of 395 combined frontobasal-midface fractures. *Arch Otolaryngol Head Neck Surg.* 1989;114:1115-1122.

9. Gruss JS. Naso-ethmoid-oribtal fractures: classification and role of primary bone grafting. *Plast and Reconstr Surg.* 1985;75:303-315.

10. Antonyshyn O, Gruss JS, Galbraith DJ, Hurwitz JJ. Complex orbital fractures: a critical analysis of immediate bone graft reconstruction. *Ann Plast Surg.* 1989;22:220-235.

11. Foster CA, Sherman JE. Naso-orbital fractures. In: Foster CA, Sherman, JE, eds. *Surgery of Facial Bone Fractures.* New York, NY: Churchill Livingstone Inc; 1987:39-65.

12. Markowitz BL, Manson PN, Yaremchuk M, Glassman D, Kawamoto H. High-energy orbital dislocations: the possibility of traumatic hypertelorbitism. *Plast Reconstr Surg.* 1991;88:20-28.

13. Farkas LG. *Anthropometry of the Head and Face in Medicine.* New York, NY: Elsevier Science Publishing Co Inc; 1981.

14. Lieberherr U. Zehn Jahre Erfahrung mit der mikrochirurgischen Versorgung fronto-basaler Liquorfisteln. *Aktuel Probl Otorhinolaryngol.* 1985;9:48-55.

15. Myers DL, Sataloff RT. Spinal fluid leakage after skull base surgical procedures. *Otolaryngol Clin North Am.* 1984;17:601-617.

16. Westmore GA, Whittam DE. Cerebrospinal fluid rhinorrhoea and its management. *Br J Surg.* 1982;69:489-492.

17. Calcaterra TC. Diagnosis and management of ethmoid cerebrospinal rhinorrhea. *Otolarygol Clin North Am.* 1985;18:99-105.

18. Park JI, Strelzow VV, Friedmann WH. Current management of cerebrospinal fluid rhinorrhea. *Laryngoscope.* 1983;93:1294-1300.

19. Samii M, Draf W. Indikation und Versorgung der frontobasalen Liquorfistel aus HNO-chirurgischer und neurochirurgischer Sicht. *Rhinol Otol.* 1978;57:689-697.

20. Manson PN, Markowitz B, Mirvis S, et al. Toward CT-based facial fracture treatment. *Plast Reconstr Surg.* 1990;2:202-212.

21. Habal MB. Clinical observations on the isolated optic nerve injury. *Ann Plast Surg.* 1978;6:603-607.

22. Fukado Y. Results in 400 cases of surgical decompression of the optic nerve. *Mod Probl Ophthalmol.* 1973;14:474.

23. Kennerdell JS, Ambaugh GA, Myers EN. Transantral ethmoidal decompression of optic nerve fractures. *Arch Ophthalmol.* 1976;94:1040-1046.

24. Stanley RB. Management of severe frontobasilar skull fractures. *Otolaryngologic Clin North Am.* 1991;24:139-150.

Otolaryngologic Manifestations of Child Abuse

Eric B. Leavitt, MD; Robert L. Pincus, MD; Roman Bukachevsky, MD

• Currently, awareness is growing of child abuse in the medical and lay communities. To familiarize otolaryngologists with the head and neck findings in abused children, we retrospectively analyzed 85 patients admitted to an inner-city hospital with the diagnosis of abuse or neglect. Forty-eight children (56%) had abnormalities within the head and neck region. Excluding coincidental findings, 31 children (36%) had findings that could be directly linked to physical abuse or neglect. The face was the region with thc most abnormal findings in our study (25 children [30%]). Soft-tissue findings were the most numerous (27 children [32%]). The literature is reviewed on the subject of otolaryngologic manifestations of abuse.

(*Arch Otolaryngol Head Neck Surg.* 1992;118:629-631)

Child abuse and neglect is a devastating and common problem. There were 2 086 000 reported cases of child abuse in 1986, and it is estimated that two thirds of child abuse goes unreported.[1] More than 200 children die annually in the country as a result of child abuse and neglect.[2] Half of the children diagnosed as being abused have had previous medical care for an abuse-related injury.[3]

Child abuse has been legally defined as "the physical or mental injury, sexual abuse or exploitation, negligent treatment, or maltreatment of a child under the age of 18 by a person who is responsible for the child's welfare under circumstances which indicate that the child's health or welfare is harmed or threatened thereby."[4]

The "battered child syndrome" was first described in 1962 by Kempe et al.[5] Although half of the injuries resulting from abuse involve the head and neck, there have been relatively few reports or literature reviews on the otolaryngologic manifestations of abuse.[6] The purpose of our study is to examine the prevalence of otolaryngologic findings in abused children and review the literature to help familiarize the otolaryngologist with child abuse and its head and neck manifestations.

Accepted for publication February 14, 1992.

From the New York Eye and Ear Infirmary, New York (NY) Medical College.

Presented at the American Academy of Otolaryngology–Head and Neck Surgery National Meeting, San Diego, Calif, September 1990.

Reprint requests to 310 E 14th St, New York, NY 10003 (Dr Pincus).

METHODS AND RESULTS

We reviewed the records of all patients admitted to an inner-city municipal hospital with the diagnosis of child abuse or neglect from January 1, 1987, to December 31, 1989. Child abuse was diagnosed by the attending pediatrician based on clinical suspicion or other evidence. All children suspected to be victims of abuse in the emergency department were admitted to the hospital. Records were examined for any abnormality within the head and neck, excluding ophthalmologic and neurologic findings. Coincidental findings such as otitis media, upper respiratory tract infection, and congenital anomalies were also noted.

There were 85 patients identified, 44 girls and 41 boys. The average age was 3.75 years, with a range of 1 month to 16 years (Fig 1). Of the 85 patients, 48 (56%) had abnormalities within the head and neck region. Excluding coincidental findings, 31 (36%) had evidence of abuse in the head and neck (Fig 2).

Otologic findings in these abused children included superficial abrasions and scarring in four patients (Fig 3). One child had an ulcer with cellulitis of the pinna, presumably due to wounds inflicted during and episode of abuse. Fifteen (18%) of 85 patients were found to have otitis media and effusion. Two patients had incidental congenital anomalies: a branchial cleft cyst and a preauricular skin tag. A total of 21 patients had otologic findings (Table 1).

Only two patients had evidence of nasal trauma. These were superficial abrasions of the nose. No nasal fractures were noted. There were 15 patients with incidental upper respiratory tract infections at the time of admission.

The oral and pharyngeal areas also showed evidence of abuse. One child had a laceration of the soft palate. Two had oral candidiasis and one had pharyngitis for which cultures were not obtained. One child had several teeth avulsed and one had severe dental caries.

Soft-tissue findings were the most numerous (Table 2). Twelve children had significant ecchymoses in the face, scalp, and neck. Ten had abrasions and four had hematomas. Two patients had impetigo. One child had parotitis due to severe dehydration. One patient had burns and one had congenital facial dysmorphism.

Four patients presented with skull fractures: three parietal, one occipital, and one frontal. One patient had two fractures. Two patients with skull fractures also had fractures in bones outside the head and neck.

There were 21 patients who were sexually abused; their average age was 6.5 years. None of these patients had evidence of oral or pharyngeal trauma or infection. Only two (10%) of the sexually abused children had trauma to the head and neck. This trauma was not of a sexual nature.

COMMENT

Ten general categories of abuse and neglect have been established, many of which may be discovered by the

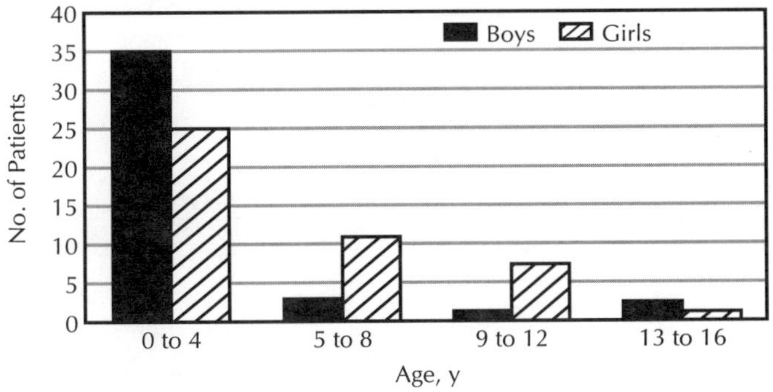

Fig 1.—*Age distribution of patients.*

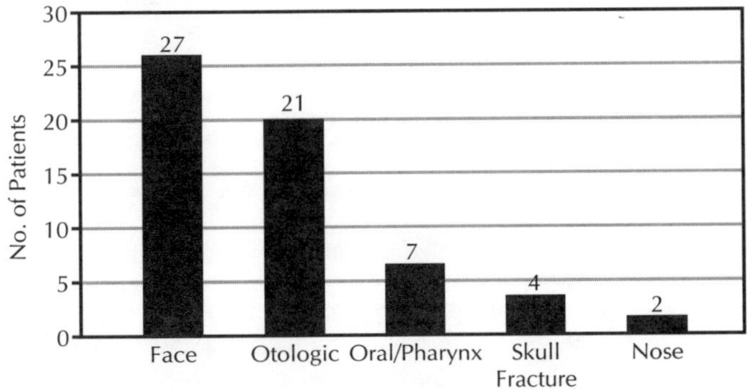

Fig 2.—*Head and neck findings by region. Includes patients with more than one finding.*

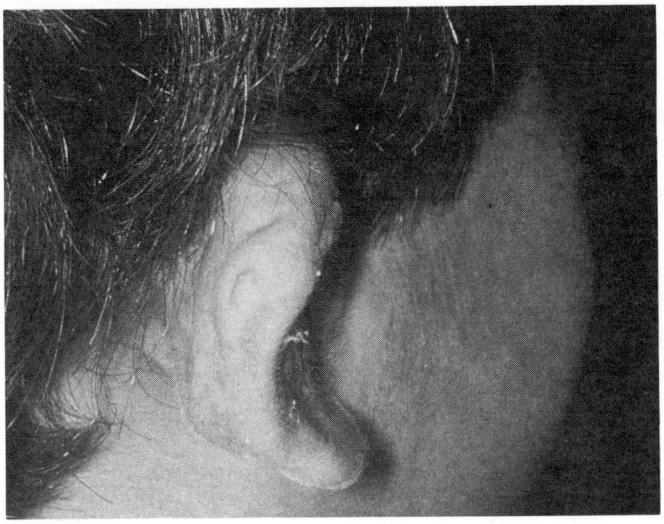

Fig 3.—*Chronic scarring of right auricle in a 3-year-old child from repeated trauma.*

otolaryngologist. These include the following: physical abuse, sexual abuse, failure to thrive, intentional drugging or poisoning, Munchausen's syndrome by proxy, health care neglect, dental neglect, safety neglect, emotional abuse and neglect, and physical neglect.[6]

Otologic trauma may be a sign of child abuse. Reported findings include pinna hematoma, laceration of the external auditory canal, ossicular discontinuity, sensorineural hearing loss, facial nerve paralysis, cerebral spinal fluid otorrhea, and tympanic membrane perforation.[7]

Pinna trauma may be a superficial manifestation of neurologic injury. Hanigen and coworkers[8] reviewed three cases of "tin ear syndrome," a triad of isolated pinna bruising,

Table 1.—Otologic Findings*

Otitis media	15
Abrasions	4
Ulcer and cellulitis	1
Congenital	2
Total	21 (25%)

*One patient had two findings.

Table 2.—Soft-Tissue Findings*

Ecchymoses	12
Abrasions	10
Hematomas	4
Impetigo	2
Parotitis	1
Total	27 (32%)

*Two patients had two findings.

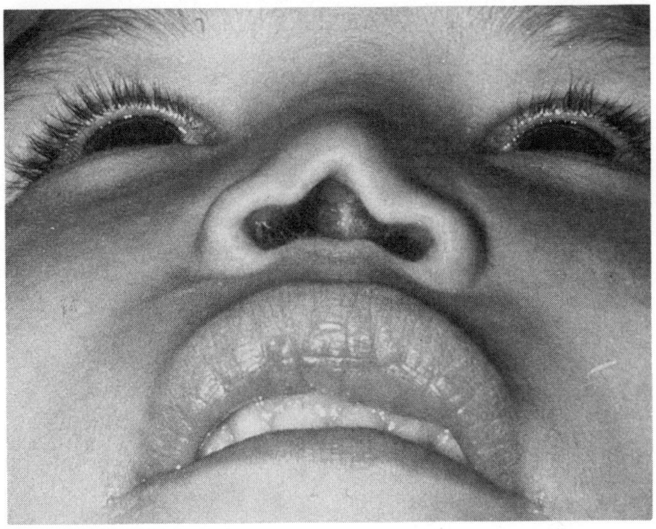

Fig 4.—*Columellar destruction from repeated trauma in child abuse.*

hemorrhagic retinopathy, and ipsilateral subdural hematoma with severe cerebral edema. Tin ear syndrome is caused by a blow to the side of the head and ear. It should be differentiated from simple bruising to the pinna.

Tympanic membrane perforations have been reported by several authors.[7,9,10] Meadows syndrome, "Munchausen's by proxy," is described as repeated trauma to the child by an adult to seek medical attention. Grace and Grace[7] reported three children whose parents caused repeated tympanic membrane perforations.

Although not supported by our study, children who are abused may be at higher risk for otitis media with effusion.[11] In our review 18% of abused children had coexisting otitis media. Additionally, deaf children may be at higher risk for sexual abuse. This was not found in our study.[12,13]

The nose is a common area to sustain trauma. Nasal perforations, foreign body insertion, hematomas, and fractures have all been reported.[7] Several reports have appeared of abuse resulting in a delayed destruction of the columella.[7,14-16] We have previously reported two patients with columellar destruction due to child abuse (Fig 4).[16]

Few reports have been published of laryngeal trauma

secondary to abuse, and there were none in our study.[7] Myer and Fitton[17] reported three cases of vocal cord paralysis due to head trauma from abuse. In each child, the vocal cord paralysis was not diagnosed until multiple attempts at extubation failed.

There are multiple ways abuse is manifest in the oral and pharyngeal regions. In one review of 260 abused children, 14 had oral trauma consisting of dental trauma, contusions, abrasions, and lacerations.[18] Most authors feel that tears of the frenulum are highly suspicious in children who are not yet ambulatory.[18-20]

Pharyngeal gonorrhea can result from sexual abuse and is often asymptomatic.[21] One study found that 10 of 16 patients with positive cultures had a normal pharyngeal appearance.[22] Pharyngeal cultures for gonorrhea should be routine in the sexually abused child.

Lacerations in the oral and pharyngeal cavities can result from a spoon or other hard object being forced into the mouth of a child.[7] One child in our study had an oral laceration. McDowell and Fielding[23] reported two cases of traumatic perforations of the hypopharynx with interstitial emphysema, a potentially lethal injury.

Caustic infection and foreign body aspiration, the third most common cause of accidental childhood death, may be due to abuse or neglect.[24] Eight percent of children who are seen for ingestion have a prior history of poisoning.[25,26] The first child described by Meadow[27] was a case of repeated poisonings. Friedman[24] reported five cases of ingestions as a result of abuse. In one of these, the mother was convicted of murder for deliberately poisoning her 1-year-old child with salt.[24]

The face was found to be traumatized in 44% of all abused children and in 25 (30%) in our study.[20] The skin is by far the most frequently traumatized system.[28-30] Ecchymoses and abrasions were the most frequent findings in our study group. Blunt facial trauma in the child should call the attention of the otolaryngologist to the possibility of abuse. However, it should be noted that cystic lymphangioma has been reported to mimic cervical bruising.[31]

Skull and facial fractures are not uncommon in the abused child. Those children who do sustain fractures of the skull and face are more likely to have other occult fractures.[32] An analysis of 429 fractures in battered children showed skull fractures were the most common fracture in children less than 1 year of age.[33]

Additionally, some severely abused children may have no evidence of external trauma as in the case of "shaken baby syndrome." This syndrome is defined as retinal hemorrhage, subdural and/or subarachnoid hemorrhage, and minimal or absent signs of external trauma, due to violent shaking in a child usually younger than 1 year of age.[34]

All 50 states have mandatory reporting laws. Each state also has laws to protect the person who files a report in good faith from recrimination. Smith[30] lists agencies in each state to whom abuse should be reported. The physician should become familiar with the protocol for investigation and reporting of potential abuse in his or her hospital. Care of the abused child should involve the close cooperation of the reporting physician, pediatrician, and social service staff.

The incidence of otolaryngologic findings in the abused child in our review was 56%. The various ways abuse manifests itself in the head and neck are numerous and have been reviewed. It is likely that the otolaryngologist will be involved in the care of the abused child. The clinician must have a high index of suspicion for abuse so that intervention can be made and repeated abuse prevented.

References

1. Monahan JA. Pulse rates. *N Y Doctor.* June 5, 1989:23.
2. Ludwig S. Child abuse. In: Fleisher G, Ludwig S, eds. *Textbook of Pediatric Emergency Medicine.* Baltimore, Md: Williams & Wilkins; 1983:1028.
3. Skinner AE, Castle RL. *Seventy-Eight Battered Children: A Retrospective Study.* London, England: National Society for the Prevention of Cruelty to Children; 1969.
4. Schmitt BD. Types of child abuse and neglect: an overview for dentists. *J Am Acad Pediatr Dent.* 1986;8:67. Special issue 1.
5. Kempe CH, Silverman FN, Steele BF, Droegemueller W, Silver HK. The battered child syndrome. *JAMA.* 1962;181:17-24.
6. Gallo LG. Child abuse: who is involved? *N Y State Dent J.* 1983;47:78-82.
7. Grace A, Grace S. Child abuse within the ear, nose and throat. *J Otolaryngol.* 1987;16:108-111.
8. Hanigen WC, Peterson RA, Wjus G. Tin ear syndrome: rotational acceleration in pediatric head injuries. *Pediatrics.* 1987;80:618-622.
9. Obiako MN. Eardrum perforation as evidence of child abuse. *Child Abuse Neglect.* 1987;11:149-151.
10. Grace A, Kalinkiewicz M, Drake-Lee AB. Covert manifestations of child abuse. *BMJ.* 1984;289:1041-1042.
11. Downs MO. Identification of children at risk for middle ear effusion problems. *Ann Otol Rhinol Laryngol.* 1980;89(suppl 68):168-171.
12. Brookhouser PE, Sul Gan CI. Loss of columella and septum from an unusual form of child abuse. *Plast Reconstr Surg.* 1975;56:345-346.
13. Brookhouser PE. Ensuring the safety of deaf children in residential schools. *Otolaryngol Head Neck Surg.* 1987;97:361-368.
14. Orton CI. Loss of columella and septum from an unusual form of child abuse. *Plast Reconstr Surg.* 1975;56:345-343.
15. Paletta FX, Van Norman RT. Total reconstruction of the columella. *Plast Reconstr Surg.* 1962;30:320.
16. Pincus RL, Bukachevsky RP. Medially based horizontal nasolabial flaps for reconstruction of columellar defects. *Arch Otolaryngol Head Neck Surg.* 1990;116:973-974.
17. Myer C, Fitton CM. Vocal cord paralysis following child abuse. *Int J Pediatr Otorhinolaryngol.* 1988;15:217-220.
18. Needleman HL. Orofacial trauma in child abuse: types, prevalence, management, and the dental profession's involvement. *Pediatr Dent.* 1986;8:71-81. Special issue 1.
19. Ambrose JB. Orofacial signs of child abuse and neglect: a dental prospective. *Pediatrician.* 1989;16:188-192.
20. Tate RJ. Facial injuries associated with the battered child syndrome. *Br J Oral Surg.* 1971;9:41-45.
21. Bernat JE. Bitemarks and oral manifestations of child abuse and neglect. In: Ellerstein MS, ed. *Child Abuse and Neglect: A Medical Reference.* New York, NY: John Wiley & Sons Inc; 1981:141-64.
22. Silber JT, Controni G. Clinical spectrum of pharyngeal gonorrhea in children and adolescents. *J Adolesc Health Care.* 1983;4:51-54.
23. McDowell HP, Fielding DW. Traumatic perforation of the hypopharynx: an unusual form of abuse. *Arch Dis Child.* 1984;59:888-889.
24. Friedman EM. Caustic ingestions and foreign body aspirations: an overlooked form of child abuse. *Ann Otol Rhinol Laryngol.* 1987;96:709-712.
25. Kersh MM, Ritter F. Caustic ingestion and subsequent damage to the oropharyngeal and digestive passages. *Ann Thorac Surg.* 1976; 21:74-82.
26. Leape L. New liquid lye drain cleaners. *Clin Toxicol.* 1974;7:109-114.
27. Meadow R. Munchausen syndrome by proxy: the hinterland of child abuse. *Lancet.* 1977;2:343-345.
28. Reece RM, Grodin MA. Recognition of non-accidental injury. *Pediatr Clin North Am.* 1985;32:41-60.
29. Altieri MF. Child abuse: when to be suspicious and what to do then. *Postgrad Med.* 1990;87:153-156.
30. Smith SF. Child abuse and neglect: a diagnostic guide for the optometrist. *J Am Optom Assoc.* 1988;59:760-766.
31. Williams CM, Spector R, Braun M. Cervical bruises: a battered child? cystic lymphangioma. *Arch Dermatol.* 1986;122:1066-1067.
32. Worlock P, Stower M, Barbor P. Patterns of fractures in accidental and non-accidental injury in children: a comparative study. *BMJ.* 1986;293:100-102.
33. King J, Diefendorf D, Apthorp J, Negrete VF, Carlson M. Analysis of 429 fractures in 189 battered children. *J Pediatr Orthoped.* 1988;8:585-589.
34. Duhaime AC, Gennarelli TA, Thibault LE, Bruce DA, Margulies SS, Wiser R. The shaken baby syndrome: a clinical, pathological, and biomechanical study. *J Neurosurg.* 1987;66:409-415.

Auricular Injury as a Presentation of Child Abuse

Ayal Willner, MD; Philip S. Ledereich, MD; Egbert J. de Vries, MD

• Child abuse causes serious physical and emotional injury. Those abused, however, are usually unable or unwilling to gain access to agencies that might help them. The otolaryngologist, while usually not the patient's primary physician, may be in the position to detect child abuse. We describe a 3-year-old boy who sustained auricular trauma as the result of child abuse. The importance of physician recognition of an abuse case and the institution of appropriate measures are discussed.

(*Arch Otolaryngol Head Neck Surg.* 1992;118:634-637)

Child abuse exacts an unacceptably high financial and human toll on society. Kempe,[1] in 1962, defined the abuse and neglect of children and the outcomes of this maltreatment in adults. Child abuse is the purposeful infliction of physical and/or emotional harm, sexual exploitation, and the neglect of basic needs, including nutritrion, housing, education, and medical care. Otolaryngologists, while usually referral physicians, may be in the position to identify cases of abuse or neglect. It is important, therefore, that the otolaryngologist be able to recognize this entity and take the appropriate steps to ensure the safety of the child. We describe a 3-year-old boy who was the victim of such abuse and who presented with an otolaryngic manifestation.

REPORT OF A CASE

A 3-year-old boy was brought by ambulance to one of our institution's hospitals for a worsening left ear infection. The parents related that 3 weeks prior to admission he had developed an "ear infection" that the mother had treated with hydrogen peroxide. She then took him to an emergency department at one hospital and subsequently to a pediatric clinic at another hospital. He was treated with sulfamethoxazole-trimethoprim and hydrocortisone cream, without improvement, and over the few days preceding admission at our institution, the infection had worsened. Two days prior to admission, according to the parents, the child had fallen against a door and lacerated his left earlobe. The parents reported that the child was "wild" and clumsy, always falling, and accident-prone.

On presentation the child was afebrile. Obvious swelling and tissue destruction of the left ear was noted (Fig 1). Eschars were present on both the lateral and medial aspects of the pinna. The ear was pushed forward and almost perpendicular to its natural plane. The pinna was indurated and had a "woody" feel, and there was a tract of fibrinous tissue from the meatus of the external auditory canal toward the area of lobule attachment. The attachment itself was missing and the edges of the defect were excoriated. The posterior aspect of the pinna was similarly involved, with erythema extending over the mastoid area. Other physical findings included an ecchymosis on the child's forehead, abrasions over the stomach, circular healed scars on the dorsum of the right hand, a right heel ulcer, and an ecchymosis in the center of his back. In addition, the child was noted to be withdrawn and small for his age.

The findings on physical examination prompted the consideration of child abuse, and a workup was initiated. The wounds were photographed, the Child Welfare Agency was notified, and further history was elicited. The patient was a third sibling and had been abandoned at birth. Repeated attempts to contact the mother had failed, and the child was to be placed in foster care. During court proceedings, however, the mother regained custody of the child, stating that she was not able to respond to hospital attempts to reach her because she had to take care of her other children. The child was later placed in the care of his paternal grandmother when his parents were both incarcerated for drug possession and sales. The parents were paroled in early 1991 and the family unit was reestablished in July 1991.

Interviews and examinations of the other siblings were carried out. The other children were found to be healthy and appeared to be well cared for. On questioning an older female sibling, inconsistencies in the parents' statements were noted. She described the patient as a quiet child who watched television and did not "fool around." She confirmed that the children were hit as part of family discipline but that the parents "did not leave any bruises or marks" on the children. On further questioning by agency caseworkers, however, she became confused and gave conflicting responses to questions. It was suspected that her answers had been previously coached.

Initial management included intravenous cefuroxime and instillation of sulfa-containing drops into the external auditory canal. Because of the "lopping" of the ear and drainage from the external auditory canal, a computed tomographic scan was obtained to rule out an acute mastoiditis. The computed tomographic scan showed soft-tissue swelling of the periotic tissues but no bony resorption, subperiostial abscess, or evidence of mastoid disease (Fig 2). Of note was the finding of marked cerebral atrophy. The antibiotic coverage was changed to ceftazidime and oxacillin to treat a severe otitis externa and pinna cellulitis. Since the initial infection had started 3 weeks prior to admission, the extent of tissue damage was similar to that of a burn, and sulfadiazine silver cream was therefore applied twice daily. The patient's condition markedly improved over the next 3 days (Fig 3), and the ear continued to improve over the next 10 days (Fig 4). During his hospital course, the child was noted

Accepted for publication February 5, 1992.

From the Department of Otolaryngology–Head and Neck Surgery, Albert Einstein College of Medicine, Montefiore Medical Center, Bronx, NY.

Reprint requests to Department of Otolaryngology–Head and Neck Surgery, Montefiore Medical Center, 3414 Bainbridge Ave, Fourth Floor, Bronx, NY 10467 (Dr Willner).

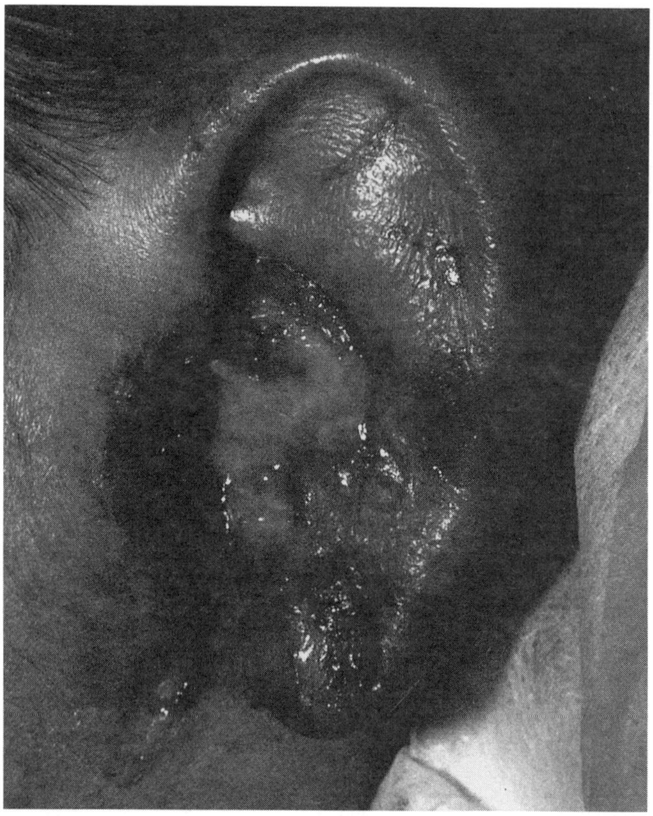

Fig 1.—*Left ear. Note destruction of earlobe attachment.*

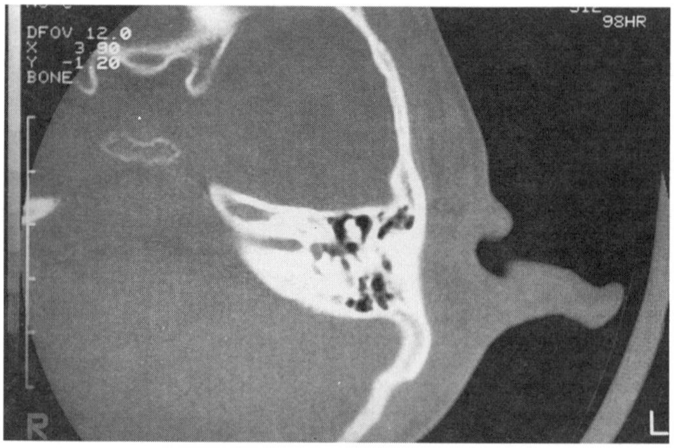

Fig 2.—*Coronal computed tomographic scan. There is extensive soft-tissue swelling, which has pushed the ear forward. There is, however, no mastoid air cell disease noted.*

to be emotionally needy, clinging to hospital staff. He was also noted to have speech delay, but audiometry performed on the uninfected ear showed normal hearing. He showed no signs of cerebellar dysfunction and no ataxia was seen. In general, he was playful and happy except when his parents visited, at which time he was noted to be apprehensive and fearful. At the time of this writing, he was awaiting foster care placement. Future reconstruction will be carried out when the child is older and able to be more active in the postoperative care of the reconstructed pinna.

COMMENT

Child Abuse

In the United States in 1989, there were approximately 2.5 million reports of child abuse to state social service agencies. These included cases of physical abuse (25%), sexual abuse (20%), and neglect (55%).[2] Information from the US Department of Health and Human Services (USDHHS) has shown that there has been a 66% increase in cases of child maltreatment from 1980 to 1988.[3] The USDHHS collected 1.1 million cases, 10% of which were classified as serious and 0.1% of which were fatal. Four thousand children die each year from physical abuse, and 10% of the children younger than 5 years who are seen in emergency departments are the victims of inflicted injuries.[4] Other experts feel that the true incidence of fatalities is higher, with estimates of 2000 to 5000 per year.[3] In addition, most authors agree that child abuse is generally underreported and that increases in incidence may be the result of increased reporting. Of note, in 81% of cases involving adolescents, the parents are the perpetrators of the abuse.[5] Also of importance is that the likelihood of child abuse, while affected by socioeconomic factors, does occur in all socioeconomic groups.[2]

In the United States, all states have laws requiring reporting of suspected child abuse.[6] In New York State, reporting is mandatory for certain professionals, including physicians, surgeons, medical examiners, coroners, dentists, osteopaths, optometrists, chiropractors, podiatrists, resident physicians, interns, registered nurses, Christian Science practitioners, day care center workers, foster care workers, child care workers, mental health professionals, peace officers, hospital personnel, district attorneys, teachers, and school officials.[4] Physicians, especially pediatricians, are well situated in the community to detect cases of child abuse. Yet, physicians account for less than 10% of abuse reports, often despite numerous visits by the patient to the private physician, the clinic, or the emergency department.[6]

There are many factors that may put a particular child at risk for abuse. Neergaard,[7] in 1990, delineated seven factors related to the mother that increase a child's risk. They are (1) the mother's family history and financial status; (2) her self-perception and the effectiveness of her support system; (3) her age when she gives birth to her first child; (4) her history of substance abuse; (5) the level of her knowledge of child growth and development; (6) her perceptions of family discipline and the pregnancy state and her feelings toward her unborn child; and (7) her labor and delivery experience.

There are, of course, many nonmaternal risk factors. For instance, a history of abuse of either of the parents when they were young increases the likelihood that they will abuse their own children. Approximately one in three parents who themselves were victims of abuse will go on to abuse their own children.[2] Other factors include a child who is handicapped, a history of poor prenatal and/or postnatal medical follow-up owing to missed appointments, a history of abuse to siblings, and repeated referrals to children's services agencies.[8]

Substance abuse deserves special mention here, since both parents in our case had a history of such abuse. Murphy et al[3] examined the incidence of substance abuse in a court sample of serious child abuse cases. They found that in these cases there was a 43% prevalence of definite drug or alcohol abuse by at least one parent and a 50% prevalence of alleged or definite drug or alcohol abuse by at least one parent. They also associated alcohol or drug abuse with a higher risk of reinjury, recidivism, danger to the child, noncompliance with treatment, and permanent removal of children by the court. Furthermore, they noted

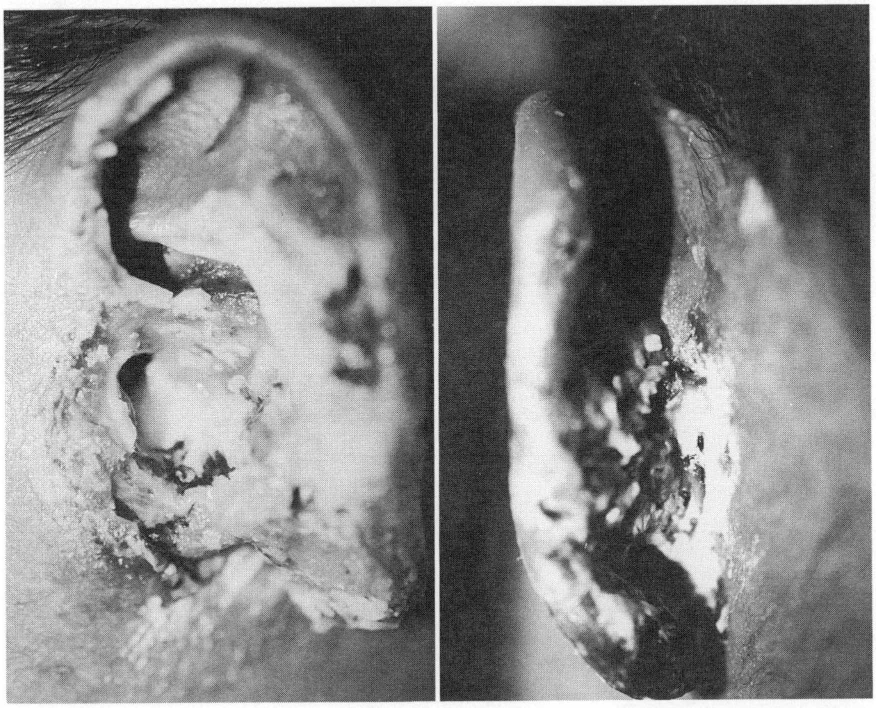

Fig 3.—*By hospital day 3, the swelling and erythema have decreased. Sulfadiazine silver (white cream) was used to treat this "burn-like" injury. Lateral (left) and posterior (right) views are shown.*

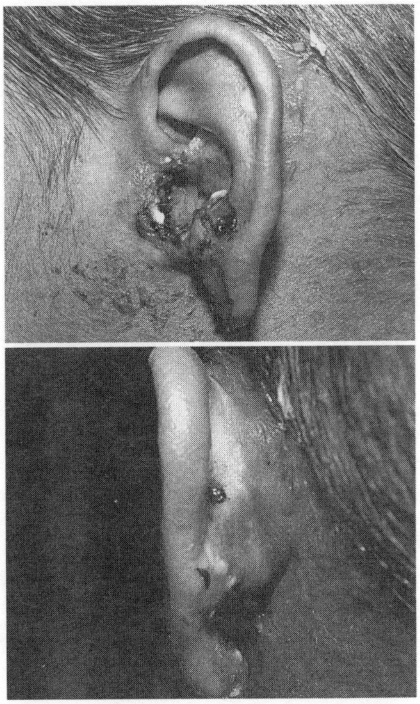

Fig 4.—*Lateral (top) and posterior (bottom) views of the patient's left ear on day 13. The infection is largely resolved, and the tissues are healing. Reconstruction will be carried out when the child is older.*

in their sample that 90% of the parents who abused hard drugs eventually had their children permanently removed. This figure was 60% for those parents who abused only alcohol.

It was pointed out, however, that while an association between drug and alcohol abuse and child maltreatment was found, no causal relationship could be established. Multiple other factors such as poverty, lack of social supports, and inadequate education were endemic.

Otolaryngological Manifestations

In general, the otolaryngologist is not the primary care provider for children. However, in cases where routine pediatric primary care is not obtained, the otolaryngologist may be in the position to identify child abuse and should be prepared to do so. Certain obvious deformities that are unusual in their presentation should alert the physician to examine the possibility of abuse more closely. Bilateral auricular hematomas, chronic draining ears that repeatedly respond to simple treatment, oral cavity/oropharynx lacerations, lacerations of the nasal vestibule, septal hematomas or perforations, and mandibular or other facial fractures have all been described as resultant from abuse.[6,9,10] While some of these presentations may be ascribed to "accidents," they should prompt a closer examination of the child's home and family setting, and repeated occurrences should prompt an evaluation by a social service agent trained in the prevention, recognition, and treatment of child abuse. More subtle manifestations that may be brought to the otolaryngologist for evaluation include headaches, chronic "sinusitis," speech and language delay, deafness, unexplained sleep apnea that occurs only in the presence of one caregiver, or enlarging head and neck masses, all of which may be indications of child abuse or neglect.[2,6]

When child abuse is suspected, further information must be sought. A complete history including other injuries, visits to the emergency department, and general pediatric care (ie, immunizations) should be elicited. In our case, the patient had been to several emergency departments under a different name prior to presentation. Parents should be questioned together and separately and other siblings should be interviewed to ascertain the extent and degree of the abuse. During these interviews, any psychological inconsistencies such as undue aggressiveness in the case of abused children and passiveness in neglect cases[5] should be noted. Inappropriate lack of separation anxiety may also be a clue to problems of abuse. A complete physical examination should then be performed with special attention to bruises in unusual places (ie, the back), circular scars that may have resulted from cigarette burns, bite marks, heel ulcers, or soreness of the palms and soles.[6] Routine blood tests, which might show signs of chronic neglect, should be performed, as well as roentgenographic evaluation to look for multiple fractures in different stages of healing. Photographic documentation of any and all injuries should be obtained, and an accurate inventory of these injuries should be entered in the chart.

Prevention

While recognition of child abuse must be aggressively pursued, prevention of abuse is of paramount importance. Social service intervention in high-risk cases should be instituted prior to the birth of the child. Programs in which a nurse visits a high-risk mother in her home during the prenatal and postpartum periods have been shown to significantly reduce the number of confirmed reports of child abuse and neglect. Other programs, utilizing mothers with effective parenting skills and foster grandparents in an effort to enhance the support system at home, have been proposed.[7] Such programs must also work to provide adequate shelter, food, drug counseling, and emotional support, using the home visitor as the conduit. In addition, the visitors must have adequate training in early recognition of home situations that may end in an episode of abuse. While this will require strong financial commitments on the part of governments and institutions, the costs incurred will not equal the economic and human toll of child abuse.

CONCLUSIONS

Child abuse is a serious social problem in the United States. The number of reports of abuse are increasing. Whether this reflects improvements in reports rather than true increase in incidents does not diminish the necessity for intervention. Our case highlights the importance of the physician's role in recognizing abuse and in initiating the necessary steps toward the protection of the child. The otolaryngologist, in his interaction with patients as either primary or referral physician, must be careful to look for signs of abuse and to refer appropriate cases for social service intervention.

References

1. Kempe CH, Silverman FN, Steele BF, Droegemeller W, Siver HK. The battered child syndrome. *JAMA.* 1962;181:17-24.
2. Rosenberg DA, Krugman RD. Epidemiology and outcome of child abuse. *Annu Rev Med.* 1991;42:217-224.
3. Murphy JM, Jellinek M, Quinn D, Smith G, Poitrast FG, Goshko M. Substance abuse and serious child mistreatment: prevalence and outcome in a court sample. *Child Abuse Negl.* 1991;15:197-211.
4. Gordon M, Palusci VJ. Physician training in the recognition and reporting of child abuse, maltreatment, and neglect. *N Y State J Med.* 1991;91:1-2.
5. Williamson JM, Borsuin CM, Howe BA. The ecology of adolescent maltreatment: a multilevel examination of adolescent physical abuse, sexual abuse, and neglect. *J Consult Clin Psychol.* 1991;59:449-457.
6. Manning SC, Margaretha C, Lammers D. Otolaryngologic manifestations of child abuse. *Int J Pediatr Otolaryngol.* 1990;20:7-16.
7. Neergaard JA. A proposal for a foster grandmother intervention program to prevent child abuse. *Public Health Rep.* 1990;105:89-93.
8. County of Los Angeles (Calif) Department of Health Services Child Abuse Prevention Program. High risk assessment criteria for high priority families. Cited by: Neergaard JA. A proposal for a foster grandmother intervention program to prevent child abuse. *Public Health Rep.* 1990;105:89-93.
9. Siegel MB, Wetmore RF, Potsic WP, et al. Mandibular fractures in the pediatric patient. *Arch Otolaryngol Head Neck Surg.* 1991;117:533-536.
10. Grace A, Grace S. Child abuse within the ear, nose, and throat. *J Otolaryngol.* 1987;16:108-111.

Toluidine Blue in the Detection at Autopsy of Perineal and Anal Lacerations in Victims of Sexual Abuse

Jan Bays, MD, Larry V. Lewman, MD

• Toluidine blue dye can be used at autopsy to aid in the detection of genital and anal injuries due to child sexual abuse. Four case examples are presented.
(*Arch Pathol Lab Med.* 1992;116:620-621)

Toluidine blue dye has been employed to document perineal lacerations following sexual assault. Toluidine blue does not stain surface layers of skin but will dye nucleated squamous cells in deeper layers of epidermis exposed by even superficial lacerations. The use of the dye in rape examinations in adult women increased the incidence of positive findings from 24% to 40% in one study.[1] In another study, application of toluidine blue increased the rate of positive findings from 4% to 28% in sexually assaulted adolescents, and from 16.5% to 33% in pediatric sexual abuse victims.[2]

We report the use of toluidine blue dye at autopsy to aid in the detection of genital and anal trauma associated with child sexual abuse.

REPORT OF CASES

CASE 1.—A 4-year-old boy was found dead in a wooded area 3 days after he disappeared while playing with his older brother in a park near his home. Autopsy revealed ligature marks around the neck and left ankle, with feces smeared around the anus, in the perineal area, and on the inside of the child's right thigh. The anus gaped open, measuring 2.5 × 1 cm (1 × 0.5 in). Two small lacerations were visible at the anal verge. There were no mucosal tears or bleeding.

The anus and lower rectum were dissected out with care and examined under a colposcope. Three lacerations were visible at the anal verge (Fig 1). After toluidine blue was applied, more than 15 lacerations became visible (Fig 2). Because of the presence of multiple injuries at the anal verge without mucosal hemorrhage, it was felt that sodomy had occurred post mortem. This was confirmed by the subsequent confession of the 28-year-old perpetrator.

CASE 2.—A 3-month-old infant was found dead on a water bed at home about 20 minutes after being put down for a nap. She was taken to an emergency department, where death was initially attributed to sudden infant death. The emergency department staff then noticed blood and apparent injuries around the anus. Roentgenograms of the body revealed a healing fracture of the left tibia. Medical records indicated the infant had been born with positive urinary toxicologic findings for cocaine and methamphetamines.

There were several tears around the anus (Fig 3). Application of toluidine blue showed deep staining at regular intervals around the anus (Fig 4). The dye also stained a previously undetected tear of the anterior frenulum of the labia minora and produced a stippled pattern of staining in the posterior fourchette and midline of the perineal body. The hymen was undamaged. Forensic specimens showed no evidence of semen. Autopsy did not reveal a cause of death, but suffocation could not be ruled out.

A forensic expert used the autopsy photographs in testimony that the stellate pattern of anal injuries matched the flanges on a plastic nozzle for filling a waterbed. The nozzle and a tube of petroleum jelly (KY) had been found on the dresser adjacent to the waterbed on which the infant's body was found. The father was found guilty in a court trial of sexual penetration with a foreign object, criminal mistreatment, and assault.

CASE 3.—A 3-year-old boy was found dead at home. The father said the boy had been vomiting for several days. At autopsy there were over a hundred injuries of different ages including burns, abrasions, lacerations, and bruises. The upper and lower lips had been avulsed from the gums. There was evidence of extensive peritonitis and a perforation of the bowel at the duodenojejunal junction. Blood cultures yielded *Escherichia coli* and *Clostridia perfringens*.

There was a 1-cm laceration of the anus and perineal body at the 6 o'clock position. After toluidine blue was applied, two smaller lacerations became visible at the 11 o'clock position (Fig 5). The father admitted he had kicked the child in the abdomen and was afraid to take the boy for medical attention because the bruises might be noticed. The father did not admit sexual abuse. The case is under investigation.

CASE 4.—A 3-year-old girl was found dead after her foster mother left her in the care of three older foster brothers. Autopsy was consistent with death due to suffocation. A foster brother admitted that he had put a pillow over the girl's face to keep her from crying. At autopsy there were old injuries, which predated her placement in foster care, fresh bruises to the head, most of which were visible only after reflection of the scalp, and a small subdural hematoma. There was no evidence of injury to the genitalia or anus. No undetected injuries were revealed with toluidine blue (Fig 6).

COMMENT

Multidisciplinary teams for the investigation of child abuse fatalities were established in Oregon in 1985. Clinicians expert in the field of child abuse are often called by the medical examiner to observe autopsies when abuse is suspected. The use of toluidine blue dye at autopsy is an example of the mutual benefit we have derived from this collaboration.

We use a 1% aqueous solution of dye applied with a cotton swab to the posterior fourchette, perineal body, and perianal area. We do not apply the dye to mucosal surfaces as results are difficult to interpret. A wet sponge

Accepted for publication March 6, 1992.
From Emanuel Children's Hospital and Healthcare Center (Dr Bays), Portland, Ore, and the Chief Medical Examiner's Office, State of Oregon, Portland (Dr Lewman).
Reprint requests to Emanuel Children's Hospital and Healthcare Center, 2801 Gantenbein St, Portland, OR 97227 (Dr Bays).

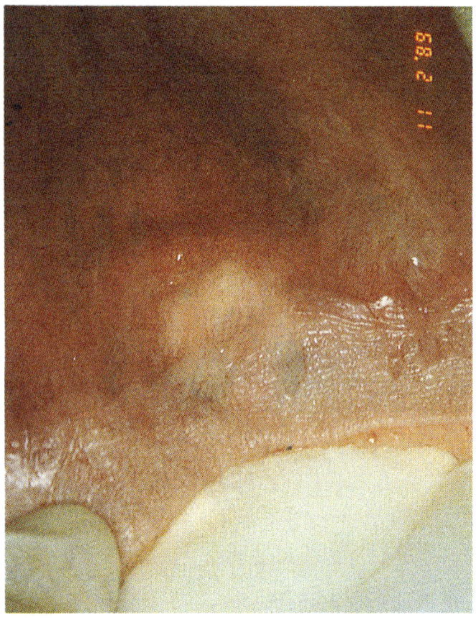

Fig 1.—*Patient 1. Portion of the anal verge before application of toluidine blue.*

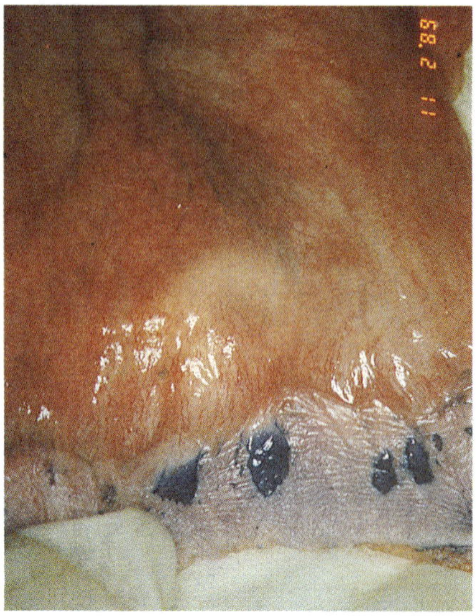

Fig 2.—*Patient 1. Toluidine blue reveals numerous lacerations.*

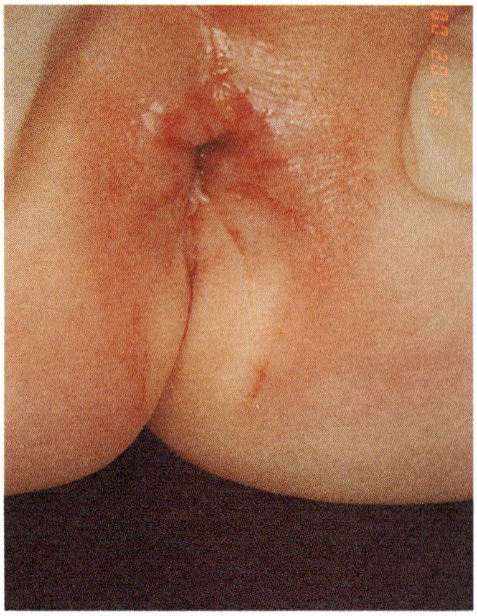

Fig 3.—*Patient 2. Anal area before application of toluidine blue. Several injuries are visible.*

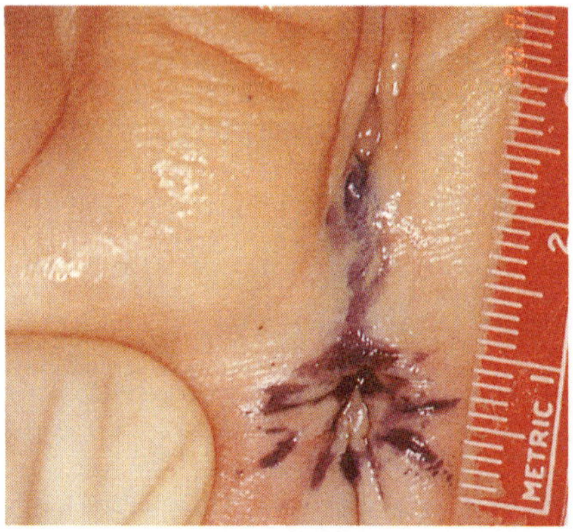

Fig 4.—*Patient 2. Toluidine blue reveals lacerations in a regular pattern around the anus.*

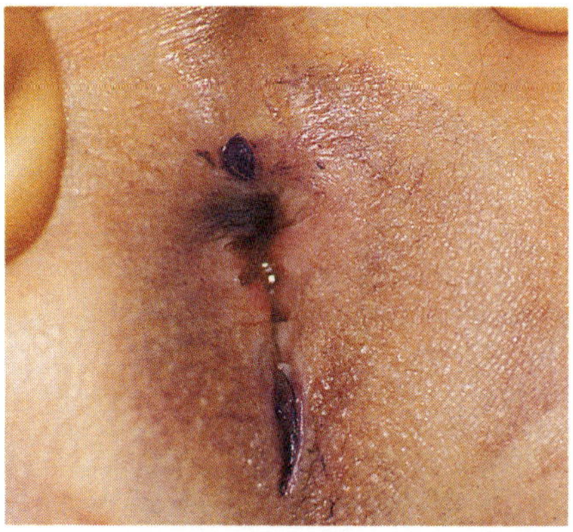

Fig 5.—*Patient 3. The smaller lacerations between 11 and 12 o'clock were visible only after application of the dye.*

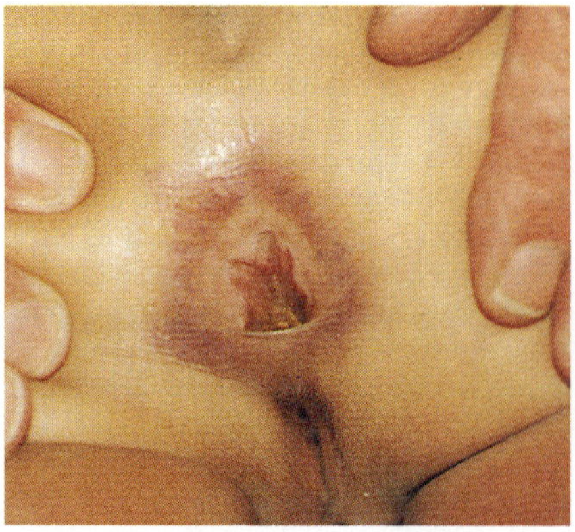

Fig 6.—*Patient 4. No injuries revealed with toluidine blue. Note postmortem anal gaping.*

or gauze with lubricating jelly is used to remove excess dye. A negative result is indicated by no uptake or light, diffusely stippled uptake of dye. A positive result is indicated by deep staining in skin defects. In patient 1, toluidine blue revealed multiple lacerations not visible to the naked eye or under the colposcope. In patient 2, the dye revealed a striking stellate pattern that was matched to an object found near the body. In patient 3, two smaller lacerations were revealed in addition to the large laceration visible on gross inspection. In patient 4, as well as many other cases, toluidine blue dye has helped confirm lack of evidence of sexual abuse.

A diagnosis of sexual abuse at autopsy may have serious implications for the criminal justice system, victims' families, and suspected offenders. Examiners should be aware of conditions that may be confused with trauma due to sexual abuse.[3] Postmortem anal dilation (Fig 6) is a common "normal" finding at autopsy, but can be alarming to clinicians accustomed to examining live patients. Staining by toluidine blue merely indicates that the skin has been broken. Inflammation due to diaper dermatitis or vulvovaginal disease may cause a diffuse or stippled pattern of uptake of dye.[1] Causes of injury other than sexual abuse, such as fissures due to constipation, perirectal abscess, surgical procedures, maceration, insect damage, or accidental injury to the body before or during autopsy[4] must be considered as well.

Toluidine blue should be used after collection of forensic evidence to avoid interference with tests for the presence of semen. The dye is spermicidal in vitro but has not been found to affect acid phosphatase levels.[1] It should be used only when an autopsy is done within a few hours to days after death and the victim's skin is relatively intact.

Toluidine blue dye is a simple, inexpensive aid in the investigation of deaths in children when sexual abuse is suspected. Its use can enhance the ability of clinicians to detect and document genital and anal injuries.

References

1. Lauber AA, Souma ML. Use of toluidine blue for documentation of traumatic intercourse. *Obstet Gynecol.* 1982;60:644-648.
2. McCauley J, Gorman RL, Guzinski G. Toluidine blue in the detection of perineal lacerations in pediatric and adolescent sexual abuse victims. *Pediatrics.* 1986;78:1039-1043.
3. Bays J, Jenny C. Genital and anal conditions confused with child sexual abuse trauma. *AJDC.* 1990;144:1319-1322.
4. Devine WA, Debich DE. Damage to the head and neck of infants at autopsy. *Pediatr Pathol.* 1990;10:475-478.

Violence and Children in the United States

Violence has become an everyday fact in our lives. From the moment we awaken and are greeted by the daily newspapers and listen to the radio or television news accounts, we are reminded of the violent society in which we live. Those of my generation know the difference between now and "then." As a youngster, I could roam the streets of my neighborhood in Philadelphia without fear of bodily harm, and could run short- and long-distance tasks walking or using public transportation without fear of theft or injury. Many of my age can recite similar nostalgic recollections. But nostalgia cannot change the current situation. We are confronted with a reality that is frightening for many of our youth.

In this issue, we publish several reports on the status of violence in some parts of the United States. This is part of the efforts of the American Medical Association's family of journals to highlight this aspect of our current societal milieu. These reports paint quite a different picture of the environment in which some children attempt to grow and develop from that of a bygone era. For example, Meehan and O'Carroll[1] describe gang-oriented culture in Los Angeles and relate it to homicide. Their data tend to dissociate drugs and drug-related crime from the deaths of youth; rather, gang-related activities appear to have an inherent violent aspect that results in death among members and those unfortunate enough to be "in the way" of gang-related activities.

Sheley and coworkers[2] report how violence is transported into the schools in 10 inner-city schools in five cities in four states. Guns, so prevalent in the surrounding neighborhoods of inner-city schools, are one of the instruments of violence and death within the schools. One frightening aspect of both reports is that of randomness; in the report by Sheley et al, one in 10 victimizations appears to involve the innocent bystander. One might expect certain precautions and behaviors to help avoid direct contact with violent persons, but one cannot protect against or avoid the random violent act that affects one irrespective of whether precautions have been taken.

These reports indicate that many of our youth live in violent surroundings. They are forced to work, play, attend school, and conduct normal activities among persons and settings that not only condone violence but have adopted it as a way of life, and this is just the tip of the iceberg. In addition to violence experienced in the school and neighborhood setting, the home is no longer a secure haven for many. Familial abuse, member against member, is also rampant. *AJDC* has published a number of reports in the past on child abuse and neglect, exploring this element of violence and its effects on growth and development.[3-9]

Further, children are exposed to violence in the media, most notably, television and cinema.[10-13] Cartoons, dramas, the news, and even comedy and musical programs project images of violent behavior, often graphically and many times gratuitously. Some have felt that the effect of these depictions is to inure the child to violence at least, and to serve as acceptable models for behavior at worst.

The picture that emerges for some of our children is that they are awash in a sea of violence—at home, in the neighborhood, in school, and in the media. It is not surprising that many resort to violence themselves, and perpetuate what has been their own experience of interpersonal interaction or modeled in the media.

Much of what has been written is descriptive, ie, it tells us what is occurring. Little has been suggested to prevent or "cure" violence in the home or in society. We almost appear to be paralyzed by the problem, without ready solutions apparent. What can be done? What can we do as physicians?

Most will admit that the problem is societal, and medical intervention is but a small fragment of the potential solutions. Poverty, drugs, unemployment, and all of the other ills rampant in our society are progenitors of violence. Until we, as a total society, successfully address these issues, violence will continue to be part of our world. However, that does not mean that we have no active role to play. As physicians we can be alert to evidence of violence in our patients. Once detected, we should not ignore the signs and should take whatever social actions are available in our community.

As pediatricians we will most often encounter violence in a family setting; child abuse, neglect, and evidence of physical abuse of our patients or their caretakers should all be reported to the appropriate social agencies, including the police departments. We can also act in concert with our professional societies. The Rochester Pediatric Society has taken a stand on gun safety. Through its Gun Safety Task Force, a report entitled *Gun Safety Guidelines* was widely circulated. This brochure offers advice to parents in an effort to protect children in that community. In 1990, during a single 10-day period, five Monroe County, New York, children were accidentally wounded by guns; three were seriously hurt and one was paralyzed. These events stimulated the Rochester Pediatric Society to play a more active role in prevention via the brochure and a comprehensive educational campaign aimed at pediatricians and, through them, parents (James Sayre, MD, personal written communication, February 1992). Other professional groups may wish to take similar actions in their own areas.

As citizens we should actively support groups in society that seek to improve the factors that contribute to violence. For example, we should be active advocates for reduced violence in children's television programming. We should advocate gun control to prevent accidental or deliberate use of handguns to kill or maim children. We can educate our communities about the dangers of guns, advocating elimination of guns in the household or, at a minimum, safe practices. We can also take a more vigorous political role in advocating gun-control legislation.

We can also instruct parents in their role in monitoring children's television-viewing habits. We can assist school boards, principals, and teachers of the schools in our districts in their attempts to reduce the violent environment in their arenas. These may seem small, even futile, steps in a problem that appears to overwhelm society, but many such small interventions may add up to effective action in a neighborhood, a school, or even an entire community.

Violence threatens to supersede illness as a cause of pediatric morbidity and mortality in some communities. We must first understand it and then take whatever actions we can as professionals and citizens to help control, and eventually eliminate, it from the lives of our patients. The American Medical Association has taken a first step in casting a light on the extent and nature of violence in our society. Let's join forces now to see if we can reduce violence and halt its impact on our youth.

VINCENT A. FULGINITI, MD
Editor, *AJDC*
Dean's Office
Tulane University School of Medicine
1430 Tulane Ave
New Orleans, LA 70112

References

1. Meehan PJ, O'Carroll PW. Youth homicide in Los Angeles: an explosive mix of drugs and gangs. *AJDC.* 1992;146:683-687.
2. Sheley JF, McGee ZT, Wright JD. Gun-related violence in and around inner-city schools. *AJDC.* 1992;146:677-682.
3. Krugman RD. Child abuse and neglect: critical first steps in response to a national emergency. *AJDC.* 1991;145:513-515.
4. Ricci LR. Photographing the physically abused child. *AJDC.* 1991;145:275-281.
5. Gutman LT, St Claire KK, Weedy C, et al. Human immunodeficiency virus transmission by child sexual abuse. *AJDC.* 1991;145:137-141.
6. Christoffel KK. Violent death and injury in US children and adolescents. *AJDC.* 1990;144:697-706.
7. Monteleone JA. Child sexual abuse and human immunodeficiency virus transmission. *AJDC.* 1991;145:847-848.
8. Baker RB. Anal fissure produced by examination for sexual abuse. *AJDC.* 1991;145:848-849.
9. Gutman LT, Herman-Giddens M, Prose NS. Diagnosis of child sexual abuse in children with genital warts. *AJDC.* 1991;145:126-127.
10. Taras HL, Sallis JF, Nader PR, Nelson J. Children's television-viewing habits and the family environment. *AJDC.* 1990;144:357-359.
11. Stiehm ER. Your child's best friend: TV or not TV. *AJDC.* 1991;145:257.
12. Bader M. Your child's best friend: TV or not TV. *AJDC.* 1991;145:963.
13. Schmitt BD. Nightmares on main street. *AJDC.* 1989;143:649.

Gun-Related Violence in and Around Inner-City Schools

Joseph F. Sheley, PhD; Zina T. McGee, MA; James D. Wright, PhD

• *Objective.*—**To assess the degree to which inner-city high school students are victimized by threat of or actual firearm attack.**

Design.—**Cross-sectional survey.**

Setting.—**Ten inner-city high schools in five cities in four states.**

Participants.—**A total of 1653 male and female inner-city high school students responding anonymously.**

Selection Procedures.—**Volunteer, convenience sample.**

Interventions.—**None.**

Measurements and Results.—**Twenty-three percent of respondents were classified as victims. Major variables predicting victimization levels were gender, number of siblings, exposure to violence outside of school, and personal violence-related attributes. Only one in 10 victimizations appeared to be random (ie, not predicted by these variables).**

Conclusions.—**Violence in school is brought into, rather than generated by, the school. Victimized students have characteristics that put them at higher risk of victimization than other students. Given the large number of victimizations and the large number of respondents with risk characteristics, intervention at the individual level seems ineffective. Instead, alteration of community social structure and culture appears to be the appropriate, although difficult, avenue of change for gun-related victimization levels.**

(*AJDC.* 1992;146:677-682)

Gun-related violence among high school youths increasingly commands the attention of the public health professions and has become a leading cause of morbidity and mortality among the young. High school–aged youths committed 7000 homicides with firearms between 1980 and 1989.[1] In 1989, 81% of the homicides of persons aged 15 to 19 years were accomplished with guns.[2] Homicide, most often committed with firearms, is now the leading cause of death of young black males.[3] Victimization survey data for 1989 indicate that 2% of the nation's students aged 12 to 19 years were victims of violent crime in or around their schools within the previous 6 months.[4]

Accepted for publication March 2, 1992.

From the Department of Sociology, Tulane University, New Orleans, La.

Reprint requests to Department of Sociology, Tulane University, New Orleans, LA 70118 (Dr Sheley).

Security has become a major difficulty for school administrators.[5] Of 11 000 eighth- and 10th-grade boys surveyed in 20 states in 1987, 3% reported having brought a handgun to school.[6] A study of 390 city high school students conducted in Baltimore, Md, in 1987 found that almost half of the boys had carried a gun at least once (*Newsweek.* January 11, 1988:18). Four percent of students in a nationally representative sample of students in grades 9 through 12 studied in 1990 reported carrying a firearm (though not necessarily in school) within the last 30 days. Twenty-one percent of the black males in the sample had carried a gun during the previous month.[1]

As enlightening as these figures are, they are too general to offer much direction for policy-making. First, they provide no information about the subpopulation of students seemingly most at risk for experiencing gun-related violence: those in inner-city high schools. What percentage of inner-city juveniles are victims of gun-related violence? Second, the research published to date reports only a few characteristics of the victims of school-related violence in general[4] and little or nothing about the victims of gun-related violence specifically. Knowledge of the characteristics of students most at risk for experiencing gun-related violence can be used to guide policy-making to reduce the risk for such violence.

Our study provides some of this information. We identified the amount of gun-related victimization, in schools and in transit to and from schools, for a sample of inner-city high school students from five US urban centers. We examined four general classes of predictors of gun-related victimization in students: (1) sociodemographic characteristics, (2) exposure to violence outside of school, (3) exposure to violence within the school, and (4) possible violence-engendering activities of the students themselves. Our aim in examining these variables was to determine whether policy designed to reduce the risk of gun-related violence among students was best directed at social and cultural institutions outside of schools or at practices and structures within schools.

Sociodemographic factors (age, race, and gender) are traditionally linked to victimization by violent crime and, especially, to victimization with handguns.[7,8] Exposure to violence outside of school implies that individuals are encouraged to behave violently. They may also be more likely to carry firearms for protection or for other reasons to be more ready to respond violently in a social world they see as hostile and dangerous.[9] A higher level of exposure to violence in school, with all else being equal, indicates a higher risk of victimization. Involvement in violence-related activities may heighten the risk for victimization. Carrying weapons, for example, raises the stakes in disputes that otherwise would have been settled less violently. Involvement in drugs (either as a user or seller) has also been linked to serious juvenile delinquency[10] and higher levels of victimization in schools in general,[4] and, thus, is a critical variable in this analysis.

METHODS

Sample

The analyses reported here are based on data derived from responses to self-administered surveys completed by 1653 students in 10 high schools in the United States in spring 1991. The schools in question were located in inner cities near state correctional facilities that were part of a related study. In all cases, local school administrators viewed the topic of gun possession and use by students as highly politically charged. They consented to our study only on the guarantee that their districts and schools would not be identified in the publication of our research results. Respecting their wishes, we note here only that we obtained responses from schools in large, prominent cities in California, Illinois, Louisiana, and New Jersey. Schools selected for study were identified by the administrators as typical inner-city schools that had experienced firearms incidents in the recent past and whose students likely encountered gun-related violence (as victims, perpetrators, or bystanders) out of school. Enrollments in these schools ranged from 900 to 2100.

The survey was introduced to students as a national study of firearms and violence among youths. Participation in the study was voluntary and anonymous. The percentage of student populations surveyed ranged from 7% to 21% (mean, 10%). The number of students surveyed per school averaged 165 (range, 109 to 229). In four of the 10 schools sampled, students were offered $5 to participate in the survey. Ultimately, neither financial inducement nor site more generally was tied to response variation across survey items. Owing primarily to respondent fatigue and varying reading skills, response rates differed by item. Average incompletion rate per survey item was 10%. The incompletion rate never exceeded 24%.

Table 1 offers a sociodemographic description of the high school students. The numbers of male and female respondents were roughly equal. Characteristic of inner-city high schools today, 75% of respondents were black; 16%, Hispanic; and only 2%, white. Most of the students were between 15 and 17 years old (mean age, 16 years). The modal grade level was 10th grade. Most respondents lived with both parents or with their mothers only. Twenty-five percent of the students had five or more siblings (mean number of siblings, 3.5). Nearly 80% of the respondents were unemployed.

Table 1.—Sociodemographic Characteristics of Inner-City High School Students

Characteristics	Males, % (n=765)	Females, % (n=829)	All Students, % (n=1594)
Gender	48	52	100
Age, y			
14	7	7	7
15	24	27	25
16	27	31	29
17	22	23	22
≥18	19	13	17
No. of students	753	829	**1582**
Race			
White	3	2	2
Black	72	78	75
Hispanic	19	13	16
Asian	5	4	5
Other	1	3	2
No. of students	756	829	**1585**
Grade			
9	25	25	25
10	32	33	33
11	21	23	21
12	22	19	21
No. of students	747	825	**1572**
Living arrangement			
With both parents	44	36	39
With mother only	36	45	41
With father only	5	4	5
With other relative	10	9	9
Other	5	6	5
No. of students	752	833	**1585**
No. of siblings			
0	5	4	4
1	14	14	15
2	21	23	22
3	20	18	19
4	14	16	15
≥5	26	25	25
No. of students	707	799	**1506**
Employment			
No	72	82	78
Yes, working less than 20 h/wk	14	9	11
Yes, working more than 20 h/wk	14	9	11
No. of students	746	825	**1571**

Measurement

The dependent variable in this study, gun-related victimization, was measured by combining responses to survey items involving (*a*) threats with guns, and (*b*) being shot at while in school or in transit to or from school in the last few years. In either case, response categories range from "never" (scored as 0) to "many times" (scored as 3). Each response to the survey item regarding gun-firing was doubled to weight it as the more serious offense. Thus, respondents could have received a gun-related victimization score ranging from 0 (never threatened or shot at) to 12 (threatened "many times" and shot at "many times").

The measurement of the sociodemographic variables was straightforward (Table 1). For correlational and regression analyses, race first was recoded as a series of dummy variables and then dichotomized as "black/nonblack." Neither coding formula produced findings different from the other. Living arrangement was coded according to degree of habitation with parents—living with both (scored as 3), living with either parent (scored as 2), and living with neither parent (scored as 1).

Exposure to violence outside of school was measured based on three items. First, respondents were asked how many males in their families carried guns habitually outside of the home. Second, they were asked the same question concerning their friends. For both items, response categories range from "none" (scored as 1) to "all" (scored as 4). Third, they were asked to what extent they strongly disagreed (scored as 1) or strongly agreed (scored as 4) that they lived in neighborhoods in which guns were plentiful and easily accessible.

Exposure to violence in school was measured in three ways. First, respondents were asked whether they agreed or disagreed with the statement that they felt scared most of the time at school. Second, they were asked whether they agreed that there was a lot of violence in their school. For both items, response categories ranged from "strongly disagree" (scored as 1) to "strongly agree" (scored as 4). Finally, respondents were asked how many students they personally knew who carried guns to school. Response categories ranged from "none" (scored as 0) to "almost all" (scored as 4).

Finally, personal violence-related activities were measured in terms of the extent to which respondents carried guns outside of school and on school property. Response categories for both items range from "never" (scored as 0) to "almost all the time" (scored as 4). Hard drug use was measured through combining responses concerning use of each of three drugs: heroin, cocaine, and crack. A respondent might have used each "never" (scored as 0) to "almost all the time" (scored as 4) in the year or two preceding administration of the survey. Combining the items produced scores ranging from 0 to 12 (used all three substances "almost all the time"). Finally, if respondents had dealt drugs (ie, been a dealer or worked for a dealer) they received a score of 1; if not, a score of 0.

RESULTS

Gun-Related Victimization

Twenty percent of the students had been threatened with a gun, and 12% had been shot at (Table 2). Twice as many males as females had been threatened with a gun, and three times as many males as females had been fired upon. Twenty-three percent of the sample had gun-related victimization scores of at least 1; 10% had scores exceeding 3. Again, males exceeded females in their combined gun-related victimization scores.

Table 2 also presents findings concerning the three independent variables in this study: exposure to violence outside of school, exposure to violence in school, and personal violence-related activity.

Exposure to Violence Outside of School

Males in the families of 39% of the respondents habitually carried guns outside of their homes. Thirty-five percent of the respondents had friends who routinely carried guns. Twenty-three percent of the respondents characterized their neighborhoods as replete with easily accessible guns. Females were slightly more likely than males to report males in their families carrying guns, although males were considerably more likely to have friends who carried guns. Perceived availability of guns in the neighborhood was roughly the same for both genders.

Exposure to Violence in School

Thirty-eight percent of students agreed that there was a lot of violence in their schools. Females were more likely to agree than males. Fifteen percent of the respondents (males and females alike) agreed that they were scared at school almost all of the time. Forty-six percent of respondents personally knew schoolmates who had carried guns to school during the last year. The value for males in this survey item was only 3 percentage points higher than for females.

Personal Violence-Related Behaviors

Twenty-two percent of the students carried a gun outside of school, and 6% carried a gun at school at least "now and then." Males were three times more likely than females to have engaged in each of these behaviors. Additionally, 4% of the students had used hard drugs during the last 2 years. Half of this subsample had drug use scores of five or more. Again, males were three times more likely than females to use hard drugs. Finally, 16% of respondents reported having dealt drugs; males' involvement in drug dealing exceeded that of females by 9 percentage points.

Table 2.—Gun Victimization, Exposure to Violence, and Personal Violence-Related Activity Among Inner-City High School Students*

Variable	Males, %	Females, %	All Students, %
Gun victimization			
Threatened with a gun	28 (n=655)	13 (n=733)	20 **(n=1388)**
Shot at with a gun	17 (n=647)	5 (n=733)	12 **(n=1380)**
Victimization score			
0	66	85	77
1	10	6	8
2	7	5	6
≥3	17	4	9
No. of students	592	732	**1324**
Exposure to violence outside of school			
Males in family carry guns			
No	63	58	61
Yes	37	42	39
No. of students	692	790	**1482**
Friends carry guns			
No	58	72	65
Yes	42	28	35
No. of students	684	784	**1468**
Access to guns in the neighborhood			
Strongly disagree/disagree	77	75	77
Strongly agree/agree	23	25	23
No. of students	630	764	**1394**
Exposure to violence in school			
Students carry guns to school			
No	52	55	54
Yes	48	45	46
No. of students	717	804	**1521**
A lot of violence in school			
Strongly disagree/disagree	65	59	62
Strongly agree/agree	35	41	38
No. of students	533	680	**1213**
Often feel afraid in school			
Strongly disagree/disagree	86	85	85
Strongly agree/agree	14	15	15
No. of students	537	682	**1219**
Personal violence related-activity			
Carry a gun outside of school			
No	65	89	78
Yes	35	11	22
No. of students	699	762	**1461**
Carry a gun to school			
No	91	97	94
Yes	9	3	6
No. of students	709	775	**1484**
Hard drug–use score			
0	93.4	97.9	95.8
1	1.0	.6	.7
2	1.0	.3	.6
3	0.3	None	0.2
4	0.5	None	0.3
≥5	3.8	1.2	2.4
No. of students	576	714	**1290**
Dealing drugs			
No	79	88	84
Yes	21	12	16
No. of students	567	718	**1285**

*Number of students indicates total number of students of each gender or total number of students of both genders for whom the given information was available.

Table 3.—Correlation Matrix of Sociodemographic Characteristics, Exposure to Violence, Personal Violence-Related Activity, and Gun Victimization Variables

	1	2	3	4	5	6	7	8	9	10	11	12	13	14	15	16	17
1. Gun-related victimization		.23*	.01	−.01	.06†	.01	.04	.26*	.21*	.15*	.19*	.10†	.02	.46*	.30*	.23*	.35†
2. Gender			.06†	.04	.01	.05†	.10*	.15*	−.05*	.06†	.03	−.06†	−.02	.28*	.12*	.09*	.13*
3. Age				−.04	.06†	−.08†	.23*	.04	−.01	.06†	.04	−.02	−.02	.05	.05†	.05	.03
4. Race					.06†	.09*	−.01	.06†	−.09†	−.07†	−.08†	−.01	.06†	−.01	−.01	.08†	−.04
5. Number of siblings						−.04	.05†	.04	.02†	.01	.05†	.08	.07†	.02	.03	.03	−.01
6. Parental living arrangement							−.02	.06†	.02	−.03	.02	.02	−.02	.06†	.01	−.02	−.01
7. Job status								.04	−.01	.05	.10*	−.03	−.03	.10*	.01	−.01	.07†
8. Friends carrying guns									.33*	.29*	.29*	.18*	.09†	.36*	.22*	.15*	.33*
9. Male relatives carrying guns										.21*	.24*	.06†	.03	.23*	.15*	.12*	.21*
10. Guns in neighborhood											.25*	.25*	.13*	.18*	.14*	.09†	.24*
11. Kids in school with guns												.16*	.04	.27*	.20*	.07†	.01
12. Violence in school													.38*	.10†	.13*	.06†	.12*
13. Afraid in school														−.02	.01	.04†	.01
14. Carrying a gun															.43*	.21*	.43*
15. Carrying a gun in school																.21*	.26*
16. Using hard drugs																	.23*
17. Drug dealing																	

*$P<.001$.
†$P<.05$.

Intercorrelations

Table 3 presents correlations among the variables examined in this study. Only two sociodemographic characteristics, gender and number of siblings, were related at the zero-order level to gun-related victimization scores. All remaining variables (except feeling scared at school) were linked to gun-related victimization. However, the coefficients in the table indicate modest interrelations among the independent variables. To ascertain which variables predicted gun-related victimization outside of the influence of the other variables, we entered all variables into regression equations. The findings presented in Table 4 reflect the model after eliminating the variables that were not associated with gun-related victimization and that, when eliminated, would not affect the adjusted explained variance.

With the exception of gender and number of siblings, none of the sociodemographic variables or survey items examining exposure to violence in school was ultimately linked to gun-related victimization score. That is, age, race, living situation, employment situation, and grade level at school did not influence gun-related victimization when examined alone and disregarding influence from other variables. This was also true for level of exposure to violence in school (amount of violence in school, feeling scared in school, and the number of persons known by the respondent to have carried guns to school).

Gun-related violence that occurs in and around inner city schools derives mainly from factors external to the schools themselves. Males and children from large families were more at risk for gun-related victimization than were females and children from smaller families. Beyond these factors, the variables associated with victimization involved exposure to violence outside of school and personal violence–related behaviors. The victims of gun-related violence in school or in transit to or from school were youths from families in which males carried guns routinely, youths who carried guns themselves (either in or out of school), and youths who used or sold drugs.

Table 4.—Regression Estimates of the Influence of Sociodemographic Characteristics, Exposure to Violence, and Personal Violence-Related Activity on Gun-Related Victimization*

Independent Variables	b	β
Gender	.391	.119†
No. of siblings	.046	.079‡
Males in family carry guns	.241	.073‡
Student carries a gun outside of school	1.246	.301†
Student carries a gun in school	.684	.089‡
Using hard drugs	.139	.103‡
Dealing drugs	.576	.130†
Constant	−.1338	Not applicable

*n=1049. $R^2=.29$; adjusted $R^2=.28$; $F=59.4825$ ($P<.001$).
†$P<.001$.
‡$P<.05$.

Random vs Nonrandom Victimization

Many discussions of violence in and around schools depict the problem as essentially random, a matter of youths being in the wrong place at the wrong time. While some victims are no doubt stricken randomly, our findings indicate that most decidedly are *not*. Indeed, of the 322 victims of gun-related violence in this study, 76% had at least one of the five nondemographic characteristics linked to victimization in Table 4; 90% of respondents with victimization scores of 3 or more had at least one such attribute.

To clarify further the risk factors for gun-related victimization, we sorted out the 77 respondents who had experienced victimization but who did *not* display any of the previously described characteristics. In this subgroup, gender was still important; beyond that, the only significant variable was the number of persons the respondent knew personally who carried guns in school. Thus, with no other risk factors present, simply knowing people who carried guns to school put one at risk for victimization. Fifty-two percent of the 77 victims knew someone who had carried a firearm to school. The exact nature of this relationship was not wholly clear. If it was a matter simply of knowing identities, the variable might reflect a risk factor of the school environment per se. However, because none of the other measures of school environment was related to victimization scores, we suspect that this variable, too, was largely behavioral; it more likely indexed the tendency of the respondent to affiliate with people who carry guns to school. If this is the correct interpretation, only 37 of the 322 victims examined lacked any apparent nondemographic attribute placing them at risk. Perhaps one gun-related victimization in 10 is the result of a youth being "in the wrong place at the wrong time." The remaining nine out of 10 result either from behavioral risk factors (eg, carrying guns, being involved with drugs, or affiliating with people who carry guns) or from environmental risk factors that exist *outside* of the schools themselves.

COMMENT

We have sought in this study to assess the degree to which inner-city high school students are victimized by the threat of or by actual gun-related violence and to ascertain the associated risk factors. Our findings indicate that gun-related victimization among inner-city school youths far exceeds that of students nationally. Whereas 2% of the nation's students report being victims of some form of violence (albeit for only 6 months[4]), 23% of inner-city students in our sample had been victims, during the last few years, of gun-related violence specifically. Males, especially, had high victimization rates (one in three males in our sample). Aside from the significant influence of gender and number of siblings, major predictors of gun-related victimization in school or in transit to or from school involved whether or not family members carried guns, the extent to which students themselves carried guns in and out of school, whether or not students used and sold drugs and, for those with none of these characteristics, whether they affiliated with others who carried guns to school. In the final analysis, 89% of the victims in this study had at least one characteristic that put them at greater risk for gun-related victimization. Gun-related victimization of youths does not "just happen"; rather, it is patterned violence.

Our results suggest that schools themselves do not generate gun-related violence as much as they represent the location where violence spawned outside of the institution is played out. Most gun-related violence that occurs in schools or on the way to and from schools occurs because many students come from social milieus where carrying and using guns is commonplace, because some pupils engage in behaviors known to breed violence (eg, drug trafficking), or simply because carrying guns (or affiliating with those who do) promotes more consequential outcomes in otherwise "normal" school-yard disputes. Apparently, only one in 10 victims (not a trivial figure in that it constitutes 2% of our entire sample of inner-city students) is involved in random gun-related violence. These, we assume, are students who become embroiled in disputes situationally rather than through higher-risk attributes or who are the random targets of robberies or the victims of gunfire meant for someone else.

Increased security in and around schools may or may not reduce levels of gun-related victimization.[6] All 10 schools in our study had histories of problems with guns and had already implemented rather tight security measures when our data were collected. Likewise, little difference has been found in rates of violent victimization between schools with and without conventional security measures such as patrolled hallways and visitor check-ins.[4] A broader policy initiative, more epidemiologic in nature, would involve some form of direct intervention in the lives of youth at risk for school-related violence.[11] However, because the predictive variables that surfaced in this analysis were either broad sociodemographic characteristics (gender and number of siblings), illegal behaviors (such as involvement in drugs), or behaviors that are not obvious before the fact (such as carrying guns or affiliating with those who do), the ability to identify those at risk before they engage in or are victims of violence is seriously limited.

Our findings point *away* from intervention at the individual level and *toward* changes in the larger familial, communal, and social situation of those most involved in gun-related violence. Inner-city youths obviously do not assume new social identities as they pass through school gates; likewise, the schools are obviously not immune to the many problems of the communities in which they are located. As we have seen, violence in and around schools is *not* predicted by factors inherent in the school environments themselves; rather, violence spills into the schools from the world outside. Given the concentration of so much of this violence (and other social ills) among inner-city inhabitants—and, by this study's account, among such high proportions of those inhabitants—structural and cultural remedies command attention.

Structurally, we are experiencing the development of an inner-city underclass unlike any in our past. In a shrinking industrial economy, we are witnessing the disintegration of the traditional family, increasing poverty and homelessness, diminishing health, and deteriorating educational institutions. The desperation of this situation is enhanced by the apparent enormity of the drug problem and the ready availability of firearms to all. Given all this, perhaps the surprising result is not that there is so much violence in the inner city, but that there is so little.

These structural ingredients have fostered a culture of violence that, unfortunately, may survive even after the structural situation has improved. Inner-city youths know they are at risk for violent victimization, and they are now accustomed to arming themselves for protection (from violence in general or from violence associated with illegal activities). They have been introduced to sophisticated weapons, including the automatic and semi-automatic firearms that currently occupy the media's attention. Even were structural elements to improve, the perceived need for protection would not disappear rapidly. Nor is it likely that, as conditions improve, youths will begin using less lethal weapons. Guns have become a part of the culture of inner city, underclass youths. As a cultural element, the desire to carry firearms will last long beyond the need to carry firearms (even assuming, perhaps unrealistically, that the need itself would be reduced by structural improvements).

It is clear that the problem of violence in inner city schools cannot be isolated from the problem of violence in larger society; violent neighborhoods and violent communities will produce violent schools whatever measures the schools themselves adopt. It is equally clear that this "larger" problem will not yield to simplistic, unicausal solutions. In this connection, it is useful to point out that nearly everything that leads to gun-related violence among youths is already against the law. What is needed are not new and more stringent gun laws but rather a concerted effort to rebuild the social structure of inner cities.

This study was funded by grants from the National Institute of Justice and the Office of Juvenile Justice and Delinquency Prevention, whose support we gratefully acknowledge.

References

1. Department of Health and Human Services. Weapon-carrying among high school students: United States, 1990. *MMWR.* 1991;40:681-684.
2. Center to Prevent Handgun Violence. *A Generation Under the Gun.* Washington, DC: Center to Prevent Handgun Violence; 1990.
3. *Homicide Surveillance: High-Risk Racial and Ethnic Groups: Blacks and Hispanics, 1970-1983.* Atlanta, Ga: Centers for Disease Control; 1986.
4. Bastion LD, Taylor BM. *School Crime: A National Crime Victimization Survey Report.* Washington, DC: Department of Justice; 1991.
5. Donahue T. *Weapons in Schools.* Washington, DC: Office of Juvenile Justice and Delinquency Prevention; 1989.
6. National School Safety Center. *Weapons in Schools.* Malibu, Calif: National School Safety Center; 1989.
7. Harlow CW. *Female Victims of Violent Crime.* Washington, DC: Bureau of Justice Statistics; 1991.
8. Rand MR. *Handgun Crime Victims.* Washington, DC: Bureau of Justice Statistics; 1990.
9. Wright JD, Rossi PH. *Armed and Considered Dangerous.* Hawthorne, NY: Aldine Publishing Co; 1986.
10. Fagan J. Social processes of delinquency and drug use among urban gangs. In: Huff CR, ed. *Gangs in America.* Beverly Hills, Calif: Sage Publishers Inc; 1990.
11. Gold MF. Epidemiologists aim at new target: health risk of gun proliferation. *JAMA.* 1989;261:675-676.

Gangs, Drugs, and Homicide in Los Angeles

Patrick J. Meehan, MD, Patrick W. O'Carroll, MD, MPH

• *Objective.*—To assess the theory that youth homicides in Los Angeles, Calif, are largely attributable to gang involvement in the trafficking or use of drugs.

***Design, Setting, and Participants.*—First, we analyzed all homicides in a police database that occurred in Los Angeles between January 1, 1986, and August 31, 1988, to examine the association between gang activity and narcotic use and trafficking. Second, we used detailed data from police files to examine the same associations for a subset of homicides in south central Los Angeles. Third, we investigated the association between gang homicide victimization and victim cocaine use for all 1987 Los Angeles homicides. Finally, we compared narcotics arrest histories for gang homicide victims with histories for other homicide victims.**

***Results.*—Gang-motivated homicides were less likely than other homicides to involve narcotics, and narcotics-motivated homicides were less likely to involve a gang member. Victims of gang-motivated homicides in 1987 were less likely than other homicide victims to have detectable levels of blood cocaine. Finally, young victims of gang-involved homicide were no more likely to have a history of narcotics arrests than other victims.**

***Conclusions.*—Our investigation does not support the theory that a substantial proportion of homicides are attributable to gang involvement in narcotics trafficking.**

(*AJDC.* 1992;146:683-687)

Between 1980 and 1988, the homicide rate in Los Angeles, Calif, was more than double the rate for the state of California (unpublished data, Los Angeles Police Department [LAPD] and the California Department of Health Services, 1989). According to the gang investigation unit of the LAPD, gang-related homicides constitute an increasingly large proportion of all homicides in Los Angeles. In 1983, 14.8% of all homicides were gang-related compared with 25.2% in 1987.

There is also objective evidence that cocaine abuse and trafficking have increased in Los Angeles. Both the number of medical encounters for problems related to cocaine abuse and cocaine seizures by law enforcement agencies have increased.[1] Furthermore, in 1987, cocaine or cocaine metabolites were detected in the blood of more than one of every five homicide victims in Los Angeles County at the time of death.[2]

Both gang activities and narcotics trafficking are inherently violent activities that are independently associated with an increased risk of homicide perpetration and victimization.[3] However, a prevalent theory in Los Angeles in the late 1980s was that a substantial proportion of the increasing incidence of homicide among the youth in that city was attributable to the increasing involvement of gang members in illicit drug trafficking, drug use, or both. According to this theory, the involvement of gangs in the narcotics trade is a particularly explosive mix, resulting in increases in violence far beyond what might be expected from the sum of the independent contributions of gang activity and narcotics trafficking. The general acceptance of this theory is reflected in both the popular media (*Los Angeles Herald Examiner*. January 14, 1989:A4; *Rolling Stone*. September 22, 1988:64-72, 114-116) and in official reports, such as the 1988 report from the California Council on Criminal Justice Task Force on Gangs and Drugs.[4] The hypothesized interaction of gangs and narcotics in causing homicide is generally thought to involve narcotics trafficking, particularly cocaine trafficking. It is also conceivable, however, that increasing *use* of narcotics by gang members could contribute to higher homicide rates, either because of direct pharmacologic effects of narcotics that promote violent behavior or because of the need of narcotics users to commit violent crimes to supply their addictions.[5]

Despite its popularity, there is little evidence to support the theory that gang involvement in the narcotics trade is responsible for a substantial proportion of homicide among youth in Los Angeles. This issue should be critically examined because it has direct relevance to the design of homicide prevention programs. If a large proportion of homicides are attributable to this intersection of gang activity and narcotics trafficking (or use), then increased efforts to prevent gangs from selling (or using) narcotics might be the most effective short-term strategy for reducing the death toll from homicide in Los Angeles. If, on the other hand, narcotics trafficking and gang activity are more important as independent contributors to homicide than as cofactors, a prevention strategy tar-

Accepted for publication March 2, 1992.

From the Division of Injury Control, National Center for Environmental Health and Injury Control, Centers for Disease Control, Public Health Service, US Department of Health and Human Services, Atlanta, GA 30333.

Reprint requests to New Hampshire Department of Health and Human Services, 6 Hazen Dr, Concord, NH 03301-6527 (Dr Meehan).

geted primarily at the intersection of these two inherently violent activities would be misdirected.

Unfortunately, no single data source is sufficient for a comprehensive examination of the various possible relationships between gangs, narcotics, and homicide. Police files, vital statistics, and medical examiner's data files provide relevant information, but each data source has limitations that prevent a straightforward epidemiologic investigation. As part of an investigation of homicides in Los Angeles, however, we were able to make use of several distinct but complementary data sources, each of which provided some evidence about the hypothesized association between gang activity, narcotics use or trafficking, and homicide.

MATERIALS AND METHODS

The available data sources permitted us to evaluate the following four hypotheses: (1) homicides due to gang rivalry (gang-motivated homicides) are more likely than others to involve narcotics; (2) homicides resulting from conflicts related to narcotics trafficking (narcotics-motivated homicides) are more likely than others to involve gang members; (3) victims of gang-motivated homicides are more likely than others to have been using cocaine before death; and (4) victims of homicides involving a gang member (gang-involved homicides) are more likely to have a history of arrests related to narcotics (possession or distribution) than are victims of homicides that involved neither gangs nor narcotics.

Each of these hypotheses posits possible associations between narcotics trafficking or use and gang involvement in homicides in Los Angeles. Because street gang members are mostly younger than 25 years, our analysis emphasizes youth homicides.

Narcotics and Gang Involvement in Homicides

We used two separate data sources to examine the first two hypotheses. The first is a database maintained by the homicide unit of the LAPD primarily for investigative purposes, which we refer to as the *LAPD database* (Table 1).

It contains information on homicide victim demographics, crime circumstances, motives, weapons, and suspects, as well as a brief summary of the incident. Information on homicides is entered by detectives at the outset of an investigation and is updated periodically. Motive was entered by the detective as a word or short phrase ("gang," "gang fight," "domestic," "narco dispute," etc). Motive was then counted by us as "narcotics-motivated" if narcotics appeared in the description of motive, "gang-motivated" if gang appeared in the description, or "motivated by one of a variety of other factors." Apart from the primary motive, "narcotics involvement" and "gang involvement" were entered by the police as separate variables. By definition, all narcotics-motivated homicides were "narcotics-involved," and all gang-motivated homicides were "gang-involved."

The LAPD defines a gang as "a group of persons working to an unlawful or antisocial end" (from LAPD intradepartmental correspondence). Operationally, gang membership is ascertained by detectives entering the data, based on whether the subject is listed in the computerized gang roster of the LAPD or based on characteristics of the event, including use of known hand signals used by gangs, gang-specific clothing, and witness statements.[3]

We verified the completeness of this database by manually comparing homicides in it with those in the master crime file housed in the LAPD data unit's mainframe computer. For the period of study, 97% of the homicides in the master file were also found in the LAPD investigative database. The determination of gang motive by the LAPD had previously been validated.[6] Further, an independent gang unit of the LAPD examined each 1988 homicide to ascertain whether it was gang-motivated. Of the 82 homicides determined to be gang-motivated by the unit, 64 (78%) were described as having a gang motive in the LAPD database. Of the 416 homicides not ascertained to be gang-motivated by the gang investigation unit, 385 (93%) were also described as other than gang-motivated in the LAPD database.

Table 1.—Study Questions and Data Sources

Question No.	Study Questions	Data Sources Used
1	Are gang-motivated homicides more likely than other homicides to involve narcotics?	LAPD database,* SCLA investigative files†
2	Are narcotics-motivated homicides more likely than other homicides to involve gangs?	LAPD database,* SCLA investigative files†
3	Are victims in gang-motivated homicides more likely than other homicide victims to have been using cocaine?	LAPD database linked with LA County Coroner's data‡
4	Are victims of gang-involved homicides more likely to have a narcotics-related arrest than are victims of homicides that were neither gang nor narcotics involved?	LAPD database (sample),§ LAPD arrest records

*Based on information from the Los Angeles Police Department (LAPD) database, 2162 homicide victims between January 1986 and August 1988 were aged 10 years or older.

†Based on south central Los Angeles (SCLA) investigative files, 114 homicide victims were aged between 10 and 19 years.

‡Based on blood cocaine levels of 74% of 618 homicide victims in the LAPD database in 1987.

§Randomly selected homicide victims in south central Los Angeles aged 15 to 24 years between January 1986 and August 1988 included 31 cases (gang-involved homicides) and 36 controls (neither gang- nor narcotics-involved homicides).

We determined that data had been reliably entered into the LAPD database for the period of January 1, 1986, through August 31, 1988. We therefore analyzed data on the victims of all homicides that occurred in Los Angeles during this period, excluding homicides due to legal intervention (during the interruption of a crime). We constructed a set of contingency tables to compare the frequency of gang involvement in narcotics-motivated homicides with that in other homicides. We also constructed contingency tables to compare the frequency of narcotics involvement in gang-motivated homicides with that in other homicides. In our analysis, we stratified the victims into two age groups: 10 to 24 years old, and 25 years and older.

Our second data source was the investigative homicide files kept in police district offices. Of 18 police districts in the city, the police had identified four contiguous districts as having the highest concentration of youths involved in gangs and homicides involving gangs. We refer to this area as *south central Los Angeles*. District office files for each homicide contain initial investigative reports and summary follow-up reports. We limited the case subjects in this analysis to a subset of the population that we studied using the LAPD database: homicide victims aged 10 to 19 years who died in south central Los Angeles from January 1, 1987, through August 31, 1988 (Table 1). We extracted demographic data, information on the weapons used, motive, relationship of victim to offender, whether narcotics were involved, and various incident characteristics.

For this part of the analysis, we defined a gang-involved homicide as one in which either the victim or perpetrator was identified as a gang member through the evidence collected. We defined a gang-motivated homicide as one that resulted from violence between rival gang factions. We defined a narcotics-involved homicide as one in which narcotics were found at the scene of the homicide or on the body of the victim or perpetrator, or in which evidence indicated that narcotic sales or use was occurring at or near the time of the homicide. Finally, we defined a narcotics-motivated homicide as one that resulted from a violent conflict over a narcotics transaction. As with the LAPD database, we used these data to look at the levels of involvement of gangs and narcotics in narcotics-motivated and gang-motivated homicides, respectively.

Cocaine Use by Homicide Victims

To examine the third hypothesis, we supplemented data contained in the LAPD database with records from the Los Angeles County Coroner's Office for 1987. The Los Angeles County Coroner's Office analyzes blood specimens from all homicide victims in Los Angeles County for the presence of cocaine and a cocaine metabolite (benzoylecgonine) according to methods described elsewhere.[2] Detection of either compound was considered evidence of recent cocaine use. Complete data were available for homicides in 1987, and we were able to link the databases from the LAPD and the Coroner's Office for 74% of the homicides that occurred in Los Angeles in 1987 (Table 1). Homicide cases that could not be linked to data from the Coroner's Office did not differ substantially from those that could in terms of the victim's age, sex, or race, the police division in which the homicide occurred, or the perpetrator's motives. The most common reason for a failed linkage was inability to match records by the common identification number.

We examined the hypothesized association between recent cocaine use and being a victim of a gang-motivated homicide by comparing the frequency of positive cocaine levels in the blood of victims of gang-motivated homicide with those in victims of homicides not motivated by gangs.

Past Narcotics Arrests Among Homicide Victims

We tested our fourth hypothesis using a case-control study design. We defined case subjects as victims of gang-involved homicides and control subjects as victims of homicides that were neither gang- nor narcotics-involved. We evaluated the prevalence of history of narcotics arrest among cases compared with controls.

We randomly selected 36 case and 36 control victims of homicide from the LAPD database of ages 15 to 24 years who resided in one of the census tracts within south central Los Angeles and were killed between January 1, 1987, and August 31, 1988 (Table 1). Correct addresses were not available for five of the sampled gang-involved homicide victims, leaving 31 case and 36 control subjects.

We assessed the decedent's history of narcotics arrests using data from computerized county arrest records. After obtaining court permission, we searched computerized law enforcement databases using the decedent's name, address, and date of birth. Any arrest history was noted, including any history of narcotics arrests (for possession or for selling). We found that 42 of the 67 study victims had arrest records. We assumed that the absence of an arrest record was indicative of a victim having no arrests for any offense. We also assumed that the possibility that a record was not found because of an incorrect name or other clerical error was equally likely for case and control subjects.

Statistical Methods

Statistical testing was done using either the Mantel-Hantzel χ^2 test or a two-tailed Fisher's exact test. Odds ratios and 95% confidence intervals (obtained from Cornfield's approximation) were calculated with Epiinfo software (Centers for Disease Control, Atlanta, Ga).

Table 2.—Narcotics Involvement in Gang-Motivated Homicides in Los Angeles from January 1986 Through August 1988

Victims	Gang Motivated	Other Motive		
10 to 24 y old				
Narcotics involved	11	135	$P<10^{-7}$	
Narcotics not involved	259	375		
Total	**270**	**510**		**780**
25 y and older				
Narcotics involved	7	281	$P<.05$	
Narcotics not involved	68	1026		
Total	**75**	**1307**		**1382**
Total 10 y and older				
Narcotics involved	18	416	$P<10^{-7}$	
Narcotics not involved	327	1401		
Total	**345**	**1817**		**2162**

RESULTS

Narcotics Involvement in Gang-Motivated Homicides

The LAPD database contained data on 2162 homicides that occurred between January 1, 1986, and August 31, 1988. Overall, it was noted that 18 (5%) of 345 gang-motivated homicides involved narcotics, whereas 416 (23%) of 1817 other homicides involved narcotics ($P\ll.01$; Table 2). For both younger and older homicide victims, gang-motivated homicides were significantly less likely to have involved narcotics than were other homicides.

Since all the narcotics-motivated homicides (conflict due to narcotics trafficking) are by definition in the "other" (comparison) homicide group when gang-motivated homicides are being examined, and since narcotics-motivated homicides are always narcotics-involved, there is an intrinsic bias toward finding more narcotics involvement in the "other" homicide group than in the gang-motivated homicide group. To account for this bias, we compared the frequency of narcotics involvement in gang-motivated homicides with that for homicides that were neither gang- nor narcotics-motivated. Gang-motivated homicides were still less likely to have involved narcotics than were other homicides. This finding held for all ages combined ($P<.005$) and for victims aged 10 to 24 years ($P<.001$). For victims 25 years and older, homicides that were gang-motivated were just as likely to involve narcotics as were homicides that were neither gang- nor narcotics-motivated (difference is not significant).

We obtained similar results from our detailed examination of investigation files for homicides among adolescents that occurred in south central Los Angeles. During the 20-month period from January 1, 1987, through August 31, 1988, there were 116 homicides in south central Los Angeles involving victims aged 10 to 19 years. We reviewed the investigative files of 114 of these homicides (records for two homicides were not available) and found that none of the 40 gang-motivated homicides involved narcotics.

Gang Involvement in Narcotics-Motivated Homicides

Overall, narcotics-motivated homicides were less likely than other homicides to have involved gangs (Table 3). Of the 281 narcotics-motivated homicides in the LAPD database, 30 (11%) were also noted to have involved gangs. Of the 1881 other homicides, 442 (23%) involved gang mem-

Table 3.—Gang Involvement in Narcotics-Motivated Homicides in Los Angeles From January 1986 Through August 1988

Victims	Narcotics Motivated	Other Motive	
10 to 24 y old			
Gangs involved	16	324	$P<10^{-7}$
Gangs not involved	81	359	
Total	**97**	**683**	**780**
25 y and older			
Gangs involved	14	118	$P=.3$
Gangs not involved	171	1078	
Total	**185**	**1196**	**1381***
Total 10 y and older			
Gangs involved	30	442	$P<10^{-5}$
Gangs not involved	251	1439	
Total	**281**	**1881**	**2162**

*Information for gang involvement was not available for one case.

bers ($P \ll .01$). When the victims were stratified by age, this negative association between narcotics-motivated homicides and gang involvement was found only for those homicides involving victims younger than 25 years. The most common motive for homicides involving gang members was a gang conflict.

Since gang-motivated homicides (involving gang conflict) are always gang-involved (include a gang member as victim or perpetrator), and since gang-motivated homicides are by definition included in the comparison group in the preceding analysis, the negative association we found between narcotics-motivated homicides and gang involvement could theoretically be due to an artifactual bias. We therefore also compared gang involvement in narcotics-motivated homicides with gang involvement in homicides that were neither gang- nor narcotics-motivated. Still, narcotics-motivated homicides were less likely to have involved gangs than were homicides that were neither gang- nor narcotics-motivated for all ages combined ($P<.05$) and for victims 25 years or older ($P=.05$). For victims aged 10 to 24 years, narcotics-motivated homicides were no more or less likely to involve gangs than were homicides that were neither gang- nor narcotics-motivated (difference is not significant).

Of the 114 homicides in south central Los Angeles for which we reviewed actual investigative files, three were found to be narcotics-motivated. None of those three homicides involved gang members.

Cocaine Use by Homicide Victims

Victims of gang-motivated homicides in 1987 were significantly less likely than victims of other homicides to have cocaine or cocaine metabolites in their bloodstreams ($P<.0001$; Table 4). This negative association between being a victim of a gang-motivated homicide and recent cocaine use was found only for homicides involving victims between 10 and 24 years old ($P<.0005$). Among those 25 years and older, no such association was found.

Past Arrest Histories of Homicide Victims

Eight (26%) of 31 victims of gang-involved homicides had a history of narcotics arrests, whereas nine (25%) of 36 control homicide victims had a history of narcotics arrests (Table 5). Thus, victims of gang-involved homicides were no more likely to have a history of narcotics arrests than were victims of homicides that were neither gang- nor narcotics-involved (odds ratio, 1.0; 95% confidence interval, 0.30 to 3.6).

Table 4.—Detection of Cocaine or Cocaine Metabolite in the Blood of Homicide Victims in Los Angeles in 1987

Victims	Gang Motivated	Other Motive	
10 to 24 y old			
Cocaine present	4	36	$P<.0005$
Cocaine not present	78	110	
25 y and older			
Cocaine present	8	119	$P=.7$
Cocaine not present	14	249	
Total 10 y and older			
Cocaine present	12	155	$P<.0001$
Cocaine not present	92	359	

Table 5.—Comparison of Narcotics Arrest Histories for Homicide Victims Between Ages 15 and 24 Years in South Central Los Angeles From January 1987 Through August 1988

Narcotic Arrest History	Homicides Involving Gangs	Homicides Involving Neither Gangs Nor Narcotics	Odds Ratio (95% Confidence Interval)
History of arrest	8	9	1.0 (0.3-3.6)
No history of arrest	23	27	

COMMENT

There is no question that a substantial proportion of homicides in urban America are attributable to gang activity and to narcotics trafficking. In Los Angeles during the period studied, 16% of the homicides among persons aged 10 years and older were gang-motivated, and 13% were narcotics-motivated (Tables 2 and 3). Thus, three out of every 10 homicide victims died from violence between rival gang factions or from violence associated with narcotics trafficking. The results of our investigation, however, do not support the popular theory that a substantial proportion of homicides are attributable to gang involvement in narcotics trafficking. Indeed, our analysis of available data sources suggests that gang-motivated homicides do not tend to involve narcotics trafficking (or victim drug use), and narcotics-motivated homicides do not tend to involve gangs.

Past research on the relationship between gangs, narcotics trafficking, and violence is inconclusive.[7] In contrast to our findings, for example, Skolnick and colleagues[8] concluded (based on a series of interviews in California with inmates of correctional institutions and police and correctional officers) that street drug dealing in California is dominated by Black gangs organized specifically for the purpose of distributing crack cocaine (institutional gangs). Such gangs are said to be distinct from the more traditional neighborhood or cultural gangs. Klein and Maxson,[3] however, have suggested that it may be tautological to define gangs in terms of the common criminal activity that brings the members together as with institutional cocaine distributing gangs. It is quite possible that violence involving traditional youth street gangs that are loosely tied together by neighborhood allegiance is a phenomenon distinct from violence involving more highly organized institutional gangs or networks that exist for the purpose of marketing narcotics.

The hypothesis that the increasing rates of gang-related homicide result from an increasing gang involvement in narcotics trafficking presupposes that gang involvement in narcotics trafficking has actually increased. There is evidence, however, that this is not the case. A 1988 study by Klein et al[9] did not show a relationship between the dramatic increase in crack cocaine sales in Los Angeles during 1983 to 1985 and gang involvement in cocaine distribution. Fagan[10] interviewed 151 gang members younger than 21 years from three inner-city, high-crime neighborhoods, including south central Los Angeles. He concluded that illicit drug use and violence were widespread among gangs but that serious drug use and dealing by individual gang members occurred regardless of the prevalence of drug dealing within the individual's particular gang. He also concluded that drug use and sales by gang members did not necessarily increase the frequency or severity of violent behavior.

Each of the four data sources we used in our analysis has certain limitations. We were concerned, for instance, that in an atmosphere of heightened concern about gang violence there might be a bias in the LAPD database toward coding homicides involving gang members as gang-motivated or gang-involved without noting the roles of narcotics or other factors. It is also possible that police may purposely downplay the role of narcotics in a homicide to avoid the introduction of mental impairment as a defense in court proceedings. Our own review of police investigation files for a subset of homicides (those occurring in south central Los Angeles and involving victims aged 11 to 19 years) helps validate the data obtained from the LAPD database; however, since the findings were similar, we cannot completely rule out such misclassification bias. We compared gang classification within the LAPD database with an independent classification provided by the gang investigation unit of the LAPD and found reasonably good agreement, and past research has provided evidence of the validity of gang involvement in homicides by the LAPD.[6] Thus, misclassification bias of gang status is unlikely. In the future, researchers who evaluate existing police data may benefit from using court records or other sources of information to check further for misclassification bias.

We were able to obtain whole blood cocaine levels on a large, representative sample of homicide victims for 1987. The hypothesized association between illicit drug use and participation in violence would clearly be better tested by using data on drug use by all crime participants, including perpetrators. Unfortunately, existing data sources did not permit us to analyze the drug use of perpetrators.

Our finding that little or no association existed between narcotics-related arrests and gang-motivated homicide victimization further supports our conclusion that gang conflicts that result in a homicide are often independent of narcotics use and trafficking. Two limitations to this part of the analysis should be noted, however. First, we used the victims' history of narcotics arrests as a marker for their involvement in narcotics use or trafficking, and an arrest history may be an insensitive measure of such involvement. Second, the power of our analysis to detect a difference is limited by the small number of homicides that we studied. A separate, larger-scale study would be useful for confirming or refuting our findings.

Despite these limitations, we believe that the consistency of our findings across these different data sets strongly suggests that if gang activity and narcotics trafficking (or use) do interact to increase the risk of homicide, this interaction does not account for a large proportion of homicides (ie, the attributable risk percent is small). In light of this, we recommend that gang activity and narcotics trafficking or use be addressed as separate, important risk factors for homicide rather than as interrelated cofactors.

References

1. McAllister D, Speckart G. Current trends and patterns of drug abuse in Los Angeles County, California 1984-1986. In: *Patterns and Trends of Drug Abuse in the United States and Europe*. Rockville, Md: National Institute on Drug Abuse; 1987;2:88-113.
2. Budd RD. Cocaine abuse and violent death. *Am J Drug Alcohol Abuse*. 1989;15:375-382.
3. Klein MW, Maxson CL. Street gang violence. In: Weiner NA, Wolfgang ME, eds. *Violent Crime, Violent Criminals*. Newbury Park, Calif: Sage Publications; 1989:198-234.
4. California Council on Criminal Justice. *Task Force Report on Gangs and Drugs*. Sacramento: Calif Council on Criminal Justice; 1989.
5. Goldstein PJ. Drugs and violent crime. In: Weiner NA, Wolfgang ME, eds. *Pathways to Criminal Violence*. Newbury Park, Calif: Sage Publications; 1989:16-48.
6. Klein MW, Gordon MA, Maxson CL. The impact of police investigations on police-reported rates of gang and nongang homicides. *Criminology*. 1986;24:489-511.
7. Clark CS. Youth gangs. *Congressional Q Res*. 1991;22:755-771.
8. Skolnick JH, Correl T, Navarro E, Rabb R. The social structure of street drug dealing. In: *BCS Forum: The Social Structure of Street Drug Dealing*. Berkeley, Calif: University of California; 1989.
9. Klein MW, Maxson CL, Cunningham L. *Gang Involvement in Cocaine Rock Trafficking: Final Report to the National Institute on Justice*. Los Angeles, Calif: University of Southern California; 1988.
10. Fagan J. The social organization of drug use and drug dealing among urban gangs. *Criminology*. 1989;27:633-665.

The Diagnosis of Child Sexual Abuse

Howard Dubowitz, MD; Maureen Black, PhD; Donna Harrington, PhD

• ***Objective.*—To examine how the history, psychological evaluation, medical examination, and child's response to the examination contributed to a diagnosis of child sexual abuse by an interdisciplinary team.**

***Design.*—Patient series.**

***Setting.*—Subspecialty clinic for evaluating prepubertal children alleged to have been sexually abused.**

***Participants.*—One hundred thirty-two children alleged to have been sexually abused and their parents or guardian, evaluated consecutively in a subspecialty clinic between September 1989 and June 1990.**

***Measurements/Main Results.*—A social worker interviewed the parents, a psychologist interviewed the child, and a pediatrician obtained a medical history and examined the child. Parents completed a Child Behavior Check list and the child's response to the physical examination was noted. Both a disclosure by the child and abnormal physical findings were significantly and independently associated with the team's diagnosis of sexual abuse, whereas the presence of sexualized behavior, somatic problems, and the child's response to the examination did not make an additional contribution to the diagnosis.**

***Conclusions.*—The findings support the need for a skilled psychological interview and a medical examination of a child alleged to have been sexually abused to make the diagnosis of sexual abuse. An interdisciplinary team appears to be a valuable approach for evaluating these children and their families.**

(*AJDC.* 1992;146:688-693)

The determination of whether a child has been sexually abused can be very difficult, and the consequences may be substantial. If child sexual abuse is not identified, there is a risk of continued abuse and serious sequelae. In contrast, if sexual abuse is erroneously diagnosed, the ramifications for the child, family, and alleged perpetrator might be very damaging. Pediatricians and other clinicians are therefore faced with a formidable challenge to make an accurate diagnosis when confronted with the possibility of sexual abuse.

The diagnosis of child sexual abuse is difficult for several reasons. There is often little or no clear history of abuse. Sexual abuse is usually committed secretly and incidents are rarely witnessed. Young children with limited verbal skills might be unable to describe their experience or their account might be questionable.[1] Even when it appears that children are describing abuse, doubts might persist about the veracity of their statements, particularly in the context of an acrimonious custody dispute.[2-4] As a result, there has been considerable controversy concerning the testimony of children as witnesses in legal proceedings.[5-8] Since many children may be unable or unwilling to discuss their abuse, anatomically detailed dolls have become a widely used adjunct to the clinical interview.[9,10] Through projective techniques children may disclose events they are unable to reveal verbally. Despite problems associated with children's disclosure, experts in the field of child maltreatment agree that the history obtained from the child is usually the most important evidence in diagnosing sexual abuse.[11]

Various behavior problems have been associated with child sexual abuse and may be useful diagnostically.[12-14] Inappropriately sexualized behavior appears to be strongly associated with a history of abuse.[12-14] However, it is often not clear what constitutes abnormal sexual behavior or knowledge.[1,15] For example, at what point is the frequency of masturbation excessive? It might also be unclear what stimulus led to the sexualized behavior; exposure to X-rated movies, observing intimate behavior between parents, or actual abuse could be responsible. In addition, highly sexualized behavior is sometimes seen in children who are not thought to have been abused.[15]

Sexually abused children have also been found to have increased psychological problems, including depression, anxiety and fears, aggression, and poor self-esteem.[12-14] However, none of these problems is unique to child sexual abuse. Even if psychosomatic disorders, such as enuresis, are more common in sexually abused children,[16] they are not specific to sexual abuse and are of limited utility in diagnosing sexual abuse. However, psychological problems and psychosomatic disorders should alert pediatricians to consider the possibility of abuse.

In addition to the history of abuse and psychological problems, the third area contributing to the diagnosis of child sexual abuse is the medical evidence. Normal examination results, however, do not rule out the possibility of sexual abuse. Indeed, many abused children have

Accepted for publication March 25, 1992.

From the Division of General Pediatrics, University of Maryland School of Medicine, Baltimore.

Reprint requests to the Department of Pediatrics, University of Maryland School of Medicine, 700 W Lombard St, Baltimore, MD 21201 (Dr Dubowitz).

been found to have normal examination results.[17-19] Although some investigators have reported high rates of abnormal physical findings among sexually abused children,[20-22] methodological problems, such as a lack of comparison groups, render many of the findings difficult to interpret.

Considerable uncertainty remains in distinguishing abnormal from normal anatomy.[11,17,19] For example, several studies of the horizontal diameter of the vaginal opening in prepubertal girls have yielded discrepant results.[17-19,23-25] Other physical findings are thought to be clearly abnormal, but might not be specific to sexual abuse: erythema in the genital area is an obvious example.[17] Only a minority of sexually abused children have unequivocal physical evidence of abuse (eg, a gonorrheal vaginal discharge).

There is a consensus in the field of child maltreatment that the state of the art in assessing possible child sexual abuse is the interdisciplinary team evaluation.[11,26-28] This approach allows for the necessary integration of the social, psychological, and medical evidence in a comprehensive assessment, and avoids relying on any single aspect of the evaluation. The interdisciplinary team still rests on the expertise of its members, and the collective misinterpretation of information remains a risk. Nevertheless, the interdisciplinary evaluation is a theoretically sound approach to the diagnosis of sexual abuse, as well as to other forms of child maltreatment.

Despite the approval of an interdisciplinary approach, many children alleged to have been sexually abused do not appear to have received an interdisciplinary evaluation. Child protective services generally have limited access to mental health and pediatric providers with expertise in the area of sexual abuse. In addition, there frequently is a reliance on the medical examination, particularly by the law enforcement and judicial systems, while the value of other relevant information might be considered less seriously. It is noteworthy, however, that there have not been any studies, to our knowledge, of how information is integrated in the interdisciplinary process.

The primary goal of the present study was to examine how the history, psychological evaluation, medical examination, and child's response to the examination contributed to a diagnosis of child sexual abuse by an interdisciplinary team.

SUBJECTS AND METHODS

Sample

The sample consisted of 132 children who were referred to an interdisciplinary outpatient clinic for evaluation of possible sexual abuse. All children seen consecutively between September 1989 and June 1990 were eligible for the study. Only one parent refused to participate. The clinic is based in an urban teaching hospital serving a low-income, inner-city, and largely minority population. All children younger than age 12 years seen in the pediatric emergency department or one of the affiliated primary care clinics with a suspicion of sexual abuse are routinely referred to the clinic for evaluation. Thirty-one percent of referrals were made from the above sources, 52% from child protective services, 3% by the police, and 14% from other sources. The children were seen several weeks following an allegation of possible sexual abuse. The case histories varied markedly, ranging from rather vague suspicions to witnessed incidents of intercourse. The referrals were screened by a nurse and all cases met the criterion of possible sexual abuse.

The Clinic

The clinic was established at the University of Maryland Hospital, Baltimore, in 1983 and the team consists of a pediatrician, child psychologist, social worker, and nurse. Background information is obtained from the referring party. The assessment is conducted in one afternoon and consists of a social worker's interview of the parent(s) or guardian, a psychological assessment of the child, and a medical evaluation. The team considers all the available information and a decision is reached about the likelihood of sexual abuse. Any inappropriate sexual contact (excluding voluntary sexual activity between peers that appears to be within the normal range for the children's age) is considered abuse, regardless of the alleged perpetrator's age or relationship to the child. The conclusions from the evaluation are communicated to the family, along with specific recommendations for appropriate interventions.

Procedure

The interdisciplinary team evaluated all the children seen in the clinic, and the data were gathered prospectively. The social work assessment included a history of the alleged abuse, the family's response to the allegation, the involvement of public agencies, and sources of support to the family. In addition, the social worker assessed the functioning of the family, parental concerns regarding the child, and access to services. During the psychological assessment, the child's emotional and developmental status were evaluated, along with the child's account of the alleged abuse. Anatomically detailed dolls were used, depending on the clinical situation. The child's sense of safety and available support were also addressed.

Following obtainment of a medical history, a brief general examination was performed by a pediatrician. The genital examinations were done in the supine frog-leg position using a halogen lamp without magnification. The anal region was examined in the supine or prone knee-chest or lateral decubitus position. Physical characteristics of the genitalia were recorded on a precoded form, following the descriptions used by Emans et al[17]; neither a colposcope nor otoscope was used in the examination. The maximum transverse diameter of the hymenal opening was measured relative to the known width of the examiner's index finger. The pediatrician rated on five-point Likert scales the response of the child to both the general and genital examination, following efforts to allay anxiety concerning the examination.

Psychosomatic Problems and Sexualized Behavior

Problem behaviors were assessed using the Child Behavior Check list (CBCL),[29] completed by each child's parent or guardian (N = 132). The CBCL is a standardized screening instrument for assessing a child's behavior. It consists of 118 items that yield scores on different scales, including psychosomatic and sexual problems. A score greater than 70 is expected among approximately 2% of children in a random sample and corresponds to a problem in the clinical range.[29]

Abuse Severity Index

To examine how the severity of the abuse might influence the team assessment, the following three variables pertaining to the alleged abuse were combined in a scale: the nature of the abuse, the relationship of the perpetrator to the child, and the proximity of the perpetrator's residence to the child. Each of these variables was rated on a three-point scale, with the most harmful characteristics (ie, intercourse, abuse by a parent, and abuse by someone living in the home) scored as a 3; a total score of 9 represented the most severe abuse. These variables were selected based on previous research suggesting that more intrusive abuse (eg, intercourse compared with fondling), abuse by someone closely related to the child, and abuse by someone living in the child's home are particularly harmful to the child.[12,30,31] Other variables of interest, such as the frequency of the abuse or the use of force, were excluded because that information was often unavailable.

Table 1.—Characteristics of Alleged Perpetrators

Characteristic	No. (%) of Subjects (n=89)
Sex	
Male	66 (74)
Female	4 (4)
Unknown	19 (21)
Age, y	
<12	9 (10)
12-19	24 (27)
20-60	33 (37)
>60	1 (1)
Unknown	22 (25)
Relationship to child	
Biological parent	9 (10)
Stepparent	5 (6)
Sibling	6 (7)
Other family member	14 (16)
Friend/neighbor	28 (31)
Sitter	7 (8)
Stranger	1 (1)
Unknown	19 (21)
Residence	
Same home	28 (31)
Elsewhere, visits	18 (20)
Other	21 (24)
Unknown	22 (25)

Table 2.—Characteristics of the Abuse

Characteristic	No. (%) of Subjects (n=89)
Type of abuse*	
Genital-genital	20 (22)
Oral-genital	11 (12)
Digital-genital	16 (18)
Fondling	20 (22)
Other	3 (3)
Unknown	31 (35)
Frequency of abuse	
Once	28 (31)
Occasionally	14 (16)
Frequently	7 (8)
Unknown	40 (45)
Location of abuse	
Child's home	31 (35)
Perpetrator's home	20 (22)
Friend's home	4 (4)
Public	8 (9)
Unknown	26 (29)

*More than one type of abuse might have occurred.

RESULTS

The mean (SD) age of the 132 children was 6.0 (3.0) years; 83% were girls and 63% were black. At the time of the clinic evaluation, 74% were living with their mother, 11% were living with both parents, 11% were living with their extended family, 2% were living with their father, and 2% were in foster care.

Based on all the available information, the likelihood of abuse was rated by the team as "low" in 30% of the 132 children (no substantial psychosocial or physical findings), "possible" in 12% (suggestive psychosocial evidence without physical findings), "moderate" in 5% (suggestive psychosocial evidence and physical findings compatible with, but not necessarily indicative of, abuse), and "high" in 52% (clear disclosure by the child or physical findings indicative of abuse). In 2% of cases the team could not assess the likelihood of abuse.

The characteristics of the alleged perpetrators and of the abuse, excluding cases that were rated as having low likelihood of abuse or that were unrated, are presented in Tables 1 and 2, respectively. A perpetrator was identified in 78% of these cases. Most of the alleged perpetrators were male, nearly one third of them lived in the same house as the child, more than one third were family members, and more than one third were younger than age 20 years.

Most of the abuse involved genital contact, although almost a quarter of the children were fondled over their clothes. Some children were subjected to more than one form of abuse. In one third of cases, the abuse was alleged to have been a single incident, and to have occurred in the child's home. Quite often, the specific details of the alleged abuse were not available, even when it seemed likely that the child had been abused.

Fourteen percent of the children scored in the clinical range (ie, a score >70) on the CBCL for somatic complaints (N=132), and 23% did so for sexual problems (n=71). Since the CBCL only includes a sexual problems score for boys aged 4 to 5 years and girls aged 4 to 11 years, data were available on only 71 children (54%). Specific somatic complaints included aches and pains (10% of children), headaches (6%), and enuresis (14%), and one child (0.8%) was described as encopretic. Parents reported that 32% of the children masturbated "too much."

Complete information was available on 99 children. Thirty-two percent of the children gave a clear verbal disclosure of abuse, and an additional 27% provided a partial disclosure. A partial disclosure included suggestive doll play or an inconclusive account of alleged abuse. The pediatricians described 59% of the children as having normal examination results, 3% as having abnormal examination results *not* due to sexual abuse, 10% as having abnormal examination results compatible with sexual abuse (eg, a thickened hymenal edge without other signs of trauma), and 28% as having abnormal examination results indicative of sexual abuse (eg, hymenal scarring). For statistical comparisons, the children having normal examination results and those having abnormal examination results *not* due to sexual abuse were combined.

Of the 28 children who had abnormal examination results indicative of abuse, *all* were rated by the team as moderately or highly likely to have been sexually abused regardless of whether or not the child disclosed the abuse (Table 3). Of the nine children with abnormal examination results compatible with abuse, eight (89%) were rated as having moderate to high likelihood of abuse. Sixty-two children had normal physical examination findings; of these, 19 (31%) fully disclosed abuse and 18 (29%) were rated as having moderate to high likelihood of abuse. The credibility of one child's disclosure was strongly doubted. Thus, given either full disclosure *or* an examination finding indicative of abuse, the probability of a rating of moderate to high likelihood of abuse approached 100%. Alternatively, the team was unlikely to conclude a moderate or high likelihood of abuse without either physical evidence or disclosure (Fisher's Exact Test; $P=.01$). Only one (3%) of the 29 children with normal examination findings and no disclosure was rated as having moderate

Table 3.—Team Rating of Likelihood of Sexual Abuse by Disclosure and Medical Examination Results

Findings	Likelihood of Abuse No. (%) of Subjects: Low to Possible (n=36)	Moderate to High (n=63)
Normal examination findings and		
No disclosure	28 (97)	1 (3)
Partial disclosure	6 (43)	8 (57)
Full disclosure	1 (5)	18 (95)
Examination findings compatible with abuse and		
No disclosure	1 (25)	3 (75)
Partial disclosure	0	5 (100)
Full disclosure	0	0
Examination findings indicative of abuse and		
No disclosure	0	7 (100)
Partial disclosure	0	8 (100)
Full disclosure	0	13 (100)

Table 4.—Physical Findings by Pediatrician's Overall Rating of the Physical Examination in Girls

Finding*	Physician Rating of Examination Findings, No. (%) of Subjects: Normal (n=50)	Abnormal (n=32)	χ^2
Vaginal opening diameter >4 mm	24 (48)	25 (78)	7.4†
Acute trauma	0	0	NA‡
Scarring	0	17 (53)	34.7†
Adhesions	1 (2)	5 (16)	5.6§
Increased friability	1 (2)	1 (3)	0.1
Discharge	3 (6)	2 (6)	0.1
Hymen symmetrical	26 (52)	8 (25)	5.9§
Hymen discontinuity	0	10 (31)	17.8†
Hymen rounded	5 (10)	16 (50)	16.4†
Hymen bumps	8 (16)	11 (34)	3.7
Hymen clefts	7 (14)	8 (25)	1.6

*More than one finding might have been present.
†$P<.0005$.
‡NA indicates that a χ^2 could not be calculated because cell size was too small.
§$P<.05$.

to high likelihood of abuse, based on other information, such as highly inappropriate sexual behavior.

The physical findings that discriminated normal from abnormal genital examination findings for girls were analyzed using χ^2 (Table 4). Individual genital findings were first noted before making an overall assessment of the genital examination. Adhesions, hymenal scarring, asymmetry, discontinuity, and rounding were more prevalent in girls with abnormal findings. Girls with abnormal findings were more likely to have a vaginal opening with a horizontal diameter of greater than 4 mm. There was a significant moderate correlation of .40 between increased size of the opening and older age; the likelihood of abuse and age were also significantly correlated ($r=.19$; $P<.05$). However, it is important to note that, with the exception of scarring and hymenal discontinuity, all other physical findings were present in both groups of girls.

Medical data were available on 17 boys. Anal scarring was found in three boys (18%), fissures in two boys (12%), and gaping in one boy (6%) (>10 mm at the mucocutaneous junction). None of the boys had abnormalities of their genitalia or a penile discharge.

There were very similar responses by the children to both the general and genital examinations. Most of the 99 children were cooperative, 88% for the general examination and 85% for the genital examination. The child's response to the examination was not related to the pediatrician's assessment of the examination, the Abuse Severity Index, the team's rating of the likelihood of abuse, the child's behavior profile on the CBCL, or the child's disclosure of abuse. Only a history of genitourinary symptoms was correlated with greater resistance to the examination ($r=.33$; $P<.01$).

COMMENT

The major finding was that both the child's disclosure of abuse and the physical examination findings significantly contributed to the team's assessment of abuse; without either kind of evidence, the team was unlikely to conclude that the child had been abused. Less direct evidence, such as the child's behavior, was unlikely to lead to an assessment of probable abuse. However, a disclosure and physical findings were often *not* both present. In this study only 21% of the children assessed as moderately or highly likely to have been abused had fully disclosed such abuse *and* had examination results indicative of abuse. Forty-four percent of the children assessed as moderately or highly likely to have been abused had normal examination results, but had disclosed abuse. This finding supports the importance of the child interview in diagnosing the likelihood of sexual abuse.[11] The importance of the disclosure makes it necessary that evaluations of suspected sexual abuse be done by clinicians trained in eliciting sensitive information from children. The value of the child's disclosure in the evaluation of alleged abuse underscores the need for professionals involved in this field to recognize the importance of the child's account, regardless of the medical evidence.

A sizable proportion of sexually abused children, however, do not disclose their abuse, even to skilled interviewers. Furthermore, the disclosure might be unclear and not allow a firm conclusion as to the likelihood of abuse; in some instances the truthfulness might be in question. This study demonstrates the added usefulness of a medical examination for determining whether a child has been abused. Of the 63 children assessed as moderately or highly likely to have been abused, 44% had examination findings indicative of abuse. Since 25% of these children with abnormal examination findings indicative of abuse did not disclose at all and 28% partially disclosed, without the examination many of these children might not have been diagnosed as abused.

Abnormal medical examination results were almost always associated with an assessment of moderate or high likelihood of abuse. Many children reported to child protective services for sexual abuse are *not* examined physically. The present study strongly supports the need for a medical examination of all children suspected of being sexually abused. Both the child's disclosure and the examination findings contributed significantly to the team's diagnosis. However, in the presence of a clear and credible disclosure, the physical examination added little in terms of assessing the likelihood of abuse. Similarly, disclosure added little when there were examination findings indicative of abuse.

Nevertheless, it is appropriate for clinical reasons that both the child interview and examination be conducted. Aside from forensic concerns, medical and mental health problems need to be identified, and reassuring the child and parent when the examination finding is normal can be very helpful. Furthermore, a comprehensive psychosocial assessment of the child and family is needed to guide an appropriate treatment plan.

It is noteworthy that the severity of the alleged abuse, the child's age, the child's response to the examination, and the child's behavior profile, including the presence of somatic problems (eg, enuresis) and sexualized behavior, did not add significantly to the team's assessment of the likelihood of abuse. Although these factors did not contribute beyond the disclosure and/or the physical examination in shaping the team's assessment, the presence of somatic and sexual problems is important for planning treatment and may have alerted the family to the possibility of abuse.

The characteristics of the perpetrators are similar to those described in other studies, particularly when pertaining to young children.[20,22,32] For example, Kendall-Tackett and Simon[32] found that 97% of perpetrators were male, and only 1% were strangers. The relative youth of the perpetrators in the present study supports the notion that a substantial number of males who molest children begin to do so at an early age.[33] Most sexually abused children are victimized by familiar males who either live in or visit the home.

Characteristics of the abuse are also similar to findings in other studies. Prepubertal children have been found to be less likely to be penetrated vaginally compared with adolescent victims.[20] Emans et al[17] reported that 5% of the girls in their study had been vaginally penetrated. The number of abusive incidents reported varies greatly in different studies and it is likely that this information is quite unreliable, particularly when young children are involved.[17,20] Possibly, the guilt and pressures that can lead abused children to retract their disclosure might also induce them to report fewer abusive incidents. In addition, young children (eg, 4-year-olds) do not have a good understanding of concepts of time and number.

The abused children in the present study had significantly higher rates of somatic complaints and sexualized behavior compared with the normative population[29] and a local comparison group of nonabused children, matched on age and gender.[34] Other research on sexually abused children has also found an increased prevalence of somatic and sexualized behavior as well as an array of psychological problems.[12,13,16,35] Lusk and Waterman[13] suggest that the sexualized behavior may be due to a lack of inhibition of sexual impulses or a way of dealing with the abuse. The somatic complaints may be rooted in the anxiety and fear that many sexually abused children experience.[12-14] It is important to note that with the probable exception of sexualized behavior, the somatic symptoms and other behavior problems are not specific to sexual abuse.

The physical findings in this study are supportive of other research in which definitive medical evidence of abuse is lacking in many cases.[17,18] Forty-three percent of the 63 children assessed as moderately or highly likely to have been abused had normal examination findings. There is a need to consider the complete genital examination rather than rely on individual findings, such as the diameter of the vaginal opening. Of the 32 girls with abnormal examination findings, 78% had a vaginal opening larger than 4 mm, and of the 50 girls with normal examination findings, 48% had a vaginal opening larger than 4 mm; 4 to 5 mm has been reported as a "normal" maximum diameter in prepubertal girls.[18,23]

Most of the children cooperated for the examination, both for the general and genital aspects. Children who have been sexually traumatized might be expected to be anxious and resistant to the genital examination; alternatively, as a result of their sexual experiences abused children might be less inhibited and resistant. We found that their response to the examination was not related to the likelihood and severity of abuse, the presence of physical findings, or their behavior profiles; only a history of genitourinary symptoms was associated with greater resistance. Possibly, children who had been symptomatic were more likely to have had genital pain and to have been examined and had cultures taken, and were therefore more resistant. Since other developmental and personality characteristics can contribute to children's responses to physical examinations, the child's response to the examination is *not* a helpful indicator of sexual abuse.

There are a few limitations to the present study. The generalizability of the findings to other sexually abused children is uncertain given the clinic's referral process. For example, it is possible that relatively ambiguous cases were more likely to be referred to the clinic by protective services. However, the clinic procedure and population are similar to many other such clinics in the United States. Since the children were not examined immediately in our clinic, we were unlikely to detect acute findings. However, information on prior evaluations was generally presented to us. In addition, there is often a delay before children disclose their abuse. Therefore, it is possible that the study findings would have been similar had the evaluations been conducted within a few days of the disclosure.

Another limitation is the use of the team's assessment as the determination of whether the child was abused. Even though the team members had considerable experience working in the area of sexual abuse, it is possible that errors in judgment were made. We cannot assume that the interdisciplinary team diagnosis of abuse is always accurate. Many cases of suspected sexual abuse are ambiguous, and a conclusive diagnosis is not always possible. However, a skilled interdisciplinary assessment is probably the optimal approach to diagnosing sexual abuse.

IMPLICATIONS

A disclosure of sexual abuse by a child and abnormal genital examination results are important determinants of the diagnosis of sexual abuse. It is therefore important that all children who are alleged to have been sexually abused be interviewed *and* examined medically by professionals trained and skilled in this area. An interdisciplinary team assessment is a useful approach for integrating the social, psychological, and medical information needed to make accurate diagnoses of child sexual abuse.

This research was supported in part by a grant from the University of Maryland, Baltimore.

We are grateful to our colleagues, Charles Shubin, MD, Yvonne Yentsch, MSW, Dee Reever, MSW, and Noreen Thomas, RN, for their assistance in this project.

References

1. Waterman J. Evaluation of young children. In: MacFarlane K, Waterman J, eds. *Sexual Abuse of Young Children.* New York, NY: The Guilford Press; 1986:16-29.
2. Paradise JE, Rostain AL, Nathanson M. Substantiation of sexual abuse charges when parents dispute custody or visitation. *Pediatrics.* 1988;81:835-839.
3. Green AH. True and false allegations of sexual abuse in child custody disputes. *J Am Acad Child Adolesc Psychiatry.* 1986;25:449-456.
4. Jones DPH, McGraw JM. Reliable and fictitious accounts of sexual abuse to children. *J Interpers Violence.* 1987;2:27-45.
5. Yates A. Should young children testify in cases of sexual abuse? *Am J Psychiatry.* 1987;7:195-205.
6. Melton G, Bulkley J, Wulkan D. Competency of children as witnesses. In: Bulkley J, ed. *Child Sexual Abuse and the Law.* Washington, DC: American Bar Association; 1985:123-129.
7. Jones DPH, Krugman RD. Case report: can a three-year-old child bear witness to her sexual assault and attempted murder? *Child Abuse Negl.* 1986;10:253-258.
8. Goodman GS, Golding JM, Helgeson US, Haith MM, Michelli J. When a child takes the stand: juror's perceptions of children's eyewitness testimony. *Law Hum Behav.* 1987;11:27-40.
9. MacFarlane K, Krebs S. Techniques for interviewing and evidence gathering. In: MacFarlane K, Waterman S, eds. *Sexual Abuse of Young Children.* New York, NY: The Guilford Press; 1987:67-100.
10. Boat BW, Everson MD. Use of anatomical dolls among professionals in sexual abuse evaluation. *Child Abuse Negl.* 1988;12:171-180.
11. De Jong AR, Finkel MA. Sexual abuse of children. *Curr Probl Pediatr.* 1990;9:495-567.
12. Browne A, Finkelhor D. Impact of child sexual abuse: a review of the research. *Psychol Bull.* 1986;99:66-77.
13. Lusk R, Waterman J. The effects of sexual abuse on children. In: MacFarlane K, Waterman J, eds. *Sexual Abuse of Young Children.* New York, NY: The Guilford Press; 1986:101-118.
14. Beitchman JH, Zucker KJ, Hood JE, da Costa GA, Akman D. A review of the short-term effects of child sexual abuse. *Child Abuse Negl.* 1991;15:537-556.
15. Friedrich WN, Grambsch P, Broughton D, Kuiper J, Beilke RL. Normative sexual behavior in children. *Pediatrics.* 1991;88:456-464.
16. Rimsza ME, Berg RA, Locke C. Sexual abuse: symptomatic and emotional reactions. *Child Abuse Neglect.* 1988;12:201-208.
17. Emans SJ, Woods E, Flagg N, Freeman A. Genital findings in sexually abused, symptomatic, and asymptomatic girls. *Pediatrics.* 1987;79:778-785.
18. Herman-Giddens ME, Frothingham TE. Prepubertal female genitalia: examination for evidence of sexual abuse. *Pediatrics.* 1987;80:203-208.
19. Muram D. Child sexual abuse: relationship between sexual acts and genital findings. *Child Abuse Negl.* 1989;13:211-216.
20. Rimza ME, Niggeman MS. Medical evaluation of sexually abused children: a review of 311 cases. *Pediatrics.* 1982;69:8-14.
21. Enos WF, Conrath TB, Beyer JC. Forensic evaluation of the sexually abused child. *Pediatrics.* 1986;78:385-398.
22. Spencer MJ, Duklee P. Sexual abuse of boys. *Pediatrics.* 1986;78:133-138.
23. Cantwell H. Vaginal inspection as it relates to child sexual abuse in girls under thirteen. *Child Abuse Negl.* 1981;7:171-176.
24. White ST, Ingram DL, Lyna PR. Vaginal introital diameter in the evaluation of sexual abuse. *Child Abuse Negl.* 1989;13:217-224.
25. Clayton RN, Barth KL, Shubin CI. Evaluating child sexual abuse. *Clin Pediatr.* 1989;28:419-422.
26. Krugman R. Recognition of sexual abuse in children. *Pediatr Rev.* 1986;8:25-30.
27. Newberger EH, Hagenbach JJ, Ebeling NB, Colligan EP, Sheehan JS, McVeigh SH. Reducing the literal and human cost of child abuse: impact of a new hospital management system. *Pediatrics.* 1973;51:840-848.
28. Hochstadt N, Harwick N. How effective is the multi-disciplinary approach? a follow-up study. *Child Abuse Negl.* 1985;9:365-372.
29. Achenbach TM, Edelbrock C. *Manual for the Child Behavior Checklist.* Burlington, Vt: University of Vermont; 1983.
30. Mrazek PB, Mrazek DA. The effects of child sexual abuse: methodological considerations. In: Kempe CH, Mrazek PB, eds. *Sexually Abused Children and Their Families.* Elmsford, NY: Pergamon Press Inc; 1981:235-245.
31. Friedrich WN, Urquiza AJ, Beilke R. Behavior problems in sexually abused young children. *J Pediatr Psychol.* 1986;11:37-57.
32. Kendall-Tackett KA, Simon AS. Perpetrators and their acts. *Child Abuse Negl.* 1987;11:237-245.
33. Marshall WL, Barbaree HE, Eccles A. Early onset and deviant sexuality in child molesters. *J Interpers Violence.* 1991;6:323-336.
34. Dubowitz H, Black M, Harrington D, Verschoore A. A follow-up study of behavior problems associated with child sexual abuse. Presented at the 32nd Annual Meeting of the Ambulatory Pediatric Association; May 5, 1992; Baltimore, Md.
35. Einbender AJ, Friedrich WN. Psychological functioning and behavior of sexually abused girls. *J Consult Clin Psychol.* 1989;57:155-157.

Evaluation of Sexually Abused and Nonabused Young Girls for Intravaginal Human Papillomavirus Infection

Laura T. Gutman, MD; Karen St. Claire, MD; Marcia E. Herman-Giddens, PA, MPH; William W. Johnston, MD; William C. Phelps, PhD

• *Objective.*—The objective of this study was to compare the prevalence of intravaginal human papillomavirus-associated disease in two groups of girls to develop information regarding the means of transmission of anal-genital human papillomavirus disease.

***Design.*—A pair of parallel studies of prevalences of human papillomavirus infections in two populations of prospectively enrolled girls.**

***Patients.*—Index patients consisted of 15 consecutive girls aged 11 years or younger who were confirmed to have been sexually abused, had signs or symptoms of vaginal disease, and required generalized anesthesia for evaluation. Selection of nonabused control patients was based on negative findings from screening evaluations and physical examinations.**

***Main Outcome Measures.*—Prevalences of cervical-vaginal human papillomavirus infections in the two populations were compared. Vaginal wash samples from index and control patients were assayed for human papillomavirus 1, 2, 4, 6, 11, and 16 by reverse-blot and Southern transfer hybridization methods. Papanicolaou smears were examined from index patients.**

***Results.*—Vaginal wash samples from five (33%) of 15 index patients were positive for human papillomavirus 6, 11, or 16, compared with none of 17 controls. The presence or absence of external anal-genital warts was not correlated with results from the assay of intravaginal samples. Blinded readings of vaginal exfoliative cytologic findings of the index patients showed koilocytosis, atypia, or inflammatory reactions in four of five human papillomavirus-positive girls, and normal cytologic findings in one human papillomavirus-positive girl.**

***Conclusion.*—These findings support other studies that indicate that sexual contact is a major route in the transmission of anal-genital human papillomavirus-related disease in children. Evaluation of intravaginal specimens was required to identify human papillomavirus-infected girls since the results of the wash samples were not correlated with the presence or absence of external anal-genital warts.**

(*AJDC*. 1992;146:694-699)

A substantial body of epidemiologic data indicates that human papillomavirus (HPV)–related diseases of the adult genital tract are transmitted primarily through sexual contact.[1] In contrast, there have been conflicting reports about the means of transmission of anal-genital warts to postneonatal children. The major area of uncertainty is whether the primary mode of transmission of genital warts to children is similar to that in adults, ie, sexual contact. This question has been studied primarily through the assessment of children who have been identified as having genital warts and were evaluated for possible sexual abuse. However, the methods of evaluating for sexual abuse have varied greatly, and, thus, reported rates of confirmed child sexual abuse in children with anal-genital warts have ranged from 0% to 91%.[2,3] Evaluation of abused girls for intravaginal HPV-related infection has not been recommended, and no data on the prevalence of intravaginal HPV infection in children have been published.

The intravaginal microbiologic findings of nonabused young girls have not been well characterized because of the social and technical limitations in acquiring samples. Prevalence studies in defined populations represent a means of investigating the relationship between sexual abuse and anal-genital HPV infection in children. However, because of the limitations on sample collection, studies to identify intravaginal HPV infection in either sexually abused girls or nonabused girls have not been reported.

The present study documents the prevalence of a selected number of HPV types from vaginal wash samples of two groups of young girls whose status regarding sexual abuse was fully characterized. The first group comprised girls who had been victims of invasive child sexual abuse, while girls in the second group had not been sexually abused. This study differs in two respects from others that have examined the means of transmission of anal-genital HPV disease in children. In this study, two

Accepted for publication March 25, 1992.

From the Departments of Pediatrics (Drs Gutman and St. Claire and Ms Herman-Giddens) and Pathology (Dr Johnston), Duke University Medical Center, Durham, NC, and the Burroughs-Wellcome Research Laboratories, Research Triangle Park, NC (Drs Gutman and Phelps).

Presented in part at the 1991 Papillomavirus Workshop, Seattle, Wash, July 23, 1991, and at the joint plenary session for the 31st Interscience Conference on Antimicrobial Agents and Chemotherapy and the Infectious Diseases Society of America, Chicago, Ill, September 30, 1991.

Reprint requests to Box 3971, Duke University Medical Center, Durham, NC 27710 (Dr Gutman).

populations of girls were compared, and the study focused on the diagnosis of intravaginal HPV disease as manifested by HPV, DNA, and cytologic findings, rather than on external genital warts.

SUBJECTS AND METHODS

Selection of Index Patients

The Duke Child Protection Team examines approximately 250 girls per year for suspected child sexual abuse, and abuse is confirmed in about 40% of examined girls. The index population comprised 15 girls aged 11 years or younger who were Tanner stage 1 or 2 in sexual development and who had been referred to the Duke Child Protection Team for evaluation of suspected child sexual abuse. The index population included all girls from a 4½-year period beginning in 1986 who fulfilled the following criteria: (1) The Child Protection Team completed the evaluation for suspected child sexual abuse. (2) The girls had a history of symptomatic vaginal disease (ie, discharge, bleeding, or pain) that required a medical examination. (3) Generalized anesthesia was used because the girls were unable to tolerate the examination while awake. (4) The girls were confirmed to have been abused by the Child Protection Team. Examinations using anesthesia were indicated when there were persistent medical signs or symptoms and the child could not tolerate the examination while awake. Index patients were referred for an examination with anesthesia for evaluation of acute injury and/or recurrent or chronic symptomatic vaginal disease manifested as bleeding, discharge, pain, or lesions (Table 1).

Table 1.—Genital Signs and Symptoms of Index Patients (n=15)

	No. of Patients
Presenting complaints	
Vaginal discharge	
Chronic or recurrent	7
Acute	2
Vaginal bleeding	5
Labial abrasions	3
Perivaginal lesions	
Perivaginal condyloma acuminatum	3
Perivaginal molluscum contagiosum	1
Perianal lesions	1
Additional findings during anesthesia administration	
Scars, tears, notches, or distortions of hymen	8
Hymenal opening transverse diameter ≥8 mm	10
Changing external examination results with serial evaluations	2
Abnormal external genital examination results	15

Selection of Control Patients

Control patients were recruited from the pediatric clinics at the Duke Eye Center, Durham, NC. They were girls aged 11 years or younger and Tanner stage 1 in sexual development who had been scheduled to receive ophthalmic examinations or procedures while receiving generalized anesthesia. Control patients underwent a screening assessment for sexual abuse because child sexual abuse is a common problem and nonabuse of this population could not be assumed.[4-6]

The median age of the index population was 59 months, with a range of 23 to 131 months. The median age of the control population was 34 months, with a range of 3 to 68 months (Table 2). The control population was significantly younger than the index population ($P=.006$; two-sample Wilcoxon's rank sum test). Eight (53%) of the index children were black and seven (47%) were white. Of 17 controls, six (35%) were black and 11 (65%) were white. The groups did not differ significantly in the percentage of black children ($P=.47$; Fisher's Exact Test).

Evaluation for Child Sexual Abuse

Methods used in evaluating the index patients for sexual abuse have been described[7] and follow currently recommended procedures, including parent interviews and child interviews and examinations.[8] Five groups of data were obtained: (1) a review of the behavioral history of the child, (2) a review of the medical history of the child, (3) multiple diagnostic interviews with the child, (4) a forensic medical examination, and (5) assessment for other sexually transmitted diseases. In the present study, "disclosure" refers to the detailed verbalization by the child or other witness of a specific sexually abusive act. Perpetrators were "identified" if the child or a caretaker had provided specific description of the person as an assailant.

Child sexual abuse was confirmed on the basis of any of the following: (1) the child or a witness disclosed the abuse; (2) genital gonorrhea or acquired syphilis was diagnosed; (3) the genital examination results were abnormal, with findings clearly indicative of abuse as outlined at the 1985 National Child Sexual Abuse Summit meeting and subsequently updated[9-12]; (4) serial genital examinations showed changing abnormalities that were indicative of active sexual abuse; or (5) there was acknowledgment by the perpetrator.

The following methods were used in evaluating control patients for concerns of sexual abuse. At an eye center clinic visit, the study and procedure were described to the parents and child by a member of the Child Protection Team and informed consent was obtained. An intake questionnaire was administered by one of us (K.S.C.) that included questions about each of the following medical areas: chronic illness and previous medical interventions (five questions asked); medications (two questions); genitourinary signs and symptoms (nine questions); gastrointestinal signs and symptoms (three questions); vaginal signs and symptoms (five questions); and behavioral disturbances (10 questions). Open questions were asked regarding any concerns the parents may have had concerning physical or sexual abuse. The physical examination of the external genitalia was performed at the time of administering anesthesia. The evaluation did not include a separate diagnostic interview with the child.

Table 2.—Study Populations

Characteristic	Index Patients (n=15)	Controls (n=17)	*P*
Median (range) age, mo	59 (23-131)	34 (3-68)	.006 (Wilcoxon's rank sum test)
Race, No. (%) of patients			
Black	8 (53)	6 (35)	.47 (Fisher's Exact Test)
White	7 (47)	11 (65)	
Assays positive for HPV6, 11, or 16, No. (%) of patients	5 (33)*	0	.015 (Fisher's Exact Test)

*HPV indicates human papillomavirus infection. The HPV types identified included HPV6 in two patients and HPV11, HPV 6/11, and HPV16 in one patient each.

The study protocol required that parents be informed of findings that raised concerns about possible child sexual abuse and the parents were aware that a report of suspected sexual abuse would be made should findings strongly indicate abuse. The study was approved by the Duke Institutional Review Board and written parental consent was obtained.

Physical Examination and Collection of Specimens

The external genital examination for both groups of children included inspection of the labia and introital area for redness, discharge, lesions, or injuries; identification of hymenal type and contour; and measurement of the horizontal diameter of the hymenal opening.[13] Samples obtained included vaginal swabs and washes. Intravaginal samples from index patients were obtained during direct visualization of the vagina and cervix, and cervical-vaginal Papanicolaou smears were obtained. Vaginal wash material was collected through a flexible, small-bore plastic catheter that was fitted to the end of a 10-mL syringe. The catheter was inserted through the hymenal opening, and 10 mL of Dulbecco's phosphate-buffered saline was washed in and out of the vagina two or three times. Direct intravaginal visualization was not attempted in the control children and therefore Papanicolaou smears were not obtained.

Virologic Diagnosis

Plasmid-cloned isolates of HPV1, 2, and 4 have been previously described.[14] The HPV6 probe consists of the Fnu4H1 (b. 509) fragment to the MstII (b. 4520).[15] The HPV16 consists of the full genome from a pUC18 clone derived from the prototype.[16] The HPV11/pUC18 was cloned from a patient specimen (L.T.G, unpublished data, 1991).

The HPV DNA fragments were isolated electrophoretically and labeled with ^{32}P using random oligonucleotide primers for use as probes.

HPV DNA Analysis

Cellular DNA was isolated from the pellet of vaginal wash material by overnight digestion, phenol extraction, and alcohol precipitation. The extracted DNA was digested with RNAse, extracted with phenol, and alcohol precipitated a second time. The concentration of DNA was determined with a spectrophotometer. The range of DNA extracted from samples from index patients was 630 ng to 2.25 μg and that from control patients was 315 to 630 ng. A minimum of 300 ng was required to complete the study protocol.

Reverse Southern Hybridization

Reverse Southern hybridization for HPV1, 2, 4, 6, 11, and 16 has been previously described.[17,18] Briefly, 200 ng of each of HPV types 1, 2, 4, 6, 11, and 16 was immobilized on a nylon filter. The probe consisted of 50 to 100 ng of patient DNA that was labeled with ^{32}P using random nucleotide primers. Hybridization was performed at 65°C. The sensitivity of this assay was less than or equal to 1 pg of HPV DNA in 1 μg of cellular DNA.

Table 3.—Type of Sexual Abuse Disclosed (n = 15)*

Site of Contact†		
Assailant	**Child**	**No. of Index Children**
Penis	Vagina	9
Penis	Anus	4
Penis	Mouth	2
Finger	Vagina	2
Mouth	Vagina	1

*Five children disclosed multiple types of abuse.
†The site of contact was unknown for two children.

Southern Transfer Hybridization

Two hundred nanograms of cellular DNA from each index and control patient was digested with the restriction endonuclease enzymes, *Bam*HI or *Pst* I, and analyzed with Southern transfer hybridization procedures.[19] Samples were separated by electrophoresis, transferred to nylon filter, and probed with ^{32}P-labeled HPV6/11 and HPV16. Hybridization produced a readily visible signal with less than 0.2 pg of HPV DNA per 200 ng of cellular DNA.

Cervical-Vaginal Cytologic Findings

Cervical-vaginal swabs were collected from index patients for cytologic examination. The preparations were interpreted by a single observer (W.W.J.), who was blinded to the results of the HPV assays. Descriptive observations were made and findings were categorized according to the Bethesda System.[20] Koilocytes are mature squamous cells characterized by a large perinuclear cavity with sharp borders. The cellular cytoplasm is dense and the nucleus shows varying degrees of degeneration. These cells are commonly present in HPV-infected lesions.

RESULTS

Control and Index Patients

Fifteen index patients met the criteria for entry into the study. Thirteen girls (87%) gave a full disclosure of sexual abuse and two (13%) gave a partial disclosure of sexual abuse. Thirteen girls had abnormal examination findings of the introital area or hymen that were consistent with healing or healed trauma from sexual abuse (Table 1). The 15 index patients came from 15 separate households and no index patient was related to any other patient.

Seventeen control patients underwent a behavioral, medical, and physical screening evaluation for child sexual abuse and had negative findings. A vaginal wash sample was obtained from each of these girls for evaluation for HPV. Two potential control patients were omitted from the study because of concerns of possible abuse that were identified during the screening evaluation. Both children disclosed their abuse and identified the perpetrators.

Perpetrators

Five (33%) of the index children had been assaulted by single perpetrators, four (27%) had been assaulted by multiple perpetrators, three (20%) disclosed abuse but did not identify a specific perpetrator(s), and three (20%) identified one perpetrator with at least one additional perpetrator suspected. All identified perpetrators were either related to the child or had access to the child because of a relationship with another member of the family.

The types of abuse that were disclosed by the index patients are listed in Table 3. Eleven children (73%) described penetrating penile-vaginal or penile-anal abuse, and two (13%) described digital abuse. Two children (13%) were unable to give details of their assault.

HPV DNA Assay

Vaginal wash samples from five (33%) of the 15 index patients were positive for HPV using Southern transfer hybridization. Four (80%) of these five were HPV types 6 or 11, and one was HPV type 16 (Table 2). The results of the reverse-blot assays corroborated the findings of the Southern transfer hybridization assays (Figs 1 and 2). Labeled DNA from index patients did not hybridize with HPV1, 2, or 4 on reverse blots. The prevalences of HPV

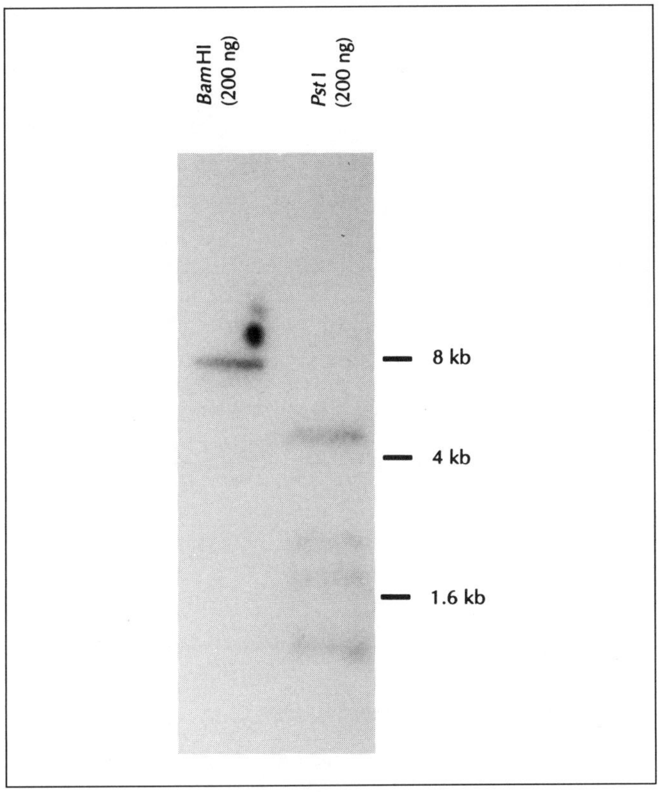

Fig 1.—*Restriction endonuclease digestion results from a cervical-vaginal wash specimen.* Bam*HI and* Pst *I demonstrated fragments characteristic of HPV6a.*

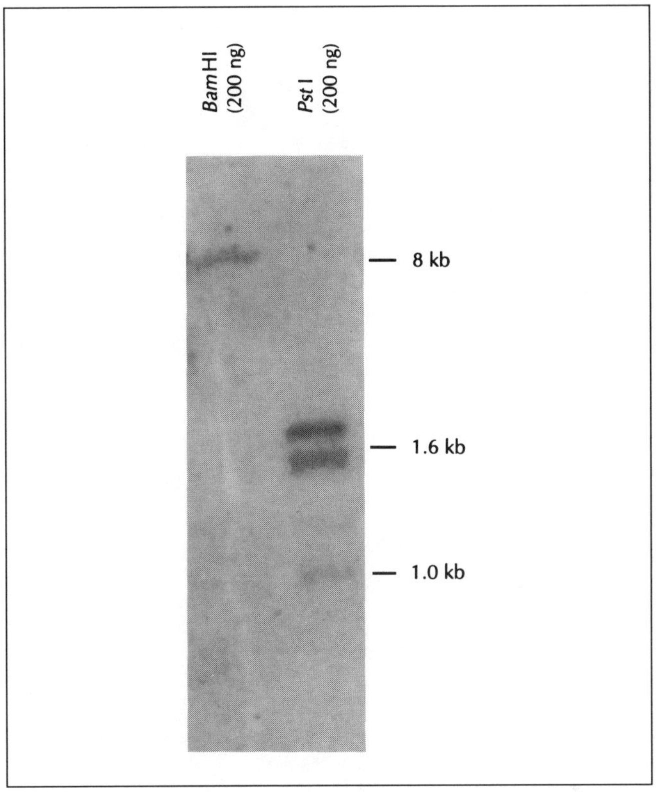

Fig 2.—*Restriction endonuclease digestion results from a cervical-vaginal wash specimen.* Bam*HI and* Pst *I demonstrated fragments characteristic of HPV11.*

DNA from the two study populations, 0 of 17 controls vs five of 15 index cases, differed significantly ($P = .015$) using Fisher's Exact Test. The 95% confidence interval for HPV positivity in the index population was 9% to 57%.

External Genital Warts

The relationship between the presence or absence of external genital lesions and intravaginal infection is shown in Table 4. Four of the index patients had clinically evident external anal-genital warts, one in the perianal area and three in the perivaginal area. Two girls also had an intravaginal specimen that was HPV positive and two did not. Three (60%) of the five girls who had HPV-positive intravaginal specimens did not have identifiable external genital warts. Biopsy material of external lesions from one patient was examined for HPV DNA, and both wash and biopsy results showed HPV6a.

Table 4.—Relationship Between Presence or Absence of External Genital Lesions and Positive or Negative Assay Results From Intravaginal Wash Samples For Index Patients With Human Papillomavirus (HPV) Infection

	Vaginal Wash Assay Results, No. of Patients		
Clinical Evaluations	HPV DNA Positive	HPV DNA Negative	Total
External anogenital warts present			
Perianal	0	1	**1**
Perivaginal	2	1	**3**
External anogenital warts absent	3	8	**11**
Total No. of index patients	**5**	**10**	**15**

Cytologic Findings

Of the five girls with HPV-positive wash specimens, only one had cytologic findings that included koilocytosis (Fig 3). Cytologic findings from a second HPV-positive child showed a severe acute inflammatory reaction in which the parabasal cells were surrounded by a dense aggregation of polymorphonuclear leukocytes. The nuclei of parabasal cells showed atypia with darkening of the nuclear chromatin, thickening of the nuclear envelope, and increased nuclear to cytoplasmic ratio. For the third child, cytologic findings were restricted to chronic inflammatory reactions showing lymphocytic and monocytic cellular predominance and relatively fewer parabasal cells. Cytologic findings for the fourth child included a severe acute inflammatory reaction with a predominance of polymorphonuclear leukocytes and parabasal cells that showed mild perinuclear clearing but not overt koilocytosis. The fifth child had normal cytologic findings, without evidence of inflammatory reaction, atypia, or koilocytosis.

Cytologic examinations from the 10 index girls who had negative HPV DNA vaginal washes showed neither cellular reactions suggestive of HPV infection nor acute or chronic inflammatory reactions.

COMMENT

The index patients represent a subpopulation of sexually abused girls who were particularly symptomatic from the trauma that they had experienced and whose abuse

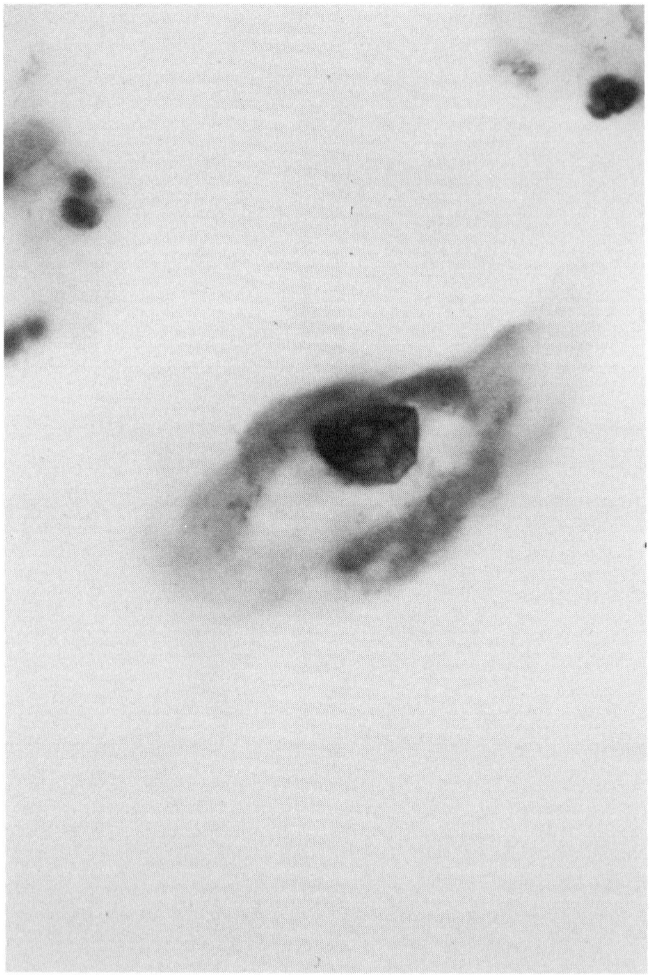

Fig 3.—*Papanicolaou smear from human papillomavirus-positive child, demonstrating koilocytic findings in squamous cell. The nucleus is marginated and condensed, the cell is enlarged, and a halo surrounds the nucleus (original magnification ×320).*

was probably unusually severe. At least four (27%) of the 15 patients had been abused by multiple perpetrators. All had signs or symptoms of intravaginal disease. Most of the types of disclosed abuse that they experienced were invasive. The 33% rate of recovery of HPV DNA from patient samples is similar to the recovery rate of HPV from a sexually at-risk adult population that was studied using a dot-blot hybridization method.[21]

Using the Southern transfer hybridization method, the recovery rate of HPV DNA from index cases was slightly higher than the 15% rate of recovery from another at-risk adult population.[22] Results from the HPV assays of the index children therefore closely resemble results from adults who are highly sexually active. Even so, the 33% prevalence rate of HPV from the index population is expected to be an underrepresentation of the true prevalence of this infection in children who have been severely abused because sample sizes were small, assays for only six HPV types were performed, and only a single sample was taken from each child.

In adults, the primary means of transmission of HPV-related genital disease is through sexual contact. Evidence of sexual transmission in adults comes from studies of couples; 90% of new sexual contacts of persons with genital warts result in the development of genital lesions.[23] In other studies, more than 60% of adults in established relationships with partners who have genital warts were concordant for the presence of lesions.[24,25] Similar data for child victims of sexual abuse are not available because, in these cases, perpetrators identified by children are rarely charged with the offense. This effectively prohibits any evaluation for sexually transmitted diseases.

Other evidence that HPV infection is sexually transmitted in adults includes data showing a relationship between prevalence of HPV infection and numbers of sexual partners. In adults, these two factors increase proportionally.[26,27] Similarly for children, a recent study has shown a significant association between the presence of multiple, other sexually associated organisms in children who have genital warts and who have been abused by multiple perpetrators.[3]

Medical literature on children with anal-genital papillomavirus disease contains conflicting information about sexual contact as the means of transmission of this infection to children. Unfortunately, many of these reports and studies were done prior to the development of currently established methods for evaluating child sexual abuse. Most of these earlier reports did not use a sexual abuse evaluation process, which must include a diagnostic interview of the child and parent by a skilled interviewer and a forensic genital examination by a qualified examiner. Rather, most of the earlier reports relied on the child to volunteer the disclosure and categorized nondisclosing children who had not received a thorough evaluation as nonabused.

Several of the more recent studies have also omitted any description of the evaluation methods and findings that they used to diagnose sexual abuse, or they have categorized children as nonabused when the child's status was inadequately documented or unknown.[2,28,29] Consequently, reported associations of sexual abuse with HPV transmission to children are likely to be inaccurately low. Despite the limitations in their diagnosis of sexual abuse, however, these earlier reports document that at least 50% of children with genital warts disclosed that they had been sexually abused.[30,31] The only published study using current diagnostic methods for child sexual abuse in girls having genital warts showed that 10 (91%) of 11 had been sexually abused. In that study disclosure of abuse was provided in 71% of cases, and in a similar study a high disclosure rate was also recorded.[3,32] Sexual abuse was confirmed in four of the five children aged 3 years or younger.[3] This strongly suggests that even in children who are preverbal or only marginally verbal the presence of genital tract lesions due to HPV is frequently associated with a confirmed diagnosis of sexual abuse.

The current study used the Southern transfer hybridization assay for several reasons. First, previous studies using this method have demonstrated that most genital papillomas of children are caused by HPV6 or 11 and only infrequently by HPV2, 16, or 18.[33,34] Other types are rarely or never identified in genital lesions of children. Consequently, our assay was designed to examine specimens for a limited number of HPV types. Second, because nonamplified DNA was measured, quantitative information was provided, and identification of the type was precise. Third, the method is the criterion standard.

In the present study, racial distribution of the index and control children did not differ significantly. The mean age of the control population, however, was significantly younger than that of the index population. The control patients were therefore closer in time to possible neonatal transmission of HPV, and they were also more likely to have difficulty in evaluations for sexual abuse due to their preverbal or poorly verbal developmental stages. These factors resulted in a conservative bias for the study.

Of particular concern for the HPV-positive children is that the long-term consequences of early exposure to this infection are unknown. Of note are reports from several medical centers about the increased incidence of genital-tract papillomavirus infections in female adolescents. Benign, dysplastic, and malignant HPV-associated lesions are also now being reported in this age range.[35-39] Because the length of time between HPV infection and progression to dysplastic and malignant stages may be quite long, some of these female adolescents may have acquired their infection prior to the legal age of consent for intercourse and through abusive sexual contact as a child.

The present data indicated that our index population of abused girls resembles populations of sexually active adults in the prevalence of intravaginal HPV DNA, in the presence of anal-genital lesions, and in cytologic findings. These children have acquired their internal genital HPV disease at very immature ages. Data regarding their prognosis and appropriate treatment are needed. Study findings also support other data that children presenting with anal-genital papillomavirus disease are at significant risk of having been abused and should be evaluated for possible sexual abuse and other sexually transmitted infections.

These studies were supported in part by a grant from the Mellon Foundation.

The authors gratefully acknowledge the active participation of Robert Machemer, MD, and Edward Buckley, MD, and the faculty and personnel of the Duke Eye Center, Durham, NC. Gerald Hajian, PhD, Burroughs-Wellcome Co, Research Triangle Park, NC, provided expert assistance with data analysis and statistical evaluation of the results, and David Barry, MD, provided editorial review. Julia Barnes, Burroughs-Wellcome Co, provided technical advice. Nancy Berson, MSW, Carmenza Salgado, PA, and Jeanne Niemeyer, MSW, Duke University Medical Center, conducted skillful interviews and examinations of index patients, and Gale Hill, PhD, Duke University, provided microbiologic support.

References

1. Koutsky LA, Galloway DA, Holmes KK. Epidemiology of genital human papillomavirus infection. *Epidemiol Rev.* 1988;10:122-163.
2. Obalek S, Jablonska S, Favre M, Walczak L, Orth G. Condylomata acuminata in children: frequent association with human papillomaviruses responsible for cutaneous warts. *J Am Acad Dermatol.* 1990;23:205-213.
3. Herman-Giddens ME, Gutman LT, Berson NL, Duke Child Protection Team. Association of coexisting vaginal infections and multiple abusers in female children with genital warts. *Sex Transm Dis.* 1988;15:63-67.
4. Russell DEH. The incidence and prevalence of intrafamilial and extrafamilial sexual abuse of female children. *Child Abuse Negl.* 1983;7:133-146.
5. Moore KA, Nord CW, Peterson JL. Nonvoluntary sexual activity among adolescents. *Fam Plann Perspect.* 1989;21:110-114.
6. Siegel JM, Sorenson SB, Golding JM, Burnam MA, Stein JA. The prevalence of childhood sexual assault: the Los Angeles Epidemiologic Catchment Area Project. *Am J Epidemiol.* 1987;126:1141-1153.
7. Gutman LT, St Clair KK, Weedy C, et al. Human immunodeficiency virus transmission by child sexual abuse. *AJDC.* 1991;145:137-141.
8. Krugman RD, Bays JA, Chadwick DL, Levitt CJ, McHugh MT, Whitworth JM. Guidelines for the evaluation of sexual abuse of children. *Pediatrics.* 1991;87:254-260.
9. Tipton AC. Child sexual abuse: physical examination techniques and interpretation of findings. *Adolesc Pediatr Gynecol.* 1989;2:10-25.
10. White ST, Ingram DL, Lyna PR. Vaginal introital diameter in the evaluation of sexual abuse. *Child Abuse Negl.* 1989;13:217-224.
11. Paradise JE. The medical evaluation of the sexually abused child. *Pediatr Clin North Am.* 1990;37:839-862.
12. Muram D. Child sexual abuse-genital tract findings in prepubertal girls, I: the unaided medical examination. *Am J Obstet Gynecol.* 1989;60:328-333.
13. McCann J, Voris J, Simon M, Wells R. Comparison of genital examination techniques in prepubertal girls. *Pediatrics.* 1990;85:182-187.
14. Heilman C, Law M-F, Israel MA, Howley PM. Cloning of human papilloma virus genomic DNAs and analysis of homologous polynucleotide sequences. *J Virol.* 1980;36:395-407.
15. Schwarz E, Durst M, Demankowski C, et al. DNA sequence and genome organization of genital human papillomavirus type 6b. *EMBO J.* 1983;2:2341-2348.
16. Durst M, Gissman L, Ikenberg H, Zur Hausen H. A papillomavirus DNA from a cervical carcinoma and its prevalence in cancer biopsy samples from different geographic regions. *Proc Natl Acad Sci U S A.* 1983;80:3812-3815.
17. deVilliers E-M, Schneider A, Gross G, zur Hausen H. Analysis of benign and malignant urogenital tumors for human papillomavirus infection by labelling cellular DNA. *Med Microbiol Immunol.* 1986; 174:281-286.
18. Webb DH, Rogers RE, Fife KH. A one-step method for detecting and typing human papillomavirus DNA in cervical scrape specimens from women with cervical dysplasia. *J Infect Dis.* 1987;156:912-919.
19. Sambrook J, Fritsch EF, Maniatis T, eds. *Molecular Cloning.* 2nd ed. Cold Spring Harbor, NY: Cold Spring Harbor Laboratory Press; 1989.
20. Solomon D. The 1988 Bethesda system for reporting cervical/vaginal cytologic diagnoses. *Anal Quant Cytol Histol.* 1989;11:291-297.
21. Burmer GC, Parker JD, Bates J, East K, Kulander BG. Comparative analysis of human papillomavirus detection by polymerase chain reaction and Virapap/Viratype kits. *Am J Clin Pathol.* 1990;94:554-560.
22. Kiviat NB, Koutsky LA, Critchlow CW, et al. Comparison of Southern transfer hybridization and dot filter hybridization for detection of cervical human papillomavirus infection with types 6, 11, 16, 18, 31, 33 and 35. *Am J Clin Pathol.* 1990;94:561-565.
23. Barrett TJ, Silbar JD. Genital warts: a venereal disease. *JAMA.* 1954;154:333-334.
24. Oriel JD. Maternal history of genital warts. *Br J Vener Dis.* 1971;47:1-13.
25. Barrasso R, DeBrux J, Croissant O, Orth G. High prevalence of papillomavirus-associated penile intraepithelial neoplasia in sexual partners of women with cervical intraepithelial neoplasia. *New Engl J Med.* 1987;317:916-923.
26. Kiviat NB, Koutsky LA, Paavonen JA, et al. Prevalence of genital papillomavirus infection in women attending a college student health clinic or a sexually transmitted disease clinic. *J Infect Dis.* 1989;159:293-302.
27. Syrjanen K, Vayrynen M, Castren O, et al. Sexual behavior of women with human papillomavirus (HPV) lesions by the uterine cervix. *Br J Vener Dis.* 1984;60:243-248.
28. Cohen BA, Honig P, Androphy E. Anogenital warts in children: clinical and virologic evaluation for sexual abuse. *Arch Dermatol.* 1990;126:1575-1580.
29. Padel AF, Venning VA, Evans MF, Quantrill AM, Fleming KA. Human papillomaviruses in anogenital warts in children: typing by in situ hybridization. *Br Med J.* 1990;300:1491-1494.
30. DeJong AR, Weiss JC, Brent RL. Condyloma acuminata in children. *AJDC.* 1982;136:704-706.
31. Shelton TB, Jerkins GR, Noe HN. Condylomata acuminata in the pediatric patient. *J Urol.* 1986;135:548-549.
32. Gilles EE, Hitchcock BS, Elvik SL. Human papilloma virus in children. Ninth National Conference on Child Abuse and Neglect; September 14-17, 1991; Denver, Colo. Abstract B.1, 55.
33. Rock B, Naghashfar E, Barnett N, Buscema J, Woodruff SD, Shah K. Genital tract papillomavirus infection in children. *Arch Dermatol.* 1986;122:1129-1132.
34. Gibson PE, Gardner SD, Best SJ. Human papillomavirus types in anogenital warts of children. *J Med Virol.* 1990;30:142-145.
35. Martinez J, Smith R, Farmer M, et al. High prevalence of genital tract papillomavirus infection in female adolescents. *Pediatrics.* 1988; 82:604-608.
36. Rosenfeld WD, Vermund SH, Wentz ST, Burk RD. High prevalence rate of human papillomavirus infection and association with abnormal Papanicolaou smears in sexually active adolescents. *AJDC.* 1989;143:1443-1447.
37. Hillard PJA, Biro FM, Wildey LS, Bradley JM, Burket RL, Rauh JL. Cervical dysplasia and human papillomavirus: evaluation in an adolescent dysplasia clinic. *Adolesc Pediatr Gynecol.* 1989;2:32-36.
38. Piver MS, Baker TR. Cervical cancer in the adolescent patient. *Pediatr Ann.* 1986;15:536-541.
39. Moscicki A-B, Palefsky J, Gonzales J, Schoolnik GK. Human papillomavirus infection in sexually active females: prevalence and risk factors. *Pediatr Res.* 1990;28:507-513.

Sexual Abuse of Children

The Detection of Semen on Skin

Tina Gabby, MD, MPH; Marilyn A. Winkleby, PhD; W. Thomas Boyce, MD; Deborah L. Fisher, MPH; Allison Lancaster; George F. Sensabaugh, D Crim

• *Objective.*—The detection of semen on the skin of children who present within 72 hours of an episode of sexual assault is critical to medical, forensic, and legal personnel. The Wood's Lamp, a UV light that causes semen to fluoresce, and four forensic laboratory techniques were compared to determine their sensitivity and decline in sensitivity over time.

Design.—A descriptive study.

Participants.—Eleven adult female volunteers.

Measurements/Main Results.—Semen was placed on the skin of the volunteers. Samples of the dried semen were assessed during a 28-hour period with the Wood's Lamp, microscopy, the acid phosphatase assay, and two assays for the prostatic protein p30 (counterimmunoelectrophoresis and enzyme-linked immunosorbent assay). The intensity of the Wood's Lamp fluorescence of semen diminished dramatically by 28 hours; in contrast, the fluorescence of urine persisted up to 80 hours. Over time, the p30–enzyme-linked immunosorbent assay technique was more sensitive than microscopy, the acid phosphatase assay, and p30-counterimmunoelectrophoresis in detecting semen on skin.

Conclusions.—The Wood's Lamp is not a sensitive screening tool and should be used with caution. To improve the detection of sexual abuse in children, we recommend that the p30–enzyme-linked immunosorbent assay be used because of its potential as a more sensitive assay than those in current clinical use.

(*AJDC*. 1992;146:700-703)

National incidence studies reveal that approximately 1% of all children will experience some form of sexual abuse in a given year.[1] It is estimated that 45% of child sexual assault cases involve acts of molestation with genital contact without penile penetration.[1] Ejaculation may occur in these cases, making the presence of semen on a child's skin diagnostically important. Unfortunately, sensitivities of the routine screening and diagnostic tests for detecting semen on skin are unknown. These tests are used in acute cases of sexual abuse, cases seen within 72 hours of an alleged assault, and are not considered to be of value after that time.

Because children often present to a medical examiner days after an episode of sexual abuse, it is important to know how increasing time affects the results of these tests.[2] It is critical that clinicians and forensic scientists, understand the limitations of the diagnostic and screening tests used during the examination of the sexually abused child. This study was conducted to evaluate the sensitivity and specificity of the Wood's Lamp (WL) and the sensitivities of four diagnostic techniques used to identify semen on a victim's skin.

The WL, a screening tool used within 72 hours of an assault, creates a UV illumination that detects semen fluorescence.[3] Detection of semen fluorescence is especially helpful in cases in which a young child's ability to give a history of sexual assault may be limited. Wood's Lamp fluorescence is not specific to semen since many other substances that may be found on skin have fluorescent properties. Despite its widespread availability and simplicity, the WL technique is not standardized, and there have been no studies to date regarding its specificity or sensitivity over time. Typically, when a fluorescent area is visualized during the examination of an abused child, a swab or scraping of the area is obtained.[4] The swab is further analyzed for semen by forensic analyses.

Three forensic techniques commonly used in the analyses of semen evidence were concurrently examined in this study: (1) sperm detection by microscopy, (2) the assay for acid phosphatase (ACP), and (3) the detection of the prostate-specific protein, p30, by counterimmunoelectrophoresis (CIE). A fourth technique, the detection of p30 by an enzyme-linked immunosorbent assay (ELISA), was also examined. These tests vary in their sensitivity and specificity. Detection of spermatozoa by microscopy is considered diagnostically specific for sexual contact.[5] Acid phosphatase is less specific since it is present in the vaginal fluid and urine of women, albeit at much lower levels than in semen.[6,7] It is not known if ACP is present in the vaginal fluid or urine of prepubescent girls; it is present at very low levels in the urine of prepubescent boys.[8] Negative ACP test results have no diagnostic value since they do not necessarily indicate the absence of semen.[9] Prostate-specific protein, p30 (also called prostate-specific antigen), is found in seminal fluid and urine of men, and under normal circumstances is absent from all other body fluids in males and from all tissues and body fluids in females.[10,11] The p30-ELISA test is approximately 100 times more sensitive than the ACP or p30-CIE tests. Although these semen markers have been studied in

Accepted for publication January 3, 1992.

From the Division of Behavioral and Developmental Pediatrics, University of California, San Francisco (Drs Gabby, Winkleby, and Boyce) and the Forensic Science Group, School of Public Health, University of California, Berkeley (Mss Fisher and Lancaster and Dr Sensabaugh).

Presented at the Maternal and Child Health Bureau–sponsored Annual Meeting of Behavioral Pediatric Training Programs, San Francisco, Calif, April 12, 1991.

Reprints not available.

postcoital vaginal samples and their specificity has been outlined, little is known about the decay in their sensitivities over time when samples are obtained from skin.

The following questions were addressed by this study: (1) How does the pattern, color, and intensity of WL fluorescence of semen change over time? (2) Do nonsemen substances, likely to be present on the skin of children referred for sexual abuse examinations, cause false-positive WL readings (thereby compromising specificity)? (3) How does the sensitivity of microscopy, ACP, and p30 techniques, analyzed from semen samples taken from the areas of WL fluorescence, change over time? (4) Can forensic tests detect semen in areas that are WL negative? Although adult subjects participated in this study, our intent was to address these questions as they specifically relate to the examination of child sexual assault victims.

SUBJECTS AND METHODS

Preliminary Testing

Preliminary testing was conducted to provide general estimates of the effects of time and body location on the WL fluorescence of semen. Since observations of semen on skin during an 80-hour period demonstrated that semen fluorescence became faint after the first 28 hours, this period was chosen for the study. There was no remarkable difference in semen fluorescence and semen analysis when semen placed on the inner thigh was compared with semen placed on the ventral forearm; therefore, the forearm was chosen for the site of study.

Preliminary testing was also conducted to identify substances that might be present in child sexual assault cases and have the potential of causing false-positive WL readings. These included infant formula, milk, cola, moisturizing lotions, petroleum jelly, a common lubricating jelly (K-Y Jelly, Johnson & Johnson, Skillman, NJ), a contraceptive foam and cream, and urine. The fluorescence of most of these substances differed from semen fluorescence in color, texture, or pattern. Urine and formula exhibited a color and pattern of fluorescence similar to semen. Moreover, urine fluorescence persisted through the preliminary observation period of 80 hours. Because urine has the potential of being present in the perineal area of young children and the fluorescence of urine could be confused with that of semen, urine was included in the study to examine its potential for generating false-positive WL readings.

Subjects and Sample Collection

Eleven women were recruited from two universities in northern California during February and March 1990, and informed consent for participation in the study was obtained. Each subject obtained a semen sample from a male partner on the evening prior to or on the morning of the study. Samples collected in the evening were promptly refrigerated after collection. (During preliminary testing, the fluorescent and forensic properties of refrigerated semen were found to be no different than those of fresh semen.) On the morning of their study participation, subjects were asked to avoid the use of lotions or creams on their arms and to collect a sample of their own urine. During the 28-hour study period, subjects were asked to avoid bathing and to wear clothing that protected their arms during the day to minimize friction against their skin.

Test Applications and Observations

Liquid semen in 50-μL aliquots was placed on eight demarcated, ventral forearm locations of each volunteer. Fifty-microliter samples of urine were also applied to two areas on the forearms. One semen area and one urine area served as sites for the measurements of fluorescence decay, as described below. The other sites were reserved for sample collection for forensic analyses. During the 28-hour test period the same examiner (T.G.) held a WL (Mineralight UVL-56 *Blak Ray* Ultraviolet Lamp, Ultraviolet Products Inc, San Gabriel, Calif) over the forearms, and the fluorescence of semen and urine was recorded as either positive, faint, or negative. The pattern of fluorescence was recorded as even or irregular, and the color was noted as yellow-green or white.

Each subject had a WL reading performed at 15 minutes and 4, 7, 11, 24, and 28 hours after semen and urine application. At each interval, specimens were taken for forensic analyses by swabbing one of the semen areas with a cotton-tipped applicator moistened with sterile water. These swabs were air dried, frozen at 20°C, and transported to the laboratory.

Control swabs, taken from areas of the skin without semen or urine applications, were collected from 10 (91%) of the 11 subjects. Because the specificities of the forensic assays were known, only three (27%) of the 11 subjects had swabs of urine collected. These samples were similarly air dried and frozen for later analyses.

Laboratory Analyses

All forensic examiners were blind to the timing of the swab sample collection. The cotton portions of the swabs were extracted in isotonic Hepes buffer and centrifuged to separate the supernatant from the cellular debris; both fractions were frozen for later analyses.

Microscopy was performed using the cellular debris from the above procedure. A so-called Christmas tree stain[12] was used that stains sperm heads red and tail structures green. Results of microscopy were recorded as positive or negative depending on the presence or absence of spermatozoa. The ACP activity was assayed with a standard quantitative assay using p-nitrophenyl phosphate as a substrate.[9] The cutoff point for significance of ACP values was defined at 0.1 IU/mL since all skin control values were below this threshold.

The CIE assay for p30 allows semiquantitation of p30 levels and is sensitive to approximately 500 ng/mL.[13] The p30-CIE results were recorded as positive or negative. The p30-ELISA assay allows detection of p30 at concentrations as low as 2 ng/mL.[14] All skin control values registered less than the 2 ng/mL detection limit for the assay configuration used (Epichrome Immunometric Assay for prostatic antigen, Cetus Corp, Emeryville, Calif); therefore, this was used as our cutoff point below which test results were considered negative. (Although the assay kit used in this study is no longer commercially available, comparable assays for prostatic antigen p30 are available from Yang Laboratories, Seattle, Wash, and Hybritech, La Jolla, Calif.)

RESULTS

Ten (91%) of the 11 subjects had WL evaluations and swabs of dried semen taken at baseline and at the five specified intervals to 28 hours after semen application; the remaining subject missed one WL reading and swab collection 4 hours after application. One subject also missed one WL reading but was instructed to collect a swab sample per study protocol. In all, 65 samples were analyzed.

The visual appearance of semen and urine spots on the subjects' skin was assessed during the 28-hour study period. Semen spots initially appeared shiny or colloid-like, then turned flaky (72% of subjects had a flaky appearance 4 hours after semen application), and finally cleared over time. After 24 hours, the skin with semen appeared clear in nine subjects (82%). In contrast, skin with urine applications appeared clear throughout the study period.

WL Findings

The color of semen fluorescence was indistinguishable from the color of urine fluorescence throughout all periods. The pattern of semen fluorescence appeared irregular in texture, while the pattern of urine fluorescence was consistently homogeneous over time. As shown in Fig 1,

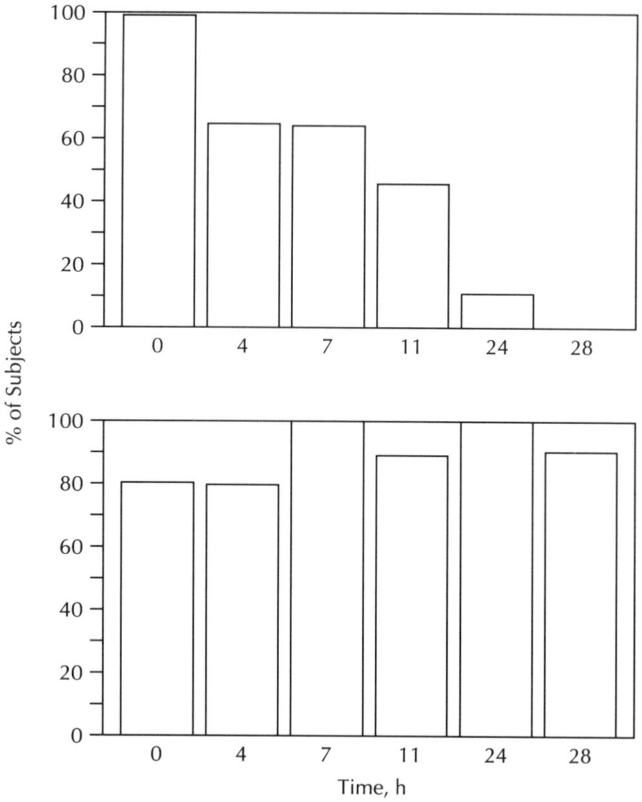

Fig 1.—*Top, Percentage of subjects with positive Wood's Lamp fluorescence of semen during a 28-hour period. Bottom, Percentage of subjects with positive Wood's Lamp fluorescence of urine during the same period.*

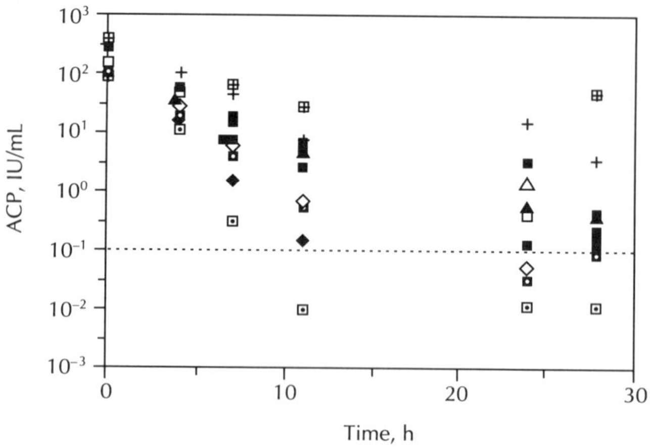

Fig 2.—*Acid phosphatase (ACP) concentrations (log base 10 scale). The broken line indicates the cutoff value below which a value is considered negative. Each symbol indicates a different subject.*

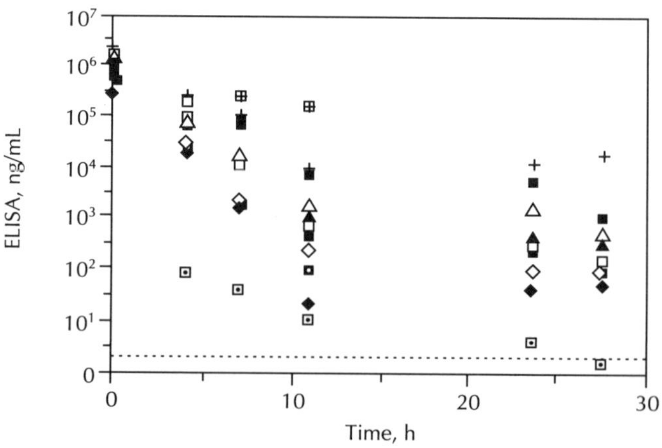

Fig 3.—*The prostatic protein p30 concentrations by enzyme-linked immunosorbent assay (ELISA) (log base 10 scale). The broken line indicates the cutoff value for a positive or negative value. Each symbol indicates a different subject.*

the intensity of semen fluorescence diminished dramatically over time. By 28 hours, six subjects (54%) exhibited faint semen fluorescence, but no subjects showed strongly positive fluorescence. In contrast, the fluorescence of 10 of the 11 urine spots remained strongly positive during the 28-hour period.

Forensic Analyses

The microscopic detection of sperm is generally considered to be the most sensitive and specific technique for semen detection.[5] By 28 hours, 55% of semen samples showed no microscopic evidence of the presence of sperm. The decline of ACP activity in the semen samples over time is shown in Fig 2. All samples were positive at the time of application, but with increasing time ACP values declined. By 28 hours, three (27%) of the 11 semen samples tested negative for ACP.

The p30 levels detected with CIE also declined with time. By 11 hours after semen application, four (36%) of the 11 samples had negative p30-CIE values, and at 28 hours seven (64%) of 11 samples had negative values. The p30-ELISA proved to be the most sensitive technique used (Fig 3). Before 28 hours no samples had negative test results. At 28 hours, only one (9%) of 11 samples had a p30 level that fell below the detection limit. Overall, the ELISA technique displayed greater sensitivity than did p30-CIE, microscopy, and ACP in detecting the presence of semen on skin. Sixty-three (97%) of 65 semen samples were found to be positive with the ELISA technique, while 47 (72%), 53 (82%), and 59 (91%) of the semen samples were found to be positive with the p30-CIE technique, microscopy, and ACP, respectively.

Regardless of the results of semen fluorescence on skin, the p30-ELISA was more frequently positive than p30-CIE, microscopy, or ACP in detecting the presence of semen. The ELISA was 100% sensitive in detecting the presence of semen when no fluorescence was seen. This was in contrast with semen samples obtained from areas of no fluorescence evaluated with p30-CIE, microscopy, and ACP, which were positive only 34%, 56%, and 69% of the time, respectively.

Control swabs from areas of skin without urine or semen and from areas with urine only were analyzed with the ELISA technique. Results of these analyses were negative.

COMMENT

Despite study findings that the WL is nonspecific and only relatively sensitive for the detection of semen on body surfaces, it remains the only screening tool currently available to detect semen traces on the skin of child sexual assault victims. The timing of the clinical examination in relation to the alleged assault and the presence of fluorescent substances other than semen are important factors to consider when using the WL on a child or adult with suspected sexual abuse. As shown in this study, the fluorescence of semen on skin significantly diminished within 28 hours. In contrast, urine on skin remained fluorescent during the 28-hour test period and persisted until 80 hours in other test series. Since urine staining might be expected in the genital and thigh regions of children, positive WL observations must be interpreted with extreme caution. Overall, positive WL findings cannot be taken as definitive indications of the presence of semen because of the many substances that were shown to cause fluorescence. More important, negative WL findings should not be interpreted as indicating the absence of semen.

It is significant to note that the forensic tests were often capable of detecting semen when the WL fluorescence results were negative or inconclusive. The most sensitive of the four tests used in this study was the p30-ELISA technique. This assay has also been found to offer improved specificity and sensitivity in detecting semen in postcoital vaginal samples.[10] Although this ELISA assay is currently used in few US crime laboratories, this study suggests it may find particular application in the investigation of child sexual assault cases.

The rapid loss of detectable sperm in the test samples was somewhat surprising. This may be an artifact of the swabbing and extraction procedure. Alternatively, it may reflect the more rapid shedding or flaking of the bulk of the semen sample from the surface of skin. Overall, factors such as friction and rubbing on the sample area would be expected to accelerate semen loss from the skin surface. Other factors, such as chemical interactions on the skin surface, may also play a role. We acknowledge that the moisture, temperature, and chemistry of an adult's forearm skin may vary from the skin of a child's perineum; thus our findings might differ if children were used as subjects.

Recommendations for Using the WL and Collecting Samples

Despite its limitations, the WL allows clinicians to identify areas of skin with suspected semen, areas that may otherwise have gone unnoticed. Although the fluorescence of most samples faded by 28 hours, some areas maintained faint fluorescence. Because faint fluorescence may persist beyond the 28-hour period studied, the WL may be useful in cases in which a child presents within 72 hours of an assault; this follows the recommendation in the California Medical Protocol for Examination of Sexual Assault and Child Sexual Abuse Victims.[15]

During the WL examination, we recommend taking a swab of any white or yellow-green fluorescent areas on the patient's skin, paying particular attention to areas the patient identifies as sites of ejaculation. In cases selected for forensic analyses, swabs of the perineal area, inner thighs, and buttocks should be obtained even when the WL results are negative.

The entire area of skin in question should be wiped with a water-moistened swab, attempting to obtain as much material as possible on one swab. Rapid air drying, preferably with a drying box, and freezing are recommended to retard deterioration of the evidence material.[16,17] Repeated thawing and refreezing of samples is to be discouraged because of the potential for enzymatic and protein decay.

Recommendations for Forensic Analyses

Microscopic analysis for sperm and a chemical test for ACP and/or p30-CIE are routine in most crime laboratories. Our work demonstrates the importance of chemical testing in the absence of microscopic findings. Positive chemical findings may be obtained with any of the three chemical tests. A positive p30 assay may be considered conclusive evidence of the presence of semen. The p30-ELISA technique, if available, should be used since it is the most sensitive chemical test. Because of the lack of specificity of the ACP assay, a positive or negative ACP result warrants further analysis.

IMPLICATIONS

The results of this study are important for the development of clinical guidelines for use of the WL and the forensic methods studied here. Through additional clinical research, it is important to confirm the value of the WL as a screening tool and the value of forensic laboratory methods, particularly the p30-ELISA technique, as definitive, diagnostic tools for detecting semen traces on skin of acutely abused children. The strengths and limitations of each test used must be understood by the medical, forensic, and legal personnel involved in the investigation of child sexual abuse. With increasing knowledge, clinicians and forensic scientists will be able to assess child sexual abuse cases with more confidence and provide more convincing evidence for their use in legal proceedings.

This study was supported by a behavioral pediatric training grant from the Maternal and Child Health Bureau of the Department of Health and Human Services and by grant 86-IJ-CX-0044 from the National Institute of Justice.

We thank Jim Norris of the San Francisco Crime Laboratory, Beth Chesterman, MA, John Jemerin, MD, Jeanne Tschann, PhD, and John McCann, MD, for their technical assistance and helpful comments.

References

1. *Study Findings, Study of National Incidence and Prevalence of Child Abuse and Neglect.* Washington, DC: US Dept of Health and Human Services; 1988. Document HE 23.1210:In 2/2; chap 4:1-8.
2. Deyoung M. Disclosing sexual abuse. *Child Welfare.* 1987;66:217-223.
3. Pollack OJ. Semen and seminal stains. *Arch Pathol.* 1943;35:140-196.
4. Krugman RD. Recognition of sexual abuse in children. *Pediatr Rev.* 1986;8:25-30.
5. Identification of semen and vaginal secretions. In: Gaensslen RE, ed. *Sourcebook in Forensic Serology, Immunology, and Biochemistry.* Washington, DC: US Dept of Justice, National Institute of Justice; 1983. Document J28.2:F 76/2:149-181.
6. Sensabaugh GF. Isozymes in forensic science. In: Rattazzi MC, Scandalios JG, Whitt GS, eds. *Isozymes: Current Topics in Biological and Medical Research.* New York, NY: Alan R Liss Inc; 1982;6:247-282.
7. Wojcieszyn JW, Wang MC, Lee CL, Murphy GP, Chu TM. Purification and characterization of a human urinary acid phosphatase. *J Appl Biochem.* 1979;1:223-234.
8. Kirk JE, Eisenstein A, MacBryde CM. The acid phosphatase concentration of the prostatic exprimate during normal puberty. *J Clin Endocrinol Metab.* 1952;12:338-345.
9. Sensabaugh GF. The quantitative acid phosphatase test. *J Forensic Sci.* 1979;24:346-365.
10. Graves HCB, Sensabaugh GF, Blake ET. Postcoital detection of a male-specific semen protein. *N Engl J Med.* 1985;312:338-343.
11. Baechtel FS. The identification and individualization of semen stains. In: Saferstein R, ed. *Forensic Science Handbook.* Englewood Cliffs, NJ: Prentice Hall; 1988;2:347-392.
12. Oppitts E. Eine neue Farbemethode zum Nachweis der Spermien bei Sittlichkeitsdelikten. *Arkiv Kriminol.* 1969;144:145-148.
13. Poyntz FM, Martin PD. Comparison of p30 and acid phosphatase levels in post-coital vaginal swabs from donor and case-work studies. *Forensic Sci Int.* 1984;24:17-25.
14. Loor R, M'Tikulu T, DeWitt SK. Individual and simultaneous monoclonal antibody-based immunoassays of prostate-specific antigen and prostatic acid phosphatase. *J Clin Immunoassay.* 1986;9:159-163.
15. *California Medical Protocol for the Examination of Sexual Assault and Child Sexual Abuse Victims.* Sacramento, Calif: State of California, Office of Criminal Justice Planning; 1987:17-26.
16. Sensabaugh GF, Bashinski JS, Blake ET. The laboratory's role in investigating rape. *Diagn Med.* 1985;8:46-53.
17. Berkowitz CD. Sexual abuse of children and adolescents. *Adv Pediatr.* 1987;34:275-312.

Make My Day

I live in a moderately sized city in upstate New York. It is conservative by usual standards. George Eastman, the industrialist and great benefactor, noted that it was a nice place to raise children. It has broad streets, nice parks, many cultural opportunities, good music, excellent medical care, and over 60 homicides a year. Two years ago we had a serial killer who brutally murdered over a dozen women. This is a city that prides itself in addressing problems by concerned citizen groups. Maybe these groups have been effective; maybe without them we would have had 100 homicides a year.

A very disquieting note is our reaction to this. In the morning paper you read about another homicide, and turn to the sports page to see what happened to the Bills. We are jaded. We have lost our sense of outrage. We suffer from violence overload. Now almost no one talks about the 66 (or was it 67 or 68?) homicides last year, or the 13 (no I think it was 14) murders by Arthur Shawcross. There is violence or aggressive behavior everywhere. Arnold, Clint, and Charles dispatch half the male population of the United States in every new picture. Admittedly, they are on the side of justice. I was driving down the road observing the speed limit, a defect in my personality occasionally manifesting itself, and was passed by an attractive, but impatient, woman, who shot me a finger in payment for my rectitude. On her rear bumper there was a sticker that read, "To Know Me Is To Love Me" (I wonder). My car, my beloved Jeep, was stolen a few weeks ago and was turned up by the police completely wrecked. My first reaction was to ask what might have happened to the occupants, but I am too embarrassed to say what I thought.

Violent and aggressive behavior is a social, educational, housing, legal, and health issue. We see it in others and we see it in ourselves. For example, the brusque handling of a patient is an aggressive act. Aggressive in that we react against someone who turns to us at their most vulnerable time.

The American Medical Association is addressing the issue of violence with the theme issue of the *Journal of the American Medical Association* and with articles in its specialty journals. The ARCHIVES is presenting four articles and a letter to the editor on this theme of special interest to our specialty. The first, by Dr Menken,[1] emphasizes the failure of our present educational system to help students understand the issues associated with violent and aggressive behavior. The second is by Elliott,[2] a neurologist, who has had wide experience in dealing with "the violent few." He points out the importance of biological factors in certain forms of violent behavior. Mahowald et al[3] look at the elusive problem of violence and sleep behavior. Ciccone,[4] a leader in the field of forensic psychiatry, describes the role of the specialist as an expert witness in cases involving violence. Finally, Deshmukh et al[5] chronicle their experience with gunshot wounds.

Neurologists have a special role to play in violence. As citizens we must necessarily have concern for this plague. As physicians we must become more aware of the problem and educate our patients and the public about this serious health problem. As neurologists we are particularly equipped to diagnose and treat these problems when they have a biological basis.

ROBERT J. JOYNT, MD, PHD
Chief Editor

References

1. Menken M. Grappling with the enigma of violence: an educational approach. *Arch Neurol.* 1992;49:592-594.
2. Elliott FA. Violence: the neurological contribution. *Arch Neurol.* 1992;49:595-603.
3. Mahowald MW, Schenck CH, Rosen GM, Hurwitz TD. The role of a sleep disorder center in evaluating sleep-violence. *Arch Neurol.* 1992;49:604-607.
4. Ciccone JR. Murder, insanity, and medical expert witnesses. *Arch Neurol.* 1992;49:608-611.
5. Deshmukh VD, Laneve L, Fallon WF. Violent brain injuries by gunshot in Duval County, Florida, 1989-1991. *Arch Neurol.* 1992;49:588.

Grappling With the Enigma of Violence

An Educational Approach

Matthew Menken, MD

As we approach the end of a millennium, it is appropriate that neurologists and other physicians link forces with the public in asking what improvements we want to achieve in health care, and how this can be done. Early in the 20th century, the population of the United States consisted mainly of children and young adults. In 1900, life expectancy at birth was 46.6 years and 48.7 years for white males and females, compared with only 32.5 years and 33.5 years for black males and females. Medical care of that period focused on acute, life-threatening illnesses, was usually ineffective, and was relatively inexpensive. Priority setting and resource allocation were not relevant issues. During the first half of this century, death rates from such disorders as diphtheria, scarlet fever, tuberculosis, pertussis, and rubeola plummeted, continuing a downward trend that started during the second half of the 19th century. This trend was largely due to the improved socioeconomic and educational status of the population, public health measures, immunizations, and the development of effective treatments. By 1950, life expectancy at birth was 66.5 years and 72.2 years for white males and females, and 58.9 years and 62.7 years for black males and females.[1]

As there is no evidence that socioeconomic factors or medical research has been able to prolong the optimum life expectancy of humans, it is understandable that life expectancy at birth has increased more slowly in recent years. As of 1989, life expectancy at birth for white males and females was 72.6 years and 79.1 years; and for black males and females, 65.2 years and 74.0 years. A life span greater than 100 years remains as elusive as ever. At the present time, chronic illness, especially among the elderly, and a variety of disorders that collectively reflect individual behavior and sociocultural values consume a major portion of our total professional effort, and society's costs.[2] Given that the resources that can be devoted to health care are always finite in the face of seemingly infinite demand, it has become evident that every society needs to identify its major health problems and to focus preventive and therapeutic efforts on them.

While we correctly call attention to the many scientifically approved and important research projects that are not carried out each year because of a lack of funding, it is also clear that not every worthy objective can be a priority, since priorities are meaningless if they include everything. For example, the Secretary of State for Health in the United Kingdom has proposed three criteria for selecting health priority areas: areas for which improvements in the health of the nation are most likely; areas for which strategies for targeted improvement in health status can be monitored; and areas for research that may increase the scope of national health priorities and targets. Using these criteria, 16 priority areas have been identified, including selected causes of substantial morbidity and mortality (stroke, trauma, and mental health), factors that contribute to these causes of morbidity and mortality (tobacco and alcohol), and areas of potential improvement or regression of national health status in the foreseeable future (rehabilitation, acquired immunodeficiency syndrome, and additional vaccines to prevent communicable diseases).[3]

VIOLENCE AS A HEALTH PRIORITY

Using criteria grounded on a population perspective, it is eminently clear that violence is currently a priority health problem in the United States, where the homicide rate alone is three to eight times higher than in other Western democracies.[4] As in the case of cocaine-related emergency department episodes, the lamentable problem of violence is greatest among minority youth and young adults. Homicides claimed 22 000 lives in the United States in 1988, and was the leading cause of death among black males in the 15- to 34-year-old age group. More than half of all homicide victims in the United States between 1986 and 1989 were in this age group, of whom about two thirds were murdered with a handgun or some other kind of firearm.[1] During the 1980s, more than 11 000 high school students died as a result of homicides with firearms. Even younger children are not infrequently affected. As a recent heartbreaking example, an 11-year-old boy, while playing in his New York City apartment less than 2 weeks before Christmas, shot his 9-year-old friend in the abdomen with his brother's .45-caliber semiauto-

Accepted for publication January 21, 1992.

From the World Federation of Neurology Research Group on Neurological Education and the Departments of Medicine and Neurology, Robert Wood Johnson Medical School, University of Medicine and Dentistry of New Jersey, New Brunswick.

Reprint requests to 1527 Highway 27, Somerset, NJ 08873 (Dr Menken).

matic weapon, believing it to be a toy; when called to the scene, the police recovered 200 vials of "crack" cocaine from the closet where the boy had discovered the gun (*The New York Times*. December 16, 1991:B2).

In the 1990 national school-based Youth Risk Behavior Survey, it was estimated that nearly 20% of all students in grades 9 through 12 carried a weapon at least once in the month preceding the survey, during which time there were an astonishing 71 weapon-carrying incidents per 100 students.[5] Just as alcohol is a contributing factor in roughly 25% of all road traffic accidents, so a range of drugs (both legally prescribed and deliberately misused), often combined with alcohol, contribute to homicides and suicides. In 1980, a Public Health Service national health objective called for a reduction of the death rate from homicide among black males aged 15 to 24 years from 70.7 homicides per 100 000 (as of 1978) to below 60 per 100 000 by 1990.[6] However, in 1988, there were 101.8 deaths per 100 000 in this age group, an increase of 44% in just one decade.

The dramatic increase in societal violence since World War II appears difficult to understand and virtually impossible to contain. There are more than 20 000 laws in the United States that deal with the sale, distribution, and use of firearms, without convincing evidence of effectiveness. Since studies of deaths in the home due to firearms show that such events are only rarely related to use of weapons in self-defense, and are 40 times more likely to be the result of accidents, suicides, and homicides, some have called for physicians to adopt a leadership role in persuading their patients and the public of the need for still further legislation to ban the private use of handguns altogether.[7] Although such proposals clearly merit our vigorous support, the failure of recent legislation to control illicit drug availability and abuse, especially among those racial and ethnic groups most affected, together with a dramatic decline in tobacco consumption in recent years that is largely unrelated to legislation, suggests that educational approaches may also be helpful. In the discussion that follows, the remedial steps proposed are directed at the problem of violence in and out of schools among our nation's youth, especially minority children and young adults. I approach this topic with the bias that educational measures are, almost always, greatly to be preferred to punitive proposals in dealing with grave and complex social issues, based in part on my activities with the World Federation of Neurology Research Group on Neurological Education.[8]

AN EDUCATIONAL MANIFESTO

Mark Twain is reputed to have said that the ancients stole all of our best ideas from us. In this context, when a prestigious study identified and examined the 102 most important ideas in *The Great Books of the Western World* in 1952,[9] violence was not included as an element of the core vocabulary of philosophical or human thought, distinct from its incorporation among such concepts as war, tyranny, good and evil, life and death, and punishment. However, when the author of the 1952 study of great ideas revisited this topic about 30 years later, he included violence among an abridged list of 64 core philosophical concepts in the great books collection.[10] Clearly, violence appears to be moving up in the lexicon of philosophically important issues, concomitant with its intrusion into all aspects of life in our society.

In my view, it is not surprising that the United States has experienced a much greater problem of violence among its youth than many other Western nations. I suggest that Draconian prison sentences and the best efforts of those who provide social services (including medical care) will probably not be much more effective in the future than they have been in the recent past, unless they are accompanied by fundamental reform of our educational system. Between 1980 and 1990, the inmate population in New Jersey's prisons increased from 86.9 to 282.5 inmates per 100 000 population, or 225%. This is not to suggest that efforts by society to prevent violence; to protect those threatened or injured; to punish those guilty of heinous crimes against their fellow human beings; and to provide a full range of diagnostic, therapeutic, and rehabilitative services to victims and perpetrators alike should not be expanded. Clearly, such deterrent and compensatory measures have the capacity to make a difference under some circumstances.

When viewed from the perspective of the World Federation of Neurology Research Group on Neurological Education, however, the problem of violence among adolescents and young adults in the United States seems inextricably linked to the failure of the nation's educational system to provide first-class basic schooling for many children. Put summarily, there is a parallel between a health system that excludes 37 million citizens from basic care and a system of local schools that labels as basic education what is all too often a gateway to a lifetime of inequality in the workplace and in society.[11] Recently, a group of 12 educators and distinguished citizens, sponsored by the Institute for Philosophical Research, presented *The Paideia Proposal* to address the need for reform of basic education, so as to achieve the goal of universal schooling of uniform quality for all children in the United States.[12]

Many of the problems identified by the Paideia group are similar to those identified by university faculties concerned with the tendency of schools of higher education (including medical schools) to emphasize highly specialized vocational knowledge, rather than the general knowledge needed by all students. *Paideia* is the Greek word (whose root is familiar in pediatrics) for the general, unspecialized learning that every child should experience, equivalent to the more familiar Latin word *humanitas*. The Paideia analysis concludes that schooling of equal length (quantity), but unequal content (quality), fails to prepare *all* children for the continuation of general learning in adult life. Moreover, a dichotomous approach to basic education is identified as a major factor contributing to a climate of disillusionment, rejection, alienation, and resentment among those children and young adults (and their families) who are denied the opportunity to travel first class in school.

By tracking some pupils along an academic, precollege path, and others along a specialized vocational path, society explicitly persists in the conviction of an earlier era that only some students are educable, and sets in place a caste system among its children. The Paideia manifesto holds that all students should receive the same quality and quantity (12 years) of basic schooling, since they all have the same three objectives in life: to take advantage of every future opportunity society offers for self-improvement; to be adequately prepared for discharging the duties and responsibilities of citizenship; and to obtain the basic skills that are necessary to earn a living in our society, no matter what specific job or career they subsequently pursue.

It is of special interest and importance for neurologists among the full-time and voluntary faculties of our nation's medical schools that the Paideia proposal also calls attention to the limitations of didactic instruction, although this format of passive learning is certainly necessary for the acquisition of organized knowledge in many fields of basic learning. There is again a parallel between the Paideia preference for the development of intellectual skills and an enlarged understanding of major ideas and issues by means of problem solving, coaching exercises, supervised practice, and particularly seminars, when these formats are compared with the renewed emphasis on problem-based learning in medical education and other fields of higher learning.[13]

CONCLUSIONS

An overview of the changing burden of illness among the industrialized Western democracies during the 20th century and the rapidly rising costs of more effective medical care suggest that each nation must target for action its priority health problems, determined by means of a population perspective. With this approach, violence is identified as a major health problem in the United States, where it is often associated with substance abuse and the culture of poverty, especially among minority children and young adults. Although medical care, social services, the judicial system, and other sectors of society can make distinct and important contributions to society's collective effort to ameliorate the enigma of violence, educational measures are likely to be the most effective (and cost-effective) steps over the longer term. This judgment arises in part from the growing awareness among many people that we have an undemocratic process of basic education in our nation's schools that must be reformed. Instead of responding to the same objectives that all children seek in their basic education by providing a uniform course of study for all, many schools support instead a program consisting of two or more tracks, only one of which goes straight ahead. The consequences of this separate and unequal approach include a process of disaffection and alienation among many children and young adults, not only toward this kind of schooling, but also toward the society that provides it.

Recently, the Paideia group of educators and concerned citizens has responded to these concerns by developing a proposal for reform of basic education in the United States. The assumption of this group is that we cannot achieve true social justice without schooling that is of uniform quantity and quality among children in all socioeconomic groups of society. All children must receive 12 years of the same course as a generic preparation for work, citizenship, and life. Didactic lectures should be supplemented with problem-solving exercises to develop intellectual skills, and especially with seminars that augment students' understanding of the essential and indispensable ideals and values of our society as reflected in our shared literary and artistic heritage. Neurologists and other physicians can respond to the enigma of violence by supporting essential reform of education in the communities where they have established medical practices.

References

1. Public Health Service. *Health, United States, 1990.* Hyattsville, Md: National Center for Health Statistics; 1991.
2. Webster JR, Berdes C. Ethics and economic realities. *Arch Intern Med.* 1990;150:1795-1797.
3. Secretary of State for Health. *The Health of Our Nation.* London, England: Her Majesty's Stationery Office; 1991.
4. Fingerhut LA, Kleinman JC. International and interstate comparisons of homicide among young males. *JAMA.* 1990;263:3292-3295.
5. Centers for Disease Control. Weapon-carrying among high school students. *JAMA.* 1991;266:2342.
6. Public Health Service. *Healthy People 2000: National Health Promotion and Disease Prevention Objectives.* Washington, DC: US Government Printing Office; 1990. US Dept of Health and Human Services publication.
7. Kassirer JP. Firearms and the killing threshold. *N Engl J Med.* 1991;325:1647-1650.
8. Menken M. Medical education for primary care. *World Health Forum.* In press.
9. Adler MJ. *The Great Ideas: A Syntopicon.* Chicago, Ill: Encyclopedia Britannica Inc; 1952;2.
10. Adler MJ. *Six Great Ideas.* New York, NY: Macmillan Publishing Co Inc; 1981:18.
11. Menken M. Caring for the underserved. *Arch Neurol.* 1991;48:472-475.
12. Adler MJ. *The Paideia Proposal: An Educational Manifesto.* New York, NY: Macmillan Publishing Co Inc; 1982.
13. Barrows HS, Tamblyn RM. *Problem-Based Learning.* New York, NY: Springer Publishing Co Inc; 1980.

Violence

The Neurologic Contribution: An Overview

Frank A. Elliott, MD

• **The role of cultural forces in either promoting or discouraging interpersonal violence is so obvious that it has been allowed to obscure the part played by biologic disorders in determining responses to endogenous and environmental challenges. Neuroscientists and clinicians have demonstrated, however, that aggression has a neuroanatomic and chemical basis, that developmental and acquired brain disorders contribute to recurrent interpersonal violence, that both biologic and sociologic factors are involved, and that to ignore either is to invite error.**

(*Arch Neurol.* 1992;49:595-603)

The term *violence* will be used in this article to indicate physical interpersonal aggression with the intent to harm or destroy. The article is not concerned with collective aggression or with the violent responses of psychotic patients to delusions, illusions, and hallucinations, or with a single episode in a normally well-controlled subject, or with the opportunistic or premeditated predatory aggression carried out for profit in street violence and in drug-related activities. Rather, it focuses on a relatively small percentage of the population who have been given to recurrent violence since childhood or early adolescence—what Hamparin et al[1] called "the violent few." Thus, in a study of 627 chronic offender delinquents from a cohort of 10 000 male individuals born in 1945, 6% were responsible for 71% of the homicides, 73% of the rapes, and 69% of the aggravated assaults.[2]

Since Kaplan[3] reported that trauma to the brain can lead to recurrent violent behavior in previously equable individuals, this has been found to occur following other disorders, including tumor, encephalitis, stroke, multiple sclerosis, Alzheimer's disease and other dementias, cysticercosis, cardiorespiratory arrest, Huntington's chorea, severe hypoglycemia, and other metabolic disorders.[4] However, such brain insults do not add greatly to the total sum of human destructiveness, and their importance lies in the fact that they demonstrate that the response of the brain to environmental or endogenous challenges can be profoundly altered by quite small lesions at specific sites, *whatever the nature of the lesion.*

A much rarer event is the abolition of a lifelong tendency to explosive behavior as a result of brain damage. A woman with a pineal tumor reported as a first symptom the loss of a lifelong tendency to explosive behavior. The tumor was found to have infiltrated the midbrain at the level of the inferior colliculus and the rostral aspect of the cerebellum.[5] A 60-year-old man who had suffered from episodic dyscontrol since adolescence had several transient ischemic attacks, which aggravated his aggressive behavior. Then, following another attack, his personality changed abruptly. He became gentle and had no further rages until his death a year later. An examination of his brain revealed multiple bilateral infarcts, but there was nothing to indicate which was responsible for his pacification (unpublished case).

THE NEURAL SUBSTRATE OF AGGRESSION AND VIOLENCE

Experimental work in animals and clinical studies in man have shown that the capacity for aggression, and for its control, is vested in a system of neuronal assemblies, both excitatory and inhibitory, which are situated bilaterally in the orbitofrontal cortex, the septal area, hippocampus, amygdala, head of caudate nucleus, thalamus, ventromedial and posterior hypothalamic nuclei, midbrain tegmentum, pons,[6,7] and in the fastigial nuclei and anterior lobe of the cerebellum. Under normal conditions, the neocortex also exerts some degree of control over this equipment, but its inhibitory capacity is fragile and can break down in the face of overwhelming endogenous drives or exogenous provocation in normal individuals. Focal lesions confined to the cortex (from bullets and shrapnel) are not as a rule followed by aggressive behavior.

The elicitation of violence by electrical stimulation at various points within the brain sheds much light on the anatomic substrate of violence and its control. The "centers" at which stimulation can give rise to affective aggression in animals are approximately the same as in man; the trigger areas for predatory aggression are slightly different. However, the results of stimulation can be difficult to interpret, because it is sometimes hard to distinguish between the effects of stimulation at one point

Accepted for publication February 17, 1992.

From The Elliott Neurological Center of the Pennsylvania Hospital, Philadelphia.

Reprint requests to The Elliott Neurological Center of the Pennsylvania Hospital, 8th and Spruce streets, Philadelphia, PA 19107 (Dr Elliott).

and the more diffuse excitation of other areas by the after discharge.[8] Again, in animals, the effects of stimulation depend, to some extent, on the presence of an appropriate prey. Care also has to be exercised in extrapolating effects of electrical stimulation from animals to man. It is much more difficult to elicit rage in man than in animals, perhaps because of differences in the mental "set" of an animal incarcerated in an operating chair or cage and a human patient undergoing the procedure in the hope of finding an answer to the burden of recurrent rages or seizures. Second, the animal's brain is presumably normal, whereas in most human patients it is not.

Little is known about the neurologic substrate of predatory aggression in man. The predatory behavior of some survivors from encephalitis, including encephalitis lethargica, with its impulsivity, lack of conscience, and egocentricity, more closely resemble a prefrontal syndrome than anything else; yet, most of the damage is in the midbrain and limbic system.

Suppressor areas for affective aggression include the prefrontal cortex, the septal area, the head of the caudate nucleus, the lateral amygdala, the cortex of the anterior lobe of the cerebellum, and the fastigial nuclei.[9-13]

From published articles[14-19] and personal observations, it seems that when small tumors or cysts have been associated with episodic violence, they have usually been situated in a position to involve the limbic system or its connections, usually in or near the midline, thus involving those portions of the brain that we have inherited from our reptilian and early mammalian ancestors. Apathy, the converse of irritability, is also a notable feature of deep midline tumors and cysts involving the anterior corpus callosum, the septum pellucidum, the cavum Vergae, the cingulate gyri, and the third ventricle.[20]

The cerebellar factor, although comparatively new to clinicians, has interested neuroscientists for some time. We do not ordinarily associate subtentorial lesions with mental and emotional disorders, and when they occur, as they did in 47% of 110 cases of cerebellar and other subtentorial tumors,[21] they are apt to be interpreted as a reaction to fear or incapacity, although this explanation is unacceptable when the mental symptoms are the first to appear and intracranial pressure is normal, or when, as in three personal cases, recurrent rages appeared for the first time after the successful removal of midline cerebellar tumors (an angioma and a grade I glioma) and following a presumed right-sided infarct.

In 1947, Moruzzi[22] reported that in thalamic cats spontaneous outbursts of sham rage were inhibited by weak electrical stimulation of the cerebellar cortex just behind and just in front of the fissura prima, but they were elicited as a rebound response if the stimulus was timed to occur during an interval of quietness. Maiti and Snider[23] reported that stimulation of the cerebellar cortex exerted a tonic inhibitory influence on the amygdala and hippocampus by way of the fastigial nuclei. This inhibitory effect could be abolished by electrocoagulation of the rostral midbrain reticular formation. In the cat, stimulation of the rostral fastigial nuclei elicits hypertension, grooming, feeding, and predatory attack behavior.[24] The results of these early experiments encouraged attempts to control both seizures and extreme violence in man by electrical stimulation of the cerebellum. Heath[25] was able to control violent aggressive behavior in schizophrenics by using a pacemaker to stimulate the anterior lobe of the cerebellum. Cooper[26] used a similar technique for the control of seizures; it also stopped attacks of rage.

Recent research has greatly expanded the conception of cerebellar affects on the forebrain. Clinical studies,[27,28] reinforced by magnetic resonance imaging and positron-emission tomographic scans, have demonstrated that the normal human cerebellum is involved in the learning process, in judging the passage of time, in the cognitive processing of words, and, perhaps, in the learning of motor skills. The effect on motor functions is provocative in that many adults with episodic dyscontrol have a history of difficulty in learning common motor skills and/or a lifelong tendency to clumsiness.

The neurochemical substrates for the instigation and control of violent behavior include excitatory and inhibitory neurotransmitters and a variety of longer lasting humeral neuromodulators, including gonadal hormones.

Although most of the work in this field has been carried out on animals of various species, there is a remarkable concordance between animal studies and human data. In man, both γ-aminobutyric acid and serotonin inhibit both predatory and affective aggression and there is a strong positive correlation between a history of angry aggressive behavior and norepinephrine levels. The antiaggressive action of serotonin is suggested by a close and consistent correlation between aggression and impulsivity and low spinal fluid levels of 5-hydroxyindoleacetic acid,[29,30] and there is a similar correlation between low serotonin level in the serum platelets of children suffering from the aggressive conduct disorder.[31]

The question arises as to whether the episodicity of both affective and predatory aggression is related, inter alia, to the diurnal, circadian, or seasonal fluctuations in the levels of many neurotransmitters and neuromodulators, fluctuations that may help to explain not only the episodicity of violence but also the seasonal fluctuations in the rates of homicide and suicide.[9,10]

THREE TYPES OF VIOLENCE

Episodic Dyscontrol

The term *episodic dyscontrol*, first used for attacks of rage resulting from neurotic conflicts, has been applied to a wider range of individuals in whom it appeared for the first time as a result of a brain insult or in whom it has been present from childhood or early adolescence in association with other developmental defects. It corresponds to the intermittent explosive disorder of the *Diagnostic and Statistical Manual of Mental Disorders, Third Edition* (*DSM-III*) and to the episodic violence of Pincus and Lewis,[32,] and it is important for its social impact as one of the causes of unpremeditated homicide, suicide, senseless attacks on strangers, spouse battery, child abuse, criminally aggressive driving, wanton destruction of property, and savage attacks on animals.[33] It occurs both in heterosexual and in homosexual partners of either sex.

Episodic violence cuts across many diagnostic boundaries, but it occurs in only a minority of cases in each disease category. It occurs in psychoses, neuroses, borderline disorders, conduct disorders in children, psychopathy, organic brain syndromes, epilepsy, mental retardation, metabolic diseases, and in developmental syndromes including attention-deficit–hyperactivity disorder (ADHD) and specific learning disorders.

Kaplan, in 1899, described what he called the *explosive diathesis* in these words,

. . . following the most trivial and impersonal causes there is the effect of rage with its motor accompaniments. They may be the most grotesque gesticulations, excessive movements of the face and a sharp explosiveness of speech; there will be cursing and outbreaks of violence which are often directed towards things; there may or may not be amnesia for these events afterwards. The outburst may terminate in an epileptic fit. There is an excessive reaction with inadequate adaptation to the situation, which is so remote from a well considered and purposeful act that it approaches a pure psychic reflex.[3]

The highly charged affect distinguishes it from the cold and callous predatory aggression of the psychopath and from the habitual aggression practiced as a means of survival in city slums and prisons.[34] Sometimes, particularly in women, the violence is verbal. The language is obscene, profane, and out of character—an elderly (60-year-old) quaker lady interrupted a social occasion by starting to villify her husband for no apparent reason. Her speech was garbled and her lips, flecked with foam, were retracted in a feline snarl. The attacks had occurred at intervals since a severe head injury at the age of 19 years. Such verbal attacks often provoke physical retaliation on the part of the male individual, who finds it easier to hit than to talk.

Physical violence often has a primitive quality, kicking, gouging, scratching, biting, and spitting. Windows are broken, doors smashed, and furniture wrecked. A young woman breaks her (female) partner's arm. The family cat is swung by its tail and smashed against the wall. A man kills another by a single stab wound to the heart and delivers 30 more to the dead body; such overkill is especially apt to occur when the aggressor is under the influence of drugs, alcohol, or extreme hatred. The attacks are usually followed by remorse except in psychopaths or in social circles where abuse of spouse and children is condoned. Individuals subject to these attacks may exhibit disinhibited behavior in other directions such as alcohol and drug abuse, rape, theft, and traffic citations. This is true of both unconvicted domestic batterers[35] and violent delinquents and criminals.[36,37]

Whatever the origin, whether the underlying problem is psychologic or neurologic, episodic dyscontrol can be triggered by small quantities of alcohol, and large amounts can produce pathologic intoxication in which the signs of drunkenness are not present but behavior is bizarre and sometimes violent, and there is complete amnesia for the episode.[38]

The Psychopath (Antisocial Personality Disorder)

Compared with other male criminals, psychopaths commit disproportionate numbers of crimes, and their crimes are also more violent and aggressive than those of other criminals.[39] The condition is marked by a retardation of social and emotional development without significant intellectual impairments, and it was described by Kraepelin[40] in 1915 as "circumscribed infantilism," a view supported by modern developmental psychology.[41] It is said to involve 3% of male and less than 1% of female individuals in the United States (*DSM-III*).

Psychopathic aggression is usually cold and callous, but the psychopaths are also capable of bouts of rage. In both cases, it appears as a disinhibitory response to minor provocation. The full personality profile includes a mask of superficial charm behind which lie inflated ideas of self-worth, a need for stimulation, impulsivity, poor self-control, shallow affect and incapacity for empathy, lack of remorse, manipulative behavior, a parasitic life-style, social irresponsibility, and multiple short-term sexual relationships.[42,43] Marginal cases, who do not display the fully fledged mosaic, present only fragments of the pattern.[44] A particularly malign combination, ie, impulsivity, aggression, lack of empathy, and lack of foresight, is not uncommon after head injury and encephalitis, and it occurs in a subset of the minimal brain dysfunction complex. It is found at all social levels, from the highest to the lowest, and in gifted individuals as well as in the mildly retarded.

A neuropathologic substrate is indicated by abnormal responses to neuropsychologic tests designed to detect "organicity," nonspecific electroencephalographic (EEG) abnormalities in the majority of aggressive cases, resistance to aversive conditioning, low levels of serotonin metabolites in the spinal fluid of adult psychopaths,[29,30] and a low level of serotonin in the platelets of children with aggressive conduct disorder.[31] Minor neurologic abnormalities are often present. In a study of 93 violent criminals, whose collective profile was that of the psychopath, 40% had EEG and/or neurologic abnormalities, including incoordination, dyspraxias, congenital stigmata, hyperactivity, hyperacousis, and photophobia.[45]

Compulsive Violence

Compulsive violence is rare in patients with the obsessive compulsive disorder. Indeed, Freud taught that such patients *never* carry out their fantasies. However, this is misleading, because it does not apply when compulsive symptoms appear following a brain insult. The epidemic of encephalitis lethargica in 1915 through 1925 produced many such cases in children and adolescents, and other types of encephalitis can also do so. In a personal case, following an attack of encephalitis associated with mumps, a previously normal 10-year-old boy showed a gross change of personality but without impairment of intelligence. He was subject to episodic attacks of rage on minimum provocation and was given to compulsive letter writing. In addition, he had an irresistible compulsion to fondle the breasts of girls and women seen in the street and to force his way into their homes where he indulged himself at knife point. As a result of this, he spent much of his time in prison.

Among my patients with cases of episodic dyscontrol, 21 exhibited concomitant compulsive features. In 18 patients, there was evidence of a neurologic disorder, ie, minimal brain dysfunction (n=8), temporal lobe epilepsy (n=4), severe head injury (n=4), and encephalitis (n=2). Denckla[46] found neurologic abnormalities in 45 of 54 children with the obsession-compulsion disorder and correlations between obsessive compulsive disorder and ADHD, the choreiform syndrome, and Tourette's syndrome. The inability to inhibit obsessions and compulsions at will suggests a failure of inhibitory mechanisms, which is supported in many cases by the favorable response to serotonin uptake blockers.

PHYSIOLOGIC CORRELATES

Age

The peak of physical violence in the home or in the street is in late adolescence and early adult life, but in the fifth decade or later pathologic violence can occur for the first time in a formerly nonaggressive individual as the result of an organic brain insult, intoxication, or a functional psychosis. Some individuals do not acquire the self-control, foresight, judgment, and social conscience that are commonly associated with the normal adult state until their 30s, and aggressive psychopaths can continue to be highly aggressive beyond middle age. It is sometimes forgotten that the cortex of the association areas of the frontal, parietal, and temporal lobes is not mature, in terms of myelination, until the third or fourth decade.[47,48]

Gender and Aggression

There are gender-determined differences between male and female brains in terms of speed of development, histology, cognitive skills (verbal IQ, for instance), and behavior.[49-51] Most normal male individuals, from cradle to grave, are more prone to physical violence than are most female individuals, and the pathologic violence exhibited by individuals in the form of episodic dyscontrol and predatory aggression is far more common in men. The physiologic differences between the two sexes seem to be the result of prenatal differentiation of the hypothalamic preoptic area as a result of the action of androgens. Another gender-related contribution to domestic violence is the premenstrual tension syndrome that, in some individuals, is accompanied by inadequate self-control or actual physical aggression. Over 60% of violent crimes committed by women occur in the premenstrual week.[52,53]

Genetics

The relationship of genetics to criminality, to violence in particular, has been widely discussed.[54,55] In animals, selective breeding to promote aggressiveness has been widely used in the production of bulls for the bullring and pit bulldogs. It has also been induced by selective breeding under laboratory conditions in mice, guinea pigs, rabbits, dogs and dingos.[56] In man, the XYY chromosome anomaly was credited with predisposing to violent criminal behavior, but some have doubts as to its importance. A more important genetic discovery is that a structural abnormality of the fragile X chromosome is often associated with mental impairment, from retardation to a low normal intelligence, learning difficulties, and behavioral problems such as hyperactivity, violent outbursts, and autistic symptoms. Large, low-set ears, large testicles, and other stigmata have also been recorded. About one fifth of the boys and two thirds of the girls who inherit the chromosome appear normal, but they act as carriers and, therefore, may have children or grandchildren with clinical symptoms.

In a study of personality variables in twins reared apart and reared together, Tellegen et al[57] found that both aggressiveness and capacity for control owed more to genetics than to common family or environmental components. Heredity also appears to have a significant role in conditions that contribute to pathologic aggression, notably the episodic dyscontrol syndrome,[58] ADHD,[59] and psychopathy.[54] Sociologic texts often conclude that when violence "runs in the family" it is necessarily something that has been learned from parents or peers. But this cannot be the entire explanation, because, in many cases, only some of the offspring in a violent household are thus affected. The generational transfer hypothesis has been sharply criticized by Stacey and Shupe[60] and others, and cannot explain the many cases of recurrent aggression that have no identifiable social origin.

NEUROPATHOLOGIC CORRELATES

Neurodevelopmental Disorders

The attention-deficit-hyperactivity disorder is a common antecedent of episodic dyscontrol and other forms of antisocial conduct, which may persist into adult life. It is viewed as a developmental condition that is generally chronic in nature, has a strong biologic and hereditary predisposition, and has a significantly negative impact on the academic and social outcomes for many children.[59]

Zametkin et al[61] have found that in adults with residual ADHD, global cerebral glucose metabolism is lower than in normal control subjects and that there was a significant reduction of values at 30 of 60 sites tested in the cerebrum—some of them subcortical.

The multiplicity of affected areas suggests a developmental defect in a diffuse system, for instance, one involving cortical and subcortical inhibitory mechanisms. This could help explain those cases of ADHD in which disinhibitory behavior occurs in behavior other than inattention and hyperactivity, such as acting on impulse without "reflective delay."[45] Disinhibition may appear in the form of substance abuse, traffic violations, theft, and sexual offenses. This is true of many prisoners convicted of violent crimes, whose histories are studded with episodes of impulsive antisocial behavior.[35-37]

The ADHD was originally linked with specific learning disorders and a heterogeneous collection of cognitive, perceptual, motor, and behavioral disorders that constituted the minimal brain dysfunction syndrome,[62,63] which was first identified by Still[64] in 1902, elaborated by others in the 1950s, and is now out of favor. Clements[65] reported that the 10 characteristics most often cited by 100 authors, in order of frequency, were: hyperactivity, perceptual-motor impairments, emotional lability, general coordination deficits, disorders of attention (short attention span, distractability, and perseveration), impulsivity, disorders of memory and thinking, specific learning disorders (reading, writing, arithmetic, spelling), disorders of speech and hearing, and equivocal neurologic signs and EEG irregularities. This complex has been subdivided into the hyperactivity disorder, the attention deficit disorder, specific learning difficulties, and minor motor disabilities that are usually lumped together as "soft signs."[4,59,62-70] However, there is much overlap between these components. Thus, in a study of developmental dyslexia, Critchley[71] found that some presented additional symptoms including disorders of spatial thought and perception, impaired perception of time, mixed cerebral dominance, defects of speech and language, disorders of motility, and poor figure-ground discrimination. Thirty-six percent showed general awkwardness in gesture, gait, and running, all of which are found in profusion in cases of episodic dyscontrol.

Fragments of the syndrome, with or without a proclivity to violence, are encountered in otherwise normal people as well as in some psychopaths, social misfits, intelligent people who have somehow failed to achieve their full potential, and even in individuals of exceptional intellectual or artistic ability.

The clinical identification of some elements of the minimal brain dysfunction syndrome is fraught with difficulties. Adults seldom volunteer accurate information about any delays there may have been in reaching the milestones of their development. Some forget, and others deny. Some who are aware of their problems do not see them as a matter for medical concern, or suppress information about details that are embarrassing to them, such as dyslexia, difficulty in spelling, an inability to catch or hit a ball, or to perform bimanual tasks such as doing up shoelaces or unscrewing the cap off a bottle. Many of these defects are only apparent in real-life situations. In many, there are motor disturbances including dyspraxias and, more often, mild forms of ataxia and clumsiness. Their spontaneous movements may be maladroit, gauche, and lacking in grace.[71] Left-right disorientation, inability to read a map, and mixed cerebral dominance are common. Many are accident prone. All of this can be present against a background of normal or high intelligence.

Multiple defects usually mean multiple sources of chronic stress. Stresses interact with each other and produce more than a simple summation of individual defects, either biologic or environmental,[72] which often lead to chronic irritability or contribute to explosive behavior. In their joint studies of violent delinquents and criminals, Pincus and Lewis[32] found that a paranoid attitude is common. It would seem to be a natural outcome in individuals who have been punished by parents, jeered at by their peers, scolded by their teachers, pursued by truant officers, rejected by members of the opposite sex, and, finally, incarcerated. The converse of these biosocial interactions is seen in the many individuals who had the benefits of a good home, understanding teachers, and good professional guidance, and who, despite their handicaps, made a good adjustment.

Epilepsy and Aggression

The majority of epileptics are not prone to violence or crime, but when we look at people who are subject to recurrent violence, the incidence of epilepsy is greater than in the general population.[32,35,44,73] This applies particularly to temporal lobe epilepsy, but, in addition to the proved cases, some patients report violent interictal episodes, with or without amnesia, that are difficult to identify on clinical grounds unless the evidence of an EEG is positive. The attacks commonly take the form of a brief disturbance in the quality or content of consciousness, with or without amnesia, and can appear without any history of identifiable seizures. To uncover the presence of these attacks is sometimes a formidable task because the violent adolescent's vocabulary is often insufficiently developed to describe their experiences.

Directed violence, with intent to harm or destroy, is a rare epileptic phenomenon; many deny its existence. A more contentious issue is whether an attack of rage associated with partial or complete amnesia can be caused by a focal limbic discharge distinct from epilepsy. Monroe[45] refers to "epileptoid" attacks, and, in the past, others used the term *epileptic equivalents*. There is evidence that epileptic discharges can produce major mood disorders, including rapid cycling depression,[74] and that an attack of rage can end in a convulsion.

Interictal attacks of aggression are not uncommon in temporal lobe epileptics, but the reported prevalence varies with the source of the cases. As is to be expected, it is higher in epileptics who have been committed to institutions, or who have been referred to neurosurgical clinics, than it is in those who have been referred to outpatient clinics. Rodin[75] recorded pathologic aggression in 4.8% of 700 epileptics. Currie et al[76] found it in 7% of 666 cases of temporal lobe epilepsy of mixed origin and type. Bingley,[77] who drew his data from the neurologic and neurosurgical practices of a general hospital in Sweden, found aggressive behavior in 17% of 90 cases. Gastaut et al[78] reported aggression in 50% of their patients with temporal lobe epilepsy. Falconer et al[79] reported interictal aggression in 38% of 50 patients with temporal lobe epilepsy, and a further 15% had a mild, but more persistent, aggressiveness associated with a paranoid outlook.

It seems that there is a relationship between aggressive behavior and temporal lobe epilepsy, but since most temporal lobe epileptics are not violent it is likely, on present evidence, that the seizures and the interictal violence are due to separate processes arising from pathologic lesions in the temporal lobe.[80,81] This is consistent with the experience that in some patients with temporal lobe epilepsy and interictal attacks of episodic dyscontrol, treatment with carbamezepine reduces the seizures, but it may require the addition of propranolol or other medication to the regimen to control the patients' interictal rages.

ENVIRONMENTAL CORRELATES

The current epidemic of both interpersonal and collective violence cannot be due to a sudden proliferation of biologic disorders. It is a result of social conditions and a decline in the power of cultural constraints.

Tidal waves of crime, many decades apart, have been happening in Europe since the 14th century and in America for 200 years[82,83]; the contemporary experience is far from unique. They have occurred during periods of social, economic, and political change, coupled with decline of cultural values. Then, as now, the escalation of violence was accompanied by an erosion of personal integrity, widespread dehumanization, a contempt for life, material greed, corruption in high places, sexual promiscuity, and increased recourse to drugs and alcohol.[84,85]

When what Eibl-Eibesfeldt[86] described as "the cultural corset" is weakened, human behavior tends to regress. The converse is seen in the relative immunity from violence and other disinhibited behaviors enjoyed by communities and nations that have maintained their social, legal, cultural, and moral constraints. The power of these cultural constraints is illustrated by the low rate of interpersonal violence in Japan. In 1980, there was only one murder in Tokyo, and there were only 48 handgun deaths in the whole country.[87] Even mental patients are not immune to the cultural corset. In relatively nonviolent nations, such as Sweden and Britain, violence is far less common in mental hospitals than in American mental institutions.[88]

Under conditions of anomie, aggression proliferates and becomes more savage.[2] Homicides, especially sex-related serial killings, are more often accompanied by mutilation, dismemberment, and cannibalism. Imitation also plays a role in adolescent violence. Thus, in a London borough, there was a small epidemic of attempted and completed adolescent suicide following the exhibition of an educational film that intended to have the opposite effect. Imitation is, of course, a normal feature of youth; but it also occurs as a symptom of prefrontal lesions in adults.[89]

Another aspect of the current epidemic is the emergence of many young people, mainly male, who, although falling short of classical psychopathy, yet exhibit some of its features. They are narcissistic, lacking in altruism and social conscience, impatient, impulsive, and impenitent. They are given to alcohol and drug abuse and to impulsive violence.[90,91] Significantly, during a period of anomie that occurred in Germany after World War I, Reich[92] encountered a similar epidemic in what he described as impulse-driven characters.

In the past, these epidemics have been brought to an end, presumably by the reimposition of the cultural corset and improvement in socioeconomic conditions.

More tangible environmental factors contributing to violence are guns, alcohol, and drugs. With regard to guns, there is little doubt that the rate of death and disablement on the streets and in the home would drop precipitously if effective gun control were introduced. Psychologically and physically, it is much easier to kill with a gun than with a knife, a two-by-four, or by strangulation.

Alcohol, the most used and abused of drugs, once described as "the solvent of the super ego" is a depressant that initially depresses inhibitors and is thus a cause of disinhibited behavior in normal people and, to a greater extent, in individuals with developmental or acquired brain defects. It plays a major role in both street and domestic violence; some women assert that it is only under the influence of alcohol that the aggressor loses control, and, in many violent confrontations, both the aggressor and the victim are under its influence. It is also recognized that the offspring of an alcoholic mother are prone to a variety of defects, including facial deformities, microcephaly, the ADHD syndrome, learning problems, minor motor defects, behavior disorders, or simply a failure to achieve their potential.

The role of street drugs is too immense a subject for this article and for its author, but a comment may be in order with reference to the possible value of marijuana in the treatment of episodic dyscontrol. Patients who have used it unofficially have said that it is much more effective than any of the drugs prescribed by doctors. Its tranquilizing effect is well known in the drug world and was confirmed by a well-documented case of rabies in an individual in whom attacks of dysphagia, terror, and "excitement" were completely brought under control by placing two grains of hashish on the tongue every hour." This was in 1838.[93]

CLINICAL STUDIES

Many studies have addressed the question of what is wrong with "the violent few." The sociologic literature has continued to blame the environment and to ignore biologic factors, whether neurologic, psychiatric, or metabolic. Indeed, Gelles and Strauss[94] listed 15 social theories of violence, none of which include the brain. But as Radzinowicz, doyen of European sociologists, wrote in 1979, after considering the international perspective, "we have no evidence to demonstrate that advances in prosperity, welfare, or education have reduced the incidence of crime or even restrained its rise."[95] However, the hegemony of sociology is being gradually replaced by the view that behavior, including violence, is the result of interactions between biological and environmental variables.[96,97]

This point of view was expressed by Bach-y-Rita et al[35] in 1971 in their landmark report on 130 violent individuals who came to emergency departments in Boston because of fear of going "out of control" and injuring somebody.[35] They presented a consistent picture of homicidal ideation, repeated acts of aggression, impulsivity, multiple traffic citations, and freqent arrests. There was a high incidence of birth injury, mental retardation, periods of unconsciousness, febrile convulsions in infancy, and head injury. Seven of those individuals had a history of temporal lobe epilepsy, and 30 others had had seizurelike episodes of loss of contact with the environment. More than half of the group had a history of hyperactivity or other features of minimal brain dysfunction. Twelve individuals had subnormal IQs, and nine others showed signs of organic impairment on neuropsychologic testing. The EEG was abnormal in 37 of 79 subjects. Their family histories revealed a high incidence of violence and alcoholism, and there was evidence of psychopathology in many. No one was judged to be psychotic.

The authors made two comments that still apply today. First, half of their patients had sought help in the past but they had not received it—they had been rejected by health professionals and by institutions. Second, the authors found themselves as psychiatrists in the invidious position of having to urge on their colleagues a more rigorous neurologic examination in this type of case.

Medical assessment of the delinquent adolescent is seldom well done. Pincus and Lewis[32] examined the pediatric, neurologic, and hospital record data on 20 adolescent boy delinquents and found that "each medical specialty had failed to identify important medical information that might have contributed to difficulties in adaptation," and they also noted that "specialists even failed to obtain data usually considered relevant to their own field of expertise."

Another uncontrolled study was carried out in a psychiatric clinic by Merikangas[98] on 128 violent patients including 16 murderers. Thirty percent were epileptic, 45% had EEG abnormalities, 23% had other neurologic defects, 25% were retarded, and the computed tomographic scan was abnormal in 9% of the patients.

A third uncontrolled study[4] of 286 recurrently violent individuals was unusual in that it involved patients seen in a private neurologic practice who were mainly of middle and upper socioeconomic status; 95% of them were white, and only 10 were incarcerated. The majority were not poor, oppressed, retarded, or uneducated. Thirteen male individuals were responsible for 18 homicides. In 96 cases, recurrent rage was accompanied by additional minor psychopathology (overt psychotics and psychopaths had been excluded from this study). Episodic dyscontrol had developed in 102 formerly stable individuals after a specific brain insult. In some, the lack of control was partial in that the violence was deflected away from its primary object to a surrogate victim—a pet, furniture, windows. There were 119 cases of the minimal brain dysfunction syndrome, 107 cases of seizures, 51 cases of serious head injury, 13 cases of cerebral tumor, 13 cases of encephalitis, 11 cases of stroke, six cases of multiple sclerosis, three cases of Alzheimer's disease, three cases of cardiorespiratory arrest, one case of Huntington's chorea, and one case of proven hypoglycemia. In two of the patients with tumor, the dyscontrol started after a biopsy of the thalamus and the subcallosal cingulate gyrus, respectively. In six others, the dyscontrol commenced some weeks after the successful removal of a benign tumor involving deep midline structures.

Double diagnoses were common (eg, head injury and

seizures). Signs of neuropathology were absent in 18 patients, but in nine of them there was a family history of "a terrible temper" involving two or three generations and affecting about half the siblings in each generation. In 139 cases there was a history of violence in one or more members of a dysfunctional family.

The large number of these patients who had had seizures at some time in their lives was within the same range as those reported by Merikangas[98] and Bach-y-Rita et al.[35] Forty patients had complex partial seizures that were linked to the minimal brain dysfunction syndrome (n=31), to head injury (n=5), to brain tumor (n=5), to encephalitis (n=3) and to multiple sclerosis (a disease in which seizures are normally expected in only 5% to 6%) (n=5/6). The computed tomographic scan was abnormal or questionable in 41% of 145 patients and EEG was abnormal in 64% of 245 patients, with a preponderance of nonspecific activity.

A high prevalence of neurologic disorders has also been found in controlled studies that were submitted to statistical analysis. Monroe[45] carried out a detailed neurologic, neuropsychologic, psychiatric, and sociologic study on 93 incorrigibly violent psychopathic criminals in a maximum security institution. The personality profile of the group was that of the psychopath. Monroe used a neurologic scale including birth data, head injury, epileptoid mechanisms, brain insults, congenital stigmata (minor physical anomalies), hyperacousis, photophobia, hypersensitivity to touch, motor strength, incoordination, and apraxia. There was a correlation at the .001 level between the neurologic scale and violent behavior, and at the .05 level and beyond with a psychiatric history for anger, violent behavior, overreactivity, emotional behavior, poor judgment, poor effort to improve self-defeating actions, lack of responsibility, grandiose illusions, hyperchondriasis, fugue states, and specific health concerns. There was a close correlation with neurotic or antisocial traits in childhood, and there were poor peer relationships in adolescence.

In another controlled study, Levine et al[99] investigated 53 delinquents aged between 11 and 16.5 years and compared them with an age-matched group from the same region to ascertain factors predisposing to delinquency including violent behavior. The mean age of the patients was 15.1 years. Twenty percent of them had been convicted for violence. The investigation covered socioeconomic deprivation, perinatal health stress, illnesses, chronic behavior disorders, family disruptions, failure in school, and neurodevelopmental difficulties interfering with learning and social adjustment. The authors found aggressive acting-out behavior in 100% of the delinquent group and in 16% of control subjects. The former also showed a high level of domestic stress and medical problems, including recurrent otitis media before the age of 3 years in 17% of the delinquents and in none of the control subjects. There was a history of socially aggressive behavior and of many developmental difficulties in communication, mathematics, and writing. They found motor problems in 8% of the delinquents and in 2% of the control subjects.

Lewis et al[100] compared 31 incarcerated delinquents and 31 nondelinquents. In the former, they found a history of abuse in childhood, exposure to family violence, severe psychiatric symptoms, many cognitive impairments, minor neurologic signs, and psychomotor symptoms, which together predicted group members for nearly 84%. The most significant variable was abuse and family violence. Paranoid ideation, loose and illogical thought processes, and suicide attempts also distinguished the delinquents from the nondelinquents. Documented seizures were present in 17% of subjects, choreiform movements in 55%, inability to skip in 26.9%, psychomotor symptoms in 67.8%, and severe head injury in 64.2% of subjects. Major neurologic impairment did not distinguish between the two groups.

Denno[101,102] conducted a unique study of the records of 987 subjects who were born at the Pennsylvania Hospital between 1959 and 1962. This group was initially part of the National Collaborative Perinatal Project. The subjects were nonwhite and predominantly of low socioeconomic status. The sample (487 male and 500 female individuals) had been followed up at intervals from birth until the age of 22 years. The study involved examination of the mothers as soon as they started attending the prenatal clinic. Their pregnancies were supervised, as were labors and deliveries. Each child was examined immediately after birth and at intervals thereafter. Researchers collected socioeconomic and family data when the mothers registered and at the child's seventh year examination. School data were available, focusing on academic achievement during the ages of 13 to 14 years and evidence of learning and behavioral disability during school attendance. Police records were collected for children aged 7 through 22 years. Much information was gathered from extensive home interviews with parents or caretakers. Each child was interviewed 16 times in all and was given pediatric examinations three times in the first 7 years. They all received selective intelligence tests at 7 years of age and achievement tests at the ages of 13 and 14 years. Serum lead level estimations, performed at the age of 7 years, were found to be high in repeat offenders.

This exercise carries with it the authority of facts recorded at the time, thus avoiding the dubious validity of retrospective questionnaires. Of 987 individuals, 151 became offenders by the age of 18 years and nearly one quarter of these were arrested for violent crimes. Five percent of the male sample were chronic offenders, a figure which jibes with those in the study by Tracy et al[2] on a cohort of 10 000 male individuals born in Philadelphia, Pa, in 1945, and with the results of a second study of 27 160 individuals born in Philadelphia in 1958,[2] approximately half of whom were male. In Denno's study,[101,102] the chronic offenders were responsible for 61% of the violent offenses. The neurologic differences between them and the control subjects included higher figures for neurodevelopmental disorders (incoordination, articulation), head injury, and serum lead levels at 7 years.

Denno concluded that "biological and environmental variables exert strong and independent influences on juvenile crime, which appeared to be directly related to familial instability and, most important, a lack of behavioral control associated with central nervous system disorders."[101]

Finally, in contrast to the above is a 15-year psychiatric study of 233 male and 66 female felons, many of whom were parolees. In addition to detailed psychiatric studies, Guze[103] carried out repeated follow-up interviews with the spouses and first-degree relatives, and the case histories included a comprehensive questionnaire on health matters including some neurologic symptoms. However, there was no neurologic examination, neuropsychologic testing, or special studies. The conclusion was: "sociopathy, alcoholism and drug dependence of the psychiatric disorders are characteristically associated with serious crimes; schizophrenia, primary affective disorders, anxiety neurosis, obsession neurosis, phobic neurosis, and brain syndromes are not."[103] Nevertheless, Guze predicted "in time neurobiology will become more influential because environmental influences can be understood completely only if biological variation is studied simultaneously."[103]

CONCLUSION

Seven of these eight samples show a much higher prevalence of overt and covert neurologic and neurophysiologic abnormalities in recurrently violent individuals than in nonviolent control subjects or in the population at large. While it is understandable that their cognitive and other handicaps might give rise to irrascibility and paranoia, it is unlikely that they could produce the intermittent Jekyl-Hyde transformation of the personality, the immense physical strength, and the primitive, even atavistic, behaviors of the dyscontrol syndrome. The latter more closely resemble sham rage resulting from gross lesions of the limbic system and midbrain in animals and man. Is it possible that a more subtle pathologic process is at work, such as the multiple developmental microdysplasias and microaneurysms that Falconer et al[79] found in the temporal lobes of some violently antisocial epileptics and that Galaburda[104] has reported in developmental learning disorders?

The increasing awareness of the close connections between recurrent interpersonal violence and anatomic, chemical, and neurologic abnormalities calls for more participation by neurologists in the assessment and pharmacologic treatment of these patients. Their intervention is particularly desirable in forensic cases, because, as pointed out by psychobiological criminologist D. H. Fishbein, ". . . The unfortunate reality for those who come into the courts by virtue of their dysfunction, however, is that the underlying causes of their disorder are inaccurately evaluated or simply unattended."[105]

References

1. Hamparin DM, Schuster R, Dinstz S, Conrad JP. *The Violent Few: A Study of Violent Offenders.* Lexington, Mass: Lexington Books; 1978.
2. Tracy PE, Wolfgang ME, Figlio RM. *Delinquency in Two Birth Cohorts.* New York, NY: Plenum Press; 1990.
3. Kaplan J. Kopftrauma und Psychosen. *Allg 2 Psychiatrie.* 1899; 56:292-297.
4. Elliott FA. Neurological findings in adult minimal brain dysfunction and the dyscontrol syndrome. *J Nerv Ment Dis.* 1982;170:680-687.
5. Netzky MG, Srobos RR. Neoplasms within the midbrain. *Arch Neurol Psychiatry.* 1952;68:115-125.
6. Cairns H. Mental disorders with tumors of the pons. *Folia Psychiatr Neurol (Netherlands).* 1950;53:193-203.
7. Lassman LP, Arjona VI. Pontine glioma in childhood. *Lancet.* 1967;1:913-915.
8. Smith JS. Episodic rage. In: Girgis M, Kiloh KG, eds. *Limbic Epilepsy and the Dyscontrol Syndrome.* New York, NY: Elsevier North Holland; 1979:255-266.
9. Moyer KE. *The Psychobiology of Aggression.* New York, NY: Harper & Row Publishers Inc; 1976.
10. Valzelli L. *Psychobiology of Aggression and Violence.* New York, NY: Raven Press; 1981.
11. Hamburg DA, Trudeau MB. *Behavioral Aspects of Aggression.* New York, NY: Alan R Liss Inc; 1981.
12. Whalen RE, ed. *The Neuropsychology of Aggression.* In: *Advances in Behavioral Biology.* New York, NY: Plenum Press; 1974;12.
13. Trimble MR. *Biological Psychiatry.* New York, NY: John Wiley & Sons Inc; 1988.
14. Alpers BJ. Relation of the hypothalamus to disorders of personality: report of a case. *Arch Neurol Psychiatry.* 1937;38:291-303.
15. MacLean PD. The triune brain, emotion, and scientific bias. In: Schmitt FD, ed. *The Neurosciences: 2nd Study Program.* New York, NY: Rockefeller University Press;1970:336-349.
16. Zeman I, King FA. Tumor of the septum pellucidum and adjacent structures with abnormal affective behavior: an anterior midbrain structure syndrome. *J Nerv Ment Dis.* 1958;127:490-503.
17. Reeves AC, Plum F. Hyperphagia, rage and dementia accompanying a ventro-medial hypothalamic neoplasm. *Arch Neurol.* 1969;20:616-624.
18. Malamud M. Psychiatric disorders in intracranial tumors of the limbic system. *Arch Neurol.* 1967;17:113-123.
19. Leslie W. Cyst of the cavum vergae. *Can Med Assoc J.* 1940;43:433-439.
20. Elliott FA. Deep midline syndromes. In: Vinken PJ, Bruyn GW, eds. *Handbook of Clinical Neurology.* New York, NY: Wiley Intersciences; 1969;2:758-775.
21. Keschner M, Bender MB, Strauss J. Mental symptoms in cases of sub-tentorial tumor. *Arch Neurol Psychiatry.* 1937;37:1-17.
22. Moruzzi G. [untitled chapter]. In: Dow RS, Moruzzi G, eds. *The Physiology and Pathology of the Cerebellum.* Minneapolis, Minn: University of Minnesota; 1958;125-126.
23. Maiti A, Snider RS. Cerebellar control of basal forebrain structures: amygdala and hippocampus. *Epilepsia.* 1978;10:521-533.
24. Reis DJ, Doba H, Nathan MD. Predatory attack, grooming, and consumatory behaviors elicited by electrical stimulation of cat cerebellar nuclei. *Science.* 1972;182:845-847.
25. Heath RG. Modulation of emotion with a brain pacemaker. *J Nerv Ment Dis.* 1970;168:300-317.
26. Cooper IS. *Cerebellar Stimulation in Man.* New York, NY: Raven Press; 1978.
27. Leiner HC, Leiner AL, Dow RS. Reappraising the cerebellum: what does the hindbrain contribute to the forebrain? *Behav Neurosci.* 1989;103:998-1008.
28. Schmahmann JD. An emerging concept: the cerebellar contribution to higher function. *Arch Neurol.* 1991;48:1178-1187.
29. Linnoila AM, Virkkunen M, Scheinin M, Nuutila A, Rimon R, Goodwin F. Low cerebrospinal fluid 5-hydroxinolol acetic acid concentration differentiates impulsive from non-impulsive violent behavior. *Life Sci.* 1983;33:2609-2614.
30. Brown GL, Goodwin FK. Human aggression: a biological perspective. In: Reid W, Dorr D, Walker SL, Bonner JW, eds. *Unmasking the Psychopath.* New York, NY: WW Norton; 1986:132-156.
31. Stoff DM, Pollock I, Vitiello B, Behar D, Bridges WH. Reduction of (3H)imipramine binding sites on platelets of conduct-disordered children. *Neuropharmacology.* 1987;1:56-62.
32. Pincus JH, Lewis DO. Episodic violence. *Semin Neurol.* 1991;11:146-154.
33. Elliott FA. Neurology of aggression and episodic dyscontrol. *Sem Neurol.* 1990;10:303-312.
34. Wolfgang ME, Ferracuti F. *The Subculture of Violence.* Beverly Hills, Calif: Sage Publications; 1982.
35. Bach-y-Rita G, Lion JR, Climent CF, Ervin FR. Episodic dyscontrol: a study of 130 violent patients. *Am J Psychiatry.* 1971;127:1473-1478.
36. Erez E. Situational or planned crime and the criminal career. In: Wolfgang ME, Thornberry T, Figlio RM, eds. *From Boy to Man, From Delinquency to Crime.* Chicago, Ill: University of Chicago Press; 1987;122-133.
37. West DG, Farrington DP. *The Delinquent Way of Life.* London, England: Heinemann Medical Books; 1977.
38. May PR, Ebaugh FG. Pathological intoxication, alcoholic hallucination, and other reactions to alcohol: a clinical study. *Q J Stud Alcohol.* 1953;14:200-227.
39. Hare RD, McPherson LM. Violent and aggressive behavior by criminal psychopaths. *Int J Law Psychiatry.* 1984;7:35-50.
40. Kraepelin E. *Psychiatrie.* 8th ed. Leipzig, Germany: Barth; 1915.
41. Kegan RG. The child behind the mask: sociopathy as developmental delay. In: Reid WH, Dorr D, Walker JI, Bonner JW, eds. *Unmasking of the Psychopath.* New York, NY: WW Norton; 1986:45-77.
42. Cleckley HM. *The Mask of Sanity.* Revised ed. St Louis, Mo: CV Mosby–Year Book; 1982.
43. Hare RD. Twenty years of experience with the Cleckley psychopath. In: Reid WH, Dorr D, Walker JI, Bonner JW. eds. *Unmasking the Psychopath.* New York, NY: WW Norton; 1986:3-27.
44. Elliott FA. Neurological aspects of antisocial behavior. In Reid WH, ed. *The Psychopath: A Comprehensive Study of Antisocial Disorders and Behaviors.* New York, NY: Brunner/Mazel; 1978:161-189.
45. Monroe RR. *Brain Dysfunction in Aggressive Criminals.* Lexington, Mass: Lexington Books; 1978.
46. Denckla MB. Neurological examination. In: Rapoport JL, ed. *Obsessive-Compulsive Disorder in Children and Adolescents.* Washington, DC: American Psychiatric Press Inc; 1989:107-118.
47. Kaes T. *Die Grosshirnrinde des Menschen in Ihren Wassen und in Ihren Fassengehalt: Ein Gehirn anatomische Atlas.* Jena, Germany: Fischer; 1907.

48. Yakovlev PI, Lecours AR. The myelogenetic cycles of regional maturation of the brain. In: Minkowski A, ed. *Regional Development of the Brain in Early Life.* Philadelphia, Pa: FA Davis; 1967:3-70.
49. Krieger DT, Hughes JC, eds. *Neuroendocrinology.* New York, NY: HP Publishing; 1980.
50. Gorski RA. Sexual differentiation of the brain. In: Krieger DT, Hughes JC, eds. *Neuroendocrinology.* New York, NY: HP Publishing; 1980:215-222.
51. Kagan J. Psychology of sex differences. In: Beach FA, ed. *Human Sexuality in Four Perspectives.* Baltimore, Md: The Johns Hopkins University Press; 1977:87-114.
52. Morton JH, Addison H, Addison RG, Hunt L, Sullivan H. A clinical study of premenstrual tension. *Am J Obstet Gynecol.* 1953;65:1182-1191.
53. Dalton K. *The Premenstrual Syndrome.* Springfield, Ill: Charles C Thomas Publisher; 1964.
54. Schulsinger F. Psychopathy, heredity and environment. In: Mednick SA, Christiansen KO, eds. *Biosocial Bases of Criminal Behavior.* New York, NY: Gardner Press Inc; 1977:109-126.
55. Wilson JQ, Herrnstein RJ. *Crime and Human Nature.* New York, NY: Simon & Schuster; 1985.
56. Ginsberg BE. The violent brain: is it everyone's brain? In: Jeffery CR, ed. *Biology and Crime.* Beverly Hills, Calif: Sage Publications; 1979:47-64.
57. Tellegen A, Lykken DT, Bouchard TJ, Wilcox KJ, Segal NL, Rich S. Personality similarity in twins reared apart and together. *J Pers Soc Psychol.* 1988;54:1031-1039.
58. Davenport CB. The feebly inhibited: violent temper and its inheritance. *J Nerv Ment Dis.* 1915;42:593-609.
59. Barcley RA. *Attention Deficit Hyperactivity Disorder.* New York, NY: Guilford Press; 1990.
60. Stacey W, Shupe A. *The Family Secret: Domestic Violence in America.* Boston, Mass: Beacon Press; 1983.
61. Zametkin AJ, Nordahl TE, Gross M, et al. Cerebral glucose metabolism in adults with hyperactivity of childhood onset. *N Engl J Med.* 1990;323:1361-1366.
62. Denhoff E, Stern L. *Minimal Brain Dysfunction: A Developmental Approach.* New York, NY: Masson Publishing USA Inc; 1979.
63. Hartocollis P. Minimal brain dysfunction in young adults. In: Bellak L, ed. *Psychiatric Aspects of Minimal Brain Dysfunction in Adults.* New York, NY: Grune & Stratton; 1979:103-112.
64. Still GF. Some abnormal psychical conditions in children. *Lancet.* 1902;1:1008-1012, 1077-1082, 1163-1168.
65. Clements SD. *Minimal Brain Dysfunction in Children.* Washington, DC: Department of Health, Education and Welfare; 1966. National Institute of Neurology and Blindness monograph No. 3.
66. Clements SD, Peters J. Minimal brain dysfunction in the school-age child: diagnosis and treatment. *Arch Gen Psychiatry.* 1962;6:185-197.
67. Wender AH. *Minimal Brain Dysfunction in Children.* New York, NY: Wiley Interscience; 1971.
68. Tupper DE, ed. *Soft Neurological Signs.* New York, NY: Grune & Stratton; 1983.
69. Cantwell DP, Baker L. *Psychiatric Developmental Disorders in Children With Communication Disorders.* Washington, DC: American Psychiatric Press Inc; 1991.
70. Gubbay SS. *The Clumsy Child: A Study of Developmental Apraxis and Agnostic Ataxia.* Philadelphia, Pa: WB Saunders Co; 1979.
71. Critchley M. *The Dyslexic Child.* 2nd ed. London, England: Heinemann Medical Books; 1970.
72. Rutter M. *Changing Youth in a Changing Society.* Cambridge, Mass: Harvard University Press; 1980.
73. Pincus JH. Can violence be a manifestation of epilepsy? *Neurology.* 1980;30:304-307.
74. Himmelhoch JM. Major mood disorders related to epileptic changes. In: Blumer D, ed. *Psychiatric Aspects of Epilepsy.* Washington, DC: American Psychiatric Press Inc; 1984:271-294.
75. Rodin EA. Psychomotor epilepsy and aggressive behavior. *Arch Gen Psychiatry.* 1973;28:210-213.
76. Currie S, Heathfield KW, Henson RA, Scott DF. Clinical course and progress of temporal lobe epilepsy: a survey of 666 patients. *Brain.* 1971;94:173-190.
77. Bingley T. Mental symptoms in temporal lobe epilepsy and temporal lobe glioma. *Acta Psychiatr Scand.* 1959;33(suppl 120):1-151.
78. Gastaut C, Morin C, LeSevre N. Etude du comportement des epileptiques psychomoteurs dans l'intervalle de leurs crises. *Ann Med Psychol.* 1955;113:1-29.
79. Falconer MA, Hill D, Meyer A, Wilson JL. Clinical, radiological and EEG correlates with pathological changes in temporal lobe epilepsy, and their significance in surgical treatment. In: Baldwin M, Bailey P, eds. *Temporal Lobe Epilepsy.* Springfield, Ill: Charles C Thomas Publisher; 1958:396-411.
80. Stevens JR, Hermann B. Temporal lobe epilepsy, psychopathology and violence: the state of the evidence. *Neurology.* 1981;31:1127-1132.
81. Fenwick P. Dyscontrol. In: Reynolds EH, Trimble MR, eds. *The Bridge Between Neurology and Psychiatry.* New York, NY: Churchill Livingstone Inc; 1989:263-287.
82. Graham HD, Gurr TR. *Violence in America.* 2nd ed. Beverly Hills, Calif: Sage Publications; 1979.
83. Cohn NR. *The Pursuit of the Millenium.* 2nd ed. New York, NY: Harper & Row Publishers Inc; 1961.
84. Tuchman B. *A Distant Mirror: The Calamitous 14th Century.* New York, NY: Ballantine Books; 1978.
85. Thompson JW. The aftermath of the black death and the aftermath of the great war. *Am J Sociol.* 1920(March):565-572.
86. Eibl-Eibesfeldt I. *The Biology of Peace and War: Men, Animals, and Aggression.* New York, NY: Viking Press; 1979.
87. Goldstein SB, Ibaraki T. Japan: aggression and aggression control in Japanese society. In: Goldstein AP, Segall MH, eds. *Aggression in Global Perspective.* Elmsford, NY: Pergamon Press Inc, 1983:313-324.
88. Lion JR, Reid WH, eds. *Assaults Within Psychiatric Facilities.* New York, NY: Grune & Stratton; 1983.
89. Lhermitte F, Pillon B, Serdaru M. Human autonomy and the frontal lobes, I: imitation and utilisation behavior: a neuropsychological study of 75 patients. *Ann Neurol.* 1986;19:326-334.
90. Wishnie HA, Nevis-Olesen J, eds. *Working With the Impulsive Person.* New York, NY: Plenum Press; 1979.
91. Sanchez J. Social crises and psychopathy. In: Reid W, Dorr D, Walker JW, Bonner S, eds. *Unmasking the Psychopath.* New York, NY: WW Norton; 1986:78-97.
92. Reich W. *The Impulsive Character and Other Writings.* New York, NY: New American Library; 1974.
93. O'Shaughnessy WB. On the preparation of the Indian hemp, or gunjah. In: Mikuriya TH, ed. *Marijuana: Medical Papers [1839-1972].* Oakland, Calif: Medi-Comp Press; 1973:1-30.
94. Gelles RJ, Strauss MA. Determinants of violence in the family: toward a theoretical integration. In: Burr WR, Hill R, Nye FJ, Reiss IL, eds. *Theories About the Family.* New York, NY: Free Press; 1979:549-581.
95. Radzinowicz L, King J. *The Growth of Crime: The International Experience.* New York, NY: Penguin Books; 1979.
96. Wilson JQ, Herrnstein RJ. *Crime and Nature.* New York, NY: Simon & Schuster; 1985.
97. Mednick SA, Christiansen KO. *Biosocial Bases of Criminal Behavior.* New York, NY: Gardner Press Inc; 1977.
98. Merikangas JR. The neurology of violence. In: Merikangas JR, ed. *Brain-Behavior Relationships.* Lexington, Mass: Lexington Books; 1981:155-186.
99. Levine MD, Karniski WM, Palfrey JS, Meltzer LJ, Fenton F. A study of risk complexes in early adolescent delinquency. *Am J Dis Child.* 1985;139:50-56.
100. Lewis DO, Pincus JH, Lovely R, Spitzer E, Moy E. Biopsychosocial characteristics of matched samples of delinquents and nondelinquents. *J Am Acad Child Adolesc Psychiatry.* 1987;26:744-752.
101. Denno DW. Human biology and criminal responsibility: free will or free ride? *Univ Penn Law Rev.* 1988;137:615-671.
102. Denno DW. *Biology and Violence: From Birth to Adulthood.* New York, NY: Cambridge University Press; 1990.
103. Guze SB. *Criminality and Psychiatric Disorders.* New York, NY: Oxford University Press; 1976.
104. Galaburda AM. Neuropathologic correlates of learning disorder. *Semin Neurol.* 1991;11:20-27.
105. Fishbein DH. Biological perspectives in criminology. *Criminology.* 1990;28:27-72.

The Role of a Sleep Disorder Center in Evaluating Sleep Violence

Mark W. Mahowald, MD; Carlos H. Schenck, MD; Gerald M. Rosen, MD; Thomas D. Hurwitz, MD

• To review the state-dependent nature of violence and present a clinically useful classification of sleep violence, this article reviews our experience with sleep-related violence, establishing a differential diagnosis, methods of evaluation, and treatment options. The study occurs in a full-service clinical sleep disorders center evaluating approximately 1000 patients annually with an active participation of 16 physicians representing seven specialties. The patients were self-, physician-, or court/social service-referred for evaluation of violent or injurious behaviors associated with the sleep period. Interventions were dependent on the final diagnosis following clinical and (usually) sleep laboratory evaluation. The main outcome measures were self-reported. During routine clinical evaluations at a multidisciplinary sleep disorder center, it has become apparent that violence is often state-dependent, occurring only during the sleep period, resulting from a number of both neurologic and psychiatric conditions (including malingering and Munchausen syndrome by proxy). In such cases, careful clinical and laboratory evaluation usually results in a specific diagnosis, with effective therapeutic recommendations. Violence may be state-dependent. It is clear that violent behaviors may arise from the sleep period, often without conscious awareness on the part of the subject. This has social, forensic, and clinical implications, and may help contribute to the understanding of violence in general.

(*Arch Neurol.* 1992;49:604-607)

Recent advances in the field of sleep medicine have permitted the identification and characterization of a wide variety of sleep-related disorders that may result in violent or injurious behaviors. The purposes of this article are to: (1) review the state-dependent nature of violence, (2) outline the various sleep-related disorders associated with violence (both cause and effect), (3) emphasize the role of the full-service sleep disorder center in the evaluation and treatment of these disorders, (4) discuss the forensic and social consequences of such behaviors, (5) offer perspectives on the neurobiologic substrates of such behaviors, and (6) underscore the fact that violence may occur in states of being other than wakefulness.

Accepted for publication February 17, 1992.

From the Minnesota Regional Sleep Disorder Center, Hennepin County Medical Center, Minneapolis, and the Departments of Neurology (Dr Mahowald), Psychiatry (Drs Schenck and Hurwitz), and Pediatrics (Dr Rosen), Hennepin County Medical Center and the University of Minnesota, Minneapolis.

Reprint requests to Minnesota Regional Sleep Disorders Center, Hennepin County Medical Center, 701 Park Ave, Minneapolis, MN 55415 (Dr Mahowald).

THE STATE-DEPENDENT NATURE OF VIOLENCE

The concept that sleep is simply the passive absence of wakefulness (W) is no longer tenable. Not only is sleep an active, rather than passive, process, it is now clear that sleep constitutes two completely different states: non-rapid eye movement (NREM) sleep and rapid eye movement (REM) sleep. Therefore, our lives are spent in three entirely different states of being—W, REM sleep, and NREM sleep. Recent studies have indicated that bizarre behavioral syndromes can occur as a result of the incomplete declaration or rapid oscillation of these states.[1] Although many "mixed states" are relatively benign (eg, narcolepsy), others may be associated with violent behaviors.

SLEEP-RELATED DISORDERS ASSOCIATED WITH VIOLENCE

Violent sleep-related behaviors have been recently reviewed in the context of automatized behavior in general.[2] There are well-documented cases of: (1) somnambulistic homicide, attempted homicide, and suicide; (2) murders and other crimes with sleep drunkenness (confusional arousals); and (3) sleep terrors/sleepwalking with potential violence/injury. A wide variety of disorders may result in sleep-related violence. These are best classified under two categories: neurologic and psychiatric, as outlined in the Table.

NEUROLOGIC

Disorders of Arousal

The disorders of arousal comprise a spectrum ranging from confusional arousals (sleep drunkenness) to sleepwalking (SW) to sleep terrors (ST).[3,4] Although there is usually amnesia for the event[5,6] vivid dreamlike mentation may be experienced and reported.[7] Contrary to popular opinion, these disorders may actually begin in adulthood, and are most often not associated with psychopathology.[7,8] The commonly held belief that SW/ST are always benign is erroneous: the accompanying behaviors may be violent, resulting in considerable injury to the individual, others, or damage to the environment.[2,7]

Sleep-Related Violent Behavior
Neurologic
1. Disorders of arousal
Confusional arousals (sleep drunkenness)
Sleepwalking/sleep terrors
2. Rapid eye movement sleep disorder
3. Nocturnal seizures
Psychogenic
1. Dissociative disorders (fugues/multiple personality disorder)
2. Malingering
3. Munchausen syndrome by proxy

Febrile illness, alcohol, prior sleep deprivation, and emotional stress may serve to trigger ST/SW in susceptible individuals.[9-11] Medications such as sedative/hypnotics, neuroleptics, minor tranquilizers, stimulants, and antihistamines, often in combination with each other or with alcohol, may also play a role.[12-14]

Confusional arousals (sleep drunkenness) occur during the transition between sleep and wakefulness and represent a disturbance of cognition and attention despite the motor behavior of wakefulness, resulting in complex behavior without conscious awareness.[15-17] These may be potentiated by prior sleep deprivation or the ingestion of alcohol or sedative/hypnotics before sleep onset.[18] These episodes of "automatic behavior" occur in the setting of chronic sleep deprivation or other conditions associated with state admixture (shoplifting has been reported during a period of automatic behavior in a narcoleptic.)[19-21] Patients suffering from obstructive sleep apnea may experience frequent arousals that may serve to trigger arousal-induced precipitous motor activity.[22]

Treatment of simple ST/SW is often not necessary. Reassurance may be sufficient. In cases of potential violence or severe disruption of other household members, effective treatment has been reported with benzodiazepines, tricyclic antidepressants, psychotherapy, progressive relaxation, and hypnosis.[7,23] The avoidance of drugs, alcohol, and sleep deprivation is also important.

REM Sleep Behavior Disorder (RBD)

Rapid eye movement sleep behavior disorder represents an experiment of nature, predicted in 1965 by animal experiments,[24] recently identified in humans.[20,25] Normally, during REM sleep, there is active paralysis of all somatic muscles (sparing the diaphragm and eye movement muscles). In RBD, there is the compromise of REM sleep atonia, which permits the "acting out" of dreams, often with dramatic and violent or injurious behaviors. The oneiric (dream) behavior displayed by these patients is often misdiagnosed as manifestations of a seizure or psychiatric disorder. The RBD is usually idiopathic, but may be associated with underlying neurologic disorders.[26] The overwhelming male predominance (90%) of RBD[27] raises interesting questions relating sex hormones to aggression and violence.[28,29] The violent and injurious nature of RBD behaviors has been extensively reviewed elsewhere.[7,20,25,26] Treatment with clonazepam is highly effective, with sustained response in 90% of patients.[27]

Nocturnal Seizures

The association between seizures and violence has been long debated. It is plain that, on occasion, seizures may be exclusively or predominantly nocturnal, and result in violent or injurious behaviors.[2,7] Of particular note is the frantic and elaborate nocturnal motor activity that may result from seizures originating in the orbital, mesial, or prefrontal region.[30-35] "Episodic nocturnal wanderings," a condition clinically indistinguishable from other forms of sleep-related motor activity such as complex sleepwalking, but that is responsive to anticonvulsant therapy, has also been described.[36,37] The treatment of nocturnal seizures is similar to that of diurnal seizures.

PSYCHIATRIC

Dissociative Disorders

Waking dissociative states may result in violence, such as genital self-mutilation.[38] It is now apparent that dissociative disorders may arise predominantly from the sleep period.[7,39,40] Virtually all patients with nocturnal dissociative disorders evaluated at our center were victims of repeated physical and/or sexual abuse beginning in childhood. Diurnal diagnoses included psychogenic amnesia, multiple personality disorder, and dissociative disorder–not otherwise specified.[41] Specialized psychiatric interventions have been developed in treating dissociative disorders.[42]

Malingering

Although uncommon, malingering must also be considered in cases of apparent sleep-related violence. Our center has recently seen a young adult man who developed progressively more violent behaviors, apparently arising from sleep, directed exclusively at his wife. This behavior included beating her and chasing her with a hammer. Extensive neurologic, psychiatric, and polysomnographic evaluations were unrevealing. It was felt that this behavior represented malingering.

Munchausen Syndrome by Proxy

In this recently described syndrome, a child is reported to have apparently serious medical symptoms, which, in fact, are induced by an adult, usually a caregiver, and often a parent. These children may present to a sleep disorders center for evaluation of apnea, seizures, unusual nocturnal spells, or excessive daytime sleepiness. Surreptitious video monitoring in a sleep laboratory during sleep (with the parent present) has provided essential documentation of the true cause for reported symptoms.[43-45] When the cause of the problem has been identified, child protection agencies should be notified and immediate psychiatric evaluation for the perpetrator should be available.

PERSPECTIVES

The fact that violent or injurious behaviors may arise in the absence of conscious wakefulness raises the crucial question of how such complex behavior can occur. Examination of extensive animal experimental studies provides preliminary answers. The widely held concept that the brain stem and other more "primitive" neural structures primarily participate in elemental/vegetative rather than behavioral activities is inaccurate. There are overwhelming amounts of data documenting that extremely complex emotional and motor behaviors can originate from these more primitive structures—without involvement of "higher" neural structures such as the cortex.[46-52]

Extrapolating from animal data to the human condition,

it has been shown that structural lesions at multiple levels of the nervous system may result in wakeful violence.[53] The animal data provide insights to violent behaviors in the disorders of arousal, RBD, and sleep-related seizures: (1) ST/SW: The behavioral similarities between documented ST/SW violence in humans and "sham rage" as seen in the "hypothalamic savage" syndrome are striking.[54] Although it has been assumed that the "sham rage" animal preparations are "awake," there is some suggestion that similar preparations are behaviorally awake, and yet (partially) physiologically asleep, with apparent "hallucinatory" behavior possibly representing REM sleep dreaming occurring during W, dissociated from other REM state markers.[55] (2) RBD: The oneiric behavior demonstrated by cats with bilateral lesions in the vicinity of the locus coeruleus and by humans with spontaneously occurring RBD clearly arises from and continues to occur *during* REM sleep.[24,26,56] (3) Seizures: Seizure activity arising in the limbic system may spread to other more "primitive" structures, with resultant clinical behaviors, without electroencephalographic involvement of the neocortex.[50]

The prosencephalic system may serve to control and elaborate, rather than initiate, behaviors originating from deeper structures.[51] In confusional arousals (sleep drunkenness) in humans that can result in confusion or aggression, there is clear electroencephalographic evidence of rapid oscillations between W and sleep.[16,17] It may be that such behaviors occurring in states other than W are the expression of motor/affective activity generated by lower structures—unmonitored and unmodified by the cortex.

Other, very important factors beyond the scope of this review include: (1) the known effect of genetics on violence and (2) the well-demonstrated effects of environmental and social factors on the structure and function of the nervous system.[57] The plasticity of the nervous system is greater than previously thought.[58,59] These factors are undoubtedly operant in both wakeful and sleep-related violence.

Keeping in mind not only that sleep is a very active process but that the generators or effectors of many components of both REM and NREM sleep reside in the brain stem and other "lower" centers, it is not surprising that, during sleep, prominent motoric and affective behaviors do occur.

CLINICAL AND LABORATORY EVALUATION OF WAKING, SLEEP/VIOLENCE

The history of complex, violent, or potentially injurious motor behavior arising from the sleep period should suggest the possibility of one of the above-mentioned conditions. Our experience with over 150 adult cases of sleep-related injury/violence has repeatedly indicated that clinical differentiation, without PSG study, among RBD, sleep terror/somnambulism, nocturnal seizures, sleep apnea, and sleep-related psychogenic dissociative states may be impossible.[1,2,7] These behaviors may also become manifest during hospitalization, particularly in the intensive care unit setting.[60]

These conditions are diagnosable and most are treatable. Clinical evaluation should include a complete review of sleep/wake complaints from both the victim and the bedpartner (if available). This should be followed by thorough physical, neurologic, and psychiatric examinations. The diagnosis may only be suspected clinically. Extensive polygraphic study employing an extensive scalp electroencephalogram at a paper speed of 15 mm/s, electromyographic monitoring of all four extremities, and continuous audiovisual recording are mandatory for correct diagnosis in cases of sleep-injury/violence.[2,3,7] Clinical and laboratory evaluations are best performed by experienced clinicians. Due to the complex nature of many of these disorders, a multidisciplinary approach is invaluable.

LEGAL EVALUATION OF SLEEP/VIOLENCE

Sleep-related behaviors may lead to accusations of domestic (spouse/child) abuse or other criminal acts. As with automatic behaviors arising from wakefulness, the identification of a specific underlying neurologic or psychiatric sleep/violence condition does not establish causality for any given act. Guidelines for the determination of the putative role of an underlying sleep disorder in a specific violent act have been outlined elsewhere.[2]

SUMMARY AND IMPLICATIONS

It is abundantly clear that violence may occur during any one of the three states of being. That which occurs during REM or NREM sleep may have occurred without conscious awareness and is due to one of a number of completely different disorders. The majority of these conditions are diagnosable and, more importantly, are treatable. The social and legal implications are obvious.

More research, both basic science and clinical, is urgently needed to further identify and elaborate on the components of both waking and sleep-related violence, with particular emphasis on neurobiologic, neuroplastic, genetic, and socioenvironmental factors. The study of violence and aggression will be greatly enhanced by close cooperation among clinicians, basic science researchers, and social scientists.

This work was supported by a grant from Hennepin Faculty Associates, Minneapolis, Minn.

We are indebted to our tireless polysomnographic technologists and to Traci Oletzke for secretarial support.

References

1. Mahowald MW, Schenck CH. Status dissociatus: a perspective on states of being. *Sleep.* 1991;14:6979.
2. Mahowald MW, Bundlie SR, Hurwitz TD, Schenck CH. Sleep violence: forensic science implications: polygraphic and video documentation. *J Forensic Sci.* 1990;35:413-432.
3. Mahowald MW, Schenck CS. Parasomnia purgatory: the epileptic/non-epileptic parasomnia interface. In: Rowan AJ, Gates JR, eds. *The Dilemma of Non-Epileptic (Pseudoepileptic) Seizures.* Stoneham, Mass: Butterworths. In press.
4. Mahowald MW, Rosen GM. Parasomnias in children. *Pediatrician.* 1990;17:21-31.
5. Fisher C, Kahn E, Edwards A, Davis DM, Fine J. A psychophysiological study of nightmares and night terrors, III: mental content and recall of stage 4 night terrors. *J Nerv Ment Dis.* 1974;158:174-188.
6. Thorn MJ, ed. *International Classification of Sleep Disorders: Diagnostic and Coding Manual.* Lawrence, Kan: Allen Press: 1990:142-150.
7. Schenck CH, Milner D, Hurwitz TD, Bundlie SR, Mahowald MW. A polysomnographic and clinical report on sleep-related injury in 100 adult patients. *Am J Psychiatry.* 1989;146:1166-1173.
8. Hartmann E, Greenwald D, Brune P. Night-terrors-sleep walking: personality characteristics. *Sleep Res.* 1982;11:121.
9. Vela Bueno A, Blanco BD, Cajal FV. Episodic sleep disorder triggered by fever: a case presentation. *Waking Sleeping.* 1980;4:243-251.
10. Bonkalo A. Impulsive acts and confusional states during incomplete arousal from sleep: criminological and forensic implications. *Psychiatric Q.* 1974;48:400-409.
11. Raschka LB. Sleep and violence. *Can J Psychiatry.* 1984;29:132-134.
12. Luchins DJ, Sherwood PM, Gillin JC, Mendelson WB, Wyatt RJ.

Filicide during psychotropic-induced somnambulism: a case report. *Am J Psychiatry.* 1978;135:1404-1405.
13. Huapaya LVM. Seven cases of somnambulism induced by drugs. *Am J Psychiatry.* 1979;136:985-986.
14. Charney DS, Kales A, Soldatos CR, Nelson JC. Somnambulistic-like episodes secondary to combined lithium-neuroleptic treatment. *Br J Psychiatry.* 1979;135:418-424.
15. Lipowski ZJ. Delirium (acute confusional state). *JAMA.* 1987;258:1789-1792.
16. Guilleminault C, Phillips R, Dement WC. A syndrome of hypersomnia with automatic behavior. *EEG Clin Neurophysiol.* 1975;38:403-413.
17. Roth B, Nevsimalova S, Sagova V, Paroubkova D, Horakova A. Neurological, psychological and polygraphic findings in sleep drunkenness. *Arch Suisses Neurol, Neurochir, Psychiatr.* 1981;129:209-222.
18. Roth B, Nevsimalova S, Rechtschaffen A. Hypersomnia with 'sleep drunkenness.' *Arch Gen Psychiatry.* 1972;26:456-462.
19. Zorick FJ, Salis PJ, Roth T, Kramer M. Narcolepsy and automatic behavior: a case report. *J Clin Psychiatry.* 1979;40:194-197.
20. Mahowald MW, Schenck CS. REM s1eep behavior disorder. In: Kryger M, Dement W, Roth T, eds. *Principles and Practice of Sleep Medicine.* Philadelphia, Pa: WB Saunders Co; 1989:389-401.
21. Parkes JD. *Sleep and Its Disorders.* Philadephia, Pa: WB Saunders Co; 1985.
22. Guilleminault C, Silvestri R. Disorders of arousal and epilepsy during sleep. In: Sterman MB, Shouse MN, Passouant P, eds. *Sleep and Epilepsy.* Orlando, Fla: Academic Press Inc; 1982;513-531.
23. Hurwitz, TD, Mahowald MW, Schenck CH, Schluter JL, Bundlie SR. A retrospective outcome study and review of hypnosis as treatment of adults with sleepwalking and sleep terror. *J Nerv Ment Dis.* 1991;179:228-233.
24. Jouvet M, Delorme F. Locus coeruleus et sommeil paradoxal. *C R Soc Biol.* 1965;159:895-899.
25. Schenck CH, Bundlie SR, Patterson AL, Mahowald MW. Rapid eye movement sleep behavior disorder: a treatable parasomnia affecting older adults. *JAMA.* 1987;257:1786-1789.
26. Mahowald MW, Schenck CS. REM-sleep behavior disorder. In: Thorpy MJ, ed. *Handbook of Sleep Disorders.* New York, NY: Marcel Dekker; 1990:567-593.
27. Schenck CS, Mahowald MW. Polysomnographic, neurologic, psychiatric, and clinical outcome report on 70 consecutive cases with the REM sleep behavior disorder (RBD): sustained clonazepam efficacy in 89.5% of 57 treated patients. *Cleve Clin J Med.* 1990;57:s10-s24.
28. Goldstein M. Brain research and violent behavior. *Arch Neurol.* 1974;30:1-34.
29. Moyer KE. Kinds of aggression and their physiological basis. *Comm Behav Biol.* 1968;2:65-87.
30. Collins RC, Carnes KM, Price JL. Prefrontal-limbic epilepsy: experimental functional anatomy. *J Clin Neurophysiol.* 1988;5:105-117.
31. Quesney LF, Krieger C, Leitner C, Gloor P, Olivier A. Frontal lobe epilepsy: clinical and electrographic presentation. In: Porter RJ, Mattson RH, Ward AA Jr, Dam M, eds. *Advances in Epileptology.* New York, NY: Raven Press; 1984:503-508.
32. Ludwig B, Ajmone Marsan C, Van Buren J. Cerebral seizures of probable orbitofrontal origin. *Epilepsia.* 1975;16:141-158.
33. Waterman K, Purves SJ, Kosaka B, Strauss E, Wada JA. An epileptic syndrome caused by mesial frontal lobe seizure foci. *Neurology.* 1987;37:577-582.
34. Tharp B. Orbital frontal seizures: an unique electroencephalographic and clinical syndrome. *Epilepsia.* 1972;13:627-642.
35. Williamson PD, Spencer SS. Clinical and EEG features of complex partial seizures of extratemporal origin. *Epilepsia.* 1986; 27(suppl 2):s46-s63.
36. Maselli RA, Rosenberg RS, Spire JP. Episodic nocturnal wanderings in non-epileptic young patients. *Sleep.* 1988;11:156-161.
37. Pedley TA, Guilleminault C. Episodic nocturnal wanderings responsive to anticonvulsant drug therapy. *Ann Neurol.* 1977;2:30-35.
38. McCaldon RJ. Automatism. *Can Med Assoc J.* 1964;91:914-920.
39. Fleming J. Dissociative episodes presenting as somnambulism: a case report. *Sleep Res.* 1987;16:263.
40. Braun BG, ed. Multiple personality. *Psychiatr Clin North Am.* 1984;7:1-198.
41. Schenck CH, Milner DM, Hurwitz TD, Bundlie SR, Mahowald MW. Dissociative disorders presenting as somnambulism: polygraphic, video, and clinical documentation (eight cases). *Dissociation.* 1989;2: 194-204.
42. Putnam FW. *Diagnosis and Treatment of Multiple Personality Disorder.* New York, NY: Guilford Press; 1989.
43. Rosenberg DA. Web of deceit: a literature review of Munchausen syndrome by proxy. *Child Abuse Neglect.* 1987;11:547-563.
44. Light MJ, Sheridan MS. Munchausen syndrome by proxy and apnea. *Clin Pediatr.* 1990;29:162-168.
45. Griffith JC, Slovik LS. Munchausen syndrome by proxy and sleep disorders medicine. *Sleep.* 1989;12:178-183.
46. Grillner S, Dubic R. Control of locomotion in vertebrates: spinal and supraspinal mechanisms. *Adv Neurology.* 1988;47:425-453.
47. Cohen AH. Evolution of the vertebrate central pattern generator for locomotion. In: Cohen AH, Rossignol S, Grillner S, eds. Neural Control of Rhythmic Movements in Vertebrates. New York, NY: John Wiley & Sons Inc; 1988:129-166.
48. Corner MA. Brainstem control of behavior: ontogenetic aspects. In: Klemm R, Vertes RP, eds. *Brainstem Mechanisms of Behavior.* New York, NY: John Wiley & Sons Inc, New York, NY: 1990:239-266.
49. Siegel A, Pott CB. Neural substrates of aggression and flight in the cat. *Prog Neurobiol.* 1988;31:261-283.
50. LeDoux JE. Emotion. In: Montcastle VB, Plum F, Geiger SR, eds. *Handbook of Physiology: The Nervous System: Higher Functions of the Brain, Part I.* Baltimore, Md: Williams & Wilkins; 1987:419-459.
51. Berntson GG, Micco DJ. Organization of brainstem behavioral systems. *Brain Res Bull.* 1976;1:471-483.
52. Bandler R. Brain mechanisms of aggression as revealed by electrical and chemical stimulation: suggestion of a central role for the midbrain periaqueductal grey region. *Prog Psychobiol Physiol Psychol.* 1988;13:67-154.
53. Weiger WA, Bear DM. An approach to the neurology of aggression. *J Psychiatr Res.* 1988;22:85-98.
54. Glusman M. The hypothalamic 'savage' syndrome. *Assoc Res Nerv Ment Dis.* 1974;52:52-92.
55. Kitsikis A, Steriade M. Immediate behavioral effects of kainic acid injections into the midbrain reticular core. *Behav Brain Res.* 1981;3:361-380.
56. Hendricks JC, Morrison AR, Mann GL. Different behaviors during paradoxical sleep without atonia depend on pontine lesion site. *Brain Res.* 1982;239:81-105.
57. Valzelli L. *Psychobiology of Aggression and Violence.* New York, NY: Raven Press; 1981.
58. Pons TP, Garraghty PE, Ommaya K, Kaas JH, Taub E, Mishkin M. Massive cortical reorganization after sensory deafferentation in adult macaques. *Science.* 1991;252:1857-1860.
59. Edelman GM. *Neural Darwinism.* New York, NY: Basic Books; 1987.
60. Schenck CS, Mahowald MW. Injurious sleep behavior disorders (parasomnias) affecting patients on intensive care units. *Intensive Care Med.* 1991;17:219-224.

Murder, Insanity, and Medical Expert Witnesses

J. Richard Ciccone, MD

• Recent advances in the ability to study brain anatomy and function and attempts to link these findings with human behavior have captured the attention of the legal system. This had led to the increasing use of the "neurological defense" to support a plea of not guilty by reason of insanity. This article explores the history of the insanity defense and explores the role of the medical expert witnesses in integrating clinical and laboratory findings, eg, computed tomographic scans, magnetic resonance scans, and single-photon emission computed tomographic scans. Three cases involving murder and brain dysfunction are discussed: the first case involves a subarachnoid hemorrhage resulting in visual perceptual and memory impairment; the second case, a diagnosis of Alzheimer's disease; and the third case, the controverted diagnosis of complex partial seizures in a serial killer.

(*Arch Neurol.* 1992;49:608-611)

For centuries, the courts have relied on the testimony of expert witnesses.[1] The expert witness is an individual, who as a result of training or specialized experience, possesses knowledge that is not available to the court through usual experience. Forensic medicine dates back to early Egyptian times. Physicians in Greece and Rome testified on medicolegal issues. In 1507, the bishop of Bamberg wrote a penal code (*Les Bambergensis*) that called for physicians to testify in cases of violent death. In 1602, Fortunatis Fidelis of Italy, a leader in the development of forensic medicine, published a text on forensic medicine.[2]

While some have suggested that physicians avoid working with the legal system, others have held that the value of the medical expert witness to the legal process justifies continuing the effort to bring medical information to the courts.[3] The medical expert provides an opinion that the court may give greater or lesser weight depending on the expert's training and experience, the nature and extent of the diagnostic process, and the quality of the reasoning used to arrive at clinical conclusions and legally relevant opinions.

The advances in diagnostic procedures to study brain anatomy and function and attempts to link the findings to human behavior have captured the attention of the legal system. An increasing number of defendants are turning to the "neurological defense" to substantiate a plea of not guilty by reason of insanity (*The Wall Street Journal*. March 4, 1992:A1, A6). One of the most public and, at times, dramatic settings for expert witness testimony is at a murder trial where the insanity defense is at issue. In the majority of cases, the medical experts agree on the diagnosis and on whether or not the accused meets the criteria required to be found lacking criminal responsibility. When the experts agree, there is no "battle." Where there is disagreement, the defense attorney tries to prove that the accused lacked criminal responsibility and the prosecution attorney tries to refute that assertion.

The courts understand that physicians use medical diagnosis as an organizing concept for clinical purposes; however, the courts are much more interested in the signs and symptoms of the disorder. The courts use this information to decide if a legal mental disease or defect exists for the purpose of determining criminal responsibility. Judge Bazelon defined a legal mental disease or defect as ". . . any abnormal condition of the mind which substantially affects mental or emotional processes and substantially impairs behavior controls."[4] The purpose of this article is to discuss the development of the modern insanity defense and to explore the role of the medical expert witness when the accused may suffer from neurologic and psychiatric disorders.

HISTORY OF THE INSANITY DEFENSE

A basic tenet of our legal system is that one must be found blameworthy before punishment may be imposed; therefore, the courts distinguish between those who are responsible for their acts and those who are excused of responsibility. A major crime has two elements. First, there must be an *actus reus* (criminal act). The act must be conscious and voluntary; an act that is the result of automatism, somnambulism, or epilepsy is technically not an act. Second, there must be a *mens rea* (criminal intent). The act must be knowingly or purposely committed.

The tests for criminal responsibility gradually evolved. Henry Bracton, in 1268, merged the strict liability of secular law with the moral intent of church law, bringing the intent component (*mens rea*) to the common law.

The English jurist William Lombarde (1536-1601) wrote, "If a madman or natural fool, or a lunatic in the time of his lunacy, or a child that apparently hath no knowledge of good nor evil do kill a man, there is no felonious act . . .

Accepted for publication March 9, 1992.

From the Psychiatry and Law Program, University of Rochester (NY) School of Medicine and Dentistry.

Reprint requests to 300 Crittenden Blvd, Rochester, NY 14642 (Dr Ciccone).

for they cannot be said to have any understanding will." In 1723, Justice Tracey wrote his criteria of responsibility, the *Wild Beast Test*. "It must be a man that is totally deprived of his understanding and memory, and doth not know what he is doing, no more than an infant, than a brute, or a wild beast—such a one is never the object of punishment."[5]

In 1843, Daniel McNaughton shot and killed Edward Drummond, secretary to the British prime minister, Sir Robert Peel. McNaughton was found not guilty by reason of insanity. In response to the public outcry at the verdict, the 15 judges of the Queen's Bench were convened. The *McNaughton Test*, the *Right and Wrong Test*, emerged.[6] For a finding of insanity, ". . . it must be clearly proved that, at the time of committing the act, the party accused was laboring under such a defect of reason, from disease of the mind, as not to know the nature and quality of the act he was doing; or if he did know it that he did not know he was doing wrong. . . ."

The nature of the act refers to the physical characteristics of the act, ie, a knife cuts, a gun fires a bullet. The quality of the act refers to the harmfulness of the act, ie, a cut can cause one to bleed to death, a gunshot can kill. These standards have a low threshold, and the issue of criminal responsibility usually turns on whether the individual could distinguish between right and wrong or knew that the particular act was considered wrong by society. Most courts have interpreted "to know" to include both cognitive and affective appreciation of the particular act.

The *McNaughton Test* was quickly and widely adopted in the United States. With some modifications, the McNaughton Test still endures in many jurisdictions. Other jurisdictions have adopted a portion of the *American Law Institute Test*: "A person is not responsible for his criminal conduct if at the time of such conduct, as a result of mental disease or defect he lacks substantial capacity to conform his conduct to the requirements of law." Throughout its history, the insanity defense has been under attack and, in repeated surveys, fewer than 25% of those polled supported the existence of the insanity defense. The American Bar Association, Chicago, Ill, and others have held that the maintenance of the insanity defense is vital to the moral integrity of the law.[3]

CASES INVOLVING MEDICAL EXPERT TESTIMONY

The study of episodic violence has sought to link brain dysfunction with the aggressive behavior. The results of positron emission tomographic scans, computed tomographic scans, magnetic resonance imaging scans, computerized electroencephalograms, and cerebral angiography may provide vivid images that may dazzle the jury. Neuropsychiatric testing may also lead to pages of seemingly "objective" evidence. However, there is substantial controversy whether a test result, eg, a computed tomographic scan, can be linked to a specific behavioral disorder. While medicine energetically moves forward in its effort to understand aggressive behavior, the courts must continue to approach new medical findings cautiously until there is "virtually certain reliability."[7] The court must determine whether the medical findings in a particular case explain and excuse the behavior at issue or whether the medical findings are not linked significantly to the crime. The court will review all the information about the defendant's history, his behavior around the time of the crime, and other relevant facts put before the court by the attorneys. Legal tests of insanity require a clear and direct link between the significant neurologic and/or psychiatric pathologic findings and the illegal act. The link must include a major impairment in the defendant's ability to undertake a conscious, voluntary, or a knowing or purposeful act.

REPORT OF CASES

CASE 1.—A 62-year-old, retired father of five, had a history of hypertension and diabetes mellitus. Five years earlier, he had a subarachnoid hemorrhage secondary to an arteriovenous malformation. A computed tomographic scan at the time of the stroke demonstrated blood in the fourth, third, and both lateral ventricles. The ventricles were of normal size, excluding the temporal horns, which were slightly dilated. There was more blood on the left side, especially in the left thalamic region. A cerebroangiogram showed an arteriovenous malformation, fed by both anterior cerebral arteries and the left middle cerebral artery involving the splenum of the corpus callosum of the left thalamus. He regained consciousness after 3 weeks, and, at discharge from the hospital, he had profound memory impairment and confusion.

He returned home, where he showed modest improvement. He had difficulty remembering things, was very concrete, and was very argumentative with his wife. He eventually decided that she was abusing him and trying to hurt him. He purchased a shotgun. A few days later, he went to the church where his wife was attending services to look for her. In the church parking lot, he spotted a woman of similar age and stature who he mistook for his wife. As he approached the woman with his shotgun, she attempted to lock the doors of the car; he shot her through the windshield. He went home and called the police to report he had killed his wife.

Only after his arrest did he learn that he had mistakenly shot another woman. Neuropsychiatric testing demonstrated a marked inability to move flexibly from one idea to another, visual perceptual impairment, and marked verbal and nonverbal memory impairment, both short term and intermediate.

The expert witnesses retained by the prosecution and the defense essentially agreed on their interpretations of clinical findings and the results of the computed tomographic scan and neuropsychiatric testing. He had a subarachnoid bleed that resulted in cognitive and behavioral changes. The court found that he was too impaired to be found fully responsible and convicted of murder but had sufficient capacity to be found responsible for the lesser charge of manslaughter.

CASE 2.—A 79-year-old married, retired businessman was charged with murdering his wife. He suffered from chronic obstructive pulmonary disease but was otherwise in good health, until approximately 4 years before his arrest. At that time, his family began to notice that he was increasingly seclusive and suspicious as well as forgetful about collecting moneys owed him and paying his bills. His family felt it was no longer safe for him to drive and took his car keys. He developed episodes of fecal and urinary incontinence. His vision was failing, and he believed that this was proof that he had colon cancer.

Early one morning, while in their kitchen, he stabbed his wife in the chest. She ran out of the house to a neighbor, who called the police. As the police arrived, he went outside to find out what was going on. Following his arrest, he was evaluated and diagnosed as having primary degenerative dementia, Alzheimer's type, with severe impairment of attention/concentration, learning and memory, and abstraction. His intact orientation and language function belied the severity and global nature of his impairment. An electroencephalogram was performed that showed a marked reduction in alpha activity with diffuse slow waves. A computed tomographic scan was within normal limits.

There was agreement that the history, clinical examination, and laboratory tests pointed to a diagnosis of Alzheimer's disease. The expert witnesses then had to apply the data to the legal test for responsibility. While the vague wording of the tests for lack of responsibility require that the expert work with uncertainty, not an unfamiliar position for the clinician when providing an opinion, the wording does provide the court with necessary flexibility to apply the law to the particular facts of the case. The expert witness disagreed as to the extent of his clinical impairments, but there was agreement that he lacked substantial capacity to meet the requirements of the law and should be found not responsible.

CASE 3.—A 44-year-old married individual was charged with the serial killing of 10 women over a period of 2 years. As an adolescent, he had three separate head injuries with periods of unconsciousness. One head injury included a right-sided skull fracture. He had academic and behavioral problems in high school and left before graduating. Soon after he burglarized a store. After serving in the army, he returned home and burglarized a gas station and committed arson. After serving time in prison he was paroled. Less than a year later he was arrested for killing two children. He served 15 years after pleading guilty to manslaughter. Within a year of being placed on parole, the killings began.

All of the women were prostitutes whose bodies were found in deserted settings. Some of the corpses had been mutilated. The patient reported little or no memory of the killings. He described uncontrollable rage. This led to an exploration of his amnesia and the possible role of a neurologic disorder. An electroencephalogram with nasopharyngeal leads was done and reported normal. A computed electroencephalogram was read by one neurologist to show paroxysmal irritative patterns in the bifrontotemporal areas, more on the right side. A computed tomographic scan showed minimal enlargement of his left lateral ventricle. A magnetic resonance scan was noted to show an old healed, right frontal skull fracture and a cystic lesion in the anterior portion of the right temporal lobe. A single-photon emission computed tomographic scan revealed bilateral scarring of the frontal white matter, more prominent on the left side.

One medical expert witness concluded that the patient's history of head injuries, lack of memory, and rage, along with the laboratory findings, indicated that the murders occurred during the automatism of a complex partial seizure.

The other medical expert witness disagreed and diagnosed malingering. In addition to a lack of history of seizures, there was evidence pointing to sexual sadism and necrophilic activity. The patient was apprehended, after months of an intensive police search, when he returned to the body of one of his victims. In addition, he resisted the urge to kill other potential victims because there were other people nearby. The court found him guilty of murder.

COMMENT

Each of the cases involved the use of medical expertise in assessing the behavior of individuals where there was a question of neurologic and psychiatric impairments. In the case of patient 1, who shot a woman he mistook for his wife, the medical expert is asked to provide an opinion, if possible, to the threshold question, "Does patient 1 suffer from a mental disease or defect?" If this patient has a significant mental disease or defect, usually of severity that psychiatrists diagnose as psychosis, the expert witness must relate patient 1's specific signs and symptoms to the specific act in question.

While the signs and symptoms of illness will remain constant for patient 1 throughout the United States, the legal test of responsibility will vary in different jurisdictions.

The medical expert must be aware of the test for criminal responsibility operative in the jurisdiction where the trial is to be held. The medical expert can expect the attorney to provide the relevant statute. The postsubarachnoid hemorrhage status with memory impairments, visual perceptual problems, concrete thinking, and an organic personality disorder in patient 1 set the stage for the second question. Did these impairments rise to a level of significance such that he could not meet the legal standard for responsibility? The expert must consider not only the clinical data but also the accounts of those who knew or saw the accused around the time of the crime. In addition, police reports, witness statements, and any statements made by the accused are important to review. If the accused flees the scene or hides the weapon, this is often seen as evidence that he "knew" what he had done. Patient 1 returned home and called the police to report he had killed his wife.

The medical expert witnesses agreed that patient 1 had had a subarachnoid hemorrhage secondary to an atrioventricular malformation involving the splenium of the corpus callosum in the left thalamus. However, in other cases, there may be disagreement on the interpretation of a computed tomographic scan or of an angiogram. Reasonable, well-trained, experienced physicians may disagree about the interpretation of both clinical and laboratory data. The expert witness essentially agreed on their clinical interpretation of the data and arrived at similar conclusions, ie, his capacity to form the requisite intent was markedly impaired. One expert witness opined, with a reasonable degree of medical certainty, that patient 1 met the criteria to be found not guilty by reason of insanity. The other expert was not as certain about the extent of patient 1's impairment. The information provided by the expert witnesses assisted the court in arriving at its verdict and was also taken into account at the time of sentencing. The court found patient 1 guilty of a lesser charge, manslaughter, and tempered that finding by sentencing him to 3 to 9 years in prison rather than the maximum 8.3 to 25 years because he had a "brain disorder."

In the second case, there was substantial clinical and laboratory data that patient 2 suffered from Alzheimer's disease when he stabbed his wife to death.[8] The obvious nature of his impairment, substantiated by careful study by the expert witnesses, provided the court with sufficient information to make a disposition that was acceptable to all. There was informal agreement between the attorneys and the court that patient 2, if he came to trial, would qualify for the insanity defense. Impairment was profound and unremitting in patient 2, and the court found him incompetent to stand trial. He was sent to a secure geriatric unit for further care and treatment.

In the third case, patient 3 was charged with being a serial killer. Since the medical experts arrived at different conclusions, a battle of the experts followed. These so-called battles rarely occur, both because the insanity defense is rarely used and, when the defense is considered, the medical experts hired by the defense and the prosecution usually find themselves in agreement. Less than 0.1% of felonies are dealt with by an insanity defense. Eighty percent of successful insanity defenses are agreed to by the prosecution. When contested, juries find the defendant not guilty by reason of insanity in less than 5% of cases.

In clinical settings, the physician's opinion is framed in the form of a diagnosis and a plan of action. In the legal setting, the physician's opinion is examined to weigh its credibility; it is the trier of fact, the judge or the jury, to arrive at a verdict and a plan of action. Patient 3 was convincing to one physician while another physician thought he was malingering.

The relationship between epilepsy and violence is of great interest to the courts, especially with the increased use of the diagnosis of epilepsy as a legal defense.[9-11] The jury heard testimony about the medical history of patient 3, the various laboratory tests, and the possible diagnosis of complex partial seizures. Efforts have been made to develop guidelines for assessing the likelihood that a crime was committed during an episode of ictal or postictal confusion.[12] The experts had to discuss complex partial seizure in terms the jury could understand. The jury found the evidence for a finding of a mental disease or defect unconvincing, and patient 3 was found guilty of murder.

These cases provide examples of violent behavior that may have arisen from organic mental disorders, epilepsy, or other neurologic conditions. As an increasing number of defendants and their attorneys explore defenses based on these disorders, medical expert witness will have the opportunity to share with the court new knowledge that links brain structure and function with violent behavior. However, the medical expert witness must use caution when bringing new research findings to courts because of the many "false dawns" that medicine has encountered in the past. Nonetheless, reasoned medical information can help the legal system better understand the defendant's actions and arrive at a just legal outcome. The participation of the medical expert witness is important to the process of bringing medical understanding to the legal system.

References

1. Clements CD, Ciccone JR. Ethics and expert witness: the troubled role of psychiatrist in court. *Bull Am Acad Psychiatry Law.* 1984;12:127-136.

2. Lande KE. Forensic medicine in Europe: legal medicine in America. *N Engl J Med.* 1936;18:826-834.

3. Ciccone JR, Clements CD. The insanity defense: asking and answering the ultimate question. *Bull Am Acad Psychiatry Law.* 1987;15:329-338.

4. McDonald v US 312 F2d 847 (DC Cir 1962).

5. Coventry CB. Medical jurisprudence of insanity. *J Insan.* 1844;1:134-144.

6. Ciccone JR. Presidential Address. Presented at the Annual Meeting of the American Academy of Psychiatry and the Law; October 1987; Ottawa, Canada.

7. Bellacosa JW. The fusion of medicine and law for *in extremis* health and medical decisions: does it produce energy and light or just cosmic dust? *Bull Am Acad Psychiatry Law.* 1990;18:5-21.

8. Chui HC. Dementia: a review emphasizing clinicopathologic correlation and brain-behavior relationships. *Arch Neurol.* 1989;46:806-814.

9. Treiman DM. Epilepsy and violence: medical and legal issues. *Epilepsia.* 1986;27(suppl 2):S77-S104.

10. Devinsky O, Luciano D. Psychic phenomena in partial seizures. *Semin Neurol.* 1991;11:100-109.

11. Porter RJ. Disorders of consciousness and associated complex behaviors. *Semin Neurol.* 1991;11:110-117.

12. Lishman WA. *Organic Psychiatry.* 2nd ed. Boston, Mass: Blackwell Scientific Publications Inc; 1987:241-242.

Severe Emotional Response to Eye Trauma in a Child: Awareness and Intervention

Posttraumatic stress disorder (PTSD) is most often associated with Vietnam veterans. However, PTSD can result from any psychologically distressing event outside the range of usual human experience, including eye trauma in children. Presented is the case of a young boy who suffered a penetrating injury to the right globe. Both he and his father experienced significant intrusive thoughts and avoidance consistent with PTSD. Patients and their families would benefit from ophthalmologists who explain the potential for psychologic sequlae of surgical intervention and provide consultation for the treatment of such symptoms.

Report of a Case.—A 4-year-old boy incurred trauma to his right eye by walking into a wall peg in a local movie rental store. His father applied pressure to decrease the bleeding, but found that contents of his son's right globe were now in his hand. An emergency surgery was performed to repair the ruptured globe. As a result of the injury, the lens was traumatically removed, the iris was irrepairably damaged, and there was a large eccentric corneal laceration. Fifteen months and six surgeries (two major and four minor) later, the patient regained best corrected visual acuity of 20/40 OD.

Fig 1.—Child's drawing showing how the injury occurred.

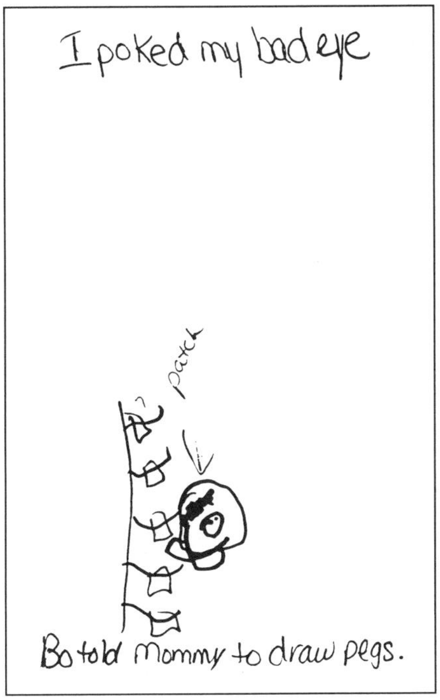
I poked my bad eye
patch
Bo told mommy to draw pegs.

After the injury, the patient began to experience nightmares (such as the video store camera man chasing and trying to kill him), rage reactions (hitting his mother and digging at his own face to cause injury), and reenactment play (bandaging the eye of his toy bear). He also demonstrated social withdrawal and requested that curtains be shut and lights be off at all times; regression (recurrent episodes of enuresis) and intrusive thoughts (thoughts of protruding video pegs) occurred. Anytime he was taken near the store, the child would exhibit specific fears, stating to family members and strangers, "You'll get hurt bad, don't go in that store." He believed something was wrong with him when asked by peers, "Why are your eyes different colors?" Finally, his fear of disapproval was expressed in a spontaneous drawing of a "clown's" mother "who did not love him [the clown] anymore."

The father also experienced symptoms of PTSD, including recurrent nightmares that his children were being cut in half. Although a clergyman, he found he could hardly control his anger about the loss of his expectations for his only son. He feared that his child's future was forever changed so that he would not be accepted socially nor become the top athlete he had envisioned. He subsequently engaged in loud outbursts or physical retaliation to persons who suggested he "should be grateful" the son's injury resulted in restored vision.

Fig 2.—Child's drawing depicting how he would solve the problem that allowed his injury to occur. Such drawings are used as therapeutic measures in children suffering posttramautic stress disorder.

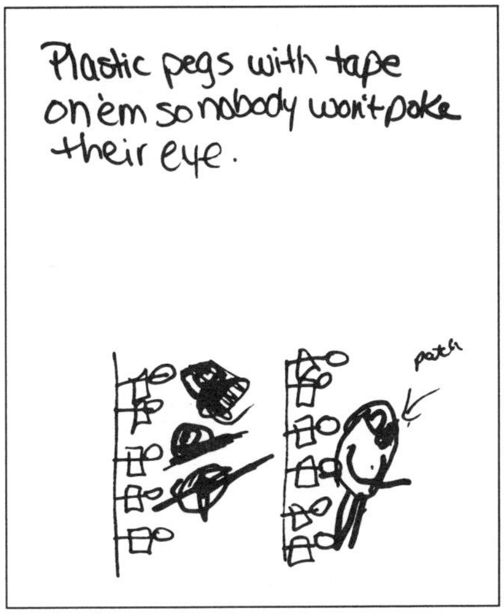
Plastic pegs with tape on'em so nobody won't poke their eye.
patch

The patient was referred to a child psychologist who concluded that the child and father were experiencing PTSD. Treatment for the child included structured reenactment[1] (through doll play designed to reenact on the doll what the child had experienced), "barb" training[2] (practice in responding to peer insults such as "old one eye," by saying, "You wouldn't talk like that if you'd been through what I've been through" and asking his parents to stop referring to his "bad" eye and to instead call it the "injured" eye), and incident resolution[3] (drawing a picture of a safer video peg that would not harm shoppers [Figs 1 and 2] and drawing a picture of the events in his nightmares in which the nightmares have better outcomes. These techniques seemed to induce 1- to 5-month periods of reduced stress for the child. Each of the surgeries, however, stimulated the reappearance of at least one symptom of PTSD that required renewed therapeutic intervention.

Comment.—This case suggests that ophthalmologists should be aware of the severity and types of symptoms of PTSD that children and parents may experience after eye trauma. With an awareness of the most important symptoms, the physician can prepare the parents and child for such symptoms by discussing the expected responses to trauma. If and when the symptoms become manifest, early recognition is more likely, and the physician can suggest the previously mentioned therapeutic measures in conjunction with proper referral. These techniques have been shown to be effective in children as young as age 4 years and can be used at home.

Most important in these situations is the recognition that a medical/surgical success, ie, restoration of 20/40 visual acuity, represents only one criterion for total success. This knowledge is crucial in the comprehensive treatment of family members who will likely believe themselves to be anything but "lucky" after such an event.

GRIFFITH C. STEINER, MD
LINDA W. PETERSON, PHD
Reno, Nev

Reprint requests to University of Louisville, Department of Ophthalmology, 301 E Muhammed Ali Blvd, Louisville, KY 40292 (Dr Steiner).

1. Terr L. *Too Scared to Cry: Psychic Trauma in Childhood.* New York, NY: Harper & Row Publishers Inc; 1990:299-303.
2. Kauffmann LM, Wagner BR. Barb: a systematic treatment for temper control disorders. *Behav Ther.* 1972;3:84-90.
3. Peterson L. Use of art in the assessment and treatment of children in wartime. In: *Proceedings of Wartime Medical Services, Second International Conference.* Stockholm, Sweden: Forsuarets Forskningsanstalt; 1990:120-129.

Eye Injury Resulting From Violence

Research and Prevention

Since one caveman poked another in the eye, little has changed over the years except the efficiency with which eye injuries may be inflicted on one person by another. For children, the range, accuracy, and injury potential of the rubber-band–propelled paper clip were greatly extended by the BB gun. In war, the progression from thrown stones to arrows, rifles, land mines, bombs, and laser weapons has made eye injury easier to inflict on more people from greater distances. The vulnerability of the eyes to newer weapons is clearly evident from the increase in eye injuries as a percentage of all wartime casualties during the century between the American Civil War (0.57%) and the Arab-Israeli Six-Day War and the Vietnam War (5% to 10%).[1]

Civilian injuries due to violence are commonly thought to be due to purposeful, criminal assault. Assault such as this accounts for only approximately 20% of the roughly 3000 penetrating eye injuries recorded in the National Eye Trauma System Registry[2] and for only 9% of eye injuries recorded in the United States Eye Injury Registry, Birmingham, Ala, in 1991. Criminal assault is only part of the total picture. Eye injuries also result from other acts that could be considered incidences of assault or violence, such as the intentional hockey foul, the tennis shot fired in anger after the point has been scored, driving recklessly or under the influence of alcohol or drugs, shooting BB guns at people, and playing war games.

Eye injuries resulting from trauma, to which purposeful violence is a significant contributor, are costly both in terms of money spent to treat the condition and in terms of the pain and disability borne by the victim. One would think that for a problem of such magnitude a significant amount of research would be dedicated to a meaningful solution, yet, this is far from being the case. Despite the fact that eye injury is second only to cataracts as the most common cause of impaired vision (according to 1991 data in the South Carolina Eye Injury Registry, Columbia), only 3% of eye research funding from the federal government is earmarked for research related to eye injuries. If a reporter from another planet attended the October 1991 American Academy of Ophthalmology meeting in Anaheim, Calif, to write a story on the most important diseases affecting the ocular health of Americans, some of the headlines might read "Scourge of myopia controlled by excimer laser" or "The heartbreak of astigmatism yields to new surgery," but certainly not, "American Academy of Ophthalmology launches campaign to prevent visual disability from trauma."

Why are scarce resources pumped into procedures of relatively little importance to public health, such as the surgical control of refractive errors, while pressing questions remain unanswered concerning the best means of preventing and treating potentially blinding traumatic eye injuries resulting from violence and other acts? One possible reason is that trauma research requires a large amount of information about factors that can be measured, including good, consistent, long-term data that can be used to monitor injury trends; data on the effects of preventive programs; and data on the efficacy of one surgical method compared with another. Data gathering is laborious and difficult to fund because analyses of decades of results are required to get meaningful answers. If we think of the relationship between trauma and refractive surgery, reasonable questions would include "Does radial keratotomy, which weakens the cornea, add to the risk of more serious eye injury from a blow to the eye?" "Is radial keratotomy dangerous for police officers, fire fighters, athletes, and military personnel who are routinely exposed to violence?" and "Is there any evidence that the corneal thinning resulting from the apparently minimal trauma of laser sculpting for treatment of myopia weakens the cornea and, thus, increases the chance of a ruptured globe if the patient is struck by a tennis ball or a fist?" As Denis O'Day, MD, discussed at an American Academy of Ophthalmology conference on trauma (oral communication, October 1991), who should record and report injuries such as the ruptured globes in a woman who underwent bilateral radial keratotomy and was then in an automobile accident in which she was not wearing a seatbelt?

The sparsity of information about the consequences of refractive surgery on an eye that is later subjected to a blow is only one reason for further research into violence and other trauma-induced eye injuries. Answers to clinical questions such as, "What is the best initial method for treatment of traumatic, total vitreous hemorrhage" require a prospective study of a large patient sample as well as accurate results.

Such a sample is beyond the capabilities and resources of most reasearchers, who have a handful of volunteers and minimal staff support. Sports injury data, for example, are typically collected by one or two volunteer ophthalmologists who devised and circulated a questionnaire and tabulated the results. It would be unwise for ophthalmology as a discipline to rely on new, young volunteers, replacing the aging cadre, to continue current studies and meet the challenges of the future. What is in it for the young ophthalmologist? If he or she develops a new technique to remove a cataract, fame and fortune are guaranteed, while organizing a data collection system will have a negative effect on income and evoke little professional recognition. We need reliable data gathered by full-time, paid professionals (with input from volunteer ophthalmologists) who make accurate reports that are available to the profession and the public. Without adequate funding, good systems, such as the once potentially powerful National Athletic Injury Surveillance System, are doomed to failure, and countless working hours and needed data may be lost.

The National Eye Trauma System Registry, which contains data on penetrating eye injuries gathered by 48 collaborating centers in 28 states, and the United States Eye Injury Registry, which contains data on all injuries resulting in significant structural or functional changes to the eye recorded by 12 state-based registries, are both worthy of long-term grant support. Data from the National Eye Trauma System Registry and United States Eye Injury Registry have the potential to reduce morbidity resulting from all traumatic eye injuries if they are used to help guide prevention, treatment, and the direction for focus of future research on eye trauma. The National Electronic Injury Surveillance System helps to identify injuries related to product use, but does not capture sufficient detail to be useful in studying injuries resulting from assaults. Neither is the surveillance system helpful in answering questions such as, "Do polycarbonate-lens eyeglasses offer eye protection to the victim of a mugging?"

Although data about eye injuries gathered thus far could be more comprehensive, progress has been made during the past few decades. Eye armor provided to the United States infantry deployed in Operation Desert Storm would almost certainly have prevented blindness for many of our troops in the event of a more prolonged ground war.[3] Protective eye wear such as polycarbonate spectacle lenses and industrial and sports eye and face protectors, which have met American National Standards Institute and American Society of Testing and Materials standards, are widely available. The greatly reduced incidence of eye injuries to industrial workers, hobbyists, and athletes who use protective gear indicates the potential for further injury reduction with more widespread use of such equipment.

While the individual ophthalmologist can do little to control the initial violent act that results in an eye injury, a good deal can be done to prevent or lessen the severity of eye injury in the event of an attack. We must keep in mind that falls in the elderly, muggings, work and sports injuries, and automobile crashes are reasonably common events that can cause eye injury. Because eye injury occurs in relatively consistent percentages in some events, it is essential that ophthalmologists obtain brief histories of the social, work, hobby, and sports involvement of each patient and prescribe protective eye wear when appropriate. Preventing blindness resulting from ocular injuries by prescribing proper eye wear is as much a part of patient care as preventing blindness by prescribing antiglaucoma therapy.

PAUL F. VINGER, MD
Lexington, Mass

References

1. Hornblass A. Eye injuries in the military. In: Vinger PF, ed. *Ocular Sports Injuries*. Boston, Mass: Little Brown & Co Inc; 1981: 121-138.

2. Dannenberg AL, Parver LM, Fowler CJ. Penetrating eye injuries related to assault: the National Eye Trauma System Registry: *Arch Ophthalmol*. 1992;110:849-852.

3. La Piana F. Development of eye armor for the American infantryman. In: *Textbook of Military Medicine*. Falls Church, Va: Office of the Surgeon General, US Army. In press.

Recognizing Child Abuse

In 1986, the Study of National Incidence and Prevalence of Child Abuse and Neglect estimated that 300 000 children are physically abused, 140 000 are sexually abused, and 700 000 are neglected or maltreated each year in the United States. This leads to at least 1100 deaths annually.[1] Approximately 15% of abused children suffer permanent physical abnormalities, while emotional deficits and learning problems are found in almost all of these children.[2]

BATTERED-CHILD SYNDROME

In 1946, Caffey[3] described the unusual association of chronic subdural hematomas and long-bone fractures in infants. The traumatic nature of this syndrome was emphasized in 1953 by Silverman,[4] who noted that a history of trauma could often be elicited from parents of these infants. Not until 1962, however, did the cause of this phenomenon become nationally recognized by the medical community. In that year, Kempe and coworkers[5] coined the term *battered-child syndrome*.

The battered-child syndrome is a clinical condition of young children who are physically abused by a parent or guardian. Affected children are usually younger than age 3 years, have injuries in different stages of healing, have histories of numerous admissions to the hospital (often to the emergency department), and suffer soft-tissue injury that is disproportionate in degree to the parent's or guardian's telling of the child's medical history.[5]

The battered-child syndrome includes the following physical manifestations: (1) intraocular and intracranial hemorrhage that often results in brain damage, mental retardation, blindness, or death; (2) body bruises in different stages of healing, with no additional bruises after hospitalization; (3) handprint bruises in which a clear area is surrounded by finger marks; (4) human bite marks or cigarette burns; (5) subgaleal hematomas caused by hair pulling; (6) genital injuries; (7) tears in the floor of tne mouth; (8) abdominal injuries, including bowel hematomas, pancreatic cysts, and ruptures of the spleen or liver; and (9) dehydration, poisoning, or unusual anxiety or jitteriness.[5] The shaken-baby syndrome is a frequently unrecognized form of child abuse that occurs when infants are shaken; intraocular and intracranial hemorrhages develop in the absence of external signs of head trauma.[6]

OPHTHALMIC MANIFESTATIONS

Forty percent of abused children will demonstrate ophthalmic manifestations of trauma. In 6% of reported cases of child abuse, an ophthalmologist is the physician primarily responsible for recognizing the abuse.[7] Olver and Hague[8] reported that four of 133 traumatized children presenting to an ophthalmology emergency department were maltreated.

The ocular manifestations of child abuse are many and include signs of periorbital trauma (eg, ecchymosis, edema, and fractures), anterior segment trauma (eg, hyphema, angle recession, and cataract), posterior trauma (eg, retinal hemorrhage and detachment, vitreous hemorrhage, and optic atrophy), and intracranial trauma (neuro-ophthalmic signs such as nystagmus, cortical blindness, and third-nerve paralysis secondary to uncal herniation).

The most frequent findings are subretinal, intraretinal, preretinal, and vitreous hemorrhages, which have been reported to signify the presence of intracranial hemorrhages in 44 of 55 patients.[9] Retinal hemorrhages unassociated with birth trauma, leukemia, or bleeding diathesis in children younger than age 3 years should be considered suggestive of child abuse unless proven otherwise.[10] Several mechanisms of retinal hemorrhages have been proposed and include (1) acute intracranial hypertension after cerebral injury, resulting in retinal venous hypertension; (2) sudden increase in venous pressure in the eyes and brain (Purtscher's angiopathic retinopathy); (3) direct eye trauma; and (4) rapid acceleration and deceleration from direct head trauma and/or shaking. Optic nerve sheath hemorrhages accompany retinal hemorrhages in 70% of cases.[11,12] Subdural optic nerve hemorrhages are caused by local rupture of dural-pial bridging vessels or by transmitted intracranial pressure.[11,12]

Retinal hemorrhages may be more sensitive indicators of intracranial hemorrhage than computed tomograms and are often markers of acute neurologic injury.[13,14] Wilkinson et al[13] found that diffuse fundus involvement, vitreous hemorrhage, or large subhyaloid hemorrhages were associated with severe neurologic injury. Giangiacomo et al[14] reported that in three of five shaken infants retinal hemorrhages *preceded* the clinical and roentgenographic recognition of subdural hematoma. Thus, recognition of these manifestations are crucial, especially when other signs of head trauma are covert.

Child abuse may also result in retinal detachment, retinoschisis, macular scars, retinal cysts, retinal gliosis, chorioretinal atrophy, and optic atrophy. Vitreoretinal traction with secondary perimacular folds may be due to shaking and/or direct head trauma.[15]

Most falls result in bruises on just one body surface. Bruises on many body planes are usually inflicted, unless a history of tumbling is present. "Falling down a stairway" is commonly offered as an explanation for bruises by the parent or caretaker. Tumbling accidents result predominantly in bruises on the elbows, knees, and shoulders; absence of bruises in these locations makes this explanation questionable. Bilateral periorbital ecchymoses and/or subconjunctival hemorrhages are frequently explained by the parent or caretaker as resulting from a fall. Absence of coexisting nasal injury should alert one to possible purposeful head injury.[2,16]

MEDICOLEGAL ISSUES

Ophthalmologists have a responsibility to learn the signs of abuse and their legal powers and obligations for protecting endangered children. Physicians and other health professionals are required, under threat of criminal and civil sanctions, to report cases of suspected child abuse and neglect to the state child protection agency. All forms of child maltreatment that might threaten the child's health or welfare must be reported. A pattern of injuries (ie, battered-child syndrome) is not necessary because *all* suspicious injuries should be reported to authorities. In some cases, ambiguous injuries or parental explanations of borderline plausibility make definitive determination impossible. As a general rule, in doubtful situations the physician or health care professional should act in favor of protecting the child and report the suspicious injuries.[2]

Twenty states require all citizens to report child abuse, regardless of professional duties. Almost all states have specific laws that make the failure to report suspected child abuse and neglect a misdemeanor crime. These laws grant immunity from civil and criminal liability to persons who report abuse.

The pathologic detection of hemosiderin in eyes at autopsy[11] and the clinical detection of perimacular retinal folds[15] may serve as markers of repeated trauma and shaking, respectively. These issues have been debated in the literature because they may help determine the guilt or innocence of caregivers. Until the mechanisms of various ocular signs of trauma are unequivocally proven, ophthalmologists must interpret these signs in the context of other pathologic and clinical findings. Further study of ocular findings in eyes of traumatized children is required.

Dennis M. Marcus, MD
Daniel M. Albert, MD
Boston, Mass

References

1. Sedlak A. *Study of National Incidence and Prevalence of Child Abuse and Neglect.* Bethesda, Md: Westat; 1987.
2. Besharov DJ. *Recognizing Child Abuse: A Guide for the Concerned.* New York, NY: Free Press; 1990.
3. Caffey J. Multiple fractures in the long bones of infants suffering from chronic subdural hematoma. *Am J Roentgenol Radiat Ther.* 1946;56:163-173.
4. Silverman F. The roentgen manifestations of unrecognized skeletal trauma in infants. *Am J Roentgenol Radiat Ther.* 1953;69: 413-426.
5. Kempe CH, Silverman RN, Steele BF, Droegemueller W, Silver HK. The battered-child syndrome. *JAMA.* 1962;181:17-24.
6. Caffey J. The whiplash shaken infant syndrome: manual shaking by the extremities with whiplash-induced intracranial and intraocular bleedings, linked with residual permanent brain damage and mental retardation. *Pediatrics.* 1946;53:396-403.
7. Friendly DS. Ocular manifestations of physical child abuse. *Trans Am Acad Ophthalmol Otolaryngol.* 1971;75:318-332.
8. Olver JM, Hague S. Children presenting to an ophthalmic casualty department. *Eye.* 1989;3:415-419.
9. Riffenburgh RS, Sathyavagiswaran L. Ocular findings at autopsy of child abuse victims. *Ophthalmology.* 1991;98:1519-1524.
10. Eisenbrey AB. Retinal hemorrhage in the battered child. *Child's Brain.* 1979;5:40-44.
11. Elner SG, Elner VM, Arnall M, Albert DM. Ocular and associated systemic findings in suspected child abuse: a necropsy study. *Arch Ophthalmol.* 1990;108:1094-1101.
12. Lambert SR, Johnson TE, Hoyt CS. Optic nerve sheath and retinal hemorrhages associated with the shaken-baby syndrome. *Arch Ophthalmol.* 1986;104:1509-1512.
13. Wilkinson WS, Han DP, Rappley MD, Owings CL. Retinal hemorrhage predicts neurologic injury in the shaken-baby syndrome. *Arch Ophthalmol.* 1989;104:1472-1474.
14. Giangiacomo J, Khan JA, Levine C, Thompson VM. Sequential cranial computed tomography in infants with retinal hemorrhages. *Ophthalmology.* 1988;95:295-299.
15. Massicotte SJ, Folberg R, Torczynski E, Gilliland MGF, Luckenbach MW. Vitreoretinal traction and perimacular retinal folds in the eyes of deliberately traumatized children. *Ophthalmology.* 1991;98:1124-1127.
16. Schmitt B. *The Child Protection Team Handbook.* New York, NY: Garland Publishing Inc; 1978.

Ocular Trauma in the United States

Eye Injuries Resulting in Hospitalization, 1984 Through 1987

Joanne Klopfer, OD, MPH; James M. Tielsch, PhD;
Susan Vitale, MHS; Lai-Chu See, MPH, MS; Joseph K. Canner, MHS

• The discharge rate for ocular trauma resulting in hospitalization and variations in rates between US census subdivisions were examined by using hospital discharge abstracts from the 1984 through 1987 National Hospital Discharge Surveys. The average annual rate of hospitalization with a principal diagnosis of ocular trauma was 13.2 per 100 000. The rate for any ocular trauma (principal or secondary diagnosis) was 29.1 per 100 000. Males were three times more likely to be hospitalized for a principal diagnosis of ocular trauma than females. Age-specific rates for principal and secondary diagnoses of ocular trauma were distributed bimodally, with the highest peak in adolescents and young adults, and another peak among those 75 years or older. This study has begun the first step in profiling ocular trauma resulting in hospitalization in the United States.

(*Arch Ophthalmol.* 1992;110:838-842)

Scant information is available on the rates of ocular trauma in the United States. National estimates range from 1 million[1] to 2.4 million eye injuries per year.[2] This variation may be due to differences in ocular trauma categories[3] or sources of data.[4] Epidemiological studies have focused on treatment of ocular trauma in different geographic regions of the country.[1,5-7] These studies have included eyes with varying severity of trauma, ranging from all medically treated eye injuries to ocular trauma resulting in hospitalization.

An accurate estimate of the magnitude and severity of ocular trauma in the United States would require a comprehensive source of eye injury data. In the absence of a centralized reporting system that represents all sections of the country, alternative sources of information need to be examined. The National Hospital Discharge Survey (NHDS) is a nationally aggregated source of data in which discharge information is abstracted from hospital medical records and collected by the National Center for Health Statistics.[8] A representative sample of eye injuries resulting in hospitalization in short-stay hospitals can be obtained for the United States by identifying records in the NHDS with either a principal or secondary diagnosis of ocular trauma.

The purpose of this study was to determine the national discharge rate of patients hospitalized for ocular trauma in the United States based on the NHDS. Discharge rates have been compared across geographic regions of the country by age and sex to determine whether there were regional variations in the incidence of serious ocular injuries.

Accepted for publication November 29, 1991.

From the Dana Center for Preventive Ophthalmology, Wilmer Eye Institute (Drs Klopfer and Tielsch and Mss Vitale and See), and the School of Hygiene and Public Health (Mr Canner), The Johns Hopkins University, Baltimore, Md.

Reprint requests to Wilmer Eye Institute, The Johns Hopkins University School of Medicine, Wilmer Room 120, 600 N Wolfe St, Baltimore, MD 21205 (Dr Tielsch).

SUBJECTS AND METHODS

The NHDS collects data on a probability sample of patient discharges from noninstitutional hospitals in all 50 states and the District of Columbia.[9] A stratified selection technique selects hospitals with six beds or more whose average length of stay is less than 30 days.[9] Approximately 84% of all sampled hospitals were represented by the NHDS in 1984 through 1987.[10] Information abstracted from the discharge summaries of the medical records contains administrative information about admission and discharge dates and patient information such as date of birth, sex, and marital status, as well as medical information about diagnoses and treatments performed. One principal (or first-listed) diagnosis and up to six secondary diagnoses are assigned to each medical record discharge sheet.[9]

The data set for this study consisted of all discharges covering the 4-year period 1984 through 1987 with a principal or secondary discharge diagnosis of ocular trauma based on the *International Classification of Diseases, Ninth Revision, Clinical Modification* (Table 1). For this study, a *principal diagnosis* was defined as an ocular trauma code recorded as the condition chiefly responsible for admission of the patient to the hospital.[9] The *secondary diagnosis* was an ocular trauma diagnosis that appeared as any one of the six secondary diagnoses listed.[9] The final sample of all ocular trauma cases contained a total of 1433 principal and secondary diagnosis discharges, with 656 being principal (or first-listed) diagnosis discharges. Hereafter, reference will be made either to the principal diagnosis discharge group or to the total diagnosis group, which includes the principal and secondary diagnoses of ocular trauma.

The study design of the NHDS allowed comparisons of rates among the nine US census subdivisions: New England, Mid-Atlantic, South Atlantic, East North Central, East South Central, West North Central, West South Central, Mountain, and Pacific. Projected numbers of principal and total ocular trauma cases were computed for each year in the subdivisions and the entire United States by using the NHDS weighting factors.[8] The mean annual number of estimated discharges was used as the numerator for the discharge rate.[11] The averaging of events over this 4-year period was justified because there was no indication that there were trends in the number of discharges over time. This approach is consistent with results previously reported from Maryland.[5] The average of the census population estimates for 1984 through 1987[12] was used as the denominator for the discharge rate. Standard errors for the numerators were based on the NHDS relative SE curves for region and other variables.[9] The SEs were calculated according the NHDS variances based on multiple years of data. Age- and sex-specific rates were calculated for the country as a whole. To examine geographic variation in the discharge rates of patients hospitalized for ocular trauma among the subdivisions, age groups were combined into the five categories of 0 to 14, 15 to 34, 35 to 64, 65 to 74, and 75+ years.

RESULTS

During 1984 through 1987, NHDS projections from the sample resulted in an average annual national estimate of 69 729 patients with ocular trauma (principal and secondary diagnoses) discharged from hospitals. Slightly more than half of these discharges, or 31 766, were for principal diagnoses of hospitalization for ocular trauma. The average annual rate of principal diagnosis of ocular trauma in the United States was

Table 1.—Ocular Trauma Discharge Diagnosis Codes From the *ICD-9-CM**

802.6-802.7	Orbital floor fractures (blow-out)
870.0-870.9	Open wounds of ocular adnexa
871.0-871.9	Open wounds of eyeball
918.0-918.9	Superficial injury of eye and adnexa
921.0-921.9	Contusion of eye and adnexa
930.0-930.9	Foreign body on external eye
940.0-940.9	Burn confined to eye and adnexa
950.0-950.9	Injury to optic nerve and pathways
951.0	Injury to oculomotor nerve

**ICD-9-CM* indicates *International Classification of Diseases, Ninth Revision, Clinical Modification.*

Table 2.—Principal and Total Diagnoses of Ocular Trauma Discharge Rates by Sex in US Census Subdivisions, NHDS, 1984-1987*

Subdivision	Total	Males	Females	M/F Ratio
Principal Diagnosis				
New England	10.3±4.1	16.1±3.5	4.9±1.6	3.3
Mid-Atlantic	11.7±3.0	17.8±5.2	6.1±2.5	2.9
East North Central	14.5±3.4	22.5±5.8	6.9±2.6	3.3
West North Central	20.4±5.7	27.5±8.8	13.7±5.5	2.0
South Atlantic	11.6±3.0	17.9±5.0	5.7±2.3	3.1
East South Central	17.0±5.3	31.4±10.2	3.5±1.2	9.0
West South Central	13.6±3.8	22.5±6.7	4.9±1.2	4.6
Mountain	13.3±4.8	23.5±8.8	3.2†	7.3
Pacific	10.9±2.9	14.5±4.5	7.4±2.9	2.0
Total	13.2±1.0	20.5±1.6	6.4±0.7	3.2
Total Diagnoses				
New England	22.1±6.7	28.3±10.2	16.4±6.9	1.7
Mid-Atlantic	30.9±6.0	41.2±9.1	21.6±5.7	1.9
East North Central	30.8±5.8	43.8±9.1	18.6±4.9	2.4
West North Central	41.0±9.1	53.8±13.9	28.9±9.0	1.9
South Atlantic	27.2±5.3	36.5±8.2	18.4±5.0	2.0
East South Central	31.2±8.0	47.9±13.4	15.6±6.3	3.1
West South Central	32.0±6.7	52.5±11.9	12.2±4.4	4.3
Mountain	27.1±7.6	43.4±13.2	11.0±2.6	3.9
Pacific	21.2±4.7	28.2±7.1	14.3±4.5	2.0
Total	29.1±1.7	40.1±2.9	17.7±1.5	2.3

*Values are mean±SE rates per 100 000 population. NHDS indicates National Hospital Discharge Survey.
†The SE did not meet National Center for Health Statistics standards of reliability or precision.

13.2 per 100 000 population (95% confidence interval [CI], 11.2 to 15.2) and 29.1 total diagnoses of ocular trauma per 100 000 population (95% CI, 25.8 to 32.4) (Table 2). Sex-specific rates in each of the nine subdivisions showed that males had consistently higher rates of principal and total diagnoses of ocular trauma, compared with females. Relative risks (male vs female) for a principal diagnosis of ocular trauma ranged from a low of 2.0 in the West North Central subdivision to a high of 9.0 in the East South Central subdivision. The highest rate for females was in the West North Central subdivision, contributing to this subdivision having the highest discharge rate for principal and total diagnoses. New England had the lowest principal diagnosis discharge rate and the Pacific subdivision had the lowest total diagnoses discharge rate. The West North Central subdivision had twice the rates of the lowest subdivisions for principal and total diagnoses. The 95% CIs for the geographic subdivisions with the lowest and highest rates for the principal and total diagnoses groups overlapped, possibly as a result of the relatively small number of subdivision-specific cases ascertained from the sample hospitals. Age and sex adjustment of the regional hospitalized discharge rates did not alter the values beyond 0.1 per 100 000 for the principal diagnosis and 0.5 per 100 000 for the total diagnoses, and pointed to the same conclusion on geographic variation. While the regional variation was not statistically significant at the 5% level, the range of observed rates suggests regional variations could exist, but larger numbers of discharges would be needed to determine such differences.

Combining the subdivisions to examine a national profile of sex- and age-specific rates revealed distinctive patterns of injury by age and sex. Males were at higher risk for ocular trauma at all ages until the age of 75+ years, when females were at an increased risk for some types of ocular trauma.

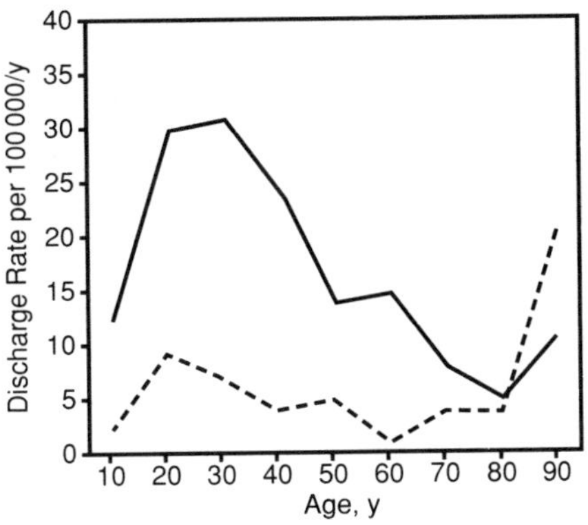

Fig 1.—Average annual hospital discharge rates for patients with a principal diagnosis of ocular trauma, by age and sex, United States, 1984 through 1987. Solid line indicates males; broken line, females.

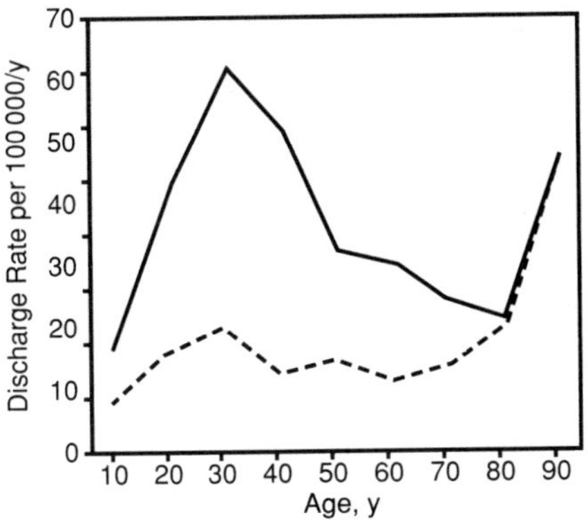

Fig 2.—Average annual hospital discharge rates for total (principal and secondary diagnoses) ocular trauma, by age and sex, United States, 1984 through 1987. Solid line indicates males; broken line, females.

Utilizing principal diagnosis (Fig 1), the peak of ocular trauma injury for males was in the "adolescent–young adult" group. Females showed a slight peak in the adolescent–young adult age group and a large increase in the principal diagnosis of ocular trauma after the age of 75 years. The overall discharge rate for the principal diagnosis of ocular trauma for males was 20.5 per 100 000 (95% CI, 17.4 to 23.6) and 6.4 per 100 000 (95% CI, 4.9 to 7.8) for females, with a relative risk of 3.2. In the 75-year-and-older age groups, the discharge rate for males was 11.4 per 100 000 (95% CI, 5.4 to 17.4) vs 21.1 per 100 000 (95% CI, 15.9 to 26.3) for females, with a relative risk of 0.5.

For total ocular trauma (Fig 2), males had a significantly higher ocular trauma discharge rate than did females at all ages until 75 years, after which the discharge rate increased similarly in both groups. The overall discharge rate for total ocular trauma cases for males was 41.0 per 100 000 (95% CI, 35.4 to 46.6) and for females was 17.7 per 100 000 (95% CI, 14.9 to 20.6), with a relative risk of 2.3. For the 75-year-and-older age groups, the discharge rate for males was 50.5 per 100 000 (95% CI, 32.8 to 68.1) and for females was 50.6 per

Table 3.—Estimated Principal Diagnosis Ocular Trauma Discharge Rates (per 100 000) by Age and Diagnosis, NHDS, 1984-1987*

	Age, y													
	0-14		15-34		35-64		65-74		75+		Total			
Diagnosis	No.	Rate	No.	Rate	No.	Rate	No.	Rate	No.	Rate	No.	Rate	(%)	M/F Ratio
Open wound, eyeball	2028	3.9	4772	5.8	2712	3.5	441	2.6	1072	9.2	11 025	4.6	(34.7)	4.4
Contusion, eyeball	2824	5.4	2416	3.0	979	1.3	61	0.4	38	0.3	6318	2.6	(19.9)	3.5
Open wound, adnexa	1429	2.7	2697	3.3	925	1.2	206	1.2	71	0.6	5328	2.2	(16.8)	3.8
Orbital blowout fracture	477	0.9	2263	2.8	1135	1.5	70	0.4	108	0.9	4053	1.7	(12.8)	2.7
Contusion, adnexa	469	0.9	558	0.7	410	0.5	76	0.4	674	5.8	2187	0.9	(6.9)	0.6
Foreign body on eye	621	1.2	191	0.2	195	0.2	0	. . .	37	0.3	1044	0.4	(3.3)	3.2
Superficial	368	0.7	267	0.3	140	0.2	0	. . .	69	0.6	844	0.4	(2.7)	2.8
Burns	0	. . .	706	0.9	35	0.05	35	0.2	0	. . .	776	0.3	(2.4)	8.4
Injury to nerve(s)	54	0.1	107	0.1	30	0.04	0	. . .	0	. . .	191	0.1	(0.01)	2.6
Total	**8270**	15.8	**13 976**	17.1	**6560**	8.5	**889**	5.2	**2068**	17.7	**31 766**	13.2	**(100)**	3.2

*NHDS indicates National Hospital Discharge Survey.

100 000 (95% CI, 36.4 to 64.8), with a relative risk of 1.0.

The rates of ocular trauma by the principal diagnoses are given in Table 3. The age distribution for "open wounds to the eyeball," "open wounds to the adnexa," and "orbital blowout fractures" showed an increase of injuries in young males 15 years and older, followed by a decline in trauma after 35 years. In the group with open wounds to the eyeball, the rate of injury increased again after the age of 75 years for males and females and exceeded the rates of the younger age groups. "Contusion to the adnexa" showed a different pattern. There was an increased rate in females over the age of 75 years, while the rate for all other age groups was low. No males older than 65 years were reported to have contusion to the adnexa. In the case of "contusions of the eyeball," young males 0 to 14 years were most likely to be hospitalized for these injuries, with the rate declining with increasing age. The small numbers in the estimated cases for "foreign body on the eye," "superficial injury," "burns," and "injury to the nerve" showed low rates of trauma that did not vary significantly by age. In the latter cases, males were at higher risk for ocular trauma than females.

Information on the "E-code," or external cause of injury, was included for 24% of the principal diagnosis data and is listed in Table 4. The major causes of injury were BB or air guns (16.6%), motor vehicle accidents (13.6%), foreign body in the eye or adnexa (12.6%), accidentally hit by a falling object or cutting instrument (12.2%), and homicide, rape, or child battering (10.4%). It is not apparent why some records were E-coded by hospitals and others were not. No significant differences were noted in whether or not the E-coding was reported when comparing age, geographic, or diagnostic categories. A slightly higher proportion of males, compared with females, had E-codes (25% vs 19%). Evaluation of this E-code information from all 4 years showed that half (50.8%) of the injuries in the 0- to 14-year-old age group were caused by BB or air guns. Several causes were identified in the 15- to 29-year-old age group, with foreign body in the eye and adnexa (19.7%) predominating, followed by motor vehicle accidents (17.0%) and accidental injury to the eye (15.0%). Fire, explosions, and excessive heat (23.3%) and homicide or rape (20.8%) were the most frequently documented causes in the 30- to 44-year-old age group, while motor vehicle accidents (28.1%) and homicide or rape (27.2%) were cited the most often in the 45- to 59-year-old age group. Abnormal reactions or later complications to surgical and medical procedures (30.8%) were the leading cause of ocular trauma reported in the 60- to 74-year-old age group. Falls accounted for half (50.0%) of the causes listed for the 75-year-and-older age group, followed by complications or reactions to surgical and medical procedures (42.8%).

Table 4.—Distribution of E-Codes for Projected Cases, Principal and Total Diagnoses of Ocular Trauma, NHDS, 1984-1987*

	No. (%)	
Cause	Principal Diagnosis	Total Diagnoses
BB or air guns	4982 (16.6)	5494 (7.9)
Motor vehicle accidents	4086 (13.6)	21 416 (30.9)
Foreign body in eye and adnexa	3800 (12.6)	4108 (5.9)
Accidentally hit by falling object or cutting instrument	3665 (12.2)	4775 (6.9)
Homicide, rape, or child battering	3137 (10.4)	9504 (13.7)
Surgical complication	1866 (6.2)	4715 (6.8)
Fire, explosions, or excessive heat	1805 (6.0)	2423 (3.5)
Accidental fall	1762 (5.9)	5812 (8.4)
Accidental poisoning or shooting	1212 (4.0)	3255 (4.7)
Animal bite	1151 (3.8)	2041 (3.0)
Other (eg, sports, suicide, adverse effect of drug)	2602 (8.7)	5737 (8.3)
Total	30 068 (100)	69 280 (100)

*NHDS indicates National Hospital Discharge Survey.

Of the total group (principal and secondary diagnoses) with ocular trauma, 26% were E-coded. The largest group of causes documented for the total ocular trauma group was motor vehicle accidents (30.9%), followed by homicide, rape, or child battering (13.7%) and accidental falls (8.4%) (Table 4). It is not surprising that skull fractures and intracranial injury (23.3%), concussion (10.9%), and open wounds to the head (6.7%) were frequently listed as the principal diagnosis among those with a secondary diagnosis of ocular trauma. Although age-related conditions such as diabetes, hypertension, carotid artery stenosis, and renal failure were principal diagnoses listed for the older population, we were unable to relate the increased ocular trauma discharge rate for the 75-year-and-older group to principal diagnoses other than head trauma. To help explain the unique patterns for the principal diagnoses of open wounds to the eyeball and contusions to the adnexa injuries in the elderly, associations of these injuries with specific secondary diagnoses that were not E-coded were examined. No consistent pattern of secondary diagnoses could be associated with the principal diagnoses of open wound to the eyeball or contusion to the adnexa in the over-75-year age group.

COMMENT

Results on national hospital discharge rates and characteristics of ocular trauma concur with data that have been reported from other hospital population-based studies. Tielsch et al[5] reported the same annual principal diagnosis rate of 13.2 per 100 000 population during 1979 through 1986, using hospital discharge abstracts in Maryland. The 29.1 per 100 000 NHDS rate (95% CI, 25.8 to 32.4) for total ocular trauma was slightly higher than the 27.3 per 100 000 rate from Maryland. The rate of 15.8 per 100 000 per year (95% CI, 12.4 to 19.4) for children 14 years old and younger was similar to the 15.2 per 100 000 incidence in 1982 estimated for children younger than 16 years in Maryland by Strahlman et al.[13]

The differences between the NHDS principal diagnosis discharge rates and the Maryland data were in the range of 0.2 to 0.9 per 100 000 for each diagnosis and occurred in similar proportions. The NHDS principal diagnosis open wounds to the eyeball rate of 4.6 per 100 000 per year (95% CI, 3.5 to 5.6) was higher than the perforating eye injury (equivalent to our open wound to the eyeball category) rate of Allegheny County, Pennsylvania, which had a mean incidence of 3.5 per 100 000 person-years from 1980 through 1986.[14] The Allegheny County series included principal and secondary diagnoses of perforating injury treated in one of 24 area hospitals. The authors from the Allegheny County study stated that the most frequent circumstance of injury (23%) was related to work with tools, but they did not show an age distribution for these types of injuries.

In the Maryland data, the incidence for the principal diagnosis of open wound to the eyeball increased to 4.2 per 100 000 after the age of 70 years.[5] The national picture for the NHDS data showed an even greater increase to 9.2 per 100 000 for the principal diagnosis of open wounds to the eyeball after the age of 75 years. Based on the E-codes, which showed falls and complications to surgical procedures (primarily ocular surgery) to be the two leading causes in the 75-year-old and older patients, we can speculate that an eye that has had a surgical procedure may be more vulnerable to further trauma. There could be a lower threshold for hospitalization, even if the trauma is minor. It is unknown whether the increased risk of ocular trauma observed in the over 75 population in the United States is related, in part, to the increase in ocular surgical procedures commonly performed on the elderly.[15]

The association of ocular trauma with age and sex has been consistently reported. Population-based studies have shown young adult males to be at significant risk, with relative risks ranging from 2 to 6 compared with females, depending on the severity of the injury.[6,7,16-18] Our study has shown a high discharge rate of the principal and secondary diagnoses of hospitalized ocular trauma in young males and an additional upswing for certain diagnoses in persons over the age of 75 years. Almost all studies[6,7,14] have reported a decline of ocular trauma with age, regardless of the type of injury incurred. We examined the NHDS data to see if the increased injury in the elderly could be related to readmissions during the 4-year period. Based on diagnoses, discharge status, and date of birth, only nine cases could be identified as possible readmissions in the total diagnosis group. With the exception of a 53-year-old man, all of these possible readmission cases were in young males younger than 30 years old.

The increase in the principal diagnosis of ocular trauma in the older population mainly was due to the two categories of open wounds to the eyeball and contusion to the adnexa. This result is consistent with the Maryland data, which were not based on weighted estimates.[5] Our study and the Maryland study have shown falls to be responsible for these types of ocular injuries in the elderly. Other studies have shown falls to be an important cause of injury in the older population.[19]

In a well-documented series of eye injuries that occurred in Northern Ireland during 1967 through 1976, Canavan et al[20] reported that road traffic accidents were the most common cause of eye injury in adults older than 56 years, particularly for females. The eye injuries examined were all in patients who were admitted to a hospital in Belfast, presumably principal and secondary diagnoses. The inclusion of both diagnoses of ocular trauma in Northern Ireland is similar to the total group of ocular trauma in the NHDS data. The major E-code that was listed for the total group of NHDS ocular trauma was motor vehicle accidents. Although chronological time, rules of the road, and types of vehicles differ in Northern Ireland and the United States, motor vehicle accidents have been shown to be an important cause of admissions to hospitals for ocular trauma.

This study is the first step in profiling patients hospitalized for ocular trauma in the United States. The most notable findings include no significant difference in the discharge rates between geographic subdivisions, the increase in principal diagnoses of "contusion of the ocular adnexa" trauma observed in women older than 75 years, and the increase in open wounds to the eyeball for males and females older than 75 years. The findings on the increased rates in the elderly could represent an increased incidence in trauma that occurs in older populations, a change in indications for hospitalization for this older population, or additional risk factors among the elderly. Reasons for this excess risk need to be elucidated to answer these questions and provide effective means for injury prevention.

Barriers to determining the causes for hospitalized ocular trauma exist because of the lack of adequate E-codes reported to NHDS. Several reasons have been given for the lack of E-code information on hospital discharge records. These include lack of financial incentive for the hospital, inadequate space on the record, and insufficient details in the medical record.[21] Lack of space did not appear to be a major obstacle to including the E-code on the hospital discharge records in this study. We also examined the positioning of the E-code, hypothesizing that placement in the last position in the secondary diagnosis slots made E-coding the last effort. This did not seem to be the case. The Centers for Disease Control has recommended that all hospital discharge summaries of injuries include the E-code as a cost-effective means to collect data needed to prevent injuries.[21] Sniezek et al[21] have suggested that health care providers become more aware of the importance of documenting information about the injury event and that the Health Care Financing Administration require the use of E-codes in a prospective payment system as well as provide two fields for E-codes on billing forms. These changes could make an important impact in making information on causes of severe ocular trauma available. Based on the 24% to 26% E-coding that was done for the NHDS data, we can only postulate that falls are an important factor for the principal diagnosis of ocular trauma in the elderly and that motor vehicle accidents play a large role in the total picture of all hospitalizations for ocular trauma.

No significant difference was found between the census subdivisions for either the principal or total diagnosis of ocular trauma. In a study by Bacon et al,[22] geographic variation was found for hip fractures among elderly whites 65 years and older. Their highest geographic region for hip fractures was in the West North Central subdivision, similar to the highest rates found in the NHDS principal and total ocular trauma series. Falls were found to be the primary cause of hip fractures in the elderly. The addition of more detailed information on the occurrence of severe ocular trauma would help to strengthen the public health messages needed to prevent unnecessary ocular trauma and blindness.

This study was supported in part by grants F32EY06279-02 and S10-RR-04060 from the National Institutes of Health, Bethesda, Md.

We appreciate the time and advice given by Helen Abbey, W. Edward Bacon, Bob Pokrus, and Iris Shimizu.

References

1. White MF Jr, Morris R, Feist RM, Witherspoon CD, Helms HA Jr, John GR. Eye injury: prevalence and prognosis by setting. *South Med J.* 1989;82:151-158.

2. Parver LM. Eye trauma: the neglected disorder. *Arch Ophthalmol.* 1986;104:1452-1453.

3. Koval R, Teller J, Belkin M, Romem M, Yanko L, Savir H. The Israeli ocular injuries study. *Arch Ophthalmol.* 1988;106:776-780.

4. Schein OD, Hibberd PL, Shingleton BJ, et al. The spectrum and burden of ocular injury. *Ophthalmology.* 1988;95:300-305.

5. Tielsch JM, Parver L, Shankar B. Time trends in the incidence of hospitalized ocular trauma. *Arch Ophthalmol.* 1989;107:519-523.

6. Karlson TA, Klein BEK. The incidence of acute hospital-treated eye injuries. *Arch Ophthalmol.* 1986;104:1473-1476.

7. Glynn RJ, Seddon JM, Berlin BM. The incidence of eye injuries of New England adults. *Arch Ophthalmol.* 1988;106:785-789.

8. Simmons WR. Development of the design of the NCHS Hospital Discharge Survey. *Vital Health Stat 2.* 1970;39:1-29.

9. Graves EJ. Detailed diagnoses and procedures, National Hospital Discharge Survey, 1987. *Vital Health Stat 13.* 1989;100:1-304.

10. American Hospital Association. *American Hospital Statistics.* Chicago, Ill: American Hospital Association; 1990.

11. Kahn HA, Sempos CT. *Statistical Methods in Epidemiology.* New York, NY: Oxford University Press Inc; 1989.

12. *Current Population Reports: State Population and Household Estimates, With Age, Sex, and Components of Change: 1981-1987.* US Bureau of the Census; 1988; series P-25, No. 1024.

13. Strahlman E, Elman M, Daub E, Baker S. Causes of pediatric eye injuries: a population-based study. *Arch Ophthalmol.* 1990;106:603-606.

14. Landen D, Baker D, LaPorte R, Thoft RA. Perforating eye injury in Allegheny County, Pennsylvania. *Am J Public Health.* 1990;80:1120-1122.

15. Stark WJ, Sommer A, Smith RE. Changing trends in intraocular lens implantation. *Arch Ophthalmol.* 1989;107:1441-1444.

16. Wilder CS, Pearson AN. Impairments due to injury, United States 1971. *Vital Health Stat 10.* 1971; No. 87.

17. Morris RE, Witherspoon CD, Helms HA, Feist RM, Byrne JB. Eye injury registry of Alabama (preliminary report): demographics and prognosis of severe eye injury. *South Med J.* 1987; 80:810-816.

18. Blomdahl S, Norell S. Perforating eye injury in the Stockholm population: an epidemiological study. *Acta Ophthalmol.* 1984;62:378-390.

19. Myers AH, Baker SP, Van Natta ML, Abbey H, Robinson EG. Risk factors associated with falls and injuries among elderly institutionalized persons. *Am J Epidemiol.* 1991;133:1179-1190.

20. Canavan YM, O'Flaherty MJ, Archer DB, Elwood JH. A ten-year survey of eye injuries in Northern Ireland: 1967-76. *Br J Ophthalmol.* 1980; 64:618-625.

21. Sniezek JE, Finklea JF, Graitcer PL. Injury coding and hospital discharge data. *JAMA.* 1989; 262:2270-2272.

22. Bacon WE, Smith GS, Baker SP. Geographic variation in the occurrence of hip fractures among the elderly white US population. *Am J Public Health.* 1989;79:1556-1558.

Penetrating Eye Injuries in the Workplace

The National Eye Trauma System Registry

Andrew L. Dannenberg, MD, MPH; Leonard M. Parver, MD; Ross J. Brechner, MD, MS, MPH; Lynn Khoo, MB, BS, MPH

• Occupational eye injuries are common and preventable. Between 1985 and 1991, there were 635 work-related penetrating eye injuries among the 2939 cases (22%) reported to the National Eye Trauma System Registry by 48 collaborating centers in 28 states and Washington, DC. The median age of the injured workers was 30 years; 75% were younger than 40 years; and 97% were male. The commonest causes of injuries were projectiles (457 cases), sharp objects (166 cases), blunt objects (60 cases), and blasts (22 cases); these terms are not mutually exclusive. Specific objects causing injuries included nails, wire, screwdrivers, and other hand tools. There was evidence of alcohol use by at least 2% of the injured workers. When they were injured, 6% of the workers were wearing safety glasses; 3% were wearing nonsafety eyewear. Posterior segment trauma, which occurred in 63% of the cases, included vitreous hemorrhage (42%), intraocular foreign bodies (35%), and retinal detachment (10%). Hyphema occurred in 35% and traumatic cataract in 32% of the cases. Initial visual acuity after injury was hand motion or worse in 43% of the cases. National Eye Trauma System Registry data are useful to identify strategies to prevent occupational eye injuries such as wider use of safety glasses and improvement in engineering controls.

(*Arch Ophthalmol.* 1992;110:843-848)

Work-related ocular injuries are common but have received little attention compared with other occupational injuries. According to one report from Finland, eye injuries account for 12% of all work-related injuries.[1] Approximately 2.4 million eye injuries are estimated to occur annually in the United States including between 20 000 and 68 000 serious vision-threatening injuries requiring hospitalization.[2,3] About one quarter of all serious eye injuries are related to activities in the workplace.[4] Workers sustaining eye injuries are typically young adult males who are in their most productive years; almost all such injuries are preventable.

The National Eye Trauma System (NETS) was formed in the early 1980s to provide for the optimal clinical management of severe eye injuries and to encourage research in eye trauma.[5] In 1985, the NETS Registry was established, with participating NETS centers agreeing to collect a standardized set of information on penetrating ocular trauma including the type of injury, circumstances of injury, treatment, and clinical outcome. Penetrating eye injuries were selected because they are vision threatening, are the most frequent trauma-related indication for hospital admission,[3] and are readily defined as injuries in which the cornea, sclera, or both are perforated.

Data are submitted to the NETS Registry by 48 collaborating NETS centers in 28 states and the District of Columbia. These centers include many of the major ophthalmologic trauma centers in the United States.

Participation in NETS is voluntary and not all eye trauma is treated in eye trauma centers. Therefore, NETS Registry data constitute a large case series and do not represent a randomly selected sample of all penetrating eye injuries. During the period covered by this article, the cases in the NETS Registry constituted approximately 6% of the total number of all penetrating eye injuries that occurred nationally, based on the estimate of 3.81 penetrating injuries per 100 000 population annually in the United States.[3]

This article describes the circumstances and initial clinical findings of 635 work-related cases identified among the first 2939 cases of penetrating ocular trauma reported to the NETS Registry. Information about the circumstances of the eye injuries is essential for efforts to prevent such injuries.

METHODS

Demographic and clinical data on eye injuries are collected on standardized forms that are completed by the attending or resident ophthalmologist treating the injured person. The 75 questions on the Preoperative Form focus on patient demographic characteristics, physical setting of injury, agent of injury, use of protective eye wear, factors contributing to injury, history of eye disease, and a detailed clinical eye evaluation. The 68 questions on the Operative Form focus on the types of surgical procedures performed and on operative findings and complications. Operative Forms are completed for each surgical operation; therefore, for some patients, data were available from more than one Operative Form.

Occupational eye injury is a positive response to the question in the Preoperative Form about whether the injury is work-related based on the history obtained by the examining ophthalmologist; no special effort is made to contact the patient's employer for confirmatory information. The questions on evidence of alcohol and illicit drug use solicit the treating physician's clinical impression of such use regardless of whether formal alcohol or illicit drug testing was done.

Completed forms are sent to the Maryland Institute for Emergency Medical Services Systems in Baltimore for data editing and entry. The Injury Prevention Center at Johns Hopkins University oversees analysis of the NETS Registry data. For this article, frequency and cross-tabulation analyses were performed using SAS software (SAS Institute, Cary, NC) on a mainframe computer. All cases were included in all analyses except where specific necessary data items were missing; therefore, the denominators varied slightly for some analyses.

RESULTS

Among the 2939 cases of penetrating eye injuries reported to the NETS Registry between 1985 and 1991, 635 injuries (22%) occurred in the work setting. The median age of the injured workers was 30 years; the mean age was 33 years. Workers younger than 40 years sustained 75% of the reported work-related penetrating eye injuries (Fig 1). Female workers sustained only 2.5% of the reported occupational eye injuries. Seven of the injuries were due to assaults and two were reportedly self-inflicted.

The most common causes of eye injuries were projectiles (457 cases), sharp objects (166 cases), blunt objects (60 cases), and blasts (22 cases); these terms are not mutually exclusive. Seventy percent of the projectiles were metal objects. Specific objects causing injury included nails (64 cases), wire (31 cases), screwdrivers (13 cases), wood chips (12 cases), pliers (eight cases), metal bands or straps (seven cases), tree branches (five cases), hammers (four cases), chisels (four cases), drill bits (four cases), staples/staple guns (three cases), and other tools (20 cases).

Accepted for publication March 19, 1992.

From the Injury Prevention Center, The Johns Hopkins University School of Hygiene and Public Health, Baltimore, Md (Drs Dannenberg, Brechner, and Khoo); and the Department of Ophthalmology, Georgetown University Medical Center, Washington, DC (Dr Parver).

Reprint requests to Injury Prevention Center, The Johns Hopkins University School of Hygiene and Public Health, 624 N Broadway, Room 539, Baltimore, MD 21205 (Dr Dannenberg).

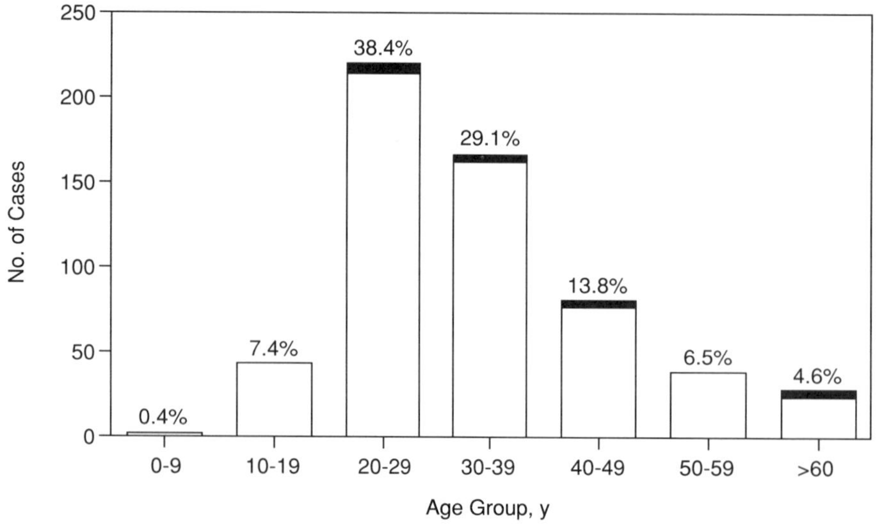

Fig 1.—Work-related penetrating eye injuries by age and gender (n=571) reported to the National Eye Trauma System Registry from 1985 to 1991. Shaded bars indicate males; closed bars, females.

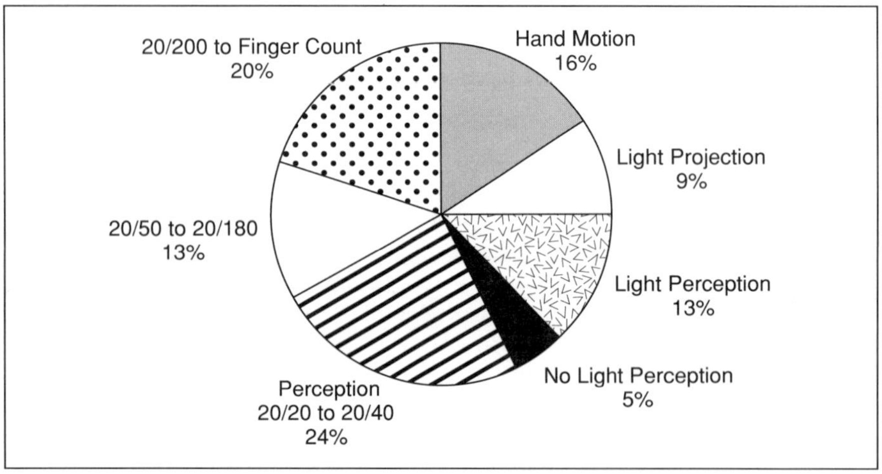

Fig 2.—Initial visual acuity of the injured eye following work-related penetrating eye trauma (n=613) reported to the National Eye Trauma System Registry from 1985 to 1991.

Among the infrequent types of injuries, one worker was injured by a live hard-shell crab in a work setting; one taxi driver was injured by a rock while driving.

Evidence of alcohol use was reported to the NETS Registry as "definite" in 1.9% and as "questionable" in an additional 1.9% of the injured workers. Evidence of illicit drug use was reported as "definite" in 0.2% and as "questionable" in 1.1% of the injured workers.

The initial visual acuity following injury is shown in Fig 2. Most penetrating eye injuries in the workplace are severe: 42.9% of such injuries presented with a visual acuity of hand motion or worse. Among the 570 cases in which laterality was reported, the right eye was injured in 50.0% of the cases, the left eye in 49.6%, and both eyes in 0.4%. Among injured workers aged 50 years and older, the injury occurred more frequently in the right eye (38 cases) than the left eye (24 cases).

Among injured workers, 20 (3.1%) were wearing nonsafety (dress) glasses and 35 (5.5%) were wearing safety glasses. Among users of nonsafety glasses, there were 16 cases of shattered lenses and three cases of broken frames. In six of the 16 cases with shattered lenses, glass or plastic was listed as the object causing or contributing to the injury. No cases of shattered lenses or broken frames were reported among users of safety glasses. While a variety of objects caused the injuries among users of nonsafety glasses, metal projectiles were the most frequent cause of injury among users of safety glasses (Table 1).

Type of tissue damage may be considered an indicator of injury severity. As shown in Table 2, 93% of the injured workers sustained anterior segment damage, including hyphema (35%) and traumatic cataract (32%). Sixty-three percent of the workers sustained posterior segment injuries, including vitreous hemorrhage (42%), retinal detachment (10%), and optic nerve damage (1%). Intraocular foreign bodies were present in 35% of the injured workers.

Treatment for most injuries included laceration closure and at least one other surgical procedure. Primary closure of the laceration of the cornea, sclera, or both was done in 465 of the 635 cases. The other common procedures were vitrectomy (279 cases), intraocular foreign body removal or inspection (228 cases), lens removal (195 cases), scleral buckle (137 cases), and cryotherapy (78 cases) (Table 3). Primary enucleation was performed in 19 cases. Intraocular infection occurred in 27 of the injured eyes.

COMMENT

Eye trauma is a common cause of work-related injury that contributes to a substantial amount of lost productivity. The National Institute of Occupational Safety and Health estimated that there were 900 000 occupational eye injuries in 1982 based on data from the National Electronic Injury Surveillance System.[6] Of these, approximately 84% were considered as minor trauma while the remainder involved more serious damage to the eye. Foreign bodies and chemical burns are among the most common types of work-related eye injuries.

Severe traumatic injuries are one of the 10 leading causes of work-related diseases and injuries in a list developed by the National Institute of Occupational Safety and Health to assist in setting priorities for efforts in the prevention of such diseases and injuries.[6] Eye injuries, including eye loss, are a major component of this category of injuries. Workers who lose vision in one eye may be restricted from operating certain motor vehicles and machinery; workers who lose vision in both eyes may be restricted from working in many industrial settings.

The NETS Registry is useful for investigating the characteristics of various types of penetrating eye injuries in the workplace and in other settings. In this analysis, work-related injuries account for 22% of all penetrating eye injuries reported to the NETS Registry from 1985 to 1991. Males aged 20 to 39 years comprise 66% of the patients with work-related eye injuries, while males in that age group constitute only 29% of the total civilian labor force.[7] The high

Table 1.—Work-Related Penetrating Injuries Occurring Despite Use of Safety or Nonsafety Glasses, National Eye Trauma System Registry, 1985-1991

	Type of Glasses	
	Nonsafety	Safety
No. of injured workers using glasses	20	35
% of all work-related injuries	3.1	5.5
Effect on glasses		
Shattered lenses	16	0
Broken frames	3	0
No failure reported	0	6
Other failure (unspecified)	2	29
Objects causing injury (No. of cases)*		
Projectiles		
	Metal (4)	Metal (21)
	Wood (3)	Nail (3)
	Glass/plastic (2)	Needle nose pliers (1)
	Chisel (1)	Screwdriver (1)
	Tree branch (1)	Unspecified (2)
Sharp objects		
	Glass/plastic (5)	Drill bit (3)
	Chisel (1)	Metal bracket (1)
	Metal (1)	Nail (1)
	...	Wire (1)
Blunt objects		
	Chain (1)	Rope (1)
	Fist (1)	...
	Metal pipe (1)	...
	Wood (1)	...
Blasts		
	Artillery device (1)	Concrete (1)
	Unspecified (3)	...

*Categories are not mutually exclusive; for example, one injury was associated with both a wood projectile and a sharp glass/plastic object.

Table 2.—Work-Related Penetrating Injuries With Selected Types of Eye Tissue Damage, National Eye Trauma System Registry, 1985-1991, n=635

Tissue Damage	No. (%) of Cases
Anterior segment injury	590 (93)
Hyphema	225 (35)
Traumatic cataract	205 (32)
Lens capsule rupture	160 (25)
Posterior segment injury	397 (63)
Vitreous hemorrhage	264 (42)
Incarceration	235 (37)
Intraocular foreign body	220 (35)
Scleral laceration/rupture	211 (33)
Prolapse	209 (33)
Retinal tear	83 (13)
Retinal detachment	61 (10)
Double penetrating injury	33 (5)
Optic nerve damage	4 (1)

Table 3.—Work-Related Penetrating Eye Injuries: Reported Surgical Procedures, National Eye Trauma System Registry, 1985-1991, n=635

Surgical Procedure	No. of Cases
Vitrectomy	279
Primary closure cornea	253
Intraocular foreign body removal or inspection	228
Lens removal	195
Scleral buckle	137
Primary closure sclera	119
Primary closure cornea and sclera	93
Cryotherapy	78
Enucleation	19

proportion of work-related penetrating eye injuries due to projectiles suggests that protective measures are needed for certain tools and machinery.

In other analyses of NETS data, there was evidence of alcohol use in a large proportion of recreational, motor vehicle, and assault-related eye injuries (A.L.D., unpublished data, 1992). In contrast, the small proportion of cases in this article in which there was evidence of alcohol or illicit drug use suggests that alcohol and illicit drugs are not major contributors to work-related eye injuries. However, these data may underestimate the actual involvement of alcohol and drugs in work-related injuries because formal alcohol and drug testing may not have been done in many of the cases reported. In studies of occupational fatalities, alcohol has not been found to be a major factor contributing to work-related injuries.[8]

Few of the injured workers wore any kind of eye protection; this finding is not unexpected because those who use safety glasses tend to be protected from eye injuries. The largest group of injuries, despite the use of safety glasses, were due to metal projectiles that presumably went around or penetrated through the safety glasses. For users of nonsafety glasses, glass or plastic fragments from shattered lenses may have contributed to some of the injuries. No information is available on the use of side shields or on the material composition of the safety or nonsafety glasses. A more intensive review of situations in which safety and nonsafety glasses failed to prevent eye injuries could be useful for improving the design of both types of glasses.

A survey by the Bureau of Labor Statistics showed that 59% of the workers were not wearing eye protection when injured, although eye protection was provided free by 70% of the employers of those workers injured while not wearing eye protection.[9] Only 5% of the injured workers who were wearing eye protection in the Bureau of Labor Statistics study reported breakage of the eye protection. Fifty-six percent of the injured workers who were wearing eye protection reported that the eyewear had reduced their injuries; 49% felt that better eye protection could have prevented or further reduced the injuries they received. While proper safety glasses should be worn by all workers at risk of eye injury, the use of polycarbonate lenses in their dress glasses could potentially have prevented some of the injuries to workers who were wearing nonsafety glasses when injured.[10]

In reviewing the literature, 23 English-language reports on eye trauma were identified that either focused entirely on work-related eye injuries or included a substantial proportion of such injuries within the report.[1,4,9,11-30] Table 4 summarizes the key findings from the NETS Registry and from reports from Brazil, Canada, Finland, Great Britain, Iceland, Israel, Spain, Sweden, and the United States published between 1956 and 1990. Comparisons of existing reports are limited due to differences in case definition, case ascertainment, and classification of setting, agent, or cause of injury.

Most reports were case series based on eye injuries treated in one or several hospitals or other clinical facilities. Other sources of reported data included workers' compensation records,[1,9] industrial medical log books,[16] a trauma registry,[4,30] and a telephone survey.[14] Population-based incidence data were available in few reports.[4,12,14,15] The studies included from 16 to 25 380 work-

Table 4.—Key Findings of Published Reports on Work-Related Eye Injuries

Source, y	Type of Report	Type of Injuries	Location	Total No. of Injuries	No. (%) of Occupational Injuries	Major Occupations	Agents of Injuries	Outcomes
Belfort et al,[11] 1972	Review of clinic records	Conjunctivitis, foreign bodies, and corneal ulcers	São Paulo, Brazil	**500**	**500 (100)**	Grinders, welders, and machine operators	Not reported	Visual acuity improved during treatment in 58% of the cases
Blomdahl and Norell,[12] 1984	Population-based registry of hospitalized patients	Perforating eye injuries	Stockholm County (Sweden)	320	87 (27)	Construction workers, building metal workers, carpenters, and technical workers	Occupational perforating injuries only: 43% metal fragments; and 14% nails	Not reported
Bureau of Labor Statistics,[9] 1980	OSHA* Survey of worker's compensation claims	Abrasions, chemical burns, lacerations, and others	19 states in United States	**1052**	**1052 (100)**	Craft workers, operatives, and laborers	52% metal items, and 18% chemicals	Not reported
Cole et al,[13] 1987	Review of hospital records	Perforating eye injuries	England	381	107 (28)	Machine operators and others	Hammer with or without chisel and operating machines	Not reported
Glynn et al,[14] 1988	Population-based telephone survey	Any eye injury needing medical attention	6 states in New England	27	16 (59)	Not reported	Not reported	10 of 16 injured workers lost at least 1 d of work
Karlson and Klein,[15] 1986	Population-based hospital records	Hospital-treated eye injuries	Dane County (Wisconsin)	1347 total; 13 severe	188 total (14); 4 severe (31)	Miscellaneous	2 chemical burns, 2 wire foreign bodies	Not reported
Kaufmann,[16] 1956	Industrial medical log books	Foreign bodies, corneal abrasions, burns, and others	Montreal, Quebec	**1107**	**1107 (100)**	Heavy industry, construction, and garment industry	Metal foreign bodies and chemical burns	26 cases required prolonged treatment
Lambah,[17] 1969	Review of hospital records	Corneal, eyelid and conjunctival injuries, penetrating injuries, and others	Wolverhampton, United Kingdom	1017	Approx 800 (80)	Heavy industry, light industry, and mining	Hammering hot metal	44% with perforating injuries were blind
Landen et al,[18] 1990	Review of hospital records	Perforating eye injuries	Allegheny County (Pennsylvania)	345	36 (10)	Not reported	Metal and wood foreign bodies	Not reported
Liggett et al,[19] 1990	Review of urban trauma center records	Blunt trauma, penetrating injuries, chemical and thermal burns, and others	Los Angeles, Calif	1132	Approx 90 (80)	Not reported	Blunt objects and sharp objects (total group)	Not reported
Macewen,[20] 1989	Review of ER records	Extraocular foreign bodies, corneal abrasions, flash burns, and others	Scotland	5671	3963 (70)	Light industry, grinding/buffing, and welding	67% extraocular foreign bodies	14 of 3963 (0.4%) hospitalized; 12 of 14 hospitalized had good visual outcomes
Maltzman et al,[21] 1976	Review of hospital records	Hyphema, traumatic cataract, perforating trauma, eyelid trauma, and others	New Jersey	468	Approx 40%	Not reported	Metal foreign bodies and other projectiles	Good outcomes reported for hyphemas (total group)
Mencía-Gutiérrez et al,[22] 1988	Review of records at one hospital	Perforating eye injuries only	Madrid, Spain	**77**	**77 (100)**	Industry, agriculture, and service trades	43% metal foreign bodies and 21% metal sharp objects	47% had acuity of 5/10 or better; 49% corneal scars

Table 4.—Key Findings of Published Reports on Work-Related Eye Injuries (cont)

Source, y	Type of Report	Type of Injuries	Location	Total No. of Injuries	No. (%) of Occupational Injuries	Major Occupations	Agents of Injuries	Outcomes
Morris et al,[4] 1987	Statewide eye trauma registry	All serious eye injuries	Alabama	736	196 (27)	Not reported	32% blunt injury; 23% sharp injury (total group)	Almost 90% of initial acuity 20/100 or better had outcomes at least as good as initially
Niiranen,[23] 1978	Review of hospital records	Perforating eye injuries	Helsinki, Finland	2015	1160 (58)	Metal workers, agriculture, and construction	Metal foreign bodies, sharp objects, and explosions	Prognosis improved from 1930s to 1950s
Punnonen,[24] 1989	Review of records at one hospital	Perforating eye injuries	Helsinki, Finland	387	139 (36)	Construction work (42%); industry (30%); and transport, commerce, and storage (15%)	Not reported	22% of injured eyes remained blind; 15% could not work or changed jobs because of injury
Saari and Aine,[25] 1984	Review of hospital records	Blunt trauma, perforating eye injuries, chemical burns, and others	Tampere, Finland	662	278 (42); 96 agricultural workers (only 70 at work)	Agriculture and construction industry	Cow horn, wood chips, metal foreign bodies, and chemical burns	Better in farming and lumbering, worse in dairying
Saari and Parvi,[1] 1984	Review of workers compensation records	Superficial injuries, radiation, burns, wounds, contusions, and others	Finland	**25 380**	**25 380 (100);** 20 102 (79) superficial; and 602 (2) wounds	Manufacturing, construction, and agriculture	Foreign bodies, machines and equipment, and chemicals	18% of all industrial injuries with 1-2 d of lost work time were due to eye injuries
Schein et al,[26] 1988	Review of ER records at one major eye hospital	Major and minor eye injuries	Massachusetts	3184 total; 161 severe	Approx 1530 (48)	Construction (63%); and automotive repair (18%)	Not reported	Ruptured globes (total group); median workdays lost, 70 d
Scherf and Zonis,[27] 1976	Review of hospital records	Perforating eye injuries	Israel	207	142 (69) includes military war injuries	Military injuries, work injuries, and agricultural injuries	Hammering, military activity	For intraocular foreign bodies, 37% had good or fair vision; and the rest were worse
Thordarson et al,[28] 1979	Review of records at one hospital	Primarily severe eye injuries	Iceland	105	43 (41)	Construction, auto repair, agriculture, and fishing	Wire, metal or wood splints, and screwdriver	Approx 2/3 of the total group had a good outcome
Vernon,[29] 1983	Review of ER records at one hospital	Nonperforating trauma	Bristol, England	3210	971 (30)	Not reported	Foreign bodies and abrasions high in total group	13% of eye injuries in total group required hospital admission
White et al,[31] 1989	Statewide eye trauma registry	All serious eye trauma	Alabama	514	144 (28)	Not reported	34% sharp object; 23% blunt object; 3% gunshot	4% enucleations; 69% return to work after rehabilitation
Present study, 1992	NETS registry	Penetrating eye injuries	48 centers in United States	2939	635 (22)	Not reported	72% projectiles; metal objects, nails, wire, and various tools	Not reported

*OSHA indicates Occupational Safety and Health Administration; ER, emergency department; and NETS, National Eye Trauma System.

related eye injuries; the larger sample sizes generally included a large proportion of minor injuries. The types of injuries varied based primarily on the source of the data and the selection criteria used by the authors. Some reports, especially those from emergency department records, included a large proportion of minor injuries such as superficial foreign bodies, corneal abrasions, and few chemical burns, thermal burns, and perforating eye injuries. Other reports, generally based on hospital records, were limited to severe penetrating trauma.

The proportion of eye injuries that were work-related ranged from 8% to 70% in the 19 reports that were not exclusively based on work-related eye injuries. In reports in which the sex ratio for work-related eye injuries was reported specifically, the proportion of males among the injured workers ranged from 83% to 99%. Workers between the ages of 20 and 40 years had the highest occurrence of occupationally related eye injuries in most reports.

The most common occupations of the injured workers were construction, manufacturing and agriculture; other eye injuries were reported for workers in the nonspecific categories of light industry and heavy industry. The most frequently reported activity at time of injury was hammering, either on metal or with a chisel. Other activities mentioned in a number of reports included handling wire, welding, grinding, drilling, and working with unspecified tools and machinery. The most common agents of injury were metal foreign bodies (including wire and nails), wood foreign bodies, and chemicals.

Other than this study, few reports mentioned the prevalence of protective eyewear use among the injured workers,[9,20] although the absence of safety eyewear was reported as the major risk factor for eye injury. Failure to use safety eyewear may relate either to not having such eyewear readily available or to a worker's decision not to wear available protective eyewear. Some cases in which protective eyewear was used but failed to prevent injury may be attributed to the use of poorly fitting safety glasses and to circumstances in which foreign material entered the eye from the side of the glasses or from falling off the glasses themselves.[9]

While some reports included information on outcomes, few results could be considered comparable. Various reports listed outcomes in terms of follow-up visual acuity, proportion of injured workers hospitalized, number of lost work days or proportion with any lost work days, and proportion able to return to the same job.

Several limitations should be considered in interpreting the NETS Registry data. The current data collection instrument identifies work-related injuries but not specific occupation or industry. The NETS Registry is implementing a revised instrument that asks for the occupation and industry of the injured worker. As a case series, NETS Registry data comprise a sample of convenience that is not necessarily representative of all penetrating eye injuries; the lack of a population-based denominator prevents the use of NETS Registry data to estimate incidence rates for such injuries. If all major eye trauma centers eventually choose to participate in the NETS Registry, it may be possible to conservatively estimate a national incidence rate for such eye injuries.

In addition, analyses are generally limited to the data collected by examining physicians. While we did not verify with employers that each injury did occur at work, treating physicians are likely to have accurate information on this item to obtain workers compensation payments for medical care costs. Additional resources would be required to do more detailed studies such as assessing workplace rules on eyewear use at the time of injury, or comparing NETS Registry data with workmen's compensation records or Occupational Safety and Health Administration files.

In the workplace, strategies to prevent eye injuries include improvements in engineering controls, education, and behavioral practices. Safety engineers can identify hazardous operations and determine the feasibility of changes to tools and machinery to reduce the risk of eye injury. For example, a shield attached to a machine with an interlock device can prevent machine operation when the shield is not in place. Safety glasses are an essential element of injury prevention in many work settings especially considering the large proportion of injuries due to projectiles such as nails and metal fragments. These data suggest it would be beneficial to routinely wear safety glasses while working with hand tools such as screwdrivers, hammers, chisels, and pliers. Management must be responsible for providing comfortable safety eyewear, educating workers on its importance, and enforcing its use.

The NETS Registry data are useful to examine the characteristics of a large case series of work-related eye injuries. The long-term objective is to identify and evaluate interventions that will reduce the incidence of occupational eye trauma.

Supported by the Division of Safety Research of the National Institute of Occupational Safety and Health, by grant R49/CCR302486 to The Johns Hopkins University Injury Prevention Center from the Centers for Disease Control, Atlanta, Ga, and by a grant to the Wilmer Eye Institute from Research to Prevent Blindness Inc, New York, NY.

The NETS Registry Investigators would like to thank the 48 National Eye Trauma System participating centers for providing the data and the Maryland Institute for Emergency Medical Services Systems for providing data management support.

For further information about the NETS Registry, contact Leonard M. Parver, MD, Director, National Eye Trauma System, Suite 607, 1145 19th St NW, Washington, DC 20036.

References

1. Saari KM, Parvi V. Occupational eye injuries in Finland. *Acta Ophthalmol Suppl.* 1984;161:17-28.
2. Feist RM, Farber MD. Ocular trauma epidemiology. *Arch Ophthalmol.* 1989;107:503-504.
3. Tielsch JM, Parver L, Shankar B. Time trends in the incidence of hospitalized ocular trauma. *Arch Ophthalmol.* 1989;107:519-523.
4. Morris RE, Witherspoon CD, Helms HA Jr, Feist RM, Byrne JB Jr. Eye Injury Registry of Alabama (preliminary report): demographics and prognosis of severe eye injury. *South Med J.* 1987; 80:810-816.
5. Parver LM. The National Eye Trauma System. *Int Ophthalmol Clin.* 1988;28:203-205.
6. Centers for Disease Control. Leading work-related diseases and injuries—United States. *MMWR.* 1984;33:213-215.
7. Bureau of Labor Statistics. *Outlook 2000.* Washington, DC: US Dept of Labor; 1990. US Dept of Labor publication 2352.
8. Smith GS, Kraus JF. Alcohol and residential, recreational, and occupational injuries: a review of the epidemiologic evidence. *Ann Rev Public Health.* 1988;9:99-121.
9. Bureau of Labor Statistics. *Accidents Involving Eye Injuries.* Washington, DC: US Dept of Labor; 1980. US Dept of Labor publication 597.
10. Davis JK. Perspectives on impact resistance and polycarbonate lenses. *Int Ophthalmol Clin.* 1988;28:215-218.
11. Belfort R Jr, Bonomo PP, Neustein I. Industrial eye injuries: analysis of 500 cases. *Ind Med.* 1972;41:30-32.
12. Blomdahl S, Norell S. Perforating eye injury in the Stockholm population: an epidemiological study. *Acta Ophthalmol.* 1984;62:378-390.
13. Cole MD, Clearkin L, Dabbs T, Smerdon D. The seat belt law and after. *Brit J Ophthalmol.* 1987;71:436-440.
14. Glynn RJ, Seddon JM, Berlin BM. The incidence of eye injuries in New England adults. *Arch Ophthalmol.* 1988;106:785-789.
15. Karlson TA, Klein BEK. The incidence of acute hospital-treated eye injuries. *Arch Ophthalmol.* 1986;104:1473-1476.
16. Kaufmann MIH. The incidence and management of common industrial eye injuries: a survey of 1,107 cases. *Can Med Assoc J.* 1956;75:284-287.
17. Lambah P. Adult eye injuries at Wolverhampton. *Eye.* 1969;88:661-673.
18. Landen D, Baker D, LaPorte R, Thoft RA. Perforating eye injury in Allegheny County, Pennsylvania. *Am J Pub Health.* 1990;80:1120-1122.
19. Liggett PE, Pince KJ, Barlow W, Ragen M, Ryan SJ. Ocular trauma in an urban population: review of 1132 cases. *Ophthalmology.* 1990;97:581-584.
20. Macewen CJ. Eye injuries: a prospective survey of 5671 cases. *Br J Ophthalmol.* 1989;73:888-894.
21. Maltzman BA, Pruzon H, Mund ML. A survey of ocular trauma. *Surv Ophthalmol.* 1976;21:285-290.
22. Mencía-Gutiérrez E, Gutiérrez-Díaz E, Gutiérrez-Díaz A, Ferro-Osuna M. Perforating ocular wounds in occupational accidents. *Ophthalmologica.* 1988;197:97-103.
23. Niiranen M. Perforating eye injuries: a comparative epidemiological, prognostic and socioeconomic study of patients treated in 1930-39 and 1950-59. *Acta Ophthalmol Suppl.* 1978;135:1-87.
24. Punnonen E. Epidemiological and social aspects of perforating eye injuries. *Acta Ophthalmol.* 1989;67:492-498.
25. Saari KM, Aine E. Eye injuries in agriculture. *Acta Ophthalmol Suppl.* 1984;161:42-51.
26. Schein OD, Hibberd PL, Shingleton BJ, et al. The spectrum and burden of ocular injury. *Ophthalmology.* 1988;95:300-305.
27. Scherf J, Zonis S. Perforating injuries of the eye. *Eye, Ear, Nose, Throat Mon.* 1976;55:32-40.
28. Thordarson U, Ragnarsson AT, Gudbrandsson B. Ocular trauma: Observation in 105 patients. *Acta Ophthalmol.* 1979;57:922-928.
29. Vernon SA. Analysis of all new cases seen in a busy regional centre ophthalmic casualty department during 24-week period. *J R Soc Med.* 1983; 76:279-282.
30. White MF Jr, Morris R, Feist RM, Witherspoon CD, Helms HA Jr, John GR. Eye injury: prevalence and prognosis by setting. *South Med J.* 1989; 82:151-158.

Penetrating Eye Injuries Related to Assault

The National Eye Trauma System Registry

Andrew L. Dannenberg, MD, MPH; Leonard M. Parver, MD; Carolyn J. Fowler, PhD,
for the National Eye Trauma System Investigators

• From 1985 to 1991, 648 cases of assault-related penetrating ocular injury were reported to the National Eye Trauma System Registry. We examined the circumstances surrounding and initial clinical findings related to this case series of injuries. Eighty-three percent of the patients were male. The median age was 28 years; 77% were younger than age 40 years, and 17% were younger than age 20 years. The ocular injury was part of multiple trauma in 34% of cases. There was evidence of alcohol and illicit drug use by at least 48% and 6% of the injured persons, respectively. Seventeen percent of the injuries involved powder or nonpowder firearms. Fists, glass fragments, metal rods or pipes, knives, and scissors were among the other objects causing injury. Posterior segment trauma, which occurred in 70% of cases, included vitreous hemorrhage (40% of cases), retinal detachment (11%), presence of intraocular foreign bodies (6%), and optic nerve damage (4%). The initial visual acuity after injury was hand motion or worse in 74% of the cases. Strategies to prevent such injuries focus on the origins of violence in general and are more difficult to devise than strategies to prevent eye injuries in other settings. Public health efforts to reduce the use of alcohol, drugs, and firearms may reduce the incidence of these injuries.

(*Arch Ophthalmol.* 1992;110:849-852)

In the United States, the number of reported physical assaults increased 56% from 1977 to 1986 according to FBI reports.[1] While assaults involving powerful weapons or extreme force may be lethal, many assaults involve nonlethal force that leaves the victim with short- or long-term disabilities. Eyes are particularly vulnerable to significant damage from assaultive blows that would cause only minor injuries if struck elsewhere on the body. Ocular injuries may be incidental to an attempt by an assailant to do general bodily harm to the victim or may result from the assailant's specific intent to damage the victim's eyes.

To examine assault-related eye injuries, we focused on penetrating eye injuries. Penetrating injuries, those in which the cornea and/or sclera are perforated, are vision-threatening and are the most frequent cause of hospital admission because of ocular trauma.[2] The National Eye Trauma System (NETS) Registry collects demographic and clinical data on persons sustaining penetrating eye injuries.[3] Between 1985 and 1991, 2939 cases of penetrating eye injuries were reported to the NETS Registry by ophthalmologists from the 48 regional eye trauma centers that participate in NETS (L.M.P., A.L.D., B. Blacklow, C.J.F., R. J. Brechner, J. M. Tielsch, unpublished data, 1992). These centers are located in 28 states and the District of Columbia. Because the reporting system is based on the voluntary cooperation of collaborating centers and because not all eye trauma is treated in eye trauma centers, the resulting data are a large case series that constitute a sample of convenience rather than a population-based sample of all penetrating eye injuries in the United States. Tielsch et al[2] estimated that approximately 3.81 penetrating eye injuries occur per 100 000 people annually in the United States. The cases in the NETS Registry constitute approximately 6% of the estimated total number of penetrating injuries nationally during the period covered by this report and represent the largest available series of such injuries.

An understanding of the circumstances surrounding assault-related injuries is the first step in developing strategies to prevent their occurrence. In this report, we describe the circumstances and presenting characteristics of 648 cases of assault-related eye injury reported to the NETS Registry and compare these cases with previously published studies.

Accepted for publication March 16, 1992.

From the Injury Prevention Center, Johns Hopkins University School of Hygiene and Public Health (Drs Dannenberg and Fowler), and the Wilmer Eye Institute, The Johns Hopkins University (Dr Parver), Baltimore, Md.

Reprint requests to The Johns Hopkins Injury Prevention Center, 624 N Broadway, Room 539, Baltimore, MD 21205 (Dr Dannenberg).

METHODS

Data are reported to the NETS Registry on standardized forms that include questions about the injured person, the injury-producing event, results of the clinical eye evaluation, and the surgical procedures performed. For each injured eye, the forms are completed by the attending or resident ophthalmologist involved in the evaluation and treatment of the injured person. Data from the completed forms are entered and edited by the Maryland Institute for Emergency Medical Services Systems. Data analyses are performed by The Johns Hopkins University Injury Prevention Center using Statistical Analysis System software (SAS Institute, Cary, NC) with a mainframe computer.

This report is based on analyses of the 648 injuries in 643 patients for whom the treating physician indicated on the Preoperative Form that the eye injury was inflicted by another person during an altercation. These analyses exclude 26 eye injuries reported as intentionally self-inflicted. Notation of alcohol and drug use by the injured person is based on information provided by the treating physician; formal testing for the use of these substances was not routinely conducted. In addition, denominators varied for analyses in which missing data were excluded.

RESULTS

The 648 cases of assault-related eye injuries constitute 22.0% of the 2939 cases reported to the Registry between 1985 and 1991. Forty-five of the 48 participating NETS centers reported assault-related eye injuries. Reports from seven of these centers, all located in areas with large urban populations, accounted for 58% of all reported assaults. and 43% of the total number of eye injuries in the NETS Registry. Patients with assault-related injuries ranged in age from 2 years to 92 years, with a median age of 28 years (Fig 1). Sixty percent of the injured persons were 20 to 39 years old, and 83% were male.

Alcohol use by the injured person was reported in at least 313 (48.3%) of the assaults, and alcohol use was suspected in another 92 cases (14.2%). In 40 cases (6.2%,) illegal drug use by the injured person was reported; it was suspected in an additional 127 cases (19.6%). The specific setting of the assault was reported for 219 cases (33.8%); of these, 173 injuries occurred in the home, 24 occurred in transportation settings, 15 occurred in recreational settings, and seven occurred in occupational settings.

The time of injury was reported in 646 cases (99.7%). Most assaultive injuries occurred at night. The distribution of

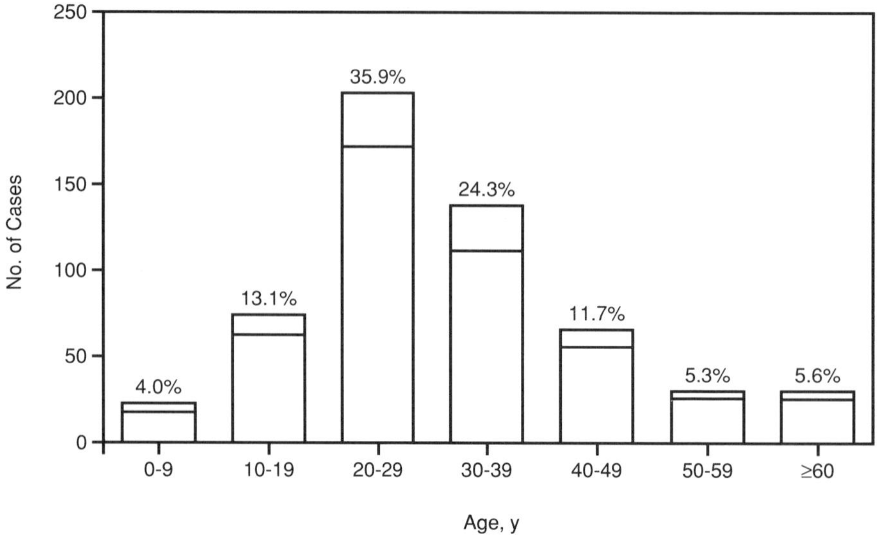

Fig 1.—Assault-related penetrating eye injuries by age and gender (n=571 [age and/or gender were not available for 77 cases]; 1985-1991 data from the National Eye Trauma System Registry). Closed areas indicate males, and open areas, females.

Table 1.—Selected Common and Unusual Objects Used as Weapons in Assault-Related Penetrating Eye Injury*

Objects Used in Five or More Cases (No. of Cases)	Objects Used in One Case
Projectiles	
Buckshot (56)	Ashtray
Bullets (43)	Block of ice
BB pellets (6)	Jumper cables
	Slingshot
	10-speed bicycle
Sharp Objects	
Glass and plastic objects† (87)	Axe
Knives and scissors (54)	Curtain rod
Wooden sticks and darts (11)	Ice pick
Metal sticks and darts (6)	Ink pen
	Jewelry chain
	Statue
	Umbrella
Blunt Objects	
Fists (120)	Axe handle
Metal rods or pipes (17)	Barbecue fork
Blunt wooden objects† (16)	Doll
Feet (12)	Fork
Butt and/or barrel of gun (9)	Hammer
Bottles (8)	Glass mug
Baseball bats (7)	Golf club
Broomstick handles (6)	Shovel
Pool cue sticks (5)	Sickle

*Data are from the National Eye Trauma System Registry for 1985-1991.
†Not otherwise specified.

cases was as follows: 9.3% from 10 AM to 4 PM, 21.1% from 4 PM to 10 PM, 63.3% from 10 PM to 4 AM, and 6.3% from 4 AM to 10 AM.

The types of objects that caused injury included projectiles (205 cases), sharp objects (200 cases), blunt objects (285 cases), and objects resulting from blasts (11 cases). These categories are not mutually exclusive. The most frequently reported causes of injuries due to blunt objects included assault with fists (120 cases), feet (12 cases), metal rods or pipes (17 cases), and unspecified blunt wooden objects (16 cases) (Table 1). The most common sharp objects causing injury were glass and plastic objects (87 cases), knives and scissors (54 cases), and metal or wooden sticks and darts (17 cases).

More than half of the injuries caused by projectiles (108 of 205 cases) were inflicted with powder or nonpowder firearms. Fifty-six assault-related penetrating injuries resulted from use of buckshot, 43 from bullets, six from BB pellets, and three from bird shot. Other types of projectiles causing injury included sharp projectiles, such as flying glass, and blunt projectiles, such as bricks and rocks. The nine cases in which the injurious object was considered both sharp and blunt involved fists with rings, brass knuckles, and a studded glove. In many cases, objects not normally considered weapons were used in assaults. These objects included beer bottles, pool cue sticks, fingernails, automobile jumper cables, belt buckles, and statues.

None of the injured persons was wearing protective safety glasses at the time of the assault. In 20 cases (3%), the injured persons were wearing nonsafety glasses at the time of the assault; in this group, 12 frames were broken and lenses from nine pairs of glasses were shattered.

Of the 641 cases for which laterality of eye injury was reported, the left eye was injured in 345 cases (53.8%), the right eye was injured in 291 cases (45.4%), and both eyes were injured in five cases (0.8%). The ocular injury was part of multiple trauma in 219 cases (33.8%). The multiple trauma involved only the head in 153 cases, and involved other body parts in 66 cases.

Initial visual acuity after assault was very poor in most cases. Initial visual acuity was better than 20/200 in only 80 (13.2%) of 608 cases (Fig 2). In 450 (74.0%) of 608 cases, initial visual acuity ranged from the ability to detect a hand moving in front of the eye (hand motion) to no light perception.

The types of tissue damage found on clinical examination (Table 2) may be considered indicators of the severity of the injuries sustained. The most frequently reported types of damage included anterior segment trauma (588 cases), such as hyphema (358 cases), and posterior segment trauma (454 cases), such as scleral laceration/rupture (367 cases), incarceration (272 cases), and vitreous hemorrhage (257 cases). Posterior segment trauma occurred in 70.1% of 648 assault-related eye injuries compared with 55.1% of the 2291 nonassault-related eye injuries recorded in the NETS Registry.

COMMENT

Assaults are an important cause of eye injuries and are responsible for 22% of all cases of penetrating injury reported to the NETS Registry. The 648 injuries described here constitute the largest reported series of assault-related ocular injuries (Table 3). The individuals sustaining these injuries were predominantly young males. The treating physician reported evidence of alcohol use (and to a lesser extent, illegal drug use) by the injured person in a large proportion of the assaults. The use of alcohol by the injured persons was probably underrepresented by our data because formal alcohol testing was not performed for

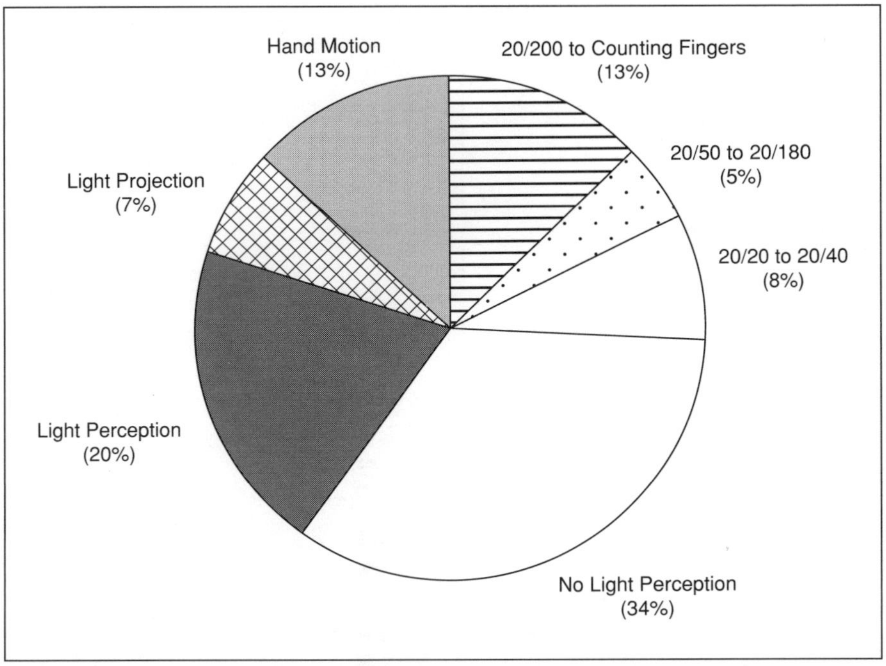

Fig 2.—Initial visual acuity of the injured eye after assault-related penetrating eye trauma (n=608 [initial visual acuity was unavailable for 40 cases]; 1985-1991 data from the National Eye Trauma System Registry).

Table 2.—Types of Eye Tissue Damage Resulting From Assault-Related Penetrating Eye Injuries*

Type of Tissue Damage	No. of Cases	% of Injured Eyes
Anterior segment injury	588	90.7
Hyphema	358	55.2
Traumatic cataract	63	9.7
Lens capsule rupture	52	8.0
Posterior segment injury	454	70.1
Scleral laceration/ rupture	367	56.6
Incarceration	272	42.0
Prolapse of intraocular tissue	309	47.7
Vitreous hemorrhage	257	39.7
Retinal detachment	69	10.6
Double-penetrating injury	47	7.3
Retinal break	41	6.3
Intraocular foreign body	41	6.3
Optic nerve damage	27	4.2

*Data are from the National Eye Trauma System Registry for 1985-1991. N=648 injuries. Some injuries involved more than one type of tissue damage.

many of the injured persons and no information was available on alcohol use by the assailants. The high proportion of injuries occurring at night may reflect the hours during which alcohol use is most common. The high proportion of eye injuries occurring in the home suggests that, as in the case of homicide,[4] many of the altercations may have been between family members or friends.

The wide diversity of objects used as weapons in assaults is particularly interesting. The object causing the most injuries was the fist, which is readily available in all settings. The use of firearms, knives, and brass knuckles in assaults suggests that in some cases the assailant was prepared to become involved in an altercation. The use of more unusual weapons (such as a doll, a bicycle, jumper cables, and a barbecue fork) suggests that in other cases the assault was a result of impulsive behavior and the weapon used was the most readily available object in that setting. In other studies, broken glass, broken bottles, fists, and knives were reported as the most commonly used weapons in assault-related eye injuries in England.[5] Fists, feet, sticks, thrown missiles, whips, and knives were reported as the most commonly used weapons causing eye injury in Lesotho.[6]

It is possible that right-handed assailants can strike a blow more easily to the left side of a victim's face than to the victim's right side. The higher proportion of injuries to the left eye is consistent with reports that facial injury after assault is more likely to affect the left side of the face.[7] The high frequency of multiple trauma suggests that the eye was often not specifically intended as the target.

The protective value of glasses during an assault cannot be estimated because no information was available on how frequently the use of glasses prevented eye injury during an assault. One would expect nonsafety glasses to provide only minimal protection against an assaultive injury. If shattered, glasses could actually contribute to the injury. Glasses with polycarbonate lenses would provide better protection,[8] although they are more expensive than the glass and plastic lenses in common use.

While a number of the published case series on ocular injuries include those related to assaults,[2,5,9-24] few reports focus specifically on assault-related eye injuries.[6,18] Assault-related injury represented between 1% and 53% of the cases reported in various series (Table 3). The proportions of assault-related injuries vary substantially by year and location. The literature suggests that assault-related eye injuries usually involve young males and frequently involve alcohol. Cole et al[5] observed regional variation in the incidence of assault-related eye injury in England and noted that higher incidence rates may "reflect more unsettled social environments" in some cities. Niiranen[20] commented that the increase in assault-related eye injuries in Finland in the 1970s compared with previous decades may have been related to increased unemployment and alcohol use during that time. The high level of ammunition-related ocular injury (17%) in the NETS data and in another report[11] is of particular concern.

While all penetrating eye injuries are severe by definition, assault-related injuries tend to be more severe than others reported to the NETS Registry. For example, in 74% of assault-related eye injuries, initial visual acuity after injury was hand motion or worse; in comparison, initial visual acuity after injury was hand motion or worse in only 43% of 613 work-related eye injuries reported to the NETS Registry.[25] Because initial visual acuity after injury is related to eventual visual outcome,[9,26] assault-related ocular injury may be expected to be associated with poor outcome relative to other causes of eye trauma. In particular, posterior segment trauma and prolapse (which are common in this series) have been shown to be associated with poor outcomes, both prospectively and retrospectively.[10,11]

Several limitations need to be considered in interpreting results of our analyses. It is not possible to calculate national incidence rates for eye trauma using NETS data because the NETS Registry is not population based. Although epidemiologically preferable, it would be both difficult and expensive to obtain a national population-based sample of assault-related eye injuries. Ocular injuries treated at eye trauma centers may differ from ocular injuries treated at general hospitals, especially with regard to severity.[27] Information in

Table 3.—Assault-Related Eye Injury as a Percentage of Reported Cases of Ocular Trauma

Source, y	Total No. of Eye Injuries	No. (%) of Assault-Related Eye Injuries	Location
Roper-Hall,[23] 1959	267	2 (1)	England
Lambah,[17] 1969	1017	75 (7)	England
Johnston,[15] 1971	295	28 (9)	Northern Ireland
Eagling,[11] 1976	237	19 (8)	England
Scherf and Zonis,[24] 1976	207	71 (34)*	Israel
Gordon and Mokete,[14] 1981	252†	134 (53)	Lesotho
Niiranen,[21] 1981	139‡	37 (27)	Finland
Vernon,[25] 1983	3210	53 (2)	England
Blomdahl and Norell,[13] 1984	318	33 (10)	Sweden
Karlson and Klein,[16] 1986	1347	201 (15)	Wisconsin
Cole et al,[6] 1987	378	42 (11)	England
Morris et al,[10] 1987	735	73 (10)	Alabama
Gilbert et al,[12] 1987	91	27 (30)	Baltimore, Md
Macewen,[20] 1989			
Total	5671	113 (2)	United Kingdom
Hospitalized	102	19 (19)	United Kingdom
Punnonen,[22] 1989	387	47 (12)	Finland
Tielsch et al,[2] 1989	2373	436 (18)	Maryland
Landen et al,[18] 1990	345	47 (14)	Pittsburgh, Pa
Liggett et al,[19] 1990	1260	511 (41)	Los Angeles, Calif
Present study, 1992	2939	648 (22)	United States

*Includes 69 military injuries.
†Excludes children.
‡Excludes children and occupational injuries.

the NETS Registry is based on voluntary reporting by ophthalmologists at 48 collaborating centers and is not independently confirmed. For example, no attempt has been made to confirm details of assault-related cases by communication with family members, witnesses, or law enforcement agencies. In some cases, the injured person may have been the instigator of the altercation; such circumstances cannot be distinguished using NETS Registry data. In addition, the NETS Registry excludes fatal injuries; for example, when a gunshot wound to the eye also involves the brain, the injured person may not survive long enough to receive treatment for the eye injury. Despite these limitations, the NETS Registry data are useful for describing the characteristics of severe assault-related eye injuries based on a large number of cases.

It is much more difficult to devise strategies to prevent assault-related eye injuries than it is to devise strategies to prevent eye injuries in the workplace or in recreational settings. Although the increased use of glasses with polycarbonate lenses may lead to a small reduction in the number of assault-related eye injuries, the most effective strategies to prevent such injuries are likely to be those focusing on the origins of violence in general. In the US Public Health Service monograph, *Healthy People 2000: National Health Promotion and Disease Prevention Objectives*,[28] a number of methods to reduce injuries related to violence are discussed. Some public health professionals have advocated teaching conflict resolution skills to adolescents to reduce the likelihood that violence will be used as the first response to interpersonal conflict. Public health interventions to reduce the use of alcohol and illicit drugs may also reduce the incidence of assaults overall.

The ready availability of firearms plays a major role in the high frequency of fatal and nonfatal injuries due to violence in the United States.[29] Our data indicate a low proportion of assault-related eye injuries involving firearms because many gunshot wounds to the head are fatal. In fatal cases, the eye injury is seldom treated or reported to the NETS Registry. Societal restrictions on access to weapons such as knives and firearms may reduce eye injuries somewhat, although our data indicate that fists and other readily available objects are commonly used in the nonfatal assaults that result in eye injuries. An awareness of the circumstances in which assault-related eye injuries occur is the first step in developing preventive strategies.

Data analysis and manuscript preparation were supported by grant R49/CCR302486 from the Centers for Disease Control.

The NETS Registry Investigators thank the 48 National Eye Trauma System participating centers for providing the data and the Maryland Institute for Emergency Medical Services Systems for providing data management support. For additional information about the NETS Registry, contact Leonard M. Parver, MD, NETS, Suite 607, 1145 19th St NW, Washington, DC 20036.

References

1. National Committee for Injury Prevention and Control. Injury prevention: meeting the challenge. *Am J Prev Med.* 1989;5(suppl):204-212.

2. Tielsch JM, Parver L, Shankar B. Time trends in the incidence of hospitalized ocular trauma. *Arch Ophthalmol.* 1989;107:519-523.

3. Parver LM. The National Eye Trauma System. *Int Ophthalmol Clin.* 1988;28:203-205.

4. Mercy JA, Saltzman LE. Fatal violence among spouses in the United States, 1976-85. *Am J Public Health.* 1989;79:595-599.

5. Cole MD, Clearkin L, Dabbs T, Smerdon D. The seat belt law and after. *Br J Ophthalmol.* 1987;71:436-440.

6. Gordon YJ, Mokete M. Ocular injuries following assault in Lesotho. *Trop Doct.* 1983;14:30-31.

7. Shepherd JP, Al-Kotany MY, Subadan C, Scully C. Assault and facial soft tissue injuries. *Br J Plast Surg.* 1987;40:614-619.

8. Davis JK. Perspectives on impact resistance and polycarbonate lenses. *Int Ophthalmol Clin.* 1988;28:215-218.

9. Morris RE, Witherspoon CD, Helms HA Jr, Feist RM, Byrne JB Jr. Eye Injury Registry of Alabama (preliminary report): demographics and prognosis of severe eye injury. *South Med J.* 1987;80:810-816.

10. Eagling EM. Perforating injuries of the eye. *Br J Ophthalmol.* 1976;60:732-736.

11. Gilbert CM, Soong HK, Hirst LW. A two-year prospective study of penetrating ocular trauma at the Wilmer Ophthalmological Institute. *Ann Ophthalmol.* 1987;19:104-106.

12. Blomdahl S, Norell S. Perforating eye injury in the Stockholm population: an epidemiological study. *Acta Ophthalmol (Copenh).* 1984;62:378-390.

13. Gordon YJ, Mokete M. Adult ocular injuries in Lesotho. *Doc Ophthalmol.* 1981;51:187-192.

14. Johnston S. Perforating eye injuries: a five-year survey. *Trans Ophthalmol Soc (UK).* 1971;91:895-921.

15. Karlson TA, Klein BEK. The incidence of acute hospital-treated eye injuries. *Arch Ophthalmol.* 1986;104:1473-1476.

16. Lambah P. Adult eye injuries at Wolverhampton. *Trans Ophthalmol Soc (UK).* 1969;88:661-673.

17. Landen D, Baker D, LaPorte R, Thoft RA. Perforating eye injury in Allegheny County, Pennsylvania. *Am J Public Health.* 1990;80:1120-1122.

18. Liggett PE, Pince KJ, Barlow W, Ragen M, Ryan SJ. Ocular trauma in an urban population: review of 1132 cases. *Ophthalmology.* 1990;97:581-584.

19. Macewen CJ. Eye injuries: a prospective survey of 5671 cases. *Br J Ophthalmol.* 1989;73:888-894.

20. Niiranen M. Perforating eye injuries treated at Helsinki University Eye Hospital 1970 to 1977. *Ann Ophthalmol.* 1981;13:957-961.

21. Punnonen E. Epidemiological and social aspects of perforating eye injuries. *Acta Ophthalmol (Copenh).* 1989;67:492-498.

22. Roper-Hall MJ. The treatment of ocular injuries. *Trans Ophthalmol Soc (UK).* 1959;79:57-69.

23. Scherf J, Zonis S. Perforating injuries of the eye. *Eye, Ear, Nose Throat Monthly.* 1976;55:32-40.

24. Vernon SA. Analysis of all new cases seen in a busy regional centre ophthalmic casualty department during 24-week period. *J R Soc Med.* 1983;76:279-282.

25. Dannenberg AL, Parver LM, Brechner RJ, Khoo L. Penetrating eye injuries in the workplace: the National Eye Trauma System Registry. *Arch Ophthalmol.* 1992;110:843-848.

26. Sternberg P Jr, de Juan E Jr, Michels RG, Auer C. Multivariate analysis of prognostic factors in penetrating ocular injuries. *Am J Ophthalmol.* 1984;98:467-472.

27. Strahlman E, Elman M, Daub E, Baker S. Causes of pediatric eye injuries: a population-based study. *Arch Ophthalmol.* 1990;108:603-606.

28. *Healthy People 2000: National Health Promotion and Disease Prevention Objectives.* Washington, DC: US Government Printing Office; 1991. US Dept of Health and Human Services publication PHS 91-50212.

29. Fingerhut LA, Kleinman JC. International and interstate comparisons of homicide among young males. *JAMA.* 1990;263:3292-3295.

Marital Aggression

Impact, Injury, and Health Correlates for Husbands and Wives

Michele Cascardi, MA; Jennifer Langhinrichsen, PhD; Dina Vivian, PhD

• The overall aim of the current study was to comprehensively evaluate the prevalence, impact, and health correlates of marital aggression in a clinic sample of maritally discordant couples seeking psychological treatment. Participants were 93 consecutively presenting clinic couples and 16 maritally satisfied matched control couples from the community. Overall, 71% of clinic couples reported at least one act of marital aggression during the past year. Although 86% of the aggression reported was reciprocal between husbands and wives, impact and injuries sustained as a function of this aggression differed between husbands and wives. Specifically, wives were more likely than husbands to be negatively affected and to sustain severe injuries (eg, broken bones, broken teeth, or injury to sensory organs). Additionally, wives who experienced marital aggression reported clinical levels of depressive symptomatology. Recommendations are offered and risk markers are identified to improve detection by physicians of patients who may be involved in violent marriages.

(*Arch Intern Med.* 1992;152:1178-1184)

In 1980, domestic violence emerged from "behind closed doors" with the national survey of family violence by Straus et al.[1] In the decade since that survey, domestic violence has been recognized as a serious health problem. In fact, former Surgeon General C. Everett Koop[2] declared violence against women as the number one health problem of American women in 1985.

Straus et al[1] assessed the prevalence of marital violence in a national random survey of more than 2000 households. These researchers used a self-report questionnaire, the Conflict Tactics Scale (CTS), which assesses the frequency of physically aggressive tactics experienced or engaged in by partners during marital conflicts. They found that 28% of the couples surveyed had engaged in either husband-to-wife (H=>W) or wife-to-husband (W=>H) aggression at some time during the marriage.[1] Husbands and wives self-reported engaging in similar frequencies of physical aggression; however, the CTS did not assess whether the injuries or impact sustained were equivalent for the two sexes.

Other researchers[3-5] have documented that the injuries sustained by women as a result of their partner's physical aggression can often be quite severe (eg, black eyes, broken teeth, broken bones, or concussions) and may require emergency medical attention. For example, Stark and Flitcraft[6] found that at any point in time, 40% of women in emergency departments were victims of wife abuse and 10% of the women repeatedly seen by emergency department physicians were victims of repeated assaults by a partner. Additionally, data collected between 1973 and 1982 by the National Crime Survey indicated that 94% of reported domestic violence incidents were committed against women; 95% of all the cases involved injuries and medical treatment for women.[7] Moreover, Cantos et al,[8] in a sample of US military couples (n=284) referred for domestic violence treatment, found that 69% of husbands and wives sustained some injury from a domestic violence incident. Of these cases, 57% of the wives and 8% of husbands reported being the sole recipient of injuries. In the remaining 35% of couples, both spouses reported sustaining some injuries. Husbands and wives also indicated on a self-report measure whether the injury necessitated medical attention. The scale ranged in severity from no medical treatment to surgery. Cantos et al[8] found that the military wives reported sustaining significantly more severe injuries that resulted in medical treatment than did their husbands.

However, the use of the emergency department or the severity of the injury are not the only measures of the impact of H=>W aggression on women's health. In fact, injury alone may not be the best index with which to evaluate the impact of physical aggression, since the majority of marital aggression may not result in injury. Stets and Straus[9] used several diverse measures of the impact of physical aggression perpetrated by either partner on a sample of women (n=336) and men (n=264) drawn from the community.[9] The participants were asked to report whether the injury resulting from marital aggression required medical treatment, time off from work, and/or days spent in bed because of illness. Significantly more women (3%) than men (0.4%) reported needing medical attention as a result of their injuries. Similarly, 9% of the women took time off from work, whereas 6% of the men did, and

Accepted for publication March 27, 1992.

From the Department of Psychology, State University of New York at Stony Brook.

Reprint requests to Department of Psychology, State University of New York at Stony Brook, Stony Brook, NY 11794-2500 (Dr Vivian).

18% of the women spent at least 1 day in bed because of illness, contrasted with 13% of the men. Although these latter gender differences were not statistically significant, they still suggest a trend for women to be more adversely affected by their partners' aggression than men.

There is also some evidence that women who have experienced H⇒W aggression are at risk for a variety of health complaints. Follingstad et al[10] documented that 65% of abused women (n = 234) solicited from the community suffered from three to seven of the following symptoms (listed in order of reported frequency): headaches, back and limb problems, frequent colds, fainting and dizziness, stomach and gastrointestinal problems, gynecologic problems, heart and blood pressure problems, lung and breathing problems, and/or skin problems. In addition, Stets and Straus[9] reported that as the severity of H⇒W aggression increased, reports of psychosomatic complaints, stress, and depression also significantly increased.

Men may also suffer adverse health consequences as a result of marital aggression. Some evidence suggests that men who engage in H⇒W aggression in fact experience more stress than do nonaggressive men.[1] Stress has been linked to a variety of chronic health problems such as high blood pressure, ulcers, chronic pain, and heart disease.[11] Moreover, anger and hostility are known correlates of heart disease in men.[12] Thus, it appears that both partners in violent marriages experience health problems that could be linked to the marital aggression.

Physicians and other health care professionals may fail to identify patients who have experienced domestic violence injuries or negative health consequences because of patients' reluctance to disclose the presence of marital aggression. For example, within the field of mental health, Hilberman and Munson[13] found that only 4% of women in marital therapy spontaneously admitted physical victimization by a partner. When these same women were asked directly about the presence of H⇒W aggression, 14% confirmed its occurrence. Even more dramatically, O'Leary,[14] in a marital clinic sample, noted that only 6% of the wives and 1.5% of the husbands spontaneously reported marital aggression as a presenting problem during the intake interview. However, 53% of these same husbands and wives (or 67% of the couples) had reported some act of H⇒W aggression on the CTS within the past year. In a related study, Riggs et al[15] examined the willingness of male and female college undergraduates to self-report relationship aggression. They documented that men and women were more likely to report having experienced, rather than having engaged in, relationship aggression, suggesting that individuals underreport their own levels of aggression.

In summary, research on domestic violence indicates that the prevalence of marital aggression is remarkably high in normative samples and even higher in clinic samples. Second, it is likely that marital aggression has a larger negative impact on women's health than on men's health in terms of injuries sustained and other, more general, emotional and somatic complaints. However, studies that have examined the impact of marital aggression have focused primarily on women. In addition, studies examining the differential effects of marital aggression on men and women are recent and not representative of the majority of marital violence research. Finally, it is clear that neither men nor women readily disclose marital aggression to helping professionals.

The overall aim of the current study was to comprehensively evaluate the impact and health correlates of physical aggression in a clinic sample of maritally discordant husbands and wives seeking psychological treatment. Findings of previous studies demonstrated that exclusive assessment of either injury or health problems related to marital aggression did not provide the most complete evaluation of the impact of marital aggression. A particularly unique aspect of this study was the multidimensional assessment of the impact of marital aggression (ie, injury, perceived impact, depressive symptomatology, past and current health problems, and current medication use).

The first goal of the study was to assess the prevalence of marital aggression in this clinic sample. Marital aggression was defined to include both H⇒W and W⇒H aggression. Based on Straus and colleagues'[1] finding of similar frequencies for men's and women's aggressive behavior, it was expected that husbands and wives in this sample would also report engaging in similar frequencies of aggression.

The second objective was to assess the impact of marital aggression on husbands and wives. It was hypothesized that experiencing marital aggression would be perceived as more negative and would result in more severe injuries for wives than for husbands. Moreover, it was expected that couples experiencing mild aggression would report the impact as less negative and would report less severe injuries than would couples experiencing severe aggression.

The documented association among marital aggression, demographic variables such as age and education, and marital distress warranted examination of these variables in this study.[16] It was expected that younger couples with less education and lower levels of marital satisfaction would be at the greatest risk for marital aggression. Finally, given the relationship between marital aggression and health complaints (eg, back pain, headaches, and depression), it was expected that wives in aggressive marriages would be more likely to report health problems and depressive symptomatology than would nonaggressive, maritally discordant wives or nonaggressive, maritally satisfied wives. In addition, based on the associations among stress, anger, aggression, and health problems, it was expected that husbands in aggressive marriages would be more likely to report health problems and depressive symptomatology than would nonaggressive, maritally discordant husbands or nonaggressive, maritally satisfied husbands.

SUBJECTS AND METHODS

Subjects

Ninety-three couples consecutively seeking therapy at the University Marital Therapy Clinic, Stony Brook, NY, from mid 1989 through late 1991 participated in this study. No couples were excluded. The University Marital Therapy Clinic is a research-based treatment facility affiliated with the Department of Psychology at the State University of New York at Stony Brook. It is known in the Suffolk County community for providing marital treatment for a wide variety of marital and individual problems including depression, sexual problems, communication problems, and physical aggression. An advertisement was used only to recruit community control couples. A telephone screening was conducted to eliminate maritally discordant or aggressive couples from the study's control group. Couples were accepted into the community control group only if both spouses agreed that they were maritally satisfied and nonaggressive throughout the duration of their marriage. Eligible couples were then matched with the overall sample of clinical couples according to age, education, years married, and income. At the time of this study, 16 community couples had been recruited. All spouses in the study gave written consent to participate in an extensive assessment procedure used for clinical and research purposes.

The clinic and community groups were compared on all demographic variables to assess the effectiveness of the matching procedure. A 2 (gender) × 2 (group) mixed-design multivariate analysis of variance was conducted on all demographic variables (ie, age, education, years married, and income) to determine overall group and gender effects. There were group and gender main effects (Rao's $R[4,61]=4.11$, $P<.01$, and Rao's $R[4,61]=3.06$, $P<.05$, respectively). Univariate analyses of variance gave evidence that age differed between the clinic and community groups and between husbands and wives ($F[1,80]=4.67$, $P<.05$, and $F[1,80]=9.90$, $P<.01$, respectively).

The mean age of the clinic husbands was 38 years (SD = 10.10 years); the mean age of the clinic wives was 35 years (SD = 11.35 years). The average age of the community husbands and wives was 44 years (SD = 8.47 years) and 39 years (SD = 7.38 years), respectively. Tukey HSD post hoc analyses revealed that the community control group was significantly older than the clinic group and husbands were significantly older than wives across groups. There were no differences in income, education, or years married between the clinic and community control groups or husbands and wives. Clinic and community control couples reported a mean family income of $48 051 (SD = $28 343), averaged 14.1 years of education, and were married 12 years on average.

Procedures

During their first visit at the University Marital Therapy Clinic, each spouse was interviewed separately for approximately an hour and a half. While one spouse was interviewed, the other spouse completed a comprehensive battery of paper-and-pencil questionnaires. The present study was derived from a subset of data that are being collected for a larger ongoing investigation of communication and cognitive patterns of maritally distressed and aggressive couples, which is being conducted by one of us (D.V.). The clinic and the community couples who participate in all aspects of the ongoing study receive $80. Examples of excluded measures pertained to psychological domains such as sexual coercion in marriage, relationship beliefs, perceived problem-solving ability, and assertion with one's spouse. This information was not germane to the health questions of interest in this study. Therefore, only the information from the following self-report questionnaires was included: the Dyadic Adjustment Scale,[17] the Modified CTS,[18] the Beck Depression Inventory,[19] and "Questions Related to Physical Illness."

Measures

Dyadic Adjustment Scale.—The Dyadic Adjustment Scale is a widely used 32-item measure of marital satisfaction.[17] The psychometric properties of this instrument are well documented. Typically a score below 100 reflects marital discord.

Modified CTS.—The Modified CTS is a 29-item questionnaire that assesses marital aggression used as a conflict tactic during the year prior to assessment. This instrument is an expanded and modified version of Straus'[20] CTS and Neidig's Modified CTS.[8] The Modified CTS assesses the frequency of 10 aggressive acts on a 7-point scale (1, never; 2, once; 3, twice; 4, three to five times; 5, six to 10 times; 6, 11 to 20 times; and 7, more than 20 times in the past year), as well as the impact and injuries sustained as a consequence of engaging in and/or experiencing mildly or severely aggressive acts.

The frequency items were dichotomized into presence/absence of any aggressive act in order to separate the aggressive and nonaggressive clinic groups. Based on past research and classification traditions within the field, items 19 through 22 (ie, pushing, grabbing, and shoving; controlling physically; throwing something; and slapping) were designated as mildly aggressive. The severely aggressive items were 23 through 29 (ie, kicking, biting, and hitting with a fist; hitting with something other than a fist; choking or strangling; forcing partner to have sex; beating up; threatening with a knife or a gun; and using a knife or a gun). This method of classification is widely accepted in the marital violence area.[1]

The impact of mildly and severely aggressive acts was assessed separately using a 7-point Likert scale (1 represents an extremely negative impact on self; and 7, an extremely positive impact on self). Five (yes/no) items were used to assess the injuries sustained because of mildly and severely aggressive acts from a spouse: (1) no injury; (2) superficial bruises, cuts, or abrasions (mild); (3) nonsuperficial cuts or abrasions (moderate); (4) broken bones, broken teeth, or injuries to sensory organs (severe); and (5) internal injuries or concussions (extreme). For some of the analyses, an injury index was formed by summing across the injury categories, weighting the injuries in order of severity (1, mild; 5, moderate; 10, severe; and 15, extreme).

While the Modified CTS is a new instrument, the CTS is the most widely used topographical measure of marital aggression. Its psychometric properties have been well documented.[1,20]

Beck Depression Inventory.—The Beck Depression Inventory[19] is a 21-item self-report measure of depressive symptomatology. It evaluates vegetative, cognitive, and behavioral signs of depression in the week prior to administration. A score equal to or greater than 14 is believed to represent moderate levels of clinical depression, while scores above 20 represent severe levels of clinical depression.[21]

Questions Related to Physical Illness.—Three health-related (yes/no) questions taken from the written intake packet were included in the study: (1) Have you ever been seriously ill? (2) Are you currently experiencing any physical problems? (3) Are you currently taking any medication? If the spouse responded yes to any of the health questions, she or he described in writing the nature of the health problem and/or the type of medication currently being used.

RESULTS

The *n*'s vary slightly across analyses because of missing data.

Marital Aggression in the Marital Clinic Sample

Husband-to-Wife Aggression.—The prevalence of H⇒W aggression was assessed based on each wife's report of her husband's behavior and/or the husband's self-report on the Modified CTS. According to the wives, 21% (n = 18) of the husbands were classified as mildly aggressive and 33% (n = 29) as severely aggressive (ie, 54% of the clinic husbands). In contrast, only 22% of the husbands (n = 19) classified themselves as severely aggressive, while 33% (n = 29) described themselves as mildly aggressive (ie, 55% of the clinic husbands). When *either/or* reporting was used (ie, reports by wives about their husbands aggression and/or reports by husbands about themselves), 27% of clinic husbands (n = 25) were classified as mildly aggressive, while 34% (n = 31) were classified as severely aggressive. Overall, 61% of couples seeking marital therapy reported at least one act of H⇒W aggression in the past year.

Wife-to-Husband Aggression.—The prevalence of W⇒H aggression was assessed based on each husband's report of his wife's behavior and/or the wife's self-report on the Modified CTS. According to the husbands, 12% (n = 10) of the wives were classified as mildly aggressive and 45% (n = 39) as severely aggressive (ie, 57% of the

Demographic Variables and Marital Satisfaction

	Group, Mean (SD)					
	Aggression		Discord Only		Community Control	
	H	W	H	W	H	W
Education, y	13.2 (2.00)	13.6 (2.09)	15.5 (3.63)	14.7 (2.56)	14.9 (3.67)	13.8 (2.14)
Age, y	35.6 (8.11)	32.4 (9.91)	44.5 (13.09)	41.8 (12.29)	48.9 (14.66)	45.4 (16.48)
Years married	9.5 (8.71)		16.1 (13.92)		18.4 (16.34)	
DAS	82.2 (19.22)	73.9 (25.87)	100.6 (16.04)	93.1 (18.75)	122.1 (9.76)	122.1 (9.95)
Total family income, $	42 788 (25 742)		61 826 (29 104)		47 846 (31 817)	

*H indicates husbands; W, wives; and DAS, Dyadic Adjustment Scale.

wives). Likewise, 9% of the wives (n=8) classified themselves as mildly aggressive, while 36% (n=31) described themselves as severely aggressive (ie, 45% of the wives). When *either/or* reporting was used, 12% of clinic wives (n=11) were classified as mildly aggressive, while 50% (n=46) were classified as severely aggressive. Overall, 62% of couples seeking marital therapy reported at least one act of W=>H aggression in the past year.

Couple Aggression.—The prevalence of couple aggression was assessed using the spouses' reports of H=>W aggression and/or the spouses' reports of W=>H aggression. This method of classification grouped the couples on the basis of the most severe tactic endorsed by either spouse. For example, if the wife reported severe aggression (either engaged in or experienced) and the husband reported mild aggression (either engaged in or experienced), the couple was classified in the severe aggression group. Accordingly, 19% (n=17) of the couples were classified as mildly aggressive, 52% (n=48) as severely aggressive, and 29% (n=26) as nonaggressive (two couples could not be classified because of extensive missing data). Of the aggressive couples, 86% reported reciprocal aggression. Only 14% of the couples reported unilateral aggression. Fifty percent (n=8) of the unidirectional violence was H=>W aggression, and 50% (n=8) was W=>H aggression. In addition, 98% of spouses in the severe aggression group also reported mild aggression. As a result of the overlap between mild and severe aggression in the severe aggression group, the analyses conducted for the impact experienced and the injuries sustained from mild aggression include both spouses who reported only mild aggression and spouses who reported both mild and severe aggression.

Mild and Severe Physically Aggressive Tactics

The most frequently reported acts of mild marital aggression were pushing, grabbing, or shoving. The most frequently reported acts of severe marital aggression were kicking, biting, or hitting with a fist.

Impact of Marital Aggression: Gender Differences

Husbands and wives were compared using paired *t* tests to determine whether experiencing aggression from a spouse had a more negative effect and resulted in more severe injuries for wives than for husbands.

Psychological Impact on Self.—Both wives and husbands were asked only to rate the perceived impact on *themselves* of their spouse's mild and/or severe aggression. When rating the impact of their spouse's mild aggression on them, the wives' mean impact rating was 1.79 (SD=.95), and the husbands' mean impact rating was 2.54 (SD=1.29) ($t[31]=3.94$, $P<.001$). The wives' mean impact rating of severe aggression was 1.79 (SD=1.05), while the husbands rated the impact at 2.45 (SD=1.18) ($t[18]=3.27$, $P<.002$). Overall then, the wives rated experiencing both mild and severe aggression as significantly more negative than the husbands did. Contrary to expectations, negativity of experienced impact did *not* differ for either husbands or wives ($t<1$, $P>.10$) depending on the level of severity of marital aggression from a spouse (ie, mild or severe).

Severity and Type of Injury.—χ^2 Analyses indicated that significantly more women than men reported sustaining injuries for each injury category. Given the low frequency of injury reports, these analyses were conducted by collapsing the mild and severe aggression acts into one group of any aggression. Moreover, since few spouses reported moderate, severe, or extreme injuries, these results must be interpreted with caution. To increase the stability and power of the findings suggested by the χ^2 analyses, an injury index was computed to transform the dichotomous data into continuous data (see "Measures" section). By transforming the data, a comparison of husbands and wives was possible on the full range of injuries sustained for mildly and severely aggressive acts separately.

As expected, for both wives and husbands, the severity of injury was significantly correlated with the frequency of marital aggression experienced ($r=.54$, $P<.05$, and $r=.30$, $P<.05$, respectively). That is, the more often a spouse reported that aggression occurred, the more likely she or he was to sustain injuries.

Consistent with our hypotheses, there were significant gender differences between husbands and wives on severity of injuries. The wives sustained significantly more severe injuries than the husbands as a consequence of mild marital aggression ($t[36]=2.27$, $P<.02$). There was also a trend for the wives to sustain more severe injuries than the husbands as a consequence of severe marital aggression ($t[15]=1.40$, $P=.09$).

Figures 1 and 2 offer descriptive information regarding the types of injuries sustained by husbands and wives who experienced mild and severe aggression. About half of the wives and two thirds of the husbands reported no injury as a result of experiencing both mild and severe marital aggression. Figure 1 shows that 15% of the wives who experienced mild aggression and 11% of the wives who experienced severe aggression reported sustaining broken bones, broken teeth, and/or injury to sensory organs. In contrast, as illustrated in Fig 2, only 2% of the

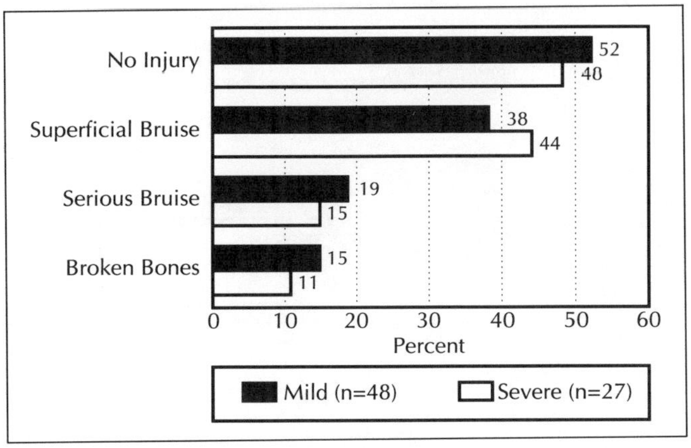

Fig 1.—*Wives' reports of injuries from mild and severe marital aggression.*

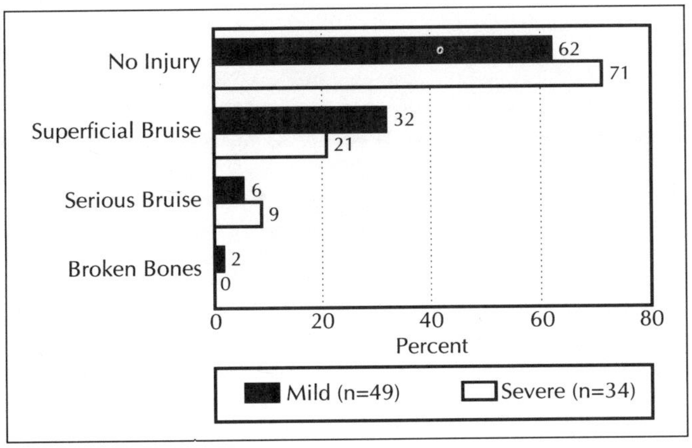

Fig 2.—*Husbands' reports of injuries from mild and severe marital aggression.*

husbands who experienced mild aggression and none of the husbands who experienced severe aggression reported sustaining broken bones, broken teeth, and/or injury to sensory organs.

Correlates of Aggression

Since injury and impact did not differ depending on the severity of aggression experienced, one aggression group was used for the remaining analyses. Membership in the aggression group was based on either the husband's or the wife's report of physical aggression because of the high degree of reciprocity in marital aggression. That is, if either spouse reported any physical aggression in the past year, he or she was included in the aggression group. The groups for the remaining analyses were as follows: marital discord/no aggression (discord only group, n=26), marital discord/any aggression (aggression group, n=65), and marital satisfaction/no marital aggression (community control group, n=16).

Demographics and Marital Satisfaction.—A 2 (gender) × 3 (group) mixed-factor multivariate analysis of variance revealed group and gender main effects (Rao's $R[8,120]=5.40$, $P<.001$), and Rao's $R[4,60]=4.36$, $P<.01$, respectively) for age, education, years married, income, and marital satisfaction. As depicted in the Table, the spouses in the aggression group were significantly younger than those in the discord only group ($F([2,79]=9.00$, $P<.001$); no significant difference emerged between the aggression and community control

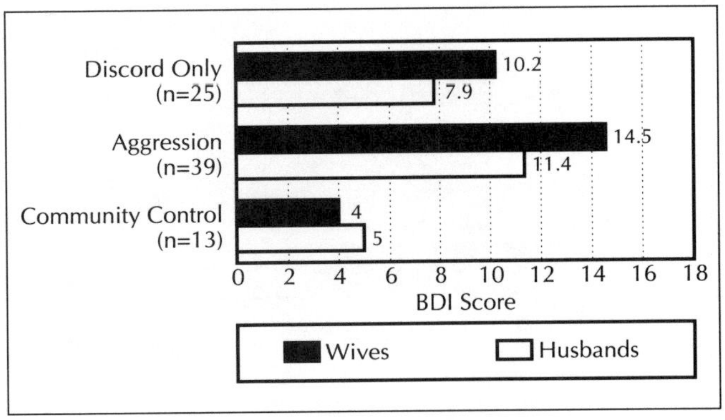

Fig 3.—*Mean Beck Depression Inventory (BDI) scores for wives and husbands.*

groups. (The reader may note that the couples in the community control group were older than the couples in the discord only and aggression groups. However, there were only significant differences in age between the discord only and aggression groups. The primary reason for the failure to find significant differences between the community control group and the aggression group is statistical power.) In addition, the wives were significantly younger than their husbands ($F([1,79]=16.27$, $P<.001$). The spouses in the aggression group reported significantly fewer years of education than the spouses in the discord only group ($F[2,99]=6.12$, $P<.005$). Finally, all of the groups differed significantly from one another on levels of marital satisfaction ($F[2,93]=38.94$, $P<.001$); and, overall, husbands were more maritally satisfied than their wives ($F[1,93]=5.83$, $P<.01$).

The three groups were then compared to determine if the aggression group also reported more depressive symptomatology and health problems than the discord only or the community control groups. Since age is correlated with depressive symptomatology and significantly differed across groups, it was used as a covariate in these analyses.

Depressive Symptomatology.—Figure 3 presents the mean Beck Depression Inventory scores for the husbands and wives in the three groups. A 2 (gender) × 3 (group) mixed-design analysis of covariance controlling for age revealed a significant main effect for group only ($F([2,57]=7.791$, $P<.001$). Using Tukey HSD post hoc analyses, both wives and husbands who experienced aggression reported significantly more depressive symptomatology than either the discord only or the community control spouses ($P<.09$ and $P<.02$, respectively). The mean amount of depressive symptomatology reported by the aggressive wives meets criteria for moderate levels of depressive symptomatology.[21]

Health Problems.—To determine specific group differences, two groups were compared at a time (eg, discord only vs aggression, discord only vs community control, and aggression vs community control) for wives and husbands on the three health questions. A z statistic based on the binomial distribution was used to assess the difference between the proportions across groups.[22] As depicted in Fig 4, 42% of the wives in the aggression group indicated that they were ill at the time of intake. Only 35% of the discord only wives and 29% of the community control wives reported being currently ill. Although the proportions were in the expected direction, these group dif-

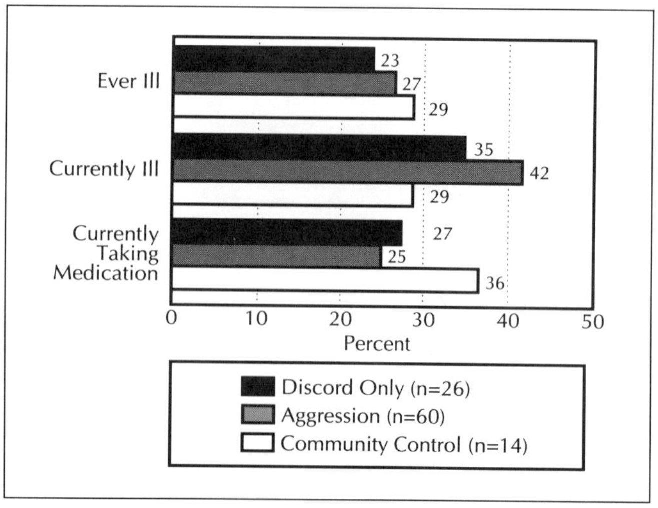

Fig 4.—*Wives' report of illness.*

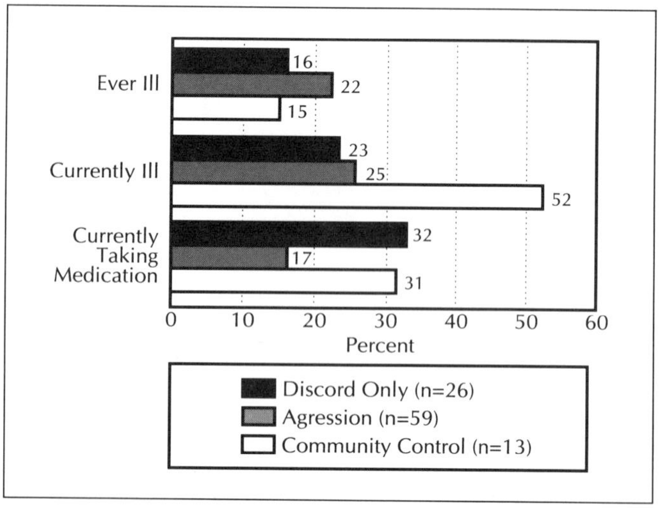

Fig 5.—*Husbands' report of illness.*

ferences were not statistically significant ($z<1.96$). The four primary current health problems reported by wives were chronic pain (33%), psychological difficulty (eg, fainting, dizziness, and anxiety) (10%), gastrointestinal and bladder (7%), and gynecologic (7%). No significant differences emerged across groups for wives for past illness or current medication use ($z<1.96$).

Figure 5 illustrates group differences on the health questions for the husbands. Twenty-five percent of the husbands in the aggression group reported being ill at intake vs 23% of the discord only husbands and 52% of the community control husbands. None of the group differences on the health questions were significantly different ($z<1.96$). The three most often reported current health problems by husbands were chronic pain (46%), coronary (17%), and gastrointestinal and bladder (12%). There were no differences among the three groups of husbands in current medication use or history of serious illness ($z<1.96$).

COMMENT

The results of this study are consistent with previous research documenting an alarmingly high prevalence of marital aggression in distressed couples seeking marital therapy. This rate was consistently high irrespective of classification method (H—>W, W—>H, or couple aggression). In fact, the most inclusive classification strategy (couple aggression) identified 71% of the clinic sample as maritally aggressive.

Also consistent with prior research,[1,9] husbands and wives reported experiencing and engaging in aggression at approximately the same rate. More specifically, the majority (86%) of aggression reported by the couples in this sample was reciprocal. That is, 56 couples reported H—>W aggression, 57 reported W—>H aggression, and 65 reported any aggression (either H—>W or W—>H). In spite of the mutuality of aggression, when impact experienced and injuries sustained were considered, a very different picture emerged. Specifically, wives were more likely than husbands to be negatively impacted by their spouse's aggression and to sustain severe injuries (eg, broken bones, broken teeth, or injury to sensory organs).

As reviewed elsewhere, a number of different models have been used to explain the gender differences in the use of marital aggression.[23] Biological models, for example, would suggest that testosterone differences between men and women result in men's greater use of aggression. According to sociological models, men use violence to maintain power and control over women, and their wives in particular. Lastly, psychological theories of marital aggression suggest that (1) men may use physical aggression to resolve conflicts; (2) gender differences in socialization processes may cause men to have greater difficulty in coping with anger; and (3) men may use physical aggression to control their aversive affective arousal during conflict.[23,24] While results from the present study do not advance any particular etiologic model, they provide strong support for our proposal that any model of marital aggression should take into account gender differences in the consequences of aggression.

Another finding in the present study was that mild and severely aggressive groups did not differ by age, income, education, or consequences of marital aggression, namely, impact or injury. One conclusion is that whenever marital violence occurs, no matter how seemingly mild or severe, it warrants attention and may be a risk factor for health consequences and distress for both partners. Another possibility is that our sample may not have included the most serious cases of wife abuse. That is, wives who are still willing to attend marital therapy with their husbands may not yet have experienced extremely negative health consequences as a result of the aggression. Couples characterized by more severe aggression and experiencing extremely severe injuries may have self-selected out of this sample. This self-selection may also have occurred because of the University Marital Therapy Clinic procedures and policies (eg, fees, acceptance of couples only, etc). Finally, the lack of differences on impact and injury between mild and severe aggression may be due to the fact that only 19% of the couples reported experiencing mild aggression alone. Therefore, the results from the mild impact ratings primarily reflect the reports of those couples who experienced both mild and severe aggression.

However, even in a sample of couples who were committed enough to their marriage to seek marital therapy, 12.8% of the wives who experienced any aggression reported a broken bone, broken teeth, and/or injury to sensory organs. Clearly, marital aggression has serious medical consequences irrespective of the level of aggression described by a patient. Further, an unfortunate consequence of addressing the correlates of marital aggression or distress (eg, depression, stress, and somatic complaints) through medical treatment alone is that one of the possible root causes of the problems, namely marital aggression, is not directly treated. This may leave women in potential danger.[3,6] Failure by professionals to address marital aggression may inadvertently perpetuate the cycle of violence.

The results of the present study highlight the need for professionals to educate patients about the impact of marital aggression. Health professionals should be prepared to discuss the negative and dangerous consequences of men's aggression on their partners. This approach is recommended even if men state that their partners are equally or more severely aggressive than they are. Likewise, women should be informed about their vulnerability to injury and marital distress when they are experiencing aggression, even if they self-report engaging in reciprocal aggression toward their husbands or are blaming themselves for the marital aggression.

The lack of demographic differences between clinic and community groups most likely indicates that successful matching occurred. As expected, however, the aggressive group differed in many significant ways both from the discord only group and from the community control group. In general, couples experiencing aggression were younger, less well educated, more depressed, and more dissatisfied with their marriages than were either of the other groups. Age differences within the clinic groups (aggression and discord only groups) indicate that young couples may be more at risk for aggression in their marriage, especially if they are experiencing marital difficulties. Contrary to our hypotheses, we did not find that the wives or husbands in the aggression group were more ill or more likely to be taking medication than were those in the discord only group or the community control group. In sum, younger, less educated, depressed, and maritally dissatisfied spouses may be at risk for marital aggression.

Overall, the group and gender differences obtained in this study make a strong case that physicians who are treating patients for injury, depression, or stress should routinely inquire about the patients' marital functioning. This is particularly important in light of past research documenting men's and women's reluctance to spontaneously disclose marital aggression.[14] For example, physicians may ask patients the following questions:

1. In general, how satisfying is your marriage?
2. What happens when you and your partner argue or fight?
3. Have you ever been physically aggressive toward your partner (ie, pushed, shoved, kicked, hit, or slapped him or her)? During the past 12 months?
4. Has your partner ever been physically aggressive toward you (ie, pushed, shoved, hit, slapped, or kicked you)? During the past 12 months?

Patients who respond affirmatively to questions about physical aggression should be asked about the frequency and severity of these acts. They also should be advised of the negative impact of physical aggression on their mental and physical health as well as the increased likelihood of further aggression taking place. Lastly, to prevent further aggression, it is extremely important to give patients a referral number to a therapist or community agency specializing in domestic violence. (The Hotline number for the National Coalition against Domestic Violence is (800)-333-SAFE.) To avoid further victimization of women, the referral source should be sensitive to gender differences regarding marital aggression.

This study was supported in part by grants MH44665 (Dr Vivian) and MH19107 from the National Institute of Mental Health, Bethesda, Md.

References

1. Straus MA, Gelles RJ, Steinmetz SK. *Behind Closed Doors: Violence in the American Family*. New York, NY: Anchor Books; 1980.
2. Koop CE. *The Surgeon General's Workshop on Violence and Public Health*. Washington, DC: Government Printing Office; 1985:i.
3. Stark E, Flitcraft A, Frazier W. Medicine and patriarchal violence: the social construction of a 'private' event. *Int J Health Serv*. 1979;9:461-493.
4. Walker L. *The Battered Woman*. New York, NY: Harper & Row Publishers Inc; 1979.
5. Cascardi M, O'Leary KD. Depressive symptomatology, self-esteem, and self-blame in battered women. *J Fam Violence*. In press.
6. Stark E, Flitcraft A. Violence among intimates: an epidemiological review. In: Van Hasselt VB, Morrisson RL, Bellack AS, Hersen M, eds. *Handbook of Family Violence*. New York, NY: Plenum Press; 1988:293-318.
7. Schwartz MD. Gender and injury in spousal assault. *Sociol Focus*. 1987;20:61-74.
8. Cantos A, Neidig P, O'Leary KD. *Fear and Injuries of Women and Men in a Treatment Program for Domestic Violence*. Stony Brook, NY: Behavioral Science Associates; 1991.
9. Stets J, Straus MA. Gender differences in reporting marital violence and its medical and psychological consequences. In: Straus MA, Gelles RJ, eds. *Physical Violence in American Families: Risk Factors and Adaptations in 8145 American Families*. New Brunswick, NJ: Transaction Books; 1990:151-166.
10. Follingstad DR, Brennan AF, Hause ES, Polek DS, Rutledge LL. Factors moderating physical and psychological symptoms of battered women. *J Fam Violence*. 1991;6:81-95.
11. Williamson D, Davis CJ, Prather RC. Assessment of health related disorders. In: Hersen M, Bellack A, eds. *Behavioral Assessment: A Practical Handbook*. 3rd ed. Elmsford, NY: Pergamon Press Inc; 1988:chap 6.
12. Roskies E, Saraganian P, Oseasohn R, et al. The Montreal Type A Intervention Project: major findings. *Health Psychol*. 1986;5:45-69.
13. Hilberman E, Munson K. Sixty battered women. *Victimology*. 1978;2:460-471.
14. O'Leary KD, Vivian D, Malone J. Assessment of physical aggression in marriage: the need for a multimodal method. *Behav Assess*. In press.
15. Riggs DS, Murphy CM, O'Leary KD. Intentional falsification in reports of interpartner aggression. *J Interpersonal Violence*. 1989;4:225-232.
16. O'Leary KD, Barling J, Arias I, Rosenbaum A, Malone J, Tyree A. Prevalence and stability of physical aggression between spouses. *J Consult Clin Psychol*. 1989;57:263-268.
17. Spanier GB. Measuring dyadic adjustment: new scales for assessing the quality of marriage and similar dyads. *J Marriage Fam*. 1976;38:15-28.
18. Vivian D. *The Modified Conflict Tactics Scale*. Stony Brook, NY: University Marital Therapy Clinic; 1990.
19. Beck AT. *Depression Inventory*. Philadelphia, Pa: Center for Cognitive Therapy; 1978.
20. Straus MA. Measuring intrafamily conflict and violence. *J Marriage Fam*. 1979;41:75-88.
21. Beck AT, Steer RA, Garbin MG. Psychometric properties of the Beck Depression Inventory: twenty-five years of evaluation. *Clin Psychol Rev*. 1987;8:77-100.
22. Fleiss JL. Assessing significance in a fourfold table. In: *Statistical Methods for Rates and Proportions*. New York, NY: John Wiley & Sons Inc; 1981:19-32.
23. O'Leary KD, Vivian D. Physical aggression in marriage. In: Fincham FD, Bradbury TN, eds. *The Psychology of Marriage: Basic Issues and Applications*. New York, NY: Guilford Press: 1990:323-348.
24. Baucom DH, Notarious CI, Burnett CK, Haefner P. Gender differences in sex-role identity in marriage. In: Fincham FD, Bradbury TN, eds. *The Psychology of Marriage: Basic Issues and Applications*. New York, NY: Guilford Press; 1990:150-171.

Cerebrospinal Fluid Monoamine and Adrenal Correlates of Aggression in Free-Ranging Rhesus Monkeys

J. Dee Higley, PhD; P.T. Mehlman, PhD; D. M. Taub, PhD; S. B. Higley; Stephen J. Suomi, PhD; M. Linnoila, MD, PhD; J. H. Vickers, DVM

• Clinical and preclinical studies involving several different mammalian species and research paradigms suggest a negative correlation between aggression and central serotonin activity. To test the generalizability of laboratory findings in rhesus monkeys that show a negative correlation between cerebrospinal fluid 5-hydroxyindoleacetic acid concentrations and aggression, we obtained cisternal cerebrospinal fluid and blood plasma samples from monkeys living in naturalistic conditions. During a semiannual trapping, 28 juvenile and adolescent male rhesus monkeys were chosen from a population of 4200 provisioned, free-ranging rhesus monkeys living on Morgan Island, a sea island located off the coast of South Carolina. Based on direct observations of participation or avoidance of aggressive behavior and examinations of apparent fight wounds, 18 monkeys were selected for cerebrospinal fluid taps and blood samples. The remaining 10 monkeys were selected at random. Descriptions of aggressive behavior and the number of old scars and recent wounds were carefully transcribed, and a photograph showing wounds and scars was obtained for each animal. Using the transcriptions and photographs, researchers experienced in rhesus monkey behavior, but blind to the subjects' monoamine and hormone concentrations, were asked to rank the monkeys from the most to the least aggressive. The results showed a significant negative correlation between high rankings for aggression and cerebrospinal fluid 5-hydroxyindoleacetic acid concentrations. There was evidence that aggression was associated with stress, in that cerebrospinal fluid, norepinephrine, and plasma corticotropin and cortisol concentrations were positively correlated with high rankings of aggression.

(*Arch Gen Psychiatry*. 1992;49:436-441)

Accepted for publication March 10, 1992.

From the Section on Neurochemistry and Neuroendocrinology, Laboratory of Clinical Studies, Division of Intramural and Clinical Biological Research, National Institute of Alcohol Abuse and Alcoholism (Drs J. Higley and M. Linnoila), and Laboratory of Comparative Ethology, National Institute of Child Health and Human Development, National Institutes of Health Animal Center (Ms S. Higley and Dr S. Suomi), Bethesda, Md, and Laboratory Animal Breeders and Services, Yemassee, SC (Drs P. Mehlman and D. Taub), and Pathobiology and Primatology Laboratory, Division of Product Quality Control, Office of Biological Product Review, Center for Biologics Evaluation and Research, Food and Drug Administration, Bethesda, Md (Dr J. Vickers).

Reprint requests to Animal Center, National Institutes of Health, Laboratory of Clinical Studies, PO Box 289, Poolesville, MD 20837 (Dr J. Higley).

A basic understanding of the etiology, chronicity, and associated risk factors involved in excessive aggression is crucial for its effective treatment and prevention. One risk factor appears to be diminished serotonin activity in the central nervous system. In humans, central serotonin functioning is frequently measured by assaying for 5-hydroxyindoleacetic acid (5-HIAA) in cerebrospinal fluid (CSF) obtained from lumbar punctures. While specific regional brain contributions cannot be identified using this method, CSF 5-HIAA concentrations are closely correlated with frontal cortex 5-HIAA concentrations.[1,2] Numerous studies have found evidence of diminished CSF 5-HIAA concentrations in violence-prone individuals who have problems of impulse control. For example, diminished CSF 5-HIAA concentrations have been found in men expelled from the marines for excessive violence and psychopathic deviance,[3] in offenders convicted for impulsive aggressive acts,[4] in sons of alcoholics arrested for violence or arson,[5] in children who torture animals,[6] in disruptive schoolchildren expressing hostility to their mothers and exhibiting aggression toward other people,[7] and in men with personality disorders who have unusually high scores for aggression, irritability, hostility, or psychopathic deviance on standardized tests.[8,9]

Direct investigation of the mechanisms producing differences in serotonin activity and aggression is difficult in humans. Investigators are limited in how well they can control the background variables hypothesized to play a role in human development, and they are limited in their capacity to measure and manipulate central nervous system activities. Animal models, however, impose fewer limitations and have been widely used to investigate central nervous system functions.[10] For example, studies with rodents have shown that drugs used to decrease or increase central nervous system serotonin increase and decrease some forms of aggression, respectively.[11,12] Phylogenic distance, however, limits somewhat the applicability of rodent studies to human biology.

Nonhuman primate models have been widely used to investigate relationships between central nervous system mechanisms producing behavioral aberrations and psychopathology. This is, in large part, due to the genetic similarity that other primates share with humans. It is estimated that one frequently studied nonhuman primate species, the rhesus monkey, shares approximately 90% to 94% of its genetic material with humans.[13,14] This genetic similarity between humans and nonhuman primates most likely underlies numerous compelling parallels in morphology, physiology, development, and complex social behaviors.[15,16] Thus, one of the major reasons for using nonhuman primates to model complex social behaviors, such as aggression, is their similarity to humans in central nervous system development and structure, and intricacies of social relationships. In addition, repeated CSF samples can be more readily obtained; in humans, CSF is generally removed from the lumbar region, whereas in monkeys, CSF can be directly removed from the cisterna magna.

Given the similarities between nonhuman primates and humans, and the numerous studies showing diminished CSF 5-HIAA concentrations in impulsive, aggressive individuals, it is somewhat surprising that, to our knowledge, no research has investigated whether highly aggressive rhesus monkeys have low CSF 5-HIAA concentrations. On the other hand, two studies of distantly related primates, squirrel and talapoin monkeys, have assessed the relationship between aggression and CSF 5-HIAA concentrations; both studies failed to detect a relationship.[11,17] The difficulty in establishing an association between CSF 5-HIAA concentrations and aggression may be due, in part, to problems in obtaining and maintaining highly aggressive monkeys in social groups in the laboratory. Laboratory colonies are generally limited in size of social groups, thus limiting the range of aggressive individuals that may be available. Perhaps most importantly, colony management procedures are usually designed to cull highly aggressive monkeys to prevent injuries to other monkeys.

Despite the absence of a clear association between diminished CSF 5-HIAA concentrations and excessive aggression in monkeys, other data suggest that nonhuman primates might provide a good model to investigate diminished serotonin activity and aggression. For example, Raleigh and McGuire[18] administered drugs to vervet monkeys to modify central nervous system serotonin activity and found that decreasing serotonin function produced the predicted increase in aggression; conversely, drugs used to increase serotonin tone produced a decrease in aggression. Similarly, increasing or decreasing tryptophan in the diet of vervet monkeys produced a decrease or an increase in aggression, respectively.[19] There is also evidence that serotonin activity may be related to social competence. Monkeys with relatively high whole blood serotonin and CSF 5-HIAA concentrations are more likely to be socially dominant; conversely, monkeys with diminished whole blood serotonin—especially when drugs are used to lower serotonin levels—are more likely to be avoided and ostracized as social companions,[18,20,21] and monkeys rated as socially deviant show diminished CSF 5-HIAA concentrations.[20,22]

An additional reason for using nonhuman primates to explore the relationship between serotonergic activity and aggression is a wealth of recent studies elucidating the variables and mechanisms involved in interindividual differences in CSF 5-HIAA concentrations. Recent data from studies with rhesus monkeys show that CSF 5-HIAA has traitlike qualities, with interindividual differences in CSF 5-HIAA concentrations showing stability over both short-term and long-term repeated samplings, even when the samples are separated in time by more than a year.[23,24] Furthermore, much is known concerning the underlying etiology of interindividual differences in CSF 5-HIAA concentrations. There are not only marked experiential contributions to CSF 5-HIAA concentrations,[24-26] but significant maternal and paternal genetic influences as well.[27,28]

A crucial step in developing a model relating central nervous system serotonergic activity to aggression in primates would be to document a clear relationship between excessive aggression and diminished CSF 5-HIAA concentrations and to show that it generalizes to a naturalistic population. The present study attempts to establish such a relationship. Rhesus monkeys were chosen for this study for several reasons: cerebrospinal fluid samples can be removed directly from the cisterna magna, allowing a more accurate estimate of central serotonergic activity than other methods of sampling, and we know more about the behavior and central nervous system function of rhesus monkeys than virtually all other primate species. Also, from a behavioral perspective, rhesus monkeys have a relatively high base rate for expressing aggression relative to many other species of nonhuman primates.[29-31]

Because highly aggressive monkeys are uncommon in most laboratory settings, we chose to collect CSF samples from adolescent males residing in a large population of 4500 free-ranging, provisioned rhesus monkeys living in a natural setting (to date, CSF samples have not been obtained from free-ranging rhesus monkeys). To generate aggressivity ratings on our subjects, we scored observable behavioral aggression when possible, combined with a technique for recording the location of canine and other tooth wounds, and scars on the torso, limbs, and head. This latter method, counting and describing wounds and scars resulting from agonistic encounters, has been widely used to assess aggression in several studies of free-ranging primates.[30,32]

In this article, we test a primary hypothesis that interindividual differences in aggressivity ratings are correlated negatively with levels of CSF 5-HIAA as a trait. We also test a second hypothesis—that stress and aggression are positively correlated—by assaying blood plasma for stress hormones. This hypothesis is based on findings by Green and colleagues[11] showing that CSF 3-methoxy-4-hydroxyphenylglycol (MHPG) concentrations are elevated in monkeys participating in aggression and other studies[33] showing a relationship between stress and aggression. Inasmuch as there are numerous studies indicating a positive relationship between testosterone concentrations and aggression[34-36] (although Johnson and Whalen[37] reported conflicting findings), we test the hypothesis that highly aggressive monkeys have elevated concentrations of testosterone. Finally, we note that this study, to our knowledge, is the first assessment of CSF monoamines from free-ranging rhesus monkeys and allows a preliminary description of the range of monoamine concentrations obtained from monkeys living in the wild.

SUBJECTS, MATERIALS, AND METHODS

Subjects and Sample Population

Twenty-eight young male rhesus monkeys (*Macaca mulatta*), ranging in age from 11 to 46 months (mean±SE, 23.1±1.8), were chosen from among 4500 rhesus macaques maintained as a free-ranging, food-provisioned breeding colony located on Morgan Island, a 475-acre South Carolina island. As in other natural populations, these monkeys are organized into matrilineal social groups (n=35; median group size, 50) and distributed in separate but overlapping home ranges. Reproductive events are reg-

Table 1.—Correlations of Time of Day and Elapsed Time With Each Biological Variable*

	ACTH	Cortisol	Testosterone	NE	MHPG	5-HIAA	HVA
Time of day	−.036	−.080	.152	−.056	.342	.034	−.001
Time to sample	−.241	−.241	−.195	.059	−.256	−.057	−.029

* Correlations of the variables time of day that sample was obtained, and the elapsed time from the technicians entering the corrals and obtaining a sample with each of the different biological variables. ACTH indicates corticotropin; NE, norepinephrine; MHPG, 3-methoxy-4-hydroxyphenylgycol; 5-HIAA, 5-hydroxyindoleacetic acid; and HVA, homovanillic acid.

ularly monitored by a staff of nine technicians who determine birth dates by field observations.

Conditions of Capture.—To perform physical examinations and routine medical procedures, the monkeys are trapped three times each year in 10 large corrals (10 to 25 m in diameter and 4 m in height) that normally serve as feeder stations. On the first day of a 5-day trapping period, all corrals are baited with food and their doors are closed. The monkeys voluntarily jump into the corrals, but are precluded from exiting by the high walls. Typically, only a portion of several social groups may jump into a corral, and they may then remain there between 1 and 5 days until the technical crew is ready to process that particular corral (the length of time monkeys spend in a corral is a function of the number of monkeys that can be processed each day during a 1-week period). All subjects used in this study were removed from the corral on the final 3 days of a 5-day trapping period. While in the corrals, monkeys have food and water ad libitum. The 10 corrals are sequentially processed. To process the corrals, the technical staff individually nets each monkey, anesthetizes it with ketamine hydrochloride (10 mg/kg), and removes it from the corral.

Selection of Subjects.—Eleven subjects in the preestablished adolescent age range were selected at random. Eight more were selected on the basis of observations of aggressive behavior in the corral and/or by their fight wounds, and nine others were selected on the basis of their display of submissive and/or fear-related behaviors in the corral.

Materials and Methods

Physiologic Measures.—All samples were obtained in a 3-day period during a routine capture in 1989, late in the breeding season during late November and early December. After each subject was captured, anesthetized, and removed from the corral, it was weighed on a commercial scale (accurate to within 0.25 kg). Immediately thereafter, CSF and blood samples were obtained from each subject. Two milliliters of CSF were obtained from the cisterna magna using a 25-gauge needle and syringe; the sample was immediately placed and maintained on dry ice. Blood samples were obtained via venipuncture and placed on ice. The blood was then transported to a laboratory on the mainland, where within 8 hours it was centrifuged, and the plasma was frozen and stored with the CSF at a temperature of −70°C. Samples were assayed for MHPG, homovanillic acid (HVA), and 5-HIAA concentrations using high-performance liquid chromatography with electrochemical detection as described by Scheinin et al.[38] All intra-assay and interassay coefficients of variation were less than 10%. All values are reported in picomoles per milliliter. Plasma samples were assayed for corticotropin (ACTH), cortisol, and testosterone concentrations by Hazelton Biotechnologies (Vienna, Va) using radioimmunoassays.[39] To control for possible influences on plasma and CSF values, records were kept of the elapsed minutes to obtain CSF and blood samples from the time when the technicians initially entered the corral; time of day was also recorded for each sample.

Assessment of Wounds and Scars.—Following the removal of CSF and blood samples, each subject was examined by the senior author (J.D.H.), and a pencil and paper record was made of the location, frequency, severity, and patterns of wounds (eg, contusions, tooth marks, nips, canine slashes, and scars). When warranted, notes were made concerning physical condition (eg, coat hygiene, weight, dandruff, teeth, missing digits, etc). A photograph was then taken of each subject. After this assessment was completed, the subject was released to the facility veterinarian or technical staff for further processing and standardized examination.

Ratings for Aggressivity.—Two primatologists, each with intensive experience observing nonhuman primate behavior (more than 1 year and more than 4 years) and blind to the monkeys' monoamine and hormone concentrations, were asked to rank the monkeys from the most to the least aggressive based on the following criteria: (1) records of direct observations of aggression, where possible; (2) frequency, severity, and patterns of wounds; and (3) a photograph of the monkey. To assess within-rater reliability, 4 months later, the same two primatologists were asked to rank the animals again. Within-rater reliability was statistically assessed by correlating the two ratings made by each primatologist ($r = .686$ and .836, $P < .0001$). Between-rater reliability was statistically assessed by correlating the mean aggressivity ratings by both primatologists using Pearson Product-Moment Correlation tests, and it was above chance level of similarity ($r = .868$). We therefore calculated the mean using the two raters' rankings for aggressivity, and all analyses reported herein use this mean rank score.

Statistical Analyses.—The data were analyzed by using Pearson Product-Moment Correlation tests to correlate the mean behavioral rating for each subject with each of the physiologic measures we obtained (CSF, norepinephrine [NE], MHPG, 5-HIAA, and HVA concentrations, and plasma ACTH, cortisol, and testosterone concentrations). Preliminary analyses indicated that there were no significant correlations between any of the CSF monoamines or plasma hormones and either the time of day or length of time from when the technicians entered the corral until the sample was obtained (Table 1). With the exception of testosterone, none of the hormones or CSF monoamines were correlated with age or weight (Table 2). Because testosterone was correlated with age ($r = .531$, $P < .005$), age was covaried out before correlating testosterone with the monoamines and hormones. There was insufficient plasma to assay for testosterone in four subjects, and CSF values from two subjects were not available. Thus, the sample sizes for each of the correlations were 26 for NE, MHPG, 5-HIAA, and HVA concentrations; 28 for cortisol and ACTH concentrations; and 24 for testosterone concentrations.

RESULTS

Table 3 displays the descriptive statistics and intercorrelations among each of the variables, and Tables 1 and 2 present the correlations among the various measures. There was a significant positive correlation between 5-HIAA and HVA concentrations ($r = .562$, $P < .003$). Testosterone was positively correlated with cortisol ($r = .40$, $P < .05$) and MHPG concentrations ($r = .53$, $P < .007$, Table 2).

There was a strong negative correlation between 5-HIAA concentrations and the rating for aggressivity ($r = -.580$, $P < .002$; Figure), and a positive correlation between aggressivity rating and NE ($r = .536$, $P < .004$) and ACTH concentrations ($r = .375$, $P < .04$). There was no significant association between testosterone and ranking for aggressivity or any of the other measures (Table 2).

COMMENT

The hypothesized negative correlation between aggression and 5-HIAA concentrations was significant, with high ratings for aggression correlating with low CSF 5-HIAA concentrations, consistent with the human studies showing that highly aggressive and violence-prone

Table 2.—Correlations of Biological Variables With Each Other and the Rating for Aggressivity*

	Age	Weight	ACTH	Cortisol	Testosterone	NE	MHPG	5-HIAA	HVA
Weight	.562†	. . .	. . .	. . .	. . .	. . .	. . .	. . .	. . .
ACTH	.020	.132	. . .	. . .	. . .	. . .	. . .	. .	. . .
Cortisol	.114	.100	.349	. . .	. . .	. . .	. . .	. . .	. . .
Testosterone	.531‡	.303	−.360	.400‡	. . .	. . .	. . .	. . .	. . .
NE	.166	−.216	.203	.369	−.310	. . .	. . .	. . .	. . .
MHPG	.140	.140	.350	.240	.530†	.160	. . .	. . .	. . .
5-HIAA	−.006	−.004	−.247	−.134	−.170	−.279	.360	. . .	. . .
HVA	−.089	.212	−.114	−.021	.050	−.036	.330	.562†	. . .
Rating	−.006	−.040	.375‡	.001	−.280	.536†	.007	−.580†	−.312

*ACTH indicates corticotropin; NE, norepinephrine; MHPG, 3-methoxy-4-hydroxyphenylgycol; 5-HIAA, 5-hydroxyindoleacetic acid; and HVA, homovanillic acid. Rating is expressed as the mean of the three ratings for aggressivity. The correlation of testosterone with the other variables was computed after removing the effect of age by partial correlation.
†=$P<.01$.
‡=$P<.05$.

Table 3.—Descriptive Statistics for Each Variable*

	Age	Weight	ACTH	Cortisol	Testosterone	NE	MHPG	5-HIAA	HVA	Aggressivity Rating
Mean	22.3	3.26	147.3	49.1	30.1	4.6	134.9	240.2	1700.7	14.2
SD	8.5	.54	102.3	6.6	17.3	1.1	17.2	41.9	324.7	7.6

*All of the hormones and cerebrospinal fluid monoamine metabolites are reported in picomoles per milliliter. ACTH indicates corticotropin; NE, norepinephrine; MHPG, 3-methoxy-4-hydroxyphenylgycol; 5-HIAA, 5-hydroxyindoleacetic acid; and HVA, homovanillic acid. Rating is expressed as the mean of the three ratings for aggressivity.

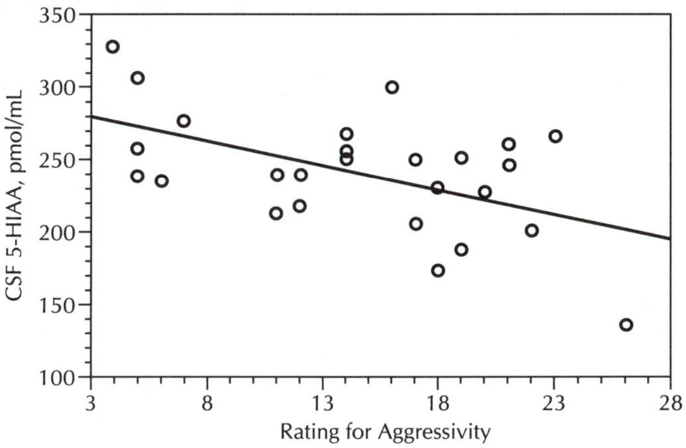

Correlation of cerebrospinal fluid 5-hydroxyindoleacetic acid (CSF 5-HIAA) concentrations and ratings for aggressivity.

individuals have low CSF 5-HIAA concentrations. Although several studies have reported a positive association between levels of aggression and plasma testosterone,[34-36] our hypothesis concerning such a positive correlation was not supported, in that there was not a significant relationship between testosterone concentrations and ratings for aggression in this study. A number of factors may have prevented detecting this relationship in the study population, including circadian changes in the samples obtained across the daily 10-hour sampling period, uncontrolled stress-induced testosterone increases, and the probability that some subjects had matured to have adult testosterone levels while others had not. In part because of the pulsatile nature of testosterone release, repeated samples of plasma testosterone from the same individual have a high degree of variability, and single-sample variability would diminish the capacity to detect traitlike testosterone and aggression relationships. Olweus et al[40,41] suggest solving this problem by obtaining repeated samples and correlating average testosterone levels with aggression. As we are in the process of repeatedly sampling the focal subjects longitudinally, many of these potential noise variables can be controlled in future studies.

Of interest was the finding that ratings for aggressivity were positively correlated with concentrations of ACTH in plasma and NE in CSF. Elevated concentrations of adrenal hormones and NE in CSF are generally considered to be manifestations of increased stress. This finding has not generally been investigated in human studies of aggression and CSF 5-HIAA concentrations. Although the present study was correlational in nature, the finding of increased stress hormones and NE in CSF in aggressive individuals has potential implications for subsequent studies of serotonin and aggression. Little is known concerning mechanisms precipitating aggression or the role that stress plays in aggression in individuals with low CSF 5-HIAA concentrations. Increased concentrations of plasma ACTH and NE in CSF in highly aggressive individuals may be a function of their diminished social skills and competence that result in diminished social support, ostracism, and increased loneliness.[3,22] Our findings suggest that future studies should assess the possible relationship between stress and aggression in individuals who have low CSF 5-HIAA concentrations. Finding increased NE concentrations in CSF in aggressive individuals is also consistent with some studies that have found increased NE activity in aggressive monkeys[36] (eg, see also Green et al as cited by Miczek and Donat[11]) and humans,[3] and illustrates that neurotransmitters other than serotonin are involved in regulating aggression.[42]

A limitation of the method used for rating aggression is that there is no way to accurately assess when a wound occurred. Thus, it is conceivable that the elevated ACTH and NE levels found in the monkeys with the most wounds might be a simple product of recent tissue trauma. While there is no way of knowing with certainty the length of time since a wound occurred, the two primate veterinarians performing examinations on the monkeys were given three subjects possessing numerous wounds to estimate the time since the most recent trauma. Both agreed that the wounds and trauma were all more than 3 days old (ie, occurred before capture). In addition, for most individuals showing wounds, there were more scars than recent trauma. This suggests that, in general, the elevated ACTH and NE levels were not merely a product of recent tissue trauma.

A second potential limitation in interpreting the present results is that the aggressivity was generally not directly observed; rather, it was largely inferred from the pattern, number, and degree of wounds and older scars. In many cases, it was clear that the trauma was a result of a bite. When recording the wounds, a half-moon shaped pattern with individual tooth depressions or bruises could be observed on the skin. In addition, others using this method have found a direct parallel between frequency of aggression received and frequency of scars and wounds.[32] Moreover, since collecting these wounding data, we have collected parallel wounding data in laboratory groups of rhesus monkeys to correlate with individual levels of aggression observed directly. In 18 monkeys, there was a strong correlation between the frequency of physical wounds and bruises and the rate of observed aggressivity ($r=.57$, $P<.01$). Thus, there are indications that the frequency and pattern of wounds is a reflection of the overall rates of aggression. Nevertheless, a limitation of this method is that it is not possible to ascertain whether the bite wounds and scars were a result of initiated or defensive aggression. However, there are indications that the animal involved was at least not running away from the fight. While specific locations could not be quantified, generally the location and patterns of wounds in the animals possessing the most wounds and scars were different from those in the monkeys possessing fewer wounds and scars. Monkeys with relatively more wounds and scars were more likely to have wounds and scars located on their faces and shoulders; on the other hand, monkeys with fewer wounds, when wounds were noted, were more likely to have wounds located on their tails, hips, and ankles. Indeed, behaviorally, most of the individuals selected as less aggressive were selected particularly because they avoided or failed to respond to aggressive encounters. We are currently collecting behavioral data on these same males as they interact within their social groups to further study this question.

While differences in early experiences, experimental setting, and capture procedures preclude a direct one-to-one comparison between samples obtained in the laboratory and the samples obtained from these subjects, it is worth noting that for 5-HIAA concentrations (which show an early age-related decline),[25] the values obtained from these feral-reared monkeys fall midway between values obtained from 18- and 50-month-old monkeys in the laboratory.[25] Nevertheless, there is a wider range in CSF 5-HIAA values in this feral population than in animals within the laboratory. For example, the two lowest values we have seen in any young male monkeys are from Morgan Island males, and while we have seen similar high-end values in the laboratory, usually they are in monkeys who have been selectively bred for high CSF 5-HIAA concentrations or in monkeys who have rearing histories atypical for the species. Concentrations of HVA were similar to those in same-aged monkeys in the laboratory. Several studies have shown an age-related decline in CSF 5-HIAA and HVA concentrations[25]; the lack of a correlation between age and these two metabolites in this population is probably because of the narrow range in age for these subjects. For MHPG, which generally shows no change from late childhood to adulthood, the values obtained from these subjects appear to be elevated over baseline values obtained in the laboratory, although not as high as those seen during acute stress, such as during the first day of a social separation (refer to Higley et al[25] and Bayart et al[43] for examples).

In summary, our findings indicate that as in human studies, excessive aggression is related to diminished CSF 5-HIAA concentrations in nonhuman primates, and that stress and aggression may be correlated. These findings, along with those by Raleigh and others,[18,19,21,44,45] which show that drugs used to deplete or increase serotonin increase or decrease aggression, respectively, indicate the potential of producing a nonhuman primate model of inappropriate aggression associated with reduced serotonin functioning. An additional long-term purpose of this study is to assess how excessive aggression and diminished CSF 5-HIAA concentrations are related to adjustment into primate society and the acquisition of social competence. We chose the present free-ranging monkeys because we plan to longitudinally follow them up to assess the long-term continuity of interindividual differences in both aggression and CSF 5-HIAA concentrations. Longitudinal assessments of these subjects will permit evaluation of how specific individuals exhibiting inappropriate aggression and diminished CSF 5-HIAA concentrations adjust to the social requirements and challenges they will face. For example, ongoing observations have revealed that the monkey rated the highest in aggressivity with the lowest CSF 5-HIAA concentrations has already left his social group, thus highlighting the potential to examine interindividual differences in social competence, life-history patterns, and future reproductive success. Continued study of this population will hopefully prove informative in assessing the role of serotonin in the acquisition of social competence and the appropriate expression of aggression.

We express our appreciation to Alan Dodson, Mariken Hasert, Ted King, and Chip Lincoln for their assistance in ranking the monkeys, data summary, and editorial assistance with the manuscript.

References

1. Stanley M, Traskman-Bendz L, Dorovini-Zis K. Correlations between aminergic metabolites simultaneously obtained from human CSF and brain. *Life Sci.* 1985;37:1279-1286.
2. Knott P, Haroutunian V, Bierer L, Perl D, Handler M, DeLeon M, Yang R, Davis K. Correlations post-mortem between ventricular CSF and cortical tissue concentrations of MHPG, 5-HIAA, and HVA in Alzheimer's disease. *Biol Psychiatry.* 1989;25:112A.
3. Brown GL, Goodwin FK, Ballenger JC, Goyer PF, Major LF. Aggression in humans correlates with cerebrospinal fluid amine metabolites. *Psychiatry Res.* 1979;1:131-139.
4. Linnoila M, Virkkunen M, Scheinin M, Nuutila A, Rimon R, Goodwin FK. Low cerebrospinal fluid 5-hydroxyindoleacetic acid concentration differentiates impulsive from nonimpulsive violent behavior. *Life Sci.* 1983;33:2609-2614.

5. Linnoila M, DeJong J, Virkkunen M. Monoamines, glucose metabolism, and impulse control. *Psychopharmacol Bull.* 1989;25:404-406.
6. Kruesi MJ. Cruelty to animals and CSF 5 HIAA. *Psychiatry Res.* 1989;28:115-116.
7. Kruesi MJ, Rapoport JL, Hamburger S, Hibbs E, Potter WZ, Lenane M, Brown GL. Cerebrospinal fluid monoamine metabolites, aggression, and impulsivity in disruptive behavior disorders of children and adolescents. *Arch Gen Psychiatry.* 1990;47:419-426.
8. Brown GL, Linnoila M, Goodwin FK. Clinical assessment of human aggression and impulsivity in relationship to biochemical measures. In: van Praag HM, Plutchik R, Apter A, eds. *Violence and Suicidality: Perspectives in Clinical and Psychobiological Research.* New York, NY: Brunner/Mazel Inc; 1990:184-217.
9. Linnoila M. Monoamines and impulse control. In: Swinkels JA, Blijleven W, eds. *Depression, Anxiety, and Aggression.* Houten, Holland: Medidact; 1988:167-172.
10. Suomi SJ. Primate separation models of affective disorders. In: Madden JI, ed. *Neurobiology of Learning, Emotion and Affect.* New York, NY: Raven Press; 1991:195-214.
11. Miczek KA, Donat P. Brain 5-HT system and inhibition of aggressive behavior. In: Archer T, Bevan P, Cools A, eds. *Behavioral Pharmacology of 5-HT.* Hillsdale, NJ: Lawrence Erlbaum Associates Inc Publishers; 1990:117-144.
12. Olivier B, Mos J, Tulp M, Schipper J, den Daas J, van Oortmerssen G. Serotonin involvement in aggressive behavior in animals. In: van Praag HM, Plutchik R, Apter A, eds. *Violence and Suicidality: Perspectives in Clinical and Psychobiological Research.* New York, NY: Brunner/Mazel Inc; 1990:79-137.
13. Sarich V. A molecular approach to the question of human origins. In: Ciochon RL, Fleagle JG, eds. *Primate Evolution and Human Origins.* Menlo Park, Calif: Benjamin/Cummings Publishing Company Inc; 1985:314-322.
14. Wilson AC, Carlson SS, White TJ. Biochemical evolution. *Annu Rev Biochem.* 1977;46:573-639.
15. Ciochon RL, Fleagle JG. *Primate Evolution and Human Origins.* Menlo Park, Calif: Benjamin/Cummings Publishing Company Inc; 1985.
16. Fleagle JG. *Primate Adaptation & Evolution.* Orlando, Fla: Academic Press Inc; 1988.
17. Yodyingyuad U, de la Riva C, Abbott DH, Herbert J, Keverne EB. Relationship between dominance hierarchy, cerebrospinal fluid levels of amine transmitter metabolites (5-hydroxyindoleacetic acid and homovanillic acid) and plasma cortisol in monkeys. *Neuroscience.* 1985;16:851-858.
18. Raleigh MJ, McGuire MT. Animal analogues of ostracism: biological mechanisms and social consequences. *Ethol Sociobiol. 1986;7:53-66.*
19. Chamberlain B, Ervin FR, Pihl RO, Young SN. The effects of raising or lowering tryptophan levels on aggression in vervet monkeys. *Pharmacol Biochem Behav.* 1987;28:503-510.
20. Higley JD, Linnoila M, Suomi SJ. Developing social competence: experiential and genetic contributions to the expression and inhibition of aggression in primates. In: Ammerman RT, Hersen M, Sisson L, eds. *Handbook of Aggressive and Destructive Behavior in Psychiatric Patients.* New York, NY: Plenum Press. In Press.
21. Raleigh MJ. Differential behavioral effects of tryptophan and 5-hydroxytryptophan in vervet monkeys: influence of catecholaminergic systems. *Psychopharmacology.* 1987;93:44-50.
22. Raleigh MJ, McGuire MT, Brammer GL. Subjective assessment of behavioral style: links to overt behavior and physiology in vervet monkeys. *Am J Primatol.* 1989;18:161-162.
23. Higley JD, Suomi SJ, Linnoila M. A longitudinal study of CSF monoamine metabolite and plasma cortisol concentrations in young rhesus monkeys: effects of early experience, age, sex and stress on continuity of interindividual differences. *Biol Psychiatry.* In press.
24. Kraemer GW, Ebert MH, Schmidt DE, McKinney WT. A longitudinal study of the effect of different social rearing conditions on cerebrospinal fluid norepinephrine and biogenic amine metabolites in rhesus monkeys. *Neuropsychopharmacology.* 1989;2:175-189.
25. Higley JD, Suomi SJ, Linnoila M. CSF monoamine metabolite concentrations vary according to age, rearing, and sex, and are influenced by the stressor of social separation in rhesus monkeys. *Psychopharmacology.* 1991;103:551-556.
26. Kraemer GW, McKinney WT. Interactions of pharmacological agents which alter biogenic amine metabolism and depression: an analysis of contributing factors within a primate model of depression. *J Affect Disord.* 1979;1:33-54.
27. Higley JD, Linnoila M, Suomi SJ. Genetic and experiential influences on CSF monoamine metabolites in a primate model of temperament and psychopathology. *Biol Psychiatry.* 1989;25:146A-147A.
28. Higley JD, Goldman D, Champoux M, Hasert MF, Linnoila M, Suomi SJ. Maternal genetic contributions to CSF monoamine concentrations in the rhesus macaque. *Biol Psychiatry.* 1990;27:71A.
29. Bernstein IS, Williams L, Ramsay M. The expression of aggression in Old World monkeys. *Int J Primatol. 1983;4:113-125.*
30. Hall KRL. Aggression in monkey and ape societies. In: Jay PC, ed. *Primates: Studies in Adaption and Variability.* New York, NY: Holt Rinehart & Winston; 1968:149-171.
31. Washburn SL, Hamburg DA. Aggressive behavior in Old World monkeys and apes. In: Jay PC, ed. *Primates: Studies in Adaption and Variability.* New York, NY: Holt Rinehart & Winston; 1968:458-478.
32. Crockett CM, Pope T. Inferring patterns of aggression from red howler monkey injuries. *Am J Primatol. 1988;15:289-308.*
33. Bernstein IS, Gordon TP, Rose RM. Aggression and social controls in rhesus monkey (*Macaca mulatta*) groups revealed in group formation studies. *Folia Primatol.* 1974;21:81-107.
34. Christiansen K, Knussmann R. Androgen levels and components of aggressive behavior in men. *Horm Behav.* 1987;21:170-180.
35. Conner RL, Levine S, Wertheim GA, Cummer JF. Hormonal determinants of aggressive behavior. *Ann N Y Acad Sci.* 1969;159:760-776.
36. Steklis HD, Brammer GL, Raleigh MJ, McGuire MT. Serum testosterone, male dominance, and aggression in captive groups of vervet monkeys (*Cercopithecus aethiops sabaeus*). *Horm Behav.* 1985;19:154-165.
37. Johnson F, Whalen RE. Testicular hormones reduce individual differences in the aggressive behavior of male mice: a theory of hormone action. *Neurosci Biobehav Rev.* 1988;12:93-99.
38. Scheinin M, Chang WH, Kirk KL, Linnoila M. Simultaneous determination of 3-methoxy-4-hydroxyphenylglycol, 5-hydroxyindoleacetic acid, and homovanillic acid in cerebrospinal fluid with high-performance liquid chromatography using electrochemical detection. *Anal Biochem.* 1983;131:246-253.
39. Abraham GE, Buster JE, Teller RC. Radioimmunoassay of plasma cortisol. *Anal Letters.* 1972;5:757-766.
40. Olweus D. The consistency issue in personality psychology revisited: with special reference to aggression. *Br J Soc Clin Psychol.* 1980;19:377-390.
41. Olweus D, Mattsson A, Schalling D, Löw H. Testosterone, aggression, physical, and personality dimensions in normal adolescent males. *Psychosom Med.* 1980;42:253-269.
42. Eichelman B. Neurochemical and psychopharmacologic aspects of aggressive behavior. In: Meltzer HY, ed. *Psychopharmacology: The Third Generation of Progress.* New York, NY: Raven Press; 1987:697-704.
43. Bayart F, Hayashi KT, Faull KF, Barchas JD, Levine S. Influence of maternal proximity on behavioral and physiological responses to separation in infant rhesus monkeys (*Macaca mulatta*). *Behav Neurosci.* 1990;104:98-107.
44. Raleigh MJ, Brammer GL, Ritvo ER, Geller E, McGuire MT, Yuwiler A. Effects of chronic fenfluramine on blood serotonin, cerebrospinal fluid metabolites, and behavior in monkeys. *Psychopharmacology.* 1986;90:503-508.
45. Raleigh MJ, Brammer GL, Yuwiler A, Flannery JW, McGuire MT. Serotonergic influences on the social behavior of vervet monkeys (*Cercopithecus aethiops sabaeus*). *Exp Neurol.* 1980;68:322-334.

Relationship Between Central and Peripheral Serotonin Indexes in Depressed and Suicidal Psychiatric Inpatients

J. John Mann, MD; P. Anne McBride, MD; Richard P. Brown, MD; Markku Linnoila, MD, PhD; Andrew C. Leon, PhD; Michael DeMeo, MD; Tammy Mieczkowski, MA; Joyce E. Myers, MD; Michael Stanley, PhD

• Serious suicidal behavior, affective disorders, and a variety of other psychopathologic behaviors and syndromes have been found to correlate with measures of the serotonin system. Clinical studies have employed a range of serotonin indexes, including the cerebrospinal fluid level of 5-hydroxyindoleacetic acid, the prolactin response to serotonin agonists, such as fenfluramine hydrochloride, and platelet serotonin-related proteins or serotonin content. Many of these indexes are correlated with suicidal behavior, but the interrelationship of these biologic measures has been uncertain. We studied the relationship of a series of serotonin indexes in patients in whom these measures were correlated with suicidal behavior. A positive correlation was found between cerebrospinal fluid 5-hydroxyindoleacetic acid and the maximal prolactin response to fenfluramine but not with platelet serotonin$_2$ receptor indexes. The fenfluramine-stimulated maximal prolactin response correlated with platelet serotonin$_2$ receptor number, particularly in older patients. We conclude that cerebrospinal fluid 5-hydroxyindoleacetic acid measurements cannot be replaced but can be complemented by less invasive procedures, such as a fenfluramine challenge test or platelet serotonin$_2$ measures, in the study of the relationship of the serotonin system to psychiatric disorders.

(*Arch Gen Psychiatry*. 1992;49:442-446)

Serotoninergic indexes correlate with suicidal behavior[1-5] and affective disorders.[2,5,6] Approaches that have been employed to study the serotonin system include measurement of cerebrospinal fluid (CSF) 5-hydroxyindoleacetic acid (5-HIAA)[5] and neuroendocrine challenge tests using a variety of precursors and direct or indirect serotonin agonists, such as serotonin reuptake inhibitors or serotonin releasing agents.[7,8] Other serotonin indexes assess peripheral tissue, of which the predominant source is the platelet.[2,3,8,9]

Little is known regarding the relationship of central measures, such as CSF 5-HIAA level and the prolactin response to fenfluramine hydrochloride, to peripheral measures, such as platelet monoamine oxidase activity, platelet serotonin content, platelet serotonin uptake, and the platelet serotonin-related receptors, namely the serotonin transporter (typical ligands are tritiated imipramine and tritiated paroxetine) and the serotonin$_2$ (5-HT$_2$) receptor. The relationship of central and peripheral serotonin indexes has theoretical and practical importance. The theoretical importance lies in studying peripheral serotonin-related proteins, because they may be abnormal due to the systematic manifestation of a genetic abnormality involving such a protein or due to the systemic effect of a humoral factor or hormone. The practical importance lies in determining what information about brain serotonin systems can be inferred from platelet indexes by studying the relationship of such indexes to brain or central serotonin indexes. For routine clinical purposes, lumbar punctures cannot be performed as readily as blood sampling, and therefore alternative approaches to a lumbar puncture would facilitate the conduct of biologic studies of the serotoninergic system.

We compared CSF 5-HIAA levels and the prolactin response to fenfluramine with platelet 5-HT$_2$ receptor indexes in psychiatric inpatients with and without a history of suicidal behavior to assess the interrelationship of these indexes, because we and others have found all of these biologic probes to be related to suicidal behavior.[1-3,5,6,9] The relationships between aspects of suicidal behavior and each of the serotonin indexes were the subject of studies that involve larger patient population in the case of each individual serotonin index. The data reported in this article are based on those subjects from these larger patient populations in whom data were available on multiple peripheral and/or central serotonin indexes. The studies of individual serotonin indexes are being reported as separate articles because they involve significantly larger pa-

Accepted for publication January 13, 1992.

From the Laboratories of Neuropharmacology, Department of Psychiatry, University of Pittsburgh (Pa) (Drs Mann and Myers and Ms Mieczkowski); Department of Psychiatry, Cornell University Medical College, New York, NY (Drs McBride, Leon, and DeMeo); Department of Psychiatry, College of Physicians and Surgeons, Columbia University, New York, NY (Drs Brown and Stanley); and Laboratory of Clinical Studies, National Institute on Alcohol Abuse and Alcoholism, Bethesda, Md (Dr Linnoila).

Reprint requests to Laboratories of Neuropharmacology, Department of Psychiatry, University of Pittsburgh, School of Medicine, Western Psychiatric Institute and Clinic, 3811 O'Hara St, Pittsburgh, PA 15213 (Dr Mann).

Table 1.—Demographic and Clinical Features of the Study Population*

	Serotonin Measures Compared		
	CSF 5-HIAA and Platelet 5-HT_2 Receptors	CSF 5-HIAA and Fenfluramine Hydrochloride	Fenfluramine and Platelet 5-HT_2 Receptors
No. of patients	24	34	22
Age, y	43.0±13.1	34.9±11.3	41.6±15.0
Male-female ratio	11/13	20/14	11/11
Suicide attempter/nonattempter ratio	17/7	24/10	12/10
Hamilton Depression Scale score (24 items)	29.2±8.3	25.9±12.0	29.9±7.4
Porportion with current major depressive episode	21/24	30/34	21/22

*CSF indicates cerebrospinal fluid; 5-HIAA, 5-hydroxyindoleacetic acid; and 5-HT_2, $serotonin_2$.

tient samples and more detailed analyses of general psychopathology and suicidal behavior.

PATIENTS AND METHODS

Patients

Patients were enrolled in the study after giving written informed consent as required by the Institutional Review Board. Eligible inpatients met *DSM-III-R* criteria for a major or minor depressive episode as independently determined by two research psychiatrists. Apart from chloral hydrate or a benzodiazepine with a short half-life, such as oxazepam, in isolated cases of distressing insomnia, 29 of 34 patients were drug free for at least 2 weeks (6 weeks in the case of fluoxetine and 3 months in the case of oral neuroleptics) and free of any active physical illness. Of the remaining five patients, four had made a suicide attempt by drug overdose within 2 weeks of study (one patient had taken nonpsychotropic drugs without effect on the brain or significant medical complications 6 days before testing; one patient had taken a benzodiazepine 4 days earlier; the third patient had taken pentobarbital sodium 11 days before testing; and the fourth patient had taken 750 mg of trazodone hydrochloride 7 days before testing). A final patient was found after the study to have received 5 mg of haloperidol 8 days before testing. The baseline prolactin level in this last patient was not above the group mean. None of the biologic measures (CSF 5-HIAA, prolactin response to fenfluramine, or platelet 5-HT_2 indexes) in this subgroup differed from those of the rest of the population, and so they were included in the data analysis. The average drug-free interval for all patients was 148±161 days. No patient had taken fenfluramine in the past. Patients were at a point in their clinical illness where they had required admission to a hospital for evaluation and treatment. They were studied immediately before somatic treatment was initiated.

The demographic and clinical characteristics of the study population are shown in Table 1. Severity of depression was assessed by means of the Hamilton Depression Scale,[10] and the suicidal behavior was characterized by the level of suicide intent according to the Suicide Intent Scale[11] and the degree of medical damage on the Medical Lethality Scale.[11] Possible gender and age effects were addressed in the analysis of the results where indicated. Of the women, five (36%) of 14 were menopausal, too few to estimate the effect of menopause on the biologic measures.

CSF 5-HIAA Measurement

Cerebrospinal fluid was drawn from the L4-5 interspace with the patient in the left decubitus position. All patients rested in bed overnight until the procedure and fasted from midnight. The CSF was spun to remove any debris, and the supernatant was stored at −70°C till assay. A 1-mL aliquot of a 15-mL sample was used for assay. The CSF 5-HIAA was assayed by high-performance liquid chromatography with an electrochemical detector as previously described.[12] The within-run and between-run coefficients of variation of the assay method were less than 10%. The level of sensitivity of the assay for 5-HIAA was 0.5 pmol per injection. All assays were done by laboratory staff who were unaware of the clinical data.

Platelet 5-HT_2 Receptor Indexes

Platelet 5-HT_2 receptor binding indexes were assessed in a membrane preparation by iodine 125–lysergic acid diethylamide binding with ketanserin to determine specific binding according to our previously published method.[8] The maximal number of binding sites per milligram of platelet membrane protein (B_{max}) and the dissociation constant (K_D) were calculated from a saturation binding isotherm. Signal transduction was assessed by measurement of serotonin enhancement of adenosine diphosphate–induced platelet aggregation (serotonin augmentation index [SAI]).[8] Receptor responsivity or sensitivity was defined as the ratio of signal transduction response and receptor number, or SAI/B_{max}. The SAI/B_{max} is a measure of the sensitivity of the individual receptor to activation and therefore provides an index of changes in receptor complex responsivity, such as supersensitivity or subsensitivity. Our analyses focused on the total number of receptors (B_{max}) and the responsivity of each receptor (SAI/B_{max}) because these two measures reflect the effects of receptor regulation.

Fenfluramine Challenge Test

Brain serotonin responsivity was assessed by means of a fenfluramine challenge test.[7] Fenfluramine is an indirect serotonin agonist in the sense that it activates serotonin receptors by increasing serotonin levels in the synaptic cleft instead of directly activating the serotonin receptors. Fenfluramine raises levels of serotonin exposed to receptors by a combination of increased release from nerve terminals and inhibition of serotonin reuptake.[13,14] The elevated serotonin levels in turn activate serotonin receptors. Fourteen of 34 patients received a single-blind placebo challenge on one day, followed by a 60-mg fenfluramine hydrochloride challenge test generally administered the next day. Twenty of the 34 patients did not receive a placebo challenge.

All patients fasted from midnight and throughout the challenge test. Patients continued to rest in bed after they awoke in the morning until they were tested. They were not permitted to sleep during the procedure. An intravenous line was inserted at approximately 8 AM, and a solution of 5% dextrose and 0.45% saline was administered. Blood samples for assay of prolactin were drawn at approximately 8:45 AM and 9 AM. Either 60 mg of fenfluramine hydrochloride or identical placebo tablets were then administered. Blood samples were drawn 1, 2, 3, 4, and 5 hours after administration of the drug. Blood samples were drawn at 3 and 5 hours to assay levels of fenfluramine and norfenfluramine by high-performance liquid chromatography as we have previously reported.[7,8] Prolactin levels were assayed by means of a purchased immunoradiometric assay kit (Hybritech Inc, San Diego, Calif).[7,8] The lower level of sensitivity of the assay was 0.3 μg/L, and interassay coefficient of variation was 4%.

Results at each time point were calculated by two methods: (1) as the difference between the prolactin response on the fenfluramine day and the prolactin level on the placebo day at each time point; and (2) as the difference between the mean of the two prolactin levels before fenfluramine was administered (−15 minutes and 0 time) and the level at 1, 2, 3, 4, and 5 hours. In both methods, the maximum increase in prolactin levels was the variable employed. The correlation between the maximal prolactin response calculated by these two methods was r=.94 (n=56, P<.0005) for our complete patient series and r=.82 (n=14, P<.0005) for the subgroup in this study. Because placebo challenge data were available for 14 of 34 patients, the results from the pooled data were calculated by the second method.

Statistical Analyses

Relationships between CSF 5-HIAA, platelet 5-HT_2 receptor indexes, and the fenfluramine-stimulated prolactin response, and the relationships of these variables to demographic and clinical variables, were analyzed by means of Pearson correlation coefficients. Spearman rank correlations (r_{sp}) were used when the sample size was relatively small. When the relationships among the serotonin indexes were analyzed, multiple regression analyses were used to control for the effects of possible confounding variables, such as age and gender. Group differences were analyzed by one-way analysis of variance. To test whether CSF 5-HIAA or the platelet 5-HT_2 receptor indexes were significant predictors of the group status of high-planning attempters vs low-planning attempters and nonattempters, logistic regression analyses were performed. All reported P values are two sided, and results are reported as mean±SD.

RESULTS

Relationship of CSF 5-HIAA to Platelet 5-HT_2 Receptor Indexes

The CSF 5-HIAA concentration did not correlate with either platelet 5-HT_2 receptor number (B_{max}; r=.09, n=24, P=.7) or platelet 5-HT_2 responsivity, defined as SAI/B_{max} (r=.09, n=24, P=.7). Even after exclusion of an outlier, the correlation between CSF 5-HIAA and SAI/B_{max} remained nonsignificant (r=.22, n=23, P=.3). When the effects of age and gender were included with SAI/B_{max} in a multiple regression analysis where CSF 5-HIAA level was the dependent variable, the relationship was nonsignificant (r^2=.03).

In a larger sample of patients that included all of the patients with CSF data reported in this study, we found lower levels of CSF 5-HIAA in those who had made highly planned suicide attempts (based on a high score on the first part of the Beck Suicide Intent Scale) compared with either suicide attempters with a low suicide intent score or nonattempters. In this article, the same result was obtained: high planners (n=5), 72.8±13.3 nmol/L, vs nonattempter patients (n=7), 119.0±40.6 nmol/L (F=5.86, df=1,10, P=.04), and vs low planners (n=10), 105.5±30.3 nmol/L (F=5.18, df=1,13, P=.04). The low planners did not differ from the nonattempter patients (105.5±30.3 vs 119.0±40.6 nmol/L; F=0.62, df=1,15, P=.44).

In a larger series of patients, we found a decrease in platelet 5-HT_2 receptor responsivity in suicide attempters (n=25) compared with nonattempters (n=18) as assessed by the SAI/B_{max} ratio (P<.05, Tukey B). The SAI/B_{max} in the high-planning suicide attempters compared with impulsive or low-planning attempters was not statistically different in the subgroup of patients described in this article (high planners [n=5], 0.05±0.03, vs low planners [n=10], 0.05±0.05 [F=0.00, df=1,13, P=.997] and vs nonattempters [n=7], 0.12±0.12 [F=1.27, df=1,10, P=0.29]). When a logistic regression analysis was performed with high-planning attempters (n=5) vs nonattempters (n=7) as the dependent variable and CSF 5-HIAA level, B_{max}, and SAI/B_{max} as the independent variables, no variable contributed significantly to the prediction of group status after CSF 5-HIAA level was entered into the model. The model with CSF 5-HIAA level as the only independent variable correctly classified 11 (92%) of the 12 subjects as being high-planning attempters or nonattempter patients. Similar results were obtained when high-planning attempters were compared with low-planning attempters, although the percentage correctly classified dropped to 67%.

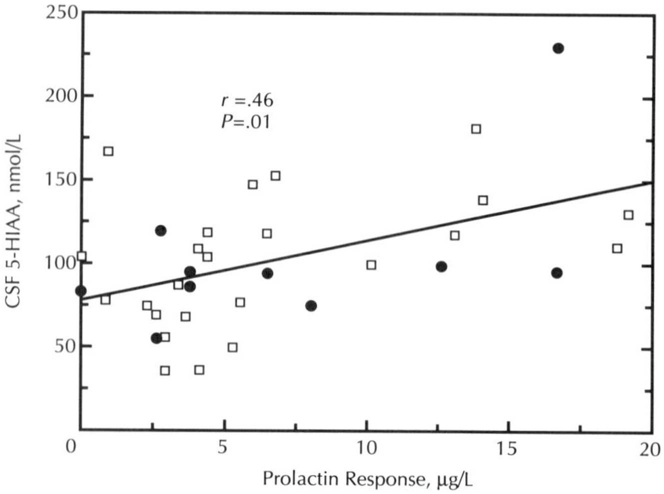

Relationship of cerebrospinal fluid 5-hydroxyindoleacetic acid (CSF 5-HIAA) to maximum fenfluramine hydrochloride–stimulated prolactin increase. Squares indicate suicide attempters; circles, nonattempters.

Severity of the medical damage caused by the suicide attempt did not correlate significantly with CSF 5-HIAA level (r=.08, n=16, not significant) or SAI/B_{max} ratio (r=.08, n=16, not significant), but it did correlate positively with B_{max} for platelet 5-HT_2 receptors (r=.6, n=16, P=.01). The presence of a major depressive episode or the severity of depression did not correlate with CSF 5-HIAA or platelet 5-HT_2 receptor indexes.

Relationship of CSF 5-HIAA to Fenfluramine-Stimulated Prolactin Release

The CSF 5-HIAA level correlated significantly with the maximum increase in prolactin level after administration of fenfluramine (r_{sp}=.46, n=34, P=.006; Figure). When patients were divided into suicide attempters and nonattempters, the CSF 5-HIAA level and the prolactin response correlated in the group of suicide attempters (r_{sp}=.50, n=24, P=.01), and although the correlation was also positive in the nonattempters, it was not statistically significant (r_{sp}=.36, n=10, P=.30). This result may be due to there being less variance in CSF 5-HIAA levels in the nonattempter group. When an outlier was removed from the nonattempter group, the correlation with prolactin response became even less significant (r_{sp}=.28, n=9, P=.46), and the variance in CSF 5-HIAA level was significantly less than in the attempter group (F=4.87, P=.03).

To determine whether age or suicide attempter status influenced the correlation between fenfluramine-stimulated prolactin response and CSF 5-HIAA level, a multiple linear regression analysis was conducted with CSF 5-HIAA as the dependent variable; the independent variables were age less than 30 years or greater than or equal to 30 years (B=14.7, t=0.97, P=.82), maximum prolactin response (B=3.9, t=3.14, P=.004), and attempter status (B=3.3, t=0.23, P=.082). Only the maximum change in prolactin response was statistically significant.

Relationship of Platelet 5-HT_2 Indexes to Fenfluramine-Induced Prolactin Release

Because of the age-related decline in fenfluramine-induced prolactin response before the age of 30 years, we compared patients under 30 years old and 30 years of age and older separately (Table 2). In patients under the age of 30 years, there was no correlation between any platelet 5-HT_2 index and prolactin levels. When prolactin responses were corrected for fenfluramine and norfenfluramine levels, the results remained nonsignificant. In patients 30 years old and older, the maximum change in prolactin response to fenfluramine was positively correlated with B_{max} (r_{sp}=.59, n=16, P=.02), and there were trends toward re-

Table 2.—Correlation of Platelet 5-HT_2 Indexes With Maximum Fenfluramine Hydrochloride–Stimulated Prolactin Release in Patients Under 30 Years of Age and 30 Years and Older*

Index	Spearman Rank Correlation Coefficient	P
Age <30 y (n=6)		
B_{max}	−.20	.70
K_D	−.37	.47
SAI	−.09	.87
SAI/B_{max}	.20	.70
Age ≥30 y (n=16)		
B_{max}	.59	.02
K_D	.44	.09
SAI	.05	.85
SAI/B_{max}	−.49	.06

*B_{max} indicates maximal number of binding sites per milligram of platelet membrane protein; K_D, dissociation constant; and SAI, serotonin augmentation index.

lationships with K_D (r_{sp}=.44, n=16, P=.09) and SAI/B_{max} (r_{sp}= −.49, n=16, P=.06). Fenfluramine and norfenfluramine levels did not differ between subjects 30 years old and older and those under 30 years of age.

When patients were also divided into attempters and nonattempters in a multiple linear regression analysis, including the effect of being under 30 years old or greater than or equal to 30 years old, there was a trend for SAI/B_{max} (receptor responsivity) to predict fenfluramine-induced prolactin release (B= −190.3, t= −1.8, P=.08). When prolactin response was adjusted for fenfluramine and norfenfluramine levels, this result became statistically significant (B= −3.2, t= −2.46, P=.02). When B_{max} was entered into a similar analyses, the results were not statistically significant. When the maximum increase in prolactin level was the dependent variable in a similar analysis, SAI/B_{max} was a significant predictor (B= −86.4, t= −2.16, P=.04), whereas B_{max} was not.

COMMENT

We have confirmed the previously reported[5] association between serious or high-intent suicidal acts and low levels of CSF 5-HIAA in this study population. Moreover, we also found a relationship between platelet 5-HT_2 receptor number and medical damage as well as between 5-HT_2 receptor sensitivity and a history of suicide attempts.[9] However, these two serotonin indexes (CSF 5-HIAA and platelet 5-HT_2 receptor binding or responsivity) did not correlate and therefore appear to explain different components of the variance in suicidal behavior. We have found that CSF 5-HIAA level correlates with degree of objective suicide intent or planning, whereas platelet serotonin indexes reflect medical damage. Although suicide intent and degree of medical damage are also correlated,[11] only CSF 5-HIAA level proved a significant discriminator of patients who had carried out highly planned suicide attempts compared with patients who had made impulsive suicide attempts or never attempted suicide. In contrast, platelet 5-HT_2 indexes correlated with the degree of medical damage but not with the degree of planning or suicide intent.

There are few studies of the relationship of CSF 5-HIAA to platelet serotonin indexes, and they generally have found no correlation. Oreland and colleagues[15] reported no difference in platelet monoamine oxidase activity in a group of patients who had histories of attempted suicide and had low CSF 5-HIAA levels compared with nonattempter psychiatric controls. Platelet imipramine binding was found not to correlate with CSF 5-HIAA level in a study of surgical patients.[16] Sarrias and colleagues[17] reported a correlation only between the ratio of platelet to plasma serotonin levels and CSF 5-HIAA levels and suggested that this correlation may be explained by the action of monoamine oxidase, which is partly under genetic control. However, human brain MAO and platelet MAO activity have been reported not to correlate,[18] so that some alternative explanation is warranted, such as a common effect on a biosynthetic enzyme. The levels of CSF 5-HIAA, brain 5-HIAA, and platelet serotonin content and uptake all appear to undergo seasonal and/or diurnal variation,[5,19-21] which suggests a common systemic effect. The mechanism of this effect is unclear. One suggestion has been that external cues, such as the dark-light cycle, drive the circadian rhythm of serotonin in brain regions, such as the hypothalamus.[21] The absence of a correlation between CSF 5-HIAA levels and platelet serotonin indexes may be due to phase differences in their biorhythms, although other explanations clearly are also possible.

We found a positive correlation between CSF 5-HIAA levels and the maximum prolactin response to fenfluramine. The prolactin response to fenfluramine is partly dependent on the level of serotonin available for release and partly on the responsivity of the postsynaptic serotonin receptor populations. Levels of CSF 5-HIAA have been reported in at least two human postmortem studies to correlate with levels of 5-HIAA in frontal cortex.[22,23] Whether levels of available serotonin in the hypothalamic neurons involved in prolactin release correlate with CSF 5-HIAA levels remains to be determined. Brewerton and colleagues[24] found that CSF 5-HIAA level was negatively correlated with the peak increase in prolactin levels after challenge with m-chlorophenylpiperazine (a serotonin agonist) in 12 low-weight anorexic patients (r= −.69) but not in weight-recovered patients. Further study of the relationship of CSF 5-HIAA level to neuroendocrine indexes of brain serotoninergic function in different patient populations is warranted. Our findings suggest that fenfluramine-stimulated prolactin release may be an indicator of brain serotonergic activity in areas other than the hypothalamus, because CSF 5-HIAA is derived from multiple brain regions, including prefrontal cortex.[22]

A blunted prolactin response to fenfluramine has been found to be associated with suicidal behavior in patients with depression as well in patients with personality disorders.[6,25] Since the prolactin response to fenfluramine and the level of CSF 5-HIAA correlate, these measures may explain similar parts of the variance in suicidal behavior. For example, CSF 5-HIAA level correlated with objective suicidal intent or planning. Insufficient data were available to determine what aspect of suicidal behavior correlated with a blunted prolactin response to fenfluramine. If it appears that fenfluramine-stimulated prolactin responses correlate with the same dimension of suicidal behavior, then the fenfluramine challenge may be an alternative to CSF 5-HIAA measurement as an investigative tool in the study of suicide attempters. Another possibility is that the two measures may be complementary.

A positive correlation was found between platelet 5-HT_2 receptor number and the prolactin response to fenfluramine. The relationship was apparent only in patients aged 30 years and older, perhaps because patients under the age of 30 years had a much greater variance in prolactin responses.[7] We previously reported the finding of a positive correlation between the prolactin response to fenfluramine and platelet 5-HT_2 responsivity as measured by serotonin augmentation of adenosine diphosphate–induced platelet aggregation (SAI) in young adults with autistic disorder,[8] indicating that this relationship extends to other patient populations. This correlation was not statistically significant in this study or in the sample of seven young normal male controls in the study of autistic patients.[8] Because the variance in SAI is less than B_{max}, larger samples will be required to determine whether age is an important factor in determining the presence of a correlation between prolactin responses to fenfluramine and platelet 5-HT_2 receptor responsivity.

We also found that another part of variance in suicide behavior, namely the degree of medical damage resulting from the suicide attempt, may be explained by platelet 5-HT_2 receptor number. Therefore, if this measure were combined with a fenfluramine challenge test, it may enhance a research approach that uses CSF 5-HIAA measurement.

It is not clear why platelet 5-HT_2 receptor number correlates with the prolactin response to fenfluramine. Studies[7,26] have attempted to determine which serotonin receptor populations mediate the prolactin response to serotonin, and the results are not entirely consistent. A role has been suggested for 5-HT_1 receptors, but some studies suggest that 5-HT_2 receptors may also be involved.[7,26] If 5-HT_2 receptors are not involved, then it is difficult to propose a common receptor regulatory effect that involves 5-HT_1 receptors mediating prolactin release and platelet 5-HT_2 receptors.

In conclusion, the concentration of CSF 5-HIAA has been found to correlate with serious suicidal behavior. The observation that suicidal behavior correlates with other indexes of serotonin activity, namely platelet 5-HT_2 receptor binding kinetics and responsivity and the prolactin response to fenfluramine, offers the possibility of employing such alternative measures for studying the serotonin system in suicidal patients. Prolactin response to fenfluramine but not platelet 5-HT_2 indexes correlates with CSF 5-HIAA level. It remains to be determined whether these measures explain the same or different components of the variance in suicidal behavior and perhaps different aspects of suicidal behavior. These studies will determine whether CSF 5-HIAA continues to be an important measure in the study of suicidal behavior.

This work was supported in part by Mental Health Clinical Research Center grant IP50-MH46745 and by MH-41847.

Donna Abbondanza, ANS, provided valuable assistance with the fenfluramine challenges and lumbar punctures. Jean Williams expertly typed the manuscript.

References

1. Mann JJ, Arango V, Marzuk PM, Theccanat S, Reis DJ. Evidence for the 5-HT hypothesis of suicide: a review of post-mortem studies. *Br J Psychiatry Suppl.* 1989;155:7-14.

2. Mann JJ, Stanley M, eds. *Psychobiology of Suicidal Behavior.* New York, NY: New York Academy of Sciences; 1986:1-357.

3. Mann JJ, Arango V, Underwood MD. Serotonin and suicidal behavior. In: Whitaker-Azmitia PM, Peroutka SJ, eds. *The Neuropharmacology of Serotonin.* New York, NY: New York Academy of Sciences; 1990:476-485.

4. Mann JJ, Marzuk PM, Arango V, McBride PA, Leon AC, Tierney H. Neurochemical studies of violent and nonviolent suicide. *Psychopharmacol Bull.* 1989;25:407-413.

5. Åsberg M, Träskman-Bendz L, Thorén P. 5-HIAA in the cerebrospinal fluid: a biochemical suicide predictor? *Arch Gen Psychiatry.* 1976;33:1193-1197.

6. Coccaro EF, Siever LJ, Klar HM, Maurer G, Cochrane K, Cooper TB, Mohs RC, Davis KL. Serotonergic studies in patients with affective and personality disorders. *Arch Gen Psychiatry.* 1989;46:587-599.

7. McBride PA, Tierney H, DeMeo M, Chen J-S, Mann JJ. Effects of age and gender on CNS serotonergic responsivity in normal adults. *Biol Psychiatry.* 1990;27:1143-1155.

8. McBride PA, Anderson GM, Hertzig ME, Sweeney JA, Kream J, Cohen DJ, Mann JJ. Serotonergic responsivity in male young adults with autistic disorder. *Arch Gen Psychiatry.* 1989;46:213-221.

9. McBride PA, Brown RP, DeMeo M, Keilp J, Stanley M, Mann JJ, Polly M. Platelet 5-HT_2 receptors: depression and suicide. Presented at the 140th Annual Meeting of the American Psychiatric Association, New Research; May 11-13, 1987; Chicago, Ill. Abstract NR157.

10. Hamilton M. A rating scale for depression. *J Neurol Neurosurg Psychiatry.* 1960;23:56-62.

11. Beck AT, Beck R, Kovacs M. Classification of suicidal behaviors, I: quantifying intent and medical lethality source. *Am J Psychiatry.* 1975;132:285-287.

12. Scheinin M, Chang W-H, Kirk KL, Linnoila M. Simultaneous determination of 3-methoxy-4-hydroxyphenylglycol, 5-hydroxyindoleacetic acid, and homovanillic acid in cerebrospinal fluid with high-performance liquid chromatography using electrochemical detection. *Anal Biochem.* 1983;131:246-253.

13. Garattini S, Jori A, Buczko W, Samanin R. The mechanism of action of fenfluramine. *Postgrad Med J.* 1975;51(suppl 1):27-35.

14. Reuter CJ. A review of CNS effects of fenfluramine, 780SE and norfenfluramine on animals and man. *Postgrad Med J.* 1975;51(suppl 1):18-27.

15. Oreland L, Wiberg A, Åsberg M, Träskman L, Sjöstrand L, Thoren P, Bertilsson L, Tubrina G. Platelet MAO activity and monoamine metabolites in cerebrospinal fluid in depressed and suicidal patients and in healthy controls. *Psychiatry Res.* 1981;4:21-29.

16. Stoff MD, Goldman W, Bridger WH, Jain AK, Pylypiw A. No correlation between platelet imipramine binding and CSF 5-HIAA in neurosurgical patients. *Psychiatry Res.* 1990;33:323-326.

17. Sarrias MJ, Cabré P, Martínez E, Artigas F. Relationship between serotoninergic measures in blood and cerebrospinal fluid simultaneously obtained in humans. *J Neurochem.* 1990;54:783-786.

18. Young WF, Laws ER, Sharbrough FW, Weinshilboum RM. Human monoamine oxidase: lack of brain and platelet correlation. *Arch Gen Psychiatry.* 1986;43:604-609.

19. Carlsson A, Svennerholm L, Winblad B. Seasonal and circadian monoamine variations in human brains examined post mortem. *Acta Psychiatr Scand.* 1980;280(suppl):75-85.

20. Wirz-Justice A. Circadian rhythms in mammalian neurotransmitter receptors. *Prog Neurobiol.* 1987;29:219-259.

21. Nicoletti F, Raffaele A, Falsaperia A, Paci R. Circadian variation in 5-hydroxyindoleacetic acid levels in human cerebrospinal fluid. *Eur Neurol.* 1981;20:834-838.

22. Stanley M, Träskman-Bendz L, Dorovini-Zis K. Correlations between aminergic metabolites simultaneously obtained from human CSF and brain. *Life Sci.* 1985;37:1279-1286.

23. Knott P, Haroutunian V, Bierer L, Perl D, Handler M, DeLeon M, Yang R-K, David K. Correlations post-mortem between ventricular CSF and cortical tissue concentrations of MHPG, 5-HIAA and HVA in Alzheimer's disease. *Biol Psychiatry.* 1989;25(suppl 7A):112A.

24. Brewerton TD, Brandt HA, Lessem MD, Murphy DL, Jimerson DC. Serotonin in eating disorders. In: Coccaro EF, Murphy DL, eds. *Serotonin in Major Psychiatric Disorders.* 21st ed. Washington, DC: American Psychiatric Press Inc; 1990:155-184.

25. DeMeo M, McBride PA, Mann JJ, Keilp J. Fenfluramine challenge in major depression. Presented at the 141st Annual Meeting of the American Psychiatric Association; May 7-13, 1988; Montreal, Quebec. Abstract NR169.

26. Cosi C, Kim HS, Wood PL. Serotonergic (5-HT_2) regulation of plasma corticosterone and prolactin. *Soc Neurosci Abstr.* 1988;14:846. Abstract.

A 2-Year Prospective Follow-up Study of Children and Adolescents With Disruptive Behavior Disorders

Prediction by Cerebrospinal Fluid 5-Hydroxyindoleacetic Acid, Homovanillic Acid, and Autonomic Measures?

Markus J. P. Kruesi, MD; Euthymia D. Hibbs, PhD; Theodore P. Zahn, PhD; Cynthia S. Keysor; Susan D. Hamburger, MS; John J. Bartko, PhD; Judith L. Rapoport, MD

• A 2-year prospective follow-up study of 100% (N = 29) of a sample of children and adolescents with disruptive behavior disorders found that the baseline lumbar cerebrospinal fluid monoamine metabolite concentration and autonomic nervous system activity predicted some subsequent outcomes. The 5-hydroxyindoleacetic acid concentration significantly predicted severity of physical aggression during follow-up. The skin conductance level significantly predicted institutionalization. Correlations were in predicted directions with lower cerebrospinal fluid 5-hydroxyindoleacetic acid concentrations and autonomic activity correlated with poor outcome. Moreover, in multivariate analyses, which included nonlaboratory measures as predictors, cerebrospinal fluid and autonomic measures still contributed significantly to the prediction. However, hypothesized predictions of cerebrospinal fluid 5-hydroxyindoleacetic acid concentrations for suicide attempts and of low autonomic nervous system activity for arrests were not supported thus far. Patients are still at risk; consequently, these results must be considered preliminary. Nonetheless, the results suggest that further investigation of relationships between biological factors and outcome of children with disruptive behavior disorders is warranted.

(*Arch Gen Psychiatry*. 1992;49:429-435)

Disruptive behavior disorders (DBDs) constitute a heterogeneous group, encompassing diagnoses (*DSM-III-R*) of attention-deficit hyperactivity disorder, oppositional defiant disorder, and conduct disorder. These overlapping groups are characterized by age-inappropriate behaviors, including hyperactivity, impulsivity, and aggression, with substantial overlap among the three disorders.[1] "Pure" conduct disorder or "pure" oppositional disorder are relatively rare in clinical samples, with most cases also qualifying for an attention-deficit disorder diagnosis.[1] Follow-up studies of hyperactive children have found a wide range of outcomes, with about half being undiscernible from that of normal controls and a substantial minority (about 25%) having antisocial outcomes.[2-4]

Conduct disorder predicts criminal[5] and substance abuse outcomes[6] of hyperactive children. However, childhood conduct disturbance is common, while only about a third have it persist into adulthood[7]; in contrast, adult antisocial personality disorder is almost always preceded by conduct disorder in childhood.[8,9] Thus, as with hyperactivity, conduct disturbance alone does not predict which disruptive individuals go on to chronicity. Aggression is an important behavioral dimension within conduct disorder, as well as for a broad range of (overlapping) poor outcomes, including subsequent aggression,[10-12] illegal drug involvement,[10] delinquency,[13] and criminal activities.[12,14-18] Aggression is an acknowledged behavioral precursor in about 75% of male chronic offenders.[19]

Follow-up studies of delinquents have concentrated primarily on psychosocial measures for prediction of outcome.[20] However, as Rutter et al[21] have argued, biological factors may well be more important than environmental factors in the subgroup of conduct disorders that persist into adult life. With the exception of a few adoption studies,[22-24] data on the predictive value of biological measures are limited, and few such variables have differentiated aggressive and antisocial subjects from controls.

Two biological measures that have most consistently differentiated adult antisocial and/or aggressive populations in independent studies, ie, cerebrospinal fluid (CSF) 5-hydroxyindoleacetic acid (5-HIAA) concentration and autonomic nervous system (ANS) activity, were selected as possible predictors. Reduced concentrations of the se-

Accepted for publication March 9, 1992.

From the Child Psychiatry (Drs Kruesi and Rapoport and Mss Keysor and Hamburger) and Child and Adolescent Disorders Research (Dr Hibbs) Branches, the Laboratory of Psychology and Psychopathology (Dr Zahn), and the Division of Applied and Services Research (Dr Bartko), National Institute of Mental Health, Bethesda, Md. Dr Kruesi is now with the Department of Psychiatry, Division of Child and Adolescent Psychiatry, Institute for Juvenile Research, University of Illinois, Chicago.

Presented in part at the New Research Program of the 144th Annual Meeting of the American Psychiatric Association, New Orleans, La, May 13, 1991.

Reprints not available.

rotonin metabolite, 5-HIAA, in lumbar CSF significantly correlated with aggression in children and adolescents with DBDs, and patients with DBDs had significantly lower CSF 5-HIAA concentrations than pediatric patients with obsessive-compulsive disorder.[25] In adults, follow-up of depressed adults has found low CSF 5-HIAA concentrations to predict suicide attempts,[26,27] while for adult offenders,[28] reduced CSF 5-HIAA concentrations are a risk factor for subsequent aggressive behavior. Similarly, Brown et al[29] reported that a reduced CSF 5-HIAA concentration predicted future discharge as unsuitable for military service.

Low autonomic activity has been related to criminal and aggressive outcomes.[30,31] The following four peripheral indexes of baseline ANS activity were found to predict outcome: (1) rate of spontaneous fluctuations of skin conductance (SFs/min), (2) mean skin conductance level (SCL), (3) mean heart rate (HR), and (4) trials to habituation of skin conductance–orienting responses to a series of brief innocuous tones. A 9-year follow-up of adolescents found that those who were sentenced for a crime during the follow-up interval had significantly lower resting base levels of SFs/min, SCL, and HR.[30] In younger children, low skin conductance activity at the age of 3 years predicted fighting at the age of 9 years.[31] Fast habituation of skin conductance responses characterized inpatients who made violent suicide attempts both retrospectively and on 1-year follow-up.[32] Thorell[33] found lower SFs/min and fewer and smaller skin conductance–orienting responses in suicidal patients compared with that in both nonsuicidal patients and normal controls.

In the present study, the predictive power of CSF 5-HIAA and ANS activity measures is examined in a group of 29 children and adolescents who initially were referred for assessment of DBDs. The patients had lumbar CSF monoamine metabolite concentrations and autonomic measures collected at the first evaluation (time 1). These laboratory measures were part of studies of CSF 5-HIAA concentrations and autonomic reactivity in relation to severity and type of aggression or DBDs (T.P.Z. and M.J.P.K., unpublished data, November 1991).[25]

The main hypothesis that drove this study was that low concentrations of CSF 5-HIAA would predict follow-up among patients with DBDs, specifically severe outcomes in the form of physical aggression and suicide attempts. Other hypothesized relationships that were based on findings from studies, as noted above, were as follows: low CSF homovanillic acid (HVA) concentrations predict suicide attempts; low SFs/min, SCL, and HR each predict arrest; and fast habituation (low trials to habituation) predicts suicide attempts. We also speculated that low 5-HIAA concentrations or ANS activity might predict other adverse outcomes, such as lower global functioning, institutionalization, and substance abuse.

SUBJECTS AND METHODS

Subjects were 29 children and adolescents, with a mean age of 11.3 years (SD, 3.6 years; age range, 6 to 17 years) with DBDs who had had lumbar CSF collected and psychophysiological studies performed during an inpatient evaluation for children and adolescents with DBDs.[25]

During the initial evaluation, we reviewed all available records from previous therapists, hospitals, residential treatment facilities, schools, etc. With the use of the previous data and structured interviews of the child and of at least one parent about the child,[34-36] *DSM-III-R*[37] diagnoses were made. Diagnoses at follow-up were made based on previous information, plus structured and clinical interviews of both patient and at least one parent. Demographic characteristics and diagnoses of the sample are listed in Tables 1 and 2, respectively.

Table 1.—Demographics of Sample (N = 29) at Time 1 Baseline Evaluation and at Follow-up*

Demographical Variable	Baseline Evaluation	Follow-up
Age, y	11.3 (3.6)	13.8 (3.9)
Wechsler IQ		
Verbal	103.9 (12.4)	. . .
Performance	103.4 (13.8)	. . .
Full scale	103.3 (12.7)	. . .
Length of follow-up, mo	. . .	26.2 (8.9)
Sex		
M	27 (93)	. . .
F	2 (7)	. . .
Race		
B	5 (17)	. . .
W	22 (76)	. . .
Other	2 (7)	. . .

*For age, Wechsler IQ, and length of follow-up, data are given as mean (SD); for sex and race, data are given as number (percentage).

At initial evaluation, parent(s) were interviewed with the Schedule for Affective Disorders and Schizophrenia.[38] The IQ was assessed with the use of the Wechsler Intelligence Scale for Children–Revised[39] or Wechsler Adult Intelligence Scale–Revised,[40] where age appropriate. Additional patient characteristics, details of CSF collection, assay of monoamine metabolites, and age correction have been described elsewhere.[25] All subjects were free of medications for at least 3 weeks before collection of the lumbar puncture and ANS activity measures.

The ANS activity measures that were performed during the baseline evaluation were the determination of the SCL and HR, which were recorded during a 3-minute rest period and a series of 10 tones (80 dB, 1000 Hz) of 1.5 seconds' duration, presented every 20 to 30 seconds to which no response was required. Skin conductance was measured via a constant (0.5-V) voltage system from 0.64 cm^2 of silver/silver chloride electrodes on the middle and ring fingertips of the left hand with the use of 0.5% potassium chloride in agar electrode paste. The HR was recorded with a tachograph from lead II. The four variables presented here are the SFs/min during the 3-minute rest period, the mean SCL, the HR during the rest period, and the number of trials to habituation of the skin conductance responses to the tones. These had minimum amplitudes of 0.02 microSiemens and onset latencies of 0.8 to 4 seconds. Habituation was defined as two consecutive tones with no elicited response.

Interim Procedure

After initial evaluation, patients were referred to community practitioners for individualized treatment, depending on the results of assessment, family needs and/or preferences, and local treatment opportunities. Follow-up interviews were scheduled after a minimum interval of 14 months.

Follow-up

All 29 patients with DBDs (100%) who had had lumbar punctures were located and interviewed in person. Parent(s) of 24 children were interviewed in person, and parent(s) of another five subjects were interviewed by telephone. The mean (±SD) follow-up interval between the lumbar puncture and subsequent interview for subjects was 26 (±8.9) months; the range was 14 to 65 months; and the mode was 24 months. The mean age at follow-up was 13.8 (±3.9) years, and the age range was 8 to 22 years.

Structured interviews of the patient and parent, including

Table 2.—Diagnoses of Sample at Time 1 Baseline Evaluation and at Follow-up*

DSM-III-R Diagnoses†	Baseline Evaluation		Follow-up	
	No. (%)	Mean Age (SD), y	No. (%)	Mean Age (SD), y
ADHD	16 (55)	9.8 (3.1)	16 (55)	13.3 (4.1)
Undifferentiated ADD	3 (10)	15.0 (1.7)	4 (14)	13.0 (3.7)
Conduct disorder/ASP	18 (62)	12.8 (3.0)	12 (41)	17.1 (2.2)
Oppositional defiant disorder	4 (14)	9.5 (5.1)	7 (24)	11.1 (2.2)
Affective/anxiety disorder	4 (14)	12.3 (4.3)	4 (14)	11.3 (1.5)
Developmental disorders	7 (24)	9.1 (3.0)	3 (10)	10.7 (1.5)
Substance abuse	2 (7)	16.0 (0)	7 (24)	17.0 (1.4)
Other disorders, including personality disorders other than antisocial	6 (21)	11.7 (4.3)	3 (10)	16.3 (3.1)
No diagnosis	0	. . .	1 (3)	. . .

*ADHD indicates attention-deficit hyperactivity disorder; ADD, attention-deficit disorder; and ASP, antisocial personality disorder.
†Total exceeds 29 as multiple diagnoses were made. Age at follow-up is, in some cases, younger because membership in a diagnostic group was not identical at follow-up.

sections of the Diagnostic Interview for Children and Adolescents and the Diagnostic Interview for Children and Adolescents–Parent version[34-36] that covered disruptive behaviors, socialization, affective disorders, and alcohol and other substance abuse, were conducted. Checklist reports about the patient's aggressive actions and their frequencies (N. E. Harnett, PhD, RN, and M.J.P.K., unpublished data, June 1991) were completed by the patient and by a custodial parent. The Child Behavior Checklist[41] was completed by a parent of all subjects who were aged younger than 17 years at follow-up.

Outcome Measures

Outcome measures were selected for aggression, suicide attempts, and arrest(s), as well as for other aspects of overall functioning during the follow-up interval. Based on interview data, as well as review of all other available information, two investigators (E.D.H. and M.J.P.K.) made diagnoses and completed ratings for the following measures to cover the interval from the time of lumbar puncture to the time of follow-up: (1) the Modified Overt Aggression Scale[42] (ie, its Physical Aggression subscale, Autoaggression subscale, and total score); (2) suicide attempt(s) (ie, from self-report of the individual and/or other sources); (3) arrest(s) during follow-up based on parent and/or patient report; (4) the Children's Global Assessment Scale,[43] which evaluates the overall functioning of a patient on a continuum of psychological health and illness; (5) institutionalization, which was defined as the child having been confined during the follow-up interval in psychiatric or substance abuse hospitalization, residential treatment, and/or correctional facilities; and (6) substance abuse diagnosis at follow-up, with the best clinical diagnosis by consensus, utilizing all available information.

Statistical Analysis

The age of the subject was anticipated to be a major confounding factor within the baseline and outcome variables. Some forms of aggression (eg, suicide and homicide) are more frequent in adolescents and young adults than in prepubertal children.[44,45] Age was also significantly (inversely) correlated with 5-HIAA, HVA, HR, and SFs/min measures at baseline. Correlations between age and all baseline measures are shown in Table 3.

Table 3.—Baseline Measures Entered Into Multiple Regression and Discriminant Function Analyses to Predict Outcome and Their Correlation With Age (n=26)*

	r	*P*
Nonlaboratory measures		
Age of child in months	. . .	. . .
Brown-Goodwin Lifetime History of Aggression	.50	.01
Socioeconomic status of the family	–.26	NS
Presence/absence of antisocial diagnoses in parent(s)	.07	NS
CBCL Aggressive subscale score	–.24	NS
CBCL Social Competence subscale score	–.28	NS
Iowa Conners' Inattention/Overactivity Ward Teacher rating	–.73	.0001
GAS lowest level of functioning—past 6 mo	–.09	NS
Full-scale IQ	.05	NS
Biological laboratory measures		
CSF 5-HIAA concentration	–.59	.002
CSF HVA concentration	–.69	.0001
SFs/min	–.31	NS
SCL	–.20	NS
Trials to habituation of skin conductance–orienting responses to a series of brief tones (trials to habituation)	–.09	NS
Resting HR	–.37	.06

*NS indicates not significant; CBCL, Child Behavior Checklist; GAS, Children's Global Assessment Scale; CSF, cerebrospinal fluid; 5-HIAA, 5-hydroxyindoleacetic acid; HVA, homovanillic acid; SFs/min, rate of spontaneous skin fluctuations per minute; SCL, skin conductance level; and HR, heart rate.

The initial analysis used Pearson Product-Moment Correlation Coefficients[46] to establish the bivariate relationships between age and the predictor (baseline laboratory and clinical measures) and outcome variables. Partial correlations, removing the effects of age from both sets of variables, were then calculated to determine whether the hypothesized relationships between predictor and outcome variables existed after the effects of age were partialed out. Although we had one-tailed hypotheses, we conservatively used two-tailed levels of significance.

If a significant relationship was found *after* accounting for the influence of age, we conducted a second tier of analyses. This was performed to explore whether baseline laboratory measures contributed to prediction above and beyond that obtained from the clinical measures. For continuous rating scale outcomes, a nonstepwise multiple regression analysis was performed in which all of the nonlaboratory variables (age, the Children's Global Assessment Scale score, socioeconomic status, IQ, aggression, parental antisocial personality disorder diagnosis, and rating scale scores) were entered as a group. This determined the amount of outcome variance that was accounted for by nonlaboratory measures alone. A second hierarchical regression analysis was then performed; this analysis included the nonlaboratory and the biological laboratory variables (5-HIAA, HVA, and ANS activity measures) as a group to determine the additional variance in the outcome measure that was accounted for by the biological laboratory variables. This was determined by the change in the R^2 from the first regression analysis to the second. A stepwise regression analysis was then performed that included *all* of the predictor variables, to determine which variable had the strongest influence on the outcome variable.

As shown in Table 3, as an exploration, a wide scope of baseline (time 1) measures were introduced into the model for the multivariate analyses.

For dichotomous outcome variables (eg, institutionalization), a BMDP[47] stepwise discriminant analysis with jackknife validation, with the use of the same nonlaboratory and biological predictor variables, was conducted to explore which baseline vari-

Table 4.—Correlation and Partial Correlations Correcting for Age of CSF Monoamine Metabolite

	CSF Predictor									
			5-HIAA Concentration				HVA Concentration			
	Age, Correlation		Correlation		Partial Correlation		Correlation		Partial Correlation	
Outcome Measure	*r*	*P*	*r*	*P*	*r*	*P*	*r*	*P*	*r*	*P*
MOAS										
Physical Aggression subscale score	.70	.0001	−.72	.0001	−.53	.006	−.53	.006	−.08	. . .
Auto-Aggression subscale score	.35	.08	−.23	. . .	−.03	. . .	−.34	.09	−.13	. . .
Total score	.69	.0001	−.60	.001	−.34	.09	−.57	.002	−.17	. . .
Suicide attempt	.37	.07	−.38	.06	−.22	. . .	−.48	.01	−.34	.09
Arrest	.63	.0005	−.42	.03	−.08	. . .	−.30	.14	.25	. . .
GAS	−.57	.002	.43	.03	.14	. . .	.52	.006	.21	. . .
Institutionalization	.80	.0001	−.47	.02	−.005	. . .	−.57	.002	−.05	. . .
Substance abuse	.59	.001	−.23	. . .	.18	. . .	−.28	.17	.22	. . .

*CSF indicates cerebrospinal fluid; ANS, autonomic nervous system; 5-HIAA, 5-hydroxyindoleacetic acid; HVA, homovanillic acid; SCL, skin conductance level; SFs/min, rate of spontaneous skin fluctuations per minute; HR, heart rate; MOAS, Modified Overt Aggression Scale; and GAS, Children's Global Assessment Scale. All *P* values are two tailed.

ables might discriminate between the presence or absence of the outcome. Discriminant function analyses utilized prior probabilities due to differing group sizes.

Patients came from a wide variety of school settings, and nine of the original 29 patients lacked ratings from their usual school—most often because of truancy, expulsion, or other conduct disturbance. So, ratings of inattention/overactivity,[48] derived from the Conners' Teacher Rating Scale,[49] utilized National Institute of Mental Health hospital schoolteacher ratings in preference to the child's usual outside teacher.

Because the repeatedly observed strong correlation of CSF 5-HIAA concentrations with concentrations of HVA, which is a dopamine metabolite, has raised questions about the possible interactions between serotonin and dopamine turnover,[50] as well as questions about the specificity of the CSF 5-HIAA concentration as a marker associated with aggression and suicide, both HVA and 5-HIAA measures were included in the correlation, multiple regression, and discriminant function analyses.

RESULTS

Clinical Course and Overall Functioning

The group continued to experience significant difficulties. For example, 12 (41%) of the 29 subjects had been hospitalized, incarcerated, and/or placed in residential treatment, and four (14%) of the 29 subjects had made suicide attempts. The mean (±SD) Children's Global Assessment Scale score at follow-up was 54 (±11.4), which was in the lower half of a 10-point range, indicating that "disturbance would be apparent to those who encounter the child in a dysfunctional setting or time but not to those who see the child in other settings."[43] This range is in between that describing "isolated or sporadic antisocial acts" and that describing "frequent episodes of aggressive or other antisocial behavior with some preservation of meaningful social relationships."

A variety of treatments had been given to the group: 24 (83%) of the 29 subjects had had medication trials or ongoing medication management during follow-up, nine (31%) of the 29 subjects had received inpatient or residential treatment, nine (45%) of 20 subjects who had not had inpatient or residential treatment had individual therapy, and three (15%) of the same 20 subjects had had family therapy. Only one of the 29 subjects could be described as not having had any formal treatment during the follow-up interval. A wide range of other interventions that were aimed at amelioration, such as out-of-home placements, new school placements, tutoring, and juvenile justice system sanctions, also occurred.

Correlational Analysis

No outliers were present. Age correlated significantly with six of eight outcome measures and with two of six baseline laboratory measures as seen in Tables and 3 and 4. Pearson and partial correlations among baseline CSF measures, baseline ANS activity measures, and outcome measures are shown in Table 4. Because of missing baseline data, the sample size was limited to 26.

As shown, 10 of 16 correlations between raw values for CSF measures and outcome were significant ($P<.05$, two tailed). After partialing out the effect of age, one of the hypothesized predictions from the CSF, ie, the inverse correlation between the 5-HIAA concentration and severity of aggression during follow-up, remained highly significant ($P=.006$). However, the hypothesized prediction of the 5-HIAA concentration for suicide attempts was not supported. Statistical trends for inverse correlations between the total score on the Modified Overt Aggression Scale and the 5-HIAA concentration, and between suicide attempts and the HVA concentration were found after partialing out the effect of age. This is a conservative approach, in that if one-tailed *P* values had been used, as hypothesized, these relationships would reach conventional levels ($P\leq.05$) of statistical significance.

Table 4 also shows correlations and partial correlations (accounting for age) between ANS activity measures and outcome variables. Three of 32 possible correlations between raw values were significant. The inverse correlation between SCL and institutionalization remained significant in the predicted direction, after the effect of age was partialed out, with the adverse outcome associated with a lower SCL. Hypothesized prediction of trials to habituation for suicide attempts and of SFs/min, SCL, and HR for arrest were not supported.

Multivariate analyses then explored whether the laboratory measures had any predictive value beyond that offered by more commonly collected clinical measures.

Because physical aggression was related to the 5-HIAA concentration after partialing out the effect of age, multiple regression analyses were carried out to explore whether the laboratory measures had any predictive import for physical aggression beyond that offered by more commonly collected clinical measures. First, a hierarchical multiple regression was carried out with the use of all the baseline nonlaboratory measures as shown in Table 3. As shown in Table 5, the multiple R^2 was .65

Concentrations and ANS Activity Measures Collected at Baseline and Outcome Measures*

	ANS Activity Predictor																	
			SCL				SFs/min				HR				Trials to Habituation			
	Age, Correlation		Correlation		Partial Correlation		Correlation		Partial Correlation		Correlation		Partial Correlation		Correlation		Partial Correlation	
	r	P	r	P	r	P	r	P	r	P	r	P	r	P	r	P	r	P
	.70	.0001	–.005	...	.19	...	–.11	...	.16	...	–.17	...	.14	...	.14	...	.28	.17
	.35	.08	.01	...	.09	...	–.17	...	–.07	...	–.35	.08	–.25	...	.05	...	.09	...
	.69	.0001	.01	...	.21	...	–.16	...	.09	...	–.31	.12	–.08	...	.07	...	.19	...
	.37	.07	–.17	...	–.11	...	–.19	...	–.09	...	–.41	.04	–.32	.12	.03	...	.07	...
	.63	.0005	–.18	...	–.07	...	–.04	...	.21	...	–.21	...	.03		.05	...	.13	...
	–.57	.002	.03	...	–.11	...	–.15	...	–.04	...	–.02	...	–.30	.14	–.24	...	–.35	.08
	.80	.0001	–.44	.02	–.47	.02	–.40	.04	–.27	.19	–.13	...	.29	.15	–.19	...	–.20	...
	.59	.001	–.24	...	–.16	...	–.19	...	–.01	...	–.10	...	.16	...	.04	...	.11	...

Table 5.—Multiple Regression Analyses*

	Cumulative R^2	Adjusted R^2
Multiple regression—hierarchical		
Nonlaboratory measures	.65	.48
Biological laboratory measures and nonlaboratory measures	.91†	.80†
Multiple regression—stepwise		
5-HIAA	.52	.52
Age	.64	.62
Antisocial diagnosis—parent	.70	.67
IQ	.75	.72

*Amount of variance (R^2) in Physical Aggression subscale of the Modified Overt Aggression Scale (outcome) that was predicted by nonlaboratory and laboratory baseline measures. 5-HIAA indicates 5-hydroxyindoleacetic acid.

†Amount of additional variance explained over model that used only nonlaboratory measures was statistically significant ($P<.02$).

Table 6.—Discriminant Analysis: Prediction of Institutionalization During 2-Year Follow-up of DBDs (n=26)*

Institutionalization, Total Group (+=11, –=15)	Cumulative R^2	Jackknife Classification, %
Age (+, older)	.64	–100
SCL (+, lower)	.72	+91†
HR (+, lower)	.84	96

*DBDs indicates disruptive behavior disorders; plus sign, the outcome occurred (eg, 11 were institutionalized); minus sign, outcome did not occur; SCL, skin conductance level; and HR, heart rate.

†Before the jackknife procedure, 100% of those who were institutionalized were correctly classified by the three predictor variables.

for the nonlaboratory measures. A second multiple regression that entered the nonlaboratory measures and the laboratory measures as a set resulted in a multiple R^2 of .91. Thus, laboratory variables significantly explained ($P<.02$)[51] an additional 26% of the variance in the physical aggression outcome variable. Adjusted R^2 values,[51] which corrected for the number of predictor variables that were entered in a multiple regression, showed a greater difference and were also significant. As an additional assessment of the relative import of laboratory and clinical measures, all predictors were competed into a stepwise multiple regression; the 5-HIAA measure was entered into the model first and accounted for 52% of the variance in physical aggression.

Another laboratory measure, ie, SCL, was significantly correlated with the dichotomous outcome of institutionalization. To explore this contribution relative to clinical measures, a stepwise discriminant function analysis was conducted by utilizing all of the baseline variables. Results are shown in Table 6.

The biological laboratory measures, ie, SCL and HR, added significantly to the prediction.

COMMENT

This 2-year prospective follow-up study found that laboratory-based biological parameters, such as the CSF 5-HIAA concentration and SCL, offered significant predictive information for severity of physical aggression and institutionalization as outcomes for children with DBDs. Hypothesized relationships among 5-HIAA concentrations, trials to habituation, and suicide attempts were not found. Low ANS activity also failed to predict arrest.

The biological laboratory measures that did predict outcome not only had significant correlations with follow-up after partialing out the effect of age, but contributed significantly in the multivariate analyses even after clinical measures, which numerous earlier studies had identified as important predictors, such as aggressivity/previous antisocial behavior[8-10,52,53] and IQ,[10,53] as well as family factors, including parental mental health[10,52-55] and socioeconomic status,[56] were forced into the model first. To our knowledge, this is the first report that has combined CSF and clinical measures in a prospective study of DBDs. The findings from this present report confirm earlier suggestions[57,58] of the predictive validity of the CSF 5-HIAA concentration in children with disruptive disorders, are generally consistent with the findings from other studies with regard to the predictive import of ANS activity,[30,59] and suggest that further study of biological factors in adverse outcomes among patients with DBDs is warranted.

Observed trends in the partial correlations are consistent with those of other studies and would have reached significance if one-tailed statistics had been used. Our results extend the findings from adult studies that lower CSF HVA concentrations can predict future suicide attempts[26,27] in children and adolescents. The trend for fast habituation to predict better global functioning at follow-up is not consistent with the idea that lower ANS activity is associated with worse outcomes. However, that trend is similar to findings in acute schizophrenia,[60,61] relating slow habituation to poor short-term outcome, and to similar findings from a recent 3- to 5-year follow-up study of children and adolescents with obsessive-compulsive disorder.[62]

Just how much laboratory measures add to the prediction by comparison with data from studies that utilized clinical variables only[9,53] is difficult to quantify. Methodological, sample, and definitional differences, and limits of data accessible from other studies, as well as limitations inherent in this study, prevent more precise quantification.

There are several other limitations to this study. Age at intake correlated with all outcome measures at a significance level of $P \leqslant .08$, and our initial wide age spread was thus unfortunate. However, even within more narrow age samples, such as that of Loney et al,[10] age at referral predicted involvement with alcohol, probably reflecting the fact that for many outcomes, there are age-related periods of risk. Thus, one perspective is that it is even more remarkable that the laboratory measures showed any predictive value. Nonetheless, future studies must focus on a more narrow age range to avoid these limitations.

The follow-up interval is relatively brief; patients are still "at risk," and ultimate outcome is still unknown. Loeber et al[63] documented continuities and discontinuities in aggressive behavior and suggested that 4-year follow-up intervals give greater accuracy. However, even briefer follow-up intervals in adult subjects found prediction of CSF 5-HIAA or HVA measures for suicide attempts during (1-year) follow-up intervals,[26,32] while Virkkunen et al[28] found significantly lower CSF 5-HIAA concentrations in those who committed a new offense during the 3 years following release from correctional facilities.

Our relatively short follow-up period may have yielded a low estimate of the predictive power of autonomic measures. Correlations between ANS activity measures and outcome measures were generally in an inverse direction, as expected. However, only one correlation between ANS activity measures and outcomes reached statistical significance after the effect of age was partialed out. The ANS activity measures did not, as hypothesized, predict which eight of 26 subjects had been arrested during the follow-up. The follow-up studies of pediatric samples that found ANS activity measures predicted later aggression or criminality[31,59] had follow-up intervals of 6 to 9 years. Yet, cross-sectional studies of relationships between ANS activity measures and aggressive or conduct disturbance in this and other pediatric samples have not consistently shown significant associations.[64]

Some synergistic risk factors have not yet entered the picture for many of these patients. Alcohol, for example, may significantly increase risk for individuals with low 5-HIAA concentrations.[27]

The consistency of findings in pediatric cases with those in adults makes the further study of relationships of CSF monoamine metabolite concentrations and autonomic activity in pediatric samples with severe intractable aggression of both clinical and research importance.

References

1. Reeves JC, Werry JS, Elkind GS, Zametkin A. Attention deficit, conduct, oppositional, and anxiety disorders in children, II: clinical characteristics. *J Am Acad Child Adolesc Psychiatry.* 1987;26:144-155.
2. Gittelman R, Mannuzza S, Shenker R, Bonagura R. Hyperactive boys almost grown up, I: psychiatric status. *Arch Gen Psychiatry.* 1985;42:937-947.
3. Weiss G, Hechtman L, Milroy T, Perlman T. Psychiatric status of hyperactives as adults: a controlled prospective 15 year follow-up of 63 hyperactive children. *J Am Acad Child Adolesc Psychiatry.* 1985;24:211-220.
4. Mannuzza S, Klein RG, Bonagura R, Malloy P, Giampino TL, Addalli KA. Hyperactive boys almost grown up, V: replication of psychiatric status. *Arch Gen Psychiatry.* 1991;48:77-83.
5. Mannuzza S, Gittelman-Klein R, Konig PH, Giampino TL. Hyperactive boys almost grown up, IV: criminality and its relationship to psychiatric status. *Arch Gen Psychiatry.* 1989;46:1073-1079.
6. August GJ, Stewart MA, Holmes CS. A four-year follow-up of hyperactive boys with and without conduct disorder. *Br J Psychiatry.* 1983;143:192-198.
7. Rutter M. Pathways from childhood to adult life. *J Child Psychol Psychiatry.* 1989;30:23-51.
8. Robins LN. *Deviant Children Grown Up.* Baltimore, Md: Williams & Wilkins; 1966.
9. Robins LN. Sturdy childhood predictors of adult antisocial behavior: replications from longitudinal studies. *Psychol Med.* 1978;8:611-622.
10. Loney J, Kramer J, Milich RS. The hyperactive child grows up: predictors of symptoms, delinquency and achievement at follow-up. In: Gadow JD, Loney J, eds. *Psychosocial Aspects of Drug Treatment for Hyperactivity: AAAS Selected Symposium.* Boulder, Colo: Westview Press Inc; 1981;44:381-416.
11. Pfeffer CR, Plutchik R, Mizruchi MS. Predictors of assaultiveness in latency age children. *Am J Psychiatry.* 1983;140:31-35.
12. Huesmann LR, Eron LD. Cognitive processes and the persistence of aggressive behavior. *Aggress Behav.* 1984;10:243-251.
13. Roff JD, Wirt RD. Childhood aggression and social adjustment as antecedents of delinquency. *J Abnorm Child Psychol.* 1984;12:111-126.
14. Stattin H, Magnusson D. The role of early aggressive behavior in the frequency, seriousness, and types of later crime. *J Consult Clin Psychol.* 1989;57:710-718.
15. Feldhusen JF, Aversano FM, Thurston JR. Prediction of youth contacts with law enforcement agencies. *Criminal Justice Behav.* 1976;3:235-253.
16. Ensminger ME, Kellam SG, Rubin BR. School and family origins of delinquency: comparison by sex. In: van Dusen K, Mednick S, eds. *Prospective Studies of Crime and Deliquency.* Boston, Mass:Kluwer/Nijhoff; 1983:73-97.
17. Douglas JWB. The school progress of nervous and troublesome children. *Br J Psychiatry.* 1966;112:1115-1116.
18. Morris HH, Escoll PJ, Wexler MSW. Aggressive behavior disorders in children: a follow-up study. *Am J Psychiatry.* 1956;112:991-997.
19. Loeber R, Stouthamer-Loeber M. Prediction. In: Quay HC, ed. *Handbook of Juvenile Delinquency.* New York, NY: John Wiley & Sons Inc; 1987:324-382.
20. Loeber R, Dishion T. Early predictors of male delinquency: a review. *Psychol Bull.* 1983;94:68-99.
21. Rutter M, MacDonald H, Le Couteur A, Harrington R, Bolton P, Bailey A. Genetic factors in child psychiatric disorders, II: empirical findings. *J Child Psychol Psychiatry.* 1990;31:39-83.
22. Mednick SA, Gabrielli WF, Hutchings B. Genetic influences in criminal convictions: evidence from an adoption cohort. *Science.* 1984;224:891-894.
23. Cloninger CR, Sigvardson S, Bowman M, von Knorring AL. Predisposition to petty criminality in Swedish adoptees. *Arch Gen Psychiatry.* 1982;39:1242-1247.
24. Crowe RR. An adoption study of antisocial personality. *Arch Gen Psychiatry.* 1974;31:785-791.
25. Kruesi MJP, Rapoport JL, Hamburger S, Hibbs E, Potter WZ, Lenane M, Brown GL. CSF monoamine metabolites, aggression and impulsivity in disruptive behavior disorders of children and adolescents. *Arch Gen Psychiatry.* 1990;47:419-426.
26. Traskman L, Asberg M, Bertilsson L, Sjostrand L. Monoamine metabolites in CSF and suicidal behavior. *Arch Gen Psychiatry.* 1981;38:631-636.
27. Roy A, DeJong RA, Linnoila M. Cerebrospinal fluid monamine metabolites and suicidal behavior in depressed patients. *Arch Gen Psychiatry.* 1989;46:609-612.
28. Virkkunen M, De Jong J, Bartko J, Goodwin FK, Linnoila M. Relationship of psychobiological variables to recidivism in violent offenders and impulsive fire setters: a follow-up study. *Arch Gen Psychiatry.* 1989;46:604-606.
29. Brown GL, Ballanger JC, Minichiello MD, Goodwin FK. Human aggression and its relationship to cerebrospinal fluid 5-hydroxyindoleacetic acid, 3-methoxy-4-hydroxyphenylglycol, and homovanillic

acid. In: Sandler M, ed. *Psychopharmacology of Aggression.* New York, NY: Raven Press; 1979:131-148.
30. Raine A, Venables PH, Williams M. Relationships between central and autonomic measures of arousal at age 15 and criminality at age 24. *Arch Gen Psychiatry.* 1990;47:1003-1007.
31. Venables PH. Childhood markers for adult disorders. *J Child Psychol Psychiatry.* 1989;30:347-364.
32. Edman G, Asberg M, Levander S, Schalling D. Skin conductance habituation and cerebrospinal fluid 5-hydroxyindoleacetic acid in suicidal patients. *Arch Gen Psychiatry.* 1985;43:586-592.
33. Thorell LH. Electrodermal activity in suicidal and non-suicidal depressive patients and in matched healthy subjects. *Acta Psychiatr Scand.* 1987;76:420-430.
34. Herjanic B, Campbell W. Differentiating psychiatrically disturbed children on the basis of a structured interview. *J Abnorm Child Psychol.* 1977;5:127-134.
35. Welner Z, Reich W, Herjanic B, Jung K, Amado H. Reliability, validity and child agreement studies of the Diagnostic Interview for Children and Adolescents (DICA). *J Am Acad Child Adolesc Psychiatry.* 1987;26:649-653.
36. Herjanic B, Reich W. Development of a structured psychiatric interview for children: agreement between child and parent on individual symptoms. *J Abnorm Child Psychol.* 1982;10:307-324.
37. American Psychiatric Association, Committee on Nomenclature and Statistics. *Diagnostic and Statistical Manual of Mental Disorders, Revised Third Edition.* Washington, DC: American Psychiatric Association; 1987.
38. Endicott J, Spitzer RL. A diagnostic interview: the Schedule for Affective Disorders and Schizophrenia. *Arch Gen Psychiatry.* 1978;35:837-844.
39. Wechsler D. *Wechsler Intelligence Scale for Children–Revised.* New York, NY: Psychological Corp; 1974.
40. Wechsler D. *Wechsler Adult Intelligence Scale–Revised.* New York, NY: Psychological Corp; 1981.
41. Achenbach TM, Edelbrock C. *Manual for the Child Behavior Checklist and Revised Child Behavior Profile.* Burlington, Vt: University of Vermont Department of Psychiatry; 1983.
42. Kay SR, Wolkenfield F, Murrill LM. Profiles of aggression among psychiatric patients, I: nature and prevalence. *J Nerv Ment Dis.* 1988;176:539-546.
43. Shaffer D, Gould MS, Brasic J, Ambrosini P, Fisher P, Bird H, Aluwahlia S. A Children's Global Assessment Scale. *Arch Gen Psychiatry.* 1983;40:1228-1231.
44. Daly M, Wilson M. Killing the competition. *Hum Nature.* 1990;1:81-107.
45. Hoberman HM, Garfinkel BD. Completed suicide in children and adolescents. *J Am Acad Child Adolesc Psychiatry.* 1988;27:689-695.
46. SAS Institute. *User's Guide: Statistics, Version 5.* Cary, NC: SAS Institute; 1985.
47. Dixon WJ, Brown MB, Engelman L, Frane JW, Hill MA, Jennrich RI, Toporek JD. *BMDP Statistical Software: 1983 Printing With Additions.* Berkeley, Calif: University of California Press; 1983.
48. Loney J, Milich R. Hyperactivity, inattention, and aggression in clinical practice. In: Wolraich M, Routh D, eds. *Advances in Developmental and Behavioral Pediatrics.* Greenwich, Conn: JAI Press Inc; 1985:113-147.
49. Conners CK. A teacher rating scale for use in drug studies with children. *Am J Psychiatry.* 1969;126:884-888.
50. Agren H, Mefford IN, Rudorfer MV, Linnoila M, Potter WZ. Interacting neurotransmitter systems: a non-experimental approach to the 5HIAA-HVA correlation in human CSF. *J Psychiatr Res.* 1986;20:175-193.
51. Draper NR, Smith H. *Applied Regression Analysis.* 2nd ed. New York, NY: John Wiley & Sons Inc; 1981:91.
52. Weiss G, Minde K, Werry JS, Douglas VI, Nemeth E. Studies on the hyperactive child, VIII: five-year follow-up. *Arch Gen Psychiatry.* 1971;24:409-414.
53. Weiss G, Hechtman L. *Hyperactive Children Grown Up.* New York, NY: Guilford Press; 1986.
54. Mendelson WB, Johnson NE, Stewart MA. Hyperactive children as teenagers: a follow-up study. *J Nerv Ment Dis.* 1971;153:273-278.
55. Barkley RA, Fischer M, Edelbrock CS, Smallish L. The adolescent outcome of hyperactive children diagnosed by research criteria, I: an 8-year prospective follow-up study. *J Am Acad Child Adolesc Psychiatry.* 1990;29:546-557.
56. Duyme M. Antisocial behavior and postnatal environment: a French adoption study. *J Child Psychol Psychiatry.* 1990;31:699-710.
57. Kruesi MJP, Linnoila M, Rapoport JL, Brown GL, Petersen R. Carbohydrate craving, conduct disorder and low 5-HIAA. *Psychiatry Res.* 1985;16:83-86.
58. Kruesi MJP. Cruelty to animals and CSF 5-HIAA. *Psychiatry Res.* 1989;28:115-116.
59. Raine A, Venables PH, Williams M. Autonomic-orienting responses in 15-year-old male subjects and criminal behavior at age 24. *Am J Psychiatry.* 1990;147:933-937.
60. Zahn TP, Carpenter WTJ, McGlashan TH. Autonomic nervous system activity in acute schizophrenia, II: relationships to short-term prognosis and clinical state. *Arch Gen Psychiatry.* 1981;38(3):260-266.
61. Frith CD, Stevens M, Johnstone EC, Crow TJ. Skin conductance responsivity during acute episodes of schizophrenia as a predictor of symptomatic improvement. *Psychol Med.* 1979;9:101-106.
62. Flament MF, Koby E, Rapoport JL, Berg CJ, Zahn T, Cox C, Denckla M, Lenane M. Childhood obsessive-compulsive disorder: a prospective follow-up study. *J Child Psychol Psychiatry.* 1990;31:363-380.
63. Loeber R, Trembalay RE, Gagnon L, Charlebois P. Continuity and desistance in disruptive boys: early fighting in school. *Dev Psychopathology.* 1989;1:39-50.
64. Garralda ME, Connell J, Taylor DC. Psychophysiological anomalies in children with emotional and conduct disorders. *Psychol Med.* 1991;21:947-957.

Marked Reduction in Indexes of Dopamine Metabolism Among Patients With Depression Who Attempt Suicide

Alec Roy, MB; Farouk Karoum, PhD; Simcha Pollack, PhD

• Cerebrospinal fluid studies have reported that low concentrations of the dopamine metabolite homovanillic acid are associated with suicidal behavior in depression. Although only a small proportion of homovanillic acid in the urine derives from the brain, we decided to examine 24-hour urinary outputs of homovanillic acid in relation to suicidal behavior in depression. Patients with depression who had attempted suicide had significantly smaller urinary outputs of homovanillic acid, dihydroxyphenylacetic acid, and total body output of dopamine (sum dopamine) than did patients with depression who had not attempted suicide. Patients with depression who reattempted suicide during 5-year follow-up had significantly smaller urinary outputs of homovanillic acid and sum dopamine than did patients who did not reattempt suicide, patients who never attempted suicide, and normal control subjects, and had significantly smaller outputs of dihydroxyphenylacetic acid than patients who never attempted suicide or control subjects. These data suggest that urinary outputs of homovanillic acid may be peripheral correlates of suicidality in depression. These data add to data on the low levels of homovanillic acid in cerebrospinal fluid in suggesting that diminished dopaminergic neurotransmission may play a part in suicidal behavior in depression.

(*Arch Gen Psychiatry*. 1992;49:447-450)

The results of cerebrospinal fluid (CSF) studies of monoamine metabolites in suicide attempters, and of postmortem neurochemical and receptor studies of suicide victims, have suggested that reduced central monoaminergic neurotransmission may be involved in suicidal behavior.[1-3] For example, Traskman et al[4] reported that suicide attempters had significantly lower CSF concentrations of both the serotonin metabolite 5-hydroxyindoleacetic acid (5-HIAA) and the dopamine metabolite homovanillic acid (HVA) than did control subjects. Most recently, we reported that patients with depression who had attempted suicide had significantly lower CSF concentrations of HVA than did patients with depression who had not attempted suicide and normal controls.[5] We followed up these patients with depression and found that patients who reattempted suicide during the 5-year follow-up had significantly lower CSF concentrations of both HVA and 5-HIAA.[6]

During index admission, these patients, not all of whom underwent lumbar punctures, had also participated in 24-hour urine collections for determination of urinary outputs of catecholamines, including dopamine and its major metabolites. Therefore, we decided to examine suicidal behavior in these patients with depression in relation to the previously published data about their urinary outputs of dopamine and its major metabolites, HVA and dihydroxyphenylacetic acid (DOPAC).[7] We hypothesized that patients with depression who attempted suicide would have significantly lower urinary outputs of HVA and DOPAC.

SUBJECTS AND METHODS

Twenty-two patients with depression seen at the National Institute of Mental Health (NIMH), Bethesda, Md, who at interview fulfilled *DSM-III* criteria for a major depressive episode and 25 normal control subjects were studied. Scores were obtained for all patients using the Hamilton Depression Rating Scale.[8] Nineteen of the patients with depression had unipolar disorder, and three, bipolar disorder. All control subjects were interviewed using the Schedule for Affective Disorders and Schizophrenia–Lifetime version[9] to exclude psychiatric disorder; none had personal or family histories of psychiatric disorder. The control subjects were physically well, were receiving no medications, and had normal results of physical examination, echocardiography, and routine blood tests. Chest roentgenograms were also normal. The control subjects were studied as outpatients.

All patients and control subjects were placed on a low-monoamine, caffeine-restricted diet that excluded alcohol for the duration of the study. All patients with depression who were receiving psychotropic medications were slowly withdrawn from all medications and were free of medication for at least 2 weeks before the study began. Two 24-hour urine samples were collected in a receptacle containing 3% sodium metabisulphite. Aliquots were kept frozen at −20°C until analyzed. Only samples of more than 900 mL were used in the study.[10] Concentrations of total urinary dopamine, HVA, and DOPAC were measured with mass fragmentography.[11] The average of both samples was considered the final value. Data comparing outputs of these substances in the urine of patients with unipolar disor-

Accepted for publication March 3, 1992.
From Hillside Hospital, Glen Oaks, NY (Drs Roy and Pollack), and the National Institute of Mental Health–Neuroscience Center at St Elizabeth's Hospital, Washington, DC (Dr Karoum), and the Department of Quantitative Analysis, St John's University, Jamaica, NY (Dr Pollack).

Reprint requests to Hillside Hospital, PO Box 38, Glen Oaks, NY 11004 (Dr Roy).

Table 1.—Clinical Data for Patients With Depression and Control Subjects*

Variable	Patients With Depression (N=22)	Control Subjects (N=25)
M/F	3/19	10/15
Age, y	47.0±14.4	44.8±13.9
Duration of depressive episode, mo	8.6±8.1	NA
Unipolar disorder	19	NA
Bipolar disorder	3	NA
Score on the Hamilton Depression Rating Scale	23.2±6.2	NA
Time without medication, wk	5.4±6.8†	NA

*Values are numbers of cases or means±SDs. NA indicates not applicable.

†n=18. Two patients had never received psychotropic medication, a third had not received it for 15 years, and a fourth had not received it for 15 months.

der and in normal control subjects have been previously reported.[7]

After NIMH index admission, all patients were discharged from the hospital and returned to the care of their referring psychiatrists. They were not subsequently readmitted at the NIMH. The 5-year follow-up was conducted for all patients via telephone interviews to determine if there had been any suicidal behavior during the years since the urine collections. Information was also obtained from telephone interviews with spouses or other relatives as well as from the referring or current psychiatrist or therapist. Only self-damaging behavior that had led to hospitalization and/or been confirmed in the patient's medical record by a treating physician was accepted as suicidal behavior, as recommended by van Praag and Plutchik.[12]

Analysis of variance was used for statistical analysis, followed by the Newman-Keuls Post Hoc Test. Because neither age nor sex was significantly correlated with any of the urinary dopamine variables in either patients or control subjects, analysis of covariance was not used. Total urinary outputs of dopamine and its major metabolites (the sum dopamine output) were also examined. Sum dopamine values were determined by adding the values for dopamine, HVA, and DOPAC.

RESULTS

Clinical data for the 22 patients with depression and the 25 normal control subjects are shown in Table 1. Before their admission to the NIMH, 12 (54.5%) of the 22 patients had attempted suicide at some time. Four (33.3%) of these 12 patients reattempted suicide during the mean follow-up of 55.1±14.8 months. Two of them committed suicide. No patient who had not previously exhibited suicidal behavior attempted suicide during follow-up.

First, data were examined in relation to the history of suicidal behavior at the time of the urinary collections at the NIMH. Patients who had attempted suicide at some time had significantly smaller outputs of HVA than did patients who had never attempted suicide ($F=5.13$; $df=2, 44$; $P<.01$) and significantly smaller urinary outputs of DOPAC ($F=7.31$; $df=2, 44$; $P<.002$) and sum dopamine ($F=4.62$; $df=2, 44$; $P<.02$) than did patients who had never attempted suicide and control subjects (Table 2).

Second, data were examined in relation to reattempting suicide during the 5-year follow-up. Patients who reattempted suicide had significantly smaller urinary outputs of HVA ($F=5.57$; $df=3, 43$; $P<.003$) and sum dopamine ($F=6.05$; $df=3, 43$; $P<.002$) than did patients who did not reattempt suicide, patients who never attempted suicide, and control subjects. They also had significantly smaller outputs of DOPAC ($F=5.96$; $df=3, 43$; $P<.002$) than did patients who never attempted suicide and control subjects (Figure).

There were significant correlations among the urinary dopamine variables. Urinary outputs of HVA and DOPAC correlated significantly among both patients with depression ($r=.79$ and $P<.0001$) and control subjects ($r=.65$ and $P<.0001$). Urinary outputs of DOPAC and dopamine correlated significantly with control subjects ($r=.55$ and $P<.005$). However, among the 13 patients who had undergone lumbar puncture, there was no significant correlation between CSF concentrations of HVA and urinary outputs of HVA ($r=-.02$), DOPAC ($r=.22$), or dopamine ($r=-.13$).

COMMENT

Our study had two main results: (1) patients with depression who had attempted suicide had significantly lower urinary outputs of HVA, DOPAC, and sum dopamine than did patients with depression who had not attempted suicide, and (2) patients with depression who reattempted suicide had significantly lower urinary outputs of HVA and sum dopamine than did patients with depression who did not reattempt suicide, patients who never attempted suicide, and normal control subjects and significantly smaller outputs of DOPAC than did patients who never attempted suicide and control subjects.

Human postmortem studies and studies in monkeys[13] have demonstrated that HVA is the major metabolite of dopamine in the brains of primates. However, the proportion of peripheral HVA derived from the brain is small. For example, Maas et al[13] estimated that approximately 25% of urinary HVA is derived from the brain. Using administration of the monoamine oxidase inhibitor, debrisoquin, which does not enter the brain, as a method of minimizing the contribution of peripheral tissues to HVA production, Kopin et al[14] estimated that about 24% of plasma HVA is from dopaminergic neurons in the brain. Kopin et al[15] also reported a striking reduction of urinary outputs of centrally derived HVA after MPTP (1-methyl-4-phenyl-1,2,3,6-tetrahydropyridine)–induced destruction of dopaminergic nigrostriatal neurons in monkeys. Most recently, Lambert at al[16] estimated that HVA overflow from the brain contributes only 12% of total body HVA. Although most urinary dopamine metabolites originate from peripheral sources, changes in dopamine turnover and metabolism in the brain that are induced by drugs (eg, antidepressants, lithium, and cocaine) and electroconvulsive therapy have been shown to positively correlate with turnover of total body dopamine (sum urinary dopamine).[17,18] Thus, it is possible that changes involving central dopamine systems may equally manifest themselves in peripheral dopamine systems. The kidney is also a source of urinary dopamine, and there was no significant difference in urinary outputs of dopamine among the groups in our study.

In the last few years, investigators have studied peripheral measures of HVA as a strategy for examining the dopaminergic system in neuropsychiatric patients. For example, in schizophrenic patients, significant relationships have been observed between plasma concentrations of HVA and features of that illness. Studies[19] of schizophrenic patients who were not receiving medication have reported positive correlations between the severity of symptoms of schizophrenia and plasma concentrations of HVA. The same studies reported that response to treatment with neuroleptic agents correlated with decreases in levels of plasma HVA.

Exogenous factors may affect peripheral measures of

Table 2.—Urinary Output of Dopamine and Its Major Metabolites in Patients With Depression Who Had or Had Not Attempted Suicide and in Normal Control Subjects*

Compound, μmol/d	Patients Who Had Attempted Suicide (n=12)	Patients Who Had Never Attempted Suicide (n=10)	Normal Control Subjects (n=25)	Significance (*df*=2, 44)
HVA	20.1±1.7	28.7±8.7	24.2±5.3	F=5.13, *P*<.01
DOPAC	5.4±2.5	8.9±3.9	9.4±2.8	F=7.31, *P*<.002
Dopamine	4.3±2.1	4.3±1.6	4.2±2.6	F=0.02, NS
Sum dopamine	29.8±9.6	42.0±12.0	37.8±8.9	F=4.62, *P*<.02

*HVA indicates homovanillic acid; DOPAC, dihydroxyphenylacetic acid; sum dopamine, the sum of HVA, DOPAC, and dopamine; and NS, not significant. Except for the last column, values are means±SDs.

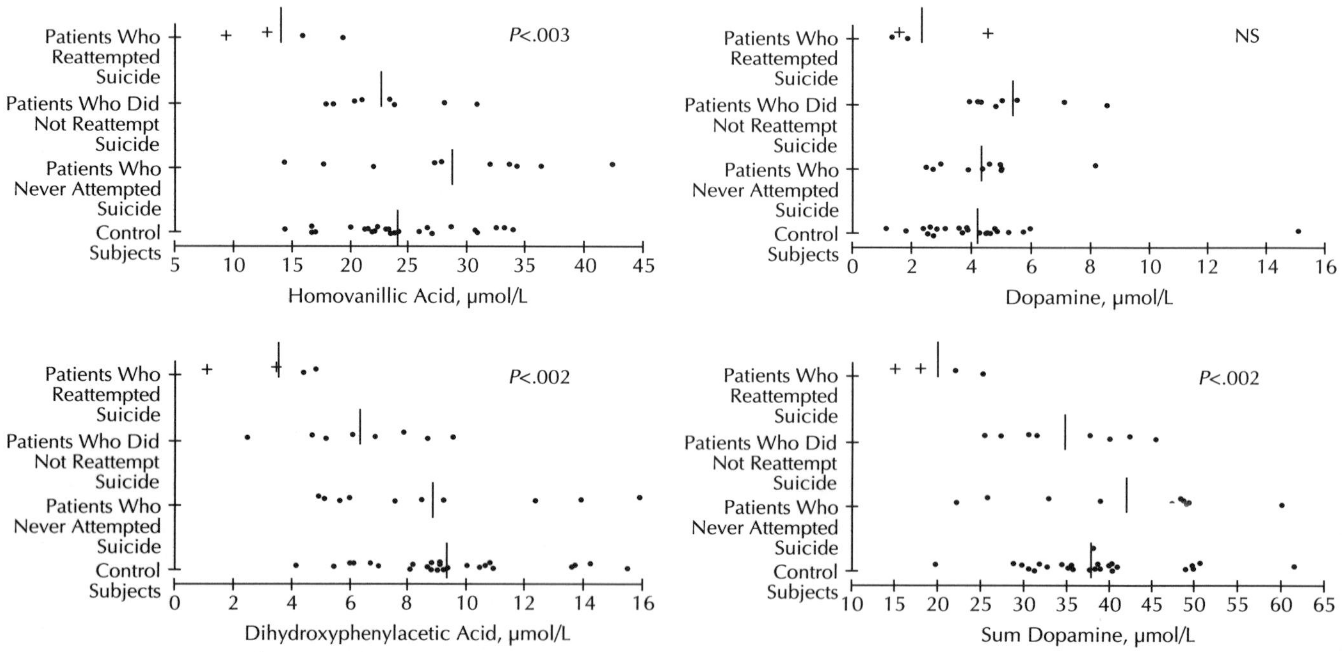

Scattergrams showing urinary outputs in patients with depression who did or did not reattempt suicide during 5-year follow-up, patients with depression who had never attempted suicide, and normal control subjects. Patients who reattempted suicide had significantly lower urinary outputs of homovanillic acid (F=5.57; df=3, 43; P<.003; *top left) and sum dopamine (F=6.05;* df=3, 43; P<.002; *bottom right) than did patients who did not reattempt suicide, patients who had never attempted suicide, and control subjects. Patients who reattempted suicide also had significantly smaller urinary outputs of dihydroxyphenylacetic acid (DOPAC) than did patients who had never attempted suicide or control subjects (F=5.96;* df=3, 43; P<.002; *bottom left). Patients who did not reattempt suicide had significantly smaller urinary outputs of DOPAC than did control subjects (*P<.05*). There was no significant difference among the groups for urinary outputs of dopamine (top right). Crosses indicate the two patients who committed suicide. Bars indicate means.*

HVA. This is noteworthy because the control subjects in our study were studied as outpatients while 18 of the 22 patients with depression were studied as inpatients. However, Davidson et al[20] demonstrated that changing position, walking for 30 minutes, or smoking two cigarettes had no effect on plasma concentrations of HVA. The patients and control subjects in our study had followed a low-monoamine diet for similar periods. Furthermore, 24-hour urine collection is a better integrated catecholamine measure than is plasma obtained at a single time point. It is also noteworthy that the urinary outputs of HVA in the 25 outpatient control subjects in our study were very similar to those of 12 control subjects studied as inpatients at the National Institutes of Health[21] (mean output, 24.2±5.3 μmol/d vs 26.7±2.3 μmol/d, respectively). Finally, that our findings were not confounded by comparison with outpatient control subjects is suggested by the fact that there were significant differences among the patients with depression. For example, patients who reattempted suicide had significantly smaller urinary outputs of HVA than did patients who did not reattempt suicide and patients who never attempted suicide.

Another possibly confounding factor is that of a depressive subgroup. For example, some studies have reported that changes in indexes of the dopaminergic system are most marked in patients with depression and melancholia. However, in our study only eight of the 22 patients with depression also had melancholia, and there was no significant difference in the number of melancholic patients in the three subgroups with depression ($\chi^2=1.28$, $df=2$). Also, there were no significant differences between melancholic and nonmelancholic patients for any of the urinary dopaminergic measures studied. Only three patients with depression had bipolar disorder, and there was no significant difference in how they were distributed among the three groups. There were no significant differences for urinary dopamine variables between patients with bipolar and unipolar disorder. None of the patients had psychotic depression.

We confirmed our hypothesis that urinary outputs of HVA and DOPAC would be associated with suicidal behavior in depression. The two patients with depression who committed suicide had the lowest urinary outputs of HVA. These data add to observations that patients with depression who attempt and reattempt suicide have significantly lower CSF concentrations of HVA than do various other groups[4-6,22-25] and suggest that diminished central dopaminergic neurotransmission may be associated with suicidal behavior in depression. However, the high degree of covariance between CSF concentrations of HVA and 5-HIAA[26] lead to the speculation that low values for HVA and 5-HIAA may be "markers" of change in some common process related to serotonin and dopamine metabolism and turnover that is associated with suicidal behavior. Nonetheless, further studies of the relationship of urinary outputs of HVA to suicidal behavior in depression are needed.

References

1. Asberg M, Nordstrom P, Traskman-Benz L. Biological factors in suicide. In: Roy A, ed. *Suicide.* Baltimore, Md: Williams & Wilkins; 1986:47-71.
2. Roy A, Linnoila M. Suicidal behavior, impulsiveness and serotonin. *Acta Psychiatr Scand.* 1988;78:529-535.
3. Roy A, Linnoila M. Monoamines and suicidal behavior. In: van Praag H, Plutchik R, Apter A, eds. *Violence and Suicidality: Perspective in Clinical and Psychobiological Research.* New York, NY: Brunner/Mazel Inc; 1990:218-241.
4. Traskman L, Asberg M, Bertilsson L, Sjostrand L. Monoamine metabolites in CSF and suicidal behavior. *Arch Gen Psychiatry.* 1981;38:631-636.
5. Roy A, Agren H, Pickar D, Linnoila M, Doran AR, Culter NR, Paul SM. Reduced CSF concentrations of homovanillic acid and homovanillic acid to 5-hydroxyindoleacetic acid ratios in depressed patients: relationship to suicidal behavior and dexamethasone nonsuppression. *Am J Psychiatry.* 1986;143:1539-1545.
6. Roy A, DeJong J, Linnoila M. Cerebrospinal fluid monoamine metabolites and suicidal behavior in depressed patients: a 5-year follow-up study. *Arch Gen Psychiatry.* 1989;46:609-612.
7. Roy A, Pickar D, Douillet P, Karoum F, Linnoila M. Urinary monoamines and metabolites in subtypes of unipolar depressive disorder and normal controls. *Psychol Med.* 1986;16:541-556.
8. Hamilton M. A rating scale for depression. *J Neurol Neurosurg Psychiatry.* 1960;23:56-62.
9. Endicott J, Spitzer R. A diagnostic interview: the Schedule for Affective Disorder and Schizophrenia. *Arch Gen Psychiatry.* 1979;35:837-844.
10. Linnoila M, Karoum F, Miller T, Potter W. Reliability of urinary monoamine and metabolite output measurements in depressed patients. *Am J Psychiatry.* 1983;140:1055-1057.
11. Karoum F, Neff N. Quantitative gas chromatography–mass spectrometry (CG-MS) of biogenic amines: theory and practice. In: Spector S, Beck N, eds. *Modern Methods in Pharmacology.* New York, NY: Alan R Liss Inc; 1982;39-54.
12. van Praag H, Plutchik R. Increased suicidality in depression: group or subgroup characteristic? *Psychiatry Res.* 1988;26:273-278.
13. Maas J, Hattox S, Martin D, Landis D. A direct method for determining dopamine synthesis and output of dopamine metabolites from brain in awake animals. *J Neurochem.* 1979;32:839-843.
14. Kopin I, Bankiewicz K, Harvey-White J. Assessment of brain dopamine metabolism from plasma HVA and MHPG during debrisoquin treatment: validation in monkeys treated with MPTP. *Neuropsychopharmacology.* 1988;1:119-125.
15. Kopin I, Bankiewicz K, Harvey-White J. Effect of MPTP-induced parkinsonism in monkeys on the urinary excretion of HVA and MHPG during debrisoquin administration. *Life Sci.* 1988;43:133-141.
16. Lambert G, Eisenhofer G, Cox H, Horne N, Kalff V, Kelly M, Jennings J, Ester M. Direct determination of homovanillic acid release from the human brain: an indicator of central dopaminergic activity. *Life Sci.* 1991;49:1061-1072.
17. Karoum F, Korpi E, Chuang L, Linnoila M, Wyatt R. The effects of desiprimanine zimelidine, electroconvulsive treatment and lithium on rat brain biogenic amines: a comparison with peripheral changes. *Eur J Pharmacol.* 1986;121:377-385.
18. Karoum F, Fawcett R, Wyatt R. Chronic cocaine effects on peripheral biogenic amines: a long-term reduction in peripheral dopamine and phenylethylamine production. *Eur J Pharmacol.* 1988;148:381-388.
19. Davis K, Kahn R, Ko G, Davidson M. Dopamine in schizophrenia: a review and reconceptualization. *Am J Psychiatry.* 1991;148:1474-1486.
20. Davidson M, Giordani A, Mohs R, Mykytyn VV, Platt S, Aryan ZS, Davis KL. Control of exogenous factors affecting plasma homovanillic acid concentration. *Psychiatry Res.* 1987;20:307-312.
21. Roy A, Adinoff B, Roehrich L, Lamparski D, Custer R, Lorenz V, Barbaccia M, Guidotti A, Costa E, Linnoila M. Pathological gambling: a psychobiologic study. *Arch Gen Psychiatry.* 1988;45:369-373.
22. Banki C, Arato M. Amine metabolites and neuroendocrine responses related to depression and suicide. *J Affect Disord.* 1983;5:223-232.
23. Palaniappan V, Ramachandran V, Somasundaram O. Suicidal ideation and biogenic amines in depression. *Indian J Psychiatry.* 1983;25:286-292.
24. Montgomery S, Montgomery D. Pharmacological prevention of suicidal behaviour. *J Affect Disord.* 1982;4:291-298.
25. Agren H. Life at risk: markers of suicidality in depression. *Psychiatry Dev.* 1983;1:87-104.
26. Agren H, Mefford I, Rudorfer M, Linnoila M, Potter W. Interacting neurotransmitter system: a non-experimental approach to the 5-HIAA HVA correlation in human CSF. *J Psychiatry Res.* 1986;20:175-193.

The Effect of Access to Lethal Methods of Injury on Suicide Rates

Peter M. Marzuk, MD; Andrew C. Leon, PhD; Kenneth Tardiff, MD, MPH; Edward B. Morgan, MPH; Marina Stajic, PhD; J. John Mann, MD

• The relationship between the availability of lethal methods of injury and suicide rates is an important, but unresolved question. We investigated this relationship by prospectively classifying lethal methods according to their accessibility in the five counties of New York City. These counties have both similarities and differences in the proportion of their populations with access to specific lethal means. We then compared the age- and gender-adjusted method-specific suicide rates of these counties. There were marked differences in overall crude suicide rates among the five counties. The counties had similar suicide rates involving methods that were equally accessible to all persons in each county (eg, hanging, laceration, suffocation, and burns) as well as methods that were accessible to a smaller, but similar proportion of the population in each county (eg, firearms and drowning in waterways). Virtually all of the differences in overall suicide risk among counties were explained by differences in rates involving methods that were differentially available in the counties, principally fall from height, overdose of prescription medications, and carbon monoxide poisoning. We conclude that differences in suicide rates between communities are, in large part, due to differences in accessibility to lethal methods of injury. Therefore, systematic studies should evaluate the effect of reducing accessibility to specific lethal means on suicide rates.

(*Arch Gen Psychiatry*. 1992;49:451-458)

Suicide rates in communities are a function of the prevalence of specific psychiatric disorders as well as socioeconomic and demographic factors associated with increased suicide risk. The effect of the access of a community to lethal methods of injury on suicide rates is controversial. For example, an association between availability of means and the suicide mortality rate has been shown for only three methods: domestic coal gas,[1-3] barbiturate poisoning,[4,5] and firearms.[6-9] The availability hypothesis suggests that differences in suicide rates between communities are due, in part, to differences in the access of their populations to lethal methods.

However, an alternative substitution hypothesis suggests that suicidal persons will use alternative methods that are more widely available if one or more means are restricted or unavailable in that community. Thus, for example, the suicide rate due to firearms and falls from height would be relatively low in a community with limited access to guns or tall structures, but the rate due to hanging would be comparatively increased.

These hypotheses have different public health implications regarding suicide prevention strategies. Both suggest that limiting access would result in a decrease in the method-specific suicide rate of the restricted method. However, the availability hypothesis suggests that limiting access would also result in an overall decrease in suicide mortality, whereas the substitution hypothesis posits a compensatory shift to other available methods and no overall decrease in mortality.

One approach that can test these two hypotheses is to compare suicide rates in communities that differ with regard to the availability of some, but not all methods. Studies comparing suicide rates of different communities are frequently limited by ascertainment bias associated with rendering a suicide verdict. To reduce this bias, we studied the five counties of New York City, which are under the jurisdiction of a single Chief Medical Examiner. These counties have both similarities and marked differences in the proportion of their populations with access to specific lethal means. Thus, we prospectively classified lethal methods into those in which the population of a county has absolute total or relatively equal proportionate access and those in which we hypothesized there were intercounty differences in accessibility. After accounting for demographic factors related to suicide risk, support for the availability hypothesis would be obtained if there were no intercounty differences in method-specific suicide rates for equal access methods *and* there were differences in suicide rates between those counties that show differences in the proportions of their population having

Accepted for publication March 3, 1992.

From the Laboratory of Psychopharmacology, Department of Psychiatry (Drs Marzuk, Leon, and Mann), and Department of Psychiatry and Public Health (Dr Tardiff), Cornell University Medical College, and the Office of Chief Medical Examiner (Mr Morgan and Dr Stajic), New York, NY. Mr Morgan is now with the Human Resources Administration, New York, NY. Dr Mann is now with the Clinical Research Center for the Study of Suicidal Behavior, Department of Psychiatry, University of Pittsburgh (Pa) School of Medicine.

Reprint requests to Department of Psychiatry, Cornell University Medical College, 1300 York Ave, New York, NY 10021 (Dr Marzuk).

Table 1.—Sociodemographic Characteristics of New York City Counties*					
	County				
Index	Manhattan	The Bronx	Queens	Staten Island	Brooklyn
1985 population†	1 455 619	1 198 598	1 917 172	371 679	2 248 139
Area, square miles	22	42	109	59	70
Population density, no. of persons per square mile	66 165	28 538	17 589	6 300	32 116
% white‡	55.4	30.8	60.9	84.8	47.0
% single§	41.9	34.6	28.6	28.2	32.8
% separated, widowed, or divorced§	23.7	23.0	18.5	14.2	20.2
Mean no. of persons per houshold§	1.96	2.66	2.63	3.00	2.67
Unemployment rate, % of civilian labor force‖	8.8	7.7	7.5	5.8	8.7
Personal income per capita, 1984 US dollars¶	20 424	10 577	14 827	14 894	11 585

*Counties are designated by their borough names.
†New York State Department of Commerce intercensal estimate.
‡1987 New York City Housing and Vacancy Survey, US Bureau of the Census.
§1980, US Bureau of the Census.
‖1985 estimate, New York Department of Labor, Division of Research and Statistics.
¶US Department of Commerce, Bureau of Economic Analysis.

access to other lethal means. Therefore, we determined and then compared the average annual method-specific, age- and sex-adjusted suicide rates of residents of each of the five counties of New York City in a 4-year period.

METHODS

Study Sites

The five counties of New York City studied include New York (borough of Manhattan), Bronx (borough of The Bronx), Kings (borough of Brooklyn), Queens (borough of Queens), and Richmond (borough of Staten Island). In this study, the counties are referred to by their borough designations. The certification of all deaths believed to be suicides in these counties falls under the jurisdiction of the Chief Medical Examiner of New York. Sociodemographic characteristics are shown for each of the five counties in Table 1. Those variables linked to suicide risk include increased age, male gender, white race, single status, recent divorce or separation, and unemployment.[10]

Eligibility

A list of all certified suicides (*International Classification of Diseases, Ninth Revision* [*ICD-9*], E950-959)[11] occurring in New York City during the calendar years 1984 through 1987 was provided by the Office of Biostatistics of the New York City Health Department. Only deaths of New York City residents occurring in that city and certified as suicides were eligible. The study specifically excluded nonresidents who committed suicide in New York City, residents who died of self-inflicted lethal injuries outside the bounds of the city, or individuals who died in a manner that was certified as "undetermined" (*ICD-9*, E980-989). Cases were individually reviewed for age, gender, location and year of suicide, county of residence, and suicide method.

Classification of Suicide Methods

All cases of suicide were classified according to one of 13 lethal methods listed in Table 2. Those few cases involving two or more distinct methods were assigned to the method considered by the medical examiner to be primarily causative of death. Suicide methods were grouped prospectively into one of three categories: absolute equal access, relative equal access, and differential access.

Absolute equal access methods include those to which the entire population of each county has unimpeded access. The population of all US communities has approximately total and therefore equal access to these methods that use instruments widely available in the home or readily transportable from one's home. These include hanging, immolation, laceration, asphyxia by plastic bag, poisoning by nonprescription medications, and "other" methods, which in this study includes drowning in bathtubs or electrocution at home.

Relative equal access methods include those for which it is assumed there is no difference in the proportion of the population exposed to those means in the five counties studied. In New York City, these methods include firearms and drowning in waterways. Although firearms are accessible to only a small proportion of the population, we assumed that the gun ownership prevalence is similar among each of the five counties since registration laws apply uniformly to all five counties. In addition, gun ownership in urban areas is related to the crime index, a composite of seven serious crimes, including murder, rape, robbery, aggravated assault, burglary, larceny, and motor vehicle theft. Manhattan, which includes the central district of the city, has an inflated daytime population and the highest crime index of the five boroughs. However, the total crime indexes of the residential areas of the five boroughs are more nearly similar when the central business district of Manhattan is excluded. Similarly, a significant proportion of the population of each county resides within 1 or 2 miles of rivers, bays, inlets, or park lakes. These two methods would be considered differential methods in the comparison of two communities with markedly different gun ownership regulations and crime indexes, or differential access to waterways (eg, New York City and Las Vegas, Nev).

Differential access methods describe those in which there were hypothesized to be substantial intercounty differences in the proportions of the population with access to lethal means. In New York City, these methods were postulated to include fall from height, asphyxia by carbon monoxide, poisoning by prescription medications, and trauma by subway or commuter rail. If both prescription and nonprescription drugs were present in a person who died of overdose, the case was classified as an overdose due to prescription drugs if the prescribed drug was ruled as causative of death by the medical examiner. Caustic agents (eg, lye) were classified as nonprescription drugs. Cyanide, which is not readily available, is considered a "prescription" drug. Subways were considered as all rail lines of the New York City Transit Authority, operating either above or below ground. Trains were considered commuter rail lines operated by the Metropolitan Transportation Authority.

Accessibility Measures

Estimates of the proportion of the population of each county that had access to lethal methods were made. These estimates

Table 2.—Annual Method-Specific Crude Rates of Suicide for New York City Counties, 1984 through 1987*

		No. per 100 000 Person-Years					
		County					
Lethal Method	*International Classification of Diseases, 9th Revision* code	Manhattan	The Bronx	Queens	Staten Island	Brooklyn	City
Absolute equal access methods	. . .	3.52	2.59	3.61	2.29	2.68	3.06
Hanging	E953.0	2.52	2.11	2.58	1.82	2.12	2.31
Suffocation by plastic bag	E953.1	0.27	0.02	0.29	0.20	0.13	0.19
Cutting and piercing	E956	0.53	0.23	0.33	0.27	0.22	0.32
Burns, fire	E958.1	0.03	0.02	0.09	0.00	0.06	0.05
Poisoning by nonprescription agents	E950	0.09	0.15	0.26	0.00	0.11	0.15
Other†	E954, E958.4	0.07	0.06	0.07	0.00	0.03	0.05
Relative equal access methods	. . .	1.99	2.19	1.73	1.48	2.05	1.95
Firearms	E955	1.60	2.02	1.58	1.21	1.75	1.69
Drowning (waterways)	E954	0.40	0.17	0.16	0.27	0.30	0.26
Total equal access methods	. . .	5.51	4.78	5.34	3.77	4.73	5.01
Differential access methods	. . .	9.67	4.53	3.96	1.82	2.68	4.70
Jumping from high place	E957	6.25	2.88	1.72	0.87	1.46	2.70
Poisoning by prescription agents	E950	2.99	0.98	1.33	0.54	0.76	1.39
Motor vehicle exhaust gas	E952.0	0.00	0.08	0.46	0.40	0.08	0.18
Lying before comuter train	E958.0	0.00	0.15	0.12	0.00	0.02	0.06
Lying on subway track	E958.0	0.43	0.44	0.34	0.00	0.37	0.37
All methods	. . .	15.27	9.43	9.44	5.58	7.48	9.81

*Counties are designated by their borough names.
†Drowning or electrocution at home.

defined a population-based accessibility measure for suicide by a particular method. For some methods in which this was not possible, more indirect estimates of accessibility were derived to allow relative intercounty comparisons.

The population at risk for absolute equal access methods and drowning in waterways in each county was assumed to be identical to the total county population. The population at risk for suicide by firearm was estimated as the product of the county population and Cook's[12] gun prevalence index for cities of the mid-Atlantic states (ie, 10% of the population is estimated to have access to guns).

Almost all suicides involving fall from height in New York City occur in residential buildings of six or more stories, usually from apartment windows. The population at risk for this method was estimated by multiplying the mean number of persons per household in each county by the number of households located on or above the seventh story, as reported by the 1980 census.[13] For Manhattan, the population at risk (ie, those living on or above the seventh floor) was calculated to be 764 357 persons. Thus, the proportion of Manhattan residents exposed directly to heights was 0.525. The proportions exposed for The Bronx, Brooklyn, Queens, and Staten Island were 0.276, 0.133, 0.130, and 0.044, respectively.

Suicides involving carbon monoxide poisoning in New York City occur almost exclusively in garages of private residences. The number of residences with garages in each county is not enumerated by any state, municipal, or private organization. However, almost all such garages are associated with one- and two-family homes. The population at risk for this method was estimated as the sum of the products of the number of owner- and renter-occupied housing units for one-detached, one-attached, and two-unit structures and the mean number of persons per household in each county. This measure estimates the total number of persons residing in one- or two-family homes for each county, as reported by the 1980 census.[13] In Staten Island, 271 521 persons were calculated to reside in such homes, representing a proportion of 0.731 of the population of the county exposed to this suicide method. The proportions exposed for Queens, Brooklyn, The Bronx, and Manhattan were 0.464, 0.298, 0.155, and 0.007, respectively.

The number of persons possessing or having access to lethal amounts of prescription medications at any time is unknown. The principal method of access to prescription medications is through physicians. In addition, the most frequent drugs identified in toxicologic assays at autopsy of suicides include psychotropic agents, particularly antidepressants, sedative or hypnotic agents, and analgesics. As an indirect population-based measure of accessibility, the number of physicians registered and practicing in each county per 100 000 residents was determined.[14] Manhattan had, by far, the greatest concentration of physicians per capita: 757 per 100 000 population. In all the other boroughs, there was a range from 187 to 263 physicians per 100 000 residents.

Suicides on New York commuter rail lines usually involve persons crossing exposed rail beds. The population at risk for this method was determined by multiplying the number of straight route miles of surface or elevated track in each of the five counties by the population density per square mile of each county. Adjustments were made for branches of rail lines within 1 mile of each other. This calculation yielded an estimate of the number of persons residing within 0.5 mile of rail lines in each county. In The Bronx, which contains Metro North Commuter rail lines, the proportion of the population exposed was 0.407. Similarly, in Queens, the proportion exposed to the Long Island Railroad was 0.228, and in Staten Island, the proportion exposed to a commuter line was 0.237. In Manhattan and Brooklyn, where most commuter lines are in tunnels, the proportion exposed to open rail beds was 0.086 and 0.029, respectively.

Subway tracks, which are largely on elevated trestles or in tunnels, are accessible only at stations. Thus, it is assumed that all subway suicides occurred among persons who had entered stations. There are no reliable population-based measures of access to subways. Annual paid ridership figures for each station are numerically redundant and are adulterated by persons who are neither county nor city residents. Nevertheless, we classified subways as a differential access method because of marked differences between the counties in number of subway lines, areas served by subways, and numbers of stations per square mile. Manhattan and Brooklyn have a large number of lines and the greatest density of stations per square mile, 6.4 and 2.1 stations per square mile, respectively. The Bronx has both an intermediate number of lines and station density (1.6 stations per square mile). Queens has few lines, with large areas that are not served by the subway, and a lower station density (0.7 stations per square mile). Staten Island has no subway service.

Determination of Suicide Rates

Annual method-specific suicide rates for each of the five counties were calculated as the number of county residents committing suicide by a particular method from 1984 through 1987 divided by the total person-years at risk expressed per 100 000. Both crude and age- and gender-adjusted rates were determined using the New York City population as a standard.[15] Person-years at risk were determined from the 1985 intercensal population estimates of the New York State Department of Commerce. A 4-year period was used to reduce the likelihood that differences in rates were due to random fluctuations or temporary anomalous factors operating during a 1-year period.

For methods in which the lethal means were readily available at home or easily transportable within or outside counties once available to the individual, rates were calculated for county residents regardless of the site of lethal injury. These methods included all absolute equal access methods, firearms, and overdoses of prescription medications.

For methods involving equipment or structures that could not be easily transported by individuals (including drowning in waterways, fall from height, lying before commuter trains or on subway tracks, or asphyxia by carbon monoxide), rates based on the site of injury were calculated separately for individuals who incurred lethal injury in their county of residence and for individuals who incurred injury in one of the other four counties of which they were not a resident. This latter category of rates, which was in practice negligible, was not included in the calculation of total equal and differential access rates, but was included in the overall county rate. Thus, the sum of total equal access rates and differential access rates is slightly less than the overall county rates.

Statistical Analysis

Data were analyzed using the Statistical Package for the Social Sciences (SPSS, Chicago, Ill) and BMDP statistical software (BMDP, Los Angeles, Calif). Age- and gender-adjusted relative risks (RRs) of suicide mortality were estimated and then compared using the Mantel-Haenszel summary odds ratio.[16] Pairwise comparisons were based on rates of four New York City counties relative to Brooklyn. Brooklyn was chosen as a standard because it had intermediate rates and no artifactual rates of zero due to complete lack of specific methods of suicide. Because of multiple comparisons (Brooklyn vs each of the other four counties), levels of significance were Bonferroni-adjusted, resulting in two-tailed α level of .0125.[17] Bonferroni-adjusted 95% confidence intervals (CIs) were calculated using the Mantel-Haenszel estimator.[18] In cases with extremely small expected values, CIs could not be reliably calculated.

RESULTS

County Suicide Rates

There were a total of 2820 suicides during the 4-year study period. The annual citywide crude suicide rate was 9.81 per 100 000 person-years-at-risk (Table 2). However, there were marked differences in overall suicide rates among the five New York counties, ranging from 5.58 per 100 000 person-years in Staten Island to 15.27 per 100 000 person-years in Manhattan (Table 2).

The countywide differences in age- and gender-adjusted rates were highly significant. For example, the age- and gender-adjusted rate in Brooklyn, which was used as the standard for determining RR, was 7.89 deaths per 100 000 person-years. The suicide rate in Manhattan was 14.04 per 100 000 (RR, 1.77; adjusted 95% CI, 1.55 to 2.00; $P<.0001$). The suicide rate in The Bronx was 10.06 (RR, 1.28; adjusted 95% CI, 1.10 to 1.48; $P<.0001$). In Queens, the rate was 9.19 (RR, 1.17; adjusted 95% CI, 1.02 to 1.34; $P=.004$), and in Staten Island, the rate was 5.92 (RR, 0.72; adjusted 95% CI, 0.54 to 0.97; $P=.0056$). Virtually all of the differences in overall countywide suicide rates were explained by differences between the counties involving specific methods with differential access (Figure).

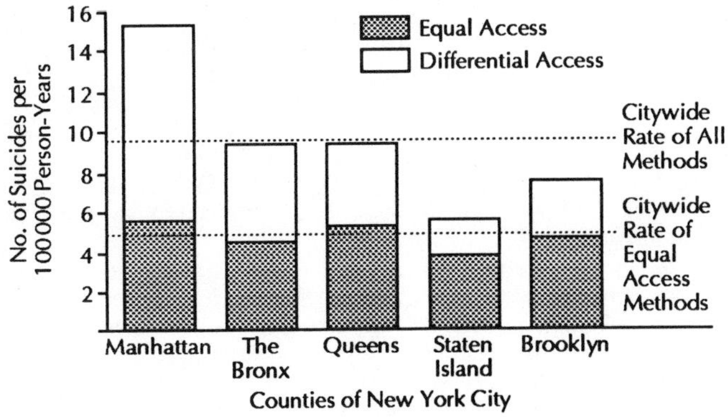

Annual crude suicide rates for each of the five counties of New York City (listed by borough name) during 1984 through 1987, grouped according to accessibility of lethal methods.

Equal Access Method-Specific Rates

The annual citywide crude rate for all absolute equal access methods was 3.06 per 100 000 person-years (Table 2). Hanging constituted the principal absolute equal access method, accounting for 75% of the method-specific mortality in this category. Firearms and drowning, which composed the relative equal access category, accounted for 1.95 deaths per 100 000 person-years (Table 2).

There were no intercounty differences in the age- and gender-adjusted rates of any of the individual absolute or relative equal access methods. For example, the age- and gender-adjusted rates for hanging per 100 000 person-years were 2.30 for Manhattan, 2.25 for The Bronx, 2.50 for Queens, 1.96 for Staten Island, and 2.25 for Brooklyn. Space considerations preclude showing the individual age- and gender-adjusted rates and RR for each of the eight equal access methods, but these data are available from the authors on request.

Overall, there was no difference between counties in the total aggregate age- and gender-adjusted rate of equal access methods, which accounted for approximately 5.0 deaths per 100 000 person-years in each county. However, they accounted for 67% of the suicide rate in Staten Island, but only 36% of the rate in Manhattan.

Differential Access Method-Specific Rates

There were marked differences between counties in both aggregate and individual rates involving differential access methods (Figure). Differential access methods accounted for approximately 9.0 deaths per 100 000 persons in Manhattan, but fewer than 2.0 per 100 000 person-years in Staten Island. Thus, in Manhattan, the RR of suicide of the aggregated differential access methods compared with Brooklyn was 3.13 (age- and gender-adjusted rate, 8.91 per 100 000; adjusted 95% CI, 2.58 to 3.79; $P<.0001$). The RR of aggregated differential access methods in The Bronx was 1.70 (rate, 4.78; adjusted 95% CI, 1.35 to 2.15; $P<.0001$), and in Queens, 1.38 (rate, 3.87; adjusted 95% CI, 1.11 to 1.71; $P=.0002$). In Staten Island, the RR of 0.66 was less than that of Brooklyn (rate, 1.94; adjusted 95% CI, 0.40 to 1.10; $P=.048$), but was not significant at the preset α level of .0125. Two methods, fall from height and overdose of prescription medications, contributed the greatest mortality rate. Fall from height was 3.75 times as likely among Manhattan residents than among Brooklyn residents (adjusted 95% CI, 2.90 to 4.84; $\chi^2=192.90$; $P<.0001$). Similarly, The Bronx, with a large proportion of its residents living in tall structures, differed significantly in this rate compared with Brooklyn (RR, 1.97; adjusted 95% CI, 1.46 to 2.68; $\chi^2=31.49$; $P<.0001$). In contrast, there was no difference between Queens and Brooklyn in this rate (RR, 1.10; adjusted 95% CI, 0.80 to 1.50; $\chi^2=.45$; $P=.50$) or in the accessibility measure for these two counties (proportion exposed in Queens, .130; in Brooklyn, .133).

Manhattan differed from Brooklyn in the suicide rate due to overdose of prescription medications (RR, 3.35; adjusted 95% CI, 2.35 to 4.79; $\chi^2=81.20$; $P<.0001$). Of note, the difference in numbers of physicians per capita was dramatically greater only in Manhattan (757 physicians per 100 000 residents) compared with other counties (187 to 262 physicians per 100 000 residents). Queens showed a more modest, but significantly elevated suicide risk compared with Brooklyn (RR, 1.66; adjusted 95% CI, 1.12 to 2.45; $\chi^2=10.05$; $P=.0015$).

Suicide rates due to carbon monoxide poisoning were highest in Queens and Staten Island, the two counties with the greatest proportion of individuals residing in one- and two-family homes with private garages (RR, 5.48; adjusted 95% CI, 1.94 to 15.49; $\chi^2=19.67$; $P<.0001$ and RR, 4.96; adjusted 95% CI, 1.25 to 19.64; $\chi^2=8.25$; $P=.0041$, respectively). In Manhattan, there were no suicides due to carbon monoxide poisoning. Less than 1% of the Manhattan population resides in private one- or two-family homes and an even smaller percentage of these homes have private garages. The Bronx and Brooklyn had similar low rates due to this method. (The Bronx RR, 1.08; adjusted 95% CI, 0.23 to 5.12; $P=1.00$).

Suicide rates by commuter train were highest for The Bronx and Queens. Although these RRs were high (6.95 for The Bronx, $P=.0152$, and 4.86 for Queens, $P=.046$), neither was significant at the prespecified α level of .0125. The Bronx, Queens, and Staten Island have the largest proportions of their populations residing within 0.5 mile of accessible track of any of the counties. Manhattan and Brooklyn have much lower proportions of their populations accessible to this method. There were no suicides by this method in Manhattan or Staten Island.

Based on the number of subway stations per square mile, it was predicted that Manhattan would have a suicide rate due to subway trauma higher than Brooklyn; The Bronx and Brooklyn would have approximately equal rates, and Queens would have a lower rate than Brooklyn. (Staten Island has a rate of zero by definition because it has no subway.) However, there were no differences between counties in suicide rates due to subway trauma.

COMMENT

This study supports the availability hypothesis that proposes that differences between communities in their access to specific lethal methods of injury, in large part, account for differences in their overall suicide rates. The five counties had, as we predicted, similar rates involving methods that were equally accessible to everyone (eg, hanging or suffocation by plastic bag). In addition, for firearms and drowning in waterways to which not all the population in a given county had access, but in which we predicted the proportion of population with access in each county was similar, there were no intercounty differences in rates. The marked differences in overall suicide rates among counties were largely accounted for by differences in rates involving methods that varied in their availability in the population (eg, tall buildings or private garages).

The availability of a greater variety of alternative lethal methods in some counties did not suppress the rates of other methods, and a relative lack of specific methods did not result in a comparative increase in the rates of the alternative methods that were available, as the substitution hypothesis would have predicted. Thus, for example, the availability of numerous lethal methods in Manhattan, particularly fall from height, did not suppress rates involving hanging, drowning, or firearms. Similarly, the limited choice of methods in Staten Island did not increase the rate due to firearms, drowning, or the ubiquitously available equal access methods, eg, hanging, cutting and piercing, or suffocation. The increase in the proportion of the population of each county that had access to different methods contributed incrementally to the total suicide rate.

Methodologic Limitations

We attempted to estimate the proportion of residents in each county who were exposed to lethal methods and thus allow relative comparisons between the counties. However, the actual access of individuals to lethal methods is unknown. Since these accessibility measures are only proxy estimates of actual exposure, we could not determine direct correlations between numbers of method-specific suicides and availability of methods. Nevertheless, our prediction of which methods would show differences in rates based on differences in accessibility were largely correct, with a few notable exceptions. We believe our failure to correctly predict certain differences in suicide rates by specific methods may reflect the imprecision of our accessibility measures or unknown factors governing method choice rather than the implausibility of the availability hypothesis. For example, we recognize that the number of physicians per capita is a coarse approximation of the availability of prescription agents. Unfortunately, data regarding prescriptions filled at retail pharmacies during the study years are not available at the county level. Similarly, gun registration data are available from the New York City Police Department only at the citywide level. However, registration rates do not accurately reflect the distribution of firearms in the community because they do not account for unregistered weapons.

It is unlikely that differences between the counties in socioeconomic and demographic variables that have been linked to suicide risk account for our findings. Suicide rates among whites are significantly higher than those for blacks or Hispanics.[19] However, Staten Island, with the greatest percentage of white residents of any of the counties, has the lowest suicide rate, and The Bronx, which has the lowest percentage of white residents, has one of the highest. The unemployment rates of the five counties, except for Staten Island, are remarkably similar. In addition, urban crowding has never been shown convincingly to correlate with suicide mortality. In fact, some of the highest suicide rates in the United States are in rural states.[19]

Suicide rates of communities are undoubtedly related to the prevalence of psychiatric disorders associated with increased suicide risk.[10] However, differences in the prevalence of these disorders among the counties, should they exist, would not necessarily account for the pattern of method-specific suicide rates observed in this study.

However, it is possible that some of the differences among counties in suicide rates may be explained by differences in family composition. The high suicide rate of Manhattan may, in part, be related to the large numbers of single persons living alone and residing in the county transiently.[20] There are larger families and more stable residency patterns in other counties. However, these factors do not account for rate differences among Queens, Brooklyn, and Staten Island.

This study does not examine factors that govern the magnitude of particular method-specific rates within a community. For example, the crude suicide rate due to hanging, a universally accessible method, is 2.31; whereas the crude rate of fall from height, a much less accessible method, is 2.70. Presumably, part of the differences in magnitudes among method-specific rates within a county are due to differences in lethality, chance of medical intervention, and cultural or personality factors governing method choice.[21,22] In addition, there are confounding factors between the access of certain methods and high-risk psychiatric disorders. The population at high risk for suicide due to mental disorders presumably has greater access, on average, to potentially lethal prescription agents.

Availability vs Substitution Hypothesis

There are two major ways in which previous studies have examined the effect of method availability on suicide rates. Most have examined temporal changes in both suicide rates and the availability of a particular method within a community. We used a 4-year period to minimize both the effect of random fluctuations or unusual method-specific suicide pacts (eg, the Jonestown suicides) of a shorter period and the confounding caused by changes in availability of methods or secular trends introduced over a longer period. Many prior studies are limited. For example, in Australia, there was a marked decline in poisoning by domestic gas accompanied by a coincident rise over a decade in poisoning by motor vehicle exhaust gas. It was concluded that the gradual elimination of one method simply resulted in substitution of another.[23,24] However, it is impossible to determine if this increase in motor vehicle exhaust suicides represents a shift in methods, which substantiates the substitution theory, or reflects the increasing possession, and therefore availability, of personal or family cars following World War II. The latter explanation is actually more likely since the decline in domestic gas poisoning did not begin until 1963, whereas the rise in motor vehicle exhaust deaths began in the 1950s. In the United States, a fall in the suicide rate due to gas poisoning occurred when gas was detoxified; however, the concomitant rise in motor vehicle exhaust suicides paralleled an increase in the per capita ownership of cars.[25] Similarly, the fall in the carbon monoxide suicide rate in the Netherlands has been reported to be compensated by a rise in the drug suicide rate.[26] However, it is not known if this rise was also accompanied by increased availability of drugs.

Alternatively, a smaller number of studies have examined the relationship between differences in suicide rates and differences in the availability of certain methods across communities. These studies, which compared international groups, are confounded by sociocultural determinants of suicide.[2] In the United States, the differences in suicide rates between communities of different geographic regions may, in part, be due to regional differences in preferred methods.[27] To reduce this bias, we examined communities within a localized region of a single nation.

Both longitudinal studies within communities and cross-sectional studies across communities have also been limited by ascertainment errors, categorization difficulties, and cross-level bias. Although the effect of ascertainment bias has probably been overemphasized,[28] the criteria for suicide can vary among jurisdictions.[29,30] In addition, certain lethal methods are more likely to receive a suicide verdict than others. Causes of death in which suicidal intent can be more definitively inferred, eg, hanging, asphyxia by plastic bag, lacerations, or firearms, are more likely to be classified as suicide than causes in which accidental circumstances are equally probable, eg, poisonings, drowning, burning, or train trauma.[31] We attempted to reduce the effect of ascertainment bias by comparing rates in counties that fall under the jurisdiction of a single Chief Medical Examiner.

Earlier studies that have investigated the availability of lethal methods and suicide mortality rates have often classified methods on the basis of their "activity" (eg, firearms) or "passivity" (eg, poisoning with sedatives). Thus, hanging, drowning, cutting and piercing, and firearms are often grouped together as "violent" means, a characteristic that is ill-defined and has little to do with actual accessibility.

Most studies have also been limited by cross-level bias due to confounding socioeconomic and demographic factors associated with enhanced suicide risk and method choice.[32] Method choice, for example, is clearly related to age and gender and, for that reason, we compared age- and sex-adjusted rates.

Despite methodologic limitations, we believe that the research literature predominantly suggests that alterations in the availability of methods within communities are associated with differences in their suicide rates. This has been most well documented for domestic coal gas, but is not without controversy. Kreitman[1] found a decline in the suicide rate in England shortly after the detoxification of domestic coal gas in the 1960s. Moreover, the rate of total decline and the decline in deaths due to carbon monoxide were approximately equal. Similar patterns have been found in other studies in England or other nations in which the carbon monoxide content of coal gas has been reduced.[2,3] However, in a study of two groups of towns, only one of which underwent detoxification, the suicide rates of both sets of towns decreased by a similar amount, suggesting that other factors were lowering the suicide rate.[26]

Studies of suicides by firearms also demonstrate the role of availability. Earlier studies noted a strong relationship between occupational exposure to guns and enhanced suicide risk.[33] Others have shown an association between firearm availability and mortality,[7,8,34-36] particularly between handgun prevalence and white male suicide rates.[9,37] While the age-adjusted rate of all other means remained the same, 5.9 in 1953 and 5.4 in 1978, the age-adjusted suicide rate by firearms in the United States increased from 4.9 to 7.1 per 100 000 population from 1953 to 1978.[6] The strictness of state gun control laws also has been shown to be related to lower suicide rates in those states.[38]

A number of other studies have noted a relationship between the availability of sedative and hypnotic agents and suicide mortality due to poisoning among young women.[4,5,39,40] Reduced prescribing of barbiturates resulted in a decline in drug-related suicides with little effect on suicide rates involving other methods.

Two recent studies support the substitution hypothesis. In Toronto, Ontario, the passage of strict gun control laws in the late 1970s resulted in a decline in the firearm suicide rate in males accompanied by a simultaneous rise in the rate of falling from height.[41] A comparison of the suicide rate due to firearms between Seattle, Wash, and Vancouver, British Columbia, the latter of which has restrictive gun ownership regulations, found that the higher suicide rate by firearms in Seattle was more than offset by a higher rate of suicide by other means in Vancouver.[42]

How then can these studies and others supporting the substitution hypothesis be reconciled with the present study and others that suggest the availability theory? One possibility, originally suggested by Lester,[25] is that neither theory adequately explains suicide rates of communities in the aggregate. Rather, different subsegments of a population are more likely to commit suicide impulsively, in which case, restricting access to methods would have a salutary effect. Other segments may engage in more planning of suicide, be more "determined" to die, and therefore likely to substitute other methods if deprived of access. For example, in the Seattle and Vancouver study, restricting access to firearms, while not reducing the overall suicide rate, was expected to reduce the rate for persons aged 15 to 24 years.[42] Similarly, the Toronto study found a substitution effect only for males.[41] Other studies of gas detoxification have found substitution effects only for males and not females.[24] Thus, it is possible that restricting access to lethal means may reduce the risk of suicide for some but not all groups. Undoubtedly, some persons who are determined will commit suicide, despite restrictions of certain methods. However, much clinical lore suggests that suicidal persons state they would kill themselves if they had certain means available to them, but would not do so otherwise. For many more individuals who are either ambivalent or impulsive or both, the presence of readily available lethal means may convert a self-destructive thought or attempt into a successful suicide.[43]

Implications

As most lethal methods are either ubiquitously available or difficult to restrict, public health initiatives to decrease the suicide rate will most certainly require strategies to decrease the prevalence of mental illnesses associated with enhanced suicide risk. Nevertheless, two lethal methods that can be controlled, firearms and prescription medications, deserve special comment because they account for a disproportionate excess of suicide mortality when accessibility is taken into account. New York City, where suicides by firearms account for approximately 1.69 deaths per 100 000 (17.2% of all suicide mortality), has some of the strictest gun control laws in the nation and among the lowest of community rates of firearm suicide. Continued tight restrictions of guns in New York and other locations will probably continue to effectively suppress suicide rates, particularly among white males of all ages and young black males. In addition, an extension of such tight gun restrictions to other areas of the nation may reduce suicide rates in those areas.[44]

Restricting the availability of medications that are lethal if taken in excess is more problematic. We believe pharmacologic management of severe mental illnesses is often an appropriate and effective treatment that should not be withheld based on physicians' fears of potential patient suicides. Nevertheless, physicians must be cautious in their prescribing practices, become knowledgeable about lethal amounts of medication, and encourage their patients to dispose of unnecessary medication or place needed medication in the hands of family members.

Suicide rates are, undoubtedly, complex functions governed by many factors associated with enhanced suicide risk. However, the result of this and other studies suggests that the availability of culturally acceptable specific lethal means is a major determinant of suicide rates, and differences in availability, to a large extent, can account for differences in overall suicide rates between otherwise closely related communities. Additional research is needed to determine the factors governing choice of method. Such research is particularly salient since other suicide prevention strategies such as suicide counseling centers or the more widespread use of antidepressants in the past 20 years have not convincingly, as yet, been shown to lower suicide rates.[45]

This work was supported by a Reader's Digest Fellowship and an American Suicide Foundation grant (Dr Marzuk), Public Health Service grant MH15774 (Dr Leon), and an Irma T. Hirschl Trust Career Scientist award (Dr Mann).

We thank Charles S. Hirsch, MD, Chief Medical Examiner of New York City, and his staff; Giselle Mery for data entry; Mary Ruth Goodley for graphics; Isadora Johnson for manuscript preparation; and members of the following agencies: the Office of Biostatistics of the New York City Health Department, the Metropolitan Transportation Authority, the New York City Transit Authority, the New York Police Department, IMS America Inc, the New York State Health Department, and the Municipal Library of New York.

References

1. Kreitman N. The coal gas story: United Kingdom suicide rates, 1960-71. *Br J Prev Soc Med.* 1976;30:86-93.
2. Farberow NL, Simon MD. Suicide in Los Angeles and Vienna: an intercultural study of two cities. *Public Health Rep.* 1969;84:389-403.
3. Hassall C, Trethowan WH. Suicide in Birmingham. *BMJ.* 1972;1:717-718.
4. Whitlock FA. Suicide in Brisbane, 1956 to 1973: the drug death epidemic. *Med J Aust.* 1975;1:737-743.
5. Oliver RG, Hetzel BS. Rise and fall of suicide rates in Australia: relation to sedative availability. *Med J Aust.* 1972;2:919-923.
6. Boyd J. The increasing rate of suicide by firearms. *N Engl J Med.* 1983;308:872-874.
7. Boyd JH, Moscicki EK. Firearms and youth suicide. *Am J Public Health.* 1986;76:1240-1242.
8. Wintemute GJ. Firearms as a cause of death in the United States, 1920-1982. *J Trauma.* 1987;27:532-536.
9. Markush RE, Bartolucci AA. Firearms and suicide in the United States. *Am J Public Health.* 1984;74:123-127.
10. Roy A. Risk factors for suicide in psychiatric patients. *Arch Gen Psychiatry.* 1982;39:1089-1095.
11. *International Statistical Classification of Diseases, Injuries, and Causes of Death, Ninth Revision.* Geneva, Switzerland: World Health Organization; 1977.
12. Cook PJ. The role of firearms in violent crime. In: Wolfgang M, ed. *Criminal Violence.* Beverly Hills, Calif: Sage Publishers Inc; 1982:236-290.
13. *Detailed Characteristics of Housing, New York.* Washington, DC: US Bureau of the Census; 1983. US Dept of Commerce publication HC80-1-B34.
14. Krasner M. *New York City Community Health Atlas 1988.* New York, NY: United Hospital Fund of New York; 1988.
15. Rothman KJ. *Modern Epidemiology.* Boston, Mass: Little Brown & Co Inc; 1986.
16. Mantel N, Haenszel W. Statistical aspects of the analysis of data from retrospective studies of disease. *J Natl Cancer Inst.* 1959;22:719-748.
17. Fleiss JL. *The Design and Analysis of Clinical Experiments.* New York, NY: John Wiley & Sons Inc; 1986.
18. Robins J, Greenland S, Breslow NE. A general estimator for the variance of the Mantel-Haenszel odds ratio. *Am J Epidemiol.* 1986;124:719-723.
19. *Vital Statistics of the United States, 1986.* Hyattsville, Md: National Center for Health Statistics; 1988. US Dept of Health and Human Services publication (PHS) 88-1122.
20. Murphy GE, Robins E. Social factors in suicide. *JAMA.* 1967;199:81-86.

21. Card JJ. Lethality of suicidal methods and suicide risk: two distinct concepts. *Omega*. 1974;5:37-45.
22. Farmer R, Rohde J. Effect of availability and acceptability of lethal instruments on suicide mortality: an analysis of some international data. *Acta Psychiatr Scand.* 1980;62:436-446.
23. Burvill PW. Changing patterns of suicide in Australia, 1910-1977. *Acta Psychiatr Scand.* 1980;62:258-268.
24. Burvill PW. The changing pattern of suicide by gassing in Australia, 1910-1987: the role of natural gas and motor vehicles. *Acta Psychiatr Scand.* 1989;81:178-184.
25. Lester D. The effects of detoxification of domestic gas on suicide in the United States. *Am J Public Health.* 1990;80:80-81.
26. Sainsbury P. The epidemiology of suicide. In: Roy A, ed. *Suicide.* Baltimore, Md: Williams & Wilkins; 1986:17-40.
27. Marks A, Abernathy T. Toward a sociocultural perspective on means of self destruction. *Life-Threat Behav.* 1974;4:3-17.
28. Sainsbury P. Validity and reliability of trends in suicide statistics. *World Health Stat Q.* 1983;36:339-348.
29. Barraclough BM. Are the Scottish and English suicide rates really different? *Br J Psychiatry.* 1972;120:267-273.
30. Atkinson MW, Kessel N, Dalgaard JB. The comparability of suicide rates. *Br J Psychiatry.* 1975;127:247-256.
31. Farmer RDT. Suicide by different methods. *Postgrad Med J.* 1979;55:775-779.
32. Morgenstern H. Uses of ecologic analysis in epidemiologic research. *Am J Public Health.* 1982;72:1336-1344.
33. Friedman P. Suicide among police: a study of 93 suicides among New York City policemen, 1934-1940. In: Shneidman ES, ed. *Essays on Self Destruction.* New York, NY: Science House; 1967:414-449.
34. Sloan JH, Kellerman AL, Reay DT, Ferris JA, Koepsell T, Rivara FP, Rice C, Gray L, LoGerfo J. Handgun regulations, crime, assaults and homicide: a tale of two cities. *N Engl J Med.* 1988;319:1256-1262.
35. Hirsch CS, Rushforth NB, Ford A, Adelson L. Homicide and suicide in a metropolitan county, I: long-term trends. *JAMA.* 1973;223:900-905.
36. Brent DA, Perper JA, Allman CJ, Moritz GM, Wartella ME, Zelenak SP. The presence and accessibility of firearms in the home of adolescent suicides. *JAMA.* 1991;266:2989-2995.
37. Boor M. Methods of suicide and implications for suicide prevention. *J Clin Psychol.* 1981;37:70-75.
38. Lester D, Murrell ME. The influence of gun control laws on suicidal behavior. *Am J Psychiatry.* 1980;137:121-122.
39. Oliver RG, Hetzel BS. An analysis of recent trends in suicide rates in Australia. *Int J Epidemiol.* 1973;2:91-101.
40. Johns MW. Self poisoning with barbiturates in England and Wales during 1959-1974. *BMJ.* 1977;1:1128-1130.
41. Rich CL, Young JG, Fowler RC, Wagner J, Black NA. Guns and suicide: possible effects of some specific legislation. *Am J Psychiatry.* 1990;147:342-346.
42. Sloan JH, Rivara FP, Reay DT, Ferris JAJ, Kellerman AL. Firearm regulations and rates of suicide: a comparison of two metropolitan areas. *N Engl J Med.* 1990;322:369-373.
43. Seiden RH. Suicide prevention: a public health/public policy approach. *Omega.* 1977;8:267-276.
44. Loftin C, McDowall D, Wiersema B, Cottey TJ. Effects of restrictive licensing of handguns on homicide and suicide in the District of Columbia. *N Engl J Med.* 1991;325:1615-1620.
45. Brown JH. Suicide in Britain: more attempts, fewer deaths, lessons for public policy. *Arch Gen Psychiatry.* 1979;36:1119-1124.

Multiple Risk Factors Predict Suicide in Alcoholism

George E. Murphy, MD; Richard D. Wetzel, PhD; Eli Robins, MD; Larry McEvoy, MA

• From a study of the lives of 50 alcoholics who committed suicide, seven nonacute clinical/historical features were identified post hoc that appear to be intimately linked to suicide. They included continued drinking, major depressive episode, suicidal communication, poor social support, serious medical illness, unemployment, and living alone. This study examined whether these features are common to alcoholics generally and/or to nonalcoholics who commit suicide or if they may be specifically predictive of suicide in alcoholics. The frequencies of these factors were compared with those in an earlier sample of 32 alcoholics who committed suicide, then with data from two St Louis studies of living alcoholics and a cohort of individuals with major depressive disorder who committed suicide. The frequency of the identified items was replicated among the 32 alcoholics in a larger community sample of individuals who committed suicide. The white men from those two samples of alcoholics who committed suicide were then combined for the advantage of sample size. Six of the seven factors could be compared with a population survey sample of 106 living alcoholics and five with a clinically identified sample of 142 living alcoholics. All compared factors were significantly more frequent among those who committed suicide than among controls. Any four of the six factors identified 46 (69%) of the 67 individuals who committed suicide with few false-positive results among the controls. Regarding all seven of the identified factors, 54 (81%) of the 67 men and 64 (83%) of the entire sample of 82 individuals who committed suicide had four or more risk factors. Alcoholic women and blacks showed the same pattern as white men. Major depression, found comorbidly in 58% of the alcoholics who committed suicide, did not account for the accumulation of other risk factors. Their distribution and frequency were significantly different from those of individuals with uncomplicated major depression who committed suicide. Seven subacute and chronic factors had a cumulative effect in identifying an increasing risk of suicide in alcoholics. Alcoholics can thus be easily monitored for increasing risk. Treatment of the accompanying depression will reduce the risk of suicide. Securing abstinence remains the goal of alcoholism treatment.

(*Arch Gen Psychiatry.* 1992;49:459-463)

Accepted for publication February 24, 1992.

From the Department of Psychiatry, Washington University School of Medicine, St Louis, Mo. Mr McEvoy is now with Anheuser-Busch Companies Inc, St Louis.

Reprint requests to 4940 Audubon Ave, St Louis, MO 63110 (Dr Murphy).

Alcoholism has been found repeatedly to account for about one fourth of the suicides that have been studied from a diagnostic perspective.[1-11] The range is wide, from 7% (in women)[11] to 54% (using multiple diagnoses and *DSM-III* criteria[9]). In those studies using hierarchical diagnoses,[1-3,5,6,11] the mean proportion of individuals committing suicide who were given the primary diagnosis of alcoholism was 23%. Among the multiply diagnosed,[4,7-10] alcoholism has been identified in 37% of subjects. Loss of a close interpersonal relationship within 6 weeks of death has been shown to be a risk factor of significance in the suicides of alcoholics, but not of persons with a primary diagnosis of major depressive disorder.[12] That finding has been strongly replicated.[13] However, recent loss was seen in only one fourth to two fifths of the suicides of alcoholics.[12-14] Can other predictors be found?

SUBJECTS AND METHODS

A reexamination of the historical data obtained retrospectively and systematically in a series of 50 consecutively studied alcoholics who had committed suicide (study 2)[14,15] brought to light a number of subacute and chronic features that seemed remarkably frequent and that had been suggested by others to be associated with suicide in alcoholics.[16-18] Data from the 32 alcoholics identified in an earlier suicide study (study 1)[1,19] were tabulated and compared on these features. Were the findings specifically characteristic of suicide or were they equally descriptive of alcoholics in the community?

The white male alcoholics in studies 1 and 2 who committed suicide (82% of all subjects in the samples) were compared with white male alcoholics from the St Louis, Mo, sample of the Epidemiologic Catchment Area (ECA) study.[20] In that large epidemiologic survey, 20 291 persons aged 18 years and older were studied in five cities across the United States from 1980 to 1984 to learn the prevalence and incidence of psychiatric disorders in the country.[21] Alcohol abuse was diagnosed in 13.5% of the population by *DSM-III* criteria.[22] A "second-wave" repeated interview was carried out 1 year after the first interview, with 84% of the original households responding.[23] Data collected in St Louis alone in the second-wave interviews lent themselves to the comparisons we made. White men having a definite diagnosis of alcoholism by stringent Washington University criteria[24] make up the comparison population. One hundred six white male ECA subjects with complete interviews met these criteria. All met *DSM-III-R* criteria[25] for definite alcohol abuse disorder as well.

A second control population consisted of 142 white male alcoholics previously identified through treatment of alcoholism or another disorder.[26] This clinical population sample also met both Washington University and *DSM-III-R* criteria for definite alcohol abuse disorder. Finally, the alcoholics who committed

Table 1.—Comparison of Findings Between Alcoholics Who Committed Suicide in Two Systematic Studies

	No. (%) of Subjects	
Characteristic	Study 1[1,19] (n=32)	Study 2[14] (n=50)
Currently drinking	31 (97)	48 (96)
Talk or threat of suicide	26 (81)	43 (86)
Comorbidity*	16 (50)	38 (76)
Major affective disorder	13 (41)	36 (72)
Other	3 (9)	2 (4)
Little or no social support	22 (69)	35 (70)
Unemployment	21 (66)	25 (50)
Serious medical problem	16 (50)	26 (52)
Living alone	16 (50)	19 (38)

*χ^2 analysis with Yates' correction=4.77; 1 *df*; $P<.05$ for comorbidity. No other row differences approached statistical significance.

Table 2.—Comparison of Frequency of Risk Factors in White Male Alcoholics Who Committed Suicide and Living Alcoholic Controls From Epidemiologic Catchment Area Study

	No. (%) of Subjects		
Risk Factor	Alcoholics Who Committed Suicide (n=67)	Living Alcoholics (n=106)	*P**
Recent heavy drinking	65 (97)	44 (42)	<.00001
Talk/threat of suicide†	53 (79)	24 (23)	<.00001
Little social support	50 (75)	28 (26)‡	<.00001
Major depressive disorder	39 (58)	5 (5)	<.00001
Unemployed	36 (54)	19 (18)	<.00001
Living alone	30 (45)	18 (17)	<.00001
Medical problem (eg, liver, pancreas)	11 (16)	7 (7)	<.080

*χ^2 with Yates' correction for continuity.
† Reported suicidal communication vs self-report.
‡No one to go to for comfort.

suicide were compared with individuals with primary major depression who committed suicide to learn if depression alone accounted for the findings.

A statistical software program (Statistical Analysis System for personal computers, version 6.03, SAS Institute, Cary, NC[27]) was used throughout.

RESULTS

All but two of a series of 50 retrospectively studied alcoholics who committed suicide[14,15] (study 2) were drinking heavily in the days, as well as the months, just prior to taking their lives. A history of talk or threat of suicide was reported in 43 (86%) of 50 subjects. Psychiatric comorbidity, the presence of another psychiatric diagnosis in addition to that of alcoholism, was found in 38 (76%) of 50 subjects. Comorbid major depressive disorder by *DSM-III-R* criteria[25] was identified in 36 (72%) of 50 subjects. Thirty-five (70%) of the 50 alcoholics who committed suicide had little or no social support by the time they took their lives. Half of the sample was unemployed. Half had serious health problems (eg, hepatic cirrhosis, duodenal ulcer, pulmonary emphysema, myocardial infarction, dementia, diabetes mellitus, and malignancy). Nineteen (38%) were living alone, a rate nearly four times that found in the general population of comparable age.

Similar categories of data had been collected in the first published systematic study of suicide 15 years earlier.[1] Of 134 consecutive suicides studied, 32 met *DSM-III-R* criteria for alcohol abuse or dependence as well as Washington University criteria for alcoholism.[24] The frequency of occurrence of these factors in the two suicide samples (study 1[1,19] and study 2[14,15]) is compared in Table 1. The findings of the two studies differ significantly in only one of the comparisons. Depressive disorder and, hence, comorbidity, was diagnosed significantly less frequently in alcoholics in study 1,[1,19] conducted in 1956 and 1957 ($P<.05$). Due to the earliness of that study, several of our current criteria symptoms were not systematically inquired about. The comorbidity estimate of 50% is thus a minimum figure. In other respects, the depth of inquiry was quite comparable. Since a lowered comorbidity rate would only weaken potential differences from comparison populations, it is not a bar to combining the two studies. Study 1 validates the findings of study 2 regarding the frequent occurrence of the factors under consideration.

White men (25 from study 1 and 42 from study 2) made up 82% of the combined suicide sample. Including the small numbers of women and blacks in the comparisons might have clouded more than clarified issues. (What is one to do statistically with 12 women or three blacks?) Consequently, the database for comparisons was white men.

A Community Sample of Alcoholics

One hundred six white male ECA subjects[23] meeting Washington University diagnostic criteria for alcoholism had complete interviews and made up a control sample from the community. Comparing them with the white male alcoholics who committed suicide on the predictor variables reveals strong differences ($P<.00001$ on six variables) (Table 2[15(p216)]). An observation substantially affected by data collection is that of serious physical illness. Half of the alcoholics who committed suicide had such a history. However, only hepatic cirrhosis and pancreatic disease were inquired about in the ECA study, rather than a broader range of serious health problems. Therefore, the broader dimension of serious medical illness cannot be compared. Little social support was defined in the St Louis ECA interview as reporting having no one to go to for comfort. The frequency of endorsement of that statement was, like the other measures, significantly lower than was poor social support described among the alcoholics who committed suicide. Major depressive disorder was diagnosed in only five (5%) of the 106 living alcoholics, but in 39 (58%) of the 67 white men who committed suicide.

The ECA population's members were, on average, 11 years younger than the alcoholics who committed suicide: their mean (±SD) age was 35.98±15.2 years, while the mean age of the alcoholics who committed suicide was 47.3±9.1 years at death. The group of living alcoholics thus included many men younger than the youngest alcoholic who committed suicide and some men older than the oldest man who committed suicide. A maximum likelihood analysis from the logistic regression procedure[27] was used, with age entered first to remove its effect. This analysis showed that current drinking ($P=.00001$), presence of major depression ($P<.0001$), suicidal thoughts or communication ($P<.0004$), poor social support ($P=.0023$), living alone ($P=.0148$), and unemployment ($P=.0474$) all contributed independently, while age did not contribute at a statistically significant level (Table available from first author on request.)

Every one of the white male alcoholics who committed suicide in our two studies had at least one of the six potential suicide risk factors being compared (Table 3[15(p219)]). Three had one factor, three had two factors, 15 had three factors, 19 had four factors, 19 had five factors, and eight had all six of these factors. In contrast, only one of the living male alcoholics had as many as four of these factors and none had more than four factors. The probability of this inverse relationship occurring by chance is extremely small (Student's $t=15.77$; $df=171$; $P<.00001$). The accu-

Table 3.—Distribution of Risk Factors in White Male Alcoholics Who Committed Suicide and Living Alcoholics*

No. of Risk Factors per Subject	No. of Alcoholics Who Committed Suicide (n=67)	No. of Living Alcoholics (n=106)
0	0	26
1	3	31
2	3	34
3	15	14
4	19	1
5	19	0
6	8	0

*Student's $t=15.77$; $df=171$; $P<.00001$. The risk factors are current heavy drinking, major depression, poor or no social support, unemployment, living alone, and suicidal thoughts or communication.

Reprinted from *Suicide in Alcoholism* (1992:219), Copyright ©1992, Oxford University Press Inc.[15]

Table 4.—Distribution of Risk Factors in White Male Alcoholics Who Committed Suicide and Treated Alcoholics*

No. of Risk Factors per Subject	No. of Alcoholics Who Committed Suicide (n=67)	No. of Living Alcoholics (n=142)
None	0	31
1	4	46
2	11	38
3	19	16
4	23	9
5	10	2

*Student's $t=10.493$; $df=207$; $P<.00001$. The risk factors are current heavy drinking, current major depressive disorder, unemployment, living alone, and suicidal communication.

Reprinted from *Suicide in Alcoholism* (1992:222), Copyright© 1992, Oxford University Press Inc.[15]

mulation of negative factors in alcoholics who committed suicide was very different from that of living alcoholics.

Only 44 (42%) of these 106 ECA subjects reported experiencing at least one symptom of alcohol abuse within the previous 6 months. These recent heavy drinkers were compared on each of the relevant variables with the 62 men meeting the diagnostic criteria but not reporting a recent symptom of alcoholism (past heavy drinkers). No difference in frequency of the pertinent characteristics between the recent and past heavy drinkers approached statistical significance.

A Clinical Sample of Alcoholics

A second control population consisted of 142 white men interviewed 8 years after having been identified as alcoholic in one of four clinical (mostly inpatient) settings.[26] Data were available on five risk factors. Neither social support nor overall medical status had been recorded. Age was again significantly different, the control group being older (mean±SD age, 50.9±12.6 years). In this control sample, 25 (18%) were identified as current heavy drinkers ($P<.0001$), 61 (43%) acknowledged suicidal ideation ($P<.0001$), and 44 (31%) had a comorbid major depressive disorder ($P<.0002$). A like proportion were unemployed ($P<.002$), and 42 (30%) were living alone ($P=.05$) (Table available on request). The frequency distribution of risk factors is again significantly different. A cutting score of three or greater identified 27 (19%) of the 142 alcoholics (Table 4[15(p222)]), a 19% false-positive rate. The point is reemphasized that the greater the number of risk factors, the greater the likelihood of a suicidal outcome.

Comparison between the 25 current problem drinkers and the remainder in the clinical sample showed no difference in the frequency of risk factors. To determine if the differences found between living and dead alcoholics were attributable to the preponderance of presumably remitted abusive drinkers, a maximum likelihood analysis was performed, comparing the 65 alcoholics committing suicide who were still drinking at the time of their deaths with the 69 alcoholics with recent alcohol-related problems in the two control samples. The difference in distribution of risk factors between the living and the dead subjects is still highly significant (Student's $t=11.69$; $df=106$; $P=.0005$) (Table available on request).

Alcoholics Who Committed Suicide vs Those With Primary Depression

Finally, we compared the pattern of accumulating risk factors among the full sample of 82 alcoholics who committed suicide in studies 1 and 2 with that of the 63 subjects who committed suicide who had a primary diagnosis of major depressive disorder in the early study of Robins et al.[1,19] Omitting major depression and current drinking, which were the primary discriminating factors of the compared groups, each of the remaining factors was significantly more frequent among the alcoholics ($P<.05$ to $P<.0001$) (Table available on request). Again, the distributions of factors run in opposite directions (Student's $t=4.50$; $df=142$; $P<.00001$) (Table 5[15(p224)]). Our finding regarding cumulative factors predicting suicide in alcoholics does not hold for depressed individuals, the group with the highest population who commit suicide in every study.[1-11]

COMMENT

Can data from a 20-year-old study and a 35-year-old study appropriately be compared with data from a more recent study? In addition to the fact that the earlier data do permit use of current research diagnostic criteria,[24] the risk factors identified in those earlier studies are exactly the ones cited more recently as characteristic of alcoholics who commit suicide.[16-18] Neither alcoholism nor suicide has changed in those respects.

The factors under consideration were not characteristically acute. Suicidal communication was usually of several years' duration. Health had deteriorated gradually as had economic and social functioning, as represented by unemployment and having little or no social support. Living alone was an expression of that lack of social support. The terminal depression ranged in duration from 2 months to 5 years, with a mean duration of 18 months and a median duration of 1 year. The suggestion that depression is the consequence of losses such as these[17] is not well supported by our findings. More often, depression impaired functioning in a variety of areas, leading to poor work performance and the growing conviction that life was unlivable.

Tables 3 and 4 indicate that as the number of risk factors increases, the likelihood of a suicidal outcome does likewise. It suggests a numerical predictor of suicide risk. If all seven factors are considered (ie, drinking, suicidal thinking, depression, poor social support, unemployment, serious medical illness, and living alone) then 54 (81%) of the 67 men and 65 (79%) of the entire sample of 82 subjects who committed suicide had four or more of these factors. Women and blacks had the same distribution of risk factors as did white men.

How appropriate were the control populations? They

Table 5.—Distribution of Risk Factors in Alcoholics Who Committed Suicide and Subjects With Primary Depressive Disorders Who Committed Suicide

No. of Risk Factors per Subject*	Alcoholics Who Committed Suicide (n=82)	Subjects With Depressive Disorders Who Committed Suicide (n=63)
0	1	11
1	8	13
2	18	15
3	27	15
4	17	5
5	11	4

*Student's $t=4.500$; $df=143$; $P<.00001$. Risk factors are communication of suicidal thoughts, little or no social support, unemployment, serious medical illness, and living alone. Current depressive episode and current drinking are selection factors for the compared groups so cannot be counted.

differed in age from the alcoholics who committed suicide. The population sample was younger, so subjects had less time to accumulate the risk factors. The clinical population was older than those who committed suicide and many of them were from deprived backgrounds. They too had significantly fewer of the risk factors. A majority of both groups denied current problems from drinking. We had no choice but to treat them as abstinent. However, there was not a significant difference in risk factors between those assumed to be abstinent and those still drinking. More tellingly, the combined groups still drinking had significantly lower risk factor counts than those who committed suicide. While these were not ideal controls, they were the best we could find. Whether a more suitably matched sample with the requisite personal data can be found remains to be seen.

Are these findings simply reflective of a major depressive episode? Does comorbid depression account for it all? Suicidal thoughts and communication are surely characteristic of depression, but are even more characteristic of alcoholics who take their lives.[28] The rate of suicidal thoughts and communication was 84% in alcoholics who committed suicide (Table 1) and only 65% in primary depressed subjects from the study by Robins et al.[1,28] Suicidal communication was both more frequent and of longer duration in the alcoholics. Drinking was not a consequence of depression in more than four or five of our alcoholics who committed suicide. Much more often, it was the other way around.

Loss of social support is not particularly characteristic of depressed individuals. When it does occur, it is more likely to be through widowhood than marital conflict or dissolution. The opposite is true of alcoholics. The serious medical conditions associated with depression are different from those in alcoholics, ie, familial and age related, not due to habitual intoxication and self-neglect. Unemployment among the alcoholics came early (mean age, 48.0 years at death) and was nearly always performance related. Among the depressed subjects, it was largely related to age and normal retirement. Thirteen (52%) of the 25 unemployed depressed subjects were aged 65 years or older (mean age at death, 66.2 years); the youngest was aged 53 years. Only two (4%) of the 50 alcoholics were aged 65 or older. Living alone was traceable to interpersonal conflict in the alcoholics; in depressed subjects, it was traceable to bereavement. The advent of depression is a highly dangerous event for alcoholics, as it is for others. However, it does not act alone in alcoholics and it cannot be held accountable for the other subacute and chronic features cited here as risk factors for suicide in alcoholics.

The low frequency of major depressive disorder in the community sample of living alcoholics (5%) is in keeping with the overall figure of 5% in men in the entire ECA study.[29] Substantially higher rates have been reported from studies of alcoholics admitted to hospitals and treatment centers.[30-33] The figure was 31% for the clinical (previously hospitalized) sample of living alcoholics. Depression is an important factor in bringing alcoholics to treatment, but it is not so characteristically a part of alcoholism in the community. Hence, the lifetime risk of suicide is nearly twice as high in previously hospitalized alcoholics as in the untreated alcoholics.[34] Depression is known to be a major risk factor for taking one's life.[1-11] It is at least as strong a risk factor for suicide in alcoholics as it is in the rest of the population.

There may well be additional factors that lower the barrier to self-destruction. These were the factors we found most strikingly frequent and most frequently associated with suicide. They are the only ones we examined. It is therefore of interest that they are also the ones that have been cited by others as characterizing alcoholics who commit suicide.[16-18] These factors are rarely found in isolation among those who commit suicide, but occur in numbers. Our data show that these factors are very much less common in living alcoholics (Table 2. Companion table for the clinical sample available on request). The clear implication of these findings is that every physician should, at frequent intervals, assess the existence and level of each of these factors in his or her alcoholic patients. As they accumulate, the risk of suicide grows. As few as four of these factors may serve to identify four fifths of those at highest risk for suicide, at a modest cost in false-positive results. False-positive results are not a problem in this circumstance, however. Efforts to treat alcoholism and depression are never inappropriate. Heightened risk of suicide is clearly linked to accumulating chronic problems.

Of particular importance is the finding that all but two of the alcoholics who committed suicide were drinking at, or near, the time of their deaths. Drinking drives the rest of the behavior, so every effort must be made to bring about and support abstinence. It is the goal of treatment for alcoholics, whether at serious risk of suicide or not. It is better if both the recognition of the alcoholism and the push for treatment come early.

Depression was found in nearly three of four of our subjects who committed suicide.[14] Whether as a complication of alcoholism or occurring alone, it is the single factor most contributory to suicide. Its recognition is straightforward and no more difficult in the presence of alcoholism than in its absence. The current pessimistic view of the efficacy of tricyclic antidepressants in this application stems from trials of these drugs to influence drinking behavior, not depression as such.[35] A recently reported study with a similar aim but much improved methods found a significant antidepressant effect of desipramine hydrochloride.[36] Pertinent to this result was recognition that "alcoholics metabolize TCAs abnormally, and may require higher doses to reach a therapeutic range."[36-38]

Study after study has shown that the depression leading to suicide has gone unrecognized and untreated (E.R., unpublished data, 1957).[7,39,40] Probably the most important single intervention that will reduce suicides overall is the recognition and vigorous treatment of major depression. That this is truly possible has been demonstrated.[41] The findings presented herein offer hope that suicides among alcoholics may be diminished.

This work was supported in part by Public Health Service research grants MH04591, MH5804, MH5938, and AA00209.

We thank Lee Robins, PhD, John Helzer, MD, and Kathleen Bucholz, PhD, for access to their data on living alcoholics.

References

1. Robins E, Murphy GE, Wilkinson RH Jr, Gassner S, Kayes J. Some clinical considerations in the prevention of suicide based on a study of 134 successful suicides. *Am J Public Health.* 1959;49:888-899.

2. Dorpat TL, Ripley HS. A study of suicide in the Seattle area. *Compr Psychiatry.* 1960;1:349-359.

3. Barraclough B, Bunch J, Nelson B, Sainsbury P. A hundred cases of suicide: clinical aspects. *Br J Psychiatry.* 1974;125:355-373.

4. Beskow J. Suicide and mental disorder in Swedish men. *Acta Psychiatr Scand.* 1979;277(suppl):1-138.

5. Hagnell O, Rorsman B. Suicide in the Lundby study: a controlled prospective investigation of stressful life events. *Neuro-psychobiology.* 1980;6:319-332.

6. Chynoweth R, Tonge JI, Armstrong J. Suicide in Brisbane: a retrospective psychosocial study. *Aust N Z J Psychiatry.* 1980;14:37-45.

7. Mitterauer B. Mehrdimensionale Diagnostik von 121 Suiziden im Bundesland Salzburg im Jahre 1978. *Wien Med Wochenschr.* 1981;9:229-234.

8. Kapamadžija B, Biro M, Sovljanski M. Socio-psihijatrijska I patomorfološka analiza 100 izvršenih samoubistava. *Soc Psihijat.* 1982;10:35-56.

9. Rich CL, Young D, Fowler RC. San Diego suicide study, I: young vs old subjects. *Arch Gen Psychiatry.* 1986;43:577-582.

10. Arató M, Demeter E, Rihmer Z, Somogyi E. Retrospective psychiatric assessment of 200 suicides in Budapest. *Acta Psychiatr Scand.* 1988;77:454-456.

11. Åsgård U. *Suicide Among Swedish Women: A Psychiatric and Epidemiologic Study.* Stockholm, Sweden: Kongl Carolinska Medico Chirurgiska Institutet: 1990.

12. Murphy GE, Robins E. Social factors in suicide. *JAMA.* 1967;199:303-308.

13. Rich CL, Fowler RC, Fogarty LA, Young D. San Diego suicide study, III: relationships between diagnoses and stressors. *Arch Gen Psychiatry.* 1988;45:589-592.

14. Murphy GE, Armstrong JW, Hermele SL, Fischer JR, Clendenin WW. Suicide and alcoholism: interpersonal loss confirmed as a predictor. *Arch Gen Psychiatry.* 1979;36:65-69.

15. Murphy GE. *Suicide in Alcoholism.* New York, NY: Oxford University Press Inc; 1992.

16. Engelbrecht GK. Alcohol as a possible variable in suicide. *Humanitas.* 1983;9:61-68.

17. Kendell RE. Alcohol and suicide. *Substance Alcohol Actions/Misuse.* 1983;4:121-127.

18. Théret L, Facy F, Pascalis JG. Le patient alcoolique suicidaire: profil, facteurs de risque et revue de la littérature de 1955 à 1988. *Ann Medico Psychologiques.* 1989;147:1092-1094. Abstract in English.

19. Robins E. *The Final Months: A Study of the Lives of 134 Persons Who Committed Suicide.* New York, NY: Oxford University Press Inc; 1981.

20. Regier DA, Myers JK, Kramer M, et al. The NIMH epidemiologic catchment area program: historical context, major objectives, and study population characteristics. *Arch Gen Psychiatry.* 1984;41:934-941.

21. Regier DA, Farmer ME, Rae DS, Locke BZ, Keith SJ, Judd LL, Goodwin FK. Comorbidity of mental disorders with alcohol and other drug abuse: results from the epidemiologic catchment area (ECA) study. *JAMA.* 1990;264:2511-2518.

22. American Psychiatric Association, Committee on Nomenclature and Statistics. *Diagnostic and Statistical Manual of Mental Disorders–Third Edition.* Washington, DC: American Psychiatric Association; 1980:494.

23. Robins LN, Helzer JE, Pryzbeck TR, Regier DA. Alcohol disorders in the community: a report from the epidemiologic catchment area. In: Rose RM, Barrett JE, eds. *Alcoholism: Origins and Outcome.* New York, NY: Raven Press; 1989:15-29.

24. Feighner JP, Robins E, Guze SB, Woodruff RA, Winokur G, Munoz R. Diagnostic criteria for use in psychiatric research. *Arch Gen Psychiatry.* 1972;26:57-63.

25. American Psychiatric Association, Committee on Nomenclature and Statistics. *Diagnostic and Statistical Manual of Mental Disorders–Revised Third Edition.* Washington, DC: American Psychiatric Association; 1987:159.

26. Helzer, JE, Robins LN, Taylor JR, Carey K, Miller RH, Combs-Orme T, Farmer A. The extent of long-term moderate drinking among alcoholics discharged from medical and psychiatric treatment facilities. *N Engl J Med.* 1985;312:1678-1682.

27. SAS Institute. *SAS/STAT User's Guide, Release 6.03 Edition.* Cary, NC: SAS Institute Inc; 1988.

28. Robins E, Gassner S, Kayes J, Wilkinson RH Jr, Murphy GE. The communication of suicidal intent: a study of 134 consecutive cases of successful (completed) suicide. *Am J Psychiatry.* 1959;115:724-733.

29. Selzer JE, Pryzbeck TR. The co-occurrence of alcoholism with other psychiatric disorders in the general population and its impact on treatment. *J Stud Alcohol.* 1988;49:219-224.

30. Smith EM, Cloninger CR, Bradford S. Predictors of mortality in alcoholic women: a prospective follow-up study. *Alcohol Clin Exp Res.* 1983;7:237-243.

31. Hesselbrock MN, Meyer RE, Keener JJ. Psychopathology in hospitalized alcoholics. *Arch Gen Psychiatry.* 1985;42:1050-1055.

32. Rounsaville BJ, Dolinsky ZS, Babor TF, Meyer RE. Psychopathology as a predictor of treatment outcome in alcoholics. *Arch Gen Psychiatry.* 1987;44:505-513.

33. Roy A, DeJong J, Lamparski D, Adinoff B, George T, Moore V, Garnett D, Kerich M, Linnoila M. Mental disorders among alcoholics: relationship to age of onset and cerebrospinal fluid neuropeptides. *Arch Gen Psychiatry.* 1991;48:423-427.

34. Murphy GE, Wetzel RD. The lifetime risk of suicide in alcoholism. *Arch Gen Psychiatry.* 1990;47:383-392.

35. Ciraulo DA, Jaffe JH. Tricyclic antidepressants in the treatment of depression associated with alcoholism. *J Clin Psychopharmacol.* 1981;1:146-150.

36. Mason BJ, Kocsis JH. Desipramine treatment of alcoholism. *Psychopharmacol Bull.* 1991;27:155-161.

37. Ciraulo DA, Alderson LM, Chapron DH, Jaffe JH, Subbarao B, Kramer PA. Imipramine disposition in alcoholics. *J Clin Psychopharmacol.* 1982;2:2-7.

38. Sandoz M, Vandel S, Vandel B, Bonin B, Allers G, Valmot R. Biotransformation of amitriptyline in alcoholic depressive patients. *Eur J Clin Pharmacol.* 1983;24:615-621.

39. Barraclough BM, Nelson B, Bunch J, Sainsbury P. Suicide and barbiturate prescribing. *J R Coll Gen Pract.* 1971;21:645-653.

40. Murphy GE. The physician's responsibility for suicide, II: errors of omission. *Ann Intern Med.* 1975;82:305-309.

41. Rutz W, von Knorring L, Walinder J. Frequency of suicide on Gotland after systematic postgraduate education of general practitioners. *Acta Psychiatr Scand.* 1989;80:151-154.

Mentally Disordered Offenders Who Push or Attempt to Push Victims Onto Subway Tracks in New York City

Daniel A. Martell, PhD, Park Elliott Dietz, MD, MPH, PhD

• Violent offenders who pushed or attempted to push victims onto the subway tracks in New York City during the 17-year period from 1975 through 1991 were studied. Forty-nine incidents involving 52 victims were identified during this period. Of 36 perpetrators who acted alone, 25 (69%) were referred for psychiatric evaluation and treatment, as was one member of an offending gang. Data concerning 20 of these 26 offenders and their crimes were collected. At the time of the offense, 19 (95%) of these offenders were psychotic, and 13 (65%) were homeless. Most of these offenders had extensive histories of psychiatric hospitalization and several prior arrests and convictions, often for violent crimes. The offenders had extensive mental health and criminal histories. The victims of these crimes were always strangers. Half of the offenders killed or seriously injured victims. Since 1986, the incidence of this offense has increased, and offenders accounting for the increase are mostly psychotic and homeless.

(*Arch Gen Psychiatry*. 1992;49:472-475)

Recent evidence[1-3] suggests that homeless persons who are mentally ill may be at greater risk for violent criminal behavior than persons who are neither mentally ill nor homeless and that, when they do commit violent crimes, they are most likely to select strangers as victims.[4] During the last 15 years, crime in the New York City subway system has also become a major public policy issue. Public fear of crime in the subways has risen significantly during this period, although data from the New York City Transit Authority suggest that the public has an exaggerated perception of the actual rate of crime in the subways. A study reported in *The New York Times* (October 2, 1988:38) indicated that about one third of riders surveyed estimated the number of felony crimes in the subways to be four times greater than the actual figure. This distorted public perception was attributed in part to the increasing numbers of aggressive panhandlers and mentally ill persons living in the city's subway stations.

More recently, public perceptions of dangers in the subway were assessed by interviewing 105 randomly selected subway riders waiting at stations throughout Manhattan (Harlem, Upper East Side, Midtown, Times Square, and Greenwich Village). Twenty-six percent of riders reported having frightening experiences in the subway system; 51% expressed fear of mentally ill persons in the subway; 77% had felt afraid of being pushed onto the tracks; and 80% regularly took specific preventive measures to avoid being pushed off the subway platform.[5]

These two studies add supportive evidence to the impression that most people who ride the subway harbor significant fears of violent crime, of the mentally ill, and of being pushed onto the tracks. Yet, the pervasiveness of the public fear is grossly out of proportion to the actual threat faced by subway riders. Pushing victims onto the subway tracks is an infrequent crime, even in New York City, which has one of the largest subway systems in the world. This crime is dwarfed by other violent crimes in the subways (*The New York Times.* October 2, 1988:38).

We attempt to provide a clearer understanding of this specific and unusual form of violent crime that so disproportionately frightens the public and affects the daily behavior of subway riders. We examined the demographic, psychiatric, and criminal background of 20 offenders referred for psychiatric evaluation who pushed or attempted to push victims onto the subway tracks in New York City during a 17-year period.

METHODS

Sample

Data were obtained from three sources. *The New York Times Index* was searched for all reports of crimes in which victims were pushed off of subway platforms or in which attempts were made to do so during the study interval. Offenses by 24 individuals or groups were reported, but not all of the offenders were identified in the stories. Offenses for which the offenders' identities were reported were cross-referenced with records maintained by the Bureau of Forensic Services of the New York State Office of Mental Health, Albany, NY, which contained files concerning four of the offenders identified in *The New York Times Index*. An additional 17 offenders were identified after interviewing ward staff members and searching patient charts at facilities that receive defendants from New York City. Finally, a search for additional cases was conducted in consultation with the Detective Bureau of the New York City Transit Authority Police. A search of their "unusual occurrence reports" failed to produce any additional cases. From these sources, we identified 41 individuals or groups who, from 1975 through 1991, were involved in 49 incidents against 52 victims. Of these 41, 36 were individuals (88%), and five (12%) were groups.

The five group offenses were perpetrated by gangs of two or more youths, three of whom victimized homeless persons and chased or pushed them onto the tracks, and two of whom victimized other vulnerable individuals. One of the gang members was referred for psychiatric evaluation. All of the 36 individuals who acted alone pushed or attempted to push their victims onto the tracks. Of the 36 individual offenders, 25 (69%) were referred for psychiatric evaluation and treatment, nine (25%) were not referred (five muggers who pushed victims onto the tracks during robbery attempts and four offenders who were never captured), and in two cases it was unknown whether psychiatric referral had occurred. We present data concerning 20 of the 26 offenders known to have been referred for psychiatric eval-

Accepted for publication March 30, 1992.

From the Nathan Kline Institute for Psychiatric Research, New York (NY) University School of Medicine (Dr Martell) and the Department of Psychiatry and Biobehavioral Sciences, UCLA School of Medicine, and the Threat Assessment Group Inc, Newport Beach, Calif (Dr Dietz).

Reprint requests to Research Department, Kirby Forensic Psychiatric Center, 600 E 125th St, New York, NY 10035 (Dr Martell).

uation. No data could be obtained concerning the other six offenders.

Procedure

Data were obtained from records maintained by the Bureau of Forensic Services of the New York State Office of Mental Health. These included police records (eg, arresting officers' reports and statements made to the police by offenders and victims around the time of the offense), criminal records, court documents, and mental health treatment records for each offender. All documentation was reviewed using a structured protocol.

Definitions

An offender was classified as *homeless* at the time of the offense if he or she was living and sleeping in the streets, a city-run shelter, an abandoned building, an abandoned car, or the subway system or if he or she was in a similar transient situation. An offender was classified as *domiciled* at the time of the offense if he or she maintained a permanent address or was residing on a permanent basis with friends or family. An offender was classified as *psychotic* at the time of the offense if the records described the presence of hallucinations, delusions, or formal thought disorder.

RESULTS

Rate of Offenses

Detectives of the New York City Transit Authority Police perceive this form of criminal behavior as rare and almost exclusively the domain of mentally ill persons. Although rare, the frequency of this offense by mentally ill persons seems to have increased substantially during the last 6 years. Among the offenders referred for psychiatric evaluation, the frequency of this offense increased from 0.9 per year from 1975 through 1985 to 2.5 per year from 1986 through 1991. (Among offenders not referred for evaluation, the frequency decreased from 1.2 per year from 1975 through 1985 to 0.3 per year from 1986 through 1991.)

Characteristics of the Offenders

Demographics.—Subjects ranged in age from 18 to 59 years (mean age, 34.8 years; SD = 10.2 years). Fifteen (75%) of the offenders were men, and five (25%), women. Seventy percent of the offenders were black; 15%, white; and 15%, Hispanic. Most were single (75%), although 15% were married, and 10% were separated or divorced.

None of the offenders was employed at the time of the offense. Twenty-five percent were financially supported by welfare; 20% were financially supported by Supplemental Security Income benefits; and 55% had no regular source of income. Fifty-five percent of subjects lacked a high school education, 30% had graduated from high school or obtained a GED, and 15% had some college education; none was known to have completed college.

Homelessness.—Sixty-five percent of these offenders were homeless, and 35% were domiciled at the time of the offense. For example, one offender had been homeless for most of the 8 to 10 years preceding his offense, except for three periods of hospitalization beginning at age 19 years, when he killed his mother's dog by throwing it into an incinerator in response to hallucinations. He was seen looking through garbage cans in the subway station just before he suddenly pushed a complete stranger onto the tracks in front of an oncoming train.

Mental Health History.—All but one of the offenders (95%) had histories of inpatient psychiatric treatment. The number of known prior admissions for psychiatric treatment ranged from 0 to 20 (mean, 7.2 admissions; SD = 5.9). Age at first admission ranged from 10 to 38 years (mean age, 21.6 years; SD = 8.5 years). Fewer subjects (nine [45%]) were known to have participated in any outpatient treatment.

Criminal History.—Data on criminal history are summarized in Table 1. Fifteen offenders (75%) had histories of prior arrest, and 13 (65%) had records of at least one prior arrest for violent criminal behavior. Eight (40%) had records of at least one prior arrest for a crime committed in the subway system. Eleven (55%) had records of prior convictions, and seven (35%) had records of prior convictions for violent crimes.

Table 1.—Criminal History of Offenders*

	Range	Mean	Median	SD
Age at first known offense, y	13-40	23.84	22.0	7.5
No. of prior arrests	0-35	6.45	4.5	8.27
No. of arrests for violent crime	0-8	2.60	1.5	2.89
No. of convictions	0-26	2.95	1.0	5.88
No. of convictions for violent crime	0-8	1.10	0.0	2.10
No. of prior arrests for subway crime	0-4	0.65	0.0	1.04

*N = 20.

Offense Characteristics

Arrest Charges.—Three offenders (15%) were charged with murder, 11 (55%) were charged with attempted murder, and six (30%) were charged with assault. One woman was not arrested or charged, but instead was brought to the psychiatric emergency department at Bellevue Hospital, New York, NY, by the police, as she was well known to them as a repeat offender with mental disorder.

Secondary arrest charges were more diverse and reveal additional information about the circumstances of specific offenses. The subway pushing occurred in the course of committing another distinct offense in seven cases (35%). The range of these offenses is reflected in the secondary arrest charges, which included sex crimes, robbery, attempted robbery, harassment, reckless endangerment, criminal sale of a controlled substance, criminal trespassing, and disorderly conduct.

Behavior After the Offense.—Behavior by the offenders after the offense varied greatly. Among the recurring patterns were (1) fleeing the scene, (2) standing and watching, and (3) attacking responding police officers. One offender went upstairs for coffee and returned to the station when he heard screaming. Another explained his delusional motive to the police and told them he would have pushed them onto the tracks, too, had they been there. One who tried to flee was caught by citizens and held for the police. One rummaged through his victim's duffle bag and tried on the Kentucky Fried Chicken uniform he found inside.

Victims.—The 20 offenders studied had pushed 24 victims. Two offenders had each pushed different victims on two separate occasions. Two other offenders had each pushed two victims in single incidents. Only limited data were available on characteristics of the victims. Age, only available for four of the victims, ranged from 13 to 58 years (mean age, 31.5 years). Of 19 victims whose sex was known, nine were male (47%), and ten, female (53%). Race was known for 14 victims, six (43%) of whom were white; two (14%), black; three (21%), Hispanic; and two (14%), Asian. One (7%) was of other racial background. All victims were complete strangers to the offenders, although in at least one case a misidentification syndrome[6] caused an offender to believe the victim was his psychiatrist from a state hospital.

Lethality.—Thirteen of the offenders (65%) succeeded in pushing a victim onto the train tracks, and all 13 pushed their victims as trains were actually entering the station. The train actually passed over four of the victims who were pushed onto the tracks. Not surprisingly, victims who were actually pushed onto the tracks were significantly more likely to be seriously injured or killed than those who were not ($\chi^2 = 4.10$; $df = 1$; $P < .05$), but one of the victims whom a train passed over sustained only minor injuries because he flattened himself between the tracks.

Table 2.—Criminal History Data by Successful and Unsuccessful Attempts to Push Victims Onto the Subway Tracks*

Data	Pushed Onto Tracks	Attempted to Push Onto Tracks
Age at first arrest, y	21.3±5.7	29.3±9.3
No. of prior arrests	8.5±9.3	2.5±3.7
No. of arrests for violent crime	3.3±3.0	1.3±2.2
No. of convictions	4.3±6.9	0.4±1.1
No. of convictions for violent crime	1.5±2.5	0.3±0.8

*n=13 for successful attempts, and n=7 for unsuccessful attempts. Values are means±SDs.

Three of the 24 victims (13%) were killed as result of being pushed onto the tracks. In one case, a 30-year-old white man was pushed onto the tracks in front of an oncoming train; he was electrocuted on the tracks and then crushed by the train. In the second and third murders, the offenders threw victims to the subway tracks where they were electrocuted on the "live" third rail. An additional seven victims (29%) were seriously injured as a result of the crime, including one woman who was pushed from the platform in front of a moving train and sustained fractures and a traumatic amputation of one arm. Eight victims (33%) suffered only minor injuries not requiring hospitalization; three victims (13%) escaped without physical injury; and four victims (17%) had nonlethal injuries of unknown severity.

Offenders were also studied according to whether they succeeded in pushing victims onto the tracks. Several statistical trends appeared when the criminal histories of successful offenders were compared with those of unsuccessful offenders (Table 2). Offenders who succeeded in pushing their victims onto the tracks were a mean of 8 years younger when first arrested than unsuccessful offenders ($t=2.35$ by a two-tailed test; $df=17$; $P<.05$), although they were not significantly older at the time of the offense studied ($t=1.06$; $df=18$; $P=.30$). Offenders who pushed their victims onto the tracks had four times as many arrests in their records ($t=-2.01$; $df=17.21$; $P=.06$) and three times as many arrests for violent crimes ($t=-1.70$; $df=16.07$; $P=.10$). In addition, offenders who pushed their victims onto the tracks had 10 times as many criminal convictions ($t=1.96$; $df=13.15$; $P=.07$) and five times as many convictions for violent crimes ($t=-1.69$; $df=15.59$; $P=.11$).

Mental State at the Time of the Offense

Psychosis.—Table 3 presents data on the offenders' psychopathology at the time of the offense. All but one (95%) of the offenders were psychotic at the time of the offense. The exception was the man who committed the offense with a partner; his only diagnosis was antisocial personality disorder. Of the 19 offenders for whom data on mental status were available, 18 (95%) were experiencing delusions, 13 (68%) were actively hallucinating, and 14 (74%) had formal thought disorder. Thirty-nine percent of offenders were intoxicated at the time of the offense.

Motives.—Except for one case that occurred during a robbery attempt by a gang of youthful drug dealers, all of the motives reported by these offenders reflected psychotic symptoms. In four cases, however, the motive was unknown.

Although 14 offenders suffered persecutory delusions, for only three offenders were these delusions the primary motive for the crime. One believed the victim and her friends had robbed his common-law wife as she was returning from buying drugs, causing him to search for and attack the victim. A second believed the victim had killed his niece and treated him poorly; also, he wanted his picture in the newspapers. A third said, "[S]he was going to stick something in my back." Grandiose delusions provided the motive for one man who gave a pregnant transit worker an inaudible message from God before pushing her onto the tracks. A man with mixed persecutory and grandiose delusions believed he was "a detective who [was] fighting against crimes," when he tried to push a police officer onto the tracks and slashed her with a straight razor. He said, "Some people here and in the streets are against me, and the person I was fighting in the subway station was in fact somebody else calling me names."

Table 3.—Mental State at the Time of the Offense*

Symptoms	No. (%) of Offenders
Hallucinations	13 (68)
Auditory	13 (68)
Command	4 (21)
Visual	2 (11)
Delusions	18 (95)
Persecutory	14 (74)
Grandiose	5 (26)
Rescuer	3 (16)
Religious	3 (16)
Being controlled	2 (11)
Reference	2 (11)
Thought insertion	1 (5)
Somatic	1 (5)
Misidentification	1 (5)
Other	7 (37)
FTD	14 (74)
Intoxication at time of offense	7 (37)

*n=19. Data were not available for one offender. FTD indicates formal thought disorder.

Three men committed offenses based on rescue delusions, according to which they were rescuing others by pushing perceived villains onto the tracks. One man with the delusion that his two victims meant to push 20 children onto the tracks said, "I knew what they were thinking." A second man believed his 13-year-old victim was a prostitute who was going to harm a younger sister who accompanied her, although he later claimed he "had a special relationship" with this stranger, whom he said was his girlfriend. A third said, "Voices told me that my wife had been killed, was taken hostage in a building, and was being raped and sexually abused. She was calling me to help her. . . . That dude was standing in my way in the subway. He called me a faggot and a motherfucker, and I couldn't take it, so we had an argument and a fight, and he tore my shirt, and I took his shirt."

Five of the offenders acted on motives derived from hallucinations, three of which were command hallucinations. One woman reported, "The baby inside me said to push her." Another offender believed the victim was a psychiatrist who had kept him hospitalized, and a voice told him to push her for revenge. Another heard voices that told him he must achieve a "victorious kill," a vendetta against the white Europeans who took his family from Africa. He knew the victim (a 30-year-old white man) was a "poor old man willing to sacrifice himself" because the spirits told him that this was his victorious kill; he was trying to help the man get to paradise. Another man said that voices told him there was a contract out on him. Yet another said that voices called him "faggot" and said, "He is dirty."

Two offenders gave less comprehensible explanations. One claimed to have done the same thing three times before, but denied the offense, saying she did not know why the eyewitnesses were harassing her. The other said her first offense was committed because the victim owed her money and that her second offense was related to her plan to take the victim to federal court.

Diagnostic Impressions.—Most offenders (14 of 19 [71%]) were diagnosed with schizophrenia (paranoid type, eight [42]%; undifferentiated type, four [21%]; and residual type, two [11%]). There was one case of bipolar disorder and one case of schizoaffective disorder. Three offenders were diagnosed as having psychotic disorders not otherwise specified. Finally, one offender was diagnosed as having antisocial personality disorder and was described as "a classic psychopath."

COMMENT

Most subway travelers say they take steps to protect themselves from being pushed onto the tracks, even though this crime occurs only a few times a year. This is consistent with research indicating that risks from dramatic or sensational causes of death tend to be greatly overestimated.[7] Some of the reasons this infrequent crime arouses disproportionate fear may include publicity attending a few sensational cases; the severity of potential harm; the seeming randomness of victim selection; and the seeming uncontrollability of mentally ill offenders.

Although our finding that the victims were all strangers to the offenders is consistent with the hypothesis that offenders select victims at random, this does not necessarily mean that travelers are powerless to prevent victimization. It could be that travelers can reduce their risk through such measures as avoiding eye contact, staying with groups, avoiding the edge of the platform, and conveying confidence and alertness toward the environment.

An increase since 1986 in the incidence of offenders pushing or attempting to push riders onto subway tracks in New York City has been entirely accounted for by an increase in the number of offenses by those referred for psychiatric examination, most of whom are psychotic and homeless. This increase is positively correlated with the increase in the number of homeless, mentally ill persons in the city during the same period.

It has been estimated that the rate of homelessness for the general population of New York City is about 1%, while the rate for mentally ill persons is approximately 2%.[2] Based on these estimates, the rate of homelessness among the subway offenders studied was 33 times that of the rest of the persons with mental disorders in the city and 65 times that of the general population. These rates exceed estimates from other studies[2,4] of crime and mental illness in New York City that suggest a rate of homelessness of 45% to 50% among offenders with mental illness.

Both the offenders we studied and the other homeless, mentally ill persons who commit crimes in the subway system can be identified by the police because of their prolonged presence in the subway stations, where they loiter or dwell. The ready identifiability of these persons makes it possible for policymakers to devise strategies of variable vigor to remove such persons from the subway system. Through the Homeless Outreach Program, the New York City Transit Police offer alternative sources of shelter. However, all such efforts to assist the homeless mentally ill face the persistent problems of providing necessary medications and support services to consenting persons as well as hospitalization for dangerous individuals in need of such care.

This study was supported in part by the Threat Assessment Group Inc, Newport Beach, Calif.

The authors thank Robert Rondinelli, Chief of Detectives, New York City Transit Authority Police, and Detective Ray Pierce, Criminal Assessment and Profiling Unit, Detectives Bureau, New York City Police Department, for their assistance with this project.

References

1. Gelberg L, Linn L, Leake B. Mental health, alcohol and drug use, and criminal history among homeless adults. *Am J Psychiatry.* 1988;145:191-196.
2. Martell DA. Homeless mentally disordered offenders and violent crimes: preliminary research findings. *Law Hum Behav.* 1991;15:333-347.
3. Pruett NS. Mental illness and homelessness as predictor of criminality: a second analysis of 728 male jail detainees. Evanston, Ill: Northwestern University; 1989. Dissertation.
4. Martell DA. Violent crime and the homeless mentally ill: base rate estimates, victimization patterns, and mental status findings. Presented at the midyear meeting of the American Psychology-Law Society, Division 41 of the American Psychological Association; March 14, 1992; San Diego, Calif.
5. Martell DA, Morrison D. Public perceptions of the mentally ill and danger in the subways: a representative survey of Manhattan subway riders. Orangeburg, NY: Nathan S. Kline Institute for Psychiatric Research, New York State Office of Mental Health; 1992. Field Study Technical Paper 92-01.
6. de Pauw KW, Szulecka TK. Dangerous delusions: violence and the misidentification syndromes. *Br J Psychiatry.* 1988;152:91-96.
7. Lichtenstein S, Slovic P, Fischhoff B, Layman M, Combs B. Judged frequency of lethal events. *J Exp Psychol (Hum Learn Mem).* 1978;4:551-578.

Mental Disorder, Intellectual Deficiency, and Crime

Evidence From a Birth Cohort

Sheilagh Hodgins, PhD

• Studies of criminality among patients in psychiatric hospitals and of mental disorder among incarcerated offenders have suggested an association between the major mental disorders (schizophrenia and major affective disorders) and crime. However, these investigations are characterized by notable methodological weaknesses, and, consequently, this conclusion has remained tentative. Little is known about the criminality of intellectually handicapped people. The present study examined the relationship between crime and mental disorder and crime and intellectual deficiency in an unselected Swedish birth cohort followed up to age 30 years. It was found that men with major mental disorders were 2½ times more likely than men with no disorder or handicap to be registered for a criminal offense and four times more likely to be registered for a violent offense. Women with major disorders were five times more likely than women with no disorder or handicap to be registered for an offense and 27 times more likely to be registered for a violent offense. These subjects committed many serious offenses throughout their lives. The criminal behavior in over half these cases appeared before the age of 18 years. Intellectually handicapped men were three times more likely to offend than men with no disorder or handicap and five times more likely to commit a violent offense. Intellectually handicapped women were almost four times more likely to offend than women with no disorder or handicap and 25 times more likely to commit a violent offense. The results of this investigation confirm and extend previous findings indicating that individuals with major mental disorders and those with intellectual handicaps are at increased risk for offending and for violent offending. However, in the United States, where rates of crime overall and crime by substance abusers are very high, the mentally disordered and intellectually handicapped would account for only a small proportion of these offenses.

(*Arch Gen Psychiatry.* 1992;49:476-483)

It has long been presumed by the general public that there is an association between mental disorder and violence and between intellectual handicap and violence. This belief has been reflected in literature and art and in both the civil and criminal laws of most countries around the world. Scientists, however, have only recently carried out investigations designed to address these issues.

Accepted for publication March 19, 1992.

From the Department of Psychology, Université de Montréal, Québec.

Reprint requests to Department of Psychology, Université de Montréal, CP 6128, Suc. "A," Montréal, Québec, Canada H1C 1H1 (Dr Hodgins).

Studies of Mentally Disordered Persons

Investigations of patients in the hospital and in the days preceding admission have revealed that many behave aggressively.[1-7] However, since aggressive individuals are more likely to be admitted than persons with symptoms of equal severity who are threatening, the observed association between mental disorder and aggressive behavior may result from sampling bias.

Follow-up studies of patients discharged from psychiatric wards[8-17] have suggested that more of these persons commit crimes than the general population of the community where they are released. The differences between the rates of conviction for the ex-patients and the general population are usually found to be greater for violent than nonviolent crimes.[9,12,13,16] There is a suggestion that men with substance abuse problems, men with schizophrenia, and those with both are at increased risk for criminality.[9,11,18,19] However, follow-up periods in these investigations were short, and samples of ex-patients rarely remained intact throughout. Consequently, patients who committed crimes would be more likely to be counted at the end of the follow-up period than patients who left treatment and had no contacts with the police. Data on criminal convictions were in many studies limited to one state or jurisdiction. Diagnoses were taken from hospital files and not validated in any way. In addition, it is difficult to compare the results from these various studies, as there is no way of knowing whether the distributions of diagnoses in the samples are similar. At the time the studies were conducted, some hospitals admitted large numbers of alcoholics, drug abusers, and patients with personality disorders, while others restricted inpatient care to psychotics.

A recent investigation,[20] which has none of these methodological weaknesses, included all inpatients in Stockholm County, Sweden, with a diagnosis of schizophrenia who were born between 1920 and 1959 and discharged in 1971. Patients underwent rediagnosis by an independent clinician, using *DSM-III* criteria, and 85% (644 patients) met the criteria for schizophrenia. These 644 patients were then followed up for 14 years. The relative risk of a criminal offense among these schizophrenics compared with the general Swedish population was 1.2 for the men and 2.2 for the women. However, the schizophrenics "committed four times as many violent offenses as the general population."[20(pp346-347)] Fifty-five percent of the schizophrenic subjects who were convicted of a crime also had a history of substance abuse.[21]

A number of investigations suggest that schizophrenics and their biological relatives are at increased risk for criminality. In a study of a cohort of 9182 consecutive live births, it was found that the offspring of schizophrenics had higher rates of registration for criminal offenses than those of parents with no disorder.[22] In the Danish high-risk schizophrenia project,[23] more of the high-risk mothers and children were registered for criminality than the low-risk mothers and children. The children's criminality was verified when they were between 21 and 31 years of age. Studies of children at increased genetic risk for schizophrenia identify an aggressive subgroup.[24] One study[22] of a cohort of 6770 male adoptees found that schizophrenia in the biological parents increased the risk of criminal behavior in the children. Furthermore, Kay[25] reports that the biological relatives of schizophrenics with positive symptoms frequently display antisocial behavior.

Studies of Offenders

Rather than looking at the criminality of identified patients, some investigators have focused on the mental disorders of criminals. Recent studies of representative samples of US prison inmates[26-29] and Canadian penitentiary inmates[30] have revealed higher prevalences of major mental disorders within these facilities than in the general population. Furthermore, two of these studies demonstrate that large numbers of the male inmates with major disorders are also substance abusers.[31,32] These five investigations all employed the same diagnostic criteria[33] and used standardized, reliable, and valid diagnostic instruments. These same instruments have been used to examine the prevalence of mental disorders in the general population,[34] and, consequently, comparisons between the prevalence of disorders among inmates and in the general population can be made with some confidence.

In addition to these studies showing that major mental disorders are more prevalent among incarcerated offenders than in the general population, three investigations suggest that the prevalence of major disorders is even higher among homicide offenders. Most investigations of homicide offenders include only compilations of assessments conducted at the request of the court. Such samples are biased and represent only a small proportion of homicide offenders.[35] In Scandinavia, all persons accused of homicide are evaluated by at least one psychiatrist, and these assessments are reviewed by panels composed of a number of other psychiatrists. A study of all homicide offenders in Copenhagen, Denmark, over a 25-year period revealed that 20% of the men and 44% of the women had a diagnosis of psychosis.[36] Among those who received a diagnoses of psychosis, 13% of the women and 41% of the men were found to be substance abusers. Lindqvist[37] studied every person who committed a homicide in Northern Sweden between 1970 and 1981. Thirty-four (53%) of 64 subjects were found to suffer from a major mental disorder, and slightly more than one third of them also received a diagnosis of substance abuse and/or dependence. Similarly, Côté and Hodgins,[38] working in Canada, have reported elevated prevalences (35%) of major mental disorders among homicide offenders.

A Population Study

To examine the relationship between mental disorder and crime, the research design with the least weaknesses is that of a longitudinal prospective study of an unselected birth cohort. This design limits any sampling bias, particularly if the cohort remains intact throughout the study. The use of central registers ensures that all convictions are compiled. Such an investigation is limited, however, by the use of hospitalization as an indicator of mental disorder. To our knowledge, only one study, a Danish thesis, has employed this design.

Ortmann[39] examined the criminal records of an entire birth cohort composed of 11 540 men born in Copenhagen in 1953 and still alive in Denmark in 1975. Data on admissions to psychiatric wards were collected from the central Danish psychiatric register in 1978 when the subjects were 25 years old. Data on offenses were collected from the central police register in 1976 when the subjects were 23 years old. While 34.8% of all the men with no disorder had been registered for at least one offense (comparable to the registration rate found in the Scandinavian countries for men[40]), 43.5% of those admitted with a major disorder, 83.2% of those admitted with substance abuse and/or dependence, and 50.9% of those with other diagnoses had been registered for an offense. Significantly more of those with psychiatric admissions had been convicted in every category of offense. While there were not many subjects within each diagnostic group, Ortmann's results suggested that the registration rates varied considerably by diagnosis.

Conclusion

The findings of studies of mentally disordered persons and of incarcerated offenders and one investigation of an unselected birth cohort suggest a relationship between major mental disorder and criminality. This relationship appears to be stronger among men, in the presence of a secondary diagnosis of substance abuse/dependence, and for violent rather than nonviolent crime.

Intellectual Capacity and Crime

Many studies have shown that offenders have lower IQ test scores than nonoffenders.[41,42] The difference in global IQ is about half an SD.[43] Prospective longitudinal investigations have demonstrated that children with lower IQ test scores are at increased risk for official delinquency and for self-reported delinquency.[44,45] This relationship has been shown to be independent of social class, race, and detection by the police.[46] Intellectual capacity is a factor that appears to protect otherwise high-risk boys from criminal involvement.[45,46]

While many studies have documented this relationship between intellectual capacity and official criminality, we were able to find only one investigation of the criminality of a population of intellectually deficient persons. Høgh and Wolf[47] investigated all 12 270 boys born in 1953 in the major urban areas of Denmark. In 1976, when the boys were 23 years of age, criminality was examined for all those still alive (94% of the original birth cohort). The IQ was assessed using a Danish adaptation of the Swedish test developed by Härnqvist. (Each subtest has scores ranging from zero to 40. The three subtest scores are summed to give a global score.) Half the sample, 7868 boys, were tested at age 12 years. One in five of the boys with an IQ score of 68 or lower had been registered for an offense by age 23 years as opposed to 8% of those with IQ scores of 90 to 120. This difference is greater for violent crimes than for nonviolent crimes. In fact, the boys who would most certainly be considered intellectually handicapped (IQ score of 1 to 44) were 13 times more likely than boys whose IQ score fell in the normal range to have been registered for a violent offense.

The Present Investigation

The present study was conducted to confirm and extend the reported findings about the relationship between mental disorder and crime and intellectual deficiency and crime. An unselected birth cohort was followed up to age 30 years. Data were collected from national psychiatric and police registers.

SUBJECTS AND METHODS

Subjects

The cohort is composed of all 15 117 persons born in Stockholm in 1953 and residing there in 1963.[48] Only subjects living in Sweden at the end of the 30-year follow-up period were included in the analyses.

Subjects who had been admitted to a psychiatric ward were divided into three groups based on the most serious discharge diagnosis: major mental disorder (schizophrenia, major affective disorders, paranoid states, and other psychoses), alcohol and/or drug abuse and/or dependence, and all other mental disorders. Among the 7362 men, 1.1% (82 subjects) were classified as having a major mental disorder, 2.1% (156 subjects) as being alcohol and/or drug abusers or dependent on alcohol and/or drugs, and 0.9% (64 subjects) as suffering from other mental disorders. Of the 7039 women, 1.1% (79 subjects) were classified as having a major mental disorder, 1.4% (98 subjects) as having alcohol and/or drug abuse or dependence, and 1.8% (124 subjects) as having another mental disorder. Studies of the schizophrenia diagnoses in this register[49] and in other Swedish registers[50] have suggested that these diagnoses are valid and closely resemble *DSM-III* diagnoses.

Intellectually handicapped subjects were defined as those who were placed in special classes for intellectually deficient children in high school and were never admitted to a psychiatric ward. Thus, 1.5% of the men (113 subjects) and 1.1% of the women (79 subjects) were considered intellectually handicapped. The comparison group was composed of all subjects who had never been admitted to a psychiatric ward or to an institution or class for the intellectually handicapped.

Procedure

In 1983, criminal records were collected from the Swedish National Police Register, and mental health records were collected from the Stockholm County register. Pregnancy and birth records, family data, school records, social welfare agency records, and military records were collected for all subjects.

RESULTS

Prevalence of Criminality

As can be seen in Fig 1, significantly more of the men with a major mental disorder, an intellectual handicap, or diagnosed substance abuse had been convicted of at least one criminal offense than men with other mental disorders or those with no disorder and no handicap. Men with major mental disorders were 2.56 (95% confidence interval [CI], 1.66 to 3.97) times more likely to have been convicted of a criminal offense than men with no disorder or handicap. The comparable odds ratio for men with other disorders was 1.15 (95% CI, 0.69 to 1.93); for intellectually handicapped men, 3.12 (95% CI, 2.17 to 4.49); and, for men

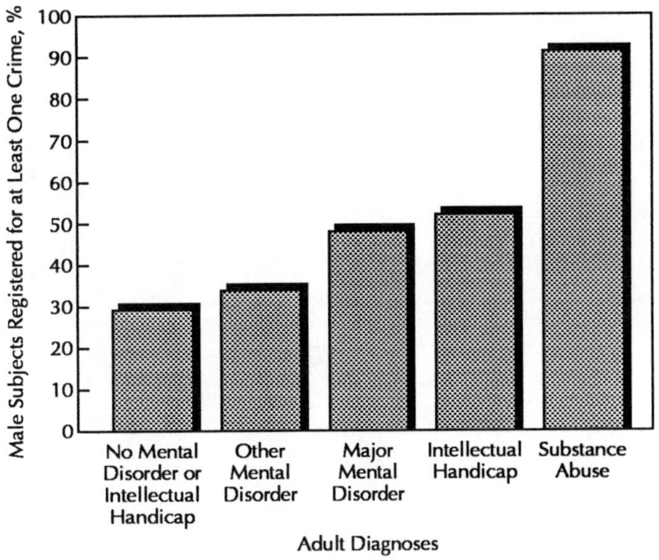

Fig 1.—*Male subjects registered for at least one crime by age 30 years by adult diagnosis status (χ^2[4, N = 7362] = 290.23, P = .00000). Compared with subjects with no mental disorder or intellectual handicap, for subjects with other mental disorder, χ^2(1, N = 7011) = 0.74 (not significant); for subjects with major mental disorder, χ^2(1, N = 7029) = 12.74 (P = .01 corrected for type I error by the Bonferroni formula, P = .0025); for subjects with intellectual handicap, χ^2(1, N = 7060) = 25.44 (P = .00000); and for substance abusers, χ^2(1, N = 7103) = 260.34 (P = .00000).*

with diagnoses of substance abuse/dependence, 20.37 (95% CI, 12.12 to 34.26).

Figure 2 presents these results for the female subjects. Proportionately more subjects with major mental disorders and substance abuse problems were convicted of crimes than women with no disorder and no handicap. Women with major mental disorders were 5.02 (95% CI, 2.78 to 9.06) times more likely to have been convicted for a criminal offense than women with no disorder or handicap. The comparable odds ratio for women with other disorders was 1.67 (95% CI, 0.91 to 3.05); for intellectually handicapped subjects, 3.73 (95% CI, 2.00 to 6.94); and, for women with diagnoses of substance abuse/dependence, 32.34 (95% CI, 21.11 to 49.53).

Age Patterns

The patterns of proportions of subjects within each diagnostic group who had been convicted of a criminal offense are relatively stable over time for both the men and the women. In fact, χ^2 values calculated separately for gender and on group differences for convictions before age 15 years, from age 15 to 18 years, 18 to 21 years, and 21 to 30 years were all highly significant. In all age groups, the percentages of subjects with a major mental disorder, intellectual handicap, or substance abuse who had been convicted of a crime exceeded those of the subjects with no disorder and no handicap.

As can be observed in Fig 3, official criminal activity appears to begin at different ages for the different groups of male subjects. Among the men with no disorder and no handicap and those with an adult substance abuse diagnosis, the proportion of subjects beginning their criminal careers decreased with age. This pattern also describes the intellectually handicapped subjects, but the decrease begins only after age 18 years. However, among the men who develop major mental disorders, the proportions who begin their criminal careers at each age are more erratic—12%, 18%, 7%, and 9% at less than 15 years, 15 to 18 years, 18 to 21 years, and 21 to 30 years, respectively.

As can be observed in Fig 4, the proportion of women with no disorder and no handicap who begin their criminal careers remains stable over time. Among the substance abusers, the proportion of subjects beginning their criminal careers increases

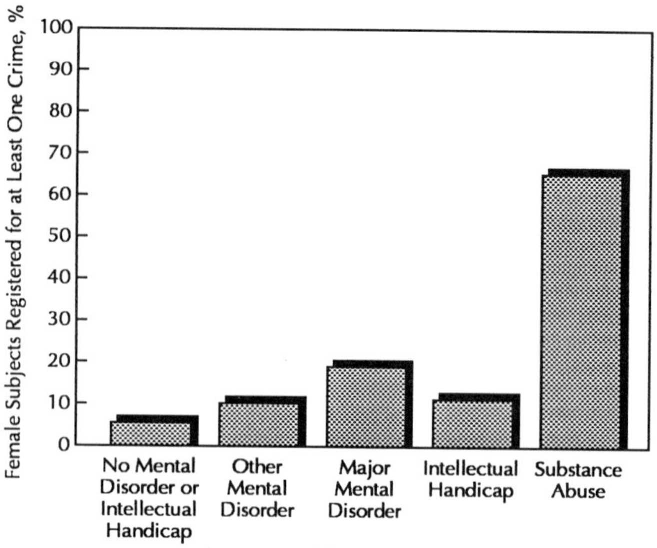

Fig 2.—*Female subjects registered for at least one crime by age 30 years by adult diagnosis status ($\chi^2[4, N=7039]=617.82$, P=.00000). Compared with subjects with no mental disorder or intellectual handicap, for subjects with other mental disorder, $\chi^2(1, N=6783)=5.57$ (not significant); for subjects with major mental disorder, $\chi^2(1, N=6738)=25.96$ (P=.00000); for subjects with intellectual handicap, $\chi^2(1, N=6738)=4.31$ (not significant); and for substance abusers, $\chi^2(1, N=6757)=617.03$ (P=.00000).*

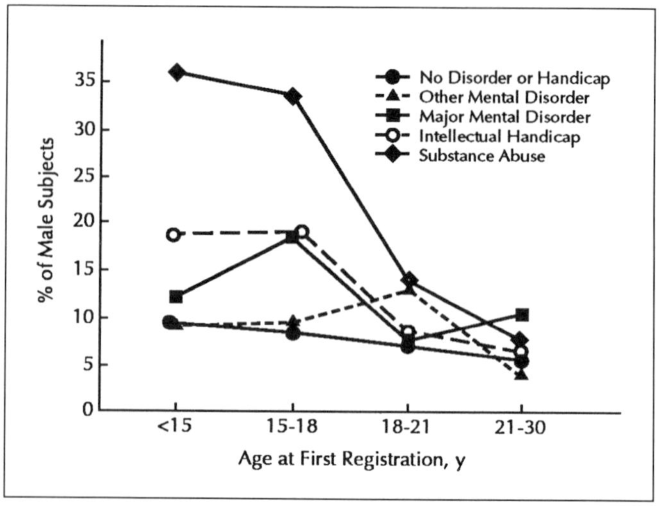

Fig 3.—*Male subjects by age at first registration. For first registration at less than age 15 years, compared with subjects with no mental disorder or intellectual handicap (NOMD), for subjects with other mental disorder (OMD), $\chi^2(1, N=7011)=0.00$ (not significant [NS]); for subjects with major mental disorder (MMD), $\chi^2(1, N=7029)=0.71$; for subjects with intellectual handicap (IH), $\chi^2(1, N=7060)=10.67$ (P=.001); and for substance abusers (SA), $\chi^2(1, N=7101)=120.75$ (P=.00000). For first registration at age 15 to 18 years, compared with NOMD, for OMD, $\chi^2(1, N=7011)=0.075$ (NS); for MMD, $\chi^2(1, N=7029)=10.12$ (P=.002); for IH, $\chi^2(1, N=7060)=14.64$ (P=.0001); and for SA, $\chi^2(1, N=7101)=118.52$ (P=.00000). For first registration at age 18 to 21 years, compared with NOMD, for OMD, $\chi^2(1, N=7011)=3.49$ (NS); for MMD, $\chi^2(1, N=7029)=0.06$ (NS); for IH, $\chi^2(1, N=7060)=0.32$ (NS); and for SA, $\chi^2(1, N=7101)=7.77$ (P=.005). For first registration at age 21 to 30 years, compared with NOMD, for OMD, $\chi^2(1, N=7011)=0.445$ (NS); for MMD, $\chi^2(1, N=7029)=3.97$ (NS); for IH, $\chi^2(1, N=7060)=0.37$ (NS); and for SA, $\chi^2(1, N=7101)=1.55$ (NS).*

up to age 21 years, then levels off. Among the intellectually handicapped, there is a burst of activity between the ages of 18 and 21 years. Among the women with major disorders, the proportions beginning their criminal careers at each age appear to be more stable, with an increase after age 21 years.

While 10.8% of the men with no disorder and no handicap were convicted in two or more age groups, 18.7% of the men with other disorders, 25.6% of those with major disorders, 32.7% of those with an intellectual handicap, and 72.4% of the substance abusers were convicted in at least two different age groups. Given the small number of female subjects in each group, patterns of convictions across age groups are difficult to verify.

Number of Convictions

Among the male offenders with no disorders and no handicap, the mean number of convictions was 7.3 (SD, 19.6); among offenders with other mental disorders, 12.0 (SD, 16.4) ($t[2066]=1.13$, $P=.261$); among offenders with a major mental disorder, 13.2 (SD, 16.4) ($t[2083]=1.87$, $P=.062$); among offenders with an intellectual handicap, 10.0 (SD, 17.2) ($t[2102]=1.03$, $P=.304$); and among substance abusers, 29.5 (SD, 39.3) ($t[143.78]=6.64$, $P=.000$). Similarly, among the female offenders, those with no disorder and no handicap had a mean number of convictions of 3.3 (SD, 7.0); among those with other mental disorders, 3.8 (SD, 3.6) ($t[14.09]=.41$, $P=.691$); among those with a major disorder, 3.8 (SD, 4.8) ($t[344]=.26$, $P=.795$); among those with an intellectual handicap, 7.9 (SD, 7.8) ($t[338]=1.83$, $P=.068$); and among substance abusers, 10.8 (SD, 19.3) ($t[65.11]=3.06$, $P=.003$). While the within-group variances are large, it appears that male and female offenders with a major disorder and those with an intellectual handicap commit as many offenses as offenders with no disorder, or even more.

Types of Offenses

Offenses were divided into seven categories by the Swedish criminologist Wikström.[51] The category "violent crimes" includes all offenses involving the use or threat of physical violence (for example, assault, rape, robbery, unlawful threat, and molestation). "Theft" includes all forms of stealing other than robbery as well as receiving stolen goods. "Fraud" includes embezzlement, crimes related to debts, and crimes of falsification. The category of "traffic crimes" does not include minor offenses, such as speeding. Drunken driving and driving without a license are the most frequent offenses in this category. The category "other" is very heterogeneous, including offenses such as defamation, sexual crimes other than rape, sexual coercion, perjury, gambling, bribery, absence without leave from the military, smuggling, and tax evasion.

As can be observed in Table 1, the various diagnoses are associated with all seven categories of crimes, as indicated by significant across-group χ^2 comparisons. Two-by-two comparisons (the percentage of subjects with no disorder or handicap compared with the percentage of subjects in each group who are convicted of a crime in each category) demonstrate that, compared with men with no disorder and no handicap, more men with other mental disorders committed fraud and vandalism, and more men with an intellectual handicap committed violent offenses, thefts, traffic offenses, and offenses classified as other. Male subjects with diagnoses of major mental disorders and substance abusers were registered for more crimes of every type than subjects with no disorder and no handicap.

The magnitude of the group differences for violent offenses was examined more closely. Men with major mental disorders were 4.16 times (95% CI, 2.23 to 7.78) more likely to have been convicted of a violent offense than men with no disorder or handicap. The comparable odds ratio for men with other disorders is 0.90 (95% CI, .33 to 2.50); for men with intellectual handicaps, 5.45 (95% CI, 3.38 to 8.80) ; and for men with diagnoses of substance abuse/dependence, 15.44 (95% CI, 11.11 to 21.44).

As can be observed in Table 2, the various diagnoses are associated with all seven categories of crimes for women, as indicated by the significant across-group χ^2 comparisons. More of the female subjects with a diagnosis of substance abuse were convicted of all types of crimes than the women with no disorder or handicap. The women with major mental disorders were 27.45 times (95% CI, 9.80 to 76.88) more likely to have been convicted of a violent offense than women with no disorder or handicap. The comparable odds ratio for the women with other mental disorders was 1.78 (95% CI, 0.43 to 7.37); for intellectually handicapped women, 24.77 (95% CI, 8.86 to 69.2); and for women with diagnoses of substance abuse/dependence, 54.58 (95% CI, 31.38 to 94.92).

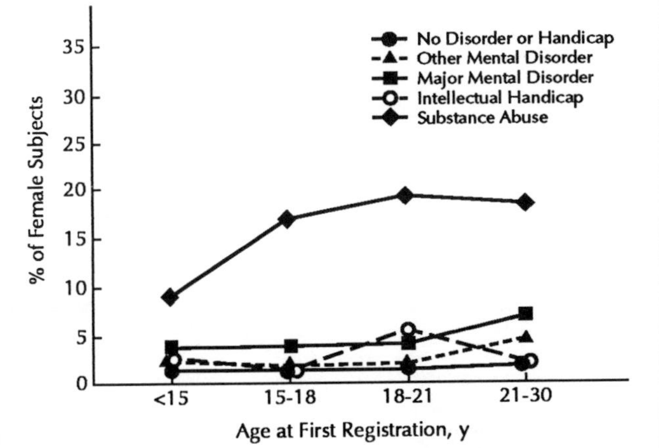

Fig 4.—*Female subjects by age at first registration. For first registration at less than age 15 years, compared with subjects with no mental disorder or intellectual handicap (NOMD), for subjects with other mental disorder (OMD), $\chi^2(1, N=6783)=0.715$ (not significant [NS]); for subjects with major mental disorder (MMD), $\chi^2(1, N=6738)=2.80$ (NS); for subjects with intellectual handicap (IH), $\chi^2(1, N=6738)=0.58$ (NS); and for substance abusers (SA), $\chi^2(1, N=6751)=30.23$ (P=.000). For first registration at age 15 to 18 years, compared NOMD, for OMD, $\chi^2(1, N=6783)=0.158$ (NS); for MMD, $\chi^2(1, N=6738)=4.22$ (P=.04); for IH, $\chi^2(1, N=6738)=0.00$ (NS); and for SA, $\chi^2(1, N=6751)=167.65$ (P=.00000). For first registration at age 18 to 21 years, compared with NOMD, for OMD, $\chi^2(1, N=6783)=0.391$ (NS); for MMD, $\chi^2(1, N=6738)=5.63$ (P=.02); for IH, $\chi^2(1, N=6738)=11.81$ (P=.0006); and for SA, $\chi^2(1, N=6751)=244.92$ (P=.00000). For first registration at age 21 to 30 years, compared with NOMD, for OMD, $\chi^2(1, N=6783)=7.38$ (P=.007); for MMD, $\chi^2(1, N=6738)=15.65$ (P=.008); for IH, $\chi^2(1, N=6738)=0.00$ (NS); and for SA, $\chi^2(1, N=6751)=206.64$ (P=.00000).*

Correlates of Criminality

The relationship between socioeconomic status and criminality within the different groups was examined. Socioeconomic status was indexed by father's occupation or, in the case of a single mother, mother's occupation. Social class was measured at the time of birth and when the subject was 10 years old. An indicator of poverty was the number of years the subject's family received social assistance. Among both the men and women with no disorder and no handicap, there are highly statistically significant relationships between socioeconomic status of the family of origin and criminality of the subject. These relationships are evident for measures at the time of subjects' births (for men, $\chi^2[4, N=6715]=123.51$, $P=.0000$; for women, $\chi^2[4, N=6648]=18.97$, $P=.002$) and when they were 10 years old (for men, $\chi^2[4, N=6947]=148.54$, $P=.0000$; for women, $\chi^2[4, N=6659]=27.31$, $P=.0001$). Also, among subjects with no disorder or handicap, significantly more offenders than nonoffenders were raised in families that received social welfare payments (for men, $\chi^2[1, N=6947]=132.77$, $P=.0000$; for women, $\chi^2[1, N=6659]=32.40$, $P=.0000$).

However, among the other groups of subjects, with one exception, there was no relationship between socioeconomic status and criminality. The exception is women with major mental disorders. At the time of these subjects' births, 43% of the families of women with a major disorder and a criminal record were upper middle class ($\chi^2[4, N=79]=11.62$, $P=.04$). When the subjects were aged 10 years, 36% of the families were upper middle class and another 36% were lower middle class ($\chi^2[4, N=79]=10.88$, $P=.05$). However, equivalent proportions of the families of those with and without a criminal record received welfare payments.

The relationship of substance abuse to criminality, both in childhood and adulthood, was examined within each group. The Child Welfare Committee records were used to index childhood substance abuse. As can be seen in Table 3, among the male subjects with no disorder or handicap, with major mental disorders, and with adult substance abuse, significantly more of those who had been convicted of a crime had a history of substance abuse in childhood. Among the women, an association between crime and childhood substance abuse is evident for subjects with adult substance abuse and for those with neither a mental disorder nor a handicap.

As adults, 48.7% of the offenders with a major mental disorder had a secondary diagnosis of alcohol and/or drug abuse and/or dependence. Among the women offenders with a major mental disorder, 42.9% had an additional diagnosis of substance abuse/dependence. No intellectually handicapped subject and,

Table 1.—Male Subjects in Each Group Convicted by Offense Type

	Male Subjects, %									All Disorders		
Type of Offense	No Mental Disorder or Handicap	Other Mental Disorder	χ^2(1,N =7011)*	Major Mental Disorder	χ^2(1,N =7029)*	Intel-lectual Handicap	χ^2(1,N =7060)*	Sub-stance Abuse	χ^2(1,N =7103)*	χ^2(4,N =7362)*	*P*	Corrected *P*†
Violent	5.7	6.3		14.6	12.03§	16.8	25.19‡	49.4	471.58‡	482.06	.001	.0001
Theft	16.6	25.0		34.1	17.86‡	34.5	25.43‡	75.0	354.44‡	383.18	.001	.0001
Fraud	4.0	14.1	16.35‡	14.6	23.17‡	7.1		42.3	485.80‡	493.52	.001	.0001
Vandalism	4.1	10.9	7.31§	12.2	13.02‖	8.8		37.2	360.60‡	364.63	.001	.0001
Traffic	13.1	14.1		22.0		25.7	15.32‡	53.2	204.71‡	218.03	.001	.0001
Narcotics	2.4	1.6		8.5	12.89‖	4.4		42.3	773.26‡	767.35	.001	.0001
Other	11.1	12.5		25.6	17.23‡	23.0	15.92‡	54.5	272.37‡	292.15	.001	.0001

*Comparisons with the group with no mental disorder or handicap; only statistically significant values are given.
†Corrected for type I error by Bonferroni's formula.
‡*P*=.001; corrected for type I error by Bonferroni's formula, *P*=.0001.
§*P*=.05; corrected for type I error by Bonferroni's formula, *P*=.007.
‖*P*=.01; corrected for type I error by Bonferroni's formula, *P*=.002.

Table 2.—Female Subjects in Each Group Convicted by Offense Type

Type of Offense	Female Subjects, %: No Mental Disorder or Handicap	Other Mental Disorder	χ^2(1,N =6783)*	Major Mental Disorder	χ^2(1,N =6738)*	Intellectual Handicap	χ^2(1,N =6738)*	Substance Abuse	χ^2(1,N =6757)*	All Disorders: χ^2(4,N =7039)*	P
Violent	0.5	1.6		6.3	50.51†	3.8	17.26†	24.5	690.43‡	643.16	.00000
Theft	3.2	5.6		12.7		6.3		46.9	501.27‡	500.04	.00000
Fraud	1.0	4.0	10.87†	3.8		2.5		27.6	501.91‡	482.15	.00000
Vandalism	0.2	0.0		1.3		0.0		15.3	601.83‡	605.30	.00000
Traffic	0.9	0.8		1.3		2.5		7.1	40.69‡	42.06	.00000
Narcotics	0.5	0.8		0.0		0.0		22.4	554.95‡	569.38	.00000
Other	0.5	0.8		1.3		1.3		23.5	597.42‡	592.10	.00000

*Comparisons with the group with no mental disorder or handicap; only statistically significant values are given.
†$P=.001$; corrected for type I error by Bonferroni's formula, $P=.0001$.
‡$P=.00000$.

Table 3.—Childhood Substance Abuse in Subjects With and Without Criminal Histories

Adult Diagnosis Status	Childhood Substance Abuse, %: Men: Crime	Men: No Crime	χ^2	Corrected P*	Women: Crime	Women: No Crime	χ^2	Corrected P*
No mental disorder or handicap	17.5	2.7	482.54 (1,N=6947)	.002	19.0	1.2	491.95 (1,N=6659)	.002
Other mental disorder	9.1	4.8	0.46 (1,N=64)	NS	0.0	5.4	0.01 (1,N=124)	NS
Major mental disorder	38.5	7.0	11.83 (1,N=82)	.002	28.6	4.6	5.49 (1,N=79)	NS
Intellectual handicap	22.4	9.1	3.74 (1,N=113)	NS	12.5	4.2	0.03 (1,N=79)	NS
Substance abuse	53.6	18.8	6.96 (1,N=156)	.01	54.0	11.4	15.41 (1,N=98)	.002

*Corrected for type I error by Bonferroni's formula. NS indicates not significant.

by definition, no subject in the group with any other mental disorder had an adult diagnosis of substance abuse/dependence.

COMMENT

An investigation of an unselected birth cohort followed up prospectively from pregnancy to age 30 years has demonstrated that, among both men and women, the proportions of subjects with at least one criminal offense vary significantly by adult mental status. Men with a major mental disorder were 2½ times more likely than men with no disorder or handicap to be registered for a criminal offense. Among women, the risk for those with a major mental disorder was five times higher than for women with no disorder or handicap. The risks of violent crime for both men and women with major mental disorders were even higher than for crime in general. The criminal behavior of subjects who eventually developed major disorders often appeared in early adolescence, well before the mental disorder would have been diagnosed. Intellectually handicapped men were three times more likely to be registered for a criminal offense than men with no disorder or handicap. Intellectually handicapped women were almost four times more likely to have been registered for an offense than women with no disorder or handicap. The risks of committing violent crime for both men and women with intellectual handicaps were even more elevated than those of committing crime generally. While criminality among the men with no disorder and no handicap decreased with age, this was not the case for those with major mental disorders. Significant numbers of these subjects began their criminal careers at all ages. The offenders with major mental disorders and those with intellectual handicaps committed multiple offenses of all types. Among both men and women, more of those with a major mental disorder and those with an intellectual handicap committed violent offenses and thefts.

These results are surprising, given that the subjects were only 30 years old when criminal offenses were documented. Investigations of persons responsible for violent crimes who were judged mentally disordered[52-57] and of inmates with major mental disorders[30] suggest that the mentally disordered commit crimes later in life than those with no mental disorder. The subjects in this cohort had not passed through the risk period for criminal behavior and had not passed through the risk period for the major mental disorders.[34] Thus, the age of the subjects would be expected to lessen the possibility of finding a difference in the proportions of mentally disordered and non–mentally disordered subjects convicted of crimes. In both the present investigation and Ortmann's study,[39] however, such differences were observed.

The association between major mental disorder and crime was weakened by excluding all subjects who died before the end of the follow-up period. A group of Swedish investigators[58] has shown increased mortality rates among mentally disordered offenders under age 30 years. Janson[59] has noted other factors that mitigated against finding such a difference in the present study. Persons sent to hospitals by the court were not counted. All had a diagnosis of psychosis, and "they would increase that male category's total offender rate by some 6% and the specific rates accordingly."[59(p49)] Men with psychoses also had less opportunity than other subjects to commit crimes because they were hospitalized, on average, for 552 days. Another factor that would also lessen the likelihood of finding higher rates of offending for those suffering from major mental disorders is the way in which admissions were documented. Patients still in the hospital at the time the data were collected were not included in the mentally disordered category.

Can we generalize from the results of this study? The specific crime rates cannot be generalized to other jurisdictions. The between-group comparisons can probably only be generalized to other countries with mental health systems, criminal justice systems, and social welfare systems similar to those in Sweden. To illustrate, the present results are similar to those of Ortmann[39] and Høgh and Wolf,[47] working in Denmark. However, consider extrapolating these results to the United States. In the United States, there is more crime and substance abuse than in Sweden but similar prevalence rates for the major mental disorders and for intellectual deficiency. Studies of mentally disordered persons would be expected to show that disproportionately more of the disordered commit crimes and violence. A sample of US offenders would be expected to include only a small proportion of subjects with major mental disorders and intellectual handicaps. Generally, that is what is reported. In other words, in the United States, given the large amount of crime and crime by substance abusers, the crimes of those with major psychiatric disorders and intellectual handicaps seem insignificant in comparison.

The within-group rates from the present investigation may be generalizable. The external validity of these findings may depend on the similarity of the ratio of crimes leading to prosecution compared with crimes committed and the similarity of the attitudes of the police and prosecuters toward the mentally disordered and intellectually handicapped.

The present findings correspond with results of studies in which significantly more subjects with major mental disorders, compared with those with no disorder, reported behaving aggressively.[60-62] The findings raise fundamental questions about these disorders, their etiology, and their treatment. A replication with a larger cohort, now under way, will allow us to examine the risk of criminality and violence by type of disorder.

This study was made possible by a grant for the author from the Enskilden Banken of Sweden to Leif Ojesjö. It was completed in collaboration with Carl-Gunnar Janson, PhD. Our thanks to Lennart Wetterberg, MD.

References

1. Convit A, Isay D, Gadioma R, Volavka J. Under-reporting of physical assaults in schizophrenic inpatients. *J Nerv Ment Dis*. 1988;176:507-509.

2. Lagos JM, Perlmutter K, Saexinger H. Fear of the mentally ill: empirical support for the common man's response. *Am J Psychiatry*. 1977;134:1134-1137.

3. Lion JR, Snyder W, Merrill GL. Under-reporting of assaults on staff in a state hospital. *Hosp Community Psychiatry*. 1981;32:497-498.

4. MacMillan JF, Johnson AL. Contact with the police in early schizophrenia: its nature, frequency and relevance to the outcome of treatment. *Med Sci Law*. 1987;27:191-200.

5. Incidence of violent patient admissions apparently stabilized at 37 percent. *Psychiatr News*. June 15, 1984.

6. Skodol AE, Karasu TB. Emergency psychiatry and the assaultive patient. *Am J Psychiatry*. 1978;135:202-205.

7. Tardiff K, Sweillam A. Assaultive behavior among chronic inpatients. *Am J Psychiatry*. 1982;139:212-215.

8. Durbin JR, Pasewark RA, Albers D. Criminality and mental illness: a study of current arrest rates in a rural state. *Am J Psychiatry*. 1977;134:80-83.

9. Giovanni JM, Gurel L. Socially disruptive behaviour of ex-mental patients. *Arch Gen Psychiatry*. 1967;17:146-153.

10. Rappeport JR, Lassen G. Dangerousness arrest rate comparisons of discharged patients and the general population. *Am J Psychiatry*. 1965;121:776-783.

11. Rappeport JR, Lassen G. The dangerousness of female patients: a comparison of the arrest rate of discharged psychiatric patients and the general population. *Am J Psychiatry*.1966;123:413-419.

12. Sosowsky L. Violence and the mentally ill. In: *Putting State Mental Hospitals out of Business: The Community Approach to Treating Mental Illness in San Mateo County*. Berkeley, Calif: University of California Graduate School of Public Policy; 1974:17-33.

13. Sosowsky L. Crime and violence among mental patients reconsidered in view of the new legal relationship between the state and the mentally ill. *Am J Psychiatry*.1978;135:33-42.

14. Sosowsky L. Explaining the increased arrest rate among mental patients: a cautionary note. *Am J Psychiatry*. 1980;137:1602-1605.

15. Steadman HJ, Cocozza JJ, Melick ME. Explaining the increased arrest rate among mental patients: the changing clientele of state hospitals. *Am J Psychiatry*. 1978;135:816-820.

16. Zitrin A, Hardesty AS, Burdock ET, Drossman AK. Crime and violence among mental patients. *Am J Psychiatry*. 1976;133:142-149.

17. Steadman HJ, Monahan J, Clark Robbins P, Appelbaum P, Grisso T, Klassen D, Mulvey E, Roth L. From dangerousness to risk assessment: implications for appropriate research strategies. In: Hodgins S, ed. *Mental Disorder and Crime*. Newbury Park, Calif: Sage Publications Inc. In press.

18. Cohen CI. Crime among mental patients: a critical analysis. *Psychiatr Q*. 1980;52:100-107.

19. Mesnikoff AM, Lauterbach CG. The association of violent dangerous behavior with psychiatric disorders: a review of the research literature. *J Psychiatr Law*. 1975;3:415-445.

20. Lindqvist P, Allebeck P. Schizophrenia and crime: a longitudinal follow-up of 644 schizophrenics in Stockholm. *Br J Psychiatry*. 1990; 157:345-350.

21. Lindqvist P, Allebeck P. Schizophrenia and assaultive behaviour: the role of alcohol and drug abuse. *Acta Psychiatr Scand*. 1989;82:191-195.

22. Silverton L. *Crime and the Schizophrenia Spectrum: A Study of Two Danish Cohorts*. Los Angeles, Calif: University of Southern California; 1985. Thesis.

23. Mednick SA, Parnas J, Schulsinger F. The Copenhagen high-risk project, 1962-1986. *Schizophr Bull*. 1987;13:485-496.

24. Asnarow JR. Children at risk for schizophrenia: converging lines of evidence. *Schizophr Bull*. 1988;14:613-631.

25. Kay SR. Significance of the positive-negative distinction in schizophrenia. *Schizophr Bull*. 1990;16:635-652.

26. Collins JJ, Schlenger WE. The prevalence of psychiatric disorder among admissions to prison. Presented at the 35th Annual Meeting of the American Society of Criminology; 1983; Denver, Colo.

27. Daniel AE, Robins AJ, Reid JC, Wilfley DE. Lifetime and 6-month prevalence of psychiatric disorders among sentenced female offenders. *Bull Am Acad Psychiatry Law*. 1988;16:333-342.

28. Hyde PS, Seiter RP. *The Prevalence of Mental Illness Among Inmates in the Ohio Prison System*. Columbus, Ohio: Dept of Mental Health and the Ohio Dept of Rehabilitation and Correction Interdepartmental Planning and Oversight Committee for Psychiatric Services to Corrections; 1987.

29. Neighbors HW, Williams DH, Gunnings TS, Lipscomb WD, Broman C, Lepkowski J. *The Prevalence of Mental Disorder in Michigan Prisons*. Ann Arbor, Mich: Michigan Dept of Corrections; 1987.

30. Hodgins S, Côté G. The prevalence of mental disorders among penitentiary inmates. *Can Ment Health*. 1990;38:1-5.

31. Abram KM. The effect of co-occurring disorders on criminal careers: interaction of antisocial personality, alcoholism, and drug disorders. *Int J Law Psychiatry*. 1989;12:133-148.

32. Côté G, Hodgins S. Co-occurring mental disorder among criminal offenders. *Bull Am Acad Psychiatry Law*. 1990;18:271-281.

33. American Psychiatric Association, Committee on Nomenclature and Statistics. *Diagnostic and Statistical Manual of Mental Disorders, Third Edition*. Washington, DC: American Psychiatric Association; 1980.

34. Robins LN, Helzer JE, Weissman MM, Orvaschel H, Gruenberg E,

Burke JD, Regier DA Jr. Lifetime prevalence of specific psychiatric disorders in three sites. *Arch Gen Psychiatry*. 1984;41:949-958.

35. Côté G. L'homicide et la recherche quantitative: aspects méthodologiques. *Rev Int Crimin Police Tech*. In press.

36. Gottlieb P, Gabrielsen G, Kramp P. Psychotic homicides in Copenhagen from 1959 to 1983. *Acta Psychiatr Scand*. 1987;76:285-292.

37. Lindqvist P. Criminal homicide in Northern Sweden, 1970. *Int J Law Psychiatry*. 1986;8:19-37.

38. Côté G, Hodgins S. The prevalence of major mental disorders among homicide offenders. *Int J Law Psychiatry*. 1992;15:89-99.

39. Ortmann J. *Psykisk ofvigelse og kriminel adfaerd en under sogelse af 11533 maend fodt i 1953 i det metropolitane omrade kobenhaun*. Copenhagen, Denmark: Rapport til Justitsministeriet, Direktoratet for kriminal forsorgen, Forksningsrapport; 1981. No. 17.

40. Reichel H. The intelligence-criminality relationship. In: Janson C-G, Janson A-M, eds. *Crime and Delinquency in a Metropolitan Cohort*. Stockholm, Sweden: Universitet Stockholms; 1989:7-29. Project Metropolitan Research Report 26.

41. Hirschi T, Hindelang MJ. Intelligence and deliquency: a revisionist review. *Am Sociol Rev*. 1977;42:571-587.

42. Wilson JQ, Hernstein RJ. *Crime and Human Nature*. New York, NY: Simon & Schuster; 1985.

43. Moffitt TE. The neuropsychology of juvenile delinquency: a critical review. In: Tonry M, Morris N, eds. *Crime and Justice: A Review of Research*. Chicago, Ill: University of Chicago Press; 1990:99-169.

44. West DJ, Farrington DP. *Who Becomes Delinquent?* London, England: Heinemann Educational Books Ltd; 1973.

45. Moffitt TE, Gabrielli WF, Mednick SA, Schulsinger F. Socioeconomic status, IQ, and delinquency. *J Abnorm Psychol*. 1981;90:152-156.

46. White JL, Moffitt TE, Silva PA. A prospective replication of the protective effects of IQ in subjects at high risk for juvenile delinquency. *J Consult Clin Psychol*. 1989;57:719-724.

47. Høgh E, Wolf P. Violent crime in a birth cohort: Copenhagen 1953-1977: Project Metropolitan: Denmark. Presented at the Symposium on Life History Research in Aggression and Antisocial Behavior; 1981; Monterey, Calif.

48. Janson C-G. *Project Metropolitan 21: A Longitudinal Study of a Stockholm Cohort*. Stockholm, Sweden: University of Stockholm; 1984.

49. Kristjansson E, Allebeck P, Wistedt B. Validity of the diagnosis schizophrenia in a psychiatric inpatient register. *Nord Psykiatr Tidsskr*. 1987;41:229-234.

50. Wetteberg L, Farmer AE. Clinical polydiagnostic studies in a large Swedish pedigree with schizophrenia. *Eur Arch Psychiatry Clin Neurosci*. 1990;240:188-190.

51. Wikström POH. Age and crime in a Stockholm cohort. In: Janson C-G, Janson A-M, eds. *Crime and Human Nature*. New York, NY: Simon & Schuster; 1989.

52. Häfner H, Böker W. *Crimes of Violence by Mentally Abnormal Offenders*. Cambridge, England: Cambridge University Press; 1982.

53. Walker N, McCabe S. *Crime and Insanity in England, II*. Edinburgh, Scotland: Edinburgh University Press; 1973.

54. Hodgins S, Webster C, Paquet J, Zellerer E. *Annual Report Year-1 Canadian Database: Patients Held on Lieutenant-Governor's Warrants*. Ottawa, Ontario; Ministère de la Justice; 1989.

55. Hodgins S, Webster C, Paquet J. *Annual Report Year-2 Canadian Database: Patients Held on Lieutenant-Governor's Warrants*. Ottawa, Ontario: Ministère de la Justice; 1990.

56. Hodgins S, Webster C, Paquet J. *Annual Report Year-3 Canadian Database: Patients Held on Lieutenant-Governor's Warrants*. Ottawa, Ontario: Ministère de la Justice; 1991.

57. Pasewark RA. Insanity plea: a review of the research literature. *J Psychiatry Law*. 1982;9:357-402.

58. Lidberg L, Wiklund N, Jakobsson SW. Mortality among criminals with suspected mental disturbance. *Scand J Soc Med*. 1988;17:59-65.

59. Janson C-G. Psychiatric diagnoses and recorded crimes. In: Janson C-G, Janson A-M, eds. *Crime and Delinquency in a Metropolitan Cohort*. Stockholm: University of Stockholm. 1989:31-55.

60. Swanson JW, Hozer CE, Ganju VK, Jono RT. Violence and psychiatric disorder in the community: evidence from the epidemiologic catchment area surveys. *Hosp Community Psychiatry*. 1990; 41:761-770.

61. Link BG, Andrews H, Cullen FT. Reconsidering the dangerousness of mental patients: violent and illegal behavior of current and former patients compared to controls. *Am Sociol Rev*. In press.

62. Steadman HJ, Felson RB. Self-reports of violence: ex-mental patients, ex-offenders, and the general population. *Criminology*. 1984; 22:321-342.

Violence (and a Message for the 90s?)

Egregious instances of violence stun the human consciousness into momentary, horrified silence. Their frequency dulls the senses. Such acts by definition abrogate discourse and the vocabulary we normally use in regulating collective and individual excesses. Thus, the challenge by George Lundberg and C. Everett Koop to the American Medical Association family of journals to address their June issues to aspects of violence that are medically relevant is timely.

Yet, the breach of norms and aspirations entailed in violence comprises a difficult complex of behaviors for the intrinsically limited sciences to disaggregate and engage. We still lack an adequate classificatory "anatomy" of different aggressive behaviors and the biosocial contexts in which they arise. Clinical and forensic psychiatry daily deal with specific problems (even though the latter's intimate experiences with aberrancies are poorly articulated for the practitioner). General psychiatry, using psychodynamic insights, often recognizes "negative identifications" in instances of impulsive "acting out." In their choreography, these acts can contain the "text" of unnoted and unmastered early experience. Without indulging the current cults of exculpatory victimology, patients may learn that such acting constitutes a search for what has not been reflectively remembered. Instead, others reflexively receive what the patient once did. And, in attempts to do better, the rigidities of zealous righteousness are often found to be projections on others (or in social causes) of fearfully disowned impulses that cannot otherwise be self controlled; in "reaction formation" the dedicated rule-enforcer is still dangerously close to the forbidden impulse. These familiar dynamics and the various arts and techniques subsumed under "conflict resolution" all have their place in the pragmatic work of psychiatry and the social sciences.

One could, in editorializing on the topic, catalog the profound reflections on human nature by philosophers, theologians, and writers, reflecting the fact that various cultures and mores exist to rationalize and implement our egoistic, affiliative, and antagonistic urges and needs. Thomas Mann referred to the necessity to face the "dark side of truth" about ourselves: the ghastly collective acts we may disown nevertheless stem from the nature of all humankind. And psychiatry is aware of Freud's ponderings about the dual instincts (Eros and Thanatos) we each must manage and, from *Civilization and Its Discontents*, of his reflections on "various schools of worldly wisdom" as they pursue different but imperfect paths to balance pleasure and pain, self and society, or "us" vs a perpetually alien "them."

Editorial columns do not lend themselves to these deeper issues, nor can the clinical sciences through philosophizing or moralizing evade the targeted, often complex specific issues with which they are charged to cope. Such tasks are more mundane, but are the focus of professional expertise in the pragmatics of biomedicine. Thus all issues of the ARCHIVES depend on the spontaneous submissions that scholars and researchers offer for our review of their treatment of quite specific problems. An exception for this issue is our invitation to Eichelman and to Tardiff to provide "summary viewpoints"—one on the psychobiology of aggressive behaviors and the other on particular problems of violence in the severe mental illnesses.

Nevertheless, anxiously scanning the mail for relevant submissions, I found myself musing on matters philosophical. I recalled a long out of print book, *Limbo*, by Bernard Wolfe, published in 1952 by Random House. Wolfe, who had studied in the Yale Psychology Department, put together what he called a "bilious rib," a "grab bag" of scientific and intellectual ideas that were around in the early 1950s. After Huxley and Orwell, he created a kind of science fiction novel and morality play as he envisaged the world of 1990—a full 18 years after a super-catastrophic World War III.

At the end of the mutual destruction, in 1972, the hero, Dr Martine, a neurosurgeon and physiologist, has barely escaped the intractable grip of the super-computers of East and West. Their algorithms' inexorable logic had not only led to the war but had replaced both societal and personal decisions. In Martine's sardonic, windy, and pun-littered diary on all this, he notes the necessity to "dodge the steamroller," and finds a home and family and continues laboratory studies on an unmapped Pacific island. There the Mandunji, in an escape from their own voracious tribal wars, have for 600 years practiced pacifism. Their name is translated "Heads without Devils" and their ceremonial practices (including occasional lobotomy) chase devils from the head. They preach that "man finds himself when he belongs to his community," yet Martine observed tribal members are almost "incognito," lacking individual expression and "confusing energy with belligerence." The tribe are discovered in 1990 by a band of touring postwar pioneers and are astonished to see them performing remarkable acrobatic feats and quotidian tasks of labor with translucent, multiwired prosthetic limbs replacing the natural ones.

To decipher where the world has come, Martine sets sail on the *SS Norbert Wiener* and finds the remnants of society totally dedicated to nonaggression in their technologically advanced underground cities. East and West are gathering for Winter Olympics to celebrate feats performed with the startlingly magnified power of the new prosthetic technologies. To mentally control these feats requires intense training in "D & D's" (discernments and dexterities); whether the brain can truly achieve steadfast perfection in managing this power is problematic. Martine's diary, abandoned on his escape, has become the bible of new societies now "mired in mission." Replacing the gideon, it and William James's *The Moral Equivalent of War* are at every bedside.

In the service of pacifism all is reverence, the wisecrack exiled and the politically correct populace constantly reminded of aggression's dangers in televised sound bites and snappy catch phrases: "No demobilization without immobilization." New heroes are the Vol-Amps (voluntary amputees), those who literally disarm. There are sharp political struggles between the elite Vol-Amps with prostheses—the "pro-pros"—and the devout "anti-pros" who believe the absence of limbs is the highest achievement, but all piously repeat "Dodge the Steamroller." Yet in marshaling against the horrors of man's aggression, an ideologically pacific statism becomes, albeit unrecognized, a new steamroller as the old is dodged. The Vol-Amps of East and West have in fact been secretly competing in a frantic search for the rare metal essential to energize their powerful limbs. That their nimble prostheses, in a denouement at the Olympics, are stealthily replaced by potent engines of destruction is not surprising. Martine reescapes to his island, but has reason to hope that a remnant—his son and a few inquiring skeptical seekers of responsible self-possession—may yet discover truths as he had from his reflections and research.

Of his sustained scientific searches on the island to remove aggression with an innovative array of depth electrodes in the brain, he says in exasperation: "Done it again . . . God damn Siamese twins. I have cut out the aggression, I have also cut out the orgasm, can't seem to separate the two." The truth of this fictional metaphor aside, Martine discerns that both excitation and inhibition are within even the single synapse and derides himself as a skilled "tailor of protoplasm" but "anything *worth* doing, I can't."

The notion that violence is a "thing," that it can be totally extirpated by drugs, surgery, science, slogans, or idealistic mass movements, Martine implies, will persist. Perhaps, he counsels, we must, individually and socially, take responsible charge of our situation and decisions. If so, we would be ever mindful of our un-untangleable complex of loving, egoistic, and ferocious urges—and above all transcend the temptations of self-justification via archenemies, over-arching rules, and deceptively simple answers (or determined denial of social challenges so starkly evident to the eye that can see).

For psychiatry, behavioral biology, brain neurocircuitry, and genetic and molecular regulatory pathways will surely throw more light on some aspects of certain dyscontrolled behaviors and their possible repair. Yet both our aspirations for this promise and the uses we can make of it face intrinsic constraints. "Science discloses," Martine observes, "but politics disposes." Further, Limbo lies forever imperfect *between* the pure and absolute polarities of our enduring visions of heaven and hell. Perhaps for an Earth so intractably located, Dr Martine had a challenge and a cautionary message for the 1990s.

DANIEL X. FREEDMAN, MD
Chief Editor

Aggressive Behavior: From Laboratory to Clinic

Quo Vadit?

Burr Eichelman, MD, PhD

• This article sets forth two theses: (1) that animal models of aggressive behavior have utility in fostering and guiding human aggression research; and (2) that clinical violence research should now focus on the severely and repetitively aggressive patients for study and therapeutic research. Animal models are reviewed in terms of typology; studies of temperament; the role of sensory cues; neuroanatomy, neurochemistry, and neuroendocrinology; studies of stress; and studies of social conditions. Examples are presented that have implications and potential utility for human research. Clinical approaches to the study of human aggressive behavior are examined and five suggestions are made to enhance the efficacy and utility of clinically relevant aggression research.

(*Arch Gen Psychiatry.* 1992;49:488-492)

This month, the journals of the American Medical Association feature violence as a relevant issue for American medicine. In addition to assembling research articles focused in this area and a clinical review of violence in psychiatric patients,[1] the chief editor has requested—assertively, not aggressively—an article about the progress of aggression research and its clinical applications for psychiatry during the past three decades, with comments about future research and clinical strategies.

Despite having studied animal models of aggression for nearly three decades, having treated both general and forensic psychiatric patients who have shown repetitively violent behavior, and having participated in innovative clinical treatment development, this is a substantial task. To accomplish this task, I have chosen to select studies from the literature as examples. This is neither a review of the biology of aggressive behavior nor of the clinical aggression literature. Other reviews of the biology,[2] the neurochemistry,[3] psychopharmacology,[4,5] and clinical management[6,7] are available elsewhere. This article will focus predominantly on patient populations rather than on societal violence for reasons addressed at the end of this article. Two theses are set forth: (1) that animal models of aggressive behavior have utility in fostering and guiding human aggression research; and (2) that clinical violence research should now focus on the severely and repetitively aggressive patients for study and therapeutic research. Both theses have several corollaries.

Accepted for publication March 18, 1992.

From the Department of Psychiatry, Temple University School of Medicine, Philadelphia, Pa.

Presented in part at the North Atlantic Treaty Organization conference on Crime and Mental Illness, Il Ciocco, Italy, August 30, 1991.

Reprint requests to Department of Psychiatry, Temple University School of Medicine, 3401 N Broad St, Philadelphia, PA 19140.

THE UTILITY OF ANIMAL MODELS OF AGGRESSIVE BEHAVIOR

Animal models of aggressive behavior have provided a strong conceptual base for approaching the study of human aggressive behavior. Several concepts have evolved from the animal literature that have focused on human aggression research and promised further guidance for research.

Typology

An understanding of the typology of a species' aggressive behaviors is essential. Moyer[8] divided aggressive animal behaviors into seven classes: predatory, intermale, fear-induced, irritable, territorial, maternal, and instrumental. Reis[9,10] regrouped Moyer's classes into two categories: affective aggression and predatory aggression. Affective aggression is characterized by marked sympathetic arousal and vocalizations, and is generally intraspecific (ie, between animals of the same species). It can be divided further into offensive and defensive behaviors.[11] Predatory aggression is without significant arousal and is generally interspecific (ie, between animals of different species). The neural circuitry of these behaviors can be separated.[12,13] Brain lesions or drugs can produce changes in one class of aggressive behavior without necessarily affecting another. For example, lesions of the septal nuclei in the rat produce an increase in shock-elicited fighting characterized by an increase in *defensive*, affective aggression (eg, bites to the snout and upright boxing posture). Lesions of the ventromedial nucleus of the hypothalamus produce an increase in *offensive*, affective aggression (eg, bites to the rump).[14] Tricyclic antidepressants enhance affective aggressive behavior,[15] but suppress predatory aggressive behavior.[16]

Little attention has been given to the development of a precise typology or ethologic study of human aggressive behaviors. The differences in the assaultive behavior patterns of patients with differing disorders such as schizophrenia, senile dementia, or particular types of mental retardation remain undifferentiated. Careful development of the typologies of patient aggressive behavior may assist in prediction, classification, and new treatment strategies for patient populations. Thus far, only preliminary attempts have been made in this regard.[17]

Temperament

From the early work by Scott and Fuller[18] with dogs, to more recent studies with rodents and feral animals, it is clear that temperament can be genetically shaped. Mice[19] and rat[20] strains differ widely in levels of aggressive behavior. In relatively few generations of selective breeding, nonaggressive and highly aggressive variants can be created in both laboratory[21] and feral[22] animals. Genetic selection for other behaviors such as performance in an open field, performance in avoidance paradigms, or neurochemical attributes produce rat strains significantly different in levels of aggressive behavior.[20,23] The strains differ in terms of neurotransmitter chemistry[24] and second-messenger systems.[25] A systematic neurochemical analysis of the differences in laboratory animals genetically bred for extremes of aggressive behavior could provide clues for the study of the neurochemistry of human temperament. This research may provide the conceptual link between low central serotonin responsivity[26] or low levels of cerebrospinal fluid 5-hydroxyindoleacetic acid (5-HIAA)[27] and measures of impulsivity. Paying more attention to temperament in aggressive clinical patients might also increase our awareness of the role of the varied typographies in aggressive behavior that appear in patients who subsequently develop disorders such as schizophrenia or senile dementia. Understanding the associated neurochemistry would provide means for specific psychopharmacologic therapies.

Sensory Cues

Animal models illustrate the importance of sensory cues in the induction and inhibition of aggressive behavior. Removal of the olfactory bulbs in rat models increases predatory aggression, but has little effect on shock-induced fighting (affective aggression).[28] Clipping rats' vibrissae suppresses affective aggression as successfully as bilateral amygdala lesions.[14] A change in sensory input affecting aggression can be induced by electrical excitation in the brain. Bandler and Flynn[29] demonstrated that the "trigger point" for eliciting predatory behavior by contact with a cat's forepaw can be enlarged with hypothalamic brain stimulation. Post[30] has documented a marked increase in irritability in kindled rats that develop generalized seizures of limbic origin following chronic treatment with lidocaine hydrochloride. Such changes in sensory thresholds or irritability strike a resonant chord with the observations by Kinzel[31] concerning "body buffer zones." *Body-buffer zones* was the term given to the physical space surrounding violent or nonviolent prisoners, that, if intruded on, induced a sense of uneasiness or threat to the subject. Prisoners convicted of violent crimes reported larger body-buffer zones than did prisoners convicted of nonviolent crimes.[31]

Perhaps kindling, subclinical epilepsy, or grand mal epilepsy in humans alter sensory perceptions or responsivity that would lead to increases in aggressive behavior. In one study,[32] 65% of habitually aggressive criminals showed abnormal electroencephalograms, whereas in the normal control population, only 12% showed abnormal electroencephalograms. In a study of children with temporal lobe and grand mal epilepsy, Nuffield[33] reported a fourfold increase over the levels of aggressive behavior in a control group with petit mal epilepsy.

With the advent of noninvasive positron emission tomography technology to assess brain metabolism, there is a need for studying repetitively aggressive patients for signs of abnormal brain metabolism that might substantiate kindling or subclinical epilepsy. Behaviorally, such central abnormalities need to be characterized as to their effect on perception and other parameters such as irritability. This type of research could well identify the patient populations for whom anticonvulsant therapies might be effective.

Neuroanatomy, Neurochemistry, and Neuroendocrinology

The animal studies regarding the neuroanatomy and neurochemistry of aggressive behavior have rapidly generated a conceptual view of the brain and aggressive behavior. Following the electrical stimulation studies by Hess,[34] the search began for an "aggression center." This search failed as it became apparent that limbic, hypothalamic, and brain stem regions, among others, all modulated aggressive behavior. After abandoning the search for a specific site, the quest began for a specific neurotransmitter. This quest also failed. Aggressive behavior may be modulated through many neuroanatomic sites and through the modulation of many neurotransmitter systems, including serotonin, norepinephrine, dopamine, acetylcholine, γ-aminobutyric acid, and the opioids.[3,35]

Despite the complexity of the neurochemistry of aggressive behavior, animal studies illustrated decisively that aggressive behavior could be markedly altered through the modification of specific neurotransmitter systems. Reviews of the animal literature in the early 1970s[10,36] presaged the subsequent human research implicating norepinephrine[37,38] and serotonin[26,27,37] in aggressive behavior disorders and the therapeutic efficacy of β-adrenergic blockers[39,40] and serotonin-enhancing drugs such as tryptophan,[41] trazodone hydrochloride,[42] and buspirone hydrochloride.[43] Animal studies also demonstrate that pharmacologic effects might only be observed in pathologically aggressive (brain-injured) animals. For example, the aggression reducing the effect of tryptophan in the rat is not seen in normal rats,[44] but only in brain-injured rats.[45] Looking ahead, a whole new chapter in the neurochemistry of aggressive behavior appears ready to unfold as research on neuromodulators such as cholecystokinin[46] identifies other potent central modulators of aggressive behavior.

Neuroendocrinologically, animal studies have demonstrated a significant role for testosterone in inducing aggressive behavior in males of a species.[47] Yet, in humans, while some studies have reported positive correlations of testosterone levels with aggressive behavior or psychological ratings of aggression,[48-50] these studies have not been solidly replicated[51] and account for a relatively small percentage of the variance in predicting aggressive behavior.[48]

There may be an interesting parallel between testosterone and serotonin. While low whole-blood levels of serotonin have been reported to be associated with aggressive behavior,[42,52] this has not been a consistent finding. What appears relevant for serotonin is the brain's response to serotonergic stimulation.[26] Central probe studies of testosterone "sensitivity" may be more productive than the measurement of peripheral levels. An animal model study[53] illustrates this point. Connor et al[53] studied the level of pain-induced fighting in normal male rats with and without exogenous testosterone treatment, in male rats castrated at weaning but tested in adulthood with and without exogenous testosterone, and in male rats castrated at birth—while significant brain development is occurring—but tested in adulthood with and without exogenous testosterone. In the group castrated at weaning, rats without exogenous testosterone treatment fought significantly less, but exogenous testosterone treatment increased their fighting to normal levels. They were "testosterone sensitive." The rats castrated at birth also fought less, but continued to fight less despite treatment with exogenous testosterone. They appeared to be "testosterone insensitive." This experiment, like the human observations with adrenogenital children[54] and children treated with female hormones in utero,[55] suggests that hormone levels in utero may affect the organization of the brain during development. The sensitivity to circulating hormones may be far more important and predictive of behavior than the actual level of hormone present at the time of a violent or aggressive act.

Stress

Environmental manipulation can alter brain chemistry and induces aggressive behavior. Isolation in the mouse[56] and sleep deprivation[57] or immobilization[58] in the rat can induce marked increases in affective aggression. Some of the neurochemical changes persist well beyond the cessation of the stressor, and the induced aggressive behavior similarly persists.[58] In the rat,[58,59] these stressors induce alterations in tyrosine hydroxylase activity and β-adrenergic receptor down-regulation, suggestive of enhanced noradrenergic activity. Similar behavioral alterations marked by increased aggressive behavior can be seen in primates that have been maternally deprived.[60] Such observations seriously raise the question of whether environmentally stressed humans (eg, physically abused children) sustain persistent central biochemical changes that induce a diathesis for aggressive behavior in adulthood.

Aggressive behavior may also serve to reduce untoward effects of stressors on the organism. Rats footshocked alone show an elevation in tail blood pressure. If shocked in the presence of another rat, there is a decrease in tail blood pressure.[61] This coincides with the observation that corticotropin release is less for a rat shocked in the presence of another rat (where fighting can occur) than for the rat shocked alone where the only possible behavior is ineffective jumping to escape footshock.[62] Thus, particular aggressive behaviors in rats reduce stress. Perhaps some of the repetitive aggressive behavior in patient populations, especially in patients who have been institutionalized long-term, actually reduces stress. This behavior then becomes a positive operant for such behavior. It is unclear, or at least untried, whether another behavior that is nonaggressive may be substituted to reduce stress.

Social Conditions

Aggressive animal behavior is often dyadic and occurs in a complex social environment. Treating the submissive member of a rat pair with a neuroleptic agent decreases the attack behavior of the dominant nontreated rat.[63] Whole-blood serotonin levels are elevated in the α-males of a primate colony,[64] but these levels drop if the α-male is removed. Furthermore, the β-male then develops the increased whole-blood serotonin levels. Alcohol given to a dominant mouse may produce sedation, but a comparable dose given to a submissive mouse can elicit increased aggressive behavior.[65]

As the animal studies indicate, it is crucial to pay attention to social factors such as hierarchy when studying aggressive behavior. Therefore, because human interaction is extremely complex and diverse, it is even more critical to pay strict attention to social conditions when studying human aggressive behavior.

THE NEED TO FOCUS ON THE SEVERELY AND REPETITIVELY AGGRESSIVE PATIENT

Psychiatry's increased understanding of the neural bases of aggressive behavior has been substantial during the past three decades, as illustrated above. Psychiatric hospitals,[66] mental retardation centers,[67] and nursing homes[68] are populated with patients displaying frequent and erratic bouts of aggressive behaviors, despite the professional "understanding" of aggressive behavior. Even with the application of many psychopharmacologic agents (lithium carbonate, benzodiazepines, neuroleptic agents, serotonin-enhancing drugs, anticonvulsants, stimulants, and β-blockers) and the potential of new agents such as the "serenics" (serotonin agonists),[69,70] psychiatry is only marginally successful in the treatment of the repetitively aggressive psychiatric patient. Certainly the episodic but dangerous behaviors can serve to dissuade researchers. Such patients pose severe strategic problems for protocol compliance, not to mention issues of research consent. Several systematic hindrances for applied research exist apart from the characteristics of the patients' behaviors. These need to be addressed to advance the clinical field of therapeutic aggression research. They are (1) the need to develop an accepted nosology that includes neutral descriptors for aggressive behaviors; (2) the need to develop and agree on standardized inpatient and outpatient rating scales to assess efficacy of interventions; (3) the need to develop alternative research strategies to demonstrate drug efficacy (single subject research design); (4) the need to effect changes in the Food and Drug Administration's policy to allow psychotropic drug "approved use" for the "symptom" of aggressive behavior after the demonstration of clinical efficacy achieved through multiple studies of single subject research rather than by studies of large, double-blind populations; and (5) the need for research agencies such as the National Institute of Mental Health to support further studies on the biological correlates of human aggressive behavior. These studies are needed to develop new, less invasive indicators of cerebrospinal fluid function. They are also necessary to establish the relationship within the same patient of various neural correlates. For example, clinicians need to know, if possible, the relationship of whole-blood serotonin levels, the amount of tritiated imipramine binding to platelets, the response to serotonin probes, and the cerebrospinal fluid level of 5-HIAA in the same patient, especially in a patient for whom one or more of these indexes is markedly abnormal.

Psychiatry continues to wrestle with the terms *aggressive, assaultive,* and *violent* behavior. These terms carry clinical and nonclinical meanings and connotations. Either a more precise clinical definition of the type of erratic, episodic violence manifested in clinical populations should be adopted, or a new term—perhaps *destructive* behavior[71]—should be adopted and reserved for clinical use and incorporated into hospital record keeping. As *DSM-III-R*[72] presently stands, a violent schizophrenic and a nonviolent schizophrenic are diagnosed and coded identically. This makes retrospective research and even the maintenance of this population of patients as an identifiable group (across psychiatric diagnosis) impossible.

At present, standardized rating scales for aggressive behavior are poorly developed compared with those available for the study of depression. Considerable effort is needed to develop and test the validity and reliability of inpatient rating scales like the Overt Aggression Scale[73] and to develop and test outpatient rating scales valid enough to allow for use in subsequent psychopharmacologic efficacy studies.

With standardized assessment tools, psychiatry needs to undertake systematic blinded studies of the various psychotropic agents currently touted as effective in attenuating aggressive behavior. Given the heterogeneity of these patients, significant effects may be lost through a homogenization of patients' individual variances while attempting to meet traditional standards of efficacy. An approach more likely to succeed in demonstrating efficacy for these compounds would be through the adoptions of single subject research designs[74] that use repetitively assaultive patients studied within an alternating control-treatment-control-treatment (ie, ABAB) design. This would need to be coupled with willingness by the Food and Drug Administration to approve drugs evaluated this way.

Intense "case study" approach may well offer a fresh and productive route for new discovery. This was a successful approach to the study of neural deficits, especially the aphasias and apraxias.[75] Such patients as the one with Cornelia de Lange syndrome as described by O'Neil et al[42] may hold significant clues in their pathology for the understanding of the biology of aggressive behavior; this patient demonstrated a very low whole-blood serotonin level associated with aggressive behavior. The behavior was attenuated by trazodone hydrochloride, which induced a ten-fold rise in whole-blood serotonin. Intense, focused study of serotonin metabolism through study of cerebrospinal fluid serotonin or 5-HIAA levels, tritiated imipramine platelet binding, and serotonin probes might point to a biological defect that could explain the role of serotonin in aggressive behavior.

Apologia

This article has not addressed the country's social epidemic of violence. It has not addressed the fact that homicides exceed deaths by emphysema, bronchitis, and asthma combined,[76] or that battery is the single most common injury for women in this country (*Time*. September 5, 1983:23). It does not address the fact that in this country, homicide is disproportionately high in the black American population. It does not address the role of drugs and drug-seeking behavior in an epidemic of violence. It does not address the role of firearms or violence on television. It does not address the role of alcohol in violence, particularly homicide both for the victim[77] and the killer.[78] Simply stated, the reason for not addressing these issues, is that they appear to this writer as more political than simply "medical" issues and beyond the scope of this article. However, this nation has the resources, technical and economic, to spend on addressing and (even) solving the myriad of social ills that plague the country. It is a political decision *not* to expend these resources in a responsible manner that will improve the human condition. Mere clinical research in medicine is not enough to overcome political narrowmindedness. Indeed, medical research, as a part of the political process, should remain ever alert not to become complacent or worse, disassociated from the social problems of our time, which it presumably tries to study.

I thank A. Hartwig, JD, PhD, for her comments and review of the manuscript.

References

1. Tardiff K. The current state of psychiatry in the treatment of violent patients. *Arch Gen Psychiatry.* 1992;49:493-499.
2. Brain PF, Benton D, eds. *The Biology of Aggression.* Alphen aan den Rijn, the Netherlands: Sijthoff & Noordhoff; 1981:637.
3. Eichelman B. Neurochemical and psychopharmacologic aspects of aggressive behavior. In: Meltzer HY, ed. *Psychopharmacology: The Third Generation of Progress.* New York, NY: Raven Press; 1987:697-704.
4. Miczek K. The psychopharmacology of aggression. In: Iversen LL, Iversen SD, Snyder SH, eds. *Handbook of Psychopharmacology, XIX.* New York, NY: Plenum Publishing Corp; 1987:183-328.
5. Eichelman B. Toward a rational pharmacotherapy for aggressive and violent behavior. *Hosp Community Psychiatry.* 1988;39:31-39.
6. Eichelman B. Psychiatric mental health nursing with the violent patient. In: Gary F, Kavanagh CK, eds. *Psychiatric Mental Health Nursing.* Philadelphia, Pa: JB Lippincott; 1990:900-920.
7. Tardiff K. *Assessment and Management of Violent Patients.* Washington, DC: American Psychiatric Association; 1989.
8. Moyer KE. Kinds of aggression and their physiological basis. *Community Behav Biol A.* 1968;2:65-87.
9. Reis D. Brain monoamines in aggression and sleep. *Clin Neurosurg.* 1971;18:471-502.
10. Reis D. Central neurotransmitters in aggression. *Res Publ Assoc Res Nerv Ment Dis.* 1974;52:119-148.
11. Blanchard RJ, Blanchard DC, Takahashi T, Kelley M. Attack and defensive behaviour in the albino rat. *Anim Behav.* 1977;25:622-634.
12. Chi CC, Flynn JP. Neural pathways associated with hypothalamically elicited attack behavior in cats. *Science.* 1971;171:703-706.
13. Chi CC, Flynn JP. Neuroanatomic projections related to biting attack elicited from hypothalamus in cats. *Brain Res.* 1971;35:49-66.
14. Eichelman B. Effect of subcortical lesions on shock-induced aggression in the rat. *J Comp Physiol Psychol.* 1971;74:331-339.
15. Eichelman B, Barchas J. Facilitated shock-induced aggression following antidepressive medication in the rat. *Pharmacol Biochem Behav.* 1975;3:601-604.
16. Katz RJ. Catecholamines in predatory behavior: a review and critique. *Aggress Behav.* 1978;4:153-172.
17. Crowner ML, Douyon R, Convit A, Volavka J. Videotape recording of assaults on a state hospital inpatient ward. *J Neuropsychiatry Clin Neurosci.* 1991;3(suppl):9-14.
18. Scott JP, Fuller J. *Genetics and the Social Behavior of the Dog.* Chicago, Ill: University of Chicago Press; 1965:468.
19. Southwick CH, Clark LH. Interstrain differences in aggressive behavior and exploratory activity of inbred mice. *Community Behav Biol.* 1968;1A:49-59.
20. Eichelman B. Variability in rat irritable and predatory aggression. *Behav Neural Biol.* 1980;29:498-505.
21. Lagerspetz KMJ, Lagerspetz KYH. Changes in the aggressiveness of mice resulting from selective breeding, learning, and social isolation. *Scand J Psychol.* 1971;12:241-248.
22. Popova NK, Voitenko NN, Kulikov AV, Avgustinovich DF. Evidence for the involvement of central serotonin in mechanism of domestication of silver foxes. *Pharmacol Biochem Behav.* 1991;40:751-756.
23. Pucilowski O, Eichelman B, Overstreet DH, Rezvani AH, Janowsky D. Enhanced affective aggression in genetically bred hyper-

cholinergic rats. *Neuropsychobiology.* 1990;24:37-41.
24. Slater J, Blizard DA, Pohorecky LA. Central and peripheral norepinephrine metabolism in rat strains selectively bred for differences in response to stress. *Pharmacol Biochem Behav.* 1977;6:511-520.
25. Orenberg EK, Renson J, Elliott, GR, Barchas JD, Kessler S. Genetic determination of aggressive behavior and brain cyclic AMP. *Psychopharmacol Commun.* 1975;1:99-107.
26. Coccaro EF, Siever LJ, Klar H, Maurer G, Cochrane K, Cooper TB, Mohs RC, Davis KL. Serotonergic studies in patients with affective and personality disorders: correlates with suicidal and impulsive aggressive behavior. *Arch Gen Psychiatry.* 1989;46:587-599.
27. Linnoila M, Virkkunen M, Scheinin M, Nuutila A, Rimon R, Goodwin FK. Low cerebrospinal fluid 5-hydroxyindoleacetic acid concentration differentiates impulsive from nonimpulsive violent behavior. *Life Sci.* 1983;33:2609-2614.
28. Bugbee NM, Eichelman B. Sensory alterations and aggressive behavior in the rat. *Physiol Behav.* 1972;8:981-985.
29. Bandler RJ, Flynn JP. Control of somatosensory fields for striking during hypothalamically elicited attack. *Brain Res.* 1972;38:197-201.
30. Post RM. Lidocaine-kindled limbic seizures: behavioral implications. In: Wada JA, ed. *Kindling 2.* New York, NY: Raven Press; 1981:149-160.
31. Kinzel AF. Body-buffer zone in violent prisoners. *Am J Psychiatry.* 1970;127:99-104.
32. Williams D. Neural factors related to habitual aggression. *Brain.* 1970;92:503-520.
33. Nuffield EJ. Neurophysiology and behaviour disorders in epileptic children. *J Ment Sci.* 1961;107:438-458.
34. Hess WR. *The Functional Organization of the Diencephalon.* New York, NY: Grune & Stratton; 1957:180.
35. Shaikh MB, Chang-Lin L, Siegel A. Affective defense behavior elicited from the feline midbrain periaqueductal gray is regulated by u and s opioid receptors. *Brain Res.* 1991;557:344-348.
36. Eichelman B, Thoa NB. The aggressive monoamines. *Biol Psychiatry.* 1973;6:143-164.
37. Brown GL, Goodwin FK, Ballenger JC, Goyer PF, Major LF. Aggression in humans correlates with cerebrospinal fluid amine metabolites. *Psychiatry Res.* 1979;1:131-139.
38. Coccaro EF, Lawrence T, Trestman R, Gabriel S, Klar HM, Siever LJ. Growth hormone responses to intravenous clonidine challenge correlate with behavioral irritability in psychiatric patients and healthy volunteers. *Psychiatry Res.* 1991;39:129-139.
39. Elliott FA. Propranolol for the control of belligerent behavior following acute brain damage. *Ann Neurol.* 1977;1:489-491.
40. Yudofsky S, Williams D, Gorman J. Propranolol in the treatment of rage and violent behavior in patients with chronic brain syndromes. *Am J Psychiatry.* 1981;138:218-220.
41. Morand C, Young SN, Ervin F. Clinical response of aggressive schizophrenics to oral tryptophan. *Biol Psychiatry.* 1983;18:575-578.
42. O'Neil M, Page N, Adkins WN, Eichelman B. Tryptophan-trazodone treatment of aggressive behavior. *Lancet.* 1986;2:859-860.
43. Ratey J, Sovner R, Parks A, Rogentine K. Buspirone treatment of aggression and anxiety in mentally retarded patients: a multiple-baseline, placebo lead-in study. *J Clin Psychiatry.* 1991;52:159-162.
44. Kantak KM, Hegstrand L, Whitman J, Eichelman B. Effects of dietary supplements and a tryptophan-free diet on aggressive behavior in rats. *Pharmacol Biochem Behav.* 1980;12:173-179.
45. Kantak KM, Hegstrand L, Eichelman B. Dietary tryptophan reversal of septal lesion and 5,7-DHT lesion elicited shock-induced fighting. *Pharmacol Biochem Behav.* 1981;15:343-350.
46. Pletnikov MV. The participation of the octapeptide cholecystokinin and beta-endorphin in the neurochemical support of the interspecific and intraspecific aggressivity of rats. *Zh Vys Nerv Dei atel Im I P Pavlova.* 1989;39:770-773.
47. Svare B, ed. *Hormones and Aggressive Behavior.* New York, NY: Plenum Publishing Corp; 1982:595.
48. Olweus D, Mattsson A, Schalling D, Low H. Circulating testosterone levels and aggression in adolescent males: a causal analysis. *Psychosom Med.* 1988;50:261-272.
49. Kreuz LE, Rose RM. Assessment of aggressive behavior and plasma testosterone in a young criminal population. *Psychosom Med.* 1972;34:321-332.
50. Rada RT, Laws DR, Kellner R. Plasma testosterone levels in the rapist. *Psychosom Med.* 1976;38:257-268.
51. Meyer-Bahlburg HFL, Boon DA, Sharma M, Edward JA. Aggressiveness and testosterone measures in man. *Psychosom Med.* 1974;36:269-274.
52. Greenberg AS, Coleman M. Depressed 5-hydroxyindole levels associated with hyperactive and aggressive behavior. *Arch Gen Psychiatry.* 1976;33:331-336.
53. Conner RL, Levine S, Wertheim GZ, Cummer JF. Hormonal determinants of aggressive behavior. *Ann N Y Acad Sci.* 1969;159:760-776.
54. Money J, Ehrhardt AA. Gender dimorphic behavior and fetal sex hormones. In: Astwood EB, ed. *Recent Progress in Hormone Research, XXVIII.* Orlando, Fla: Academic Press Inc; 1972:735-754.
55. Yalom I, Green R, Fisk N. Prenatal exposure to female hormones. *Arch Gen Psychiatry.* 1973;28:554-561.
56. Valzelli L. The 'isolation syndrome' in mice. *Psychopharmacologia.* 1973;31:305-320.
57. Morden B, Conner R, Mitchell G, Dement W, Levine S. Effects of rapid-eye-movement (REM) sleep deprivation on shock-induced fighting. *Physiol Behav.* 1968;3:425-432.
58. Lamprecht F, Eichelman B, Thoa NB, Williams RB, Kopin IJ. Rat fighting behavior: serum dopamine-β-hydroxylase and hypothalamic tyrosine hydroxylase. *Science.* 1972;177:1214-1215.
59. Eichelman B, Hegstrand L. Stress-induced alterations in aggression and brain biochemistry. Presented at the 13th Collegium Internationale Neuropsychopharmacologicum; June 15, 1982; Jerusalem, Israel.
60. Higley JD, Suomi SJ, Linnoila M. CSF monoamine metabolite concentrations vary according to age, rearing, and sex, and are influenced by the stressor of social separation in rhesus monkeys. *Psychopharmacology.* 1991;103:551-556.
61. Williams RB, Eichelman B. Social setting: influence on the physiological response to electric shock in the rat. *Science.* 1971;174:613-614.
62. Conner RL, Vernikos-Danellis J, Levine S. Stress, fighting and neuroendocrine function. *Nature.* 1971;234:564-566.
63. Powell DA, Francis J, Braman MJ, Schneiderman N. Frequency of attack in shock-elicited aggression as a function of the performance of individual rats. *J Exp Anal Behav.* 1969;12:817-823.
64. Raleigh MJ, McGuire MT, Brammer GL, Yuwiler A. Social and environmental influences on blood serotonin concentrations in monkeys. *Arch Gen Psychiatry.* 1984;41:405-410.
65. Krsiak M. Effect of ethanol on aggression and timidity in mice. *Psychopharmacology.* 1976;51:75-80.
66. Lion JR, Reid W, eds. *Assaults Within Psychiatric Facilities.* New York, NY: Grune & Stratton; 1983:322.
67. Hill BK, Balow EA, Bruninks RH. A national study of prescribed drugs in institutions and community residential facilities for mentally retarded people. *Psychopharmacol Bull.* 1985;21:279-284.
68. Rovner BW, Kafonek S, Filipp L, Lucas MJ, Foltein MF. Prevalence of mental illness in a community nursing home. *Am J Psychiatry.* 1986;143:1446-1449.
69. Bradford LD, Olivier B, Van Dalen D, Schipper J. Serenics: the pharmacology of fluprazine and DU 28412. In: Miczek KA, Kruk MR, Olivier B, eds. *Ethopharmacological Aggression Research.* New York, NY: Alan R Liss Inc; 1984:191-208.
70. Olivier B, Van Dalen D, Hartog J. A new class of psychotropic drugs: serenics. *Drugs Future.* 1986;11:473-494.
71. Eichelman B, Hartwig A. The Carolina nosology of destructive behavior (CNDB). *J Neuropsychiatry Clin Neurosci.* 1990;2:288-296.
72. American Psychiatric Association, Committee on Nomenclature and Statistics. *Diagnostic and Statistical Manual of Mental Disorders, Revised Third Edition.* Washington, DC: American Psychiatric Association; 1987.
73. Yudofsky SC, Silver JM, Jackson W, Endicott J, Williams D. The Overt Aggression Scale for the objective rating of verbal and physical aggression. *Am J Psychiatry.* 1986;143:35-39.
74. Guyatt G, Sackett D, Tayler DW, Chong J, Roberts R, Pubsley S. Determining optimal therapy: randomized trials in individual patients. *N Engl J Med.* 1986;314:889-892.
75. Geschwind N. Disconnection syndromes in animals and man. *Brain.* 1965;88:237-294.
76. *Monthly Vital Statistics Report (Final Data).* National Center for Health Statistics. June 1984;33(suppl 22):27-28.
77. Wolfgang ME. Victim precipitated criminal homicide. In: Wolfgang ME, ed. *Studies in Homicide.* New York, NY: Harper & Row Publishers Inc; 1967:35-70.
78. Wolfgang ME. *Patterns in Criminal Homicide.* Philadelphia, Pa: University of Pennsylvania Press; 1958:413.

The Current State of Psychiatry in the Treatment of Violent Patients

Kenneth Tardiff, MD, MPH

• **During the past 2 decades psychiatry has made great progress in describing patterns of violence by psychiatric patients and developing standards for the evaluation and treatment of these patients. Studies have found that roughly 10% of patients were violent toward other persons just prior to psychiatric hospitalization. Young male patients and patients in certain diagnostic groups had higher rates of violence. This report describes the proper evaluation of violent patients and proposes a model for the short-term potential of violent behavior. Psychiatry has developed guidelines for the acute treatment of violent patients using verbal intervention, physical restraint, and emergency medication. Long-term treatment relies on medication for the underlying disorder. Beyond their traditional indications, carbamazepine, propranolol hydrochloride, and lithium carbonate may be effective in diminishing violence. Some violent patients respond to long-term psychotherapy.**

(*Arch Gen Psychiatry*. 1992;49:493-499)

This report describes the current state of our specialty in the diagnosis and treatment of violent patients. The term *patients* rather than *persons* points to a basic premise of this report, namely that psychiatrists as physicians have expertise in the management of violence for a group of persons defined as patients but not for violence at large in society. Violence in society is related to factors such as economics, culture, criminal behavior, drug dealing, mass media, and the availability of weapons. These factors are not within the usual realm of psychiatric expertise, although such factors must be considered in the treatment of an individual patient. Psychiatric and medical techniques of assessment, diagnosis, and treatment of patients with violent behavior parallel the techniques used for other clinical problems of patients.

During the past 2 decades, psychiatry has made great progress in developing standards for the evaluation and treatment of violent patients. There has been exponential growth in research on the psychopathology of violence and on more specific treatments to fit the psychopathology manifested by individual patients. Prior to 1970, psychiatry's involvement with the problems of violence was often diffuse and sometimes more on the level of philosophy than science. Violence was discussed in terms of aggressive drives, as part of human nature, or as the product of vague social forces.[1] Needless to say, this was of little practical use to the clinician who was responsible for treating violent psychiatric patients.

Systematic studies of the characteristics of violent patients done in the beginning of the 1970s looked at patients seen at special clinics.[2,3] The interests of the researchers and the types of patients presenting to these clinics were often skewed toward neurophysiologic causes of violent behavior.[4,5] However, soon the scope of study of violent psychiatric patients broadened to include a variety of diagnostic groups as well as clinical settings.[6-8] Researchers began to study large numbers of patients admitted to psychiatric hospitals. The first large study looked at 9365 patients admitted to public hospitals on Long Island in New York in the mid 1970s.[9] Ten percent of these patients had been physically violent toward other persons just before admission to these hospitals. Young men and some diagnostic groups had higher rates of violence. An important point made by the study was that violence was not uncommon. Subsequent studies of large patient populations in a variety of psychiatric hospitals found similar percentages of patients who were physically violent toward other persons.[9-14]

CHARACTERISTICS OF VIOLENT PATIENTS

What became apparent from these studies was that violent patients are not a homogeneous group. There were many types of patients who were violent, suggesting that for purposes of treatment psychiatrists and other clinicians must evaluate the underlying psychopathology causing violence in each individual case. A review of the types of violence in relation to diagnosis may be instructive.

A number of studies have found that schizophrenic patients are overly represented in groups of patients who are violent toward other people just before and/or during psychiatric hospitalization. Studies in the United States and in other countries, such as Great Britain and Sweden, link violence to paranoid delusional thinking and hallucinations in schizophrenia.[9,11,12,15-19] These patients believe that people are threatening, persecuting, or in some other way trying to harm them. Violence is a reaction to these

Accepted for publication March 12, 1992.
From the Department of Psychiatry, Cornell University Medical Center, New York, NY.
Reprint requests to the Payne Whitney Clinic/New York Hospital, 525 E 68th St, New York, NY 10021 (Dr Tardiff).

perceived threats. Often, the theme of the delusion is consistent over time.

However, when one looks at groups of patients in less acute settings or in hospital settings in which patients stay for long periods, the nonparanoid schizophrenic is even more likely than the paranoid schizophrenic to be violent.[10,20-23] In these cases, rather than from paranoid delusional thinking, violence comes from psychotic disorganization or general excitability. Some patients may have difficulty delaying gratification and have low frustration tolerance, with violent consequences. Sometimes violence is due to factors other than the schizophrenic process per se. For example, I have observed that violence can be an indirect complication of neuroleptic medication when patients with akathisia restlessly move around on the inpatient unit and bump into other patients. It is important to keep in mind that schizophrenic patients may have another disorder primarily responsible for violence, such as neurologic impairment or mental retardation.[24]

Finally, violence by schizophrenic patients may be due to personality disorders, alcohol or drug abuse, or reasons not related to psychiatric impairment (for example, retaliation or self-defense). Keeping this in mind it is apparent that not all violence by schizophrenics should be treated with neuroleptics and that violence due to psychosis should be distinguished from violence due to other causes in the treatment of violent schizophrenic patients.

Manic patients have been found to have sudden severe violent episodes.[9,12,23,25,26] Often violence erupts in the early phase of treatment of the acute manic state. Such a patient may respond violently to any form of containment or limit setting, be it physical or otherwise, as when a nurse insists that the patient take a dose of medication.

Substance abuse is associated with violence. Alcoholism as a primary disorder or in conjunction with other psychiatric disorders can result in violence.[18,22,27-30] This is often the result of "disinhibition," particularly in the early phase of intoxication, as well as emotional lability and impaired judgment. A number of other substances also have been associated with violence.[27,29-32] Stimulants, particularly cocaine, can be dangerous. The early phase of cocaine intoxication is manifested by euphoria that can quickly turn to irritability, agitation, suspiciousness, and violence, especially with crack or intravenous cocaine. With continued use of cocaine in a binge as well as chronic amphetamine use, suspiciousness may turn to paranoid delusional thinking and violence. Heavy cocaine use has caused manic-like delirium with severe violence. The craving for cocaine also may result in violence, as the addict desperately seeks more cocaine or the money to purchase it.

Hallucinogens, particularly phencyclidine, which is a dissociative anesthetic, are known to cause violence, suicide, and bizarre behaviors.[33] Hallucinogens can produce impaired judgment and cause perceptual changes and delusional thinking. However, one review of the literature concluded that the risk of violence from phencyclidine is overstated and is often related to alcohol or other substances.[34] There are no reliable data linking lysergic acid diethylamide (LSD)–like substances to such violence. Benzodiazepines and sedatives do not commonly produce violence through intoxication.[35] Short-acting barbiturates can produce assaultive behavior similar to that found with alcohol use during serious violent crimes by adolescents.[36] However, abrupt discontinuation of the short-half-life benzodiazepines may result in irritability and agitation so that the risk of violence may be increased. Withdrawal from alcohol may produce violence by similar mechanisms or by the delirious state.

There are many studies demonstrating that organic brain disease can result in violence.[4,5,9-12,22,24,37,38] Violence in temporal lobe epilepsy is not frequent, but when it occurs it may occur during the ictal period and, if so, is often purposeless.[39,40] Violence has been found rarely in the interictal period among patients with temporal lobe epilepsy.[41] Some researchers have maintained that temporal lobe epilepsy or more subtle neurophysiologic dysfunction is responsible for violence in some patients.[42,43] They point out that electroencephalography (EEG) is an insensitive measure of subcortical activity and that some patients with episodic violence respond to anticonvulsants. Others stress the effect of head trauma and other neurologic and medical disorders that can impact on the brain and produce violent behavior.[44,45] Infections of the brain, including viral encephalitis, acquired immunodeficiency syndrome, tuberculosis, fungal meningitis, syphilis, and herpes simplex, can be associated with violent behavior. Other diseases of the brain associated with violence include normal pressure hydrocephalus, cerebrovascular diseases, tumors, Huntington's chorea, multiple sclerosis, Pick's disease, multi-infarct dementia, Alzheimer's disease, Parkinson's disease, and Wilson's disease, as well as postanoxic or posthypoglycemic states with brain damage.

Clinically, it has been observed that organic impairment of the brain may produce violence through general dyscontrol or through psychosis, as in the case of senile dementia in which there are paranoid delusions or misidentifications.[46,47] These elderly patients can be quite dangerous, and armed with weapons resist what they perceive as forces that will hurt them or deprive them of property or other possessions. In the future, with imaging and other new laboratory techniques, mechanisms through which organic factors produce violence will become clearer.

For example, persons with bifrontal damage to the brain detected with magnetic resonance imaging and sociopathic behaviors have defective skin conductance responses to socially significant stimuli.[48] Thus, they may not be able to appreciate the consequences of their behavior. In contrast, patients with temporal lobe dysfunction, as in temporal lobe epilepsy, are said to be excessively concerned with morality and the social consequences of their actions.[49] There is evidence that more subtle damage to the amygdaloid nucleus and adjacent structures, as detected with magnetic resonance imaging, is associated with violent behavior.[50] However, all such reports require extensive and intensive research to ascertain the mechanisms and frequencies of behaviors attributed to structural changes in the brain.

A wide range of medical illnesses have been found to be associated with violent behavior.[9,10,45] Many of these are treatable and reversible. These disorders include hypoxia; electrolyte imbalances; hepatic disease; renal disease; vitamin deficiencies, such as B_{12}, folate, or B_1; systemic infections; hypoglycemia; Cushing's disease; hyperthyroidism; hypothyroidism; systemic lupus erythematosus; poisoning by heavy metals, insecticides, and other substances; and porphyria.

Personality disorders have been found to be associated

with increased risk of violence, particularly in antisocial and borderline patients.[5,9,12,28,51,52] In the case of the borderline personality disorder, in addition to frequent displays of anger and recurrent physical violence toward others, the patient with borderline personality disorder manifests a number of other behavioral problems and severe psychological problems. Violence manifested by persons with antisocial personality disorder is just one of many antisocial behaviors. These patients repeatedly get into physical fights and manifest a number of other antisocial behaviors, such as stealing, lying, and reckless driving. The patient shows no guilt or remorse for violence and other antisocial behavior. These disorders should be distinguished from another nonpsychotic episodic violence disorder, which has a better prognosis in regard to treatment. Intermittent explosive disorder is manifested by recurrent outbursts of violence that are grossly out of proportion to any precipitating psychosocial stressor. Following a violent episode there is often remorse. In the intervening period between these violent episodes, there is little evidence of other behavioral problems.

Episodic nonpsychotic violence usually involves family members, usually a man battering a woman, and less often a parent abusing a child. The pattern of violence repeats itself in a predictable way. Spouse battering characteristically involves a man who has low self-esteem with financial, sexual, or other conflicts that are expressed physically rather than verbally. The female victim feels helpless, guilty, ashamed, and afraid to take action to stop the violence. Arguments escalate in a repetitive fashion, often fueled by alcohol, and culminate in physical violence toward the woman.

Children and adolescents may be violent due to disruptive behavioral disorders or mental retardation.[10,12,52,53] There can be physical violence toward others, cruelty to animals, stealing, robbery, and other antisocial behaviors. This violence and other antisocial behaviors usually are not accompanied by guilt or remorse. Children with conduct disorders may grow up to be antisocial violent adults.[54] Children and adults with mental retardation are at greater risk of violence than the general population.[10,55] Violence in the mentally retarded is associated with hyperarousal, frustration, and anger when the patient is unable to achieve goals and cannot verbalize conflicts, concerns, and feelings adequately.

It has been noted that a history of violent behavior regardless of diagnosis indicates an increased risk of subsequent violent behavior.[9,21,22,56,57] This emphasizes the need to ask patients about past violence in great detail, as will be described further in terms of evaluation of patients. Other past impulsive behaviors, such as suicide attempts, may reflect future increased risk of violence as well as suicide.[9,10,58-60] Low cerebrospinal fluid 5-hydroxyindoleacetic acid concentration and responses to fenfluramine challenge in impulsive violent individuals suggest that serotonin may be important in self-control vs impulsive behaviors.[61-64]

There are demographic differences between violent and nonviolent psychiatric patients. Violent patients are more likely to be male.[3,9,12-14,22,23,30] However, when long-term chronic inpatients are studied, there is no significant difference in the rate of violence and gender of the patient.[10,23] In long-term hospitalization, sex role expectations may not be as important as psychopathology in violence. Being young increases the risk of violence.[3,9,12,21,22,30] However, some studies have found an increase in violence at the other age extreme.[9,46,47] This appears to be the consequence of dementia and other organic brain deficits. Perhaps unexpectedly, given racial differences in violent crime in society at large, black psychiatric patients are no more likely than white psychiatric patients to manifest violent behavior.[9,27,30] Presumably, psychopathology per se is more important.

EVALUATION OF THE VIOLENT PATIENT

Before one decides on treatment, a complete evaluation of the patient is essential. When faced with a patient who speaks of violence and/or has been violent, clinicians may become fearful or anxious or experience other emotions that cause them to veer from the assessment routine followed for other psychiatric problems.[65] Recent writings on the evaluation of violent patients should remind clinicians of standard clinical practice. These principles will be summarized herein.[45,66]

The evaluation of the patient who presents with problems of violence should include an assessment of the chief complaint, history of the present illness, family history, personal and developmental history, medical history, mental status, and results of physical examination, laboratory tests, and imaging. In gathering information about the patient the clinician should use as many sources of information as possible. This includes information from the patient, the police, relatives, the patient's therapist, and the primary care physician, as well as previous medical and criminal records.

The clinician should record the patient's stated reasons for being in the clinical setting at that time. Even though the patient's stated chief complaint may not agree with other sources of information, the clinician should evaluate the complaint as stated by the patient. The clinician will more fully evaluate the violence later, but it is important in the early phase of evaluation to let the patient present his or her view of the problem to assess the patient's perspective of what the problem is, to ascertain the patient's accuracy and reliability, and to avoid confrontation in the early phase, which would impede subsequent evaluation.

All aspects of the patient's present psychiatric illness should be assessed in the interview, but the focus here is on the history of violence as a symptom. There should be a determination of the time of onset of the first violent episode and of the occurrence of violence since then. Questions should be asked about the frequency and target of violent behavior, with attempts made to identify recurring patterns of escalation and violence. Severity of injury or intended injury should be determined. Associated symptoms preceding, during, or following the violent episode should be explored.

The clinician should inquire about prior evaluations of violent behavior, including tests done. A history of treatment, including medication and hospitalizations related to violence, as well as to other disorders, should be obtained. Records of prior evaluations and treatment should be requested. The clinician should inquire about other types of impulsive behavior. These include past suicidal behavior, reckless driving, destruction of property, fire setting, reckless spending, and sexual acting out.

There should be an extensive review of the patient's medical history because, as was pointed out earlier, a number of medical and neurologic diseases may be associated with violent behavior. The physical examination may reveal signs of underlying medical disorders that have been mentioned earlier as sometimes being associated with violence. Signs of alcohol or drug intoxication may be present, as in slurred speech, incoordination, unsteady gait, nystagmus, dilated or constricted pupils, and elevated blood pressure and heart rate. Withdrawal from alcohol and some drugs may produce tremors, increased autonomic activity, and even seizures.

In addition to the usual laboratory testing and procedures, I believe that EEG should be part of the routine evaluation of the violent patient. The routine EEG should be augmented with nasopharyngeal leads as well as a sleep EEG. Blood and urine for alcohol and drug assays should be monitored. One should use imaging for violent patients, with a preference for magnetic resonance imaging because of its superiority over computed tomography in detecting temporal lobe pathology. If a specific disorder is suspected other laboratory tests are indicated, such as a determination of arterial blood gas levels, testing for human immunodeficiency virus antibodies, glucose tolerance tests, determination of ceruloplasmin and copper levels in urine and serum, determination of urine porphobilinogen levels, heavy metal screening, determination of antinuclear antibodies, and lumbar puncture, if intracranial pressure is not elevated.

The mental status examination must be complete to enable the clinician to determine the cause of violence. For example, the role of delusions and hallucinations must be assessed and distinguished from other factors. Sensorium must be assessed for delirium due to alcohol withdrawal, drug intoxication, and a wide range of medical and neurologic disorders. Higher integrative functions must be assessed for organic disorders affecting the brain. More subtle themes in thought content, as in issues of self-esteem or problems with authority, must be assessed. The clinician must decide which aspects of psychopathology are linked to which forms of violence, keeping in mind that there may be more than one cause of violence for the patient.

PREDICTION OF VIOLENCE BY PATIENTS

Psychiatrists have debated whether they can predict violence by patients, yet the law expects them to protect intended victims of violence from their patients.[67] Since psychiatrists must make decisions about whether to hospitalize a potentially violent patient, when to discharge a previously violent patient, or whether to warn a potential victim, some guidelines have been formulated.[66,68] A model that is simple, practical, and analogous to the prediction of suicide potential is suggested until definitive research on prediction is done. This model is limited to prediction in the short term, that is for days or a week at most. It incorporates many of the factors discussed earlier in this report.

As with the evaluation of suicide potential, evaluation of violence potential includes assessment of how well planned is the threat or idea. Vague threats of killing someone are not as serious as well-formulated threats against a specific person. As with suicide, the availability of means of inflicting injury is important. If the patient has recently purchased or owns a gun, one should obviously take the threat more seriously. A history of violence or other impulsive behavior is often predictive of future violence.

One should assess the degree of past injuries as well as toward whom the violence has been directed and under what circumstances. Often there is a repetitive pattern of violent behavior and escalation between family or friends or in similar settings, for example, in bars. Alcohol and other drug abuse should be assessed. Central nervous system disorders have been associated with violent behavior and have been described earlier, as have some systemic disorders affecting the central nervous system. As with suicide, the presence of psychosis should make one take threats of violence very seriously and makes the assessment of violence potential essential, even if threats are not apparent.

All of these factors are weighed in the final assessment of whether the patient poses such a significant risk to others that some action is necessary. Thus, a vague threat such as "one day I am going to kill my wife" by a man who has no history of violence, does not drink heavily, and is not psychotic is not as serious as the same threat by an alcoholic with a history of violence. On the other hand, a paranoid schizophrenic with no history of violence or alcohol abuse who reluctantly describes a detailed plan of how to kill a specific doctor because of a delusional belief that a prescribed drug poisoned him should be taken very seriously.

Action may include changing the treatment plan, hospitalizing the patient, or warning the intended victim and/or the police and distancing the victim from the threatening patient. All of the data on which the decision about violence is based should be documented in writing and the rationale in arriving at the decisions should be evident in written documentation. Reassessment of violence potential should be made at short intervals, for example, from visit to visit within a few days, if the patient is to continue to be treated outside of the hospital or other institution. In general, clinicians have not been faulted for inaccurate prediction, but they have been faulted for failure to collect relevant data and to use those data to make a prediction.[67]

TREATMENT OF THE ACUTELY VIOLENT PATIENT

The treatment of a patient who is actively attacking others, breaking objects, or on the brink of violence is an emergency that must be approached with as much calm and professional demeanor as possible. One or more of the three means of controlling violence can be used, namely, verbal de-escalation, medication, and/or physical restraint. The intervention used depends on the individual case, but utmost care must be given to ensure the safety of staff and the patient. Psychiatry's recognition that professionals are frequently injured by patients is reflected by a recent American Psychiatric Association (APA) Task Force on Clinician Safety that will issue its report during 1992. The basics of safety in the treatment of acutely violent patients include the following: (1) know when verbal means of de-escalation are appropriate, (2) have adequate manpower to subdue a patient, (3) be familiar with physical restraint techniques, and (4) dress appropriately if participating in physical restraint maneuvers.

This report cannot cover the details of the acute treatment of violence. Another APA Task Force developed guidelines that are covered in its report as well as in a book.[69,70] These guidelines have become minimal standards across institutions and in the legal arena. These publications have been supplemented with more details on the use of medication and verbal techniques in recent publications.[66,71,72]

A decision to attempt to de-escalate aggression by talking to the patient is made on an individual basis, but it is unusual for a psychotic or grossly organic patient to respond to verbal interventions. One must turn to restraint, seclusion, and/or emergency medication. Which control is used is based on the clinical needs of the individual case. For example, if the cause of the violent behavior is unknown, restraint may be indicated to maintain the patient drug free for purposes of evaluation. In addition, a violent patient may be preferentially treated in seclusion and restraint because of medical illness or drug allergies that would preclude the use of certain medications to control violent behavior.

There are contraindications to the use of seclusion and restraint. They should never be used for punishment, that is, for seeking retribution for an act when no danger exists to the patient or others. Seclusion may be contraindicated because of the patient's clinical or medical condition, for example, if the patient is suicidal or is in medically unstable condition so that close monitoring and physical proximity to staff is a necessity. Restraint may be preferable in cases of delirium in which reduced sensory input may lead to worsening of the clinical state in seclusion. Other situations representing relative contraindications to seclusion include those in which patients have just taken overdoses and require close monitoring, those in which patients present with the symptoms of serious and uncontrollable self-mutilation, and those in which seclusion rooms cannot be sufficiently cooled on hot days for patients receiving drugs, such as neuroleptics, that impair thermoregulation.

Restraint or seclusion is an emergency procedure usually initiated by nursing staff, but a physician must see the patient as soon as possible and write an order to continue these procedures. Orders are time limited and must be renewed periodically, depending on the institution's guidelines. The APA Task Force outlined standards for the monitoring and care of a patient in restraint and seclusion by nursing staff to ensure the patient's safety.

Emergency medication may be used instead of or in addition to seclusion or restraint. Neuroleptic medication should be used primarily for the treatment of violent patients who manifest psychotic symptoms. It may be indicated for patients who are not psychotic but who are violent, as in the case of patients with organic brain dysfunction whose clinical picture may be worsened with benzodiazepines.

Much has been written about the use of neuroleptics and the acute treatment of the violent patient.[73] It is important to distinguish the procedure of rapid "tranquilization" using low doses of neuroleptic medication during 30- to 60-minute intervals with the specific goal of attentuating violence, agitation, and excitement from the procedure of rapid "neuroleptization," which uses high doses of neuroleptics for several days in the misguided goal of trying to accelerate the decrease of psychotic symptoms.[74] A range of neuroleptics can be used and there is general safety and efficacy with rapid tranquilization. They have been demonstrated to be effective with schizophrenia, mania, and other psychotic disorders.

Benzodiazepines can be used very effectively in emergency situations. Benzodiazepines may be used with the neuroleptic medications for schizophrenics, manics, and patients in other psychotic states or they may be used alone for the treatment of nonpsychotic patients. For patients who appear to have some degree of control, they may be offered as an oral medication. However, in most emergency situations intramuscular medication is necessary. Lorazepam is preferred since it is reliably and rapidly absorbed from intramuscular injection, unlike diazepam or chlordiazepoxide.[75] Diazepam administered intravenously is effective, but this is a difficult maneuver with a struggling patient and may lead to respiratory arrest.[66] Lorazepam is more appropriate in the long-term treatment of violence than in emergency situations.

LONG-TERM TREATMENT OF THE VIOLENT PATIENT

Much progress has been made in formulating the long-term treatment of violent patients with medication, behavioral therapy, and psychotherapy. Medication is used to treat the underlying disorders, for example, schizophrenia, mania, or an organic state. Anticonvulsants, β-blockers, and lithium have been used to treat violence in the absence of disorders these medications were designed to treat.

Carbamazepine is effective in managing aggression and irritability in patients with overt seizures, in schizophrenic patients with and without EEG abnormalities, and in other types of patients with episodic violence, particularly personality disorders without gross brain damage or mental retardation.[76-79] Valproic acid is used usually after an unsuccessful trial of carbamazepine or in cases in which the hematologic status of the patient precludes the use of carbamazepine. Clonazepam can be used for episodic violence on a long-term basis, with relatively few side effects.

There have been a number of reports on the effectiveness of β-blockers, particularly propranolol hydrochloride in the management of aggressive behavior.[71,80-89] Most of the patients who responded to propranolol were those with organic brain disease, often with gross impairment secondary to trauma, alcoholism, encephalitis, Huntington's disease, dementia, Wilson's disease, or Korsakoff's psychosis. In addition, some patients with minimal brain dysfunction or attention-deficit disorder have also been reported to respond to propranolol. Nearly all the patients in these studies were refractory to other medications, including neuroleptics, anxiolytic agents, anticonvulsants, and lithium. In a number of cases, concurrent neuroleptic medication was used. Other β-blockers, such as pindolol, nadolol, and metoprolol tartrate have been used successfully to treat aggressive behavior.[85-87]

Lithium has been used to treat a number of different types of violent patients. In a double-blind trial lithium was effective in the treatment of aggression in adult mentally retarded patients.[88] The administration of lithium was the same as that for the treatment of bipolar patients. There have been other reports of the use of lithium for patients with other disorders, including those with organic brain syndrome and head injury; aggressive schizophrenics; nonpsychotic, aggressive prisoners and delinquents; and children with conduct disorders and attention deficit.[89-91] Finally, buspirone hydrochloride has been reported to diminish aggression as well as anxiety in developmentally disabled patients.[92]

Behavioral therapy has been used in programs for the management of violent behavior in severely impaired institutional populations. This approach may be used for chronic schizophrenics or mentally retarded patients in conjunction with other treatment approaches. The basic principles have been described elsewhere.[93,94] In setting up a behavioral treatment program on an inpatient unit, the services of a trained, experienced behavioral analyst should be obtained. It is the responsibility of the behavioral analyst to plan the treatment program in conjunction with the interdisciplinary staff and to train and supervise staff in the implementation of the treatment program. Behavioral treatment programs should be reviewed periodically by persons other than the ward personnel to ensure their quality and ethical standards. In addition, the patient should be involved as much as possible in the formulation of the plan, and informed written consent should be obtained if the patient is competent to offer it.

The goals and techniques of long-term psychotherapy have been described for violent patients.[95] These patients are nonpsychotic and have primarily personality disorders or intermittent explosive disorders. If spouse abuse is the problem, couple's sessions may be indicated as long as the spouse's safety can be ensured. The treatment of spouse abuse has a long tradition.[96] The first goal of therapy is to evaluate whether the patient is really motivated in situations in which divorce or job loss is pending. Next, the patient must identify patterns of escalation in violence and learn to disengage at the early phase of escalation. Often, the early phase involves a physiologic sensation as anger builds, for example, flushing of the face.

The therapist must closely monitor transference and be prepared to deal promptly with negative thoughts or threats by the patient. Countertransference must be monitored since violence can evoke inappropriate feelings and reactions to patients. Psychotherapy should provide insight as to why the patient must use violence as a means of expression. Often, these patients have difficulty verbally expressing their feelings and conflicts. Issues common in the treatment of violent patients often involve low self-esteem in terms of money, sex, and authority.

COMMENT

Psychiatry has made progress in the treatment of violent patients. The domain of psychiatry has focused on patients and not on problems of violence in society. Having done this, it was possible to study violence in a systematic, scientific manner. Different types of violence have been described and treatment has been targeted to the cause of violence, be it delusions or other aspects of psychosis, intoxication, organicity, or psychodynamic factors. Standards for the acute treatment of violent patients using restraint, seclusion, and medication have been formulated for the safety of staff and patients. With more sophisticated imaging and biochemical analyses in the future, one can look forward to continued progress in the assessment and treatment of the causes of violence by patients.

This study was supported in part by grant DA 06534 from the National Institute of Drug Abuse and a grant from the Aaron Diamond Foundation.

References

1. Chodorkoff B, Baxter S. Psychiatric and psychoanalytic theories of violence. In: Mulvihill DJ, Tumin MM, eds. *Crimes of Violence: A Staff Report to the National Commission on the Causes and Prevention of Violence.* Washington, DC: US Government Printing Office; 1969:1118-1162.

2. Bach-y-Rita G, Lion JR, Climent CE, Ervin FR. Episodic dyscontrol: a study of 130 violent patients. *Am J Psychiatry.* 1971;127:1473-1478.

3. Climent CE, Ervin FR. Historical data in the evaluation of violent subjects. *Arch Gen Psychiatry.* 1972;27:621-624.

4. Mark VH, Ervin FR. *Violence and the Brain.* New York, NY: Harper & Row Publishers Inc; 1970.

5. Monroe RR. *Episodic Behavioral Disorders.* Cambridge, Mass: Harvard University Press; 1970.

6. Lion JR, Bach-y-Rita G, Ervin F. Violent patients in the emergency room. *Am J Psychiatry.* 1969;125:1706-1711.

7. Kalogerakis ME. The assaultive psychiatric patient. *Psychiatr Q.* 1971;45:372-381.

8. Tardiff K. A survey of psychiatrists in Boston and their work with violent patients. *Am J Psychiatry.* 1974;131:1008-1011.

9. Tardiff K, Sweillam A. Assault, suicide, and mental illness. *Arch Gen Psychiatry.* 1980;37:164-169.

10. Tardiff K, Sweillam A. Assaultive behavior among chronic inpatients. *Am J Psychiatry.* 1982;139:212-215.

11. Craig TJ. An epidemiological study of problems associated with violence among psychiatric inpatients. *Am J Psychiatry.* 1982;139:1262-1266.

12. Tardiff K. Characteristics of assaultive patients in private hospitals. *Am J Psychiatry.* 1984;141:1232-1235.

13. Rossi AM, Jacobs M, Monteleone M. Violent or fear-inducing behavior associated with hospital admission. *Hosp Community Psychiatry.* 1985;36:643-647.

14. Mc Niel DE, Binder RC, Greenfield TK. Predictors of violence in committed acute psychiatric patients. *Am J Psychiatry.* 1988;145:965-970.

15. Planansky K, Johnston R. Homicidal aggression in schizophrenic men. *Acta Psychiatr Scand.* 1977;55:65-73.

16. Addad M, Benezech M, Bourgeois M, Yesavage J. Criminal acts among schizophrenics in French mental hospitals. *J Nerv Ment Dis.* 1981;169:289-293.

17. Yesavage JA. Inpatient violence and the schizophrenic patient. *Acta Psychiatr Scand.* 1983;67:353-357.

18. Taylor PJ, Gunn J. Violence and psychosis. *BMJ.* 1984;288:1945-1949.

19. Lindquist P, Allebeck P. Schizophrenia and crime: a longitudinal follow-up of 644 schizophrenics in Stockholm. *Br J Psychiatry.* 1990;157:345-350.

20. Shader RI, Jackson AH, Harmatz JS, Appelbaum PS. Patterns of violent behavior among schizophrenic patients. *Dis Nerv Sys.* 1977;38:13-16.

21. Karson C, Bigelow LB. Violent behavior in schizophrenic inpatients. *J Nerv Ment Dis.* 1987;175:161-164.

22. Kay SR, Wolkenfeld F, Murrill LM. Profiles of aggression among psychiatric patients. *J Nerv Ment Dis.* 1988;176:547-557.

23. Binder RL, Mc Niel DE. The relationship of gender to violent behavior in acutely disturbed psychiatric patients. *J Clin Psychiatry.* 1990;51:110-114.

24. Krakowski M, Convit A, Jaeger J, Lin S, Volarka J. Neurological impairment in schizophrenic patients. *Am J Psychiatry.* 1989;146:849-853.

25. Yesavage JA. Bipolar illness: correlates of dangerous inpatient behavior. *Br J Psychiatry.* 1983;143:554-557.

26. Binder RL, Mc Niel DE. Effects of diagnosis and context on dangerousness. *Am J Psychiatry.* 1988;145:728-732.

27. Convit A, Isay D, Gadioma R, Volarka J. Underreporting of physical assaults in schizophrenic patients. *J Nerv Ment Dis.* 1988;176:507-509.

28. Bland R, Orn H. Family violence and psychiatry. *Can J Psychiatry.* 1986;31:129-137.

29. Holcomb WR, Anderson WP. Alcohol and multiple drug use in accused murderers. *Psychol Rep.* 1983;52:159-164.

30. Swanson JW, Holzer CE, Ganju VK, Jono RT. Violence and psychiatric disorder in the community: evidence from the Epidemiologic Catchment Area surveys. *Hosp Community Psychiatry.* 1990;41:761-770.

31. Lowenstein DH, Massa SM, Rowbotham MC, Collins SD, McKinney HE, Simon RP. Acute neurologic and psychiatric complications associated with cocaine abuse. *Am J Med.* 1987;83:841-846.

32. Honer WE, Gewirtz E, Turey M. Psychosis and violence in cocaine smokers. *Lancet.* 1987;1:451.

33. Budd RD, Lindstrom DM. Characteristics of victims of PCP-related deaths in Los Angeles County. *J Toxicol Clin Toxicol.* 1982;19:997-1004.

34. Brecher M, Wang WB, Wong H, Morgan JP. Phencyclidine and violence: clinical and legal issues. *J Clin Psychopharmacol.* 1988;8:397-401.

35. Dietch JT, Jennings RK. Aggressive dyscontrol in patients treated with benzodiazepines. *J Clin Psychiatry.* 1988;49:184-187.
36. Tinklenberg JR, Murphy PL, Murphy P, Darley CF, Roth WT, Kopell BS. Drug-involvement in criminal assaults by adolescents. *Arch Gen Psychiatry.* 1974;30:685-689.
37. Tupin J. The violent patient: a strategy for management and diagnosis. *Hosp Community Psychiatry.* 1983;34:37-40.
38. Weiger B, Bear D. An approach to the neurology of aggression. *J Psychiatr Res.* 1988;22:85-98.
39. Delgado-Escueta AV, Mattson RH, King L, et al. The nature of aggression during epileptic seizures. *N Engl J Med.* 1981;305:711-716.
40. Leicester J. Temper tantrums, epilepsy and episodic dyscontrol. *Br J Psychiatry.* 1982;141:262-266.
41. Hermann BP, Whitman S. Behavioral and personality correlates of epilepsy: a review, methodological critique and conceptual model. *Psychol Bull.* 1984;95:451-497.
42. Devinsky O, Bear D. Varieties of aggressive behavior in temporal lobe epilepsy. *Am J Psychiatry.* 1984;141:651-656.
43. Monroe RR. Episodic behavioral disorders and limbic ictus. *Compr Psychiatry.* 1985;26:466-479.
44. Lewis DO, Pincus JH, Shanok SS, Glaser G. Psychomotor epilepsy and violence in a group of incarcerated adolescent boys. *Am J Psychiatry.* 1982;139:882-887.
45. Reid WH, Balis EU. Evaluation of the violent patient. In: Hales RE, Frances AJ, eds. *American Psychiatric Association Annual Review.* Washington, DC: American Psychiatric Press; 1987;6:491-509.
46. Petrie WM, Lawson EC, Hollender MH. Violence in geriatric patients. *JAMA.* 1982;248:443-444.
47. Deutsch LH, Bylsma FW, Rovner BW, Steele C, Folstein M. Psychosis and physical aggression in probable Alzheimer's disease. *Am J Psychiatry.* 1991;148:1159-1163.
48. Damasio AR, Tranel D, Damasio H. Individuals with sociopathic behavior caused by frontal damage fail to respond autonomically to social stimuli. *Behav Brain Res.* 1990;41:81-94.
49. Bear D, Schenk L, Benson H. Increased autonomic responses to neural and emotional stimuli in patients with temporal lobe epilepsy. *Am J Psychiatry.* 1981;138:843-845.
50. Tonkonogy TM. Violence and temporal lobe lesion: head CT and MRI data. *J Neuropsychiatry.* 1991;3:189-196.
51. Hare R, Mc Pherson L. Violent and aggressive behavior by criminal psychopaths. *Int J Law Psychiatry.* 1984;7:35-50.
52. Tardiff K, Koenigsberg HW. Assaultive behavior among outpatients. *Am J Psychiatry.* 1985;142:960-963.
53. Pfeffer C, Plutchnik R, Mizruchi M. Predictors of assaultiveness in latency age children. *Am J Psychiatry.* 1983;140:31-35.
54. Monahan J. *The Clinical Prediction of Violent Behavior.* Rockville, Md: US Dept of Health and Human Services; 1981:41-43.
55. Kuehnel TG, Slama KM. Guidelines for the developmentally disabled. In: Tardiff K, ed. *The Psychiatric Uses of Seclusion and Restraint.* Washington, DC: American Psychiatric Press; 1984:87-101.
56. Convit A, Jaeger J, Lin S, Volarka J. Predicting assaultiveness in psychiatric inpatients: a pilot study. *Hosp Community Psychiatry.* 1988;39:429-434.
57. Kroll J, Mackenzie T. When psychiatrists are liable: risk management and violent patients. *Hosp Community Psychiatry.* 1983;34:29-37.
58. Apter A, Bleich A, Plutchik R. Suicidality, depression and conduct disorder. *J Am Acad Child Adolesc Psychiatry.* 1988;27:696-699.
59. Brown GL, Ebert MH, Goyer PF, et al. Aggression, suicide and serotonin: relationship to CSF amine metabolites. *Am J Psychiatry.* 1982;136:741-746.
60. Lidberg L, Tuck JR, Asberg M, Scalia-Tomba P, Bertilsson L. Homicide, suicide, and CSF 5-HIAA. *Acta Psychiatr Scand.* 1985;71:230-236.
61. Linnolia Am, Virkkunen M, Scheinin M, Nuutila A, Rimon R, Goodwin FK. Low cerebrospinal fluid 5-hydroxyindoleocetic acid concentration differentiates impulsive from nonimpulsive violent behavior. *Life Sci.* 1983;33:2609-2614.
62. Apter A, Kotler M, Sevy S, et al. Correlates of risk of suicide in violent and nonviolent psychiatric patients. *Am J Psychiatry.* 1991;148:883-887.
63. Fishbein DH, Lozovsky D, Jaffe JH. Impulsivity, aggression and neuroendocrine responses to serotonergic stimulation in substance abusers. *Biol Psychiatry.* 1989;25:1049-1066.
64. Coccaro EF, Siever LJ, Klar HM, et al. Serotonergic studies in patients with effective and personality disorders. *Arch Gen Psychiatry.* 1989;46:587-599.
65. Lion JR, Pasternak SA. Countertransference reactions to violent patients. *Am J Psychiatry.* 1973;130:207-210.
66. Tardiff K. *Assessment and Management of Violent Patients.* Washington, DC: American Psychiatric Press; 1989:44-63.
67. Beck JC. *The Potentially Violent Patient and the Tarasoff Decision in Psychiatric Practice.* Washington, DC: American Psychiatric Press; 1985.
68. Brizer DA. Crowner M. *Current Approaches to the Prediction of Violence.* Washington, DC: American Psychiatric Press; 1989.
69. American Psychiatric Association. *Seclusion and Restraint: The Psychiatric Uses.* Washington, DC: American Psychiatric Association, Task Force No. 22; 1985.
70. Tardiff K, ed. *The Psychiatric Uses of Seclusion and Restraint.* Washington, DC: American Psychiatric Press; 1984.
71. Brizer D. Psychopharmacology and the management of violent patients. *Psychiatr Clin North Am.* 1988;11:511-568.
72. Eichelman B. Toward a rational pharmacotherapy for aggressive and violent behavior. *Hosp Community Psychiatry.* 1986;39:31-39.
73. Soloff PH. Emergency management of the violent patient. In: Hales RE, Frances AJ, eds. *American Psychiatric Association Annual Review.* Washington, DC: American Psychiatric Press; 1987;6:510-536.
74. Dubin WR, Weiss KJ, Dorn JM. Pharmacotherapy of psychiatric emergencies. *J Clin Psychopharmacol.* 1986;6:210-222.
75. Garza-Trevino ES, Hollister LE, Overall JE, Alexander WF. Efficacy of combinations of intramuscular antipsychotics and sedative-hypnotics for control of psychotic agitation. *Am J Psychiatry.* 1989;146:1598-1601.
76. Evans RW, Gualtieri CT. Carbamazepine: a neuropsychological and psychiatric profile. *Clin Neuropharmacol.* 1985;8:221-241.
77. Luchins DI. Carbamazepine in psychiatric syndromes: clinical and neuropharmacological properties. *Psychopharmacol Bull.* 1984; 20:569-571.
78. Mattes JA, Rosenberg J, Mays D. Carbamazepine versus propranolol in patients with uncontrolled range outbursts: a random assignment study. *Psychopharmacol Bull.* 1984;20:98-100.
79. Neppe VM. Carbamazepine as adjunctive treatment in nonepileptic chronic inpatients with EEG temporal lobe abnormalities. *J Clin Psychiatry.* 1981;44:326-331.
80. Yudofsky SC, Williams D, Gorman J. Propranolol in the treatment of rage and violent behavior in patients with chronic brain syndrome. *Am J Psychiatry.* 1981;138:218-220.
81. Silver JM, Yudofsky SC. Propranolol for aggression: literature review and clinical guidelines. *Int Drug Newsletter.* 1985;20:9-12.
82. Greendyke RM, Kanter DR, Schuster DB, Verstreate S, Wooten J. Propranolol in the treatment of assaultive patients with organic brain disease. *J Nerv Ment Dis.* 1986;174:290-294.
83. Whitman JR, Maier GJ, Eichelman B. Beta-blockers for aggressive behavior in schizophrenia. *Am J Psychiatry.* 1987;144:538-542.
84. Kuperman S, Stewart M. Use of propranolol to decrease aggressive outbursts in younger patients. *Psychosomatics.* 1987;28:315-319.
85. Greendyke RM, Kanter DR. Therapeutic effects of pindolol on behavioral disturbances associated with organic brain disease. *J Clin Psychopharmacology.* 1986;6:423-426.
86. Mattes JA. Metroprolol for intermittent explosive disorder. *Am J Psychiatry.* 1985;142:1108-1109.
87. Sorgi PJ, Ratey JJ, Polakoff S. Beta-adrenergic blockers for the control of aggressive behaviors in patients with chronic schizophrenia. *Am J Psychiatry.* 1986;143:775-776.
88. Craft M, Ismail A, Krishnamurti D, Regan A, Seth V, North PM. Lithium in the treatment of aggression in mentally handicapped patients. *Br J Psychiatry.* 1987;150:685-689.
89. Williams KH, Goldstein C. Cognitive and affective responses to lithium in patients with organic brain syndrome. *Am J Psychiatry.* 1979;136:800-803.
90. Sheard MH, Marini JL, Bridges CI, Wagner E. The effect of lithium on impulsive aggressive behavior in man. *Am J Psychiatry.* 1976; 133:1409-1413.
91. Siassi I. Lithium treatment of impulsive behavior in children. *J Clin Psychiatry.* 1982;43:482-484.
92. Ratey JJ, Sovner R, Parks A, Rogentine K. The use of buspirone in the treatment of aggression and anxiety in mentally retarded patients. *J Clin Psychiatry.* 1991;52:159-162.
93. Liberman RP, Wong SE. Behavioral analysis and therapy procedures related to seclusion and restraint. In: Tardiff K, ed. *The Psychiatric Uses of Seclusion and Restraint.* Washington, DC: American Psychiatric Press; 1984;35-67.
94. Wong SE, Woolsey JE, Innocent AJ, Liberman RP. Behavioral treatment of violent psychiatric patients. *Psychiatr Clin North Am.* 1988;11:569-580.
95. Lion JR, Tardiff K. In: Hales RE, Francis AJ, eds. The long-term treatment of the violent patient. *The American Psychiatric Association Annual Review.* Washington, DC: American Psychiatric Press; 1987:537-548.
96. Straus MA, Gelles RJ, Steinmetz SK. *Behind Closed Doors: Violence in the American Family.* New York, NY: Doubleday/Ancho; 1980.

Index

I

T

U